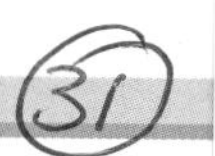

Tidy's Physiotherapy

Dedication

To Alison, Claire and Jessica, my daughters, who may outgrow my lap but who will never outgrow my heart.

For Elsevier

Commissioning Editor: Heidi Harrison
Associate Editor: Siobhan Campbell
Development Editor: Veronika Watkins
Project Manager: Frances Affleck
Design Direction: George Ajayi
Illustrators: Marion Tasker, Graeme Chambers, Antbits
Illustration Manager: Merlyn Harvey

Tidy's Physiotherapy

FOURTEENTH EDITION

Stuart Porter BSc (Hons), Grad Dip Phys, MCSP, SRP, Cert MHS

Lecturer in Physiotherapy, School of Health Care Professions, University of Salford

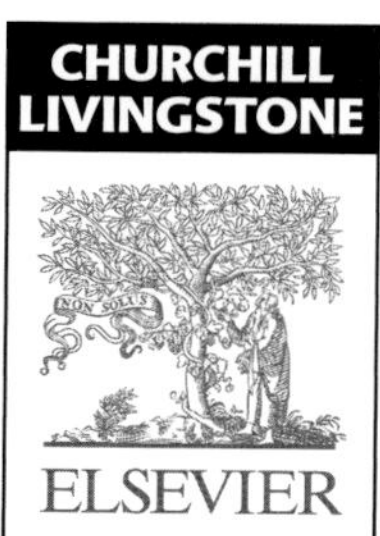

EDINBURGH LONDON NEW YORK OXFORD PHILADELPHIA ST LOUIS SYDNEY TORONTO 2008

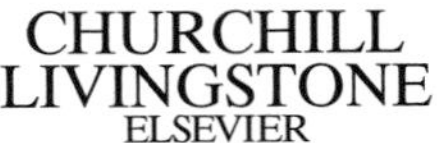

ISBN 978 0 443 10392 6

British Library Cataloguing in Publication Data
A catalogue record for this book is available from the British Library

Library of Congress Cataloging in Publication Data
A catalog record for this book is available from the Library of Congress

Note
Knowledge and best practice in this field are constantly changing. As new research and experience broaden our knowledge, changes in practice, treatment and drug therapy may become necessary or appropriate. Readers are advised to check the most current information provided (i) on procedures featured or (ii) by the manufacturer of each product to be administered, to verify the recommended dose or formula, the method and duration of administration, and contraindications. It is the responsibility of the practitioner, relying on their own experience and knowledge of the patient, to make diagnoses, to determine dosages and the best treatment for each individual patient, and to take all appropriate safety precautions. To the fullest extent of the law, neither the publisher nor the editor assume any liability for any injury and/or damage.

The Publisher

Printed in China

Contents

Contributors

Julie Barlow
Professor of Health Psychology and Director, Interdisciplinary Research Centre in Health, Faculty of Health and Life Sciences, Coventry

Ann Birch MSC MCSP
Clinical Specialist Physiotherapist

Gill Brook MCSP
Physiotherapy Co-ordinator, Bradford

Kirsty Carne RGN
National Osteoporosis Society, Camerton, Bath

Yvonne Coldron PHD MSC MCSP MMACP
Clinical Specialist, Thornton Health, London

Dr Elaine N. Court
Department of Biological Sciences, University of Central Lancashire, Preston

Sally Dean GRAD DIP PHYS MCSP
Clinical Specialist, Hand Therapy, Burns and Plastics Unit, Whiston Hospital, St Helens and Knowsley Hospital Services NHS Trust and Knowsley PCT

Anne Dyson GRAD DIP PHYS MCSP
Deputy Manager Physiotherapy, Cardiothoracic Centre, Liverpool

Dr Stephanie Enright PHD MPHIL MSC CERT HE MCSP
School of Biology and Life Sciences, Cardiff University

Georgina Evans MCSP
Senior Physiotherapist, Oxford

Dr Sally French BSC MSC PHD DIP TPF
Freelance Researcher and Writer; Associate Lecturer, Open University

Lynne Gaskell MRES MCSP GRAD DIP PHYS
Lecturer in Physiotherapy, University of Salford, Greater Manchester

Professor John Goodacre MD PHD FRCP
Director of Clinical Research and Honorary Consultant in Rheumatology, Lancashire School of Health and Postgraduate Medicine, University of Central Lancashire, Preston

Dr Lynne Goodacre PHD DIP COT
Senior Lecturer, Lancashire School of Health and Postgraduate Medicine, University of Central Lancashire, Preston

Janette Grey MSC (RESEARCH) MCSP PGCE
Professional Lead in Physiotherapy, Department of Allied Health Professions, University of Central Lancashire, Preston

Georgie Gulliford MCSP
Specialist Physiotherapist in Women's Health, Chichester

Carolyn A. Hale MSC GRAD ASSOC PHYS MCSP HPC REGISTERED
Clinical Specialist Physiotherapist, Pace Rehabilitation Ltd, Cheadle, Cheshire

Ralph Hammond MCSP
Professional Advisor, Chartered Society of Physiotherapy, London

Jeanette Haslam MPHIL MCSP
Honorary Lecturer, University of Bradford

Ruth Hawkes FCSP
Women's Health Physiotherapist, Lincoln

Lester Jones MSCMED(PM)
Senior Lecturer, School of Physiotherapy, Faculty of Health and Social Care Sciences, St George's, University of London and Kingston University, London

Annie Karim MCSP
Physiotherapy Manager, Princess Grace Hospital, London; Executive Committee, Association of Orthopaedic Chartered Physiotherapists

Dr Robert W. Lea
Department of Biological Sciences, University of Central Lancashire, Preston

Judith Lee MCSP
Clinical Specialist Women's Health Physiotherapist, Nottingham

Alison Lewis MCSP
Senior Physiotherapist Women's Health (Retired), Swindon

Melanie Lewis MCSP
Lead Macmillan Lymphoedema Physiotherapy Specialist, Swansea

Duncan Mason BSC (HONS) SRP MCSP
Lecturer in Physiotherapy, University of Salford, Manchester
www.athletematters.com

Dr Jonathan P. Moore BSC (HONS) PHD
Department of Chemical and Biological Sciences, University of Huddersfield

G. Lorimer Moseley PHD BAPPSC (PHYSIOTHERAPY) (HONS)
Department of Physiology, Anatomy and Genetics, University of Oxford

Juliette O'Hea MCSP MSC PGDIP (RHEUM)
Physiotherapy Advisor, National Ankylosing Spondylitis Society

Sue Pieri-Davies MSC PGCILTH MCSP
Respiratory Clinical Specialist, North West Regional Spinal Injuries Centre, Southport and Ormskirk NHS Trust, Southport

Ann Price
Superintendent Physiotherapist, Wrightington Hospital, Lancashire

Dr Chandini Rao MBBS MSC FRCP (UK)
Consultant Rheumatologist, Blackpool, Fylde and Wyre NHS Trust, Blackpool Victoria Hospital, Blackpool

Gillian Rawlinson BSC (HONS) MSC MCSP
Senior Lecturer in Physiotherapy, Department of Allied Health Professions, University of Central Lancashire, Preston

Professor Jim Richards PHD MSC BIOENGINEERING BENG (HONS) MECHANICAL ENGINEERING
Department of Allied Health Professions, Faculty of Health, University of Central Lancashire, Preston

Julie Rigby MSC BSC (HONS) MCSP
Consultant Therapist, Community Neuro-Rehabilitation, Salford Primary Care Trust, Manchester

Sushma Sanghvi MSC MA MCSP
Lecturer Practitioner, Physiotherapist Lecturer in Physiotherapy Studies, Mary Seacole Building, Brunel University, Uxbridge, Middlesex

Daphne Sidney MCSP
Women's Health Physiotherapist, Retford

Christine Smith MSC GRAD DIP PHYS CERT ED
Co-director of Physiotherapy, Senior Lecturer in Physiotherapy, University of Salford, Manchester

Professor John Swain PHD
Professor of Disability and Inclusion, Faculty of Health, Social Work and Education, University of Northumbria, Newcastle-upon-Tyne

Ros Thomas MCSP
Extended Scope Practitioner, Women's Health, Bath

Jacquelyne Todd MCSP PGCE (FE)
Physiotherapist Consultant in Lymphoedema, Leeds

Kathleen Vits MSC MCSP
Clinical Specialist Physiotherapist, Southampton

Pauline Walsh MCSP
Clinical Specialist Physiotherapist in Women's Health, Guildford

Anita Watson BSC (HONS) MCSP SRP
Lecturer in Physiotherapy, University of Salford, Manchester

Professor Tim Watson
School of Health and Emergency Professions, University of Hertfordshire

Joan M. Watt MA MCSP MSMA
Chair of Chartered Physiotherapists in Massage and Soft Tissue Therapy; Honorary President, Sport Massage Association; Commonwealth Games Physiotherapist, Great Britain Athletics; Head Physiotherapist, Olympics, World and European Championships

Julie Dawn Wheeler DIPCOT
Head of Research and Clinical Effectiveness, Chartered Society of Physiotherapy, London

Preface

'If there's a book you really want to read but it hasn't been written yet — then you must write it.' Toni Morrison (Pulitzer and Nobel Prize Winner).

This key textbook returns for its 14th edition, for which experts from a wide range of clinical and academic backgrounds have produced chapters that give physiotherapy students a clearly laid out reference guide whilst at the same time encouraging them to problem-solve and facilitate their learning in the process.

This extensive yet readable textbook is grounded in the clinical world and presented in an extremely clear format with state-of-the-art illustrations, web links and case studies. This time, the textbook includes an exciting new DVD containing demonstrations of musculoskeletal tests, massage and exercise.

The myriad contributors, each a specialist within his or her own field, also add significantly to the overall content of the textbook. They increase the diversity between chapters and consequently overall readability. The case studies are an excellent means of consolidating the information and new knowledge gleaned and give students out in practice the confidence to apply their skills.

Forenote

The importance of a skilled physiotherapist can never be under-estimated. It takes great skill and application to fully understand how to accurately diagnose and treat an athlete who has suffered an injury. It would have taken me a lot longer to recover from the injury that I sustained during the 2006 World Cup without the help from my club, a supportive family and, crucially, a group of skilled and knowledgeable physiotherapists.

Michael Owen

Michael has recently teamed up with Richie Partridge and Mark Browes to open 10bridgeclinic, a health and wellbeing clinic based just outside Chester, UK. For further information, please visit www.10bridgeclinic.co.uk.

Acknowledgements

I would like to thank Heidi Harrison, Veronika Watkins and Siobhan Campbell at Elsevier in Oxford for their support and faith in entrusting me with the task of editing this book.

The following people have been an invaluable source of opinions and comments: Marc Hudson, Joanne Fawcett, Hannah Cushion, Laura McLeod, Eleanor Ford, Robert Hodgkiss, Kezia Purdie, David Wilkes, James Baldwin, Vicky Platt, Jamie Murphy, Paul Sparrow, Mark Eales, Steve Morris, Candice Olliver, Amy Glasgow, Chris Hodson, Laura Hay, all undergraduate physiotherapy students who formed the focus group.

I am grateful to Patricia Lambert-Zazulak DCR(T) BA PhD, Research Associate at the Mummy Tissue Bank of the Egyptology Department of Manchester Museum for her advice on ancient diseases and trauma.

My great friend of 35 years, Mark Hothersall, provided some of the digital image manipulation.

My thanks also go to: Paula-Jayne McDowell, Guidelines Initiative Officer, Royal College of General Practitioners; Nick Goudge, Kate Slingsby, Kay Hack, Simon Crozier, David Dean and Sharon Baines, Lecturers, University of Salford; Judith Chapman, Lecturer, University of Southampton; Sue Barnard, Lecturer in Physiotherapy, University of Southampton; Rod Moore, Medical Dynamics; Pauline Davey, Assistant Communications Manager, National Osteoporosis Society; Mr RF Adam FRCS MCh Orth, Consultant Orthopaedic Surgeon; Fiona Cobbold, Senior Physiotherapist, Mike Somervell and Julie Butler, Senior Occupational Therapists, Southport and Ormskirk Hospital NHS Trust; Reinier van Mierlo, Superintendent Physiotherapist, Royal Preston Hospital; Carol Barnes, Senior Physiotherapist, Stepping Hill Hospital, Stockport, Manchester; Medical Photography Department, Whiston Hospital. Thanks also go to Andrew and Justine Arlow for their encouragement and advice; Jackie Moore; Joanne Tarrant, Graphic Designer, Blatchford Products Ltd, Lister Road, Basingstoke, Hants RG22 4AH; Nadia Khan, Student Physiotherapist, Brunel University; Jacinta Lynch, Chartered Physiotherapist; Kat Green, Paul Williamson, Claire Coop, Joanne Kenyon, Sandra Barton, Jennifer Brown, Christine Parker; Laura Hitchcock, EMPICS, a PA Group Company; Winifred Porter, Lynn Jackson, Martin George, Laura Jane Cowdell, Caroline Unsworth, Dr Peter Gill and Amelia Didsbury.

Chapter 1

The responsibilities of being a physiotherapist

Ralph Hammond and Julie Dawn Wheeler

CHAPTER CONTENTS

INTRODUCTION

This chapter aims to provide the reader with an insight into what it means to be a professional (in the context of this chapter, a physiotherapist), focusing on the responsibilities, both ethical and practical, that are inherent in claiming to be a professional working in the UK.

The current status and privilege of physiotherapists as autonomous professionals will be placed in the context of the history of the profession, and the impact of autonomy on clinical practice will be explored. The chapter will reflect on the implications for physiotherapists of the increasing expectations of both the general public and the government for health professionals to deliver high-quality health services. Explanations of how physiotherapists can meet these expectations through clinical governance will be provided. Finally, the reader will be offered a look at the possible future of the profession in light of the changing shape of health services in the UK.

Physiotherapists come into the profession because they have an underlying sense of — and commitment to — helping others and improving their quality of life. Indeed, Koehn (1994) argues that professionals can be thought of as being defined by a distinctive commitment to benefit the client. Physiotherapists want to be able to use their acquisition of knowledge, skills and attributes from qualifying programmes to benefit people, in whatever specialty or with whichever patient group they wish to work once qualified — for example, elite athletes, older people, people with developmental or acquired conditions, people with mental health problems. This chapter will help readers understand how they can make benefiting patients a reality in the context of the expectations of society for the provision of high-quality, safe and effective care.

While earlier editions of *Tidy's Physiotherapy* may have been popular for their prescriptive descriptions of what physiotherapists should do in particular situations or for specific conditions, this edition demands more from the reader. No two patients are quite the same; each requires the skills of the physiotherapist to carry out a full and accurate assessment, taking account of the individuality of the patient, and then to use clinical reasoning to problem-solve and offer appropriate options for treatment, on which the patient will make a decision. A professional is required to have the maturity to take full responsibility for the privilege of autonomy. This will be by maintaining a competence to practise through career-long learning and through self-evaluation, as well as through the evaluation of present practice; by keeping up to date with the most effective interventions; and by maintaining the trust of patients by doing good. Readers should realise that while this approach is more challenging, it will also be more rewarding.

CHARACTERISTICS OF BEING A PROFESSIONAL

Becoming a professional requires an acceptance, often implied, of certain responsibilities, in return for certain privileges. These responsibilities require certain behaviours and attitudes of individuals in whom professional trust is placed. Broadly, professionalism requires these attributes:

- a motivation to deliver service to others
- adherence to a moral and ethical code of practice
- striving for excellence, maintaining an awareness of limitations and scope of practice
- the empowerment of others (Hodkinson 1995 and Medical Professionalism Project 2002, both cited in CSP 2005b).

To practise in the profession of physiotherapy in the UK, registration with the statutory regulator is required. The Health Professions Council (HPC) sets standards of professional training, performance and conduct for thirteen professions, including physiotherapy (HPC 2006). It keeps a register of health professionals that meet its standards, and it takes action if registered health professionals do not meet those standards. It was created by the Health Professions Order 2001 (HPC 2002). Only those registered with the HPC may call themselves a physiotherapist/physical therapist (HPC 2006). It is the duty of registrants to keep up to date with the processes and requirements decreed by the Regulator; this is particularly important currently because of the changing attitudes to, and legislation of, healthcare professions in recent times.

The professional body for physiotherapists, the Chartered Society of Physiotherapy (CSP), provides a framework for the curriculum of physiotherapy education and approves those physiotherapy programmes that meet the requirements of the framework on behalf of the profession.

The CSP also publishes rules of professional conduct and standards of physiotherapy practice derived from within the profession, which are in harmony with those of the HPC. Anyone on the HPC physiotherapist register may call themselves a physiotherapist; only those who are members of the CSP may call themselves a *chartered* physiotherapist.

The breadth of activity and resources that the CSP undertakes and provides seek to establish a level of excellence for the profession. Its education and professional activity is centred on leading and supporting members' delivery of high-quality, evidence-based patient care. This activity emanates from its status as the professional body for physiotherapy in the UK and therefore as the primary holder and shaper of physiotherapy practice. The CSP works on behalf of the profession to protect the chartered status of physiotherapists' standing, which is one denoting excellence. It is worth noting that the relationship with the HPC is one of *registrant*; with the CSP it is one of *membership*.

While the principles of professionalism should be aspired to by physiotherapists anywhere in the world, the existence and/or role of regulators and professional bodies and the way these characteristics are manifested may vary, depending on political, social and financial factors.

Belonging to an organisation that sets standards and ideals of behaviour

The *Rules of Professional Conduct* (the *Rules*) were endorsed at the very first council meeting of the CSP in 1895 (Barclay 1994) and have been revised and updated at intervals since. The *Rules* define the professional behaviour expected of chartered physiotherapists. The current *Rules* set out a number of principles, the basis for all of which is to safeguard patients (CSP 2002a). They include requirements that chartered physiotherapists should:

- respect the dignity and individual sensibilities of every patient
- work safely and competently
- ensure the confidentiality of patient information
- report circumstances that might otherwise put patients at risk
- not exploit patients
- act in a way that reflects credit on the profession and does not cause offence to patients.

Although the CSP has had *Rules of Professional Conduct* since its inception, agreed national standards were not published until 1990. The CSP *Standards of Physiotherapy Practice* provides statements about the practical application of the ethical principles set out in the *Rules*. The fourth edition (CSP 2005a) has evolved to place more emphasis than in earlier editions on practitioners:

- involving patients in decision-making
- being fully abreast of the evidence of effectiveness in order to inform patients and offer the most effective interventions
- evaluating their practice and measuring a patient's health gain as a result of treatment.

This reflects the increasing expectations of the public to be active partners in their healthcare, the expectations of clinical governance to provide more effective care, and the growing demands of funders of services, as well as patients, to be able to demonstrate the benefits or 'added value' of physiotherapy. All these will be discussed later in the chapter.

Standards of Physiotherapy Practice is written in a way that offers a broad statement of intent (the Standard statement), which is followed by a number of measurable statements about expected performance or activity by the physiotherapist, student or assistant (known as 'criteria'). For example, Core Standard 2 states 'Patients are given relevant information about the proposed physiotherapy procedure, taking into account their age, emotional state and cognitive ability, to allow informed consent.' The criteria for this standard include the following:

- The patient's consent is obtained before starting any examination/treatment.
- Treatment options, including significant benefits, risks and side-effects, are discussed with the patient.
- The patient is given the opportunity to ask questions.
- The patient is informed of the right to decline physiotherapy at any stage without that prejudicing future care.
- The patient's consent to the treatment plan is documented in the patient's record.

These measurable criteria allow performance to be assessed against them, through clinical audit, described in more detail later.

The content of this standard and accompanying criteria set out the specific actions required in order to conform, in this case, to an aspect of Rule 2 of *Rules of Professional Conduct*: 'Chartered physiotherapists shall respect and uphold the rights, dignity and individual sensibilities of every patient,' which includes guidance on informed consent. This is a good example of how the *Standards* and *Rules* complement each other. They should be used together to ensure compliance with the characteristics and actions required of members of the physiotherapy profession.

Commitment to discipline other members

As of 15 October 2006 the CSP no longer handles complaints concerning the professional conduct or fitness to practise of its members, except those described in the next paragraph. The HPC considers all complaints of this nature.

The Society does however, handle complaints or consider matters of fitness to practise concerning members of the Society who are not regulated by the HPC. (This includes physiotherapist's physiotherapy treatment of animals, students and the CSP's associate members (CSP 2006).)

Possessing knowledge and skills not shared by others

Any profession possesses a range of specific knowledge and skills that are either unique, or more significantly developed than in other professions. The World Congress for Physical Therapy (WCPT) has described the nature of physiotherapy as 'providing services to people and populations to develop, maintain and restore maximum movement and functional ability throughout the lifespan' (WCPT 1999).

It adds, in a detailed description, that physical therapy is 'concerned with identifying and maximising movement potential, within the spheres of promotion, prevention, treatment and rehabilitation' (ibid, p28).

WCPT identifies the interaction between 'physical therapist, patients or clients, families and care givers, in a process of assessing movement potential and in establishing agreed upon goals and objectives' as crucial and acknowledges that this requires knowledge and skills unique to physical therapists (ibid, p28).

In the UK, one approach to conceptualising physiotherapy has been to focus on three core elements: massage, exercise and electrophysical modalities (CSP 2002a). For physiotherapy, the roots of the profession can be found in massage, the founders of the profession having been a group of nurses who carried out massage. The significance of therapeutic touching of patients still sets physiotherapy aside from other professions. Physiotherapists continue to use massage therapeutically as well as a wide range of other manual techniques such as manipulation and reflex therapy. Therapeutic handling underpins many aspects of rehabilitation, requiring the touching of patients to facilitate movement.

Another description of the profession's knowledge and skills can be found in the *Curriculum Framework for Qualifying Programmes in Physiotherapy* (CSP 2002b). This sets out the underpinning knowledge and skills required of newly qualifying physiotherapists, setting this in the context of their application in professional practice areas and environments. These are, in turn, underpinned by a set of professional attributes, identity and relationships, such as understanding the scope of practice and active engagement with patient partnership. Finally, the framework sets out the outcomes that graduates should be able to demonstrate: for example, 'enable individual patients and groups to optimise their health and social well-being' and 'respond appropriately to changing demands'.

Definition

Physiotherapy is a healthcare profession concerned with human function and movement and maximising potential. It uses physical approaches to promote, maintain and restore physical, psychological and social well-being, taking account of variations in health status. It is science-based, committed to extending, applying, evaluating and reviewing the evidence that underpins and informs its practice and delivery. The exercise of clinical judgement and informed interpretation is at its core (CSP 2002b).

Cott et al. (1995) have proposed an overarching framework for the profession: the movement continuum theory of physical therapy, arguing that the way in which physiotherapists conceptualise movement is what differentiates the profession from others. They suggest that physiotherapists conceive of movement on a continuum from a micro (molecular, cellular) to a macro (the person in his or her environment or in society) level. The authors argue that the theory is a unique approach to movement rehabilitation because it incorporates knowledge of pathology with a holistic view of movement, which includes the influence of physical, social and psychological factors in an assessment of a person's maximum achievable movement potential. They argue that the role of physiotherapy is to minimise the difference between a person's current movement capability and his or her preferred movement capability.

Exercising autonomy

Autonomy, or 'personal freedom' (*Concise Oxford Dictionary*, 7th edn) is a key characteristic of being a professional. It allows independence, but is mirrored by a responsibility and accountability for action. Central to the practice of professional autonomy is clinical reasoning, described as the 'thinking and decision-making processes associated with clinical practice' (Higgs and Jones 2000). Clinical reasoning requires the ability to think critically about practice, to learn from experience and apply that learning to future situations. It is the relationship between the physiotherapist's knowledge, his or her ability to collect, analyse and synthesise relevant information (cognition), and personal awareness, self-monitoring and reflective processes, or metacognition (Jones et al. 2000).

This professional autonomy has, however, to be balanced with the autonomy patients have to make their own decisions. Patient-centred decisions require a partnership between patient and professional, sharing information, with patients' values and experience being treated as equally important as clinical knowledge and scientific facts (Ersser and Atkins 2000). Higgs and Titchen (2001) describe the notion of the professional's role as a 'skilled companion'. The professional is characterised as a person with specialised knowledge which can be shared with the patient in a reciprocal 'working with' rather than 'doing to' relationship, and as someone who 'accompanies the patient on their journey towards health, adjustment, coping or death'. This patient-centred model facilitates the sharing of power and responsibility between professional and patient.

A history of how the physiotherapy profession's autonomy evolved in the UK can be found later in this chapter.

Licensed by the state

As previously mentioned, physiotherapists in the UK have to be registered with the HPC in order to use the title *physiotherapist* and therefore to work in any setting in the UK. This is a government measure to protect patients from unqualified or inadequately skilled healthcare providers.

In 2006, the HPC put in place a system requiring re-registration at intervals of two years, linked to an individual's commitment to Continuing Professional Development (CPD), whereby individuals must undertake and maintain a record of their CPD activities and, if required, submit evidence of this and of the outcomes of their CPD on their practice, service users and service. Re-registration is in response to a lessening of public confidence in the National Health Service (NHS) following, for example, the report into children's heart surgery in Bristol (Bristol Royal Infirmary Inquiry 2001). Equally disturbing were the revelations about the murders of so many patients by Harold Shipman, a man who had been a previously trusted general practitioner, where health systems failed to detect an unusually high number of deaths (Department of Health 2004).

This has led the government to introduce a number of measures, including the requirement for all health professionals to re-register at specified intervals, in order to be seen to be protecting the public through a more explicit and independent process (Department of Health 2002). It aims to identify poor performers who may be putting the public at risk, as well as providing an incentive for professionals to keep up to date, maintaining and further developing their scope of practice and competence to do their job. Disciplinary processes are in place to remove, ultimately, an individual from the register (HPC 2005). The means by which individuals can maintain their competence are discussed later in the chapter.

Making a commitment to assist those in need

As stated earlier, one of the characteristics of a professional is to want to 'do good'. This is reflected in the ethical principles of the physiotherapy profession, where there is a 'duty of care' incumbent on the individual towards the patient, to ensure that the therapeutic intervention is intended to be of benefit, as set out in Rule 1 (CSP 2002a). This is a common-law duty, a breach of which (negligence) could lead to a civil claim for damages.

More generally, Koehn (1994) suggests, professionals are perceived to have moral authority, or trustworthiness, if they:

- use their skills in the context of the client's best interests and 'doing good'
- are willing to act as long as it takes for assistance to achieve what it set out to achieve, or for a decision to be made that nothing more can be done to help the client
- have a highly developed internalised sense of responsibility to monitor personal behaviour: for example, by not taking advantage of vulnerable patients
- demand from the client the responsibility to provide, for example, sufficient information to allow decisions to be made (compliance)
- are allowed to exercise discretion (judgement) to do the best for the client, within limits.

Koehn (1994) argues that trustworthiness is what stands out as a particularly unique characteristic of being a professional — to do good, to have the patient's best interests at heart and to have high ethical standards. Physiotherapists not prepared to maintain such ethics, even in difficult and stressful situations, run the risk of losing the respect as well as the trust of their patients and the public.

RESPONSIBILITIES OF BEING A PROFESSIONAL

Physiotherapists in the UK are granted the right to make their own decisions, in partnership with patients, about meeting needs. Being a professional is a privilege — in particular the trust that is bestowed by the public which underpins the patient's ability to benefit from treatment. However, this brings with it weighty responsibilities.

Doing only those things you are competent to do

Every physiotherapist has her or his own personal 'scope of practice' (CSP 2002a) — that is, a range (or scope) of professional knowledge and skills that can be applied competently within specific practice settings or populations.

When a person is newly qualified, this scope will be based on the content of the pre-qualifying Curriculum Framework, but will also be informed by the individual's experience in clinical placements, and the amount of teaching and reflective learning that has been possible as part of those placements.

As a career progresses, and as a result of CPD, some physiotherapists will become competent in highly skilled areas such as intensive care procedures, or splinting for children with cerebral palsy, which are unlikely to have been taught before qualification. Others will extend their skills in areas in which they already had some experience: for example, dealing with people with neurological problems. Others will enhance their communication and life skills, as well as refining their physiotherapy skills by, for example, working with elderly people or people with learning difficulties.

It is the responsibility of the professional to understand his or her personal scope of practice as it changes and evolves throughout a career. To practise in areas in which you are not competent puts patients at risk and is a breach of the CSP's *Rules of Professional Conduct*, and the standards of the profession's regulator, the HPC (2003).

Maintaining competence to practise

An individual's scope of practice and competence are constantly evolving, based on professional and life experiences, learning from reading, from evaluating practice, from reflecting on practice, or more formal ways of learning. It includes undertaking programmes of structured CPD. Clinical reasoning skills are continually refined and further developed throughout a career through evaluative and reflective practice, leading to the ability to deal with increasingly complex and unpredictable situations.

Physiotherapists have a duty to keep up to date with new information generated by research, with what their peers are thinking and doing, and by formally evaluating the outcome of their practice. The responsibility for this is dictated by the HPC (2003) and reflected in the *Standards of Physiotherapy Practice* (CSP 2005a). In particular, Core Standards 19–22 are concerned with a requirement that individuals assess their learning needs, then plan, implement and evaluate a programme of CPD based on that assessment.

Responsibility to patients

This chapter has already discussed the importance of the individual physiotherapist as well as the profession as a whole in maintaining the attributes of professionals. Trust is perhaps the most essential characteristic with which to develop a sense of partnership with patients; in turn, this will optimise the benefits of intervention. For physiotherapy, many of the other hallmarks for building and securing trust are set out in the profession's *Rules* and *Standards*. For example:

- to provide safe and effective interventions (safety of application as well as safe and effective) — Rule 1 and Core Standards 4, 8, 16
- to treat patients with dignity and respect — Rule 2 and Core Standard 1
- to provide patients with information about their options for treatment/interventions — Rule 2 and Core Standard 2
- to involve patients in decisions about their treatment (informed consent) — Rule 2 and Core Standard 2.

Responsibility to those who pay for services

Physiotherapists have an ethical responsibility to those who finance services, whether these are commissioners of healthcare, taxpayers or individual patients, to provide efficiently delivered, clinically and cost-effective interventions and services, in order to give value in an era when resources for healthcare are limited. This is embedded within Rule 1 of the CSP's *Rules of Professional Conduct* in relation to the establishment of a 'duty of care' towards the patient (CSP 2002a).

Responsibility to colleagues and the profession

A profession has legitimate expectations of its members to conduct themselves in a way that does not bring the profession into disrepute, but rather enhances public perceptions. Physiotherapists have a duty to inform themselves of what is expected of them. Indeed, the *Rules of Professional Conduct* state that knowledge of and adherence to the *Rules* are part of the contract of membership of the CSP. The *Standards of Physiotherapy Practice* make it clear there is an expectation that all physiotherapists should be able to achieve all the core standards (CSP 2005a). Where they do not, programmes of professional development should be put in place to facilitate full compliance, as part of the individual's professional responsibility.

Physiotherapists should not be critical of each other, except in extreme circumstances. However, they do have a duty to report circumstances that could put patients at risk. In the NHS, there are procedures and a nominated officer within each trust from whom advice can be sought. Outside the NHS, advice can be sought from the CSP. Physiotherapists are encouraged to be proactive in supporting each other's professional development and in promoting the value of the profession in local workplace settings, in policy-making forums and in the media.

BECOMING AN AUTONOMOUS PROFESSION

The CSP was founded in 1894, under the name of the Society of Trained Masseuses. This section will not attempt to relate the history of the profession, except in the context of developing autonomy. However, more about the early days of the profession can be found in the book *In Good Hands* (Barclay 1994).

For many years, doctors governed the profession. One of the first rules of professional conduct stated 'no massage to be undertaken except under medical direction' (ibid). Even in the 1960s doctors were asserting that they must take full responsibility for patients in their charge and 'professional and technical staff have no right to challenge [the doctor's] views; only he is equipped to decide how best to get the patients fit again' (ibid). It is hard to believe now that it took more than 80 years to escape the paternalism of doctors, on whom physiotherapists were dependent for referrals. The first breakthrough came in the early 1970s, when a report by the Remedial Professions Committee, chaired by Professor Sir Ronald Tunbridge, included a statement that while the doctor should retain responsibility for prescribing treatment, more scope in application and duration should be given to therapists.

The McMillan report (DHSS 1973) went further, by recommending that therapists should be allowed to decide the nature and duration of treatment, although doctors would remain responsible for the patient's welfare. There was recognition that doctors who referred patients would not be skilled in the detailed application of particular techniques, and that the therapist would therefore be able to operate more effectively if given greater responsibility and freedom.

Eventually, a Health Circular called *Relationship between the Medical and Remedial Professions* was issued (DHSS, 1977). This acknowledged the therapist's competence and responsibility for deciding on the nature of the treatment to be given. It recognised the ability of the physiotherapist to determine the most appropriate intervention for a patient, based on knowledge over and above that which it would be reasonable to expect a doctor to possess. It also recognised the close relationship between therapist and patient, and the importance of the therapist interpreting and adjusting treatment according to immediate patient responses.

Autonomy was only achieved by being able to demonstrate competence to make appropriate decisions, building up the trust of doctors and those paying for physiotherapy services. The need to acquire skills of assessment and analysis became a key component of student programmes from the 1970s. Today, qualifying programmes stress even further the development of skills, knowledge and attributes required for autonomous practice.

CLINICAL GOVERNANCE

So far, this chapter has explored the responsibilities of being a physiotherapist from a professional perspective. The focus has been on the individual's personal responsibility as a professional. This section will put all that in the context of a professional's responsibilities to the employer organisation, whether it be in the public or the independent sector.

In the NHS, responsibility for the clinical safety of patients and the quality and effectiveness of services is maintained via a system of clinical governance. It seems probable this will apply equally to the independent sector in the near future. However, even though clinical governance is the responsibility of NHS trusts, its foundation is based on 'the principle that health professionals must be responsible and accountable for their own practice' (Secretary of State for Health 1998). The individual's professional responsibility is therefore still paramount.

What is clinical governance?

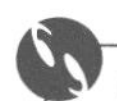

Definition

Clinical governance is a framework through which NHS organisations are accountable for continuously improving the quality of their services and safeguarding high standards of care by creating an environment in which excellence in clinical care will flourish (Secretary of State for Health 1998). (While this definition has been used in England, similar interpretations of the term have been made in Scotland, Wales and Northern Ireland.)

A number of key themes were introduced as part of clinical governance.

The accountability of chief executives for quality

Although some chief executives of NHS trusts claim they were always responsible for quality, this had not been a statutory responsibility in the way it was for a trust's finances. Chief executives now have a statutory responsibility for quality.

The introduction of a philosophy of continuous improvement

One-off improvements are not enough — the NHS has to move to a culture of continuous improvement to achieve excellence. In addition, the emphasis has shifted from improving a particular aspect of care in isolation, to examining the whole system of care, crossing professions, departments, organisations and sectors, to ensure the whole process meets the needs of patients through an integrated approach to healthcare.

An aspiration to achieve consistency of services across the NHS

This is founded on two principles:

- If one trust can provide excellence in a service, then so can all trusts.
- Local services should, where possible, be based on national standards: for example, National Service Frameworks or nationally developed clinical guidelines.

There is some evidence to suggest that nationally developed standards or clinical guidelines are likely to be more robustly developed (Sudlow and Thomson 1997) and that their universal implementation locally will ensure consistency and effectiveness.

An emphasis on continuing professional development (CPD) and life-long learning (LLL)

Clinical governance acknowledges the importance of CPD/LLL for all healthcare workers, in order to keep up to date and deliver high-quality services.

Is clinical governance something new?

Yes and no. Its component parts are all familiar activities, but there is also an underpinning philosophy in clinical governance to reduce risks for patients, a new and more focused emphasis that was not previously articulated. It can be argued that clinical governance is, at least in part, a response to a loss of public confidence in the NHS, as discussed earlier, which has undermined people's perceptions of the NHS as an organisation they can rely on to 'do good' and of the government as a protector of the public. In addition, the public has become more litigious, suing doctors and trusts more readily for mistakes, thus drawing money away from front-line clinical services. So clinical governance is about rebuilding the public's confidence in health services, providing high-quality and effective care and, above all, reducing the risk of harm through negligence, poor performance or system failures.

The components of clinical governance

Although clinical governance should be seen as a package of measures that together ensure excellence and a reduction in risk, it can also be viewed as a number of component parts, some of which have been in place for a number of years and are already familiar (Figure 1.1). They include:

- evidence-based practice and clinical effectiveness
- applying national standards and guidelines locally
- evaluating the effectiveness and quality of services
- continuing professional development/life-long learning
- having the right workforce and using it appropriately.

The following sections deal with these aspects.

EVIDENCE-BASED PRACTICE

At the beginning of this chapter, it was asserted that people who want to become physiotherapists have an inherent desire to 'do good'. But how do we know what works — what interventions have been shown to be effective? It is hard to comprehend that health professionals have not always sought evidence for the effectiveness of the treatments they use. Perhaps they did — but until the early 1990s this 'evidence' was based on personal experience and on opinions derived from that experience, together with the experience of colleagues, or those perceived to be experts and opinion leaders. Is that good enough?

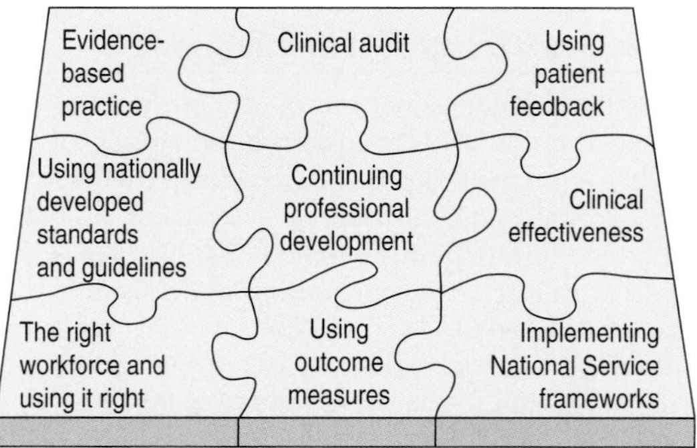

Figure 1.1 Components of clinical governance.

In 1991, Sir Michael Peckham, then Director of Research and Development for the Department of Health, noted that 'strongly held views based on belief rather than sound information still exert too much influence in healthcare. In some instances the relevant knowledge is available but is not being used, in other situations additional knowledge needs to be generated from reliable sources' (Department of Health 1991). At about the same time, a relatively small group of doctors began to write about evidence-based medicine.

Definition

An early definition of evidence-based medicine stated that it is the 'conscientious, explicit and judicious use of current best evidence in making decisions about the care of individual patients' (Sackett et al. 1996).

A recent definition has updated this, drawing on criticisms of the initial position and stating that evidence-based practice requires that 'decisions about health care are based on the best available, current, valid and relevant evidence. These decisions should be made by those receiving care, informed by the tacit and explicit knowledge of those providing care, within the context of available resources' (Dawes et al. 2005).

What do we mean by evidence? Is research the only form of evidence? Certainly for some questions, such as the efficacy of particular drugs, or a particular modality such as exercise programmes for the management of back pain, research studies which compare one intervention with another or a placebo (randomised controlled trials) can provide reliable information about the degree to which an intervention is effective. But other forms of evidence are also important (Figure 1.2). What patients tell us about their condition, which treatments they find effective, the degree to which interventions improve their ability to get on with their lives also provides important evidence. The physiotherapist also contributes evidence in the form of clinical expertise, derived from clinical reasoning experience. Thinking and reflecting on what you are doing, as a practitioner during or after a clinical encounter, will develop such expertise (Jones et al. 2000). Knowledge which arises from and within practice (practice-based and practice-generated knowledge) will become part, along with research evidence, of your rationale for practice (Higgs and Titchen 2001). Sackett and colleagues reflected this in concluding their definition that evidence-based practice requires integration of 'clinical expertise with best available external clinical evidence from systematic research' (Sackett et al. 1996).

A hierarchy of evidence is often described or used in the literature. This ranges from (1) systematic reviews, in which evidence on a topic has been systematically

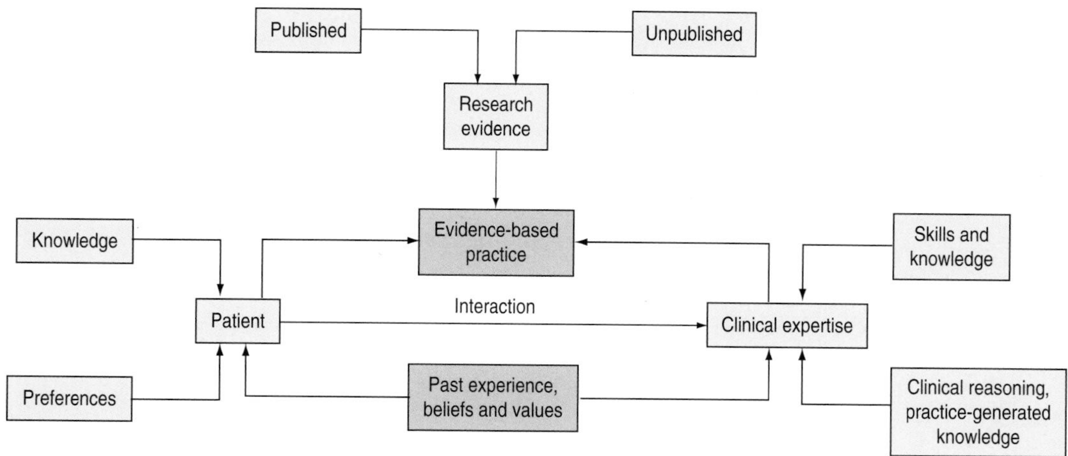

Figure 1.2 What do we mean by 'evidence'? (Adapted from Bury 1998, with permission.)

identified, appraised and summarised according to predetermined criteria (usually limited to randomised controlled trials) — said to be the strongest evidence (the most reliable estimate of effectiveness) to (2) expert opinion, perceived as the least reliable. An example is shown in Table 1.1.

However, such a hierarchy fails to recognise that different research methods are needed to answer different types of question and that, while a qualitative study may be the best research method for a particular question, it still receives a low rating. The hierarchy also fails to recognise the importance of expertise derived from clinical reasoning experience, discussed above. Physiotherapists need to contribute to an ongoing debate to develop a hierarchy that reflects more appropriately a patient-centred approach to practice.

Table 1.1 A hierarchy of evidence

Level	Type of evidence
Ia	Evidence obtained from a systematic review or meta-analysis of randomised controlled trials
Ib	Evidence obtained from at least one randomised controlled trial
IIa	Evidence obtained from at least one well-designed controlled study without randomisation
IIb	Evidence obtained from at least one other type of well-designed quasi-experimental study
III	Evidence obtained from well-designed non-experimental descriptive studies, such as comparative studies, correlation studies and case studies
IV	Evidence obtained from expert committee reports or opinions and/or clinical experience of respected authorities

Adapted from National Institute for Health and Clinical Excellence (2001).

So what does evidence-based practice mean for physiotherapists? Core Standard 4 (CSP 2005a) states that: 'In order to deliver effective care, information relating to treatment options is identified, based on the best available evidence.' A range of sources of information the physiotherapist may need to draw on, including research evidence, patient organisations and clinical guidelines, is listed. What practical steps need to be taken to identify and use research evidence?

- Think about the clinical question you are trying to answer in your information search. Identify the population (e.g. people with multiple sclerosis with symptoms of urinary incontinence), the intervention you are looking for (e.g. neuromuscular electrical stimulation) and the outcome (e.g. a reduction in symptoms), and use this information to formulate a search strategy.
- Work in partnership with an information scientist to get the best results from a literature search (his or her information skills and knowledge combined with your clinical skills and knowledge).
- Look first for evidence that has already been synthesised — systematic reviews, nationally developed clinical guidelines or standards. This saves a lot of effort searching for individual studies. If it is a high-quality synthesis, it will also provide a more reliable estimate of effectiveness.
- Know your databases well enough to know which will have the most relevant information on any particular topic.

- Check the titles and abstracts for relevance.
- Critically appraise any relevant papers you have found to assure yourself of their quality and of the reliability of their conclusions. (A list of appraisal instruments can be found at the end of this chapter.)
- When you find the 'best available evidence', think about it in relation to your patient and your past experience. Is it appropriate for that patient, will you be able to quantify for the patient the degree of likely benefits and harms (if any)?
- Discuss the evidence with the patient and agree the preferred intervention(s) together.
- Implement the preferred intervention(s).
- Evaluate the effect of the intervention(s) and act accordingly.

Weblink

More information about evidence-based practice can be found in Herbert et al. (2005) or at www.nettingtheevidence.org.uk/, a catalogue of useful electronic learning resources and links to organisations that facilitate evidence-based healthcare. See also 'Sources of Critical Appraisal Tools' towards the end of this chapter.

CLINICAL EFFECTIVENESS

Clinical effectiveness, as defined by the Department of Health, sounds very much like evidence-based practice — doing things you know will be effective for a particular patient or group of patients. But the fact that an intervention has been proved to work in research studies, in a relatively controlled environment, does not necessarily mean that it will work for a particular patient. Both patients and practitioners are unique beings, and there are many additional factors, practical and behavioural, that need to be considered to ensure the patient gets the maximum benefit from an intervention.

Definition

Clinical effectiveness was defined by the Department of Health in 1996 as 'the extent to which specific clinical interventions, when deployed in the field for a particular patient or population, do what they are intended to do – that is, maintain and improve health and secure the greatest possible health gain from the available resources' (NHS Executive 1996).

- Is the practitioner sufficiently skilled to apply the intervention safely and effectively?
- Is the practitioner an effective communicator?
- Does the practitioner give the patient an opportunity to describe the symptoms fully, to explain the impact of the problem on daily life, and to ask questions?
- Does the patient have enough information to be able to give informed consent?
- Are other options discussed that may have been more acceptable to the patient, even if less effective?
- Would treatment in a hospital setting mean a long, exhausting and expensive journey for the patient?
- Would the patient feel intimidated by a hospital environment?
- Would treatment be more effective if it were provided closer to home: for example, in the GP's surgery or health centre?
- Would treatment be more relevant if it were given in a patient's own home, to be able to develop a programme tailored to the person's lifestyle and environmental needs?
- Wherever treated, does the patient have adequate privacy, warmth and comfort?
- How long has the patient had to wait for treatment and will a delay alter the effectiveness of the interventions?

The answer to each of these questions can have an impact on the patient's ability to benefit from an intervention, however effective the research evidence might suggest an intervention is. This also illustrates the complexity of the clinical reasoning process, where highly skilled judgements have to be made based on a consideration of the whole person, physically, emotionally and within society, as well as the environment, practitioner skills and resources available, in order to provide truly effective treatment.

So while evidence-based practice is a key component of clinical effectiveness, clinical effectiveness also takes account of a range of other influences that could affect the patient's ability to benefit from an intervention based on high-quality research evidence.

APPLYING NATIONAL STANDARDS AND GUIDELINES LOCALLY

Standards

One of the tenets of clinical governance is consistency — for the public, being confident that they will experience the same quality of care and have access to the most effective interventions, regardless of where they live. There should be no postcode lottery, where some treatments might be available in some parts of the country

1

and not others; the quality of the average and worst services should be raised to that of the best. Where there are high-quality national standards, therefore, these should be used locally. Two examples are set out below.

Nationally developed standards

The CSP's *Standards of Physiotherapy Practice* provides a universal framework for the delivery of services throughout the UK, to which it is expected all physiotherapists will conform. So, for physiotherapy, patients can expect similar values and processes within a healthcare experience.

National Service Frameworks (NSFs)

This government initiative aims to provide the NHS with explicit standards and principles for the pattern and level of services required for a specific service or care group. The NSFs aim to address the 'whole system of care' and each will set out where care is best provided and the standard of care that patients should be offered in each setting. They provide 'a clear set of priorities against which local action can be framed' and seek to ensure that patients will get greater consistency in the availability and quality of services, right across the NHS (Secretary of State for Health 1998).

Table 1.2 lists the NSFs that have been developed. They provide broad statements of expected services. For example, the NSF for older people states: 'Older people who have fallen receive effective treatment and rehabilitation and, with their carers, receive advice on prevention through a specialised falls service.'

Physiotherapists will therefore need to address the implementation of this standard in any services they provide to older people. Implementation will also provide opportunities to promote the value of physiotherapy to this patient population and highlight the contribution physiotherapists can make to a trust's compliance with this particular standard.

Table 1.2 National service frameworks developed by the Department of Health

- Coronary heart disease (including cardiac rehabilitation)
- Cancer
- Paediatric intensive care
- Mental health
- Older people (including falls, osteoporosis and stroke)
- Diabetes
- Long-term conditions
- Renal
- Children
- Chronic obstructive pulmonary disease (2008)

Clinical guidelines

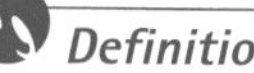

Definition

Clinical guidelines are 'systematically developed statements to assist practitioner and patient decisions about appropriate healthcare for specific circumstances' (Field and Lohr 1992).

The key factors in the development of clinical guidelines are the systematic process for identifying and quality-assessing research evidence, and the systematic and transparent process used for the interpretation of the evidence in the context of clinical practice, in order to formulate reliable recommendations for practice.

National Institute for Health and Clinical Excellence (NICE)

NICE is a Special Health Authority for England and Wales, established by the government in 1999 to provide health professionals and the public with authoritative information about the clinical effectiveness and cost-effectiveness of healthcare. One of its work programmes is to develop clinical guidelines, which are carried out by a series of collaborating centres. The Department of Health and the Assembly for Wales have given NICE the remit for developing 'robust and authoritative' clinical guidelines, taking into account clinical effectiveness and cost effectiveness. More information about the key principles that underpin the way NICE approaches clinical guideline development can be found on its website.

Weblink

National Institute for Health and Clinical Excellence (NICE): www.nice.org.uk.

Scottish Intercollegiate Guidelines Network (SIGN)

SIGN was formed in 1993. Its objective is to improve the quality of healthcare for patients in Scotland by reducing variation in practice and outcome, through the development and dissemination of national clinical guidelines containing recommendations for effective practice based on current evidence. Further information can be found on its website.

Weblink

Scottish Intercollegiate Guidelines Network (SIGN): www.show.scot.nhs.uk/sign.

1

Professionally led clinical guidelines

The physiotherapy profession has developed national, physiotherapy-specific clinical guidelines. To ensure quality and provide confidence for users, the CSP has established a process for the endorsement of these clinical guidelines. The criteria for assessing whether the quality of a guideline warrants CSP endorsement can be found in an appraisal questionnaire developed by a European consortium, known as the AGREE instrument. For users of clinical guidelines, CSP-endorsed clinical guidelines can be considered of high quality and should be implemented locally. Further information about the process for the development of clinical guidelines in physiotherapy is available from the CSP website.

Weblink

AGREE Collaboration (Appraisal of Guidelines Research and Evaluation):
www.agreecollaboration.org.
Chartered Society of Physiotherapists (CSP):
www.csp.org.uk.

EVALUATING SERVICES

How do you know whether you are being effective? Knowing whether you are or not is part of your professional responsibility as a physiotherapist. Rule 1 of *Rules of Professional Conduct* (CSP 2002a) describes the responsibility a physiotherapist has to ensure that any intervention offered to a patient is intended to be of benefit. Several of the CSP's standards of physiotherapy practice include criteria that relate to evaluation, including:

- As part of the assessment process, physiotherapists consider and critically evaluate information about effective interventions relating to the patient's condition (Core Standard 4.1).
- A published, standardised, valid, reliable and responsive outcome measure is used to evaluate the change in the patient's health status (Core Standard 6).
- All physiotherapists participate in a regular and systematic programme of clinical audit (Service Standard 3.2).
- Physiotherapists use the results of audit to assess their learning needs (Core Standard 19.1) and/or as a means to achieve their personal learning objectives (Core Standard 20.3h).

All evaluation is about learning which leads to improvements in the quality and effectiveness of practice. It should be carried out, and the results used, in the context of CPD and reflective practice, to improve an individual practitioner's personal practice and/or the delivery of a whole service. Set out below are four means by which physiotherapists can evaluate their practice. They are not mutually exclusive.

Evaluating the process of care (clinical audit)

In order to evaluate the *process* of care, it is necessary to have a reliable benchmark with which to compare your practice. Earlier, the importance of the local implementation of nationally developed standards and evidence-based clinical guidelines was discussed. These provide such a reliable benchmark. Clinical audit is a tool with which to measure your own performance (or more often, the performance of the service) against standards or criteria based on the 'best available evidence' of effectiveness. This will enable you to identify the extent to which you adhere to those standards or criteria, from which recommendations can be put in place to improve adherence, if necessary.

Definition

Clinical audit is a cyclical process involving the identification of a topic, setting standards, comparing practice with the standards, implementing changes, and monitoring the effect of those changes (CSP 2005a). Further information about clinical audit can be found in an information paper published by the CSP (2002d) and in *Principles for Best Practice in Clinical Audit* published by NICE (2001).

Evaluating the health outcomes of care

This will determine the *impact* of the process of care on the patient's life by using specific measures before and after treatment. The use of a test, scale or questionnaire which records what it aims to record (*is valid and responsive*) and is sufficiently well described to ensure that everyone who uses it does so in the same way (*is reliable*) will help to give physiotherapists the chance to see whether the aims of their intervention have had the impact intended.

A database of outcome measures can be found on the CSP website. This will facilitate the selection of the most appropriate measures for a specific patient or patient group. More information on using measures can be found in a CSP information paper (CSP 2001a).

As well as patients themselves having an interest in an objective assessment of their improvement, it is increasingly important for managers and team leaders to present such information to commissioners of healthcare, to demonstrate the benefits of physiotherapy services and their value for money.

Using patient feedback

Another mechanism for evaluating practice is to ask the patient for feedback. This could be through the use of a validated patient-assessed outcome measure to provide information about the patient's perception of health gain, or through the use of a structured questionnaire to determine the patient's perception of the quality of the treatment. The CSP's *Standards of Physiotherapy Practice* pack includes a ready-made Patient Feedback Questionnaire, designed to measure criteria in the core standards, for which only patients can judge compliance. Patients are asked to respond to statements that mirror the criteria (Table 1.3).

Responses from the feedback questionnaires can be used by individuals or services to reflect on the extent to which the criteria are being met, and to introduce new processes or development opportunities to secure greater conformance, if necessary.

Another valuable source of patient feedback is patients' complaints. These should be considered positively as opportunities to address the issues contained within them, in order to introduce a service improvement. Any issue that becomes a problem for a patient is a problem for the service, which should be analysed. The involvement of the patient making the complaint in this process, if willing, will facilitate the finding of a solution that can then be embedded into systems and processes.

Peer review

Peer review provides an opportunity to evaluate the clinical reasoning behind your decision-making with a trusted peer. It can be applied most effectively to the assessment, treatment planning and evaluative components of physiotherapy practice, where the reasoning behind the information recorded in the patient documentation can be explored. Guidance on peer review can be found in the clinical audit tools document contained in the *Standards of Physiotherapy Practice* pack (CSP 2005a).

CONTINUING PROFESSIONAL DEVELOPMENT

Definition

Continuing professional development (CPD) is the work-oriented aspect of life-long learning and should be seen as a systematic, ongoing structured process of maintaining, developing and enhancing skills, knowledge and competence both professionally and personally in order to improve performance at work (CSP 2003).

Definition

Life-long learning (LLL) is a theme the government promulgates across all sectors of the population, in order to ensure the workforce is equipped to do the jobs that will contribute to high-quality public services and promote prosperity in the UK.

In healthcare, the connection between CPD/LLL and the quality of services is at the centre of the government's view of a new, modernised NHS. Physiotherapists have always had a strong commitment to CPD evidenced by the clear statement in Rule 1 of *Rules of Professional Conduct*: 'Chartered physiotherapists shall only practise to the extent that they have... maintained... their ability to work safely and competently.' The *Core Standards of Physiotherapy Practice*, with which all physiotherapists should conform, include

Table 1.3 Extract from a patient feedback questionnaire

Criteria	Patient feedback questionnaire	Response option
Core Standard 5.3 The findings of the clinical assessment are explained to the patient	By the end of your first visit, were the results of the assessment explained?	Yes, no, don't know
Core Standard 8.1 Physiotherapists ensure that the patient is fully involved in any decision-making process during treatment planning	I felt involved in deciding about my treatment plan	Strongly disagree, disagree, uncertain, agree, strongly agree
Core Standard 12.3 All communication, written and verbal, is clear, unambiguous and easily understood by the recipient	The physiotherapists used words I didn't understand	Strongly disagree, disagree, uncertain, agree, strongly agree

(Adapted from CSP 2000.)

standards for the assessment, planning, implementation and evaluation of a CPD programme. Service Standards 6 and 7 require that all physiotherapy services should have a programme of CPD/in-service training for staff.

The requirement for re-registration of physiotherapists and other healthcare professionals, discussed earlier, makes CPD an essential component of professional life. A philosophy of LLL and individual responsibility for this will be introduced in qualifying programmes, equipping students for a lifetime of learning in order to maintain and continually improve their competence to practise. Written evidence of learning and development, and its impact on improving practice, is now an essential requirement. Every physiotherapist must establish a portfolio containing such evidence, which will need to be maintained throughout a career. Guidance on this can be found in *Developing a Portfolio: a Guide for CSP Members* (CSP 2001b).

Some key characteristics of continuing professional development (CSP 2003)

- It should comprise a broad range of learning activities (courses, in-service education, reading, supervision, research, audit, reflections on experience, peer review — this is not an exhaustive list).
- It is based on individual responsibility, trust and self-evaluation.
- It links learning with enhancement of quality of patient care and professional excellence whilst ensuring public safety.
- It should recognise the outcomes of CPD with a focus on achievement.

The emphasis on the importance of CPD/LLL within clinical governance is a welcome development. The challenges for physiotherapists in keeping up to date are huge, with the fast pace of change in healthcare — in particular the rapid increase in the volume of information that has to be evaluated and incorporated into practice. It is hoped that protected time for CPD, including time in the workplace, will become a reality in the NHS, as recommended by the Kennedy Report (Bristol Royal Infirmary Inquiry 2001) and the CSP (2003).

Another form of professional development is reflective practice, a process in which practitioners think critically about their practice and as a result may modify their action or behaviour. 'Reflection enables learning at a sub-conscious level to be brought to a level where it is articulated and shared with others' (CSP 2001b). Learning from experience requires the development of skills such as self-awareness, open-mindedness and critical analysis.

Definition

Reflective practice is the process of reviewing an episode of practice to describe, analyse, evaluate and inform professional learning; in such a way, new learning modifies previous perceptions, assumptions and understanding, and the application of this learning to practice influences treatment approaches and outcomes (CSP 2002b).

HAVING THE RIGHT WORKFORCE (AND USING IT APPROPRIATELY)

Physiotherapists have a professional responsibility to use their skills appropriately. This reflects Rule 1 of *Rules of Professional Conduct*, which states that physiotherapists should 'only practise to the extent that they have established, maintained and developed their ability to work safely and competently'. But there is also a professional responsibility to use resources (human as well as financial) appropriately in delivering healthcare. This means giving consideration as to whether you need to refer a patient on, either because he or she requires a higher level of skill than you possess, or needs a specialist in a different clinical area. Equally, consideration should be given as to whether there are elements of the treatment programme that can be delegated to a physiotherapy assistant or other support worker. (The word 'assistant' is used in the following section to mean both of these.)

The decision about whether to delegate, and which tasks or activities to delegate, is entirely the responsibility of the physiotherapist making that decision. The physiotherapist also takes full responsibility for the application of the tasks or activities carried out by the person who has been delegated. So choosing tasks to be undertaken by an assistant is a complex element of professional activity, which depends on an informed professional opinion.

- *What to delegate?* Physiotherapists need to use their own skills and knowledge to carry out an assessment of a patient in order to formulate a clinical diagnosis and a programme of treatment derived from those findings. This process requires skills of analysis and clinical reasoning, key professional attributes. However, an appropriately trained assistant may well have the attributes required to be able to carry out some or all elements of the treatment programme, based on existing knowledge and skills. This would include the monitoring of the patient's

condition and progress with the plan, and advising the physiotherapist of any variations in either of these. As there are no hard and fast rules about what to delegate, the physiotherapist should consider carefully the scope and nature of the task and ensure that these are clearly defined and communicated to the assistant.
- *Who to delegate to?* The factors to be considered here are the competence of the assistant and the nature of the task. The competence of the assistant will be affected by the person's length of service, prior experience and training received, coupled with judgements by the physiotherapist about the assistant's ability to deal with that particular patient in those particular circumstances.

The decision about what to delegate and who to delegate to is one that, while ultimately the responsibility of the physiotherapist, also requires the active involvement of the person to whom the task is being delegated. The assistant, therefore, must be allowed to make an assessment of his or her own competence in relation to the particular task. The task should *not* be delegated if either the physiotherapist *or* the assistant is concerned about the assistant's competence. The physiotherapist will then need to decide whether training is required.

Newly qualified physiotherapists should recognise and value the skills and knowledge many assistants possess, particularly those who have long service within the profession, so that effective partnerships between physiotherapists and assistants can contribute to the efficient and effective delivery of physiotherapy services. Physiotherapy assistant members of the CSP have a *Code of Conduct* (CSP 2002c) to which they are expected to adhere in the same way physiotherapists are to the *Rules*. Users of physiotherapy services have a right to expect those who deliver them to be competent to do so. The physiotherapist has the ultimate responsibility to the patient for ensuring this is the case, but also needs to consider competence in the context of effective resource use, in terms of both finance and skills.

MONITORING CLINICAL GOVERNANCE

NHS physiotherapy managers are responsible for devising, implementing and reporting on a departmental clinical governance programme, which should reflect all the aspects of clinical governance discussed in this chapter. Physiotherapists should play an active part in contributing to physiotherapy clinical governance programmes and also participate in relevant multiprofessional clinical governance activities such as clinical audit or local protocol/clinical pathway design.

The Healthcare Commission is an independent statutory body established to raise standards throughout England and Wales. In Scotland a similar function is provided by NHS Quality Improvement Scotland, the Health and Personal Social Services Regulation and Improvement Authority (HPSSRIA) undertakes regular reviews of the quality of services in Northern Ireland. The Healthcare Commission is tasked with assessing the implementation of clinical governance in every NHS trust and making its findings public. Teams of trained reviewers visit trusts every 3–5 years (and can be called in at any time should concerns be raised) to review trust information and data, talk to staff and patients, and consider the trust's performance in specified categories. The Healthcare Commission has added to its existing responsibilities those for inspecting hospitals and care homes in the private sector and carrying out value-for-money studies and performance management within the NHS.

Examples of a physiotherapy manager's responsibilities within a clinical governance programme

- Check staff are currently on the state register.
- Deal with and learn from complaints.
- Carry out programmes for quality improvement, including clinical audit and evaluation, and report how these have led to improvements for patients.
- Ensure that nationally produced, high-quality standards and clinical guidelines are implemented locally.
- Have an appropriate skill mix and staffing level to ensure the safety of patients, making appropriate use of human and financial resources, in order to provide effective care.
- Have a process for identifying and supporting staff members whose competence is in question.
- Provide an in-service training programme and time for individual CPD activities.
- Ensure appropriate participation in multiprofessional clinical audit and quality improvement activities.

So, being a competent physiotherapist who displays the essential characteristics of a professional in the current climate is a complex and demanding process. Figure 1.3 attempts to summarise the elements of professionalism described in this chapter.

THE FUTURE

The health service continues to be a high priority for the government. Change is constant and a key challenge for

Patient-focused practice, underpinned by sound clinical reasoning and professional judgement, ongoing reflection, and critical application of the evidence base
Professional responsibility, manifested in adherence to a professional code of conduct/standards of practice, undertaking structured, evaluated CPD to meet identified learning needs, and engagement with the full implications of clinical effectiveness
Professional privilege, expressed through professional autonomy and self-regulation

Figure 1.3 Elements of professionalism. (With thanks to Dr Sally Gosling.)

physiotherapists is to respond to the opportunities and risks presented to ensure that high-quality services are delivered to patients. Many of the government's priority health programmes will be dependent for their success on the provision of effective rehabilitation in order to ensure people can continue to lead independent lives, including services for older people, children and those with long-term conditions. Physiotherapists also have a key contribution to make to keeping people fit for work through, for example, the effective management of musculoskeletal problems or the delivery of cardiac rehabilitation programmes. Ensuring ergonomically safe environments in the workplace and offering a rapid work-based response when treatment is needed provide other examples of the value of the profession.

Structural changes

Continued investment in healthcare will bring with it an increase in the expectations of the public whose money is being used, and challenges from the government and the public about the need to change and modernise the way in which healthcare is delivered. Services will need to be more responsive to patients' needs, provided in settings closer to patients' own environments, and delivered more speedily to maximise health benefits and utilise available resources more effectively.

Many more physiotherapy services will be provided in primary care and community settings. Primary Care Trusts (PCTs) will hold 60 per cent of the total budget for healthcare in their local area, and local people will have a much stronger voice in the decision-making process about how those funds are used. In addition, the government has committed itself to increasing integration between health and social care, through Care Trusts, where budgets are pooled in order that they can be used more flexibly to meet the needs of the local population.

More services delivered in primary care and community settings

Physiotherapy already has a track record of delivering responsive and effective services in primary care and community settings. The success of domiciliary and community-based physiotherapy services in avoiding hospital admissions and allowing speedier discharges will be further reinforced through the introduction of intermediate care. The musculoskeletal physiotherapy services delivered in GP practices and health centres, where trust is already established between doctors and physiotherapists, has facilitated more direct access to patients and better referrals, making services more efficient as well as effective.

The challenges, however, will lie with greater team working and delegation of tasks, with physiotherapists having to be prepared to be more flexible, often taking on teaching roles in order to allow other staff such as rehabilitation assistants to deliver services. There will be a need to take on some non-physiotherapeutic roles, such as key worker or case manager, in order to deliver a more consistent approach to care to vulnerable people living in the community.

Another challenge will be the experience of working in more isolated settings, with less easy access to peer support, supervision or shared CPD with colleagues. At a time when clinical governance, the requirement for re-registration and the need for systems to assure patients of practitioners' competence and safety are to the fore, physiotherapists will need to work hard to create systems to support their ongoing learning, while also ensuring their managers accept their responsibilities too. Networking with colleagues with similar interests and case mix at a local and national level will become more important. Where face-to-face contact is not possible, the use of electronic networks for communication and accessing learning resources will need to be embraced.

Delivering clinically effective and cost-effective services

The profession can thrive only if it can clearly demonstrate the 'added value' it offers to patients through increasing their independence, shorter hospital stays, fewer work days lost and so on. In order to achieve this, the profession needs a two-pronged approach. First, it needs to increase its knowledge base about the effectiveness of specific interventions, through research. Second, it needs to use information from the evaluation of practice to demonstrate the benefit to patients of those interventions. The profession urgently requires high-quality researchers who can access NHS and other funding in order to increase the knowledge base of the profession. Challenges from commissioners of services, to provide evidence of the effectiveness of physiotherapy for particular patient or diagnostic groups, will not go away and physiotherapy services are in increasing jeopardy without it.

The profession must be brave enough to look critically at the outcomes of interventions. Where research evidenceshows that particular interventions are ineffective, these should cease to be provided. Where patient outcomes are used as a determinant and demonstrate little or no effect, consideration should be given to possible alternative strategies for securing benefit to those patients which may lie outside physiotherapy. For physiotherapists to continue to provide services in areas where there is little benefit weakens the image of the profession to the public and to colleagues from other professions.

There is a growing emphasis in the NHS on working smarter, looking at systems of care from a patient's perspective, breaking down what are perceived as tribal boundaries between professions, and redesigning patient-centred delivery systems rather than 'doing things that way because we always have'. Physiotherapists will need to embrace new ways of working without feeling defensive or appearing to be protectionist. Opportunities will emerge from redesign for physiotherapists to adopt new and highly skilled roles in just the same way as the successful creation of extended-scope practitioner and physiotherapy consultant roles.

Influencing the agenda

To make any of this work, physiotherapists need to be confident about their roles and able to articulate to others the value of physiotherapeutic interventions or approaches from a science-based as well as a holistic point of view. Physiotherapists must adopt a political astuteness that makes them aware of the wider national and local drivers for change in order that opportunities for the profession and for services can be identified and seized positively. They need to be seen to be engaged with and responsive to current agendas through contacts with patient and public representatives as well as senior managers and local politicians.

Characteristics of the profession required to maximise the opportunities being presented

One thing is certain. The delivery of healthcare within organisations, whether funded by the state or privately, will continue to be highly complex, ever-changing and resource-challenged. Qualifying programmes are tasked with equipping physiotherapy students 'with the attitude, aptitude and capacity to cope with change, uncertainty and unpredictability and with a commitment to the concept of quality improvement' (CSP 2002b). Qualifying physiotherapists of today will therefore be better equipped than ever to cope. The NHS is increasingly looking for leaders who are innovative, clear, lateral thinkers and problem-solvers. Physiotherapists are well placed to adopt such roles and should be proactive in looking for opportunities to do so. The skill is to turn challenges and pressures into opportunities to demonstrate the 'added value' of physiotherapy, which in turn will provide job satisfaction, recognition and benefit for patients and the profession.

SOURCES OF CRITICAL APPRAISAL TOOLS

Critical Appraisal Skills Programme

Weblink

Qualitative research:
www.phru.org.uk/~casp/resources/qualitative.pdf
Randomised controlled trials:
www.phru.org.uk/~casp/resources/rct.pdf
Systematic review:
www.phru.org.uk/~casp/resources/reviews.pdf

Scottish Intercollegiate Guidelines Network

Weblink

Case-control study:
www.sign.ac.uk/guidelines
Cohort study:
www.sign.ac.uk/guidelines
Diagnostic study:
www.sign.ac.uk/guidelines
Randomised controlled trial:
www.sign.ac.uk/guidelines
Systematic review:
www.sign.ac.uk/guidelines

Users' guide series

Guyatt GH, Sackett DL, Cook DJ 1993 Users' guides to the medical literature. II: How to use an article about therapy or prevention, pt A. JAMA 270(21): 2598–2601

Guyatt GH, Sackett DL, Cook DJ 1994 Users' guides to the medical literature. II. How to use an article about therapy or prevention, pt B. JAMA 271(1): 59–63

Oxman AD, Cook DJ, Guyatt GH 1994 Users' guides to the medical literature. VI: How to use an overview. JAMA 272(17): 1367–1371

Books

Bury T, Mead J (eds) 1998 Evidence-Based Healthcare: a Practical Guide for Therapists. Butterworth–Heinemann: Oxford

Greenhalgh T 2000 How to Read a Paper: the Basics of Evidence-Based Medicine. BMJ Books: London

Clinical Guidelines

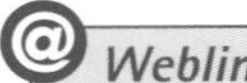

Weblink

Appraisal of Guidelines for Research and Evaluation (AGREE) instrument:
www.agreecollaboration.org

ACKNOWLEDGEMENTS

With thanks to Judy Mead who created the original chapter in the 13th edition. We are also grateful to a number of colleagues who commented on an earlier draft of this chapter and whose thoughts have improved its content, in particular Sarah Fellows and Sally Gosling.

REFERENCES

Barclay J 1994 In Good Hands. Butterworth–Heinemann: Oxford

Bristol Royal Infirmary Inquiry 2001 The Report of the Public Inquiry into Children's Heart Surgery at the Bristol Royal Infirmary 1984–1995. Stationery Office: London

Bury T 1998 Evidence-based healthcare explained. In: Bury T, Mead J (eds) Evidence-Based Healthcare — a Practical Guide for Therapists. Butterworth–Heinemann: Oxford

Cott CA, Finch E, Gasner D et al. 1995 The movement continuum theory of physical therapy. Physiother Can 47(2): 87–95

CSP (Chartered Society of Physiotherapy) 2000 Clinical Audit Tools. CSP: London

CSP 2001a Outcome Measures. CSP: London

CSP 2001b Developing a Portfolio: a Guide for CSP Members. CSP: London

CSP 2002a Rules of Professional Conduct. CSP: London

CSP 2002b Curriculum Framework for Qualifying Programmes in Physiotherapy. CSP: London

CSP 2002c Physiotherapy Assistants Code of Conduct. CSP: London

CSP 2002d Clinical Audit. CSP: London

CSP 2003 Policy statement on Continuing Professional Development (CPD). CSP: London

CSP 2005a Standards of Physiotherapy Practice. CSP: London

CSP 2005b Demonstrating Professionalism through CPD. CSP: London

CSP 2006 website. http://tinyurl.com/ydbr7d; accessed 18 October 2006

Dawes M, Summerskill W, Glasziou P et al. 2005 Sicily statement on evidence-based practice. MBC Med Educ 5: 1

DHSS (Department of Health and Social Security) 1973 McMillan Report: The Remedial Professions (report by a working party set up in March 1973 by the Secretary of State for Social Services). HMSO: London

DHSS 1977 Health Services Development: Relationship between the Medical and Remedial Professions [HC(77) 33]. DHSS: London

Department of Health 1991 Research for Health: an R&D Strategy for the NHS. DoH: London

Department of Health 2002 Health Professions Order Statutory Instrument 2002 No. 254. HMSO: London

Department of Health 2004 The Shipman Inquiry: Fifth Report — Safeguarding Patients: Lessons from the Past, Proposals for the Future. HMSO: London. Website: www.the-shipman-inquiry.org.uk/home.asp; accessed 4 December 2006

Ersser SJ, Atkins S 2000 Clinical reasoning and patient-centred care. In: Higgs J, and Jones M (eds) Clinical Reasoning in the Health Professions. Butterworth–Heinemann: Oxford

Field MJ, Lohr KN (eds) 1992 Guidelines for Clinical Practice: From Development to Use. National Academy Press: Washington, DC

Herbert R, Mead J, Jamtvedt G, Birger Hagen K 2005 Practical Evidence-based Physiotherapy. Butterworth–Heinemann: Oxford

Higgs J, Jones M (eds) 2000 Clinical Reasoning in the Health Professions, 2nd edn. Butterworth–Heinemann: Oxford

Higgs J, Titchen A 2001 Rethinking the practice–knowledge interface in an uncertain world: a model for practice development. Br J Occup Ther 64(11): 526–533

HPC (Health Professions Council) 2002 The Health Professions Order 2001: Stationery Office: London; www.hpc-uk.org/publications/ruleslegislation/index.asp?id=89

HPC 2003 Standards of conduct performance and ethics. HPC: London

HPC 2005 What Happens if a Complaint is Made about me?. HPC: London

HPC 2006 About Us; www.hpc_uk.org/, accessed 1 December 2006

Jones M, Jensen G, Edwards I 2000 Clinical reasoning in physiotherapy. In: Higgs J, Jones M (eds). Clinical Reasoning in the Health Professions. Butterworth–Heinemann: Oxford

Koehn D 1994 The Ground of Professional Ethics. Routledge: London

NHS Executive 1996 Promoting Clinical Effectiveness. Department of Health: London

NICE (National Institute for Health and Clinical Excellence) 2001 The Guideline Development Process — Information for National Collaborating Centres and Guideline Development Groups. NICE: London

Royal College of Nursing, University of Leicester, National Institute for Clinical Excellence 2002 Principles for Best Practice in Clinical Audit. Radcliffe Medical: Oxford

Royal College of Physicians 2005 Doctors in society: medical professionalism in a changing world: Report of a Working Party of the Royal College of Physicians of London. RCP: London

Sackett DL, Rosenberg WMC, Gray JAM et al. 1996 Evidence-based medicine: what it is and what it isn't. BMJ 312: 71–72

Secretary of State for Health 1998 A First Class Service: Quality in the New NHS. Department of Health: London

Sudlow M, Thomson R 1997 Clinical guidelines: quantity without quality (editorial). Qual Health Care 6: 60–61

World Congress for Physical Therapy 1999 Declaration of Principles and Position Statements. London: WCPT. www.wcpt.org; accessed 29 November 2006

Chapter 2

Musculoskeletal assessment

Lynne Gaskell

CHAPTER CONTENTS

INTRODUCTION

Students are often in awe of qualified clinicians who assess and make complex clinical reasoning decisions in real time with apparently little effort. Becoming competent in patient assessment, like most things in life, takes practice, refinement and reflection, and it looks easy when performed by an expert. The ability to examine and assess patients effectively is an essential skill for physiotherapists to possess. This chapter introduces some important principles of musculoskeletal assessment. It provides an illustrated guide to many of the important techniques and tests that are valuable tools in the arsenal of the chartered physiotherapist. Furthermore it provides some assessment templates for specific joints of the body. The objectives of this chapter are:

- to identify the appropriate questions to include in a subjective musculoskeletal assessment
- to discuss the use of regional and special questions for particular joints
- to explain the use of appropriate subjective and objective markers
- to explain the use of specific and regional tests at particular joints
- to recognise the need for continuous reassessment.

This chapter includes templates for assessment of the lumbar spine (including a biopsychosocial assessment), the cervical spine, the shoulder, the hip, the knee, the ankle and the foot.

GENERAL ISSUES

Since 1977, chartered physiotherapists in the UK have been able to work as autonomous practitioners, making treatment decisions independently of other medical professionals. This professional autonomy makes the profession stimulating and exciting but with it comes a great deal of responsibility. Upon qualifying, physiotherapists are legally responsible for their actions and treatments. Increasing numbers of physiotherapists now work in the primary care setting and this trend is likely to continue. Allowing patients direct access to physiotherapists could relieve other medical practitioners of considerable workload.

Recent years have seen the introduction of extended-scope practitioners, clinical specialist and consultant physiotherapy posts. Physiotherapists in these roles are assessing patients usually referred by GPs who would otherwise have been examined by a consultant orthopaedic surgeon. These practitioners are required to possess excellent assessment skills and a wide experience of different clinical conditions and pathologies, and to be able to recognise the appropriate course of action for that particular patient. Audits of these interventions have been encouraging; Gardiner and Turner (2002) found that the extended-scope practitioners showed more consistency between clinical diagnosis and arthroscopic findings in the knee than did their medical counterparts. In the present climate these posts, along with the newly established consultant physiotherapist role, are likely to expand and in doing so will deservedly raise the profile of the physiotherapy profession.

When should physiotherapists assess patients?

- On first patient contact, it is essential to perform an initial assessment to determine the patient's problems and to establish a treatment plan.
- During treatment, assessment is particularly appropriate whilst performing interventions such as mobilisations and exercises when the patient's signs and symptoms may vary quite rapidly. Be aware of any improvement or deterioration in the patient's condition as and when it occurs.
- Following each treatment, the patient should be reassessed using subjective and objective markers in order to judge the efficacy of the physiotherapy intervention. Assessment is the keystone of effective treatment, without which successes and failures lose all of their value as learning experiences. Subjective and objective markers are explained later in this chapter.
- At the beginning of each new treatment, assessment should determine the lasting effects of treatment or the effects that other activities may have had on the patient's signs and symptoms. In reassessing the effect of a treatment, it is essential to evaluate progress from the perspective of the patient, as well as from the physical findings.

Format of the assessment

- *Listen* – history and background.
- *Look* – observation.
- *Test* – individual structures (range of movement, strength).
- *Record* – an accurate account of findings.
- *Assess* – and remember to involve the patient.

Aims of the subjective assessment

A subjective assessment aims to gather all relevant information about the site, nature, behaviour and onset of symptoms, and past treatments, and to review the patient's general health, along with any investigations, medication and social history. This should lead to a formulation of the next step: physical tests.

Definition

Symptoms are what the person complains of (e.g. 'my knee hurts'). Signs are what can be measured or tested (e.g. the patient has a positive patellar tap test).

Aims of the objective assessment

The objective assessment aims to seek abnormalities of function, using active, passive, resisted, neurological and special tests of all the tissues involved. This may be guided by the history. However, it is important to conduct all tests objectively and equally and to resist the temptation to bias the findings in an attempt to make the hypothesis fit.

Objective examination is concerned with performing and recording objective signs. It aims to:

- reproduce all or parts of the patient's symptoms
- determine the pattern, quality, range, resistance and pain response for each movement
- identify factors that have predisposed to or arisen from the disorder
- obtain signs on which to reassess the effectiveness of treatment, by producing reassessment 'asterisks' or 'markers' (Jull 1994).

SUBJECTIVE ASSESSMENT

Initial questioning

Subjective assessment needs to include the name, address and telephone number of the patient, and the patient's hospital number if appropriate. Both the age and the date of birth of the patient should be recorded.

The medical referrer's name and practice should also be recorded for correspondence, discharge letters and so on.

It is also essential for the physiotherapist to obtain sufficient details of the patient's employment. Is the patient currently working? If not, determine the reasons for this. Is it because the person is unable to cope with the physical demands of the job? Do heavy lifting, repetitive movements or inappropriate sustained postures increase the symptoms? These factors may be precursors of poor posture and muscle imbalance, which may accentuate degenerative disease and increase symptoms. However, it is equally important to recognise that withdrawing from normal activities of daily life can result in deconditioning of musculoskeletal structures that may lead to degenerative disease and an increase in symptoms (Waddell 1992; Frost et al. 1998).

Identify patients' hobbies or interests. Are they able to participate in a sport if desired? If not, determine the reasons. Identify the length of time the patient has been off work or has been unable to participate in physical activities. Evaluate the progression of symptoms. If the person has not been participating in physical activities and if no improvement has occurred, it may be appropriate to advise a return to light training in order to prevent devitalisation of tissues and fear avoidance issues.

Present condition

Area of the symptoms

It is useful to record the area of the pain by using a body chart, because this affords a quick visual reference (Maitland 2001). The patient may complain of more than one symptom, so the symptoms may be recorded or referred to individually as P1 and P2 and so on. Areas of anaesthesia or paraesthesia may be recorded differently on the pain chart — they may be represented as areas of dots, in order to distinguish them from areas of pain (Figure 2.1).

Severity of the symptoms

The severity of the pain may be measured on a visual analogue scale (VAS) (Figure 2.2), or on a numerical scale of 0–10 to quantify the pain, where 0 stands for no pain at all and 10 is perceived by the patient as the worst pain imaginable. The mark on a VAS can then be measured and recorded for future comparisons

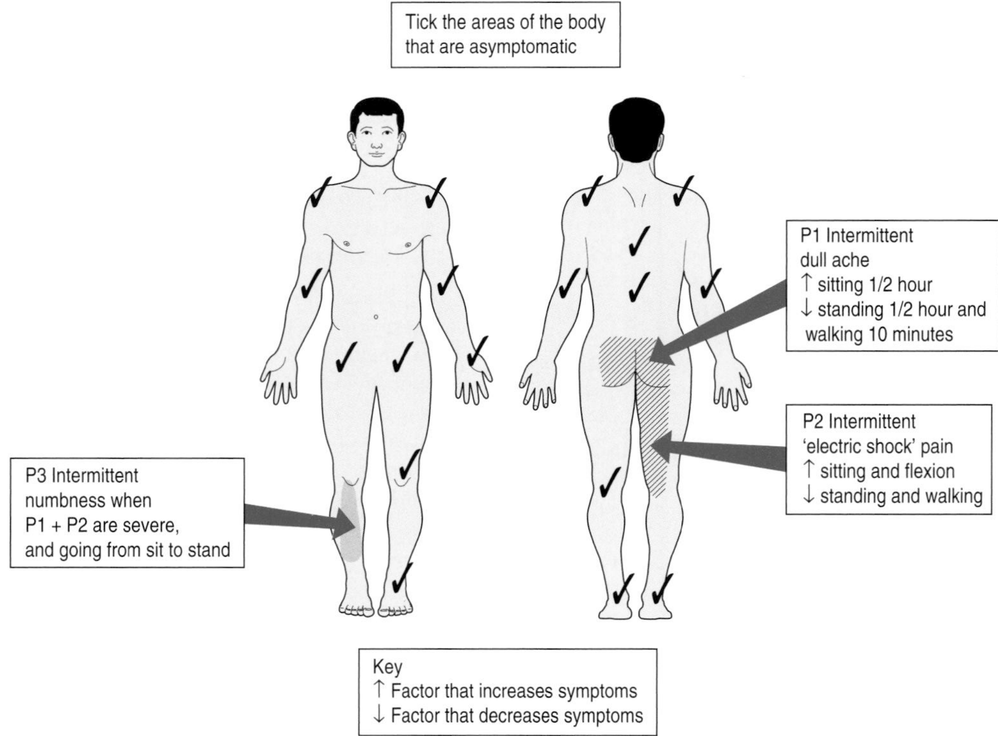

Figure 2.1 Typical body chart. In this example the patient's details have been recorded.

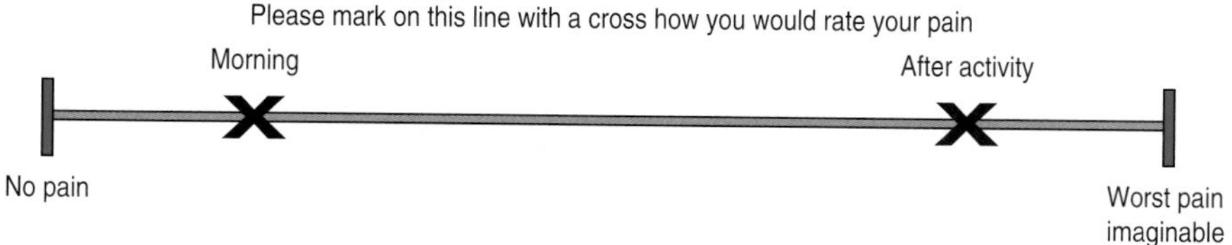

Figure 2.2 The visual analogue scale (VAS).

using a ruler. Although these measures are not wholly objective, they do allow changes to be monitored as the treatment progresses.

Duration of the symptoms

Establish whether the pain and symptoms are intermittent or constant. Is the pain present all of the time or does it come and go depending on activities or time of day?

Aggravating and easing factors

Positional factors

Most musculoskeletal pain is mechanical in origin and is therefore made better or worse by adopting particular positions or postures that either stretch or compress the structure that is giving rise to the pain. Moreover, aggravating and easing movements may provide the physiotherapist with a clue as to the structure that is causing the pain. Various body or limb positions place different structures on stretch or compression and the resultant deformation produces an increase in severity of the pain. The aggravating and easing factors can be recorded on the pain chart, as in Figure 2.1. It is also necessary to record the length of time it takes for engaging in aggravating activities to produce an increase in symptoms or alternatively the time it takes to settle down. This indicates the irritability of the patient's condition.

Time factors

It is useful to record the behaviour of signs and symptoms over a 24-hour period — the diurnal pattern. Do the symptoms keep the patient awake, or awaken the person regularly during the night? Is this due to a particular sleeping posture or to other unrelated factors? On arising, how are the symptoms for the first hour or so of the day, and moreover, do the symptoms vary from the morning to the afternoon and into the evening? Does this follow a particular pattern? This information can be included on the body chart.

Be careful not to confuse time of day with the performance of particular activities that the patient may undertake at that time. Certain pathologies tend to be more painful at characteristic times of the day. For example, chronic osteoarthritic changes are characteristically painful and stiff initially on arising from sleep; intervertebral disc-related pain is often worse on arising owing to the disc imbibing water during sleep and thus exerting pressure on pain-sensitive structures. Prolonged morning pain and stiffness, which improves only minimally with movement, suggests an inflammatory process (Magee 1992).

Determining the SIN factors

Once the severity of the symptoms and the aggravating and easing factors have been noted, it is then possible to determine the SIN factor of the condition: **s**everity/**i**rritability/**n**ature. SIN factors are used to guide the length and firmness of the objective assessment and subsequent treatment.

Severity

This can be quantified on the VAS, numerical scale or other valid pain questionnaire. It can be recorded as high (pain score of around 7–10), moderate (score around 4–6) or low (score around 1–3).

Irritability

This is the length of time for which the person has to perform the activity to increase the pain, and conversely how long it takes before the pain settles to its former intensity. It can be measured as either high (the aggravating factor causes the pain to increase very quickly or instantly and then the pain takes a long time to settle back), moderate (the aggravating factor takes longer to increase the symptom) or low (the aggravating factor can be performed for a long time before exacerbating the patient's symptoms and then on stopping the activity the symptoms subside rapidly). An example of the latter would be knee pain that is aggravated after jogging for 1 hour and then subsides after 1 minute of rest.

Nature

It is possible to hypothesise the nature of the condition following the subjective history — that is, whether the patient's condition has a predominantly inflammatory, traumatic, degenerative or mechanical cause.

History of the present condition

Insidious onset

Insidious onset means that the patient's symptoms appear without any obvious cause. An example of this would be a degenerative condition such as osteoarthritis. These types of condition often begin with a small amount of stiffness and pain, which is characterised by exacerbation and remission but is none the less progressive.

Traumatic onset

Can the onset of symptoms be related to a particular injury? Identify if there was a definite cause for the patient's symptoms. The mechanism of injury may be indicative of the structures damaged. For example, a valgus strain of the knee may stretch the medial collateral ligament of the knee, whereas forced rotation of the knee joint when in a semi-flexed weight-bearing position may tear the menisci.

Progression of the condition

Are the patient's symptoms getting better or worse? Acute soft-tissue injuries normally undergo a period of inflammation and repair, and symptoms may subside rapidly within a few days or weeks. However, progressive arthritic diseases may have a history of exacerbation and remissions, with a general increase in the severity or frequency of their symptoms as the disease progresses.

Progression of the condition may indicate how quickly the patient's symptoms will subside.

Chronicity or age of the condition

How long has the patient experienced the symptoms? Is the condition acute or chronic? If the injury is chronic or has not resolved completely, this may indicate a number of different causes, such as mechanical instability from a ligament disruption, functional instability due to weakened muscles, loss of proprioception (and therefore the loss of an inherently protective reflex mechanism at the joint), or malalignment. Furthermore, it may be developing into a degenerative condition. The physiotherapist should identify the following:

1. Is this the first episode?
2. Is it recurrent?
3. Is it getting better or worse?

Previous treatments

Has the patient received any treatment for this condition in the past; if so, was it effective? Was the improvement partial or total, and did it provide permanent or temporary relief? If the treatment has been effective in the past, it may well help again. Be careful not to repeat unsuccessful interventions, as they are unlikely to be therapeutic.

Investigations

Record the results of any investigations that the patient has undergone. Case notes, radiographic films and reports can be ordered and read, as patients may not always be a reliable source of the results of their investigations.

X-Rays, MRI scans, CT scans and bone scans

Scans are now commonly used to aid the diagnosis of musculoskeletal disorders. X-rays are useful in that they show the degree or extent of arthritis present at a joint. They are also useful in determining the extent of osteomyelitis (bone infection), some malignancies and osteoporosis. Moreover, they are valuable following trauma to identify fractures or dislocations. Be aware, however, that there is a poor correlation between X-rays and spinal symptoms, for non-specific low back and neck pain. What is identified as pathological on these tests may not always be the structure responsible for the patient's signs and symptoms. Routine X-rays are not helpful in non-specific degenerative spinal disease (CSAG 1994).

Computed tomography (CT) may be used to identify the precise level and extent of disc prolapse and subsequent nerve impingement prior to discectomy. Magnetic resonance imaging (MRI) may be used to identify ligamentous and muscular injuries, particularly in athletes, as well as discogenic prolapse. Bone scans are sensitive to 'hot spots' or areas of inflammation present in bone and may detect malignancy or diseases such as ankylosing spondylitis, some fractures and infection sites.

Blood tests

These are used extensively for the confirmation of the diagnosis of particular diseases, such as rheumatoid arthritis, ankylosing spondylitis, osteomyelitis and malignancy.

Other investigations

The patient may be undergoing investigations for other pathologies that could possibly relate to the musculoskeletal condition. These should be noted and recorded.

Past medical history

Determine whether or not the patient is suffering or has suffered any major operations or illnesses. These might affect the vitality of the tissues and be a contraindication to particular treatments. Examples are respiratory or cardiac disease, diabetes, rheumatoid arthritis and epilepsy.

The prolonged use of oral steroid medication should be noted, since this affects bone density and produces a tendency towards bruising. This is commonly found in patients suffering with chronic respiratory diseases, inflammatory bowel diseases or rheumatoid arthritis. Always identify cases of unexplained weight loss and general debility.

> *Clinical note*
>
> Unexplained weight loss, general debility or the patient looking generally unwell – unremitting pain that is unrelieved by changing position or medication – may suggest a non-mechanical basis for the pain. Feeling unwell or tired is common in neoplastic disease affecting the spine (O'Conner and Curner 1992). In these cases, malignant disease should be suspected and the patient should be sent back to the referring GP or consultant immediately with a full report of your findings. Physiotherapy management may well be contraindicated in this situation and may be wasting valuable time for the patient.

Medication

Record the type and dosage of medication prescribed for or taken by the patient. Commonly prescribed drugs for use in musculoskeletal conditions are:

- analgesics (painkillers) such as paracetamol and co-codamol
- non-steroidal anti-inflammatory drugs (NSAIDs) such as ibuprofen
- skeletal muscle relaxants such as diazepam and baclofen.

The medications currently prescribed should alert you to pathologies that the patient may have forgotten to inform you about. For example, people may tell you that they have no significant medical history, but then later in the assessment say that they are currently taking anticoagulation therapy for a recent deep vein thrombosis!

OBJECTIVE ASSESSMENT

Following the subjective assessment it is important to highlight the main findings and determine the SIN factor. A hypothesis may be reached as to the cause of the patient's symptoms and the testing procedures are performed in order to support or refute the physiotherapist's hypothesis.

General Observation

Observe the person's gait and general demeanour on entering the department.

Local Observation

Note any localised swelling at the joint. This may be measured with a tape measure around the joint or limb circumference. Note any asymmetry of joint contours, redness of the overlying skin suggesting local inflammation, atrophy and asymmetry of musculature, deformity, and malalignment of the joint or joints. Compare one joint closely with the other side whenever possible.

Posture

Observe any asymmetry of posture in standing, walking and sitting. Poor posture is frequently a precursor to muscle imbalance, selective tightness and weakness through over- or underuse of specific muscles. The result of prolonged poor postural habits may lead to an acceleration of certain pathologies such as adhesive capsulitis, shoulder impingement syndrome, spinal pain and arthritis. Poor posture is frequently the cause of aches and pains and may be correctable in the early stages, and improved in later stages. Correction may prevent recurrence or acceleration of specific pathologies.

Palpation

Palpate for the following:

- tenderness
- heat (use the back of your hand, which is more sensitive to heat changes)
- swelling
- muscle spasm.

Assessment of movement

Active movements

These are movements performed by the patient's voluntary muscular effort.

Passive movements

These are movements performed by an external source, such as the physiotherapist or a pulley system. There are two types of passive movement:

- Physiological movements can be performed actively by the patient (e.g. flexion of the knee or abduction of the shoulder joint).

- Accessory movements cannot be performed actively by the patient (e.g. they incorporate glide, roll or spin movements that occur in combination as part of normal physiological movements). An example of an accessory movement is an anterior–posterior glide at the knee joint.

Resisted movements

These are performed against the resistance of the physiotherapist or weights by the patient's own effort.

> **Clinical note**
> Passive, active and resisted movements are used in the assessment and in the treatment of musculoskeletal disorders, and specific examples of these are included later in the individual joint assessment formats.

Assessment of range of movement

Measurement of joint range using a goniometer

Active movement may be assessed by the use of a goniometer (Figure 2.3) or alternatively by visual estimation. It is measured in degrees. It is useful to practise using the goniometer by measuring the hip, knee and ankle joints in various positions. Either the 360 degree or 180 degree universal goniometers may be used. Ensure adequate stabilisation of adjacent joints prior to taking the measurements and locate the appropriate anatomical landmarks as accurately as possible. For details on specific joint measurements using the goniometer, refer to the appropriate joint assessment. Physiological and accessory passive movements are measured respectively in terms of the above and by the end-feel.

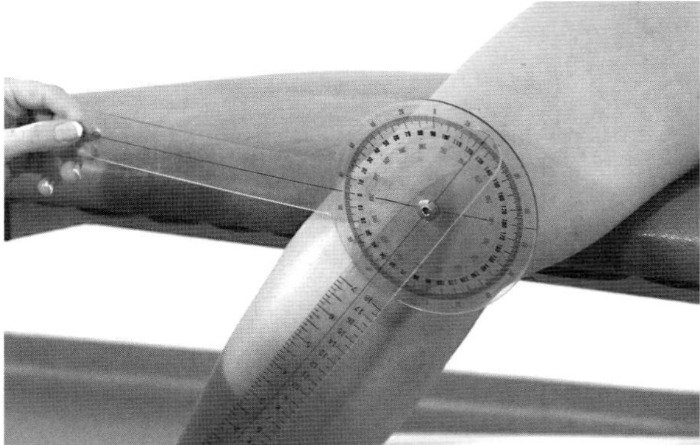

Figure 2.3 Using the goniometer to measure hip joint medial rotation with the hip in 90 degrees of flexion.

Differentiation tests

If a lesion is situated within a non-contractile structure such as ligament, then both the active and passive movements will be painful and/or restricted in the same direction. For example, both the active and passive movement of inversion will produce pain in the case of a sprained lateral ankle ligament. However, if a lesion is within a contractile tissue such as a muscle, then the active and passive movements will be painful and/or restricted in opposite directions (Cyriax 1982). For example, a ruptured quadriceps muscle will be painful on passive knee flexion (stretch) and resisted knee extension (contraction).

> **Clinical note**
> Remember that it is insufficient to measure only the range of movement occurring. The quality of movement should also be observed, along with limiting factors to the movement. Is it the pain, muscle spasm, weakness or stiffness that is limiting the movement? This is determined by noting the differences between active, passive and resisted movements.

End-feel

During passive movements, the end-feel is noted. Different joints and different pathologies have different end-feels. The quality of the resistance felt at the end of range has been categorised by Cyriax (1982). For example:

- Bony block to movement or a hard feel is characteristic of arthritic joints.
- An empty feel, or no resistance offered at the end of range, may be due to severe pain associated with infection, active inflammation or a tumour.
- A springy block is characterised by a rebound feel at the end of range and is associated with a torn meniscus blocking knee extension.
- Spasm is experienced as a sudden, relatively hard feel associated with muscle guarding.
- A capsular feel shows a hardish arrest of movement.

Assessment of muscle strength

Symptoms arising from resisted contractions

The Oxford scale is relatively quick and easy to use and is employed widely in clinical practice. However, it is not very objective, functional or sensitive to change since the movements resisted are concentric contractions and the spaces between the grades are not linear. Nevertheless, it provides a guide to muscle strength and is somewhat sensitive to change.

The Oxford classification

0 = no contraction at all.
1 = flicker of contraction only, movement of the joint does not occur.
2 = movement is possible only with gravity counterbalanced.
3 = movement against gravity is possible.
4 = movement against resistance is possible.
5 = normal functional movement is possible.

Measurements using isokinetic machines

Objective measurements of strength throughout different joint angles and at different velocities are made more accurately using isokinetic machines such as Cybex or Kin-Com. These machines are particularly valuable in rehabilitative regimens such as anterior cruciate rehabilitation programmes, and can determine the strength ratio of the quadriceps to the hamstrings or the ratios of the operated versus the non-operated leg. Objective markers such as percentages of strength ratios or ratios of operated versus non-operated leg may be used in setting discharge protocols. Isokinetic machines have been found to be reliable and valid in measuring muscle torque, muscle velocity and the angular position of joints (Mayhew et al. 1994). However, they are limited in their use, and Wojtys et al. (1996) suggest that agility and functional exercises may be more beneficial than isokinetic machines in the strengthening of muscle.

Clinical note

Tests of specific structures are performed in order to reproduce the patient's symptoms or signs, i.e. to reproduce the comparable sign. Differentiation tests are useful to distinguish between two or more structures that are suspected to be the source of the symptoms.

Differentiation tests of muscles and tendons

These are contractile structures and are therefore tested by performing a contraction against resistance. A pain response and/or apparent weakness may indicate a strain of the muscle at any particular point of the range of movement. Full range should be checked since the muscle may be weak only at a particular point in the range. Muscle length may also be tested, particularly those muscles that are prone to become tight and then lose their extensibility. Muscles that pass over two joints and have mobiliser characteristics are particularly prone to tightness. Examples of these are the hamstrings, rectus femoris, gastrocnemius and psoas major. The length of the muscle is tested by passively moving the appropriate joints. The stretch is compared to the other side to determine reproduction of pain and/or restriction of movement.

Passive insufficiency of muscles

This occurs with muscles that act over two joints (Figure 2.4a). The muscle cannot stretch maximally across both joints at the same time. For example, the hamstrings may limit the flexion of the hip when the knee joint is in extension since they are maximally stretched in this position. However, if the knee is flexed passively, then the hip will be able to flex further since the stretch on the hamstrings has been reduced.

Active insufficiency of muscles

This, too, occurs with muscles that act over two joints (Figure 2.4b). The muscle cannot contract maximally across both joints at the same time. An example is the finger flexors. If you are to make a strong fist, you may notice that the wrist is in a neutral or an extended position when you do this action. Now, if you attempt to flex your wrist joint actively whilst keeping your fingers flexed, you will find that the strength of the grip is greatly diminished. This is because the wrist and finger flexors are unable to shorten any further and so the fingers begin to extend or lose grip strength.

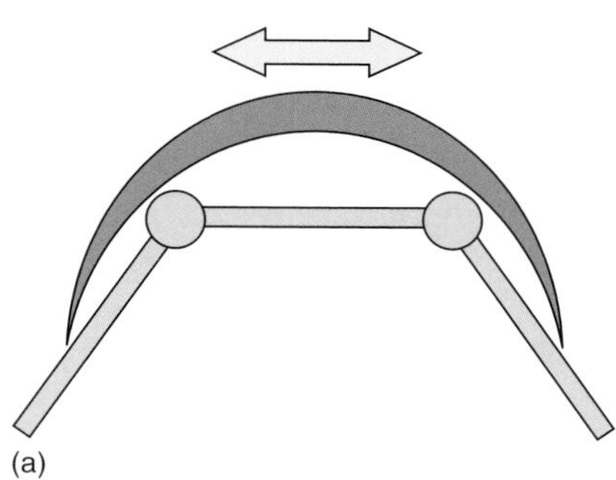

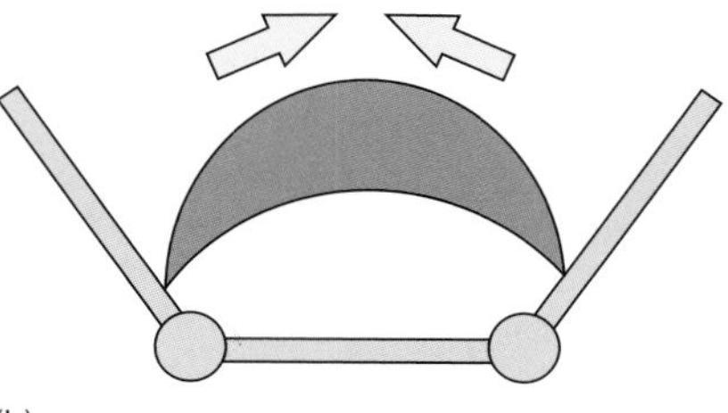

Figure 2.4 (a) Passive insufficiency: the muscle cannot simultaneously stretch maximally across two joints. (b) Active insufficiency. The muscle cannot simultaneously contract maximally across two joints.

2

Differentiation tests of ligaments

Ligaments are non-contractile structures and are tested by putting the structure on stretch. Examples are a valgus strain of the knee, to stretch the medial collateral ligament of the knee; or passive inversion of the subtalar joint, to stretch the lateral ligament of the ankle. A positive test would be a pain response or observation or feel of any excessive movement of the joint when compared to the other side.

Differentiation tests of bursae

Bursae are sacs of synovial fluid. Inflammation of these (bursitis) results in tenderness and/or heat on palpation. The tenderness is often very localised to the site of the inflamed bursa.

Differentiation tests of menisci

The history and mechanism of injury, combined with anterior joint tenderness and inability to passively hyperextend the knee, are useful diagnostic markers of meniscal injury. Rotation on a semi-flexed weight-bearing knee is a common cause of injury.

A history of locking, whereby the joint momentarily locks and is unable to release itself actively or passively from the position, is also common. Objectively, the knee joint is unable to fully flex/hyperextend passively.

Characteristics of degenerative joint disease

Signs and symptoms may include:

- pain that increases on weight-bearing activities (standing and walking, particularly walking downstairs)
- insidious onset of symptoms followed by progressive periods of relapses and remissions
- pain and stiffness in the morning
- stiffness following periods of inactivity
- pain and stiffness that arise after unaccustomed periods of activity
- bony deformity (e.g. characteristic varus deformity may follow from collapse of the medial compartmental joint space)
- reduction of the joint space observed on X-ray, with bony outgrowths or osteophytes.

Writing up the assessment

It is imperative to record the assessment immediately following the physical testing. Patient notes should be completed on the day of the assessment for legal reasons.

Ensure that your assessment findings are clear and concise and that they highlight the main points. (It may be useful to include one subjective and one objective marker.) Formulate a problem list, in agreement with the patient. Agree and record SMART goals (**s**pecific, **m**easurable, **a**chievable, **r**ealistic, **t**imed) with the patient. Use the **p**roblem-**o**rientated **m**edical **r**ecords (POMR) system.

Remember, if you have insufficient time to conduct a full and thorough assessment, you can always continue with this when the patient attends for his or her subsequent appointment.

SPINAL ASSESSMENTS

THE LUMBAR SPINE

Posture

Normal alignment

Posteriorly, the shoulders, waist creases, posterior superior iliac spines, gluteal creases and knee creases should be horizontal (Figure 2.5). The spine should appear to be vertical. There should be no rotation, side flexion, scoliosis (lateral curvature) or shift (lateral deviation). Laterally, you should observe a normal lordosis in the lumbar spine. *Anteriorly*, the anterior superior iliac spines should be horizontal.

Common deviations from normal posture (Figure 2.6)

- *Creases* in the posterior aspect of the trunk and particularly adjacent to the spine may indicate areas of hypermobility or instability of that motion segment.
- *Sway back* comprises hyperextension of the hips, an anterior pelvic tilt and anterior displacement of the pelvis.
- *Flat back* consists of a posterior pelvic tilt and a flattening of the lumbar lordosis, extension of the hip joints, flexion of the upper thoracic spine and straightening of the lower thoracic spine.
- *Kypholordosis* consists of a forward-poking chin posture, elevation and protraction of the shoulders, rotation and abduction of the scapulae, an increased thoracic kyphosis, anterior rotation of the pelvis and an increased lumbar lordosis.
- *Shifted posture* (lateral shift) commonly arises from disc herniation, or acute irritation of a facet joint. The shift is thought to result from the body finding a position of ease, whereby the shoulders are displaced laterally in relation to the pelvis. Most commonly the shift occurs away from the painful side (Figure 2.7).

Movements

Assess not only the range of movement and the pain response, but also localised areas of give and restriction at specific motion segments.

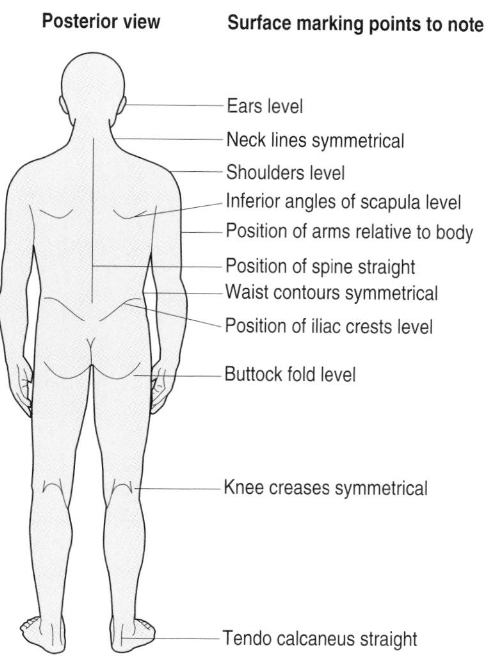

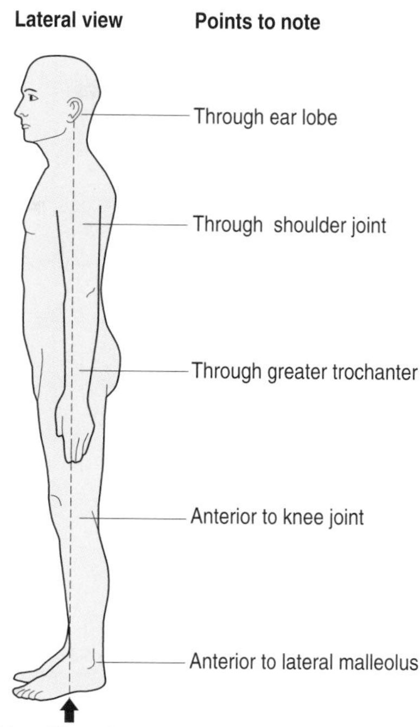

Figure 2.5 Examination of the spine.

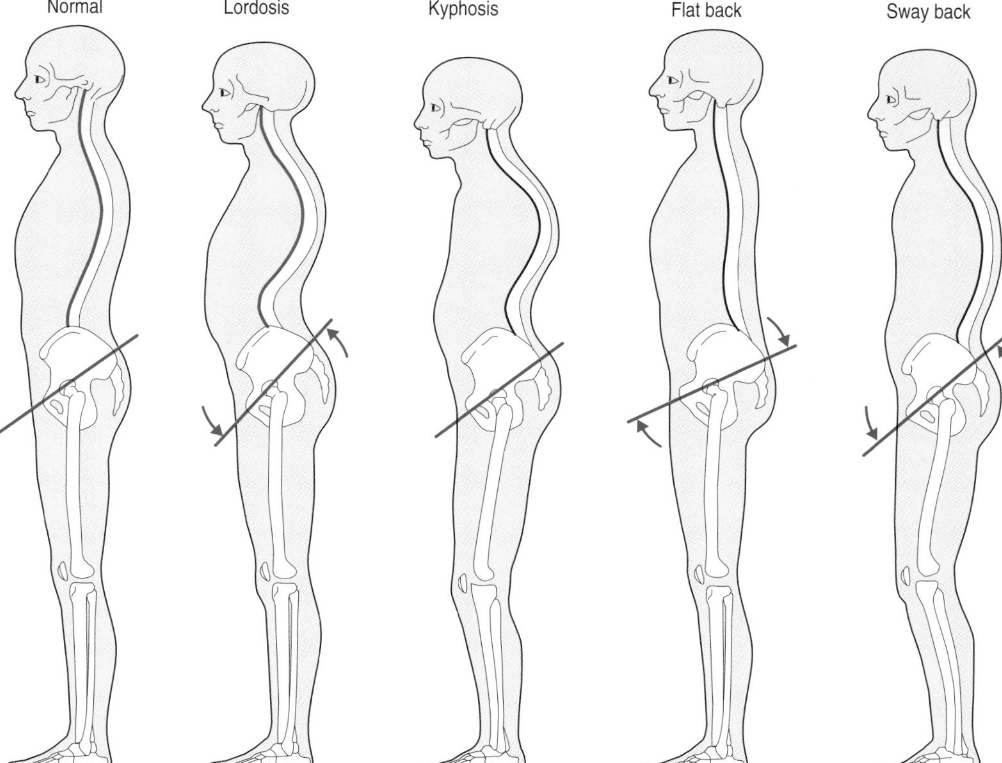

Figure 2.6 Abnormal postural curves of the spine.

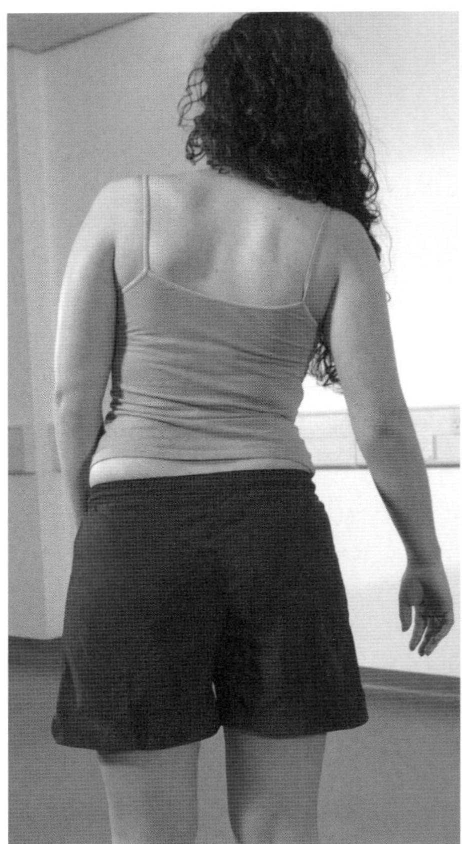

Figure 2.7 Lateral shift.

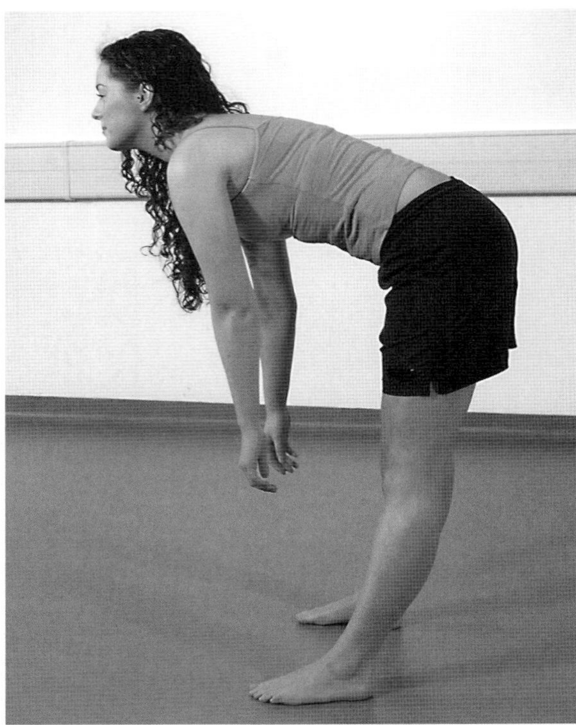

Figure 2.8 A faulty lumbar flexion pattern. All movements occur at the hip joint while the lumbar spine remains in an extended position.

Active movements

Flexion

Flexion should result in a smooth curve. Segmental areas of give or restriction appear as hinging (segmental hypermobility). Lack of movement in the lumbar spine may be compensated by flexion at the hips or thoracic spine. The gross movement may be measured as fingertip to floor distance with a tape measure. Note any limitation of movement, lateral deviation and pain response (Figure 2.8).

Extension

Observe extension in relation to areas of give or restriction. Observe for hinging at specific motion segments indicating areas of hypermobility. This may appear as horizontal lines appearing across the hypermobile segment. Note any limitation of movement and pain response.

Side flexion (Figure 2.9)

Normal movement should be observed as a smooth curve. Areas of give or restriction will be observed as hinging (segments of hypermobility) or plane lines (areas of hypomobility). Compare with the other side for symmetry. Note any 'coupling' of movements, i.e.the trunk may flex or rotate to compensate for restriction of side flexion.

Passive physiological intervertebral movements (PPIVMs)

These can be used to confirm any restriction of motion seen on active movement tests, and to detect restriction of movement not discovered by the active movement tests. PPIVMs also detect segmental hypermobility (Magarey 1988; Maitland 2001).

Overpressure

If the plane movements have full range and are pain-free, then overpressure applied slowly and with care can be administered. At the end of the available range the physiotherapist may apply a small oscillatory movement to assess the quality and end-feel of the movement. Also the range of further movement should be noted, as well as the pain response.

Repeated movements

Repeating movements several times may alter the quality and range of the movement and may give rise to latent pain. McKenzie (1981) advocates the use of repeating

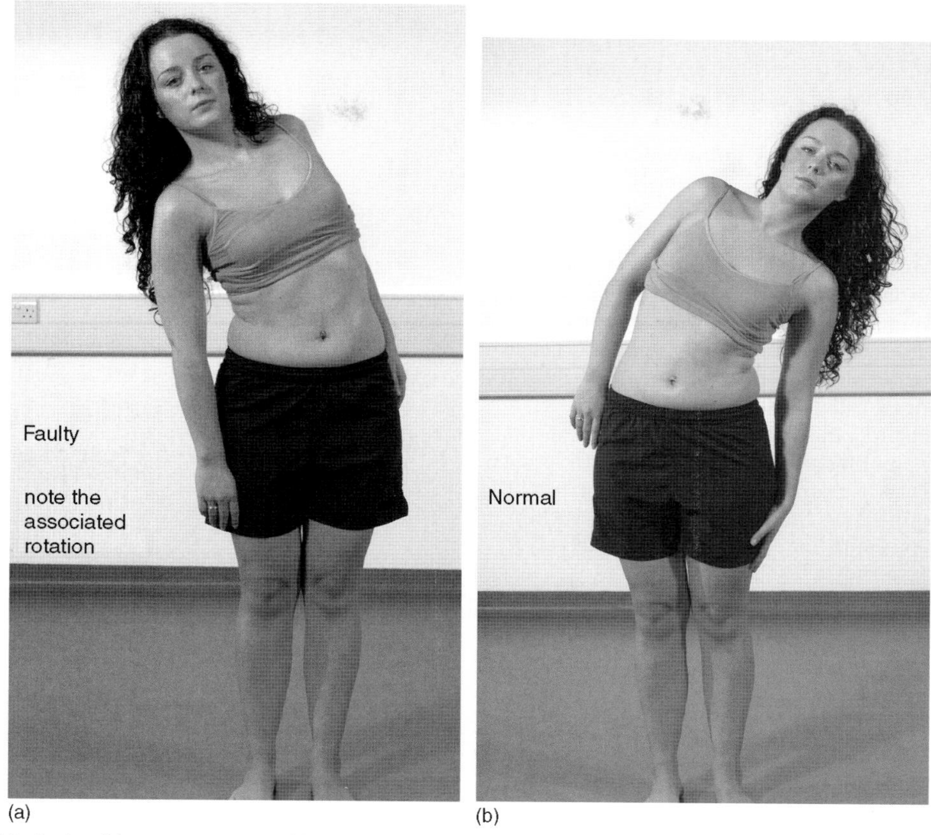

Figure 2.9 Side flexion (a) to the right, and (b) to the left. Note the difference, and the pain response.

flexion and extension in both standing and lying to determine the movement that may centralise patient's symptoms (Figure 2.10). According to Palmer and Epler (1998), progressive worsening of pain on repeated movements indicates a disc derangement, the pain either becoming more intense or spreading more distally. Centralisation of symptoms means that the referred pain becomes more proximal, i.e. pain experienced at the medial aspect of the shin may centralise to the buttock. Thus, the exercise is believed to be reducing the patient's symptoms and the disc derangement.

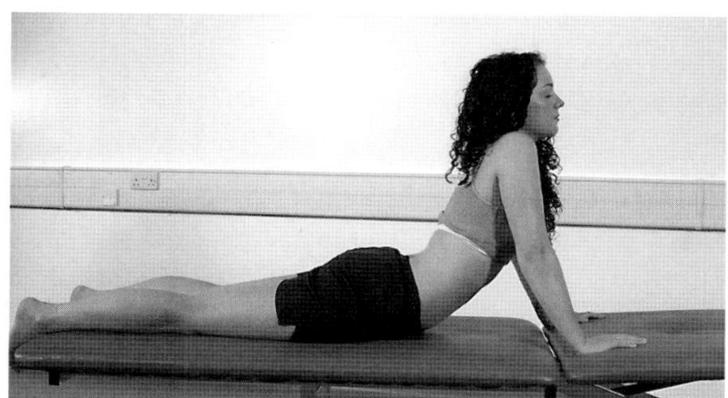

Figure 2.10 Repeated extension in prone.

Combined movements

According to Edwards (1992): 'Although the use of combining movements is not always necessary — adequate results being obtained by standard examination procedures — there are times when they are helpful. Often, with the more difficult mechanical problems, their use is essential.'

For example, lumbar spine extension may be performed and, whilst maintaining that extension, side flexion may be added. Symptoms are likely to vary with the addition of a second movement and this may indicate whether or not there is a regular or irregular stretch component to the signs and symptoms. For example, if a disc prolapse is aggravated by flexion, it would be reasonable to hypothesise that the addition of contralateral side flexion would also further increase the symptoms, because both of the movements are stretching the posterior component of the disc and posterior longitudinal ligament. Combining ipsilateral side flexion with flexion would be expected to lead to a reduction in the patient's symptoms, since the ipsilateral side flexion is reducing the stretch component.

Differentiation between the hip and lumbar spine as a source of symptoms

The hip joint may give rise to pain in the buttock or groin, and in order to differentiate between pain arising as a result of spinal or hip pathology it is important that the therapist discounts the hip joint as a possible source of symptoms. With the patient supine, full flexion, medial and lateral rotation are performed actively and passively at the hip joint. These are the movements that are commonly painful or restricted by degenerative joint conditions such as osteoarthritis. If these movements are pain-free and full-range, then it is unlikely that the hip is a source of symptoms. Compare both sides.

Assessing the sacroiliac joint

Sitting flexion (Piedello's sign)

The seated patient is asked to flex forwards. The physiotherapist palpates the sacral dimples bilaterally. Both sacral dimples should move equally in a *cephalad* direction (i.e. towards the head). (This tests the movement of the sacrum on the ilium.) Excessive rising of one side indicates hypomobility at that sacroiliac joint.

Standing flexion (stork test)

With the patient standing, the physiotherapist locates the sacral dimples (level of S2) and places the other hand centrally at the sacrum. The patient is instructed to stand on one leg whilst flexing the non-weight-bearing hip and knee. The sacral dimple on the non-weight-bearing side should appear to move *caudally* (towards the floor) by approximately 1 cm as the ilium rotates posteriorly. Hypomobility is observed if the dimple does not move distally in relation to the sacrum.

Compression tests

Posterior ligaments

These test the integrity of the *posterior* sacroiliac ligaments. The patient lies supine and the hip is passively flexed towards the ipsilateral shoulder (Figure 2.11). A downward thrust is applied along the line of the femur. Observe for pain response, clunk and difference in end-feel between both sides. The test is repeated for (oblique) hip flexion towards the contralateral shoulder, and (transverse) hip flexion towards the contralateral hip.

Anterior ligaments – FABER test (DVD)

Flexion plus **ab**duction plus **e**xternal **r**otation (the FABER test) assesses the integrity of the anterior sacroiliac ligaments. The test is also described as the 'four test' because of the position of the patient's limb, a combination of flexion, abduction and external rotation. The physiotherapist pushes the leg downwards, just proximal to the knee joint, whilst stabilising the opposite hip with the other hand. A normal finding would be for the patient to lower the leg to the level of the opposite leg. Observe for pain response or limitation of movement (Figure 2.12).

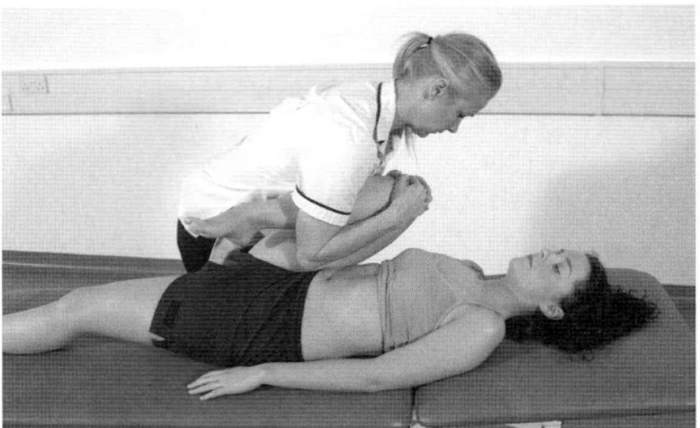

Figure 2.11 Compression testing of the posterior sacroiliac ligaments.

Neurological testing

Compression or traction of spinal nerve roots by disc trespass and/or osteophytes may give rise to referred pain, paraesthesia and anaesthesia and also provoke positive neurological signs. Neurological signs should be carefully monitored as deterioration may indicate worsening pathology.

Dermatomes

A dermatome is an area of skin supplied by a particular spinal nerve. Dermatomes may exhibit sensory changes for light touch and pin prick. Test each dermatome individually, on the unaffected and then the affected side.

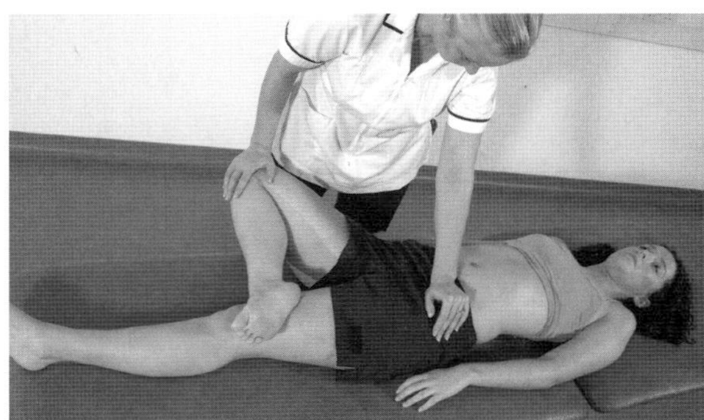

Figure 2.12 The FABER or four-test. Normal range of movement.

Myotomes

A myotome is a muscle supplied by a particular nerve root level. These are assessed by performing isometric resisted tests of myotomes L1–S1 in middle range, held for approximately 3 seconds. Test the unaffected side, then the affected: LI–L2 for the hip flexors (Figure 2.13), L3–L4 for knee extensors (Figure 2.14), L4 for foot dorsiflexors and invertors, L5 for extension of the big toe, S1 for plantar flexion (Figure 2.15) and knee flexion, S2 for knee flexion and toe standing, and S3–S4 for muscles of the pelvic floor and the bladder.

Reflexes

- Test the non-affected side first and the affected side second. Note dull reflexes may indicate lower motor neurone dysfunction. Brisk reflexes may indicate an upper motor neurone dysfunction.
- L3 corresponds to the quadriceps. The patient sits with the knee flexed and the therapist hits the patellar tendon just below the patella (Figure 2.16).

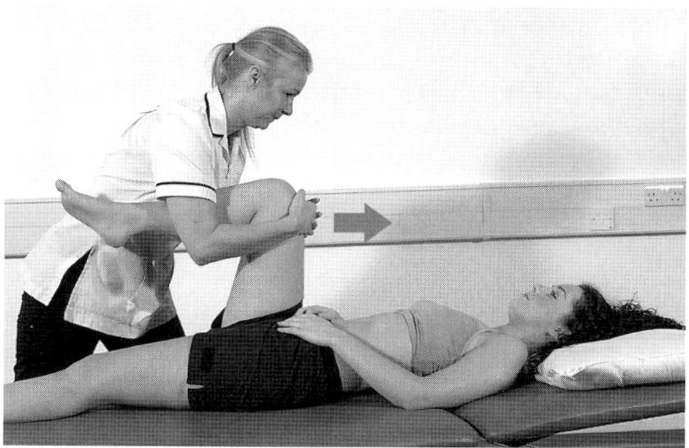

Figure 2.13 Resisted hip flexion to test myotome L1–L2.

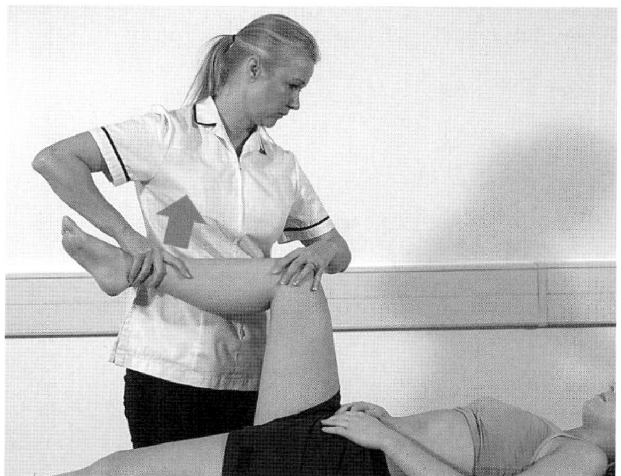

Figure 2.14 Resisted knee extension to test myotome L3.

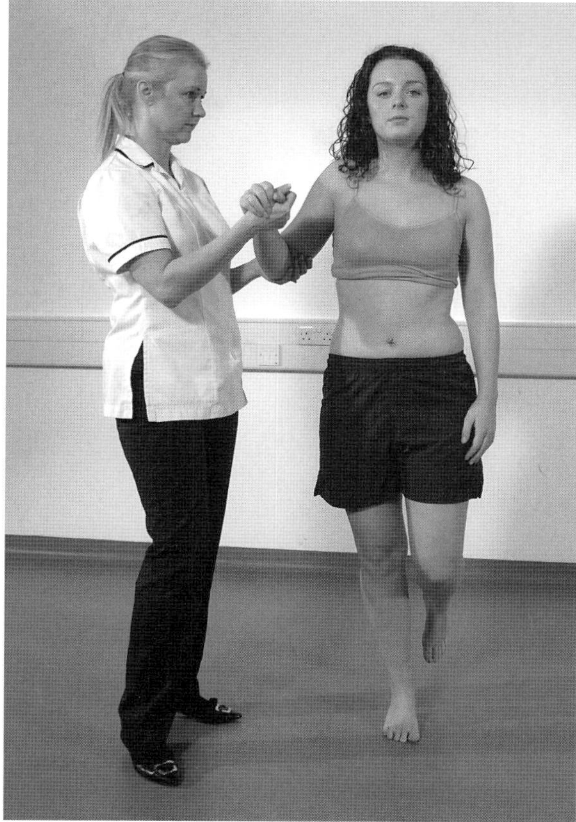

Figure 2.15 Toe standing (plantar flexion) to test myotome S1.

- S1 corresponds to the plantar flexors. Dorsiflex the ankle and strike the Achilles tendon. Observe and feel for plantar flexion at the ankle (Figure 2.17).

Clinical note

The Babinski reflex (or plantar response) is an abnormal response and occurs when a blunt object is drawn up the lateral aspect of the sole of the foot. Normally the great toe (big toe) flexes. Abnormally the great toe extends, indicating upper motor neurone damage. Note that this primitive reflex is seen in the newborn but disappears with time.

Adverse mechanical tension

Passive neck flexion

The patient is supine. The physiotherapist passively flexes the patient's neck. Observe for any low back pain response, which may suggest disc pathology.

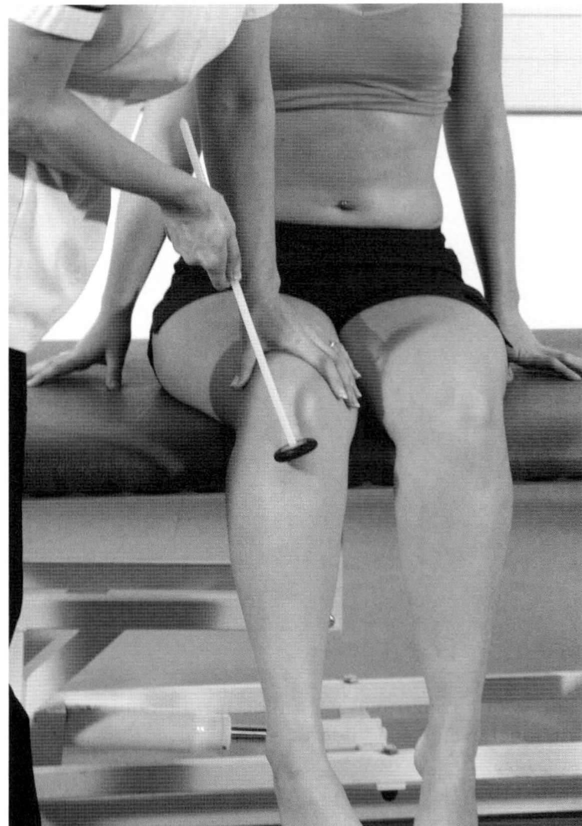

Figure 2.16 The quadriceps reflex (L2, L3, L4).

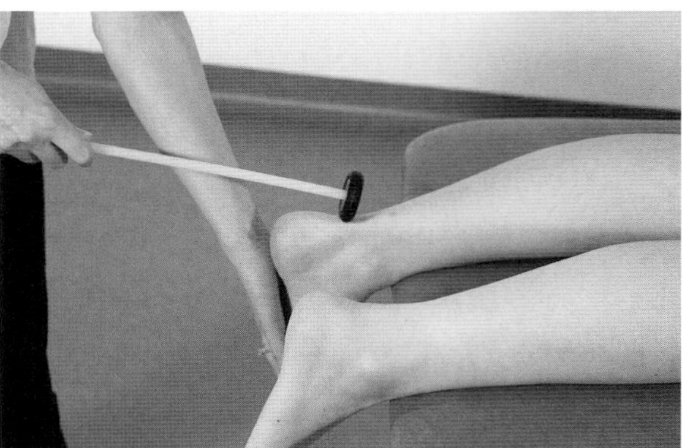

Figure 2.17 The Achilles tendon reflex (S1, S2).

Straight leg raise (SLR)

This is also known as Lasègue's test. The patient is supine. The physiotherapist lifts the patient's leg whilst maintaining extension of the knee (Figure 2.18). An abnormal finding is back pain or sciatic pain. The sciatic nerve is on full stretch at approximately 70 degrees

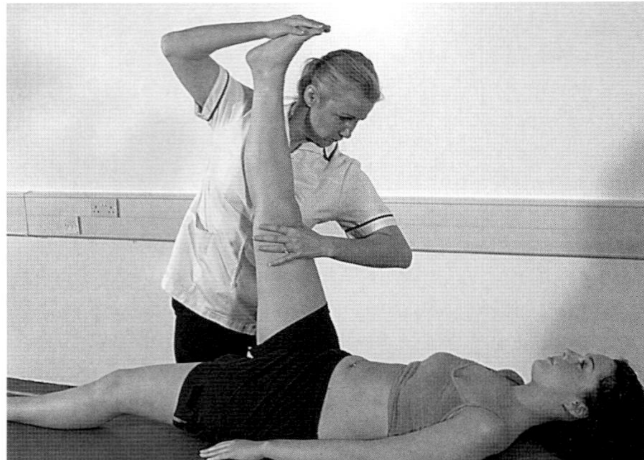

Figure 2.18 Straight leg raise (SLR) test adding dorsiflexion of the ankle joint.

of flexion, so a positive sign of sciatic nerve involvement occurs before this point (Palmer and Epler 1998). Any pain response and range of movement are noted and comparison made with the other side. Factors such as hip adduction and medial rotation further sensitise the sciatic nerve; dorsiflexion of the ankle will sensitise the tibial portion of the sciatic nerve; plantar flexion and inversion will sensitise the peroneal portion of the nerve.

Prone knee bend (femoral nerve stretch) DVD

The patient lies prone and the physiotherapist flexes the person's knee and then extends the hip (Figure 2.19). Pain in the back or distribution of the femoral nerve indicates femoral nerve irritation or reduced mobility. Comparison is made with the other side.

Slump test

This tests the mobility of the dura mater. The patient sits with thighs fully supported and hands clasped behind the back. The patient is instructed to slump

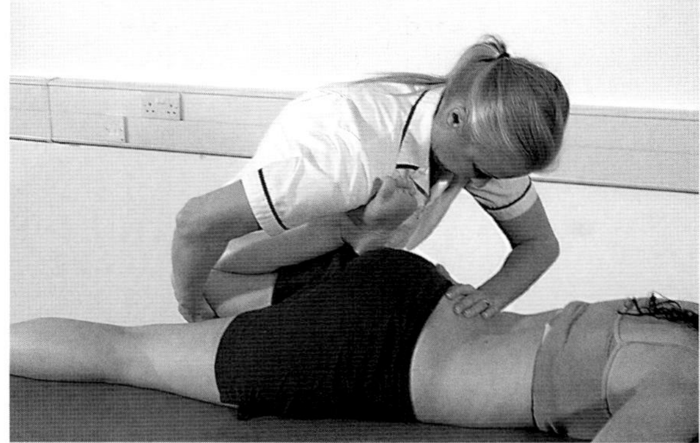

Figure 2.19 Femoral nerve test.

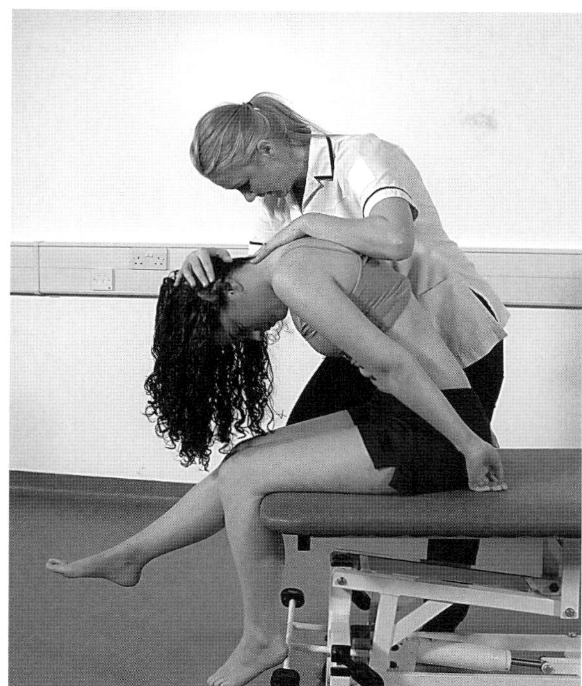

Figure 2.20 Slump test with single knee extension.

the shoulders towards the groin (Figure 2.20). The physiotherapist applies gentle overpressure to this trunk flexion. The patient adds cervical flexion, which is maintained by the therapist. The patient then performs unilateral active knee extension and active ankle dorsiflexion. The physiotherapist should not force the movement. The non-affected side should be assessed first.

Any symptoms are noted, along with the particular part of the range at which they occur. If the dura mater is tethered, symptoms will increase as each component is added to the slump test. The patient is instructed to extend the head. A reduction in symptoms on cervical extension is a positive finding, indicating abnormal neurodynamics.

Testing for lumbopelvic stability

Stability of the lumbar spine is necessary to protect the lumbopelvic region from the everyday demands of posture and load changes (Panjabi 1992a). It is essential for pain-free normal activity (Jull et al. 1993) and should always be assessed.

With the patient in crook lying with the hips at 45 degrees flexion, he or she is instructed to maintain a neutral spine. (It may be useful to tell the patient to maintain such a lordosis that an army of ants could just crawl through!) The person then performs an abdominal in-drawing by contracting the transversus abdominis muscle whilst attempting to maintain the spine in neutral. To challenge the transversus abdominis and multifidus stabilising muscles (and consequently the spinal position), the patient adds the leg load by alternately lifting the heels from the floor and sliding out the leg whilst maintaining a neutral spine position. The maintenance of a neutral spine posture can be assessed by using a biofeedback device. An inability to maintain the spine in neutral will result in the lumbar spine extending as the leg is lifted. The intra-abdominal pressure mechanism is controlled primarily by the diaphragm and transversus abdominis, which provides a stiffening effect on the lumbar spine (Hodges and Richardson 1997).

Palpation

Soft-tissue thickening over the articular pillar at one or more spinal levels is a common finding in cases of degenerative disease of the lumbar spine, as is hard bony thickening and prominence over the apophyseal joints. Note any general tightness, or localised thickening of muscular tissue or ligamentous tissue. In general, the older the soft-tissue changes, the tougher they are; the more recent, the softer they are. However, a thickened or stiff area is not necessarily painful or the source of a patient's symptoms (Maitland 2001).

Accessory spinal movements

The physiotherapist applies central postero–anterior (PA) pressures on the spinous processes, and unilateral (one-sided) pressure over the articular pillar (Figure 2.21), noting areas of hyper- and hypomobility. Record any

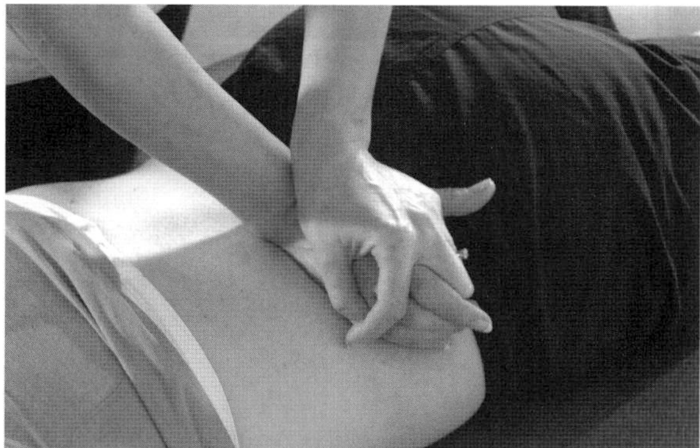

Figure 2.21 Unilateral pressures applied to the lumbar spine over the articular pillar. Note the pressure is applied through the physiotherapist's pisiform bone.

pain experienced by the patient, and the corresponding spinal level.

Biopsychosocial assessment (lumbar spine)

Although historically there has been no change in the pathology or prevalence of low back pain (LBP), disability due to non-specific LBP has increased dramatically in modern western societies. Medical interventions for chronic LBP using a limited biomedical approach have been relatively unsuccessful and the cost to NHS physiotherapy services has been estimated to be £151 000 000 per annum (Maniadakis and Gray 2000). LBP has been described as a twentieth-century healthcare disaster (Waddell 1992). In 80 per cent of cases of LBP no significant pathology is ever found despite considerable disability. Recent guidelines based on systematic reviews of contemporary literature have recommended a biopsychosocial approach in the assessment and treatment of LBP (CSAG 1994; RCGP 1999).

Fundamental differences between acute and chronic pain

It is not satisfactory to view chronic pain simply as acute pain that has persisted for a long period. Acute pain and chronic pain are different clinical entities. We now acknowledge that there are many different mechanisms and processes involved in the genesis of chronic pain states which are not relevant in acute pain. The diversity of these elements has led to the use of a biopsychosocial approach to indicate that there are biological, social and psychological factors relevant within an individual that can be either causing or maintaining the chronic pain state.

Acute pain is basically a protective mechanism to reduce the possibility of increasing the injury. It is usually self-limiting, and lasts until the tissues are healed. It is usually associated with increased sympathetic nervous activity. This may be associated with feelings of anxiety, panic, nausea, etc. and may be observed during traumatic injuries to the bones and soft tissues.

Chronic pain is detrimental because it lasts long after the injury has healed. Tonic self-sustaining neural loops are set up to perpetuate the pain. Decrease in sympathetic activity may cause depression and apathy. Chronic pain outlasts the normal time of healing, and has no recognisable end-point (Grichnik and Ferrante 1991).

Predictors of chronic incapacity

Can disability from LBP be predicted? Psychosocial researchers in the last decade have found common psychosocial and social traits in people who have developed chronic disability due to LBP. Many subjects with chronic LBP have been reported to have a psychological profile that predisposes them to develop chronic pain (Burton et al. 1995; Carrageen 2001). Additionally, people aged between 50 and 60 years are more likely to become disabled due to LBP (Burton et al. 1995).

Further major predictors are:

- people who have unrealistic beliefs about their pain and the nature of their disease (Waddell 1992)
- people whose occupation involves heavy manual work and sustained postures
- people with a previous history of sickness absence
- people who seek multiple investigations and treatments (Waddell 1992; Harding and Watson 2000)
- people with low educational achievement or low-status occupations (Cats-Baril and Frymoyer 1991; Frymoyer 1992)
- people who have pending compensation issues (Tait and Chibnall 2001)
- people with fear-avoidance beliefs, i.e. that a fear of activity may be more disabling than the original injury (Vlaeyen et al.1995; Fritz et al. 2001)
- people who exhibit 'illness behaviour', which may include attention-seeking, grimacing, catastrophising about their problems or LBP, inappropriate coping strategies, excessive use of splints, braces, walking aids, over-reliance on the NHS, and passive rather than active treatment modalities.

In view of the above factors, it is necessary to screen patients with LBP in order to attempt to reduce the likelihood of chronic disability. It is important to note that a patient's general physical fitness may be a poor predictor of chronic incapacity (Deyo and Weinstein 2001). The identification of the patients at risk of progression to chronicity (failure to respond to treatment) is by means of psychosocial questionnaires, because clinical variables contribute practically nothing to our predictive ability (Burton et al. 1995). The psychosocial traits concerned (coping strategies, depressive tendencies, inappropriate beliefs about pain and activity) are present in the acute phase — they are not just the result of persistent symptoms (Burton et al. 1995).

Management guidelines for LBP (CSAG 1994; RCGP 1999)

In the early management of acute LBP, analgesia with NSAIDs should be administered immediately following an acute onset. Manipulative therapy is advised in the early stages, and active exercise and physical activity should be encouraged. Bed rest is ineffective as treatment for back pain, but is acceptable in moderation in the acute situation for 1–2 days.

Encourage physical activity and an early return to work and sport whenever possible. Practise psychosocial management; educate the patient of the importance of good postural habits and activities of daily living. Challenge the patient who has unrealistic beliefs about the LBP condition and prognosis.

Biopsychosocial assessment

The biopsychosocial assessment differs from the physical assessment in that it incorporates psychological and social issues in more depth. This gives the physiotherapist a good overview of the patient's circumstances, his or her overall mood state, beliefs, attributes and thoughts about the problem, about therapy and about the future.

Psychological factors

A previous history of anxiety and depression, general attitudes and expectations are noted. The patient's perceived level of control over the pain is also assessed with particular regard to the use of active or passive coping strategies. (These are often referred to as 'internalised' or 'externalised' locus of control.)

Social factors

Identify social areas, including work issues, pending compensation, a history of injury, sickness benefits and daily functioning, because these may affect the outcome.

Physical examination

A body chart and physical examination may or may not be compiled/conducted, as the physiotherapist deems necessary. However, if red flags are noted then a neurological examination is indicated. Assessments may include functional tests such as:

- the distance that can be walked in 5 minutes
- the number of times the person can stand from sitting in 1 minute
- the number of times the person can step up and down in 1 minute.

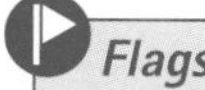

Flags

'Yellow flags' are psychosocial factors including a previous history of anxiety and depression, impending compensation, absence from work, sickness benefit, invalidity benefit, passivity and high levels of dependency, and poor coping skills. 'Red flags' are clinical features that should alert the therapist to the possibility of severe pathology. They include bladder and bowel malfunction, saddle anaesthesia, bilateral paraesthesia, neurological signs, unexplained weight loss, a past history of carcinoma, general debility and fever.

Outcome measures questionnaires

The following questionnaires and tools are validated, reliable and sensitive. They can be used prior to and following intervention to determine efficacy:

- the Oswestry Disability Index (Fairbank et al. 1980)
- the visual analogue scale
- the Present Pain Index
- the short-form McGill Pain Questionnaire (Melzack 1987)
- the Hospital Anxiety and Depression Questionnaire (Zigmond and Snaith 1983)
- the locus of control questionnaire (Fear Avoid Beliefs Questionnaire, FABQ).

Treatment of biopsychosocial aspects of LBP disability

Many studies have reported decreases in pain levels and disability following intensive back rehabilitation programmes combining exercise and cognitive therapy (e.g. Frost et al. 1998; Guzman et al. 2001). The aims of chronic spinal rehabilitation programmes are to:

- reduce the patient's pain if possible, or enable the patient to cope more effectively with the pain
- reduce the patient's disability
- encourage a return to work and hobbies, when possible, to promote better physical functioning (by challenging the unhelpful belief that pain always equates to harm)
- encourage an active patient-centred approach to LBP management.

Von Korff and Saunders (1996), in a survey of LBP sufferers in the USA, found that patients wanted to understand the following four things:

1. the likely course of their back problem
2. how to manage the pain
3. how to return to normal activities of daily living
4. how to minimise recurrences of back pain.

Example of the content of a back rehabilitation programme

- Pre-intervention questionnaire and physical tests for outcome measures.
- Circuit training, including aerobic and strengthening regimes, with emphasis on postural control, spinal stability, back extensors and deep abdominal musculature.
- Patient-centred discussions, seminars on anatomy, pathology, medication, self-help measures, posture and exercise, etc.
- Relaxation workshops.
- Post-programme questionnaire and physical tests.
- Follow-up questionnaires at 1 and 12 months to determine how patients are managing their LBP.

2

CASE STUDY LUMBAR SPINE 

A 30-year-old labourer was referred for physiotherapy following a lifting injury at work. He complained of left-sided low back and medial shin pain and intermittent paraesthesia affecting his left great toe. The pain was aggravated by flexion and eased by standing and walking. On examination he had a marked shift to the right. Flexion was reduced to fingertips to knees and his left SLR was reduced to 50 degrees.

Owing to the rapid onset of symptoms associated with a lifting injury in a flexed posture, and the pain being aggravated by flexion and eased by extension activities, the injury was hypothesised to be discogenic. Clinical trials suggest that the most usual sources of low back pain are the intervertebral disc, the zygapophyseal (facet) joint and the sacroiliac joint (Maitland 2001).

The patient was treated by rotations to the right (as demonstrated on another patient in Figure 2.22), which centralised his pain. His shift was manually corrected on the first visit. He was prescribed repeated extension exercises in prone, as advocated by McKenzie (1985), to do at home every 2 hours. By the third visit his pain had centralised to left low back pain, and his SLR was 80 degrees. He was then treated by unilateral mobilisations on the left at grade 4. This alleviated his symptoms and he regained a full range of all movements.

Prior to discharge, he was given a programme of abdominal and multifidus exercises. He was also given postural and ergonomic advice prior to his return to work. The multifidus and the transversus abdominis muscles have been found to be primarily responsible for imparting local stability to the lumbar spine in the joint's neutral zone (Wilke et al. 1995; Goel et al. 1993; Panjabi 1992; Hodges and Richardson 1996).

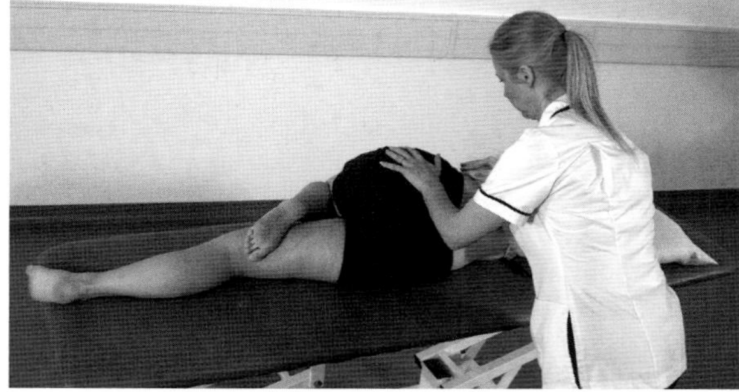

Figure 2.22 Right-sided lumbar rotation, used to treat left-sided back and leg pain.

THE CERVICAL SPINE

Following on from the subjective assessment, the physiotherapist should highlight the main findings and formulate a hypothesis regarding the clinical diagnosis. The SIN factors will determine the vigour of the examination. The physiotherapist will attempt to find the patient's comparable sign by means of movement or palpation.

Clinical note

Patients presenting with disorders of the cervical spine may also complain of headaches, dizziness, nausea and vertigo. Record this in your assessment. These may be symptoms of vertebrobasilar insufficiency (VBI).

Posture

Note the symmetry of the head on the neck, and the neck relative to the thorax. The chin should be at 90 degrees to the anterior aspect of the neck. There should be no obvious horizontal skin creases posteriorly. A plumbline from the tragus of the ear should fall behind the clavicle.

Assess the cervical lordosis. A decreased lordosis predisposes the vertebral bodies and discs to bear more weight. An increased lordosis increases the compressive loads on the zygapophyseal (facet) joints and posterior elements. Observe for muscle hypertrophy, hypotrophy, spasm, tightness or general asymmetry.

An acute wry neck (torticollis) presents as a combination of flexion and rotation or side flexion away from the painful side. Patients with chronic pathology often have a poking chin posture which consists of excessive upper and middle cervical extension and lower cervical/cervicothoracic flexion. This results from a weakness of the deep cervical flexors and overactivity of sternocleidomastoid and levator scapulae muscles (Figure 2.23).

Note that cervical posture is influenced by lumbar posture, and hence the poking chin posture is exaggerated by lumbar and thoracic flexion (Figure 2.23). Cervical and shoulder posture should therefore be viewed in both the sitting and standing postures.

The shoulders should ideally be level, but this is often not the case because of handedness. For example in a right-handed person the right shoulder is often held slightly lower than the left.

Movements

It is important to assess not only the range of movement occurring in the cervical region but also the quality of that movement. Note in particular the motion segments

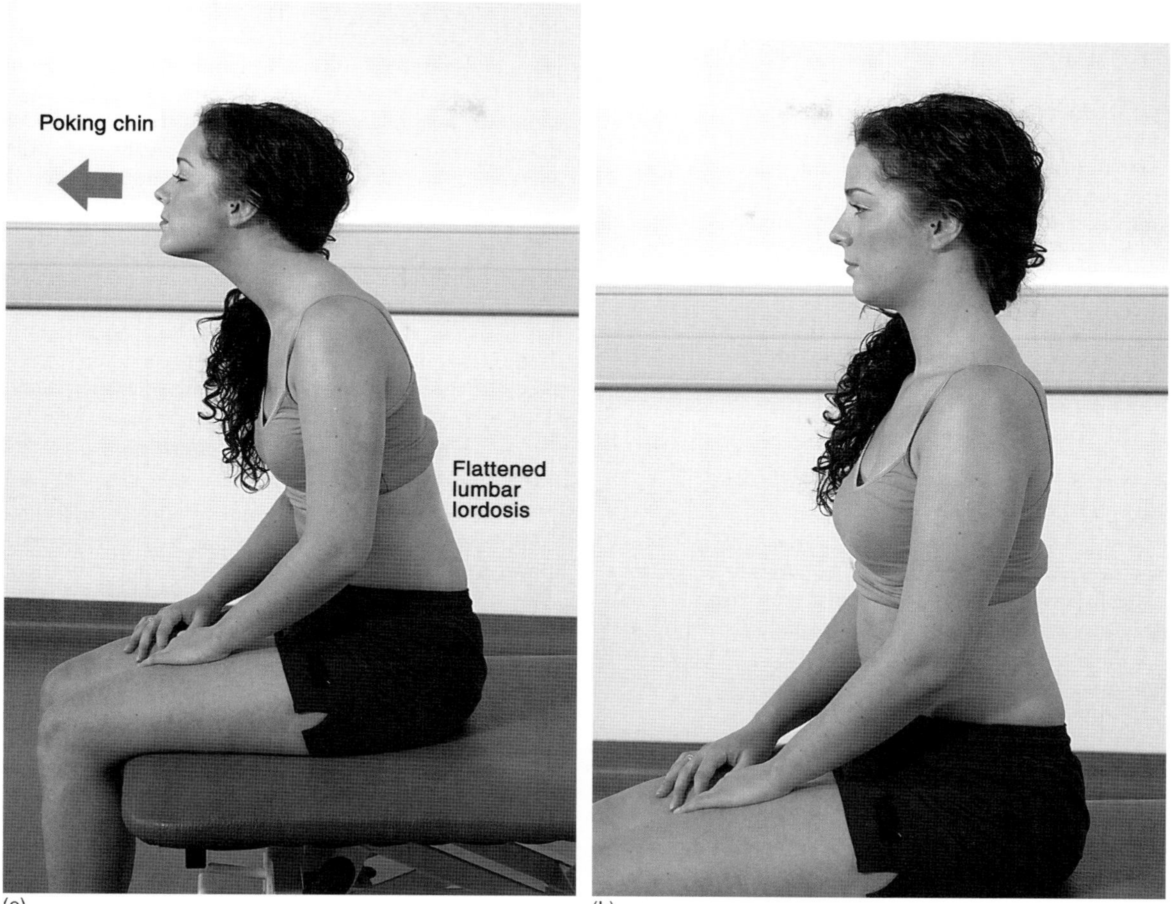

Figure 2.23 (a) Poking-chin posture, exaggerated by thoracic and lumbar flexion. (b) Correction of cervical posture by maintaining the lumbar spine in a neutral position.

where the movement is occurring. Hinging may be observed which indicates areas of hypermobility or instability. Conversely, areas of hypomobility or stiffness are observed as areas of plane or straight lines.

Key point

For consistency and reliability of reassessment, the same order of active movements should be carried out each time.

Active movements

Flexion

The movement should be performed to either the patient's pain or the limit of movement. During flexion the cervical lordosis should be obliterated, and the spine appears to be flexed or neutral. The spinous process of C7 should be the most prominent, C6 and T1 less so. The chin should approximate the chest. Common faulty patterns are the upper cervical spine remaining in extension or chin poke. Loss of range and areas of give and restriction should be noted, as well as the pain response, muscle spasm and crepitus.

Extension

The entire cervical spine should extend, and the face should be almost parallel to the ceiling. A vertical line should be observed from chin to sternum. Common faulty movement patterns include a loss of lower cervical extension and the head not moving posteriorly to the shoulders. Furthermore, excessive hyperextension of the upper and mid-cervical spine may occur earlier on in the movement and the chin pokes forwards.

Side flexion

Often this movement is the most restricted in degenerative spinal pathologies. Tightness in the contralateral sternocleidomastoid and trapezius may be observed. Common faulty patterns include coupling with rotation due to tightness in anterior flexor musculature. Observe range, pain response and areas of give or restriction. Compare the sides for symmetry.

Right and left rotation

Observe the range of movement available and the patient's pain response, muscle spasm and crepitus. Common faulty patterns include coupled movements with side flexion and the eyes not moving in a purely horizontal plane (Figure 2.24). Compare the right and the left sides.

Overpressures in repeated and combined movements

If the plane movements are full-range and pain-free, then overpressure may be applied. At the end of the available range the physiotherapist may apply a small oscillatory movement to assess the quality and end-feel of the movement, and the range of further movement. The pain response is also noted. Combined movements may be examined in an attempt to reproduce the patient's pain or restriction of movement. The patient should, if possible, perform repeated movements, since this may alter the quality and range of the movement and may give rise to latent pain (McKenzie 1990).

The shoulder complex

Observe full shoulder elevation through flexion and abduction for the shoulders bilaterally, because during the last few degrees of elevation the thoracic spine extends to allow for full shoulder elevation. A stiff kyphotic thoracic spine will limit shoulder elevation.

Passive physiological intervertebral movements (PPIVMs)

PPIVMs may be used to confirm any restriction of motion seen on active movement and to detect restriction of movement not discovered by the active movements. They are also used to detect segmental hypermobility (Magarey 1988; Maitland 2001).

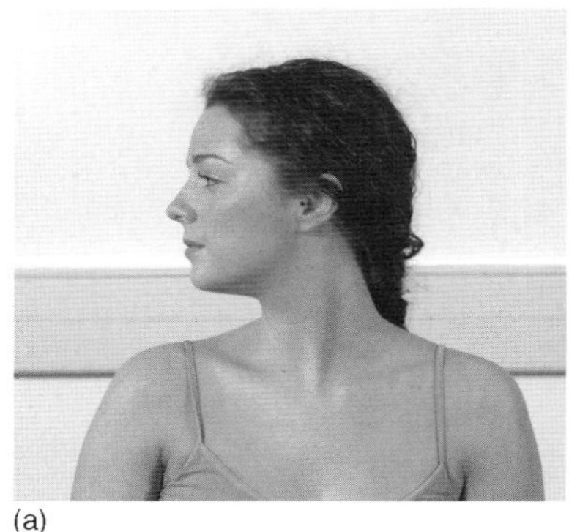

(a)

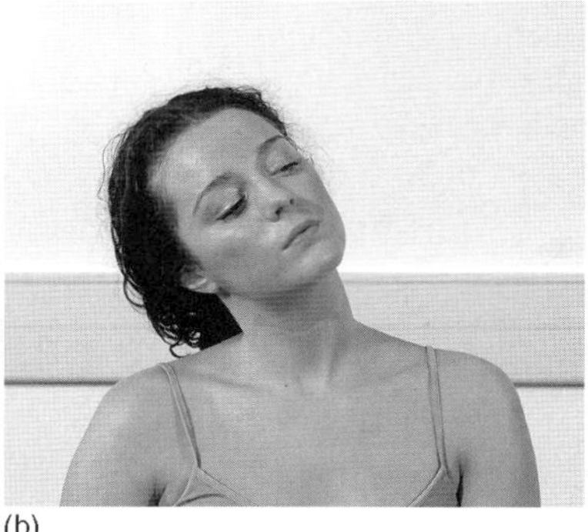

(b)

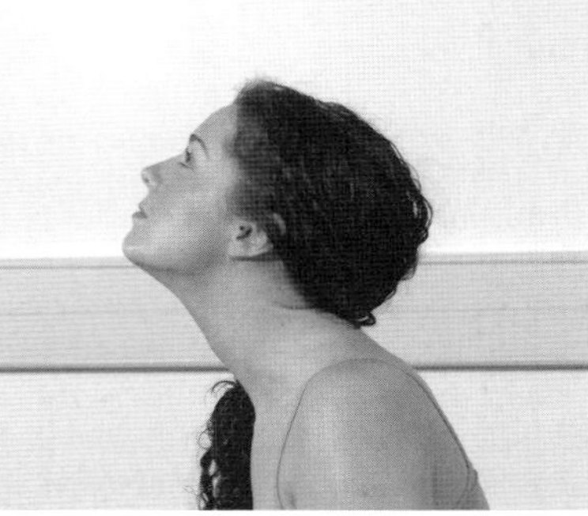

(c)

Figure 2.24 (a) Normal right cervical rotation. (b) Faulty position: right side flexion limited and completed with contralateral rotation. (c) Faulty position: extension with chin poke, upper cervical extension, lower cervical spine remaining flexed.

Vertebral artery testing

See DVD for a detailed account of how to perform these tests. (DVD)

Key point

Vertebrobasilar insufficiency (VBI) is a contraindication to cervical manipulation and high-grade mobilisations, particularly rotations, extensions or longitudinal distractions and traction.

Differentiation test to determine between vestibular and VBI symptoms

The patient stands and rotates the cervical spine to the right and left. Note is taken of symptoms such as dizziness or nausea. Either vertebrobasilar artery insufficiency or the vestibular apparatus could cause symptoms produced as a result of this manœuvre. In order to differentiate between these two structures, the physiotherapist fixes the patient's head and the patient keeps the feet static and facing forwards. The patient then rotates his or her body to the right and to the left whilst maintaining the head in a static position

If symptoms such as dizziness or light-headedness are produced with this manœuvre, then they are due to vertebrobasilar pathology, because the head remains still (and the vestibular apparatus will be unaffected) and the cervical spine is rotating, affecting the artery.

Vertebrobasilar testing (Maitland 2001) (DVD)

This test is performed in both sitting and supine positions.

1. Sustained rotation for 10 seconds is performed to each side. Note any symptoms.
2. Sustained extension for 10 seconds is performed. If the patient is asymptomatic then:
3. Combined rotation and extension to each side is sustained for 10 seconds. Note any symptoms. A positive test would induce feelings of dizziness and nausea.

Key point

If the patient has grossly restricted range of movement, then the test for VBI is not valid.

Neurological testing

Dermatomes

Test for normal sensation, the cutaneous area supplied by a single posterior root of each spinal segment, light touch with the dorsal aspect of the hand or cotton wool and pin-prick sensation for each dermatome, C1 to T1.

Myotomes

Isometric testing of the muscles supplied by a spinal segment in mid-range for a few seconds is performed at each level from C1 to T1 (Figure 2.25). Weakness may indicate a lower motor lesion from a prolapsed disc, or another space-occupying lesion.

Reflexes

Test for normal reflexes: biceps (C5–C6), triceps and brachioradialis (C7). Compare one side with the other. Note brisk reflexes which may be indicative of an upper motor neurone lesion, and dull reflexes which may be indicative of a lower motor neurone lesion.

- C5–C6 corresponds to biceps brachii. The person's arm should be semi-flexed at the elbow with the forearm pronated. Place your thumb or finger firmly on the biceps tendon and hit your finger with the hammer (Figure 2.26).

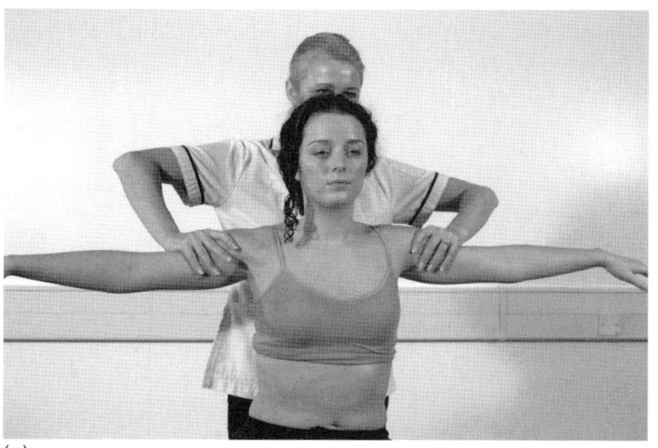

(a)

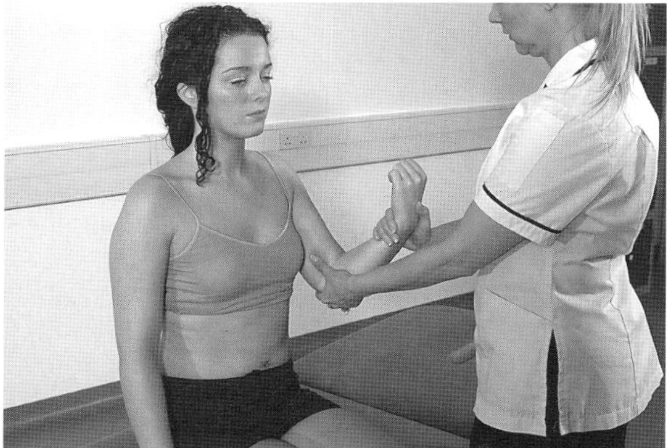

(b)

Figure 2.25 (a) Resisted shoulder abduction (C5) myotome. (b) Assessment of C6 myotome in resisted biceps.

- C6–C8 correspond to triceps. Support the person's upper arm and let the forearm hang free. Hit the triceps tendon above the elbow (Figure 2.27).

Mechanical tension tests (DVD)

The upper limb tension test (ULTT) is referred to as the SLR test of the cervical spine. This test mobilises the brachial plexus and particularly biases the median nerve to determine the degree to which neural tissue is responsible for producing the patient's symptoms. Certain movements of the arm, shoulder, elbow, wrist and hand, and similarly the neck and the lower limb, can cause neural movement in the cervical spine. These tests are so important that all physiotherapists should know and use them (Butler 1991).

The physiotherapist depresses the patient's shoulder, then adds in 90 degrees abduction, 90 degrees lateral rotation of the shoulder, elbow extension, forearm supination, and wrist and finger extension to the supine patient (Figure 2.28a). Sensitising manœuvres such as ipsilateral (same side) or contralateral (opposite side) cervical rotation and side flexion are added (Figure 2.28b). Symptoms of pain, paraesthesia and restriction are noted, and compared with the other side. Common findings will be reduced range or the reproduction of symptoms on the affected side.

Palpation

Palpate the soft tissues, noting the positions of vertebrae and myofascial trigger points (localised irritable spots within skeletal muscle). These trigger points produce local pain in a referred pattern and often accompany chronic musculoskeletal disorders. Palpation of a hypersensitive nodule of muscle fibres of harder than normal consistency is the physical finding typically associated with trigger points (Alvarez and Rockwell 2002).

Observe for local or referred pain, thickening of structures or stiffness. Remember that anomalies of the bifid spinous processes of the cervical vertebrae and differences in their spacing are not uncommon and may not be clinically significant (Maitland 2001).

Soft-tissue changes including suboccipital thickening and shortening in the extensors, and prominence and thickening of the articular pillar of C2–C3 facet joints are common in degenerative disorders. Soft-tissue changes around the cervicothoracic junction are also

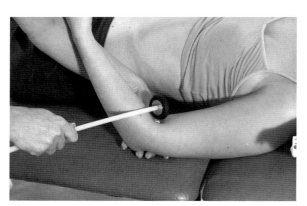

Figure 2.26 The biceps reflex (C5, C6).

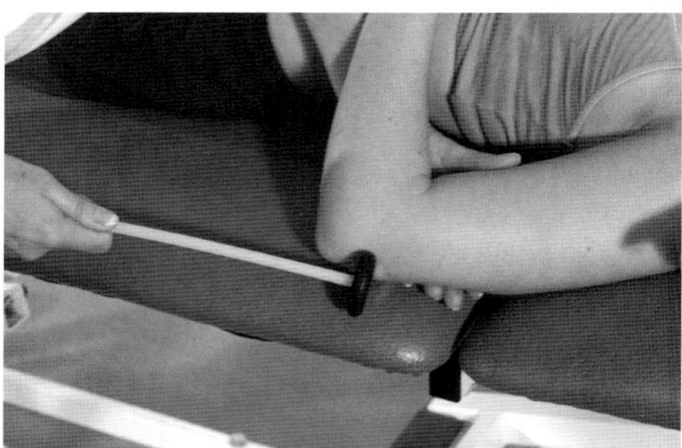

Figure 2.27 The triceps reflex (C6, C7, C8).

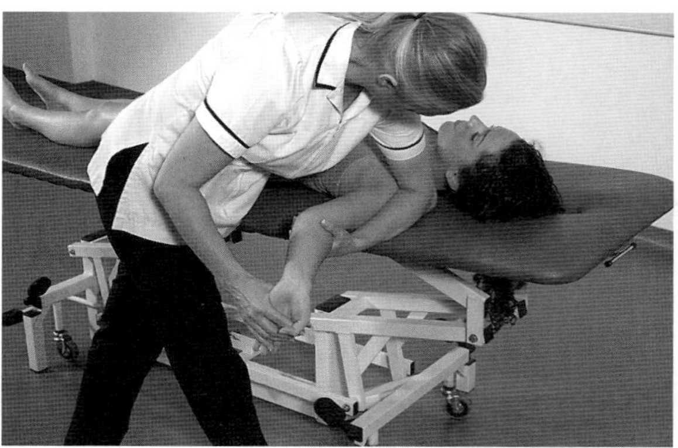

(a)

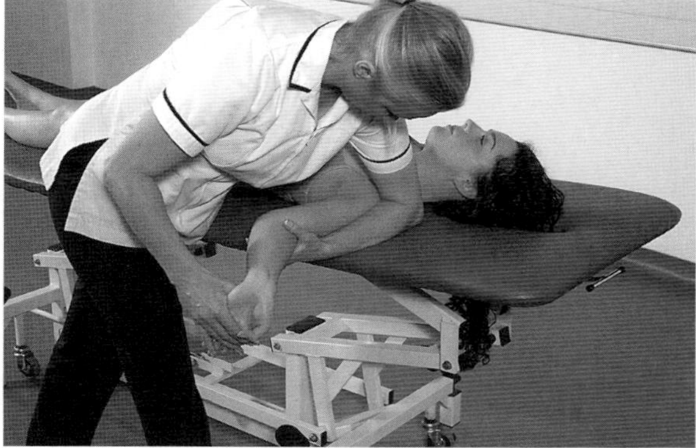

(b)

Figure 2.28 (a) Upper limb tension test (ULTT). (b) ULTT with contralateral right side flexion of the cervical spine.

commonly found, and may be referred to as a dowager's hump.

Bony anomalies

Osteophytes may be palpable at the C2–C3 facet joints, in patients with pre-existing spinal pathology (Maitland 2001). Approximation of the spinous processes of C6–C7 is also a common feature.

Accessory spinal movements

With the patient prone, central pressure on the spinous processes C2–T6 and unilateral pressures on the articular pillars C2–T6 are applied by the physiotherapist, noting levels of stiffness, pain response, muscle spasm and areas of hypermobility (Figure 2.29).

CASE STUDY — CERVICAL SPINE

A 50-year-old woman with a 2-year history of central neck and occasionally bilateral shoulder pain (4 on the VAS) was referred for physiotherapy. On examination she had a marked protracted cervical spine (poking chin posture) which could, however, be corrected by the patient on demand. Her cervical range of movement was approximately two-thirds on all movements. Neurological testing was normal. Palpation revealed stiffness at levels C5 and C6 to central PA pressures over the spinous processes.

The patient was treated with grade III PA central pressures (as in Figure 2.29) and was given postural correction exercises: priority one cervical neutral shin slides against a wall. Following three treatment sessions her pain was reduced to 1 on the VAS and her range of movement was almost full. She was given deep flexor exercises on the fourth visit, along with exercises for normal range of movement. On the fifth visit she was asymptomatic, and was discharged to continue with the exercises at home.

Both manipulations and mobilisations aim to reduce pain and increase the joint range of motion for spinal conditions (Johnson and Rogers 2000; Maitland 2001). Studies have shown that cervical mobilisation produces a hypoalgesic (pain-relieving) effect and can decrease visual analogue scores (Sterling et al. 2001). The majority of studies conclude that spinal mobilisations have a positive short-term effect on pain (Bronfort et al. 2001; Coulter 1996). Koes et al. (1992) observed an improvement in physical functioning when compared to other physiotherapy modalities, placebo or GP involvement. It could be argued that, by improving pain in the short term, the patient will return to normal activities more quickly and thus avoid the potential for deconditioning and chronicity.

Muscle imbalance procedures were instituted into the woman's programme to improve her postural awareness, to increase the strength of the deep cervical flexors, and to stretch out the tight suboccipital extensors. According to Heimeyer et al. (1990), it is important for the therapist to differentiate between people who have protracted chin posture but who

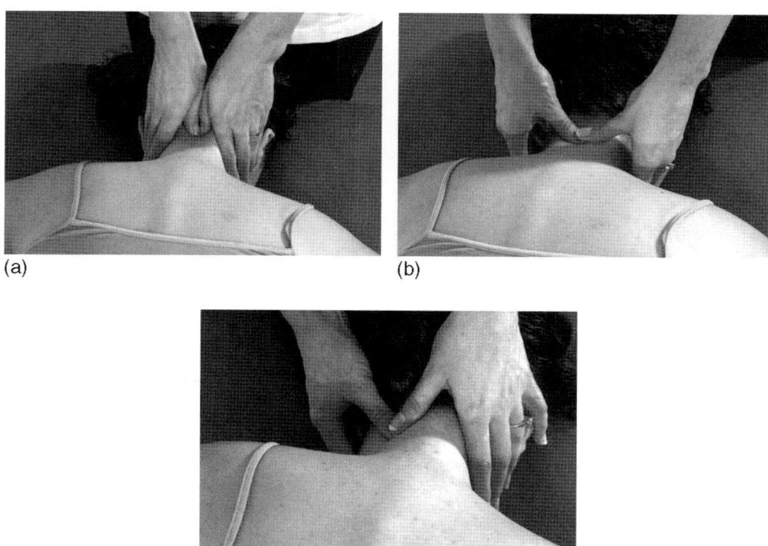

Figure 2.29 Accessory movements: (a) central PA pressure on spinous process; (b) central PA with thumbs superimposed; (c) unilateral pressure on the left articular pillar.

2

can voluntarily correct it, and those who cannot. For the person in this case study, the posture was correctable, so the role of the physiotherapist as adviser was paramount. Repeated sessions of electrotherapy, for example, would have been inappropriate or would have provided only a short-term solution to the pain. Treatment should be geared towards behaviour modifications — the change of bad postural habits. In this case the combination of manipulative therapy, corrective exercises and advice was employed with success.

PERIPHERAL JOINT ASSESSMENTS

THE SHOULDER JOINT

Key point

The patient should be suitably undressed to view the cervical spine, thoracic spine, shoulder girdles, shoulders and both arms.

Posture

It is important to assess the posture of the cervical and thoracic spine because a scoliosis, kyphosis or poking chin posture will affect the mechanics of the shoulder, by altering the plane of the glenohumeral joint. The spinal and shoulder complex postures should be observed with the patient in both sitting and standing.

Posterior alignment

The shoulders should ideally be level, but for a right-handed person the right shoulder is often held lower than the left, and vice versa. Elevation of the shoulder girdle may be due to tightness or overactivity in the levator scapulae or the upper fibres of trapezius, and lengthening or weakness in the lower fibres of trapezius.

Observe the symmetry of the scapulae. They should lie flat against the thoracic wall and the medial borders lie approximately 50–75 mm lateral to the spine. Winging of the scapulae is observed when the whole length of the medial border of the scapula is displaced laterally and posteriorly from the wall of the thorax. This may result from weakness in the serratus anterior muscle or a lesion of the long thoracic nerve. Pseudo-winging of the scapulae occurs when the inferior angle of the scapula is displaced from the thoracic wall.

Observe the soft-tissue contours of the shoulder for symmetry and for areas of atrophy and hypertrophy. The acromion processes should be horizontal to, or slightly higher than, the point at the root of the scapula. If the root of the scapula is higher, this indicates tightness or overactivity of the levator scapulae and rhomboid musculature, which causes a downward rotation of the glenoid fossa. This may be a precursor to impingement syndromes and rotator cuff pathologies. Moreover, the levator scapulae may cause anterior shear on the cervical spine and give rise to cervical and scapula pain.

Anterior alignment

Note any irregularities of the clavicle and sternoclavicular and acromioclavicular joints resulting from previous fractures or dislocations. Note the soft-tissue contours with respect to symmetry, atrophy and hypertrophy, particularly in the deltoid, upper trapezius and sternocleidomastoid muscles.

Lateral alignment

Note the relative positions of the humeral head; no more than one-third of the humeral head should lie anteriorly to the acromion process. Excessive forward translation may result from tightness in the pectoral muscles and elongation of the posterior shoulder capsule. The patient's arms should lie comfortably at the side with the thumbs facing almost forwards. Excessive medial rotation of the shoulders will result in the thumbs facing inwards towards the body. Excessive protraction of the shoulders with an increased thoracic kyphosis and tightness in the pectoral muscles is a common faulty posture.

Palpation

Palpate the local skin temperature, noting any increase suggestive of underlying inflammation. Palpate the acromioclavicular and sternoclavicular joints, observing for pain or tenderness. Palpate the supraspinatus and infraspinatus tendons for tenderness associated with tendonitis, calcification and strain. Palpate the upper trapezius and levator scapulae for tenderness and trigger points. These hyperirritable areas within the muscle and connective tissue are thought to be due to a secondary tissue response to disc or joint disorders (Hubbard and Berkhoff 1993). They are painful to compression and may cause referred pain.

Muscle length tests

Levator scapulae

With the patient supine, flex and lateral flex the cervical spine away to resistance and add ipsilateral rotation (rotation to the same side as side flexion). Depress the shoulder girdle and compare range and pain response on both sides.

Pectoralis minor
With the patient supine, the lateral border of the spine of the scapula should be within 25 mm of the plinth. If pectoralis minor is shortened, the lateral border of the spine of the scapula is more than 25 mm from the plinth since the shoulder girdle is protracted.

Movements

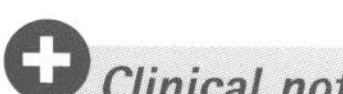

Clinical note

Since the cervical and thoracic spines may refer pain to the shoulder and scapula areas, full active movements and accessory movements of these areas should be assessed. Note any increase or referral of pain around the shoulder or scapula areas. Overpressure may be used if the movements are pain-free. Furthermore, the ULTT may be performed to rule out referral of pain from neural structures. Refer to the objective assessment of the cervical spine for descriptions of these techniques.

Active movements

Full active movements of the shoulder girdle and joint are performed, noting any restriction, asymmetry and pain response. Note the capsular pattern for the glenohumeral joint is limitation of lateral rotation, abduction and medial rotation (Cyriax 1982).

Shoulder girdle movements
Assess shoulder girdle elevation, depression, protraction and retraction, observing for pain asymmetry and crepitus.

Shoulder joint flexion
Observe flexion through to elevation and return of movement, assessing the scapulohumeral rhythm. Normal should be in the ratio of 2:1 (humerus:scapula). Reversed scapulohumeral rhythm occurs in conditions causing restriction of the glenohumeral joint, such as adhesive capsulitis ('frozen shoulder').

Shoulder joint abduction
Observe abduction through to elevation and return (Figure 2.30), again noting the scapulohumeral rhythm.

Key point

A painful arc of movement is observed in patients suffering from impingement syndromes, whereby the superior aspects of the rotator cuff, biceps tendon and bursae are impinged by repetitive overarm activities. Pain is experienced between 90 and 130 degrees of abduction.

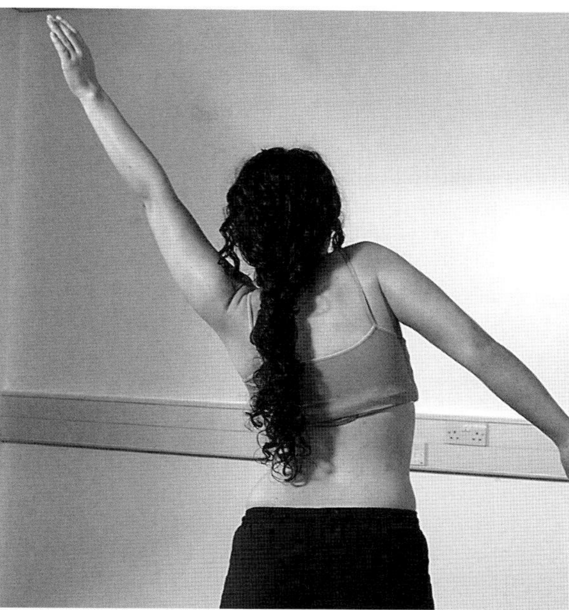

Figure 2.30 Reversed scapulohumeral rhythm of the right shoulder.

Impingement may be caused by loss of scapular stability. Faulty patterns of scapula motion include early rotation and elevation of the scapula (reversed scapulohumeral rhythm). This may implicate weakness in the stabilisers (e.g. lower fibres of trapezius, rhomboids and serratus anterior), or shortness and overactivity in the upper trapezius and levator scapulae.

Impingement may also be caused by weakness or inhibition of the rotator cuff muscles that produces a superior translation of the humeral head (i.e. subscapularis, teres minor and lower infraspinatus). There may also be late timing of lateral rotation during abduction which may cause impingement.

Tightness of pectoralis minor can cause increased protraction of the scapula which decreases the subacromial space.

Repetition of the movement may induce an element of fatigue, and abnormal movements may derive from that. A juddering movement of the scapula on return from elevation implicates poor eccentric control.

Differentiation. If abduction reproduces the person's pain, then differentiation between the glenohumeral and subacromial structures may be required.

1. If the movement is repeated and compression applied to the glenohumeral joint causes an increase in symptoms, then the glenohumeral joint is implicated.
2. If the movement is repeated and a longitudinal force in a cephalad direction is applied (increasing compression on the subacromial structures), with an increase in pain, the subacromial structures are implicated.

2

Failure to initiate or maintain abduction when placed passively into abduction is a sign of rotator cuff rupture, and the patient should be referred to a consultant for a repair/further investigations.

Shoulder joint rotation
Test medial and lateral rotations, both beside the trunk and at 90 degrees of abduction. Note pain response and limitation of movement.

Clinical note (Figure 2.31) 

The medial kinetic rotation test assesses movement dysfunction and impingement and instability risk at the shoulder.
The patient is supine with the arm at 90 degrees of abduction and off the plinth. The therapist stands above the patient's right shoulder facing his feet and places her left index finger on the patient's humeral head and her left middle finger on the coracoid process. Passively she medially rotates the patient's shoulder using the forearm to 70 degrees.
In an ideal situation or negative test the therapist's fingers on the left hand should not move whilst rotating the shoulder joint medially to 70 degrees.
Early movement of the humeral head (index finger) suggests an anterior instability of the glenohumeral joint. Early movement of the coracoid (middle finger) suggests scapula instability and a potential impingement risk at the glenohumeral joint.

Shoulder joint horizontal flexion and extension (Scarf test)
Pain on these movements implicates the acromioclavicular joints as the source of pain or restriction.

Shoulder joint extension
Compare both sides for range and pain response.

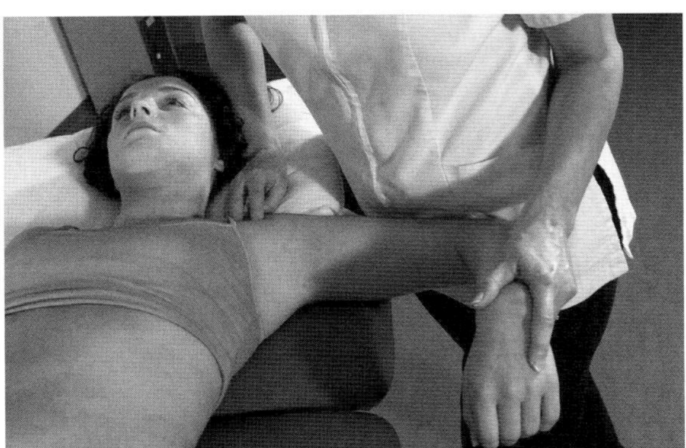

Figure 2.31 Medial kinetic rotation test.

Shoulder functional movements
Functional movements, such as hand behind the back (HBB) and the hand behind the neck (HBN), should also be assessed. These movements are grossly restricted in patients with adhesive capsulitis.

Other shoulder joint abnormalities
Sporting activities that give rise to symptoms, such as the late cocking stage of throwing a ball overhead, should also be assessed to determine faulty mechanics.

Passive movements

All movements performed actively can be repeated passively, noting the differences in range. Observe the differences in end-feel and compare these with the unaffected side.

Key point

Note that the capsular pattern for the glenohumeral joint is limitation of lateral rotation, abduction and medial rotation (Cyriax 1982).

Accessory movements

Acromioclavicular and sternoclavicular joints
Test AP and PA draw, and caudal glide.

Glenohumeral joint
Test AP and PA draw, caudad and cephalad glide, and lateral distraction (Figure 2.32).

Further tests (Maitland 2001)

The following tests should be performed only in shoulders of low irritability, and when no comparable sign has been found. They stress a number of different structures around the shoulder and are therefore not diagnostic:

- locking test of the shoulder
- quadrant test of the shoulder (Figure 2.33).

Resisted muscle testing
This provides a guide to strength ratios and pain response. Test abduction and flexion at around 30–60 degrees; internal and external rotation beside the trunk and at 90 degrees of elevation in the plane of the scapula; and resisted muscle testing in positions of function and/or pain (Figure 2.34).

Muscle length tests
It may be useful to test the length of muscles that are prone to shortness — latissimus dorsi, pectoralis major and minor, upper fibres of trapezius, levator scapulae and sternocleidomastoid.

Acromioclavicular joint compression and distraction
End-of-range overpressure into horizontal flexion compresses the acromioclavicular joint and may give rise to

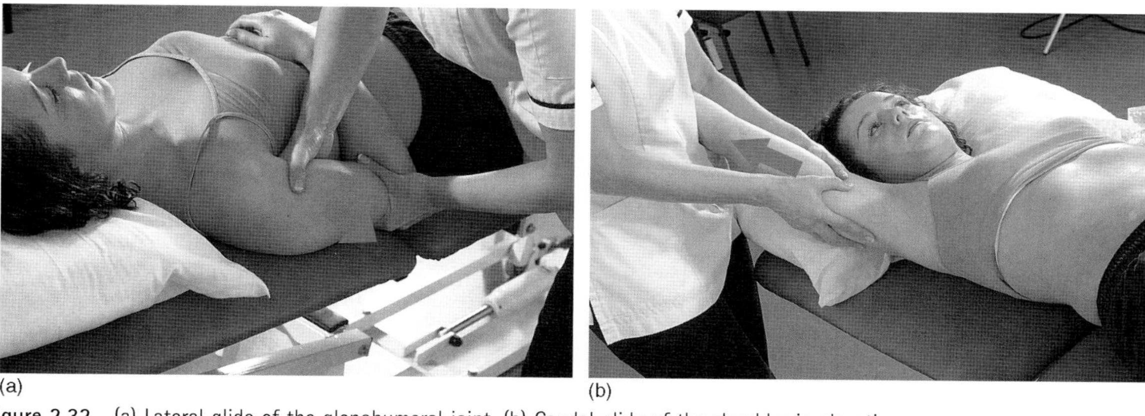

(a) (b)

Figure 2.32 (a) Lateral glide of the glenohumeral joint. (b) Caudal glide of the shoulder in elevation.

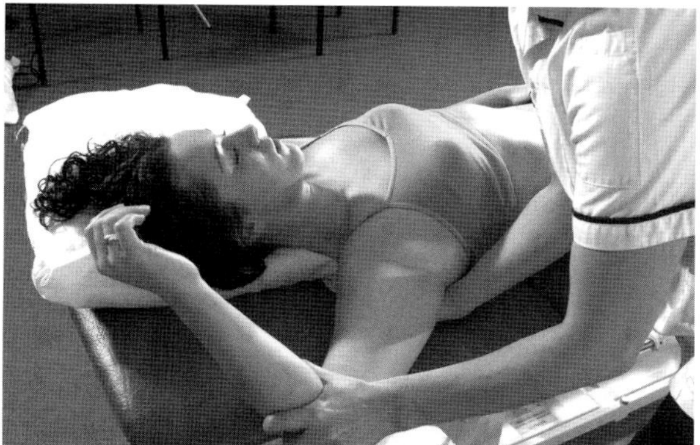

Figure 2.33 Quadrant test of the shoulder.

pain arising from this joint. Acromioclavicular distraction tests the instability of the acromioclavicular joint, by applying a downward traction on the arm whilst palpating the joint line. Reproduction of pain or palpable separation of the joint line is a positive test.

Tests for shoulder instability

Anterior draw/translation (Lachmann's of the shoulder)

This is performed in supine with the patient's arm at around 30 degrees of abduction, 45 degrees of lateral rotation and slight flexion. The physiotherapist grasps the humeral head with one hand, and the medial hand is used to stabilise the shoulder girdle. The lateral hand applies the anterior translation force in the same way as the anterior draw test of the knee. Laxity of the joint (excessive anterior translation) is a positive sign (Figure 2.35).

Posterior draw test

This is performed in supine with the patient's glenohumeral joint at the edge of the examination couch in abduction not exceeding 90 degrees. Posterior pressure is applied on the anterior aspect of the humeral head. Excessive movement compared with the other side is a positive sign.

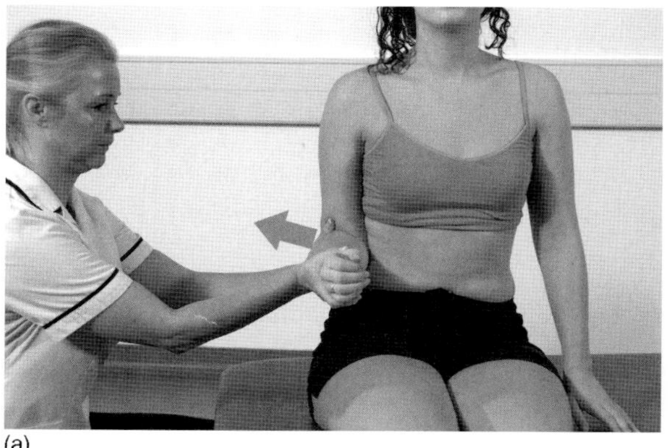

(a)

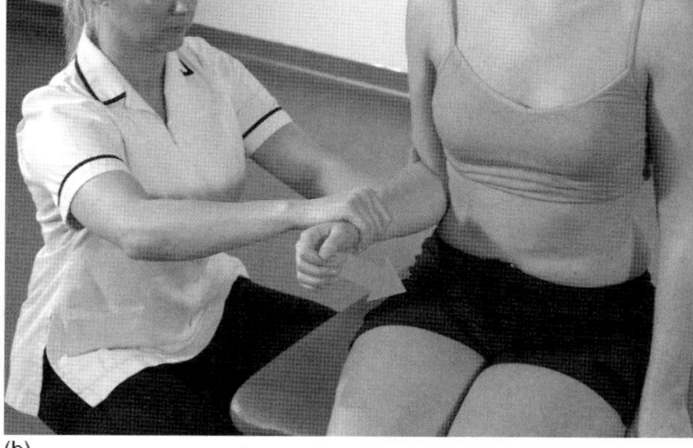

(b)

Figure 2.34 (a) Resisted lateral rotation at the shoulder. (b) Resisted medial rotation at the shoulder.

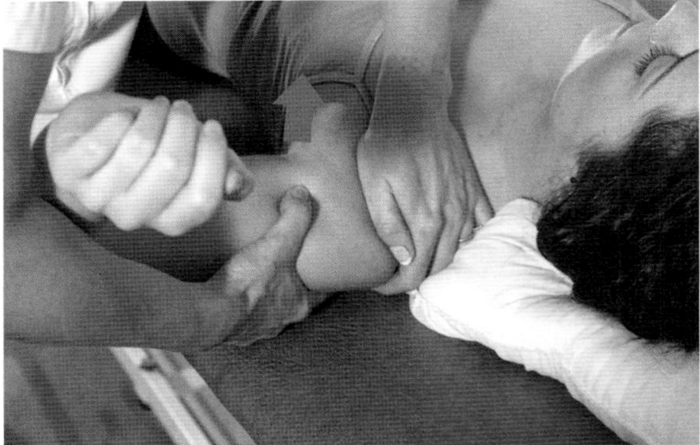

Figure 2.35 Anterior draw of the glenohumeral joint in abduction with stabilisation of the shoulder girdle.

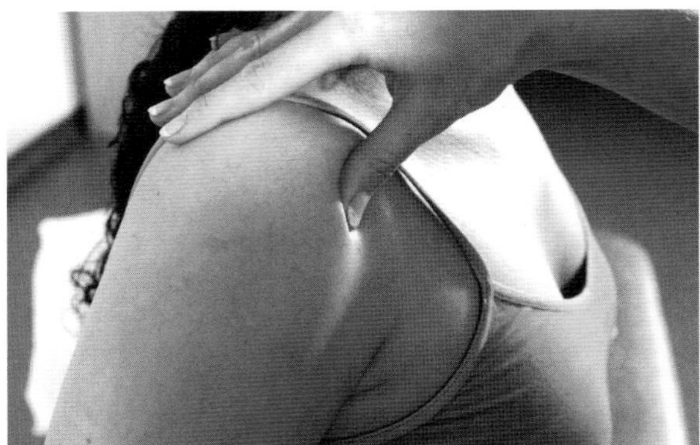

Figure 2.37 Palpation of the supraspinatus tendon. The patient's hand is behind the back.

Inferior draw (sulcus) test (DVD)

This is performed in sitting or supine, arm by the side. The physiotherapist exerts a strong downward traction force on the arm, grasping the head of the humerus with both hands, to the limit of movement, pain or apprehension, whilst monitoring the superior contour of the shoulder joint. Excessive inferior glide or a significant depression or sulcus distal to the acromion is a positive sign.

Impingement test (DVD)

Supraspinatus (empty can test)

This is performed in sitting or standing with 90 degrees of abduction bilaterally, full available medial rotation, and 30 degrees of horizontal flexion (Figures 2.36 and 2.37). Supraspinatus is the main support for the suspended arm in this position. The physiotherapist resists abduction of the shoulder. Pain on resistance is a positive test for a lesion of the supraspinatus muscle or tendon. Following the objective assessment record your findings clearly and asterisk objective findings.

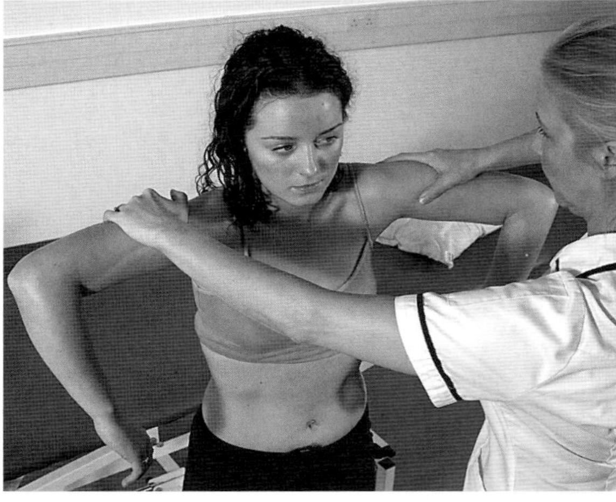

Figure 2.36 The empty can test position. Resistance to abduction is applied by the therapist.

TEST YOURSELF

Match these five scenarios to the likely pathology:

1. reduced range of movement, particularly on active and passive rotations and abduction
2. painful arc of movement between 90 and 120 degrees
3. inability to abduct the arm actively away from the body and maintain the position when the arm is placed there passively
4. pain and weakness on resisted elbow and shoulder flexion
5. excessive movement on passive anterior, posterior and sulcus draw tests of the shoulder.

THE HIP JOINT

Key point

The patient should be suitably undressed to view the hip, pelvis and spine. Note that the hip joint is too deep to observe an effusion or palpate the joint line.

Answers

(1) Frozen shoulder (adhesive capsulitis). (2) Impingement of supraspinatus under the acromion. (3) Rupture of the rotator cuff musculature. (4) Ruptured biceps brachii muscle. (5) Global instability.

Gait

Observe the person's gait from the front, back and side. Assess the patient with and without a walking aid, as deemed appropriate. Ask the patient to walk forwards and backwards, whilst you observe:

- stride length symmetry
- the time spent on the single leg support phase on each leg
- corresponding factors of pain, stiffness and/or weakness during the cycle.

Posture

Standing

With the patient standing, view from the front, rear and sides. Note:

1. Pelvic tilting: a line joining the two anterior sacroiliac joints should be horizontal (the same applies posteriorly).
2. The relative levels of the posterior superior iliac spine to the ipsilateral anterior superior iliac spine viewed from the side: differences may be suggestive of sacroiliac rotatory asymmetry.
3. Rotational deformity of the hips: this may be observed as in-toeing or out-toeing.
4. Leg length discrepancy: this may be observed from the differences in the horizontal levels of the gluteal and knee creases.
5. Scoliosis of the lumbar spine: this may be structural or a compensation for a leg length discrepancy.
6. Inequality of weight distribution: the patient may reduce the amount of weight borne on the painful side.
7. Increased lumbar lordosis: this may suggest a fixed flexion deformity of the hip(s).
8. Bruising in the abdominal or groin area: this is suggestive of a sportsman's hernia.
9. Muscle wasting: wasting, particularly of the quadriceps and gluteal muscles, is common and may appear as hollowing posteriorly or laterally at the buttocks.

Supine

With the patient supine, note the following:

1. leg rotation, through observing the relative positions of the patella and/or the feet
2. pelvic rotation
3. leg length discrepancy, through observing the relative position of the medial malleoli or heels.

Leg length discrepancy

Apparent leg length discrepancy is measured from the xiphoid of the sternum to the tip of the medial malleolus using a tape measure. (Compare with the other leg.) *True leg length discrepancy* is measured, using a tape measure, from the ASIS to the tip of the medial malleolus. A difference in leg length of up to 1–2 cm is considered normal by some clinicians. If there is a leg length difference, measure the length of the individual bones — i.e. thigh and leg.

Key point

From the movement of supine to sitting, one leg may appear to be longer in supine and shorter in sitting. This is caused by anterior rotation of the innominate bone on the affected side and is a sacroiliac joint dysfunction.

Muscle length assessments

The Thomas test DVD

This test determines the presence of a fixed flexion deformity at the hip. With the patient supine, the hip is fully flexed passively, and the lumbar lordosis is obliterated. If the contralateral (opposite) hip rises off the bed, this indicates a fixed flexion deformity of that hip. This may be due to tightness or restriction in the capsule, iliopsoas or rectus femoris.

To differentiate between the iliopsoas and rectus femoris as the source of restriction, the patient's knee is passively extended (Figure 2.38). If this results in the patient's hip dropping down into less flexion, then the restriction is in the rectus femoris muscle because by extending the knee an element of stretch has been removed. If the hip is unaffected and remains, in the same degree of flexion, independently of the knee extension, then the restriction is in the iliopsoas muscle. This is measured and recorded.

The length of the following muscles may be tested since they are prone to shortening: quadratus lumborum, tensor fascia lata and the hamstrings.

Modified Ober's test (iliotibial band) DVD

With the patient in side-lying, the uppermost hip fully rotated laterally and the knee joint in unlocked extension, the uppermost leg should drop (adduct) to the plinth (Figure 2.39). A tight iliotibial band would result in the leg not being able to adduct to the plinth.

Piriformis test

With the patient supine or side-lying and the hip at 90 degrees flexion, adduct maximally to resistance and externally rotate. (Note piriformis is a medial rotator in flexion.) Pain in the buttock or in the distribution of the sciatic nerve may signify compression of the sciatic nerve by the piriformis muscle (Figure 2.40).

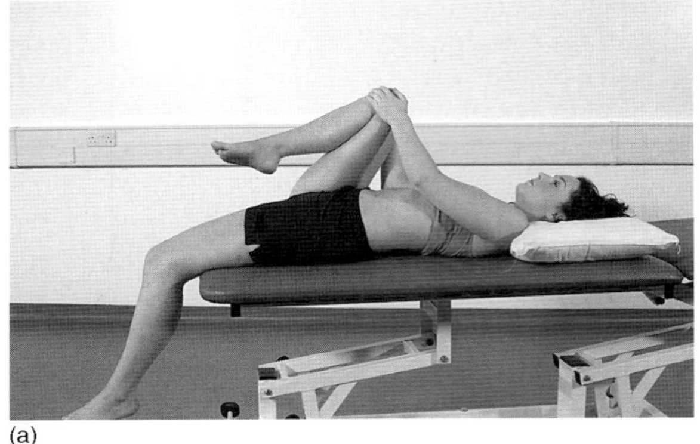

(a)

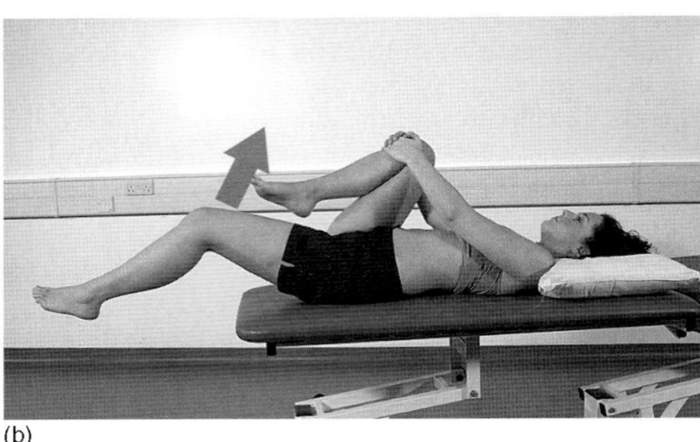

(b)

Figure 2.38 The Thomas test: (a) normal; (b) abnormal.

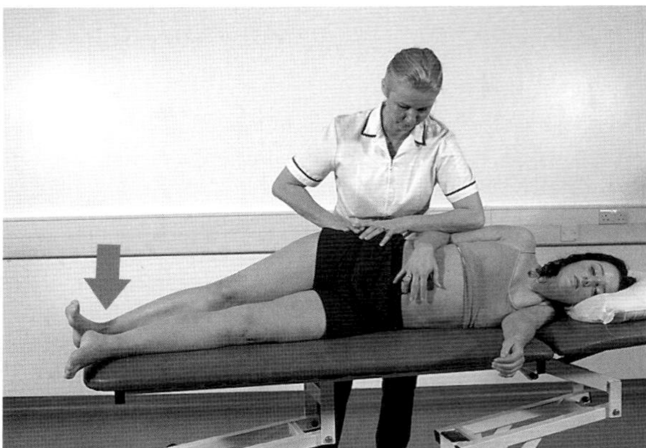

Figure 2.39 Modified Ober's test.

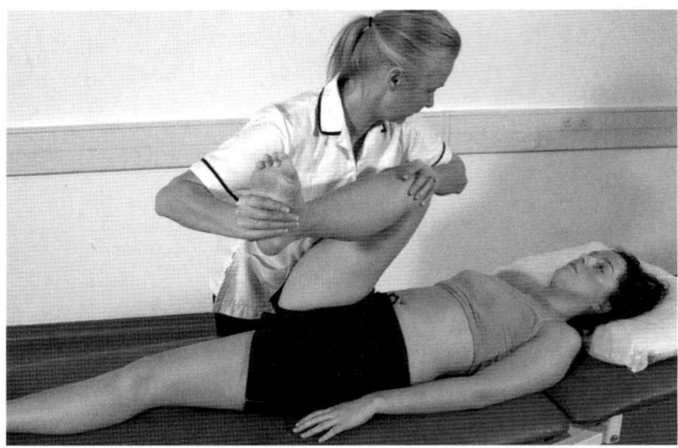

Figure 2.40 Piriformis stretch. Note that, in the flexed position, piriformis becomes a hip medial rotator.

Hamstrings

With the patient sitting, spine in neutral and the hip at 90 degrees, he or she should be able to extend the knee to within 10 degrees of full extension (Figure 2.41).

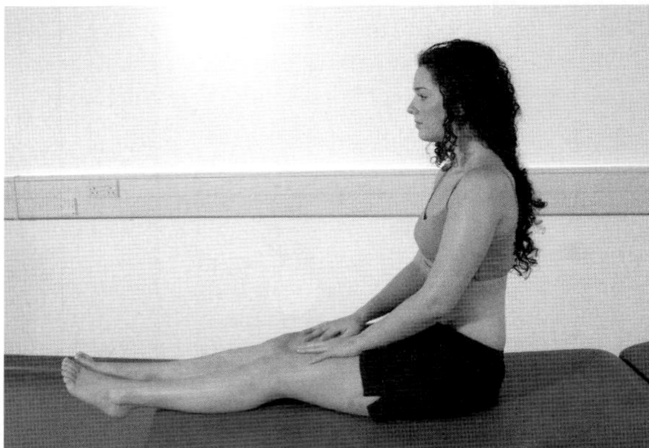

Figure 2.41 Assessment of hamstring length. Note that the lumbar spine remains in neutral. This picture shows normal hamstring length.

Quadratus lumborum

Test side flexion against a wall without associated flexion or rotations. Compare the two sides. A shortened quadratus lumborum will result in limitation of contralateral side flexion.

Movements

Allow the patient to demonstrate functionally his or her aggravating movement in order to determine the likely structures implicated in producing the symptoms.

Lumbar spine differentiation

The lumbar spine may give rise to referred pain in the region of the hip or groin, so it is important to exclude the lumbar spine as a possible cause of symptoms arising at the hip joint. Flexion, extension and bilateral side flexion should be observed actively in standing. Loss of range of motion and pain response should be noted, particularly if these movements reproduce the patient's hip pain or the patient's comparable sign. If the movements are pain-free and full-range, then overpressure may be applied to observe whether this reproduces the patient's symptoms. Accessory movements of the lumbar spine, femoral nerve stretch and SLR should also be screened.

Trendelenburg test DVD

A positive Trendelenburg test demonstrates that the hip abductors are not functioning owing to weakness or pain inhibition and are unable to perform their role of stabilising the pelvis on the weight-bearing leg. To perform the test the patient stands on the unaffected leg and flexes the other knee to a right angle. The pelvis should remain level or tilt up slightly on the non-weightbearing side. The patient then stands on the affected leg and flexes the knee of the other leg. If the pelvis drops on the NWB side, this signifies a positive Trendelenburg test (Figures 2.42 and 2.43).

Palpation

- Palpate the head of the femur lateral to the femoral artery.
- Rotate the hip passively to elicit crepitus or tenderness at the joint.
- Palpate the psoas major and adductor longus tendons to localise strains and contractures of these structures.
- Palpate the greater trochanter of the femur for tenderness associated with bursitis. Palpate the ischial tuberosity for suspected hamstring strains.
- Tenderness located over the ASIS may indicate a strain of the sartorius muscle or contusion of the

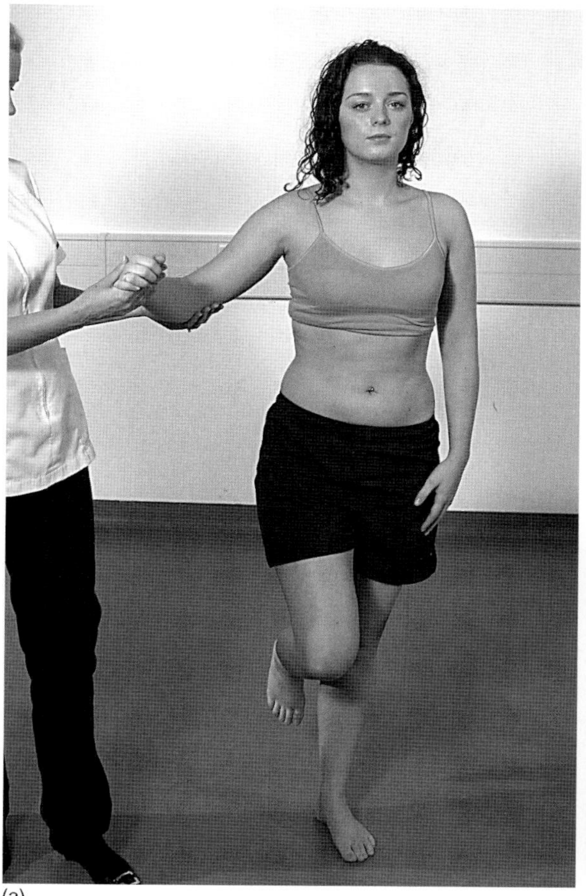

(a)

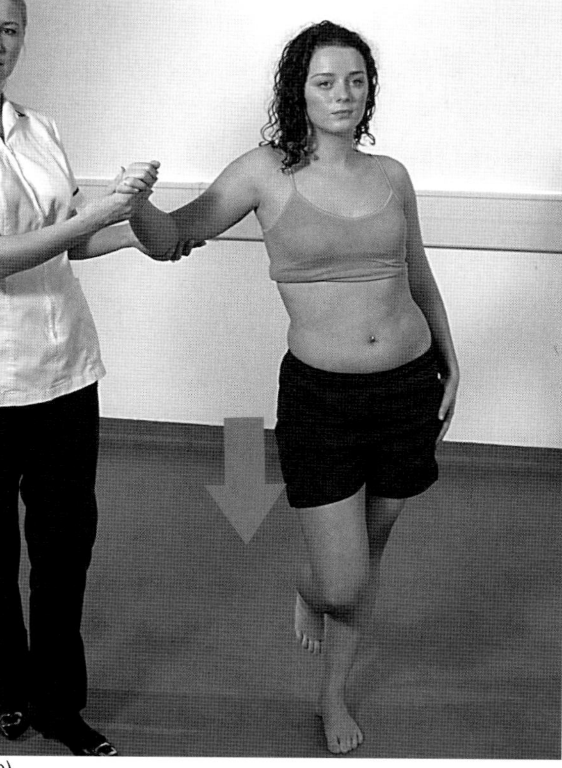

(b)

Figure 2.42 Trendelenburg test of right hip abductors: (a) normal; (b) abnormal or positive sign.

2

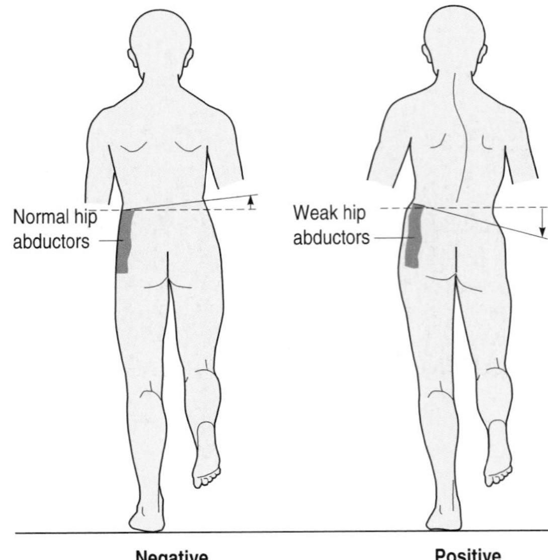

Figure 2.43 Schematic of Trendelburg's sign.

spine following contact sports. This is referred to as a 'hip-pointer'.

- Palpate the lower abdominal musculature for suspected inguinal or sports hernias.

Active movements

Key point

Note pain, crepitus and/or limitation of movement. Apply overpressure to the movement if it is pain-free to see whether this reproduces the symptoms not elicited on other movements. Measure both the normal and affected hip for comparison.

Hip flexion/extension

The patient is supine or side-lying. The axis of the goniometer is placed directly over the greater trochanter of the femur. The static arm should be parallel to the patient's trunk. The dynamic arm should be placed parallel to the femur. Note loss of range or pain response.

Hip abduction/adduction

The patient is supine. The axis of the goniometer is placed over the ASIS. The static arm should be in line between the left and right ASIS. The dynamic arm should be parallel to the long axis of the femur. Note loss of range or pain response.

Hip rotation

Hip rotation can be easily measured with the patient sitting. Note that the hip joints are flexed to approximately 90 degrees (Figure 2.3). The axis of the goniometer is placed at the mid-point of the patella. The static arm is perpendicular to the floor. The dynamic arm should be parallel to the anterior midline of patella. If active movements are full-range and pain-free, then gentle overpressure can be applied, noting any reproduction of symptoms.

The normal ranges of movement at the hip joint should be approximately:

- 0–120 degrees for unilateral flexion, 0–150 for bilateral flexion
- 10–15 degrees for extension
- 0–40 degrees for abduction
- 0–25 degrees for adduction
- 0–35 degrees for medial rotation
- 0–45 degrees for lateral rotation (Figure 2.44).

Key point

Note that the capsular pattern for the glenohumeral joint is limitation of lateral rotation, abduction and medial rotation (Cyriax 1982).

Passive movements

Flexion, extension, abduction, adduction, and internal and external rotation should be performed passively by the therapist (Figure 2.45). Note any differences between active and passive ranges and identify reasons for this.

Muscle strength testing

Test the muscles both isometrically and isotonically through range to detect weakness at any particular point

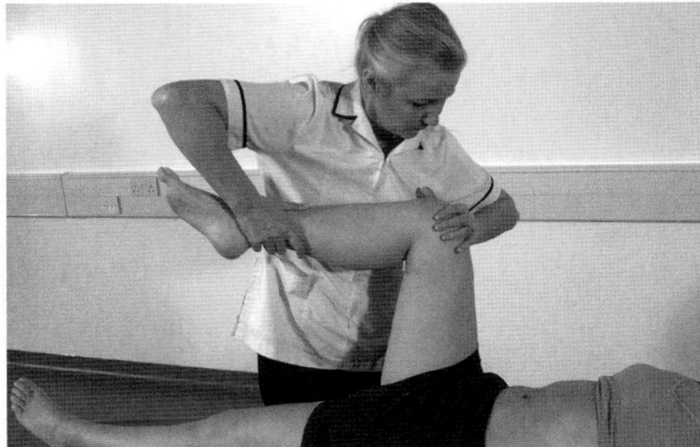

Figure 2.44 Resisted lateral rotation of the hip in flexion.

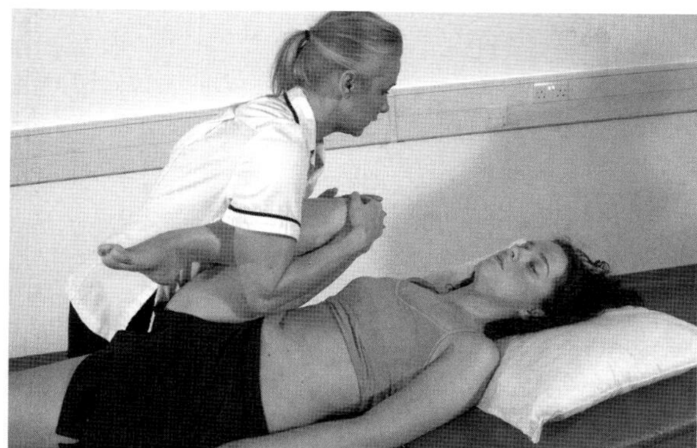

Figure 2.45 Passive hip and knee flexion.

in the range. Compare with the opposite side. Pain inhibits muscle contraction and it is therefore important to differentiate between true weakness and pain-induced inhibition.

With the patient side-lying, test the strength of the hip abductors and adductors (weakness of adductors is a common finding in recurrent groin strains). With the patient supine, test the strength of the hip adductors, flexors and medial/lateral rotators (Figure 2.44).

Accessory movements

Test:

- cephalad longitudinal accessory movement (Figure 2.46)
- caudad longitudinal accessory movement
- lateral transverse movement (joint distraction).

Flexion/adduction combination and the hip quadrant test may be performed on non-irritable hips when all plane movements are clear with overpressure (Figure 2.47; Maitland 2001).

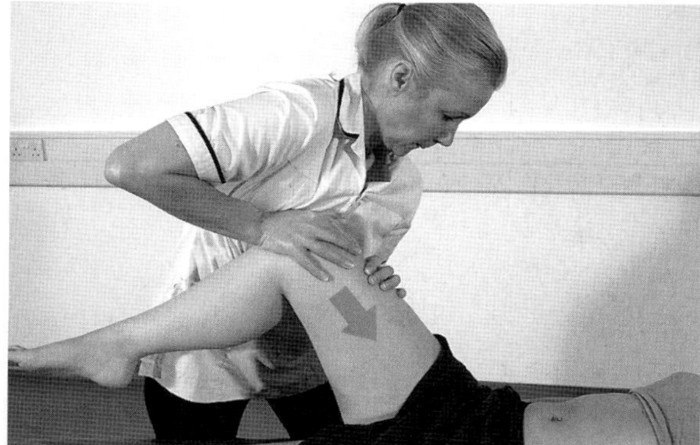

Figure 2.46 Compression applied through the hip joint.

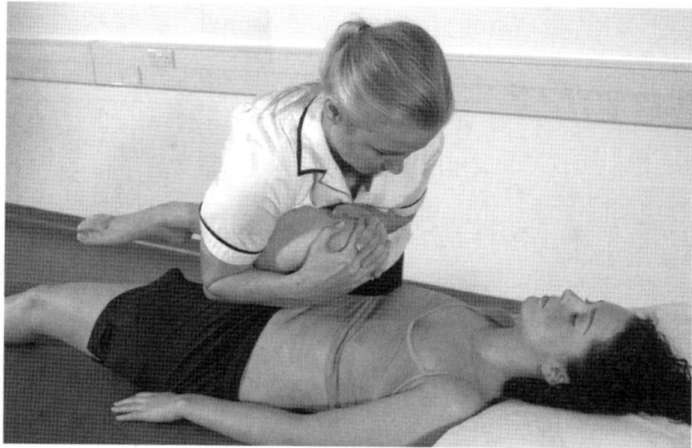

Figure 2.47 Quadrant test of the hip (flexion and adduction).

Neural tests

Neural tests may be performed if the symptoms produced at the hip appear to be originating from neural or spinal structures:

- femoral nerve stretch test (prone knee bend)
- sciatic nerve stretch test (straight leg raise)
- slump test.

For descriptions of these tests refer to the objective assessment of the lumbar spine.

Functional tests

Observe patients performing activities that reproduce their pain. If appropriate, assess activities such as hop, squats, walking forwards, backwards, sideways, etc.

Key point

On completion of the assessment, specific objective signs that reproduce the patient's symptoms should be marked with an asterisk (*) or highlighted. This is commonly referred to as a 'comparable sign' and needs to be reassessed at each treatment, to determine the effectiveness of the physiotherapy intervention. Record your findings clearly.

TEST YOURSELF

Match these five scenarios to the likely pathology:

1. local tenderness at the ischial tuberosity and pain on resisted knee flexion
2. pain in the groin on coughing, resisted adduction sit-ups and weight-bearing
3. a 3-year history of pain and stiffness, particularly on medial rotation

4. local tenderness and heat palpated in the area of the greater trochanter having an insidious onset
5. increased or exaggerated lumbar lordosis and a positive Thomas test.

THE KNEE JOINT

Key point

The patient should be suitably undressed to view the hip, knee and ankle joints.

Gait

Observe the gait as the person walks forwards and backwards. Make particular note of the equality of stride length, dwell time on each leg, reluctance to bear weight, and any pain responses.

Clinical note

The hip joint may refer pain to the knee. To differentiate between the hip and knee joints as a source of symptoms, the hip joint is tested by observing full flexion of the hip joint and then medial and lateral rotation in 90 degree flexion passively. Observe for any pain response or limitation of movement compared with the other side. If the movements are full-range and pain-free, it is unlikely that the hip joint is the source of pain (Figure 2.44).

Knee examination

Posture with patient standing

Observe any deformities such as genu varum, genu valgus or genu recurvatum (Figure 2.48). Note any evidence of muscle atrophy, particularly evident in the vastus medialis muscle. Observe the relative positions and size of the patellae. 'Patella alta' is the term used to describe a small-high riding patella.

Note any foot, ankle or subtalar deformity, such as foot pronation which will cause medial rotation of the tibia and hence affect the mechanics of the knee joint.

Swelling and discoloration

Swelling that extends beyond the joint capsule may suggest an infection or a major ligamentous injury, and the suprapatellar pouch will appear distended.

Answers
(1) Hamstring strain. (2) Sportsman's hernia. (3) Osteoarthritic (OA) hip. (4) Trochanteric bursitis. (5) Tightness in the hip flexors (iliopsoas.)

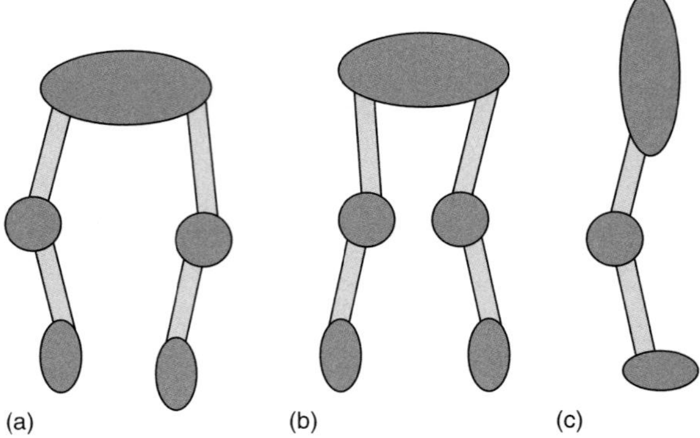

Figure 2.48 Leg posture deformities: genu varum (bow legs); (b) genu valgus (knock-knees); (c) genu recurvatum (hyperextending knees).

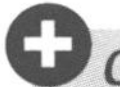

Clinical note

On your patient, draw a straight line across the middle of the patella. From the centre of this, draw a straight line going downwards through the centre of the tibial tuberosity, and another going upwards towards the ASIS (Figure 2.49). Normal values are approximately 12 degrees for males and 15 degrees for females. An increase in the Q angle is a predisposing factor in anterior knee pain and lateral dislocation of the patella.

Bruising may suggest trauma to superficial tissues or ligaments. Redness of the skin suggests an underlying inflammation. Palpate the temperature around the knee joint with the back of the hand; heat is indicative of an underlying inflammatory disorder.

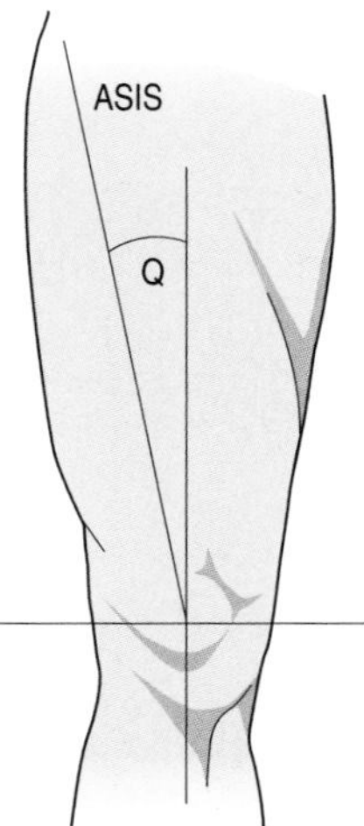

Figure 2.49 Measuring the Q angle.

Observe scar tissue that may be indicative of previous surgery or trauma.

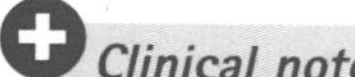

Clinical note

An effusion (swelling confined within the joint capsule) will appear to obliterate the natural hollows at the sides of the patella. The synovial membrane of the knee is expansive, and extends the width of 3–4 fingers above the superior aspect of the patella.

Loss of muscle bulk

Observe loss of bulk in the quadriceps muscles, particularly in the vastus medialis which atrophies earlier than vastus lateralis following trauma, degenerative diseases and pain episodes. With a tape measure check the circumference of both thighs at 5, 8, 15 and 23 cm above the upper pole of the patella to obtain an objective marker (Magee 1992).

Ask the patient to perform a static quadriceps contraction. Palpate the tone and compare left and right sides of the musculature. Inability to extend the knee actively may result from rupture of the quadriceps tendon or quadriceps weakness, patella fractures, rupture of the patellar ligament, or avulsion of the tibial tubercle. Note any loss of tone in the anterior and posterior tibial muscles and again measure if appropriate at specific recorded distances below the patella.

Patellar tap (DVD)

Patellar tap is a simple test to determine the presence of an effusion at the knee joint. It is performed with the patient supine. Any excess fluid is squeezed out of the suprapatellar pouch by sliding the index finger and thumb from 15 cm above the knee to the level of the upper border of the patella (Figure 2.50). Then place the tips of the thumb and three fingers of the free hand squarely on the patella and jerk it quickly downwards. A 'click' sound indicates the presence of effusion. The test will, however, be negative if the effusion is gross and tense, such as with a haemarthrosis of the knee (blood within the joint) following an anterior cruciate rupture.

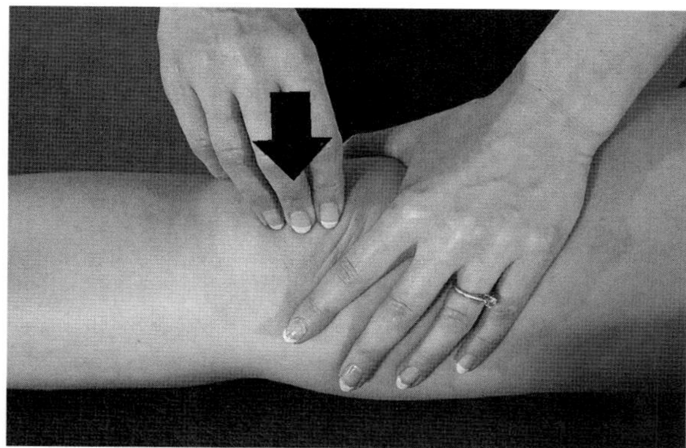

Figure 2.50 Patellar tap test.

Fluid displacement test

This is performed as above, by squeezing excess fluid out of the suprapatellar pouch and then stroking the medial side of the knee joint to displace any excess fluid in the main joint cavity to the lateral side of the joint. Repeat this procedure by stroking the lateral side of the joint. Any excess fluid will be seen to move across the joint and distend the medial side of the knee.

Tenderness at the knee (tibiofemoral joint)

Identify the joint line clearly by flexing the knee and observing for hollows at the sides of the patella ligament — these lie over the joint line.

1. Tenderness at the joint line is common in meniscal and fat pad injuries.
2. Tenderness along the line of the collateral ligaments of the knee joint is common at the site of a lesion following a tear, particularly at the upper and lower attachments and at the ligament's midpoint. Associated bruising and oedema may also be a feature of acute injuries.
3. Tenderness at the tibial tubercle — in children and adolescents, tenderness and hypertrophy of the tibial tubercle prominence — is associated with Osgood–Schlatter's disease. Tenderness is also found following acute avulsion injuries of the patella ligament and its tibial attachment.
4. Tenderness and swelling in the popliteal fossa may indicate the presence of a Baker's cyst. This condition is associated with degenerative changes or rheumatoid arthritis involving the knee joint.
5. Tenderness at the adductor tubercle may indicate strain in the adductor magnus muscle.
6. Femoral condyle tenderness may indicate the presence of osteochondritis dissecans.

Patellofemoral joint assessment

A knee assessment should include assessment of both the tibiofemoral and patellofemoral joints. Observe the position of the patella and compare both sides.

- Determination of a high or small patella (patella alta) is made by calculating the ratio of the length of the patellar tendon to the longest diagonal length of the patella. The normal value for this ratio is 1.02 plus or minus 20 per cent (Simmons and Cameron 1992). Patella alta is a predisposing factor in anterior knee pain and recurrent dislocation of the patella.

- Observe any tilting, lateral glide and rotation of the patella during a quadriceps contraction. Compare this with the other side.
- McConnell (1996) described a 'critical test' for the patellofemoral joint. Resisted inner-range quadriceps contraction is performed with the patient sitting at various degrees of knee flexion to determine whether this reproduces the patient's symptoms. Compare both sides (Figure 2.51).
- The McConnell critical test may be repeated with the patella taped in the corrected position. This will determine whether the taping is effective and should be incorporated into the treatment programme. Taping is believed to enhance activation and earlier timing of vastus medialis in quadriceps contractions and thus restore patellar tracking to normal.
- Observe any excessive pronation of the feet which may increase the Q angle (Figure 2.49).
- Test for tightness in the following structures: lateral retinaculum, iliotibial band, hamstrings and calves. Tightness of the above structures will increase dorsiflexion, and therefore pronation of the foot and ankle during the gait cycle. All of this will increase the Q angle (Olerud and Berg 1984).
- Perform passive accessory movements to test the mobility and pain response of the patella in all directions. Observe pain, laxity or muscle spasm.
- Perform Clarke's test. The patient is asked to contract the quadriceps whilst the patella is pressed firmly down against the femur. Pain is produced in conditions such as chondromalacia or osteoarthritis affecting the patellofemoral joint.

Movements

Active movements

The patient is in half-lying. Measure the active range of flexion and extension on each leg. The normal range of movement at the knee joint is approximately *minus* 5 degrees to 135 degrees of flexion. Note limitations of pain, stiffness or spasm. Overpressure the movement if full active movement is pain-free.

The axis of the goniometer should be positioned over the lateral femoral condyle. The static arm should be parallel with the long axis of the femur towards the greater trochanter. The dynamic arm should be positioned parallel to the long axis of the fibula and lateral malleolus (Figure 2.52). Hyperextension is present if the knee extends beyond 0 degrees (i.e. when the tibia and femur are in line).

Failure to hyperextend or lock out the knee fully may be a sign of a meniscal tear, which is blocking the movement of the joint. Moreover, a springy end-feel may be indicative of a bucket-handle tear of the meniscus. A rigid block to extension is common in arthritic conditions affecting the knee.

Passive movements

Check the range of extension and flexion passively. If there is a difference in active and passive range determine reasons for this.

Valgus Stress test (medial collateral ligament of the knee) DVD

With the patient supine, the physiotherapist applies a valgus force to the knee joint (i.e. the femur is pushed medially and the leg pulled laterally) whilst the joint is held in extension (Figure 2.53a). A positive sign is observed as excessive opening up on the medial side

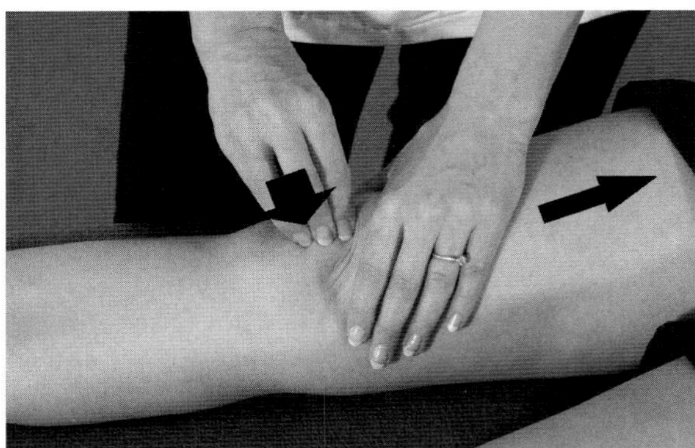

Figure 2.51 Critical test for patellofemoral pain. The test works because of the different contact areas of the patella against the femoral condyles in varying degrees of knee flexion.

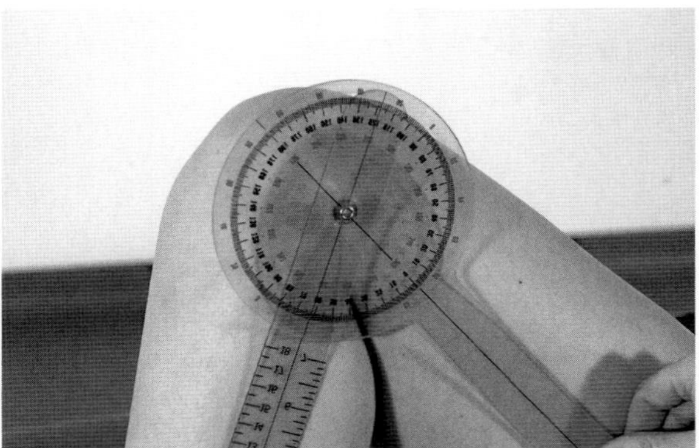

Figure 2.52 Measuring knee flexion using a 360 degree goniometer.

2

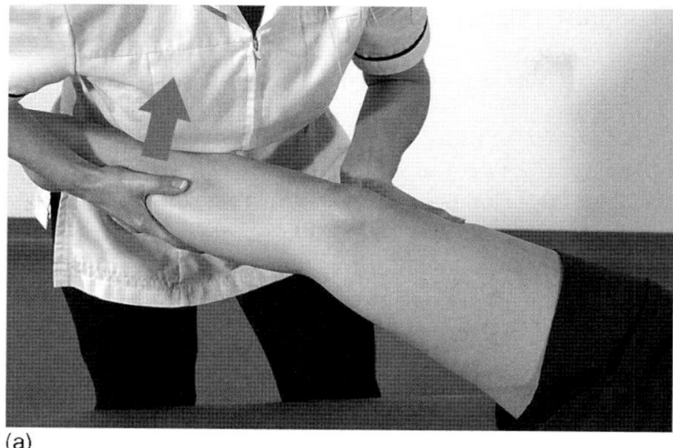
(a)

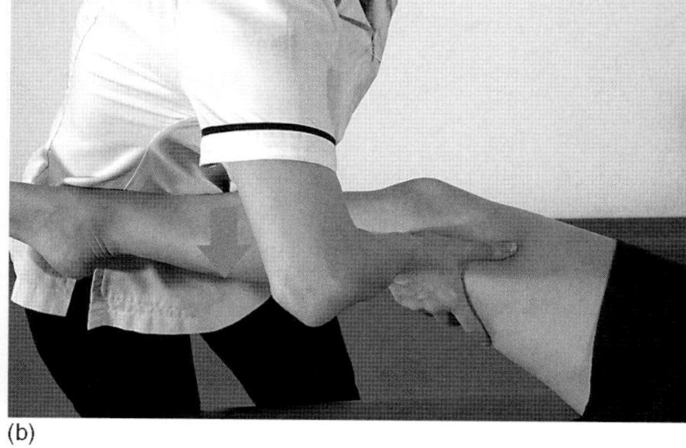
(b)

Figure 2.53 Stress tests: (a) valgus; (b) varus.

of the joint. With the knee held in extension, a positive sign suggests major ligamentous injury involving the medial collateral, posterior cruciate and potentially the anterior cruciate. The test is performed again with the knee in 20–30 degrees of flexion.

Varus Stress test (lateral collateral ligament of the knee) DVD

With the patient supine, the physiotherapist applies a varus force to the knee joint (i.e. the femur is pushed laterally and the leg pulled medially) whilst the joint is held in extension (Figure 2.53b). A positive sign is observed as excessive opening up on the lateral side of the joint. As with the valgus stress test, with the knee held in extension a positive sign suggests major ligamentous injury involving the lateral collateral, posterior cruciate and potentially the anterior cruciate. The test is performed again with the knee in 20–30 degrees of flexion.

Anterior draw test (anterior cruciate ligament) DVD

With the patient crook-lying, the physiotherapist sits on the patient's foot to stabilise the leg, grasps around the proximal tibia and tibial tuberosity and pulls the tibia forwards (Figure 2.54a). A positive sign is elicited by excessive translation of the tibia anteriorly. (The normal translation is approximately 6 mm.) Translation of 15 mm confirms rupture. Compare this with the other side. This test also stresses the posterior joint capsule, the medial collateral ligament and the iliotibial band (Magee 1992).

Clinical note

Figure 2.55 illustrates the positive PA draw following rupture of the anterior cruciate ligament.

Posterior draw test (posterior cruciate ligament) DVD

With the patient crook-lying, the physiotherapist sits on the patient's foot to stabilise the leg, grasps around the anterior aspect of the proximal tibia and pushes the tibia backwards (Figure 2.54b). A positive sign is elicited by excessive translation of the tibia posteriorly. Compare this with the other side. This test also stresses the

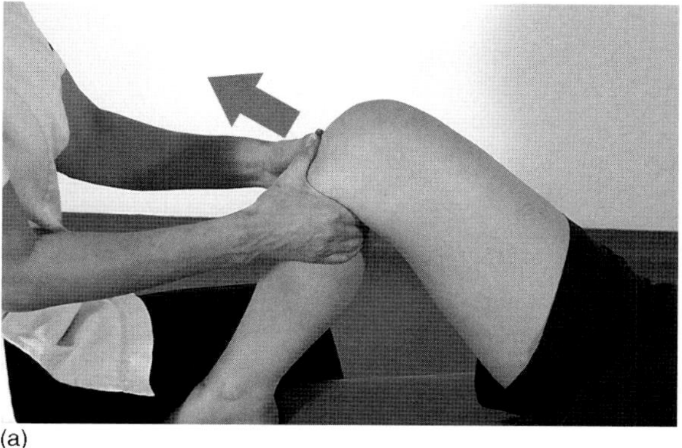
(a)

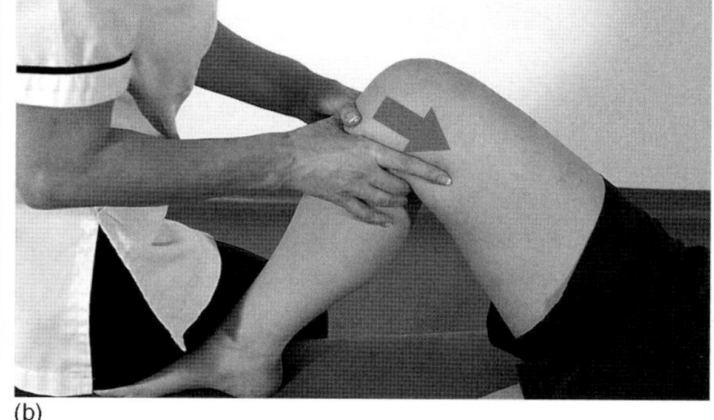
(b)

Figure 2.54 Draw tests: (a) anterior; (b) posterior.

2

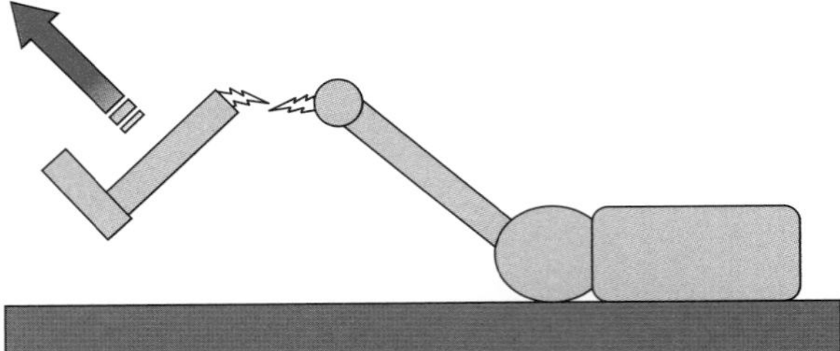

Figure 2.55 Schematic of positive PA draw following rupture of the anterior cruciate ligament (ACL).

arcuate–popliteus complex, posterior oblique ligament and anterior cruciate ligament (Magee 1992).

> **Clinical note** (DVD)
> A 'sag sign' is observed with the patient in crook-lying, whereby the tibia is posteriorly displaced in relation to the femur. Posterior displacement may give the false impression that the patient has a rupture of the anterior cruciate ligament since, when an anterior draw test is performed, a considerable amount of movement is noted. This is due to the tibia returning to its normal position, however.

Lachmann's test (modified anterior draw test) (DVD)

The patient is supine with the knee resting over the physiotherapist's thigh at around 20–30 degrees of flexion (Figure 2.56). The physiotherapist grasps around the medial proximal aspect of the tibia with the right hand. The lateral aspect of the patient's femur is stabilised by the therapist's left hand. Anterior and posterior translation of the tibia is produced by the physiotherapist's right hand. This tests the anterior cruciate ligament, the posterior oblique ligament and the arcuate–popliteus complex (Magee 1992). The Lachmann test has been shown to be sensitive for the diagnosis of anterior cruciate injury (Kim and Kim 1995).

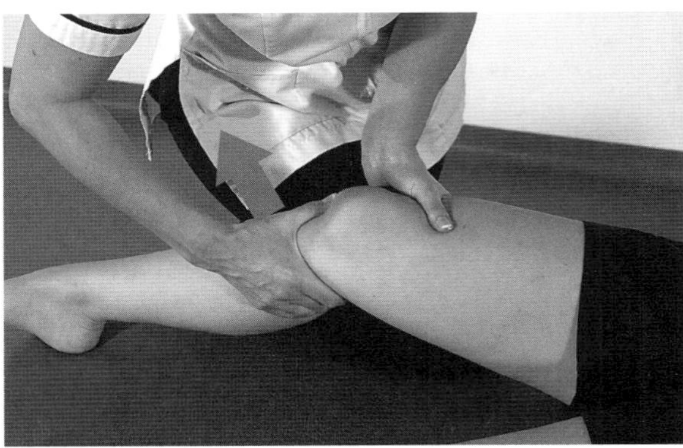

Figure 2.56 Lachmann's test.

The pivot shift test

This is a test for anterolateral instability of the knee joint. With the foot in medial rotation and the knee in 30 degrees of flexion, a valgus stress is applied to the knee whilst simultaneously extending it. A 'clunk' indicates a positive test and suggests anterior cruciate ligament pathology (McRae 1999).

> **Key point**
> Peripheral tears of the menisci can now be sutured arthroscopically. Many authorities believe that McMurray's tests (described below) may be of limited value (Evans et al. 1993).

McMurray's medial and lateral meniscus tests

The physiotherapist palpates the medial aspect of the joint line, and passively flexes and then laterally rotates the tibia, so that the posterior part of the medial meniscus is rotated with the tibia. The joint is then moved back from a fully flexed position to 90 degrees of flexion, to test for the posterior part of the meniscus. A positive test occurs if pain is elicited, or a snap or click of the joint will occur if the meniscus is torn. The test is then repeated for the lateral meniscus by medially rotating the tibia.

Note that the examiner may be able to detect clicking or snapping sounds when performing this test, since there are various structures in the knee joint that can produce these signs. It is thus easy for this test to produce a false positive result (Palmer and Epler 1998).

Apley's compression/distraction test (for differentiation between meniscus and ligament)

The patient is prone with the knee flexed at right-angles. The physiotherapist medially and laterally rotates the tibia whilst applying a distraction force through the knee joint. The test is repeated by applying a compressive force through the knee joint. If the patient's symptoms are worse on compression, then the symptoms are likely to be arising from a meniscal injury. Conversely, if they are worse on distraction, then they are likely to be arising from a ligamentous injury.

Proprioception

Proprioception is tested with the patient standing on the unaffected leg and then on the affected leg whilst maintaining balance. Progressive adaptations may include standing on one leg with the eyes closed, standing on a wobble board, catching and throwing a ball, etc.

Accessory movements

Patellofemoral joint

- Medial, lateral, cephalad and caudad glides.
- Medial and lateral rotation.
- Compression and distraction.

Superior tibiofibular joint

- AP and PA glides.
- Compression.

Tibiofemoral joint

- AP and PA glides.
- Medial and transverse glides.

Quadrant tests

These are performed on non-irritable knees when plane movements are pain-free:

- flexion/adduction quadrant
- flexion/abduction quadrant
- extension/adduction quadrant
- extension/abduction quadrant.

Following the objective assessment record your findings clearly and asterisk objective markers.

TEST YOURSELF

Match these six scenarios to the likely pathology:

1. The knee is stiff and painful for about half an hour in the morning, aches at the end of the day, and has been like that for a long time.
2. The knee locks and has to be jiggled around to unlock it.
3. Since a tackle last week the knee keeps giving way and becomes very swollen.
4. The knee is very red and swollen. The person also feels feverish and generally unwell.
5. When the person walks downstairs he feels pain behind his kneecap.
6. There is pain on the inside of the knee and it hurts performing sideways movements.

THE ANKLE AND FOOT

Key point

The patient should be suitably undressed to view the legs, ankles and feet.

Answers

(1) Osteoarthritis. (2) Torn meniscus. (3) Ruptured anterior cruciate. (4) Infective arthritis. (5) Chondromalacia patella. (6) Torn medial collateral ligament.

Gait

Observe the patient's gait both barefoot and with shoes. Ask the patient to walk backwards and forwards. Assess the normal heel-to-toe pattern and stride length, rhythm, the posture of the longitudinal arch and weight-bearing on both feet. Note any pain, stiffness and weakness. Inspect the patient's footwear for areas of uneven or greatest wear.

Foot and ankle examination

Pulses (leg circulation)

Palpate the posterior tibial and dorsalis pedis pulses, to establish the state of the distal circulation. Circulation is often poor in patients suffering from peripheral vascular disease or diabetes. Compare both sides.

Oedema

Note any oedema, suggesting a systemic rather than a local cause for the patient's symptoms. This may indicate heart failure or excessive water retention. Bruising is suggestive of muscle or ligament injury. This is commonly situated on the lateral aspect of the foot beneath the lateral malleolus, following lateral ligament tears.

General condition

Note the skin texture, colour and nail condition, which identifies the state of the peripheral circulation.

Temperature

Feel for any increase in temperature around the joint and compare with the opposite foot. A foot with impaired arterial circulation is colder than normal and may appear cyanosed (blue). Conversely a warm foot may be indicative of an inflammatory response: for example, following an injury or associated with conditions such as rheumatoid arthritis.

Tenderness

- Tenderness localised over and just proximal to the malleoli often occurs following a fracture.
- Tenderness and pain in the area distal and inferior to the lateral ligaments is common following inversion sprains. The anterior talofibular ligament (ATF) is the most commonly injured since the ligament is most often torn in the combined position of inversion and plantar flexion. This is the loose-packed position and one in which the anterior band of the lateral ligament is particularly placed on stretch.
- Tenderness along the line of the long flexor tendons and/or the peroneal tendons may indicate the presence of tenosynovitis. This may be accompanied by local thickening.
- Tenderness at the articular surface of the talus is common in osteoarthritic conditions.

- Tenderness at the heel is found in conditions such as calcaneal exostosis (bony spurs), tendocalcaneal bursitis and plantar fasciitis.
- Diffuse tenderness under the metatarsal heads may be a sign of Morton's neuroma. This is a condition characterised by inflammation and pain around 3rd and 4th digital nerves. Pain is reproduced on squeezing the medial and lateral sides of the forefoot together.
- Diffuse tenderness and swelling on both the plantar and dorsal surfaces of the forefoot is a common finding in rheumatoid arthritis.
- Tenderness on the mid-posterior aspect of the calcaneus may be a sign of a calcaneus bursitis.
- Tenderness along the Achilles tendon may be a sign of a sprain or tendonitis in the Achilles tendon.

Clinical note

A *pronated* foot has the appearance of rolling in on the medial side with bulging of the navicular bone medially. Additionally, the longitudinal arch appears flattened.
A *supinated* foot has the appearance of rolling outwards with the inner border raised.

Alignments

Observe the posture of the heel relative to the leg. The heel and lower leg should be parallel and the calcaneus should rest squarely on the ground. Note any postural misalignment such as excessive supination or pronation.

Excessive pronation may cause posteromedial shin splints, plantar fasciitis, hallux valgus or Achilles tendonitis. Excessive supination may cause anterolateral shin splints, dropped first ray (metatarsal) or plantar fasciitis.

Note whether the heel is inverted or everted. Posteriorly the Achilles tendon and the calcaneus should be vertically aligned. *Calcaneal varus* is observed as the calcaneus being inverted relative to the leg; *calcaneal valgus* is observed if the calcaneus is everted relative to the leg.

Is the foot splayed or flattened? This may be due to weakness of the intrinsic muscles and subsequent flattening of the longitudinal arch. Observe the posture of the medial arch and assess its height in comparison with the other.

Note any wastage of the calf musculature. Compare both sides. Measure the circumference of the leg with a tape measure at specified points below the patella.

The leg and hindfoot

With the patient prone, the physiotherapist bisects the calcaneus by drawing a vertical line through the posterior aspect of it, then bisects the lower leg by drawing a vertical line on the posterior aspect of the lower third, and places the subtalar joint in a neutral position. If the lines are parallel there is correct alignment of the leg and hindfoot (Figure 2.57b). *Rear foot varus* is observed as the calcaneus appearing to invert relative to the leg (Figure 2.57a); *rear foot valgus* is observed as the calcaneus appearing to evert relative to the leg.

Key point

Complex foot misalignments may require referral to a podiatrist.

The hindfoot and forefoot

As above, observe the position of the whole foot. Correct alignment is observed if the hindfoot and forefoot are in line and perpendicular to the floor. *Forefoot varus* is observed if the first toe is superior to the lateral toes. *Forefoot valgus* is observed if the fifth toe is superior to the medial toes.

The toes

Look for:

- clawing (hyperextension of the metatarsophalangeal joints and flexion of the other phalanges)

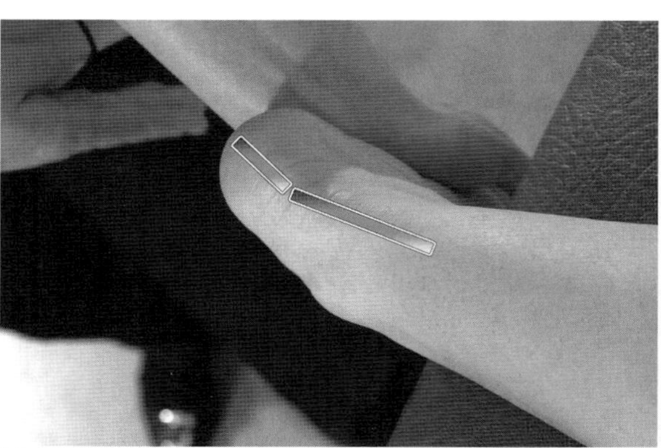

(a)

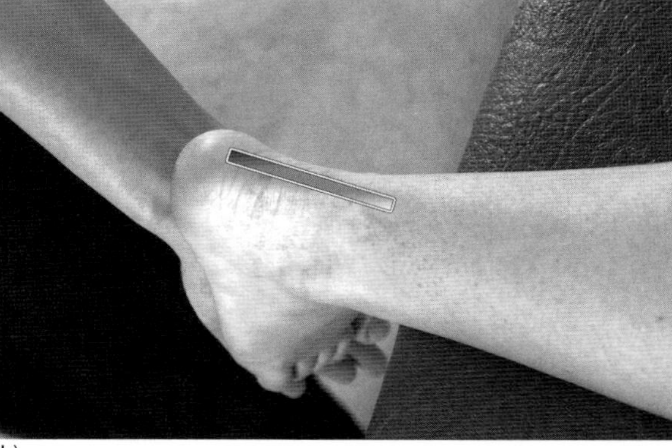

(b)

Figure 2.57 Alignment of the right leg and hindfoot: (a) calcaneal varus; (b) normal.

- mallet toe (flexion of the distal interphalangeal joints)
- hammer toe (hyperextension of the metatarsophalangeal and flexion of the proximal interphalangeal joints)
- hallux valgus (lateral deviation of the first interphalangeal joint)
- hallux rigidus (stiffness of the first interphalangeal joint).

Functional activities

Assess the patient's ability to stand on heels, toes and the inner and outer borders of the feet. Test the patient's proprioception. This may be performed with the patient standing on one leg or on a wobble board, with the eyes open and then closed. To make this more difficult the patient can catch and throw a ball whilst trying to maintain balance. Balance on the unaffected leg is assessed and then compared with the affected side. Also, when appropriate, test the patient's ability to hop, squat and jump, noting any stiffness or pain response.

Movements

Active movements

Ankle joint

The patient is in supine or sitting. Measure plantar flexion and dorsiflexion. Movement occurring at the tarsal joints is easily mistaken for movement at the ankle, and vice versa. Note pain or stiffness compared with the other side. Overpressure the movement if it is full-range and pain-free.

The axis of the goniometer is placed 15 mm inferior to the lateral malleolus. The static arm should be parallel to the fibula. The dynamic arm should be parallel to the long axis of the fifth metatarsal (Figure 2.58).

- Normal range of plantar flexion is approximately 50–55 degrees.
- Normal range of dorsiflexion is approximately 10–15 degrees.

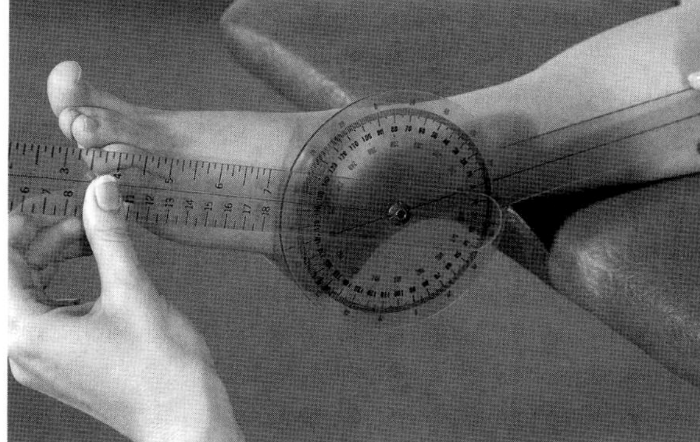

Figure 2.58 Measurement of ankle plantar flexion/dorsiflexion.

Note that the knee needs to be in slight flexion if full dorsiflexion is to be achieved. This takes the stretch off gastrocnemius.

Definition

Inversion is the movement whereby the soles of the feet face inwards towards one another. Eversion is the movement whereby they face outwards.

Subtalar and mid-tarsal joints

In the normal foot, 80 per cent inversion and eversion occurs at the subtalar joint. Most of the remainder occurs at the mid-tarsal joints, with a little at the tarsometatarsal joints. Determine the range by percentage of the abnormal to the normal. Test:

- combined inversion and adduction (supination)
- combined eversion and abduction (pronation).

Toe movements

Observe flexion and extension at all the toes and compare with the opposite side.

Passive movements

All the movements measured actively can be measured and tested passively. Note any difference between active and passive ranges and identify possible reasons for discrepancies.

Muscle strength

The dorsiflexors, plantar flexors, invertors and evertors are tested by isometric and isotonic resisted movements. Assess any weakness or pain elicited at any part of the range.

Ligament tests

Lateral ligament stress test. The patient lies supine and the physiotherapist grasps the heel and passively inverts the foot, feeling for any opening at the lateral side of the foot (Figure 2.59). A positive test may reveal increased inversion movement, a sulcus dimple on the lateral side of the foot or a pain response.

To differentiate between the three bands of the lateral ligaments, the test should be performed in:

- plantar flexion and inversion to strain the anterior band
- inversion only to strain the calcaneofibular band
- a combination of dorsiflexion and inversion to strain the posterior band.

Medial ligament stress test. The patient lies supine and the physiotherapist grasps the heel and passively everts the foot. A positive test may reveal increased movement of eversion compared with the other side and/or may elicit a pain response.

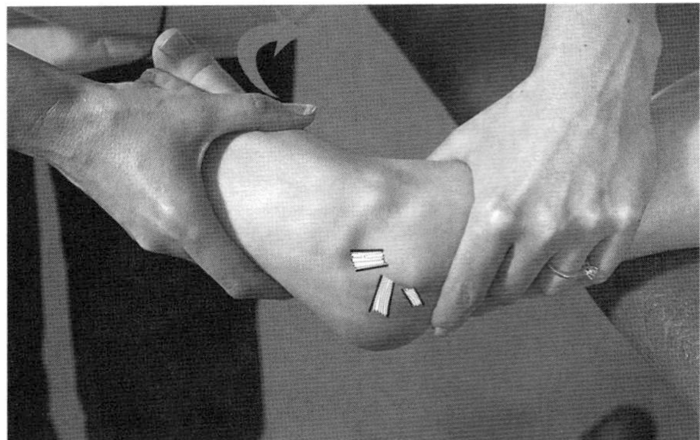

Figure 2.59 Passive inversion of the plantar flexed foot to test the anterior talofibular ligament.

Anterior draw test at the ankle. This detects the integrity and stability of the anterior talofibular and calcaneofibular components of the lateral ankle ligaments. The patient lies supine. The physiotherapist stabilises the distal leg, grasps around the talus and pulls it forwards. A positive test reveals an anterior displacement of the talus in the mortise of the lower end of the tibia and fibula and suggests major lateral ligament disruption. Observe for laxity, an audible 'clunk' or the presence of a lateral suction dimple.

Accessory movements (Maitland 2001)

Inferior tibiofibular joint

Perform PA and AP glides (Figure 2.60).

Ankle joint

Perform:

- PA and AP glides
- longitudinal movement cephalad and caudad
- medial and lateral rotation.

Subtalar joint

Perform medial and lateral glides.

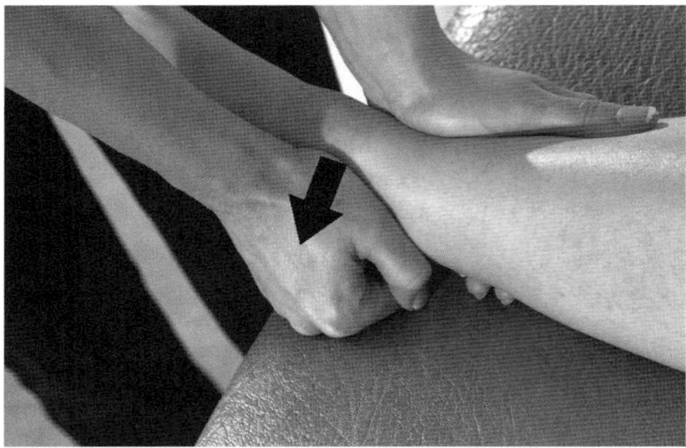

Figure 2.60 AP glide at the inferior tibiofibular joint.

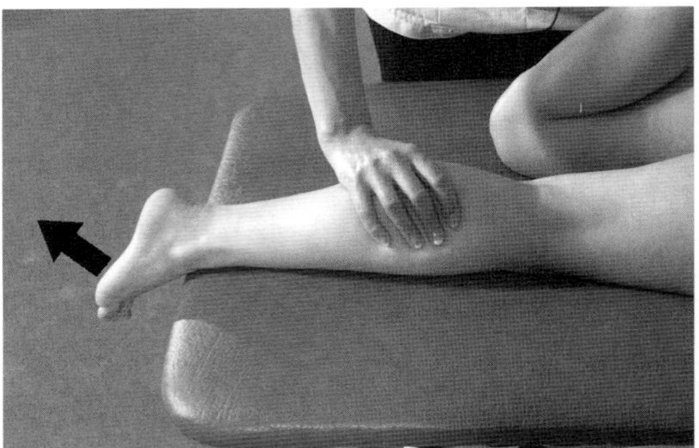

Figure 2.61 Thompson's test of the right calf. Slight plantar flexion of the ankle suggests an intact Achilles tendon.

Metatarsophalangeal and interphalangeal joints

Perform:

- PA and AP glides
- rotations and distractions.

Thompson's squeeze test 

This tests the integrity of the gastrocnemius/soleus/Achilles tendon complex. With the patient prone, the physiotherapist squeezes the calf firmly just distal to its maximum circumference (Figure 2.61). If the tendon is intact, the foot will plantar-flex. A positive test will occur if the tendon or muscle is ruptured and the ankle will not plantar-flex. A palpable gap in the tendon or muscle belly may sometimes be observed if the tendon is ruptured.

Following on from the objective assessment write up your findings clearly and asterisk an objective marker.

TEST YOURSELF

Match these five scenarios to the likely pathology:

1. One ankle keeps giving way and feels unstable. There is poor proprioception on one leg.
2. There is pain in the plantar aspect of the heel on weight-bearing, or toe extension.
3. There is pain under the medial malleolus, increasing on resisted inversion.
4. There is longstanding, insidious pain and stiffness in the ankle, increasing on weight-bearing.
5. The patient has a history of an inversion strain combined with swelling and bruising under the lateral malleolus.

Answers

(1) Lengthened lateral ligaments. (2) Plantar fasciitis. (3) Tendonitis of tibialis posterior. (4) Osteoarthritis of the ankle. (5) Lateral ligament sprain.

REFERENCES

Alvarez DJ, Rockwell PG 2002 Trigger points: diagnosis and management. Am Fam Phys 65(4): 653–660

Bronfort G, Evans R, Nelson B et al. 2001 A randomized clinical trial of exercise and spinal manipulation for patients with chronic neck pain. Spine 26(7): 788–799

Burton K, Tillotson M, Main C, Hollis S 1995 Psychological predictors of outcome in acute and chronic low back trouble. Spine 20(6): 722–728

Butler DS 1991 Mobilisation of the Nervous System. Churchill Livingstone: Edinburgh

Carrageen EJ 2001 Psychological and functional profiles in select subjects with low back pain. Spine 1(3): 198–204

Cats-Baril W, Frymoyer J 1991 Identifying patients at risk of becoming disabled because of low back pain: the Vermont Rehabilitation Engineering Centre Predictive Model. Spine 16(6): 605–607

Coulter I 1996 Manipulation and mobilization of the cervical spine: results of a literature survey and consensus panel. J Musculoskel Pain 4(4): 113–123

CSAG (Clinical Standards Advisory Group) 1994 Back Pain Management Guidelines. HMSO: London

Cyriax J 1982 Textbook of Orthopaedic Medicine: Diagnosis of Soft Tissue Lesions, 8th edn. Baillière Tindall: London

Deyo RA, Weinstein JN 2001 Low back pain. N Engl J Med 344: 363–370

Edwards BE 1992 Manual of Combined Movements. Churchill Livingstone: Edinburgh

Evans PJ, Bell GD, Frank C 1993 Prospective evaluation of the McMurray test. Am J Sports Med 21(4): 604–608

Fairbank J, Davies J, Coupar J, O'Brian JP 1980 Oswestry Low Back Pain Disability questionnaire. Physiotherapy 66: 271–273

Frost H, Lamb S, Klaber E et al. 1998 A fitness programme for patients with chronic low back pain: 2-year follow-up of a randomised controlled trial. Pain 75: 273–279

Fritz JM, George SZ, Delitto A 2001 The role of fear-avoidance beliefs in acute low back pain: relationships with current and future disability and work status. Pain 94(5): 7–15

Frymoyer JW 1992 Predicting disability from low back pain. Clin Orthopaed Rel Res 221: 101–109

Gardiner J, Turner P 2002 Accuracy of clinical diagnosis of internal derangement of the knee by extended scope physiotherapists and orthopaedic doctors: retrospective audit. Physiotherapy 88(3): 153–157

Goel VK, Kong W, Hans JS et al. 1993 A combined finite element and optimisation investigation of the lumbar spine with and without muscles. Spine 18: 1531–1541

Grichnik KP, Ferrante FM 1991 The difference between acute and chronic pain. Mt Sinai J Med 58(3): 217–220

Guzman J, Esmail R, Karjalainen K et al. 2001 Multidisciplinary rehabilitation for chronic low back pain: systematic review. BMJ 322: 1511–1516

Harding V, Watson P 2000 Increasing activity and improving function in chronic pain management. Physiotherapy 86 (12): 619–630

Heimeyer K, Lutz R, Menninger H 1990 Dependence of tender points upon posture: a key to the understanding of fibromyalgia syndrome. J Man Med 5: 169–174

Hodges PW, Richardson CA 1996 Inefficient muscular stabilisation of the lumbar spine associated with low back pain: a motor control evaluation of transverse abdominis. Spine 21(22): 2640–2650

Hodges PW, Richardson CA 1997 Contraction of the abdominal muscles associated with movement of the lower limb. Phys Ther 77: 132–144

Hubbard DR, Berkhoff GM 1993 Myofascial trigger points show spontaneous needle EMG activity. Spine 18: 1803–1807

Johnson D, Rogers M 2000 Spinal manipulation. Phys Ther 80(8): 820–823

Jull JA, Richardson CA, Topperberg R et al. 1993 Towards a measurement of active muscle control for lumbar stabilisation. Aust J Physiother 39: 187–193

Jull GA 1994 Examination of the articular system. In: Grieve's Modern Manual Therapy, 2nd edn. Churchill Livingstone: Edinburgh, p. 511

Kim SJ, Kim HK 1995 Reliability of the anterior drawer test, the pivot shift test, and the Lachmann test. Clin Orthop 317: 237–242

Koes BW, Bouter LM, Van Maeren H et al. 1992 A blinded randomised clinical trial of manual therapy and physiotherapy for chronic back and neck complaints: physical outcome measures. J Manip Physiol Therap 15(1): 16–23

Magarey ME 1988 Examination of the cervical and thoracic spine. In: Grant R (ed.) Physical Therapy of the Cervical and Thoracic Spine, pp. 81–109. Churchill Livingstone: New York

Magee DJ 1992 Orthopaedic Physical Assessment, 2nd edn. WB Saunders: Philadelphia

Maitland G 2001 Maitland's Vertebral Manipulation, 6th edn. Butterworth–Heinemann: Oxford

Maniadakis N, Gray A 2000 The economic burden of back pain in the UK. Pain 84: 95–103

Mayhew TP, Rothstein JM, Finucane SD, Lamb RL 1994 Performance characteristics of the Kin-Com dynamometer. Phys Therap 74(11): 56–63

McConnell J 1996 Management of patellofemoral problems. Man Ther 1: 60–66

McKenzie RA 1981 The Lumbar Spine: Mechanical Diagnosis and Therapy. Spinal Publications: New Zealand

McKenzie RA 1985 Treat Your Own Back. Spinal Publications: Raumati Beach, New Zealand

McKenzie RA 1990 The Cervical and Thoracic Spine: Mechanical Diagnosis and Therapy. Spinal Publications, New Zealand

McRae R 1999 Pocketbook of Orthopaedics and Fractures. Churchill Livingstone: Edinburgh

Melzack R 1987 The short-form McGill Pain Questionnaire. Pain 30(2): 191–197

O'Conner MI, Curner BL 1992 Metastatic diseases of the spine. Orthopaedics 15: 611–620

Olerud C, Berg P 1984 The variation of the Q angle with different positions of the foot. Clin Orthop 191: 162–165

Palmer ML, Epler ME 1998 Fundamentals of Musculoskeletal Techniques, 2nd edn. Lippincott: Philadelphia

Panjabi MM 1992 The stabilising system of the spine. 1: Function, dysfunction, adaptation and enhancement. J Spinal Dis 5(4): 383–385

RCGP (Royal College of General Practitioners) 1999 Clinical Guidelines for the Management of Low Back Pain. RCGP: London

Simmons E, Cameron JC 1992 Patella alta and recurrent dislocation of the patella. Clin Orthop 274: 265–269

Sterling M, Jull G, Wright A 2001 Cervical mobilisation: concurrent effects on pain, sympathetic nervous system activity and motor activity. Man Therap 6(2): 72–81

Tait RC, Chibnall JT 2001 Work injury management of refractory low back pain: relations with ethnicity, legal representation and diagnosis. Pain 91(1/2): 47–56

Vlaeyen JW, Kole-Snijders AM, Boeren RG, van Eek H 1995 Fear of movement/(re)injury in chronic low back pain and its relation to behavioral performance. Pain 62(3): 363–372

Von Korff M, Saunders K 1996 The course of back pain in primary care. Spine 21: 2833–2837; discussion 2838–2839

Waddell G 1992 Biopsychosocial analysis of low back pain. Baillière's Clinical Rheumatology 6(3): 523–555

Wilke HJ, Wolf S, Claes LE et al. 1995 Stability increase of the lumbar spine with different muscle groups: a biomechanical in-vitro study. Spine 20: 192–198

Wojtys EM, Huston LJ, Taylor PD 1996 Neuromuscular adaptations in isokinetic, isotonic and agility training programmes. Am J Sports Med 24: 187–192

Zigmond AS, Snaith RP 1983 The Hospital Anxiety and Depression Scale. Acta Psychiatr Scand 67(6): 361–370

Chapter 3

An introduction to fractures

Annie Karim and the Executive Committee of the Association of Orthopaedic Chartered Physiotherapists

CHAPTER CONTENTS

INTRODUCTION

This chapter looks at some basic facts and concepts about fractures but should not be seen as a definitive guide to fracture management. Suggested further reading is included at the end of the chapter.

DEFINITION AND CLASSIFICATIONS

Definition

A fracture is an interruption in the continuity of bone. The terms fracture and break mean the same thing in medicine. The symbol # (hash) represents a fracture.

Classification of fractures

There are numerous ways of classifying fractures and this will vary depending on country, hospital or consultant preference. Although it is helpful to categorise common fracture types and mechanisms, any bone may break in a variety of ways, so no two fractures will be exactly alike. The type of fracture will obviously affect the initial management and treatment.

Fractures may be classified as *open* or *closed* (Figure 3.1). Open or *compound* types of fracture occur when the bone end or some other object has pierced the skin. These fractures are an additional cause for concern because of the possibility of the introduction of micro-organisms leading to bone infection (osteomyelitis). With closed fractures the skin remains intact. Another common classification refers *displaced* or *undisplaced* fractures.

Figure 3.2 shows a further classification. *Spiral* fractures commonly occur from a twisting injury. A direct blow could give a *transverse or oblique* fracture, depending on the angle of the force and whether the limb is

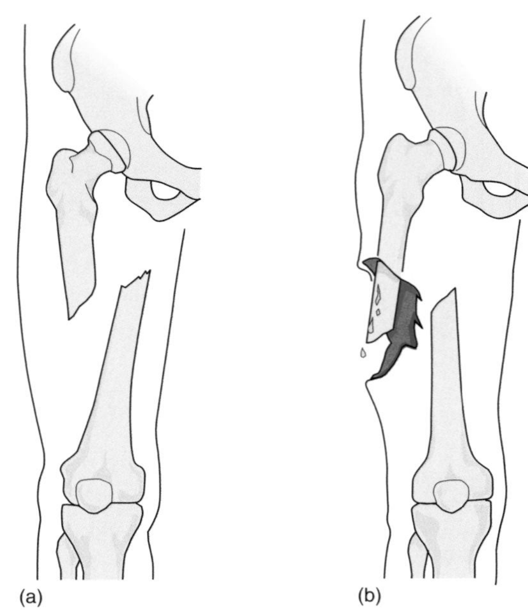

Figure 3.1 (a) Closed fracture. (b) Open or compound fracture. (Adapted from Dandy and Edwards 1998, with permission.)

fixed or moving at the time of the trauma. Longitudinal forces tend to result in *compression* or *crush* fractures. In some cases there are a number of fragments of bone and this is termed a *comminuted* fracture (not to be confused with *compound*). Loose fragments of bone are known as 'butterfly fragments'.

A *greenstick* fracture is a type of fracture sustained by young children; their bones are still relatively malleable and fractures are therefore more likely to present as an incomplete or greenstick fracture. (The analogy is that of attempting to break a green twig, which will bend and split but not snap.) *Avulsion* fractures occur when a bit of bone is pulled off due to its attachment to soft tissues (e.g. ligaments). *Impacted* fractures are generally compressed and therefore more stable.

THE CAUSES OF FRACTURES

Trauma

Most fractures are due to some form of injury. This might be a *direct* blow, a fall from a height, or a weight falling on to a part of the body. Other fractures may be caused by *indirect* trauma, such as falling on an

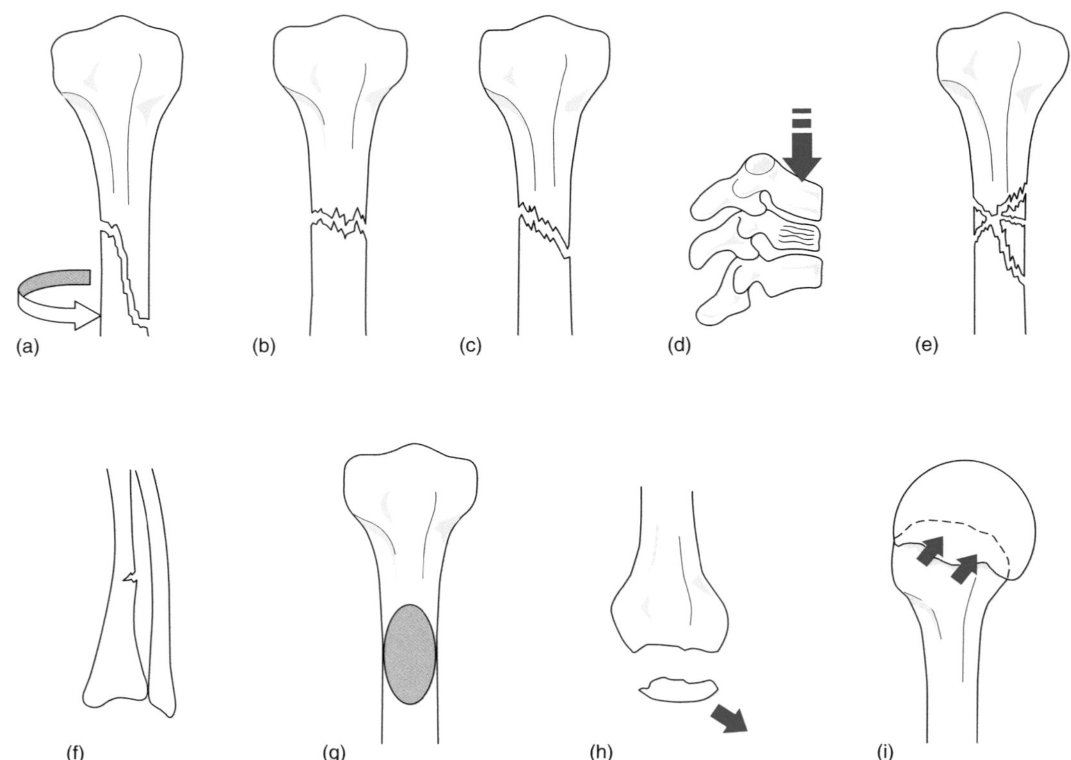

Figure 3.2 Classification: (a) spiral; (b) transverse; (c) oblique; (d) compression; (e) comminuted; (f) greenstick; (g) pathological; (h) avulsion; (i) impacted.

outstretched hand, leading to the transmission of force up the arm and a fracture of the clavicle. *Twisting* forces may result in fractures of the tibia and fibula: for example, during soccer or skiing, when the weight of the body rotates on a fixed foot. *Stress* or *fatigue* fractures are caused by repeated minor trauma, which can occur after walking or running long distances, and often affect the foot metatarsals.

Pathological fractures

These occur as the result of a disease that weakens the composition of the bone itself, making it liable to fracture after a relatively trivial injury. There are a number of such diseases but those most commonly seen clinically are osteoporosis, Paget's disease, carcinoma, osteomyelitis and osteogenesis imperfecta (brittle bone disease).

CLINICAL FEATURES OF FRACTURES

Clinical features vary, depending on the cause and nature of the injury, and range from unconsciousness to the patient being able to use the limb although complaining of pain — such as following fatigue fractures and some impacted or crack fractures. Most will be diagnosed by X-ray. Some fractures — for example, fractures of the scaphoid bone — are sometimes not detected upon initial X-ray and can be misdiagnosed as wrist sprain. The clinical features of fractures are summarised below.

Pain

This may be immediate from the local inflammatory reaction and trauma, but the cause may not be obvious in some cases. There will be marked tenderness around the site of the fracture. Once reduced, a fracture is remarkably painless.

Deformity

This is noticeable when there is displacement of the bone fragments. Some fractures exhibit classical deformities — for example, the 'dinner fork' deformity that occurs following a Colles' fracture of the distal radius, caused by displacement of the distal fragment, and also shortening of the leg with a fractured neck of femur.

Oedema

This is localised immediately after the injury and becomes more extensive with time. It may be necessary to apply a temporary cast or splint and then reapply the plaster as soon as the swelling has subsided.

Muscle spasm

Muscle spasm is an attempt by the body to stop things from moving. It often affects powerful muscle groups such as the quadriceps and may cause displacement or overriding of the bone ends. Traction may be needed to counteract this.

Abnormal movement/crepitus

There may be grating between the broken ends of the bone. Do not deliberately attempt to elicit this, though, because that might result in further damage.

Loss of function

This may be complete following severe fractures but some activity may be possible when the injury is less severe, such as with a stress, impacted or crack fracture. Sometimes normal function can be regained very quickly with appropriate assessment, advice and treatment, whereas in other cases there are a number of problems for which more intensive treatment may be required. Modern orthopaedics is now geared towards early mobilisation with minimal surgical trauma, and physiotherapy needs to complement this.

Shock

Hypovolaemic shock is a possibility following fractures. A fractured shaft of femur may haemorrhage as much as 3 pints (1.7 L).

Limitation of joint movement

Joint mobility can be affected by many factors: adhesion formation, tight muscles, pain, spasm, fear, mechanical obstruction or swelling. Movement may also be limited because of weak muscles, in which case it will be possible to move the joint passively through total range. If the fracture involves the articular surface of the joint, this may also cause limitation of movement and future cartilage degeneration. For this reason, certain fractures are now treated aggressively with almost immediate movement (aggressive in this context meaning soon, not rough).

Muscle atrophy

There will be a loss of strength in disused muscle groups.

FRACTURE HEALING

Healing of compact bone

Bone has the incredible ability to replace itself with new bone, not scar tissue. Healing starts within seconds of a fracture being sustained and will still be ongoing years later. This makes ascribing a healing timescale difficult.

Wolff's law states that bone responds to the stresses that are imposed upon it by rearranging its internal architecture in the best way to withstand the stresses.

In other words, bone is laid down where it is needed and absorbed where it is not. It is important to understand this concept when dealing with people who have sustained fractures. Bone is a living tissue, not the brittle, chalky specimens that students may be familiar with. It is continually in a dynamic equilibrium of growth and reabsorption. Figure 3.3 shows the process of fracture healing in compact bone taken through five stages.

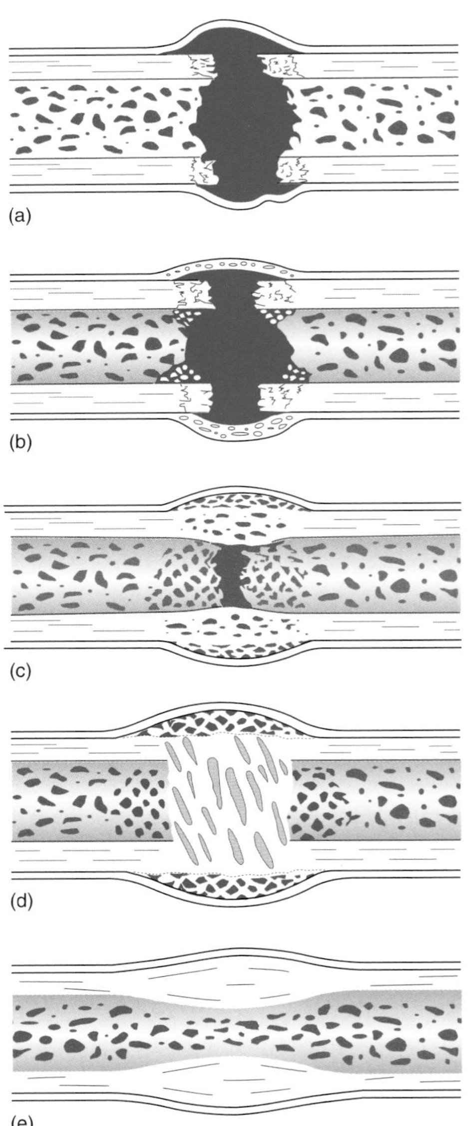

Figure 3.3 Fracture healing: (a) haematoma; (b) periosteal and endosteal proliferation; (c) callus formation; (d) consolidation; (e) remodelling.

Haematoma

As a result of the tearing of blood vessels, within seconds of the injury a haematoma forms at the fracture site. Very small portions of bone immediately adjacent to the fracture die and are gradually absorbed.

Periosteal and endosteal proliferation

There is a proliferation of cells from the deep surface of the periosteum adjacent to the fracture site. These cells are precursors of the osteoblasts and form around each fragment of bone. At the same time cells proliferate from the endosteum in each fragment and this tissue gradually forms a bridge between the bone ends. During this stage the haematoma is gradually reabsorbed.

Callus formation

The proliferating cells mature as osteoblasts or, in some instances, as chondroblasts. The chondroblasts form cartilage and are found in varying amounts at a fracture site. Osteoblasts lay down an intercellular matrix of collagen and polysaccharide which then becomes impregnated with calcium salts, forming the immature bone called callus or woven bone. This is visible on X-ray and provides evidence that healing is taking place.

Consolidation

Osteoblastic activity results in the change of primary callus to bone, which has a lamellar structure, and at the end of this stage union is complete. New bone forms a thickened mass at the fracture site and obliterates the medullary cavity. The amount of this new bone varies for a number of reasons. It tends to be more extensive if there has been a large haematoma or it has been impossible to obtain exact apposition of the bone fragments.

Remodelling

The lamellar structure is changed and the bone adapts by strengthening along the lines of stress imposed upon it. The surplus bone formed during healing is gradually removed and eventually the bone structure appears very similar to the original. In children, healing is usually very good and it is difficult to see the fracture site on an X-ray. In adults there may be a permanent area of thickening, which might be felt or seen, in a superficial bone.

Healing of cancellous bone

This follows a different pattern from that described above. As with compact bone, a haematoma will form, but since there is no medullary cavity, the second stage differs. Cancellous bone has a greater area of contact between the fragments of bone, and penetration of the bone-forming tissue is facilitated by the open arrangement of trabeculae as it grows out from both fragments.

Osteogenic cells lay down intercellular matrix, which calcifies to form woven bone. The process of remodelling then continues to form the cancellous bone.

When is a fracture healed?

One of the most common questions asked by patients is 'When will my fracture be healed?' Unfortunately the answer to this question is not always straightforward and depends upon many factors, including the type of bone fractured, the type of fracture sustained, the person's age, the treatment undergone, and the person's nutritional status.

The current mainstay for evaluating when a fracture is healed is still based upon a combination of clinical judgement, X-ray evaluation and historical knowledge of specific fracture behaviours. A fracture is considered to be clinically healed judging from the combination of physical findings and symptoms over time.

The following suggest complete healing:

- absence of pain on weight-bearing, lifting or movement
- absence of tenderness on palpation at the fracture site
- blurring or disappearance of the fracture line on X-ray
- full or near-full functional ability (Hoppenfeld and Urthy 1999).

Time for a fracture to unite

This depends on a number of factors.

- *Type of bone.* Cancellous bone heals more quickly than compact bone. Healing of long bones depends on their size, so that bones of the upper limb unite earlier (3–12 weeks) than do those of the lower limb (12–18 weeks).
- *Revascularisation* of devitalised bone and soft tissues adjacent to the fracture site.
- The *mechanical environment* of the fracture (Marsh and Li 1999).
- *Classification of the fracture.* It is easier to obtain good apposition of bone ends with some fractures than with others. This may depend on the initial position of the fragments before reduction and the effect of muscle pull on the fragments.
- *Blood supply.* Adequate blood supply is essential for normal healing to take place. Certain fractures can be notoriously slow to heal (e.g. fractures of the lower third of tibia). This part of the bone has a poor blood supply due to the fact that under normal circumstances it does not require one; there is little muscle bulk here, and therefore little demand for nutrients and oxygen.
- *Fixation.* Adequate fixation prevents impairment of the blood supply, which may be caused by movement of the fragments. It also maintains the reduction, thus preventing deformity and consequent loss of function. Interestingly, if a fracture is rigidly immobilised, the stimulus for callus to form is lost, so a small amount of movement at a fracture site actually encourages fracture healing.
- *Age.* Union of a fracture is quicker in children and consolidation may occur at between 4 and 6 weeks. Age makes little difference to union in adults unless there is accompanying pathology.
- It has been suggested that certain *drugs* such as NSAIDs may interfere with fracture healing; however, evidence remains inconclusive (Bandolier 2004)
- *Smoking.* There are increased rates of delayed union and non-union in smokers who have sustained open tibial fractures (Adams et al. 2001).
- *Ultrasound.* Recent work has suggested that low-intensity ultrasound may accelerate fracture healing (Azuma et al. 2001).

COMPLICATIONS OF FRACTURES

Critical blood disorders

Pulmonary embolism and *deep vein thrombosis* are two possible complications of a fracture. *Shock* may be caused by hypovolaemia or loss of blood. Femoral shaft fractures may bleed as much as 3 pints (1.7 L) and pelvic fractures may lose 6 pints (3.4 L). Clinical signs of this are tachycardia (rapid heart rate), pallor from reduced peripheral perfusion, hypoxia (decreased oxygen saturation), confusion and a state of semi-consciousness.

Infection and *tetanus* are threats, especially following open or compound fractures. Most people are now immunised against tetanus or given booster tetanus injections if they have a large open wound. Bone infection (osteomyelitis) can be stubborn to respond to treatment.

Fat embolism (Acute Respiratory Distress Syndrome – ARDS)

If a person sustains multiple fractures of large bones or crushing injuries, or if large amounts of marrow become exposed, there may be leakage of microscopic fat globules into the circulatory system. These may become trapped in the lungs. Symptoms include respiratory distress, shortness of breath, drowsiness, decrease in saturation of oxygen levels and petechiae (tiny haemorrhages which appear on the chest). ARDS is potentially fatal.

Skin plaster sores

Reassure the patient that large amounts of dry flaky skin following removal of plaster is normal. Reddened areas or sores caused by plaster or splints must be reported to the relevant team member.

3

Muscle damage and atrophy

Muscle fibres may be torn, crushed or ruptured as a result of the injury, and this will cause additional bleeding and swelling. Tendons may be severed, particularly in the case of open fractures, or sometimes there may be a rupture following a fracture. Surgical intervention is usually necessary to repair a rupture.

Compartment syndrome

If muscles become damaged or inflamed at the time of injury, and intramuscular pressure builds up with no means of release, necrosis (death) of the tissues from ischaemia (lack of blood supply) may result. It is defined as the condition in which high pressure within a closed fascial sheath reduces capillary blood perfusion below the level necessary for tissue viability. Compartment syndrome is seen most commonly in the anterior tibial muscles or forearm muscles.

Clinical signs of a limb with compartment syndrome may be remembered using the five Ps:

- pale
- painful
- pulseless
- paraesthesiae
- paralysed.

Treatment revolves primarily around accurate diagnosis. Check colour, sensation and movement after any injury or surgery; elevate and cool the limb. Surgical decompression (fasciotomy) may be necessary as an emergency procedure.

Avascular necrosis

Bone receives its blood supply via the soft-tissue structures attached to it or via intra-osseous vessels (within the bone). In certain instances one part of the bone is very dependent on the intra-osseous vessels for its blood supply, and if this is interrupted because of a fracture, avascular necrosis may occur (that is, part of the fractured bone may die). It can arise in fractures of the neck of femur, leading to avascular necrosis of the head, and in fractures of the scaphoid bone, where the proximal pole may be affected. This may be a cause of non-union of the fracture, and as the fragment usually includes an articular surface, it can lead to osteoarthritis.

Problems with union

Delayed union may occur if the gap between the bone ends is too big, the blood supply is poor (lower third of the tibia), the area is infected or internal fixation is used. (This sometimes removes the stimulus for callus formation.)

There may be distinct pathological changes and radiological evidence of *non-union*. There appears to be no callus formation and the fractured ends of bone become dense and the outline clear-cut. The gap between the bone fragments may be filled with fibrous tissue and form a pseudo-arthrosis. The lower third of the tibia has notoriously poor healing capabilities, even occasionally in the young and healthy.

A fracture may heal in a less than perfect position — *malunion*. Overlapping of the fragments could lead to shortening and this would affect function. Angulation or rotation of the fragments may impair function because of the resulting alteration in biomechanics.

Growth disturbance

In younger people there may be growth disturbance if the fracture includes the epiphysis (growth plate).

Complex regional pain syndrome I (CRPS I)

This is also be known as Sudeck's atrophy, reflex sympathetic dystrophy — RSD, algodystrophy or causalgia. The term CRPS is now being used to describe these pathological states. This is a complication where the patient complains of severe pain on movement, or at rest, out of proportion to the initial injury. The limb is swollen. The skin appears shiny and discoloured and feels cold; in extreme cases this may lead to the limb becoming exquisitely tender and discoloured. Osteoporosis and permanent contractures may follow.

Management is difficult. Sympathetic nerve blocks and active physiotherapy management programmes are often employed with varying degrees of success (Viel et al. 1999). Vasodilator drugs such as guanethedine are occasionally successful. Pain may also respond to nerve blocks, local analgesia, transcutaneous electrical nerve stimulation (TENS), and other local therapies, but recovery is slow and may take several months. Fortunately this complication is comparatively rare.

Intra-articular fractures

Fractures involving the articular cartilage (e.g. fractures of the tibial plateau) predispose the joint to osteoarthrosis in the future. This is due to the area of roughness that inevitably results after a fracture, and also because the immobilisation of the fracture results in cartilage death (see below). For the latter reason, some fractures are now treated aggressively by physiotherapists from an early stage.

Another problem with intra-articular fractures is that, if callus is attempting to form within a joint cavity, it is constantly being washed away by synovial fluid — for example, after a fractured neck of femur.

Visceral injuries

A fractured pelvis may damage the bladder or urethra. A fractured rib may cause a pneumothorax. A skull fracture may cause brain injury. These are just three examples.

Adhesions

These may be within the joint (intra-articular) or around the joint (periarticular). Adhesions are the price paid for immobilising a fracture. Intra-articular adhesions may occur when the fracture extends into the joint surface and there is a haemarthrosis or bleeding within a joint cavity. If this is not absorbed, fibrous adhesions may form within the synovial membrane. Periarticular adhesions may occur if oedema is not reduced and is allowed to organise in the surrounding tissues. This leads to adhesion formation between tissues such as the capsule and ligaments, and results in joint stiffness; this is less of a problem now that new techniques of fixation allowing early mobilisation have been developed.

Capsular adhesions are common: for example, in the capsule of the shoulder joint, which possesses dependent folds on its inferior aspect to permit a huge range of motion. These may stick together after fracture or injury, causing limitation of movement.

Injury to large vessels

If a large artery is occluded in such a position as to cut off the blood supply to the limb, this may lead to gangrene; if there is partial occlusion, an ischaemic contracture may develop. These injuries must be dealt with as an emergency by the surgical team.

Thrombosis of veins may occur in the area of the fracture. This presents as a sudden development of a cramp-like pain in the part, as an increase of swelling, and as marked tenderness along the line of the vein. Anything that appears to be abnormal in the circulatory system must be reported to the surgeon immediately. Blood vessels may sustain damage; for example, following supracondylar humeral fractures the brachial artery may be damaged.

Nerve injury

Certain fractures (e.g. mid-shaft humerus) may lead to radial nerve palsy; hence the importance of a knowledge of functional anatomy when treating. If a plaster is too tight, it may cause nerve damage. The common peroneal nerve is vulnerable to this if a plaster cast is moulded too tightly around the fibular head, resulting in foot drop as the tibialis anterior muscle is affected and unable to perform its function of decelerating the foot upon heel strike, and permitting toe clearance during the swing-through phase of gait.

Oedema

Oedema may be apparent below the level of the plaster and it is often necessary to elevate the limb, exercise the fingers or toes not encased in plaster, and perform isometric contractions of the muscles within the cast in an attempt to encourage muscle pump activity (Sheriff and Van Bibber 1998; Tschakovsky et al. 1996). Once the plaster has been removed, atrophied muscles may not provide an adequate muscle pump on the veins, in which case swelling may reappear, especially after activity or non-elevation.

PRINCIPLES OF FRACTURE MANAGEMENT

Once a fracture has been diagnosed, the most suitable treatment must be decided upon. This should be the minimum possible intervention that will safely and effectively provide the right environment for healing of the fracture. As already mentioned, nature has devised a system by which a slight amount of movement at a fracture site is useful in stimulating callus formation, and if a fracture is plated or immobilised in such a way that practically eliminates motion between the bone ends, callus will not form (Figure 3.4; Cornell and Lane 1992).

This is a common dilemma in orthopaedics. In the same way that there is no recipe for the physiotherapy treatment of a fracture, there is no single recipe for the surgical management of fractures. This 'see-saw' will be referred to in the case study later in this chapter.

Reduction

Reduction means to realign into the normal position, or as near to the normal anatomical position as possible (Figure 3.5). Reduction of a fracture may be either open or closed. *Closed reduction* means that no surgical intervention is used, the fracture being manipulated by hand under local or general anaesthesia. *Open reduction* means that the area has been surgically opened and reduced.

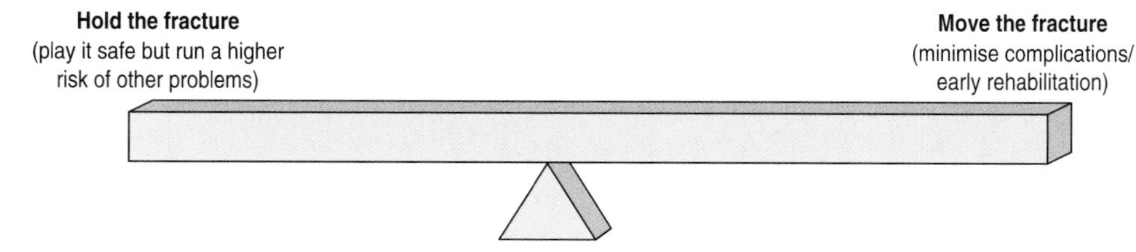

Figure 3.4 The mobilisation see-saw.

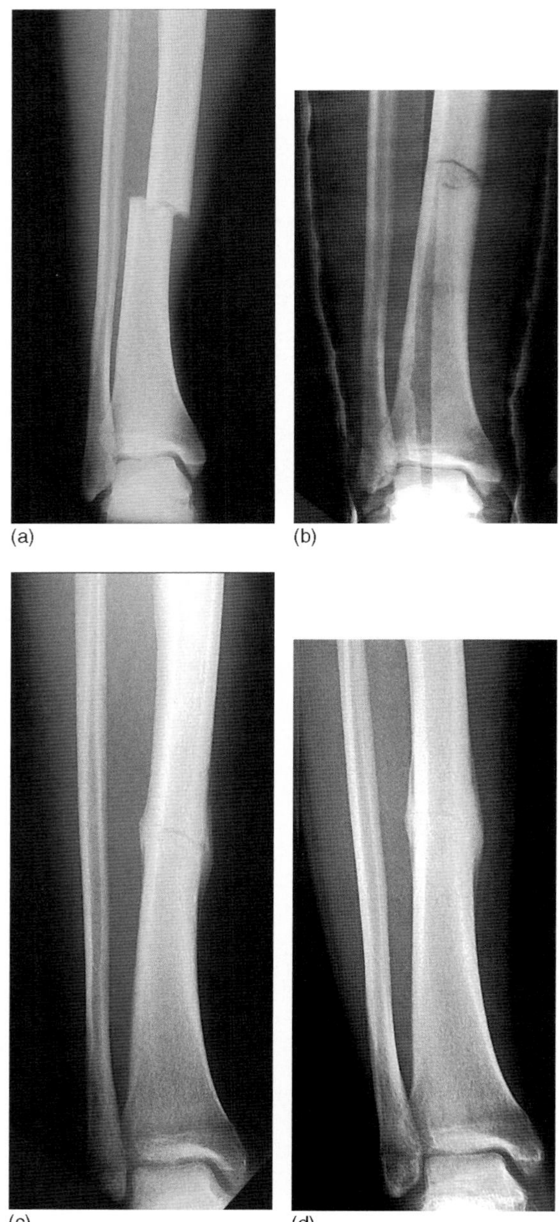

Figure 3.5 Reduction and healing of a fractured shaft of tibia showing the developing callus formation: (a) injury; (b) reduction; (c) at 8 weeks; (d) at 12 weeks. (With thanks to Martin George, Superintendent Radiographer, Sue Evans, Senior Radiographer, and Lynn Jackson, Sonographer, Southport and Ormskirk Hospitals.)

Reduction may not always be necessary, even when there is some displacement. For example, fractures of the clavicle may heal with a bump, which may be a problem only in the cosmetic sense; function is the most important end-point.

However, when there is poor alignment of the fragments or the relative positions of the joints above and below the fracture are lost as a result of angulation or rotation of the bone ends, or if there is loss of leg length, then accurate anatomical reduction is necessary.

X-rays are used to ascertain the exact position of the fragments before and after reduction. Real-time X-rays can now be taken using image intensifiers so that the surgeon can more accurately reduce. Improvements in CT and MRI mean that complex fractures can be studied in great detail pre-operatively, which assists the planning of surgery.

Immobilisation

The objectives of immobilising a fracture are:

- to maintain the reduction
- to provide the optimal healing environment for the fracture
- to relieve pain.

In some fractures where there is no likelihood of displacement, fixation may not be necessary, or minimal fixation will suffice: for example, buddy strapping for some finger fractures (Figure 3.6).

Common methods of fracture immobilisation

Plaster of Paris (PoP)

This is a plaster-impregnated bandage which can be moulded to the part when wet and sets in time. The standard method of external splinting is still PoP (Figure 3.7).

Synthetic materials are now used for splinting some fractures because of their light weight and waterproof qualities. Custom-made lightweight thermoplastics can be moulded to the limb and remoulded if swelling or atrophy causes changes in the limb contour. Some synthetic casting materials, however, are less malleable and cannot be moulded as effectively as PoP. They can occasionally cause allergies.

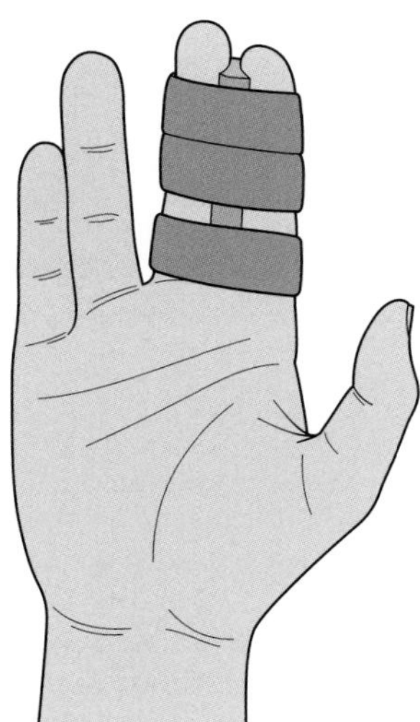

Figure 3.6 Double buddy strapping applied to both sound and damaged fingers to assist movement of the latter.

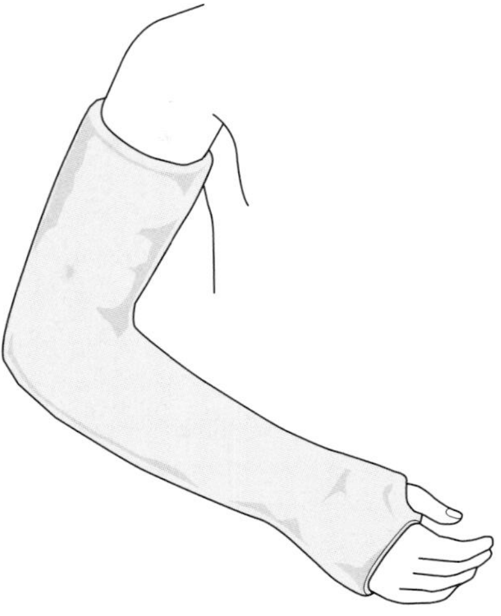

Figure 3.7 Plaster of Paris immobilisation.

A plaster saw is needed to remove a cast. This special tool has an oscillating blade that will cut through the hard cast without damaging the skin.

The advantages and disadvantages of using PoP are listed in Table 3.1.

> ***Clinical note***
>
> Medical advice should be sought if any of the following occur to a limb that is in a plaster of Paris or similar splint:
>
> - pale or blue coloration of the skin on the injured part
> - numbness, tingling or throbbing of the injured part
> - inability to move the fingers or toes
> - excessive pain in the injured part
> - swelling, bulging or puffiness around the edges of the cast
> - a foul smell from under the cast
> - if it becomes loose and slides around.

Functional bracing (cast bracing)

It has been found unnecessary to fix some fractures as rigidly as was thought necessary in the past, and an example of this type of fixation is cast bracing (functional bracing). Functional braces have hinges to allow movement. (See the case study towards the end of the chapter — Figure 3.25.)

3

Table 3.1 The advantages and disadvantages of plaster of Paris

Advantages	Disadvantages
▪ No surgery or its complications ▪ No infection risk ▪ Quick to apply ▪ Rapid patient discharge ▪ Cheap and relatively easy to apply with training ▪ New lightweight casts are an alternative ▪ Radio-translucent (bones can be X-rayed through the cast) ▪ May absorb fluids or bleeding. The extent of bleeding can be traced on the cast itself and monitored daily ▪ Can be moulded for several minutes before hardening	▪ It may not be possible to reduce the fracture correctly or maintain reduction ▪ May require surgery at a later date ▪ Plaster needs removal or windowing (removal of a piece of the cast) to inspect the skin ▪ May need removal in case of increased swelling or reapplication once swelling has subsided ▪ Smelly if it becomes wet ▪ Heavy ▪ May crack ▪ May rub the skin and cause sores

The soft tissues of the limb squeeze against the inside of the brace and, in conjunction with the use of a heel cup, permit weight to be taken through the substance of the brace. This has reduced many of the problems that were seen as a direct result of prolonged immobilisation. Another benefit of allowing movement of joints, provided that it does not unduly stress the fracture site, is that it may promote union by improving the area's blood supply.

Internal fixation

Surgical intervention by applying a plate and screws to the fracture is known as *open reduction and internal fixation*, often abbreviated to ORIF (Figure 3.8).

Advantages of ORIF. It permits a detailed inspection and accurate surgical assessment of the site of injury and procedure to be undertaken.

Disadvantages of ORIF.

- Surgery inevitably causes additional trauma and potential exposure to micro-organisms.
- It can convert a closed fracture into an open fracture.
- It requires surgery with all its sequelae and potential complications. Ironically, rigid fixation may remove the stimulus for callus formation. The implants may be removed 12–18 months in the future or if they start to become a problem. For example, the screws may become an irritant. In the young, they will be removed, as whilst they are in place, bone will not grow and respond to stress normally, as some of the stresses will be taken by the implants themselves.

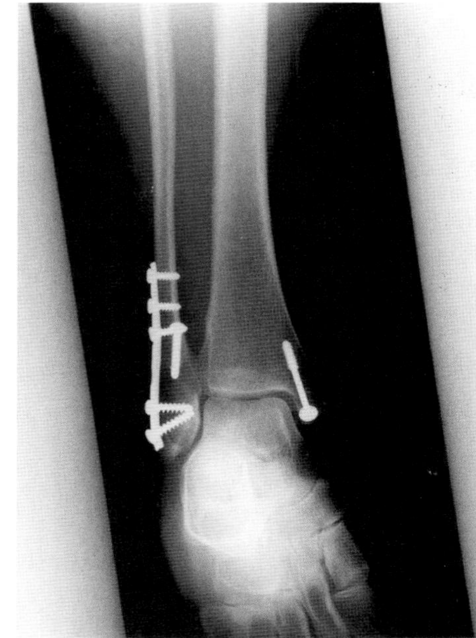

Figure 3.8 Fracture of the tibia/fibula fixed by plate and screws.

Intramedullary (IM) nailing

A hollow metal rod is introduced at one end of a long bone, travels down the medullary canal and may be locked with screws distally and proximally (Figure 3.9a). The proximal aspect of the nail is threaded and this permits a tool to be threaded on to the nail at a later date for its removal.

IM nailing for fractures of long bones has revolutionised management of many fractures, which historically would have been managed by prolonged bed rest. The trauma is less than with open techniques and results in decreased hospital stay, more rapid patient

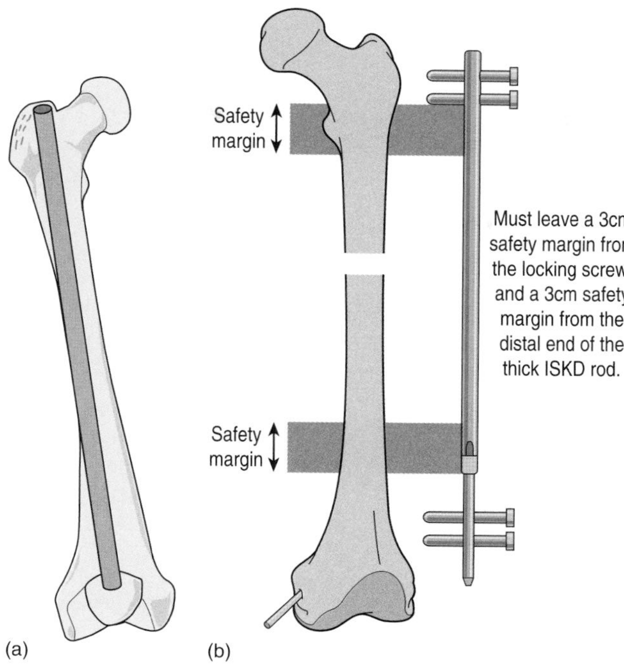
Safety margin
Safety margin
Must leave a 3cm safety margin from the locking screw, and a 3cm safety margin from the distal end of the thick ISKD rod.
(a)
(b)

Figure 3.9 (a) Intramedullary nailing; (b) intramedullary skeletal kinetic distractor (ISKD) nail. (With thanks to Dania Sorio, Customer Service International, and Grit Soboll, Communications Manager, Orthofix SRL, for 3.9b; www.orthofix.it)

mobilisation, and rehabilitation with minimal risk of complications associated with immobility. The implant rather than the bone may take stresses and strains and for this reason the surgeon may choose to remove the locking screws at a later stage. This permits the nail to move slightly and cause compaction of bone ends (dynamisation). It allows the bone to take its normal stresses and strains once again and to adapt in accordance with Wolff's law. The endosteal proliferation which occurs as part of the normal fracture healing process may be lost with certain types of internal fixation. Fractures of the shaft of tibia and humerus may also be nailed in this way.

Intramedullary skeletal kinetic distractor (ISKD). The ISKD (Figure 3.9b) is a two-part metal rod that can be used for tibial or femoral lengthening. An osteotomy is performed to allow distraction to take place. The device can only rotate in one direction and requires the patient to perform a rotational movement to cause lengthening. A hand-held monitor that contains a magnetic sensor is able to detect a small magnet sealed inside the ISKD. As the ISKD lengthens, the magnet rotates through 360 degrees. The monitor detects these changes and is able to record measurements so that lengthening can be very accurately controlled. Patients take measurements regularly throughout the day. Duration of lengthening depends on how much length needs to be achieved. The average desired rate is usually 1 mm per day. Patients are generally non-weight-bearing during the distraction phase.

External fixation

Figure 3.10 shows fixation of a fractured tibia using an external fixator. Pins or wires are driven into the fragments and held by a piece of apparatus on the outside of the body. Figure 3.11 shows an external fixator for a comminuted intra-articular fracture of the distal radius. Figure 3.12 shows an external fixator for an unstable pelvic fracture.

The advantages and disadvantages of external fixation are listed in Table 3.2.

The *Ilizarov method* of fracture fixation had its origins in Russia in the 1940s. It incorporates an axial system of wires or pins fitted through the bone and connected to a circular ring. It has proved successful in cases of non-union (Schwartsman et al. 1990). This method also incorporates the principle of 'distraction osteogenesis', and can be used in the restoration of large skeletal defects, limb lengthening, and the correction of skeletal deformities (Figure 3.13).

In *skeletal traction* a Steinman pin is inserted through the bone and a weight system attached to allow localised, effective traction. Common sites for this are the tibial plateau or the calcaneum. Pin sites must be kept

3

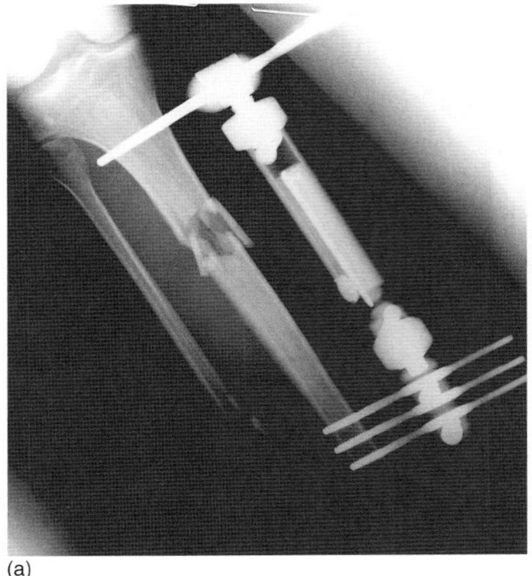

(a)

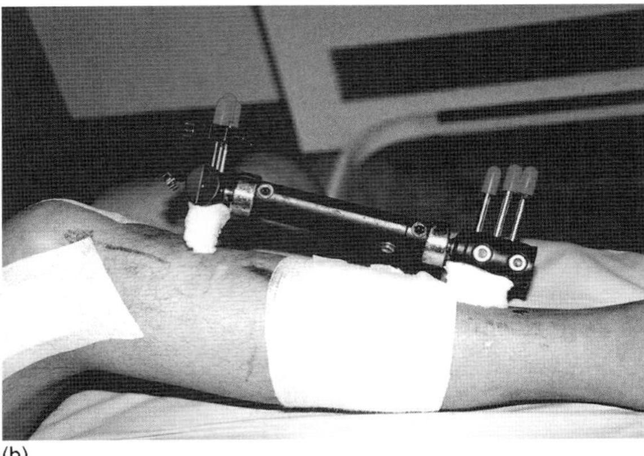

(b)

Figure 3.10 Fixation of a fractured tibia using an external fixator. (a) Pins or wires are driven into the fragments; (b) they are held by a piece of apparatus on the outside of the body. (Reproduced by kind permission of Mr RF Adam.)

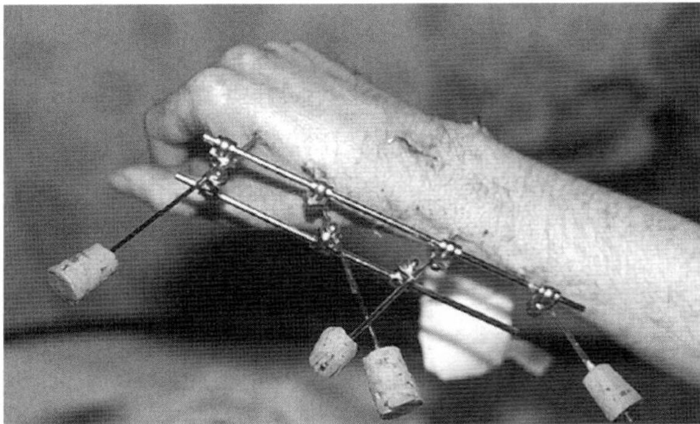

Figure 3.11 Fixation of a comminuted intra-articular fracture of the distal radius. (Reproduced by kind permission of Ms Fiona Cobbold, ©.)

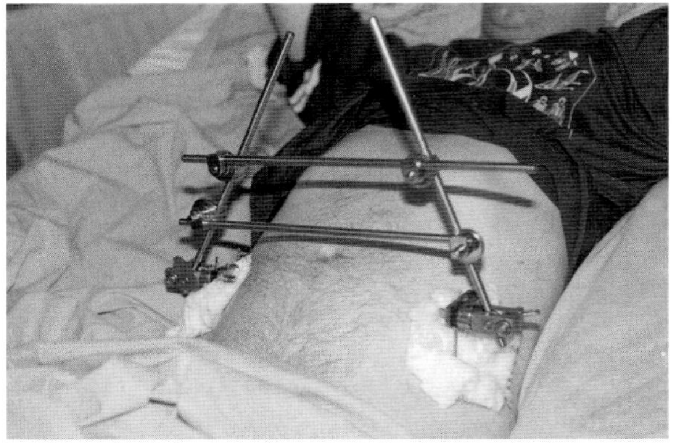

Figure 3.12 External fixator for an unstable pelvic fracture.

clean and free of infection. These pins are usually well tolerated and are not as painful as they appear.

Traction

Traction is the application of a pulling force to a part of the body; it may be either a direct or an indirect pull. Traction is less common on the orthopaedic ward nowadays, although it still has its place. Uses include:

- restoration of bone or limb length if this has been reduced by fracture or disease
- maintenance of correct limb length and the overcoming muscle spasm, which may be the cause of limb shortening after a fracture
- correction of deformity in a joint
- reduction of a dislocated joint
- immobilization of a joint
- pre-operative relief of pain
- promotion of rest and healing postoperatively.

Figure 3.14 shows an example of skin traction. The traction force is applied through the skin instead of through the bone.

PHYSIOTHERAPY AND FRACTURES

General issues

The physiotherapist's role is to identify the cause of the problem and to select the appropriate procedure to alleviate or eliminate the cause of the loss of movement — 'the right tool for the right job'. For example, there is

Table 3.2 Advantages and disadvantages of external fixation

Advantages	Disadvantages
▪ Minimal disruption to the fracture site ▪ Enables inspection of the wound and fracture ▪ Can be adjusted with minimal trauma ▪ Can be used for limb-lengthening procedures ▪ Can be used to pin multiple fragments (e.g. comminuted fractures) ▪ Allows preservation of tissues in open or compound fractures, degloving injuries or burns	▪ Infection risk at pin sites ▪ Needs meticulous wound care ▪ Cosmetically ugly ▪ Functional impairment (e.g. adjacent joints may be restricted or soft tissues pierced by fixator) ▪ Anaesthetic risk and its associated complications ▪ Patient will need several days in hospital ▪ Stresses taken by implant, so decreased stimulus for callus formation ▪ Heavy

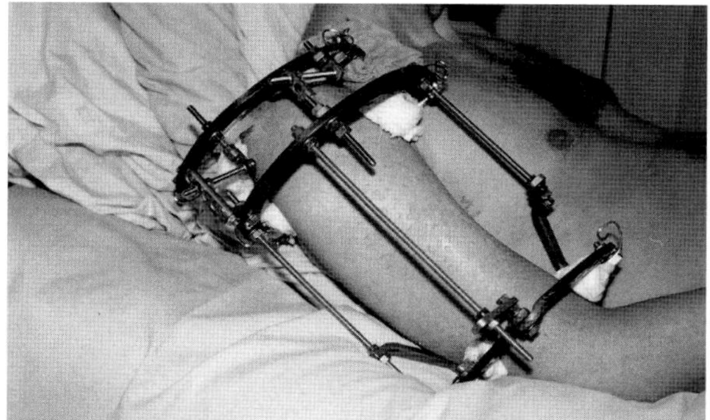

Figure 3.13 Ilizarov fixation for fractured humerus and scapula.

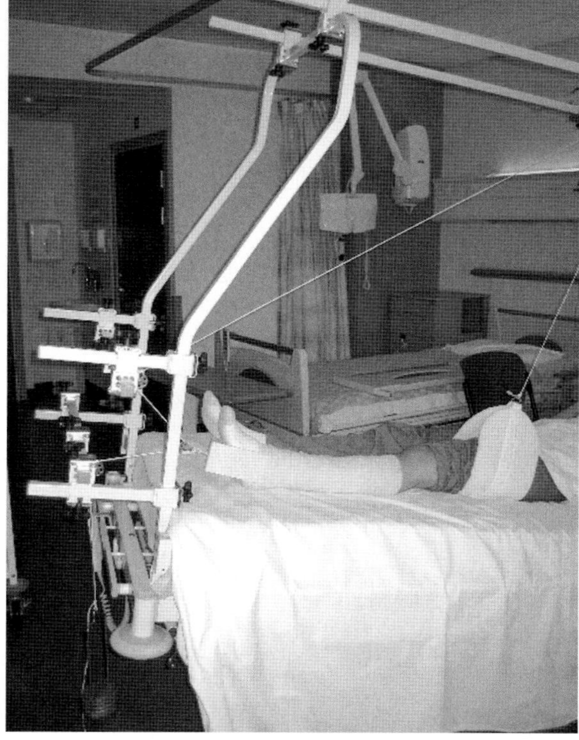

Figure 3.14 Skin traction. This woman sustained a fractured shaft of femur; owing to her general health, surgery was not indicated and she was managed conservatively. (With thanks to K Macgregor.)

little point in using accessory joint mobilisations if muscle spasm is the limiting factor, and a hot pack would not be appropriate if there were a bony block to movement.

Assessment of each individual will dictate the rehabilitation programme; there is no standard 'recipe' for the treatment of fractures. Any exercises given to a person must be realistic, attainable, adaptable, functional and memorable since patients often become confused about their exercises.

Most orthopaedic units have in place standardised protocols/guidelines and postoperative care plans for particular surgical or orthopaedic interventions, and the physiotherapist should adhere to these. Providing the best possible treatment to orthopaedic patients will take many years of practice, reflection and fine-tuning of clinical reasoning skills.

Clinical reasoning is not an abstract concept; it is applying common sense to your knowledge base. Your knowledge will improve every time you assess a patient and it evolves with experience. The following section gives pointers to assessing patients who have sustained fractures.

How physiotherapists assess and treat fractures depends very much on the time elapsed since the fracture

3

and the stage of rehabilitation at which they are performing the assessment. For example, students are often dismayed on their clinical placement to find that they are unable to perform a complete assessment of a patient who has just been put into plaster of Paris. Their treatment plan may now consist of:

1. Attain safe non-weight-bearing on elbow crutches.
2. Negotiate stairs safely.
3. Plan for safe discharge home.
4. Advise on isometric exercises.

The principles of orthopaedic assessment and treatment are summarised in Table 3.3.

Initial patient assessment

An assessment is essential if you are to plan a safe and appropriate treatment. Assess a fracture like any other condition, but be aware of any specific instructions or limitations. For example, is the patient allowed to bear weight fully or partially? Take time to think about what you are doing. If you omit something, make a note and remember to follow it up next time. Your assessment will vary considerably, depending on the clinical setting.

The problem-oriented medical record (POMR)

The POMR system is based on a data collection system that incorporates the acronym SOAP:

- *Subjective*. Any information given to you by the patient: allergies, past medical history, past surgical history, family history, social history (living arrangements, social conditions, employment, medication), review of systems.
- *Objective*. All information obtained through observation or testing: e.g. range of joint movement, muscle strength.
- *Analysis*. A listing of problems based on what you know from a review of subjective and objective data. For patients with multiple problems, number and list each problem consecutively, putting the most important first.
- *Plan*. As the name implies, this refers to the plan of forthcoming treatment.

Key point

Documentation is developing and many hospitals now use multidisciplinary integrated care pathways (ICPs) or electronic records. Documentation of your clinical reasoning and adherence to both your local and CSP Core Standards of Practice is paramount.

The subjective assessment

Basic background information to record

- Occupation.
- Drug history.
- X-rays/scans/other tests.
- Family history.
- Date of next clinic appointment.
- Specific surgical instructions.

History of present condition

Include the date of onset, mode of onset, course, and treatment to date. Note specific instructions: for example, partial weight-bearing for the next 3 weeks. If the patient cannot tell you what postoperative instructions he or she was given, do not guess. Speak to the other team members to establish treatment parameters.

Previous medical history

Are there any warning signs or findings that might affect your treatment options? For example:

Table 3.3 Physiotherapy and fractures: summary of general issues

Statement	Consequence for the physiotherapist
No two orthopaedic patients are alike	Do not ask for a 'treatment recipe'. Your approach should be flexible and dynamic and will change as a result of many factors
No two assessments are alike	Learn the basic assessment framework but tailor your assessment slightly to each individual
No two treatment courses are alike. Patients do not always do what the textbook says!	Keep an open mind, recognise when a treatment is not working and change or modify it
No single assessment can predict the outcome of the problem	Experienced physiotherapists are able to 'assess as they treat'. This means that the patient is continually receiving the most appropriate attention and the situation is dynamic. Treatment goals may need modification and should not be totally inflexible

- A person with internal fixation in place would not be considered for certain electrotherapy treatments.
- A patient with advanced osteoporosis would not be considered for high-impact gym work.
- Diabetic patients may have neurovascular complications that impact on the skin and healing.
- Patients with a history of chronic obstructive pulmonary disease (COPD) may have limited mobility and exercise tolerance.

Social history

Do not underestimate the importance of asking these questions:

- Is the patient living alone?
- Does the person need to climb stairs?
- Is the person losing money through non-employment?
- What are the person's hobbies?
- Does the person care for sick relatives?
- What does that person need to be able to do to be 'normal'?

The most effective physiotherapists are able to listen to what the patient tells them and incorporate this into the treatment plan. Do not ask leading or multiple questions, but keep your questioning on track and relevant and do not lose sight of why you are there. Set long- and short-term goals as you would with any other patient, but be prepared to adapt them if necessary.

Pain

It is not sufficient to ask merely whether or not the patient has pain. Ask the person about the location, type, duration and radiation of the pain. Is it related to time of day or certain activities, and does it have alleviating or aggravating factors? Visual analogue scales may be used as an attempt to quantify pain (Ch. 2). Remember that dull aching of the fracture site may be considered normal, especially after activity. This may signify bone remodelling. Sharp pain of a prolonged nature is greater cause for concern — hence the need to understand the physiology underlying healing.

The objective assessment

From the subjective assessment you should be able to devise a plan for your objective testing. The symptoms will act as a guide to the structures that will be examined: articular, muscular, vascular or neural. The painful areas should all be assessed, including areas other than the fracture site with associated soft tissue injuries. The tests used will be adapted to the stage in the healing process and the individual. By remembering the fundamental principles of fracture treatment — reduction, immobilisation and preservation of function — the assessment can be completed effectively and without damage. With an unstable fracture, for example, muscle contraction across the site could cause further damage. Fixators immobilise a fracture but are not as stable as union and should be treated with care.

Convenient subheadings for your assessment are: look, feel and move (Table 3.4).

Look

The observational skills you develop over time will be very important. A physiotherapist is often the first to pull back the bed covers to find overnight changes. Alterations in swelling, bruising, deformity, spasm, oedema and atrophy will indicate the progression of the pathology. Leg length discrepancies, posture alignment and gait patterns can be seen and then converted into objective measurements.

Feel

The palpation of swelling, pulses, heat, spasm and tenderness may be the main substance of your objective assessment in the acute unstable fracture. They are also essential for the detection of complications. Sensation changes will indicate the extent of your neural testing.

Move

This section is used to design your exercise programme for the preservation of function. A patient will be fearful of movement and will rely on you to indicate what

Table 3.4 Objective examination

Look	Feel	Move
Swelling Spasm Deformity Bruising Oedema Atrophy	Swelling Heat Sensation Tenderness on palpation Spasm	Active first Then passive Then overpressure (care – this may be inadvisable depending upon the stage of fracture healing) What are the quality and amount of movement and what is the end-feel?

and how to get moving. Therefore it is essential to test joints above and below the site to establish for patients the limitations of their condition. Local to the acute unstable fracture passive or assisted active movements would be less painful and harmful. However, in later stages of the pathology, active, passive and then overpressure testing is required. What is the quality and amount of movement and what is the end-feel? In answering these questions you will be able to diagnosis the nature of the damage.

The stage of fracture healing will dictate the extent of strength testing. Muscles that do not cross the fracture site but move the limb should be assessed. Their role as an agonist, antagonist, synergist or fixator will influence the choice of test and the maintenance exercises prescribed.

Functional movement tests are essential to tailor your treatment to individuals, whose abilities may be influenced by their injury, age or comorbidities. Measuring their ability to move about the bed, to get in and out of bed, to maintain weight-bearing status and to tackle stairs will indicate discharge suitability. In the later stages the tests may relate more to occupational or leisure needs.

Setting goals for orthopaedic patients

The assessment described above allows you to pull together the subjective and objective findings to form a clinical diagnosis. You may need to discuss this with your supervisor initially to help clarify your reasoning, and to aid goal setting and treatment planning. To complete the planning stage it is necessary to inform the patient of your findings and agree the treatment plan.

Without goals we have nothing to measure our performance against. This simple summary should help you plan goals for patients. When you set goals for any patient (orthopaedic or otherwise) the goals need to be SMART:

- **s**pecific
- **m**easurable
- **a**chievable
- **r**ealistic
- **t**imely.

Typical examples of orthopaedic goals possessing all the SMART characteristics are:

1. Goal — Mr X will be able to negotiate stairs safely, partial weight-bearing with two elbow crutches in 4 days' time.
2. Goal — Mrs Y will have attained 50 degrees of active knee flexion by 1 week from today.
3. Goal — Mrs Z will be able to transfer safely from bed to chair within 2 days.

TEST YOURSELF

Each of these goals fails to achieve one or more of the SMART criteria:

1. Mr X will be totally pain-free within 1 day of sustaining his fractured femur, tibia and humerus.
2. Mr X will be able to walk in 8 months' time.
3. Mr X will be much better in 1 week.
4. Mr X will mobilise full weight-bearing on his unstable fracture within 1 week.
5. Mr X will have more knee flexion within 1 week.

General points

Think about how you will realistically progress your treatment and how you will measure any progression (e.g. grip strength, isokinetic machine, goniometry). Work as part of the multi-disciplinary team (MDT) and think about who else needs to have input into the case — but at the same time do not forget your own role. Be aware of potential complications, and reassure and encourage your patient — who is the most important member of the MDT. Make the patient responsible for his or her own recovery — a partner, in fact. Home exercises should be clear, practical and monitored. Reassess progress as necessary. Are you attaining your goals? If not, change or modify your goals or your treatment. Before you discharge the patient remember that a normal limb needs:

- full active movement
- accessory movement
- full strength
- full function
- anything else specific to that patient.

Does the patient need follow-up appointments or domiciliary physiotherapy? Membership and relative roles of the MDT change according to the nature of the injury and the stage of treatment, but the physiotherapist must liaise and work with the other team members throughout the rehabilitation period. Initially, if the patient is in hospital, the members of the team will include: the patient, medical staff, nurses, occupational therapist, pharmacists, radiographers, district nurse and corresponding domiciliary staff.

Answers

(1) Not realistic: it is extremely unlikely that Mr X will be totally pain-free 1 day after three such major fractures. (2) Not timely; the end-point of this goal is too far in the future. (3) Not specific: what does 'much better' mean? (4) Not achievable: the orthopaedic protocol does not permit this. (5) Not measurable and not specific: what does 'more' mean?

COMMONLY ENCOUNTERED FRACTURES AND SOME PRINCIPLES OF MANAGEMENT

Fractures of the upper limb

Fractures of the clavicle and scapula

Scapular fractures are not particularly common and usually occur as a result of direct trauma. The clavicle often fractures following a fall on to the side or as a result of a fall on an outstretched hand. The fracture is usually in the middle or the junction of the outer and middle thirds of the bone. The pull of sternocleidomastoid muscle can cause displacement.

These fractures are usually immobilised by a brace, a sling, or a collar and cuff. Complications include a restricted range of movement in the shoulder girdle or shoulder joint since the two work together, and associated muscle weakness.

Fractures of the proximal humerus

These may be classified using the Neer classification:

- Group 1 — minimal displacement
- Group 2 — anatomical neck fracture with less than 1 cm displacement
- Group 3 — displaced or angulated surgical neck
- Group 4 — displaced fracture of greater tuberosity
- Group 5 — fractures of the lesser tuberosity
- Group 6 — fracture dislocations.

Fractures of the surgical neck of the humerus

These usually occur in elderly people as the result of a fall on the outstretched hand. There may or may not be displacement of the fragments, but in a large number of cases the fragments are impacted. This means that one bone fragment has been driven into the other, often stabilising the fracture at the time of injury. Displaced fractures, and particularly those occurring in the elderly, are not usually reduced for a number of reasons:

- Lack of good alignment does not affect union.
- It is preferable to avoid surgery in the elderly unless essential.
- Early movement is important to avoid a stiff shoulder.

Fractures of the shaft of the humerus (Fig. 3.15)

These fractures usually occur in the middle third of the bone and may be due to direct or indirect trauma. *Direct trauma* may give rise to transverse or oblique fractures and sometimes presents as a comminuted fracture. Displacement may result due to muscle pull, and if the fracture is below the insertion of deltoid the upper fragment will be abducted. *Indirect trauma* tends to give a rotational force resulting in a spiral fracture.

In stable fractures the fixation can be minimal and consist of a sling alone or with a posterior slab from below the shoulder to the wrist with the elbow at 90 degrees. This allows the weight of the arm to maintain reduction. If the fracture needs sturdier fixation, IM nailing is possible, or a complete plaster from the shoulder to the wrist or hand may be applied.

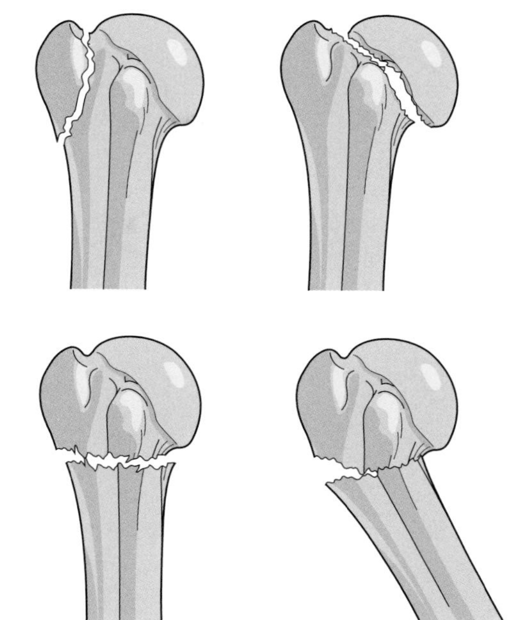

Figure 3.15 Neer classification of proximal humeral fractures.

Because the fracture usually occurs in the middle part of the shaft, the radial nerve may be affected as it winds through the radial groove. Since the radial nerve supplies the wrist and forearm extensor muscles, a wrist drop may result. The injury may compress the radial nerve and cause a neuropraxia, or if it is stretched it may result in axonotmesis. Normally these will recover spontaneously, although an axonotmesis will take longer as degeneration of the nerve has occurred within the sheath. In an open fracture the radial nerve may be severed, resulting in a neurotmesis and this will require surgical suturing.

Delayed union or non-union can be complications but are not very common.

Fractures of the condyles of the humerus

These fractures are common in children following a fall. A supracondylar fracture is the most common type (Figure 3.16). After reduction the arm may be immobilised in one of the following ways depending on the type of fracture:

- plaster with the elbow at approximately 90 degrees or a little more and extending from below the shoulder down to the wrist or hand (the plaster should

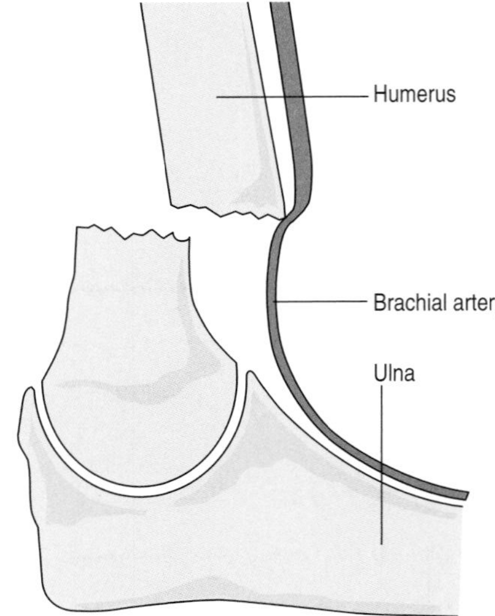

Figure 3.16 Supracondylar fracture of the humerus.

be cut so that it is possible to feel the radial pulse at the wrist)

- a posterior slab plus a collar and cuff
- a collar and cuff.

Some fractures of the condyles may extend on to the articular surfaces and thereby cause additional problems. One of the most serious complications that can occur is damage to the brachial artery, which could be severed or contused owing to its close proximity to the fracture site. Therefore circulation must be monitored. Impairment of the circulation requires emergency treatment as occlusion can lead to irreversible ischaemic effects within a few hours. If the circulation is not restored, Volkmann's ischaemic contracture may develop. This affects the flexor muscles of the forearm, which are replaced by fibrous tissue that contracts and produces flexion of the wrist and fingers. The skin and nerves will also be affected by the diminished blood supply.

Another problem following elbow fractures is post-traumatic ossification, sometimes known as myositis ossificans. If there is a severe injury, the periosteum may be torn from the bone, resulting in bleeding and the formation of a haematoma. Osteoblasts invade this blood clot and new (ectopic) bone forms. This can also occur as the result of forced extension of the elbow. First indications that this is developing may be pain and loss of movement. The elbow should be rested in a sling or collar and cuff for about 3 weeks to allow the haematoma to be absorbed. If this does not occur and bone is formed, it may be necessary to remove the bone tissue surgically. If deformity develops at the elbow — such as a cubitus valgus — this may cause a stretch on the ulnar nerve, which may require surgical intervention with a transposition of the nerve from the posterior to the anterior aspect of the elbow. Fractures that extend on to the articular surfaces and cause disruption of the joint may cause a permanently stiff elbow, lead to the development of osteoarthritis, or both.

Fractures of the radius

Management of radial head fractures ranges from no immobilisation at all in undisplaced fractures, to screw fixation, excision or replacement arthroplasty.

With fractures of the radius and/or ulna, both bones may be fractured as a result of direct or indirect violence such as a fall on the outstretched hand. The resulting displacement may be difficult to correct and in some instances may require open reduction. Accurate anatomical reduction is very important because loss of the normal relationship between the two bones may result in impairment of pronation and supination — a very important component of hand function. In children the damage may not be so severe and they may sustain a greenstick fracture with minor angulation, which normally will heal without any complications. Fracture of the ulna with radial head subluxation is called a *Monteggia fracture*, while fracture of the radius and subluxation of the lower end of ulna is called a *Galeazzi fracture*.

Colles' fractures of the distal radius are very common, particularly in the elderly, as a consequence of osteoporosis. They are usually caused by a fall on the outstretched hand. This may result in the typical dinner-fork deformity due to the backward (towards the dorsum) displacement of the distal fragment (Figure 3.17).

After reduction the Colles wrist may be immobilised with a complete plaster from just below the elbow to the hand, ending just above the proximal crease on the palm, or alternatively a plaster slab. The position of the wrist and whether or not there is a complete plaster will depend on the pattern of the displacement. If there is gross swelling it may be necessary to use a plaster back slab and then a complete plaster when the swelling has reduced. Fixation is usually maintained for 4–6 weeks.

A less common fracture is the *Smith's fracture*, similar to a Colles but with volar (towards the palm) as opposed to dorsal displacement of the distal fragment.

Fractures of the proximal radius are less common and tend to occur in younger people following either a direct blow or a fall on the outstretched hand, which causes a fracture through the head of the radius. Fractures of the ulna alone are not as common as those of the radius.

There are a number of complications that can occur with fractures of the lower end of the radius, although these are rare considering the numbers of fractures dealt

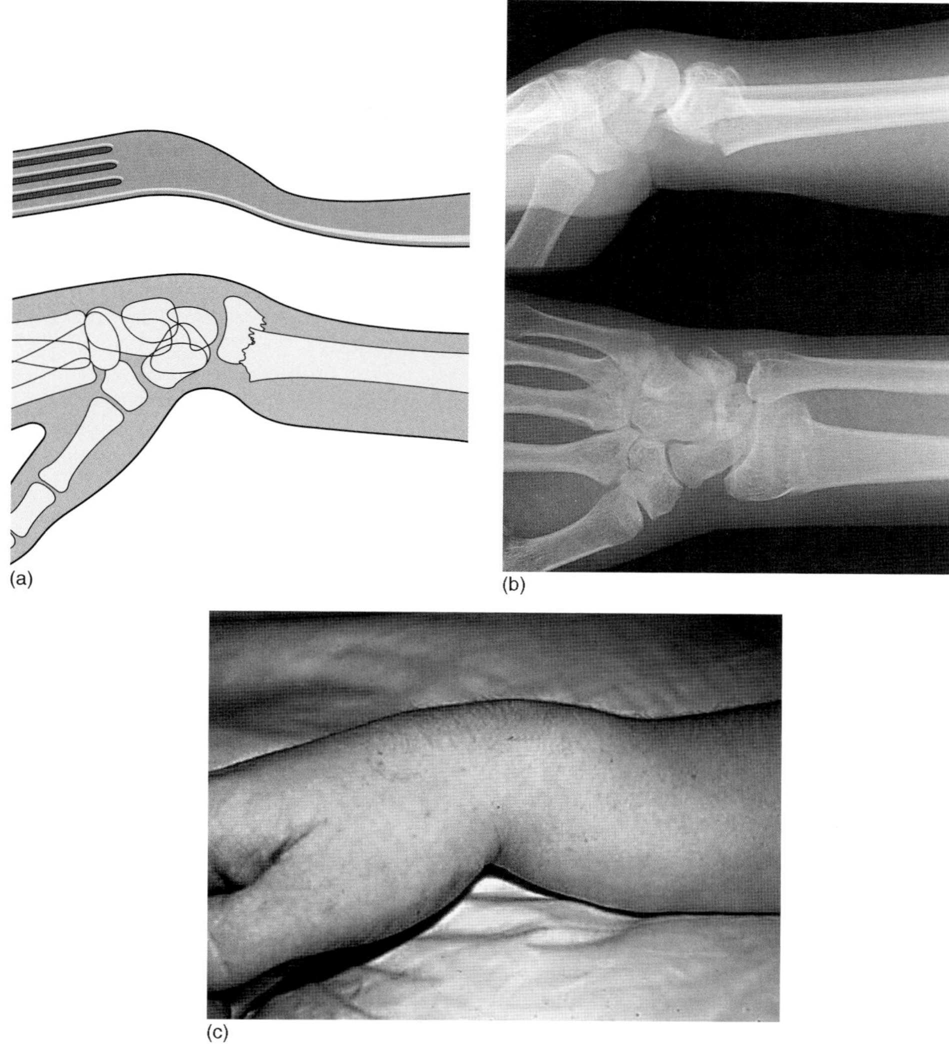

Figure 3.17 Colles' (dinner-fork) fracture.

with in fracture clinics. Loss of shoulder movement may occur, as it could be injured when the person falls or be a consequence of wearing a sling or collar and cuff. Rupture of the extensor pollicis longus may be noted, occurring 4–8 weeks after the fracture. A late complication can be that of Sudeck's atrophy. Median nerve neuritis can also be a complication if displacement causes stretching or compression of the nerve.

Fracture of the scaphoid

This fracture tends to occur in young adults as the result of falls on the outstretched hand. It may be overlooked either because the person considers it to be a strain, or because the fracture may not be visible on the initial X-ray. Healing is often slow in this fracture and in some instances there may be non-union. In the latter case the arm is usually placed in a so-called 'scaphoid plaster' as a precaution and X-rayed again after a couple of weeks. If these fractures are accurately diagnosed within 1 week followed by plaster immobilisation, non-union could be prevented (Roolker et al. 1999).

If the fracture occurs through the waist of the bone, the blood supply to the proximal part of the bone will be impaired and avascular necrosis may develop. Long-term complications include the development of osteoarthrosis.

3

Fractures of the phalanges or metacarpals

Accurate anatomical reduction and fixation are essential, but it is also important to keep the period of immobilisation as short as possible if a good functional result is to be obtained. The position of the fixation will vary, depending on which phalanx or phalanges are fractured and on the subsequent stability of the reduced fracture. This can be very important in relation to regaining function of the hand, and the team has to decide on the priorities in each case. The optimal splinting position for the hand ensures that the metacarpophalangeal (MCP) joints are held in 90 degree flexion with the interphalangeal (IP) joints in neutral. This ensures that the MCP collateral ligament length is maintained, preventing contractures and loss of range of motion and function.

In stable fractures, a buddy strap splint may be used, which fixes the injured finger to the adjacent finger and gives some support while encouraging some movement.

Bennett's fracture

This is a fracture dislocation affecting the carpometacarpal joint of the thumb.

Fractures of the lower limb

Weight-bearing (WB) status

The patient's WB status is dependent on many factors, including the type of fracture, quality of bone, age of the patient and the orthopaedic management undertaken.

Fractures of the pelvis

The pelvis may be thought of as a ring; like a ring, it will often break in two places at once. An isolated fracture is not serious as a rule, unless it is complicated by damage to the internal organs. The same is true of double or even multiple fractures, provided that there is no fracture or dislocation in the iliac segment. But if there are two or more fractures or dislocations with at least one in each segment, then the displacement may be considerable.

The majority of pelvic fractures are caused by direct violence or falls, or following crushing injuries. In major pelvic trauma the blood loss sustained by the patient at the time of the injury, or from damage to the internal organs, may be a life-threatening complication. When the pelvic ring is severely disrupted, then rapid reduction and fixation is necessary. If it is possible to reduce the displacement manually, then fixation may be by means of a plaster spica, but otherwise another method of external fixation may be used, placing pins through the iliac bones and fixing them to a transverse bar. Skeletal traction may be used for certain pelvic fractures. Complications may include injuries to the bladder or urethra and possibly to other tissues within the pelvis.

More common fractures include *pubic ramus* fractures (secondary to osteoporosis), which are managed conservatively with analgesia and gradual mobilisation. These fractures can be very painful as the hip adductors have their origin in this area, so walking is understandably painful.

The skill as a physiotherapist in this situation is to gain the confidence and respect of patients and gradually mobilise them to recovery. It also highlights the need for teamwork when coordinating analgesia with mobilisation.

Avulsion fractures occasionally occur in the pelvis at the anterior iliac spines, more specifically at the attachment of rectus femoris and sartorius. They are caused by forcible contraction of the muscle, pulling off the tip of the bone.

Fracture of the neck of femur

This is probably the most common and most significant fracture in terms of morbidity, mortality and socioeconomic impact in developed countries (Reginster et al. 1999). Mortality after fractured neck of femur is high; Schurch et al. (1996) found that the 1-year death rate was as high as 23.8 per cent.

The following is the Garden classification of femoral neck fractures:

- Type 1 — inferior cortex is not completely broken.
- Type 2 — cortex is broken but there is no angulation.
- Type 3 — some displacement and rotation of the femoral head.
- Type 4 — complete displacement.

In addition, femoral neck fracture is classified by its location (Figure 3.18):

1. subcapital
2. transcervical
3. basicervical
4. intertrochanteric
5. subtrochanteric.

Femoral neck fractures are extremely common in the elderly, often following falls, and most orthopaedic units will have a number of these fractures at any one time. The bone's architecture may have been so weakened that patients state they 'heard a crack' before they hit the ground. In other words, the fracture caused the fall, not the fall the fracture. Osteoporosis is often referred to as the silent epidemic as it may not present any clinical signs until fracture. It is discussed elsewhere in this textbook.

The resulting fracture is usually displaced with lateral rotation of the femoral shaft so that the leg will

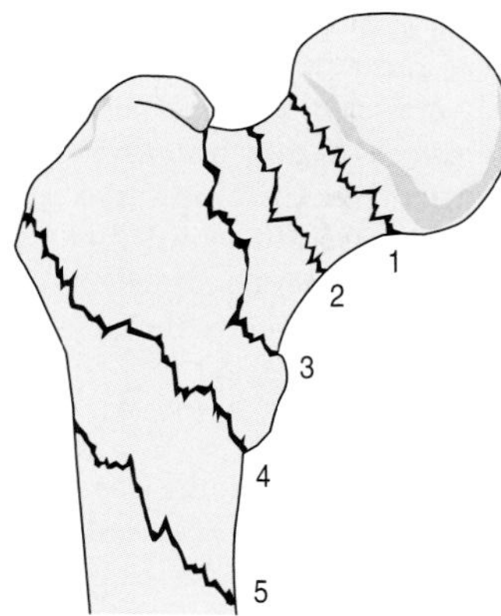

Figure 3.18 The Garden classification of femoral neck fractures: (1) subcapital; (2) transcervical; (3) basicervical; (4) intertrochanteric; (5) subtrochanteric.

be laterally rotated in comparison with the other limb. Occasionally the fragments are impacted in slight abduction and the patient may be able to get up and walk after the injury. Displaced fractures will need operative fixation (Figure 3.19). The usual method is to excise the head and perform replacement arthroplasty using one of the metal prostheses available (e.g. Thompson's hemiarthroplasty — Figure 3.20). This is the method of choice for displaced fractures because of the dangers of avascular necrosis, and because of the benefits of early mobilisation, which is so important in the frail.

An alternative method of fixation is a compression screw plate called a 'dynamic hip screw' — so called because it permits dynamic movement at the fracture site, which stimulates healing. Minimally displaced (e.g. Garden type 1) fractures may be managed by cannulated screw fixation.

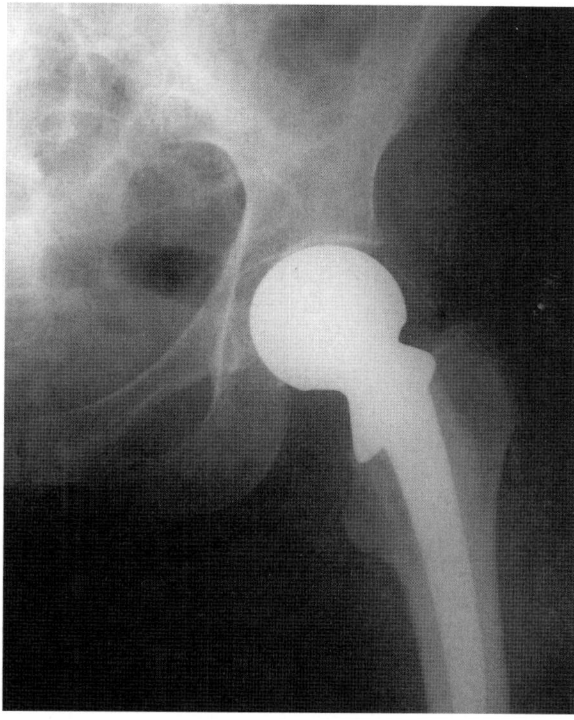

Figure 3.20 Thompson's hemiarthroplasty.

Complications

The blood supply to the femoral head is predominantly via a periarticular anastomosis (Palastanga et al. 1998). Avascular necrosis (death of part of the bone owing to lack of blood supply) can occur, as the blood supply to the head of the femur may be impaired following a fractured neck of femur (Figure 3.21).

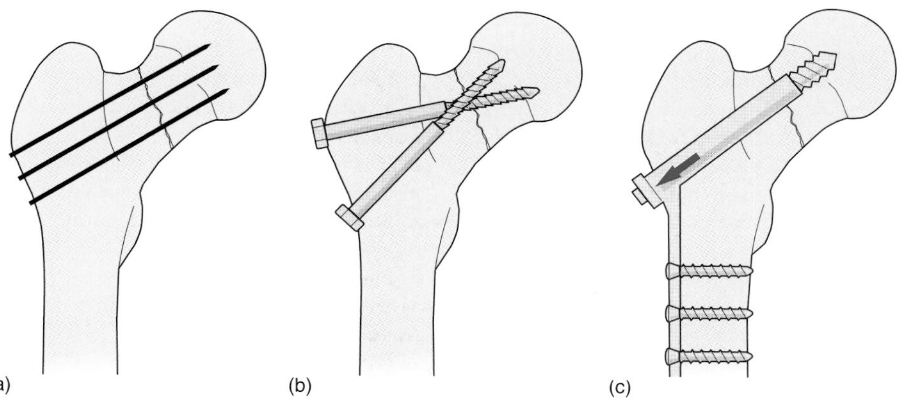

Figure 3.19 Methods of fixation for femoral neck fractures. (Reproduced from Dandy and Edwards 1998, with permission.)

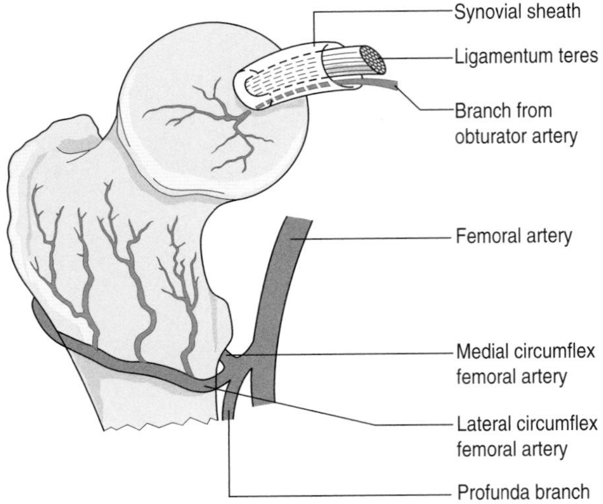

Figure 3.21 Arterial supply to the hip. (Reproduced from Palastanga et al. 2002, with permission.)

Fracture of the shaft of the femur

These fractures are usually the result of severe violence. They may occur at any part of the shaft and be of any type — transverse, oblique or spiral; they may be comminuted. Usually there is marked displacement with overlap of the fragments, which could lead to limb shortening if not corrected. Angulation may occur, depending on the injury and on powerful muscle spasm pulling the fragment in the direction of the attached muscles.

For children under the age of 3 years 'gallows' traction may be used. A modern, more acceptable alternative to traction is the use of IM nailing (Figure 3.9), which can be performed by the closed technique. The nail is passed through the greater trochanter, down the medullary canal of a long bone and through the fracture site. This is preferable to the previously favoured method of prolonged traction or open reduction, as there is less risk of infection and of the complications of bed rest and immobility.

If the fracture is an open fracture, there is a risk of infection. Delayed union or non-union is occasionally a complication of this injury, as is malunion. If the overlap of the fragments is not reduced or there is redisplacement, this can occur with consequent shortening of the femur. When the fracture has been fixed internally with an intramedullary nail, mobilisation can occur more rapidly.

Fractures around the knee

These include fractures of the tibial condyles, the patella (see below) and the femoral condyles.

Injury to the tibial condyles may comprise either a comminuted compression or a depressed plateau fracture. In the former, reduction is not usually attempted and early mobilisation is encouraged. Depressed plateau fractures require reduction to try to achieve an anatomically correct articular surface. Continuous passive motion (CPM, see below) may be used immediately after the fracture or after surgery to preserve synovial sweep and maintain articular cartilage nutrition.

Fractures of the femoral condyles are not very common but a supracondylar fracture occurs more frequently.

Complications

- Stiff knee could occur as the result of adhesions or because of disruption of the articular surfaces in fractures of the tibial condyles or patella.
- Secondary osteoarthritis may occur as a late complication following disruption of the articular surfaces.
- Genu valgum may develop following depression of the lateral tibial condyle.
- Haemarthrosis may be a problem after fractures of the tibial condyles. This may need to be aspirated (drained) and bandaged, but the swelling that occurs as a result of a synovitis will gradually absorb. If other soft-tissue structures are damaged there may be further swelling, in which case the limb should be elevated to assist drainage.

Continuous passive motion (CPM)

Use of the CPM machine is variable in the orthopaedic setting (Figure 3.22). Like any other modality in medicine, it has its place and its limitations. Salter (1993) has made an interesting study of the uses of CPM.

The benefits of CPM are as follows:

- There is maintenance of synovial sweep and thus hyaline articular cartilage nutrition. This is useful after certain intra-articular fractures (e.g. tibial plateau).
- Regular rhythmical motion can act as an analgesic, can stimulate circulation, and may assist in reduction of swelling.
- CPM has been used following anterior cruciate reconstruction, particularly following patellar tendon graft. It is possible that this encourages more rapid revascularisation and therefore strength of the donor graft.
- It is possible to increase flexion/extension in a controlled manner that is immediately obvious to the patient and can assist in giving the patient a goal to strive for.
- Some units have counters so that the healthcare team can tell exactly how long the patient has been using the unit.
- CPM units are now available for shoulder, wrist and other joints.
- CPM units may now be used in the patient's home.

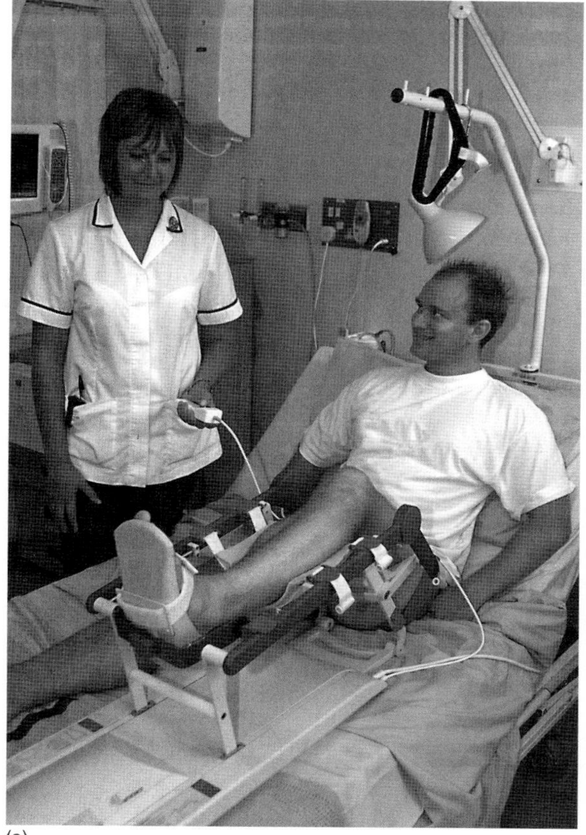
(a)

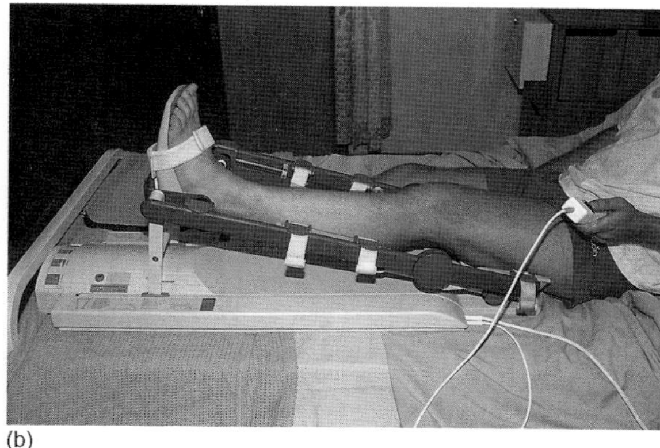
(b)

Figure 3.22 A demonstration of a continuous passive motion (CPM) machine. (With thanks to Joanne Kenyon.)

The disadvantages of CPM are as follows:

- It is passive, and therefore by definition will not build muscle strength. Some patients mistakenly neglect active exercises in the belief that they no longer need to undertake them. It is the responsibility of the physiotherapist to ensure that this situation does not occur.
- Some patients are distressed by the appearance of the unit and feel threatened. Most units have a panic button so the patient can stop the unit for rest, meals or toileting.
- The units can be bulky and expensive.
- If incorrectly positioned, they can cause pressure problems and be uncomfortable.

They pose an infection risk if not properly cleaned and if policies for their use are not followed.

Fracture of the patella

This can be caused by a direct blow on the knee or a sudden violent contraction of the quadriceps, resulting in an avulsion fracture. The former tends to cause a crack or comminuted fracture, whereas the latter may produce a transverse fracture. Internal fixation may be required if there is separation of the fragments.

Fractures of the tibia and fibula

These fractures are common and occur at all ages, as a result of direct or indirect violence. Often they are open fractures, either because of the direct violence or because the anterior tibia is very close to the surface and the fragments may extrude through the skin.

Direct violence, commonly due to road traffic accidents or soccer, is likely to give an oblique or transverse fracture. It may be comminuted and further complicated by soft-tissue damage. Fractures caused by a rotatory force, such as may occur in skiing, are usually spiral and the fractures of the two bones are at different levels.

Fixation will depend on the type of fracture and the amount of soft-tissue damage. A functional brace with a hinge at the ankle may be used and this has the advantage of allowing more movement and a better walking pattern. If there is a lot of soft-tissue damage and consequent swelling, a split plaster may be applied and the leg elevated on a Braun frame. This is replaced with a plaster once the swelling has subsided.

Another method that is used to immobilise this fracture is external fixation. Sometimes internal fixation is employed, with either an IM nail or plate and screws. It is common practice now to commence active movement in elevation immediately after surgery and delay the application of a plaster until movements are sufficiently regained.

Complications

Fractures of the tibia or fibula alone are not very common. The tibia can be the site of a stress fracture due to repeated minor trauma probably associated with sport. Infection is a possible complication, as many of these are open fractures; fortunately the problem is less serious these days with the advent of antibiotics and improved wound care.

Vascular impairment can occur due to damage to a blood vessel or a plaster cast that is too tight. Great care must be taken by all concerned with the management of these patients to monitor for any signs of circulatory deficiency.

Compartment syndrome is common, as is delayed union or non-union. Occasionally these fractures are very slow to heal or there may even be non-union owing to the lower third of the tibia having such a poor blood supply.

Fractures around the ankle

Figure 3.23 shows fractures resulting from an abduction/lateral rotation force or an adduction force. Complications include limitation of movement in the ankle joint and foot resulting from periarticular and intra-articular adhesions or from disruption of the articular surfaces. The latter may also lead to the later development of secondary osteoarthritis.

For fractures without displacement, a below-knee walking plaster may be applied for 3–6 weeks. When there is displacement it is important for the surgeon to try to ensure that reduction establishes the normal anatomical relationship at the ankle joint. If reduction cannot be attained by manipulation and plaster immobilisation, it may be necessary to have an open reduction with internal fixation (ORIF) and use a screw or screws to maintain a good position of the fragments followed by immobilisation in a below-knee plaster. The modern trend is towards immediate postoperative

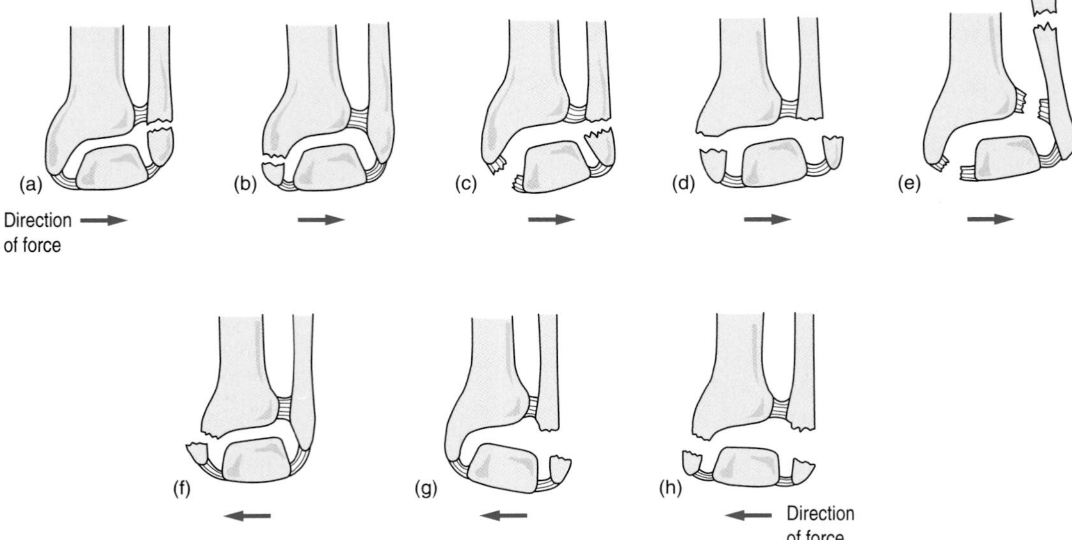

Figure 3.23 Parts (a)–(e) show fractures resulting from an abduction/lateral rotation force: (a) fracture of lateral malleolus; (b) avulsion fracture of medial malleolus; (c) fracture of lateral malleolus, rupture of medial ligament, and lateral shift of talus; (d) fracture of lateral and medial malleoli and lateral shift of talus; (e) tibio-fibular diastasis – rupture of tibio-fibular and medial ligaments, fracture of shaft of fibula, and lateral shift of talus. Parts (f)–(h) show fractures resulting from an adduction force: (f) fracture of medial malleolus; (g) avulsion fracture of lateral malleolus; (h) fractures of lateral and medial malleoli plus medial shift of talus.

active exercise (with adequate analgesia), then subsequent application of a cast once good movement (particularly dorsiflexion) is attained.

A tri-malleolar fracture involves fractures of both the medial and lateral malleoli as well as fracture of the posterior tibial malleolis. Tri-malleolar fractures are generally unstable.

Fractures in the foot

Fractures of the calcaneum usually occur as the result of a fall from a height on to the feet, fracturing the calcaneum in one foot or sometimes both feet. It may well be accompanied by a fracture of one of the lower thoracic or upper lumbar vertebrae. (Take note if a patient with a fractured calcaneum complains of back pain.) Calcaneal fractures can be extremely painful and carry a poor functional prognosis if inversion and eversion are not regained, since their movements are essential for normal function of the foot in such activities as adapting to uneven surfaces. These may be managed either conservatively or by open reduction and internal fixation.

The emphasis of physiotherapy management is on the reduction of the oedema and mobilisation. Once the patient is allowed to bear weight it is important to re-educate gait, as well as concentrating on strengthening muscles and regaining range of movement in the ankle and foot. It may not be possible to regain any movement at the mid-tarsal joints and the patient will have to learn to adapt to this loss of movement. The arches of the foot may have flattened and this could be the result of weak muscles, deformity of the foot, or both. In the former case the muscles can be strengthened, but if the latter is the case the arches will not reform; the patient may continue to have persistent pain and tenderness for a long time after the fracture has healed and it is difficult to relieve.

Generally speaking, it is advisable to commence early active mobilisation in elevation. Cryotherapy/TENS, Flowtron boot, and patient-controlled analgesia (PCA) have all been used with success. In later stages, accessory mobilisations to the affected joints may be appropriate.

The phalanges and metatarsals are most likely to be fractured by a heavy object falling on the foot. This will also cause soft-tissue damage and consequently swelling is likely to be severe. These fractures do not as a rule require reduction or immobilisation. However, a below-knee walking plaster is usually applied for fractures of the metatarsals to relieve pain and enable the patient to walk. If swelling is severe, the patient will need to rest in bed with the leg elevated for a few days.

Another type of fracture that occurs in the metatarsals is a stress fracture, often known as a 'march' fracture. It is caused by repeated minor trauma that may arise from prolonged walking, particularly on hard surfaces, and usually in someone who is unaccustomed to walking long distances. It is usually a crack fracture affecting the shaft or neck of the second or third metatarsal. No fixation is required but a walking plaster may be applied if the pain is severe.

Complications

Complications include stiffness, particularly if there has been disruption of the subtalar joint articular surfaces. Secondary osteoarthritis may develop later as a result of the disruption of the joint surfaces.

Spinal fractures

These are not dealt with in this text.

CRYOTHERAPY

This is regularly used in the orthopaedic setting and is covered in Chapter 13.

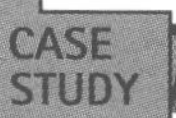

FRACTURED SHAFT OF THE FEMUR

Note that the material in this section does *not* represent a recipe for the management of all fractures of the femur.

BACKGROUND

Ms Jones is a 25-year-old law student who was involved in a road traffic accident. She was driving, and as a result of a head-on collision, the dashboard was pushed backwards into her knees. She sustained a fractured shaft of the left femur (Figure 3.24a). She was treated by intramedullary fixation (Figure 3.24b). Ms Jones spent 10 days in hospital and has now come to the outpatient physiotherapy department. She did not sustain any other injuries.

ON EXAMINATION

Ms Jones is partial weight-bearing, and is mobilising with two elbow crutches and wearing a functional (cast) brace. She is independently mobile, although she needs help to remove her training shoe and sock. The brace was custom-made by the occupational therapists (Figure 3.25) and it is unlocked to permit 0–90 degrees of knee flexion. The physiotherapist may unlock the brace by a further 10 degrees each

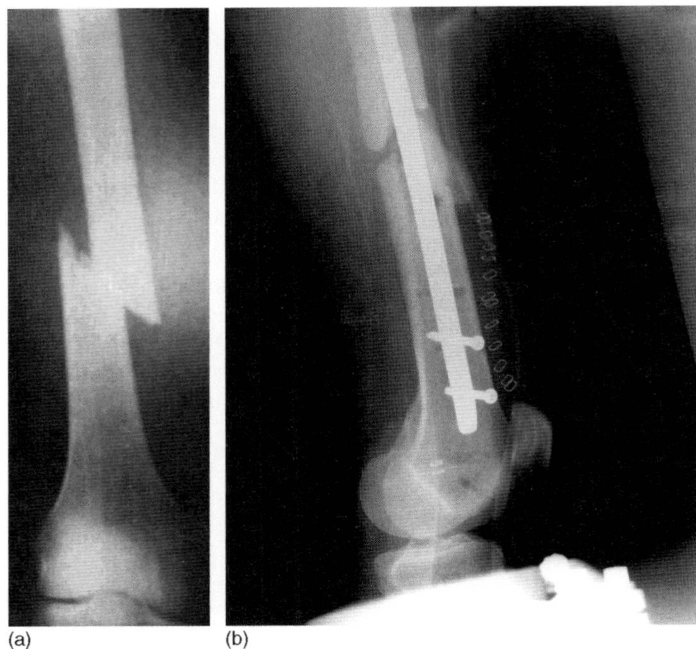

Figure 3.24 (a) The femoral fracture. Note that spasm in the quadriceps has resulted in overriding of the fracture fragments. (b) Note the locking screws and skin staples visible on X-ray.

week. The patient must wear the brace when walking but is permitted to remove it to perform knee flexion exercises and to take a shower.

She is extremely anxious about what is going to happen to her and confused about how much or how little she should be doing. The only exercise she can remember is straight leg raise (SLR). She is articulate, cooperative and keen to take advice. She cannot currently attain heel strike and she states that this is because it causes her calf to be painful — although deep vein thrombosis has been excluded. She has been told to keep moving, and as a result, she is walking long distances every day. Her leg aches badly at bedtime and she is worried that the fracture has 'moved', although X-rays show that it has not displaced since the time of surgery.

OBJECTIVE EXAMINATION

There are two incisions: one proximal to the greater trochanter, one lateral to the knee joint. These have healed. The patient has a reddened area over the lateral malleolus, which is due to the brace rubbing her skin.

Knee joint

The range of movement of the knee joint with the brace removed is shown in Table 3.5.

Patello-femoral joint

All accessory movements are reduced by approximately 50 per cent on the left side.

Ankles

There is full active-range plantar flexion in both ankles. Terminal dorsiflexion of the affected side causes calf 'tightness' when the left knee is in the fully extended position. The range of plantar and dorsiflexion is full, however. Small joints of the foot, intertarsal and tarso-metatarsal, have some loss of accessory movement of the subtalar and intertarsal joints of the affected side. There is some oedema of the ankle. Capillary filling is poor.

Muscle strength

Oxford grade — left and right — is shown in Table 3.6.

Pain

Figure 3.26 shows the pain recorded using a visual analogue scale.

Limb girth

See Table 3.7.

3

Table 3.5 Features of the patient's knee Joint

	Left knee			Right knee		
	Passive[a]	Active[b]	Overpressure[c]	Passive	Active	Overpressure
Flexion	0–60	0–40	–	130	130	–
Extension	Full extension possible but causes posterior knee discomfort			Full 0-degree extension painless		
Lateral rotation	Full			Full		
Internal rotation	Full			Full		

[a]Limited by apprehension. [b]Limited by aching at the fracture site and quadriceps spasm. [c]Not tested in view of fracture status and patient apprehension. The units are degrees.

Table 3.6 Features of the patient's muscle strength (Oxford Grade)

	Left	Right
Quadriceps	4	5
Hamstrings	4	5
Tibialis anterior	4	5
Gastrocnemius	4	5

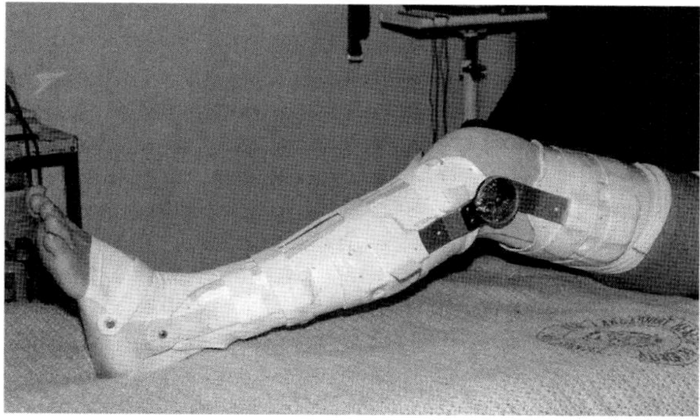

Figure 3.25 The functional brace. The heel cup is essential for correct off-loading of weight from the fracture. (Courtesy of Mike Somervell and Julie Butler.)

SHORT-TERM PROBLEMS

Do not underestimate the impact of apprehension and confusion. If a person is nervous, frightened or confused, whatever you plan to tell, teach or ask of them will be adversely influenced. Do not think only of the fracture; take a holistic approach. Physiotherapists are not technicians; they are also educators. It is perfectly valid to undertake a teaching session on fracture healing with this patient and to discuss the aims of treatment. This might seem time-consuming but consider your aims and your role as her physiotherapist. The quality of your communication and subsequent discussion of your management plan will influence her eventual health outcome. There is now strong research evidence suggesting a positive correlation between effective professional–patient communication and improved patient health outcomes (Lorig 1982; Lorig et al. 1984).

The sore caused by the brace is a high priority. The physiotherapist needs to refer the patient to the occupational therapist for adjustment of the brace. If the sore develops to the point where she cannot tolerate the brace, your ability to progress her treatment will be adversely affected.

Pain and aching at the end of the day are normal. Your goal here is to explain *why* the pain is happening and that it signifies bone healing. Do not assume that your patient will automatically know this. Some patients equate pain with progress ('no pain no gain') and see it as a positive factor, whereas others will be frightened by it. In this person's case it seems likely that too much walking is being undertaken; she needs advice on going for smaller, more frequent walks with attainable goals. For example, she could be told to walk the length of her home every hour. Knee flexion may be painful, in which case your role as her physiotherapist is to identify the specific cause and to minimise or reduce it prior to active exercise. This might consist of asking the patient to take her analgesia 1 hour before commencing her exercises, or the application of TENS or hydrotherapy as a supplement to exercise.

The current exercise regimen is unacceptable. Repeated straight leg raising will do nothing to provide functional quadriceps strength and at worst it will cause backache. Straight leg raising is probably one of the most abused exercises in physiotherapy. It will strengthen the hip flexors but little else. This patient needs functional exercises such as inner-range quadriceps, hamstring, gastrocnemius and anterior tibial and hip abductor work within the permitted limits of the fracture rehabilitation. These

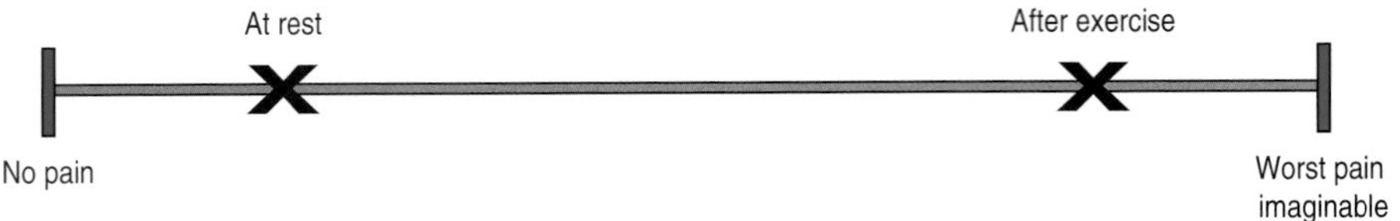

Figure 3.26 The patient's pain scale.

Table 3.7 The patient's limb girth

	10 cm above patella apex	20 cm above patella apex
Left leg	48 cm	44 cm
Right leg	56 cm	52 cm

must be taught and explained clearly, written down if possible and the rationale behind them explained to the patient. Patients often become confused about their exercises; keep them simple and understandable. Patient compliance with exercise is poor in general (Campbell et al. 2001), and the more you can do to make home exercises simple and practical, the more success you will have in educating and rehabilitating your patient.

Loss of knee flexion due to callus may be impeding soft tissue mobility. Pain, fear or muscle spasm might also be causes of limited mobility; since she has more passive than active range, something other than the joint is limiting her movement. Your role is to identify the cause and treat it accordingly. Heat pack or massage may relieve spasm. The brace limits flexion to 90 degrees but there is no reason why you should not aim for 90 degrees at this time.

With regard to the oedema, an inefficient muscle pump is a likely cause. She is not attaining heel strike but is walking great distances; these will both exacerbate dependent oedema. Little and often is the key, with elevation during periods of rest, and a graduated increase of walking distance. Massage might be used to relieve oedema but can be time-consuming.

This person has a loss of limb girth on the affected side. This will be due to disuse atrophy. Decreased limb girth is not as important as muscle function but may be distressing to the patient; reassure her that function will come first, then bulk. Whilst function is not a true reflection of quadriceps girth or strength, it does give the person something specific to aim for.

Loss of accessory movement needs to be addressed in the treatment plan: for example, to the small joints of the foot and mid-tarsal joints. The loss of accessory motion at the patello-femoral joint should also be addressed; the function of this joint cannot and should not be isolated from the function of the knee joint itself.

It is relatively easy to identify immediate problems, but unfortunately this alone is insufficient; you also need to be aware of potential or longer-term complications.

POTENTIAL AND LONG-TERM PROBLEMS: THE BIGGER PICTURE

- Adaptive shortening of the Achilles tendon, leading to permanent soft tissue contracture may occur if the patient's gait is not corrected as a consequence of her not attaining heel strike. She currently does not have any soft-tissue contracture since her measurements are full.
- Encourage her to walk shorter distances with a normal gait.
- Check that her pain is being controlled adequately so that she is not afraid to attain heel strike.
- Explain this to the patient so that she can take an active role in her own rehabilitation.
- Make sure that a potential problem does not become a real one.
- Fixed flexion deformity of the knee joint is also a possibility if the importance of attaining full knee extension is not explained to the patient.
- Fibrous adhesions may occur if oedema is allowed to organise.
- Retro-patellar adhesions may form as a result of immobility of the knee's expansive synovial membrane and might become a cause of stiffness. The likelihood of this happening might be reduced by isometric contractions of the quadriceps and articularis genus muscle, whose task it is to retract the synovium of the knee joint (Ahmad 1975).
- Degeneration of hyaline articular cartilage occurs if a joint is not subjected to movement. The patient should be encouraged to undertake general mobility and exercise little and often.
- Generalised osteopenia, or a reduction in bone mineral density, may result if weight is not placed through the limb. The see-saw needs careful consideration here — see earlier in this chapter.

TREATMENT PLAN

- The patient must effectively become involved in the management of her condition.
- Commence partial weight-bearing gait and progress within protocol guidelines.
- Re-educate normal gait — i.e. heel strike.
- Mobility of all unaffected joints must be maintained during the period of immobilisation.
- Return movement and function to normal. This is person-specific and full function might not be attained until removal of the nail in 1 or 2 years' time.
- Draw up a thorough and fully understood home exercise programme, which can be monitored and progressed as needed. It is better to teach two exercises well and have the patient thoroughly understand them than teach ten exercises that are too complex and confusing to the patient.
- Strengthen appropriate muscles, depending on your assessment findings.
- Progress to full weight-bearing within rehabilitation guidelines; check any protocols and specific guidelines.

OVERALL PROGRESS AND DISCHARGE

Study the simplified graph in Figure 3.27. If we plot a hypothetical 'improvement versus time' graph, the student might *hope* for this pattern. ('Improvement' may mean different things to different people. For purposes of clarity it has been shown as a single item.) If this were the case, recovery could always be predicted, all patients could use the same treatment regimen, one assessment would be sufficient, a discharge date could be predicted many weeks in advance, and undergraduate training would take about a month! Unfortunately this is not the case.

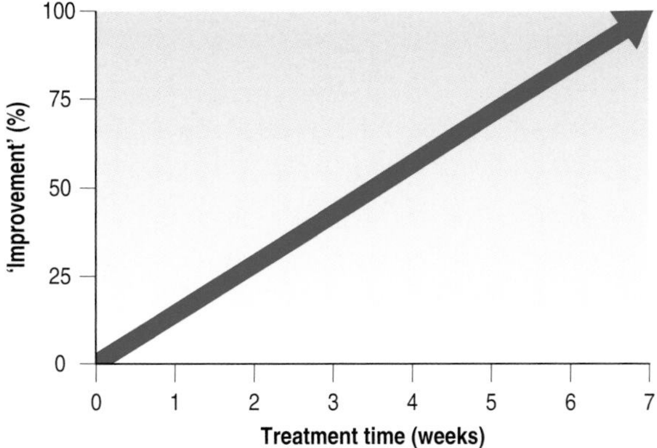

Figure 3.27 A hypothetical improvement chart.

It is more likely that you will see a pattern of peaks, troughs and plateaus, with a general trend towards recovery. The overall shape of the real improvement curve displays the gradual attainment of a plateau in improvement.

This pattern of recovery is common. The patient may gain 10 degrees of knee flexion per week for the first 3 weeks of treatment, then improvements will slow to the point where it takes a further 3 weeks to attain an additional 5 degrees. This presents the physiotherapist with a constantly changeable situation — which is one of the reasons why the profession is so stimulating. It also poses the problem of when to discharge the patient. The final decision must be a mutually agreed decision between physiotherapist and patient, and it is at this point that previously agreed goals are essential. It may be the case that 95 per cent 'improvement' is the maximum possible improvement attainable whilst the IM nail remains in situ. For example, there may be some residual discomfort on running or squatting. Experienced physiotherapists will be able to integrate their knowledge of anatomy, physiology and biomechanics and explain to the patient that now is the time for discharge and that the further 5 per cent will occur following implant removal. Without a sound prior assessment and formulation of goals, appropriate patient discharge may be jeopardised, resulting in discharge that is too early or treatments that become repetitive, non-adaptive and inappropriate. The advantage of physiothera-pists being autonomous practitioners is that, with a little thought and a sound initial assessment, one can avoid the situation where the patient is seen 'twice a week for 8 weeks' with no change in treatment or progression. The patient and physiotherapist 'own' the process.

ACKNOWLEDGEMENTS

With thanks to Grit Soboll, Communications Manager, Orthofix SRL; Dania Sorio, Customer Service International, Orthofix SRL; Annie Karim, Association of Chartered Physiotherapists Executive Committee Officer.

FURTHER READING

Association of Orthopaedic Chartered Physiotherapists Guidelines of Good Practice in Orthopaedics: www.aocp.co.uk

Atkinson K, Coutts F, Hassenkamp AM 1999 Physiotherapy in Orthopaedics — A Problem-Solving Approach. Churchill Livingstone: Edinburgh

Barker KL, Lamb SE, Simpson AH 2004 Functional recovery in patients with nonunion treated with the Ilizarov technique. J Bone Joint Surg Br 86-B: 81–85

Barry S, Wallace L, Lamb S 2003 Cryotherapy after total knee replacement: a survey of current practice. Physiother Res Int 8(3): 111–120

Bruckner P, Bennell K 1997 Stress fractures in female athletes: diagnosis, management and rehabilitation. Sports Med 24(6): 419–429

Duckworth T 1995 Lecture Notes on Orthopaedics and Fractures. Blackwell Science: Oxford

McRae M 1999 Pocketbook of Orthopaedics and Fractures. Churchill Livingstone: Edinburgh

Scottish Intercollegiate Guidelines Network (SIGN) 1997 Management of Elderly People with Fractured Hip: A National Clinical Guideline (no. 15). SIGN: Edinburgh

Stewart MA 1995 Effective physician–patient communication and health outcomes: a review. CMAJ 152(9): 1423–1433

Tidswell M 1998 Orthopaedic Physiotherapy. Mosby: New York

REFERENCES

Adams CI, Keating JF, Court-Brown CM 2001 Cigarette smoking and open tibial fractures. Injury 32(1): 61–65

Ahmad I 1975 Articular muscle of the knee — articularis genus. Bull Hosp Joint Dis 36(1): 58–60

Azuma Y, Ito M et al. 2001 Low-intensity pulsed ultrasound accelerates rat femoral fracture healing by acting on the various cellular reactions in the fracture callus. J Bone Miner Res 16(4): 671–680

Bandolier Evidence-Based Healthcare 2004 NSAIDs, Coxibs, Smoking and Bone. March:www.jr2.ox.ac.uk/bandolier/booth/painpag/wisdom/NSAIbone.html

Campbell R, Evans M, Tucker M et al. 2001 Why don't patients do their exercises? Understanding non-compliance with physiotherapy in patients with osteoarthritis of the knee. J Epidemiol Commun Health 55(2): 132–138

Cornell CN, Lane JM 1992 Newest factors in fracture healing. Clin Orthop 277: 293–311

Dandy DJ, Edwards DJ 1998 Essential Orthopaedics and Trauma, 3rd edn, p. 94. Churchill Livingstone: New York

Lorig K 1982 Arthritis self-management: a patient education program. Rehabil Nurs 7(4): 16–20

Lorig K, Laurin J, Gines GE 1984 Arthritis self-management. A five-year history of a patient education program. Nurs Clin North Am 19(4): 637–645

Hoppenfeld S, Urthy VL 1999 Treatment and Rehabilitation of Fractures. Lippincott Williams & Wilkins: Baltimore

Marsh DR, Li G 1999 The biology of fracture healing: optimising outcome. BMJ 55: 856–869

Palastanga N, Field D, Soames R 2002 Anatomy and Human Movement, 4th edn. Butterworth–Heinemann: Oxford

Reginster JY, Gillet P et al. 1999 Direct costs of hip fractures in patients over 60 years of age in Belgium. Pharmacoeconomics 15(5): 507–514

Roolker W, Maas M et al. 1999 Diagnosis and treatment of scaphoid fractures: can non-union be prevented? Arch Orthop Trauma Surg 119(7–8): 428–431

Salter RB 1993 Continuous Passive Motion (CPM) — A Biological Concept for the Healing and Regeneration of Articular Cartilage, Ligaments and Tendons. Williams & Wilkins: Baltimore

Schurch MA, Rizzoli R et al. 1996 A prospective study of socioeconomic aspects of fracture of the proximal femur. J Bone Miner Res 11(12): 1935–1942

Schwartsman V, Choi SH, Schwartsman R 1990 Tibial nonunions: treatment tactics with the Ilizarov method. Orthop Clin N Am 21(4): 639–653

Sheriff DD, Van Bibber R 1998 Flow-generating capability of the isolated skeletal muscle pump. Am J Physiol 274(5:2): H1502–H1508

Tschakovsky ME, Shoemaker JK et al. 1996 Vasodilation and muscle pump contribution to immediate exercise hyperemia. Am J Physiol 271(4:2): H1679–1701

Viel E, Ripart J et al. 1999 Management of reflex sympathetic dystrophy. Ann Med Interne (Paris) 150(3): 205–210

Chapter 4

Management of burns and plastic surgery

Sally Dean

CHAPTER CONTENTS

This chapter introduces the reader to current practice and physiotherapy management in the field of burns and plastic surgery. Towards the end of the chapter there is a case study of a person with burns, and a selection of further reading.

INTRODUCTION TO BURNS

An external burn injury comprises damage to the skin, and there can be loss of skin and underlying tissues with impairment of skin functions. The effects of a burn depend on its cause and on the extent and site of damage. If serious, a burn injury is thought to be the most severe trauma that is survivable. If patients do survive, their injuries will alter their life as well as that of their families for many years; the disfigurements are for life and will alter their physical function and affect them psychologically. The results of such an injury can be reduced by reconstructive surgery, a high standard of rehabilitation and other therapies. With adequate and appropriate support these patients can and do learn to live their lives to the full again.

Classification of burns

Erythema

The skin remains intact, the erythema lasts for a few days, and the patient does not normally seek medical help unless the problem is extensive, as can occur with sunburn.

Superficial

The tissue damage results in seepage of fluid in between the layers of epidermis, causing a blister, which is surrounded by a dark red erythema. Movement of the burned areas can be very painful. Blisters will continue to appear over the first 24 hours after burning.

Partial-thickness

- In a superficial partial-thickness burn the epidermis is destroyed.
- In a deep dermal burn both the epidermis and part of the dermis are destroyed.

There are blisters, patches of white destroyed tissue, and red areas (Figure 4.1). Sensation varies according to the depth of dermal damage and the sensory nerve endings involved.

Full-thickness

The epidermis, dermis and other underlying tissues are destroyed. The presenting surface may be black, white or yellow. It is inelastic and unable to stretch (the eschar).

If the burn is circumferential (e.g. around the forearm, chest or finger) the damaged skin can have a tourniquet effect as swelling develops. In these cases the tension must be released by longitudinal incisions through the eschar along its full length (escharotomy; Figure 4.2). This procedure will be performed within the first hours of admission to hospital. The skin is dead; therefore no analgesia is required.

Aetiology of burns

The most common causes of injury are fire, chemicals, scalding, electricity and inhalation.

- *Fire burns.* These occur when the patient is caught by fire. Because the clothes ignite, the burns are often partial- or full-thickness. Flash flames tend to cause partial-thickness burns.
- *Chemical burns.* Caustic substances (e.g. cement) can cause deep burns. The depth of tissue involved can be limited by prompt action.
- *Scalding.* Hot water is the most common cause of scalds. It may be in the form of a hot drink, or boiling fluid from a pan or kettle. Scalds are common in the elderly, often caused when climbing into a hot bath and being unable to climb out again. These burns will vary in depth relative to the exposure time.
- *Electrical burns.* Burns will appear on the skin where there has been contact with a live wire. There will be a burn at the entry and exit site of the electric current. Neither the depth nor the size of the burn is predictable. There can be extensive damage to deep structures with little external evidence. Often this type of injury is complicated by cardiac and respiratory arrest.
- *Inhalation burns.* Direct thermal injury can be sustained by inhalation of flames, hot gases or steam. This constitutes a major threat to the upper airway, causing oedema of the larynx, pharynx and trachea. Early diagnosis of an inhalation injury is essential. The patient must be intubated before the oedema becomes extensive, as this will prevent the passing of the endotracheal tube.

Prevention of burns

There have been a number of studies relating to burn prevention, but from these there emerges no clear method for effective prevention (British Burns Association 2001, p. 62). A large number of burns result from domestic accidents in the home, young children and the elderly being particularly vulnerable. It is essential to ensure that:

- kettles and hot pans are out of the reach of children
- electrical sockets have shutters, and electrical cables are secure with the insulation intact

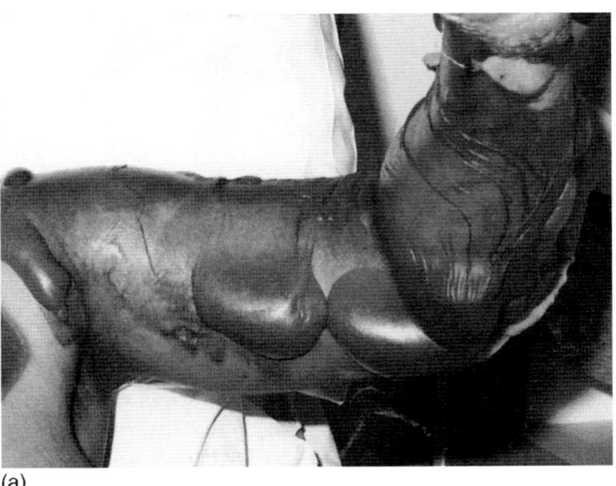

(a)

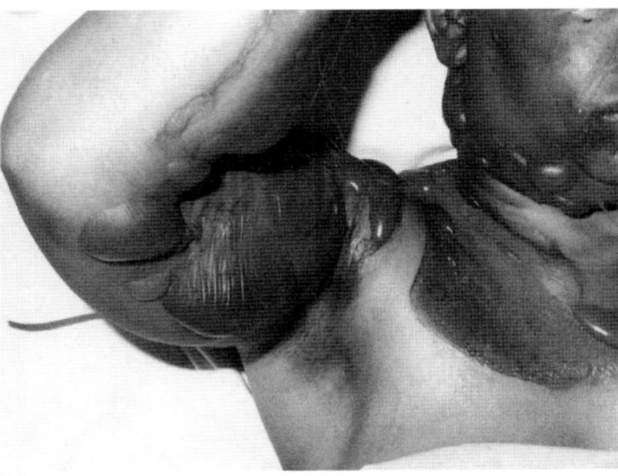

(b)

Figure 4.1 Partial-thickness burns to both upper limbs and neck with extensive blister formation.

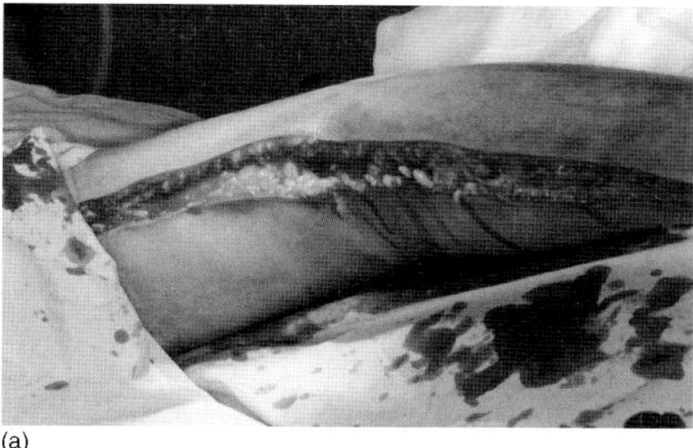
(a)

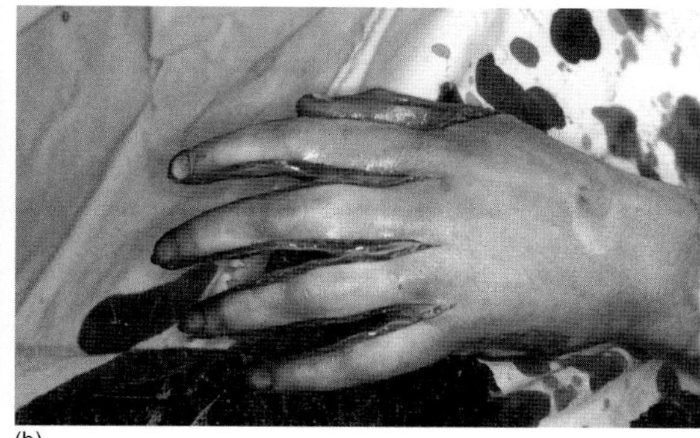
(b)

Figure 4.2 Full-thickness burns: inelastic leather-like skin with escharotomies to (a) lower limb and (b) fingers.

- circuit breakers are in use with external appliances
- matches and cigarette lighters are stored safely
- thermostatic valves are fitted to bathroom taps
- smoke alarms are fitted
- clothes, especially children's, are flameproof.

A number of burns are industrial, caused by chemicals, electrical accidents, molten metals, friction burns or blowbacks. The Health and Safety at Work Act 1974 and other legislation have gone some way towards preventing such accidents by enforcing rising standards of safe working practices.

PATHOLOGICAL CHANGES WITH BURNS

Shock

Definition

The inability of the circulatory system to meet the needs of tissues for oxygen and nutrients and the removal of their metabolites (Dietzman and Lillehei 1968; cited by Settle 1986).

Shock can last for 2–3 days, and longer in the elderly. Within minutes of the burn being sustained, oedema gathers beneath the damaged areas, a result of increased capillary permeability of the affected tissues. There is loss of protein and electrolytes from the blood. The main changes are:

- reduced plasma volume — hypovolaemia
- increased ratio of red blood cells to plasma in the blood vessels — resulting in increased blood viscosity and slowing of the circulation
- reduction of cardiac output
- increased heart rate.

During this stage the main dangers are from pulmonary oedema, occlusion of arteries, cardiac failure, renal failure, liver failure, and permanent brain and vital organ damage.

Inhalation injury

Thermal pulmonary damage will result from the inhalation of steam, or from flames igniting a fuel/oxygen gas mixture in the airways. Injury to the alveoli will be caused by the inhalation of corrosive and toxic fumes released as products of combustion. It may be difficult to diagnose such an injury when the patient is first admitted and further investigations are required.

Carboxyhaemoglobin (COHb) levels are raised in patients with smoke inhalation and the level of blood COHb can be used in diagnosis. A level of COHb of over 15 per cent at 3 hours after the incident is strong evidence of smoke inhalation.

Hypoxia can result from alveolar damage, causing ventilatory insufficiency, impairment of the circulation and reduced oxygen transport (COHb). A Pao_2 of less than 10 kPa when inspired oxygen concentration is 50 per cent is suggestive of an inhalation injury.

The airway will have mucosal oedema in the bronchi, carbonaceous sputum and possible bleeding or ulceration of the lining of the bronchial tree. To find diagnostic evidence of these a fibreoptic bronchoscopy can be carried out.

None of the above physiological changes would give rise to alteration of a normal X-ray of the lung fields in the early post-burn period, so X-rays are of no value in the initial diagnosis of an inhalation injury.

Complications of burns

See Table 4.1.

Table 4.1 Complications of burns

- Heart problems
- Inhalation injuries
- Pneumonia
- Acute respiratory distress syndrome – ARDS (shock lung)
- Infection of the wound site
- Infection of the urinary tract
- Septicaemia
- Renal and liver failure
- Joint effusion and periarticular swelling
- Calcification of periarticular tissues
- Contraction of scar tissue causing joint deformity
- Psychological trauma to the patient

PROGNOSIS OF THE BURNS PATIENT

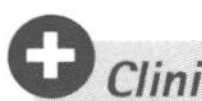

Clinical note

Burns in people aged over 60 years or under 5 years carry a poor prognosis.

Total burn surface area (TBSA)

The greater the total burn surface area, the poorer the prognosis. A formula for gauging outcome is: percentage chance of survival = [100 – (age in years + percentage TBSA)]. For example, a 60-year-old with 30 per cent TBSA has a 10 per cent chance of survival [100 – (60 + 30)]. A 20-year-old with the same TBSA has a chance of survival of [100 – (20 + 30)], or 50 per cent.

It is interesting to note that if both legs are burnt, 36 per cent TBSA is affected. Therefore, a 50-year-old with such extensive burns has [100 – (50 + 36)] or 14 per cent chance of recovery. A method for gauging the total body surface area is the 'rule of nines'. This rule divides the body surface into 11 areas, each constituting 9 per cent of the total (Figure 4.3). The perineum is counted as 1 per cent. Other charts may be used (e.g. the Lund and Browder chart).

An experienced doctor should carry out the assessment of the TBSA, as the correct percentage area will determine the correct volume of fluid replacement required for the resuscitation process. It must be noted that the TBSA cannot be considered alone, as the site and depth of the injury will affect the prognosis. For example a 4 per cent TBSA superficial burn on the back of a young fit male will lead to a full recovery, where as a 4 per cent TBSA of the face with an inhalation injury could lead to complications or even death. The level of hospital care will also differ with the above injuries.

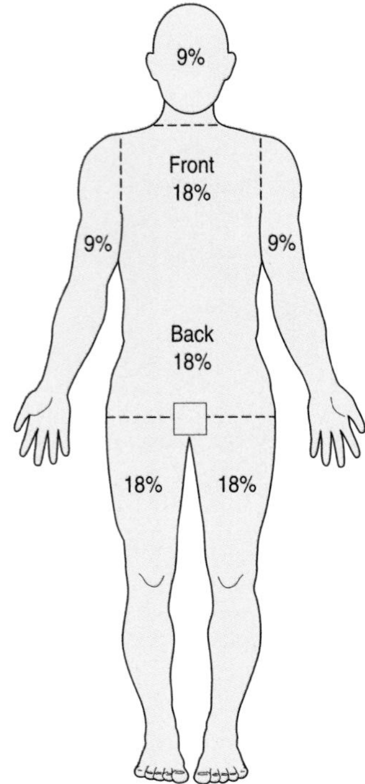

Figure 4.3 The 'rule of nines'.

The accuracy and variability of burn size calculations using the Lund and Browder charts currently in clinical use and the rule of nines diagrams have been evaluated. The study showed that variability in estimation increased with burn size initially, plateaued in large burns, and then decreased slightly in extensive burns. The rule of nines technique may overestimate the size of the burn, but it is somewhat faster than the Lund and Browder method (Wachtel 2000).

Key point

Patients with a poor prognosis must be treated with the same care and attention as any other.

Inhalation burns

A high percentage of patients with facial burns develop pneumonia. Where there are inhalation burns as well, the mortality rate is very high.

CLINICAL FEATURES OF BURNS

The following signs and symptoms may be present, depending on the extent of the burn.

At the site of the burn

- Redness — erythema.
- Blisters.
- Weeping of plasma — straw-coloured.
- Yellow/white skin — leathery in nature.
- Blackened crispy tissues — exposed blackened structures.

Inhalation injury

- Burnt lips and nose.
- Soot in the nostrils and mouth.
- Singed nasal and facial hair.
- Hoarseness of the voice.
- Sore throat.

During shock (up to 3 days post-burn)

- Restlessness and disorientation.
- Coldness and paleness of the skin.
- Collapsed veins and rapid pulse.
- Sweating.
- Thirst.
- Hypotension.
- Tachycardia.
- Rapid breathing — later becoming gasping.
- Cyanosis.

Post-shock phase

- Separation of the burned skin (eschar).
- Formation of scar tissue.
- Contraction of scar tissue, causing (a) pain due to traction of the sensory nerve endings; (b) limitation of joint movement; (c) joint deformities; (d) loss of function.

Long-term

The severity of dysfunction and disfigurement depends on the site and extent of burn:

- possible amputation of a limb
- disabling damage to the hands
- possible loss of independence
- loss of employment
- facial damage, making rehabilitation of the patient and family very difficult
- social rejection
- emotional trauma for both patient and relatives.

MANAGEMENT OF BURNS

First aid

A friend, relative or stranger may rescue the victim of a serious burn accident. The decisions made and the treatment given at the scene of the accident — especially the quality of the first aid — has often had a profound effect on mortality and morbidity (British Burns Association 2001, p. 17).

- *Flame burns* must be smothered. Cold water applied continuously over the burnt area relieves pain and limits the depth of the burn, because heat is conducted to the deeper tissues for several minutes after the flames have been extinguished.
- With *chemical burns*, contaminated clothing must be removed and copious quantities of running water applied to the area. Neutralising agents need to be identified and applied accordingly.
- With *scalds*, thorough and continuous dousing with cold water can limit the extent of the damage and reduce the pain.
- With *electrical burns*, the patient may require cardiopulmonary resuscitation (CPR) before attention can be paid to the injury. Unlike heat burns, these injuries do not spread and it is sufficient to cover the area with a clean cloth that has been soaked in clean cold water.

4

Hospital referral

Referral guidelines

The determining criterion for admission to a burns unit was traditionally the area of skin injured. Now it is based on the complexity of the injury. Guidelines for burn injury referral have been set (British Burns Association 2001, pp. 68–69).

Minor burns

These are defined as less than 10 per cent surface area in a child or less than 15 per cent in an adult. If the injury is non-complex, these injuries are cleaned with chlorhexidine and covered with a bactericidal non-stick dressing. The patient can rest at home and, depending on local circumstances, the dressings are changed every 2–3 days by a district nurse or at the hospital dressings clinic.

Major burns

These are injuries that involve 10 per cent or more of the body surface area in children and 15 per cent or more in an adult. If the injury is complex, the patient will be admitted to the burns unit or intensive care unit.

Medical management

Early hospital management (including the shock phase) involves:

- maintenance of a clear airway
- pain relief
- assessment of TBSA

- maintenance of fluid balance (see below)
- removal of adherent clothing and covering of the burns with sterile cotton dressings
- application of neutralising agents for chemical burns
- reassurance and explanation to the patient
- transfer to a burns unit or admission for an intensive care unit.

Whether the person is sent to the operating theatre for shaving of burns and grafting depends on the depth of the burns, the age of the patient and whether he or she is fit for surgery.

Resuscitation

Fluid replacement is administered over a 36-hour period (from the occurrence of the burn, not the time of arrival at hospital).

The volume of plasma required by the burns patient is related to the TBSA and the size of the patient (Evans et al. 1952; cited by Settle 1986, p. 14). To calculate the volume of fluid required for resuscitation, the following formula is used (Muir and Barclay 1962): mL of plasma = {1/2} TBSA × age of patient.

Management of the wound areas

All injuries to the skin need to be repaired, either by dressings alone or by some form of skin replacement.

Management of wound areas varies according to the experience of the staff and facilities available. The two main themes are 'open' or 'closed'.

Open method

This method leaves the wound exposed. If exudate is cleaned away regularly, the area dries out and bacterial growth is inhibited. This method is used for areas that are difficult to dress, such as the face. Healing of the epithelium tends to be slower than with the closed method.

Closed method

The primary layer of dressing is non-adherent: for example, petroleum jelly gauze. This is then covered with layers of absorbent cotton gauze or gamgee, held in place by crêpe bandages or net. With bandages securing the dressings the patient may be able to begin to mobilise about the ward with the aid of the physiotherapist (see below).

Dressings may need to be changed frequently (daily). For the patient this can be very painful and distressing. In order to achieve the process with this in mind, the use of general anaesthesia and sedatives for dressing changes is becoming the practice.

Surgical intervention

If the skin is so damaged that it prevents spontaneous healing using the above methods, then it will require skin grafting. This must be carried out at the earliest possible opportunity following the initial injury. A burn that requires surgical intervention may first require tangential excision. The wound is gradually debrided until all necrotic tissue is removed and only healthy tissue remains. This process is carried out progressively until the wound bed is bleeding, thus indicating healthy tissue.

Healing and reconstruction

After superficial burns, the skin heals and can be normal. Following burns that have destroyed the epidermis, there is scar tissue. Over a number of weeks this tissue can become contracted and bound down or may have excessive growth, as in keloid scarring.

Where there is extensive destruction of the skin, the patient undergoes grafting and reconstructive surgery, which may take months. In the case of children there may have to be episodes of surgery for many years.

Surgical management of full-thickness burns

Escharectomy is removal of the dead, burnt skin by a method of excision or shaving. This may be carried out on the day of admission, depending on the stability of the patient. A bleeding surface remains, which has to be grafted.

Grafting involves covering the open tissues with a layer of split skin (see under plastic surgery below). This may be from an uninjured area on the patient (an autograft) or from another person (allograft). Temporary and permanent skin replacements such as pig skin, skin banks, cadaver skin, laboratory-cultured skin cells and synthetic skin replacements may be used where there are extensive areas to be covered. Grafts other than autografts do not give permanent cover but provide protection for 2–3 weeks.

Donor sites (for autografts) take 10–14 days to heal and can be very painful during the first few days. Where there is a shortage of available donor sites on the body owing to the area of the burn, the 'split-skin' that is removed for grafting purposes has to be extremely thin so that the donor area can be used again after 14 days. Unfortunately these very thin grafts have a greater tendency to contract.

Extensive burns require considerable excision and grafting carried out every 1–2 weeks. This is a long and distressful period for the patient, who has to have repeated anaesthesia and operations.

Grafts are kept in position with petroleum jelly gauze and bandages, and splints can be applied to immobilise the joints adjacent to the grafts.The dressings are taken down at 24 hours after grafting to look for any formation of haematoma or a seroma (space filled with serum). The change of dressings can be very painful and the process may be carried out on the ward, under a general anaesthetic or with the use of Entonox.

Permanent skin substitutes

Epidermal cells

Epithelial cells can be cultured from a small skin biopsy. The process forms sheets of epithelial cells, which are then attached to a petroleum gauze carrier to ease handling. Although the use of these in treatment of burns has increased, the outcomes have many imperfections, thought to be attributable to the absence of a dermal element (Herndon 2002).

Dermal analogs

The characteristics of flexibility, strength, lubrication, sensation and heat dissipation are provided by the dermis in normal skin. Integra™ was the first dermal substitute to be developed and used successfully in a clinical situation in the treatment of widespread burns. It consists of an inner layer of collagen fibers and glycosaminoglycan chondroitin-6-sulphate. This layer allows fibrovascular ingrowth, after which it is designed to biodegrade. The outer layer of the membrane is a polymer with characteristics similar to normal epithelium. This product is designed to be placed on freshly excised full-thickness burns and the outer silicone layer is replaced with a very thin epithelial autograft 2–3 weeks later (Herndon 2002).

Composite substitutes

The ideal skin replacement would have both dermal and epidermal layers. Work on such a product has been going on for years, with some success in animals, and products are presently undergoing clinical pilot trials.

THE BURNED HAND

The hand accounts for only 3 per cent TBSA, yet it is involved in a large percentage of treated burn injuries. The hand is commonly burned in isolation and rarely escapes injury in burns of 60 per cent TBSA or more. The hands are often burned when used in a reflex action to protect the face or extinguish a fire. Dorsal burns are far more common than palmar, the skin of the palm being much thicker; burns to the dorsum may be full-thickness where a palmar burn will be less thick. Burns of the hand will often indicate referral to a regional burns unit for specialist care.

Most hand burns occur in employed males who sustain injury at work, including flame, electrical or chemical burns. Injuries at home are more likely to be caused by scalds or open fires. Contact burns are most common in small children.

Treatment of the burned hand

To allow free movement of the hands they are placed in a polythene bag containing chlorhexidine, an antibacterial agent, and the bag is bandaged to the forearm (Figure 4.4).

The patient is able to exercise the hand freely through full range of motion at regular intervals. The bag is changed daily, or more frequently if indicated by large amounts of exudate collecting in the bag. The bag is changed to dry dressings at the nurse's discretion. The physiotherapist must be aware of the change and encourage the patient to maintain the range of motion, as this becomes more difficult when the wounds begin to dry.

Exercise of the hand

The exercise regime will depend on the extent of injury and the severity of the burn.

For superficial and partial-thickness burns, full range of active movement is encouraged, including isolated flexion and extension of individual joints as well as composite movement. Thumb abduction, extension

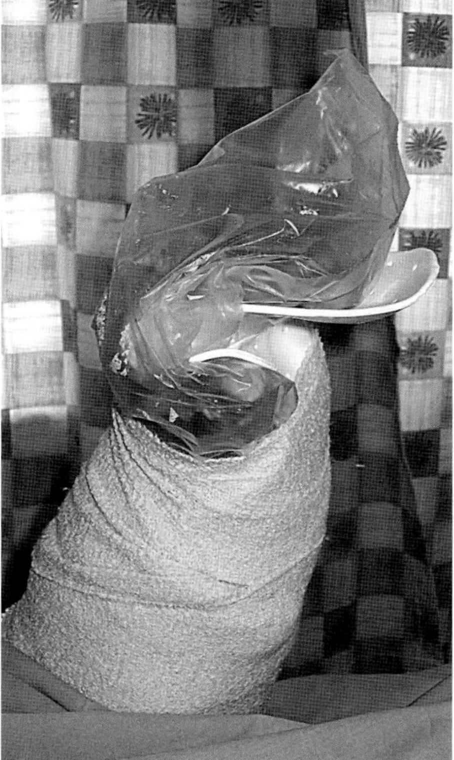

Figure 4.4 Mixed-depth burns 2 days after injury, wrapped in a plastic bag with a volar resting splint.

4

and opposition are encouraged, as are fist-making, hooking of the fingers and lumbrical stretches.

For deep dermal and full-thickness burns care must be taken if it is thought the extensor apparatus is involved in the damaged tissues. When moving the IP joints care must be taken to avoid extensor tendon rupture. To avoid excessive stretches of these structures passive flexion is not carried out, and fist-making must be supervised by the physiotherapist.

Splints are to be worn at all times, and are only removed for dressing changes and physiotherapy sessions.

Where a deeper burn has disrupted the mechanics of the proximal IP joint in a finger, i.e. tendon rupture, exposed or joint damage, this will give rise to a boutonnière deformity (PIP joint flexion with distal IP joint hyperextension). This must be managed by static splinting to hold the PIP joint in extension, allowing healing; secondary reconstruction of the extensor may be carried out at a later date.

Complications of the burned hand

Oedema develops very quickly post-burn and poses a serious threat to hand mobility and function. Elevation is therefore of the utmost importance very early on and a flow pulse machine may be of use.

The burned hand will adopt a poor posture with the wrist in flexion, metacarpal joint extension, IP joint flexion and thumb in adduction.

The common challenges of a burn injury to the hand may include contractures of the thumb web, PIP joints of the fingers and dorsal skin, and little finger boutonnière deformity.

In the acute phase treatment may be impaired by poorly fitting splints due to frequently changed dressings and fluctuation in swelling, prolonged immobilisation and delays in commencing active mobilisation.

During the rehabilitation phase progress may be affected by poor compliance with garments and splints, and poor attendance as an outpatient after hospitalisation.

A comprehensive treatment plan must be engaged for patients with these injuries in order to return the hands to as near normal function as possible. The physiotherapist will be responsible for oedema control, patient positioning, splint maintenance, progression of functional tasks and strengthening of both fine pinch and power grip.

REHABILITATIVE PHYSIOTHERAPY OF A BURNS PATIENT

Therapy is dependent upon, and should be tailored to, the stage of tissue healing (Glassey 2004).

The rehabilitation process commences on the day of admission. The ultimate goal for the burns team is to return the individual to society with unaltered appearance, abilities and potential. This is very often impossible owing to the nature of the burn, but the goal remains the same. The process of rehabilitation involves healthcare professionals, support groups and the individual's family and friends. The burns care team consists of a multidisciplinary team of professionals who specialise in the care of the burns patient. In addition to medical, nursing and therapy staff, a dietitian, psychologist, cosmetologist and plastic surgery prosthetist (to name a few) may be involved in the rehabilitation process.

It is impossible to say exactly what intensity of treatment a burns patient should receive, as this depends on the complexity and extent of the injury. The more complex burns require intensive physiotherapy and an experienced therapist to assess their needs and develop a treatment plan (CSP Therapy Standards Working Group 2000).

Inpatients may be treated in a special ward, intensive care unit or regional burns unit. The latter is most advantageous because the patient receives specialist attention, but difficulties can arise for relatives needing to undertake long journeys to visit. The physiotherapist and other team members must recognise the devastating effect a bad case of burning can have on the family. It is important to recognise mood changes — guilt, depression, anger, bewilderment and bitterness — which can arise in the patient and family. The cause of the accident clearly has a bearing on these moods. The physiotherapist has to gauge what the appropriate reaction is — sympathy, cajoling, encouragement or optimism — whilst achieving the aims of treatment.

Aims

The aims of physiotherapy are to:

- achieve a clear airway and so prevent respiratory complications
- maintain joint range of movement, and prevent contractures or deformities
- maintain soft-tissue length
- maintain muscle strength
- regain maximum function
- minimise scarring
- help the patient to gain independence and return to an active lifestyle.

Respiratory care

Chest physiotherapy consists of vibrations, percussion, postural drainage, coughing and suction to clear secretions. Patients with infection must be treated several times a day. If it is very uncomfortable for the patient to have hand pressure applied to a chest burn, then a piece of foam may be used under the hands. If the patient has chest burns and no respiratory complications, vibrations and percussion should be kept to minimum where possible, as further trauma to the already burned tissue may lead to superficial burns becoming deeper.

Tipping is contraindicated if there is facial oedema but the patient may lie supine or on either side. A ventilated patient usually requires suction and humidification. A little treatment is often the most effective. Humidification may be necessary for the non-ventilated patient, especially when there has been inhalation of smoke or fumes. Breathing (expansion) exercises are also important to maintain ventilation of all lung areas. When the patient has respiratory problems, the physiotherapist must not be afraid to treat with the vigour required to achieve these aims, even when the chest skin is burnt.

Intensive respiratory care is required in the following situations:

- for the elderly patient
- for burns affecting face, mouth and respiratory passages
- for immobile patients
- where there is a history of a chronic respiratory condition
- pre- and postoperatively
- for patients with a full-thickness burn to the chest to keep the eschar mobile.

Joint range of movement

Positioning, splinting and exercise are used for maintaining and improving joint range.

Positioning

The position of comfort for the patient is usually that of joint flexion. Unfortunately, this allows scar tissue to contract and cause deformities. Therefore, it is essential that joints be held in the correct position during recovery. The correct positions to be maintained are described below.

Head and neck

A small roll (towel) behind the neck and/or a pillow under the shoulders will help to maintain extension of the cervical spine. The patient may be in lying (chest and leg burns) or in half-lying (with facial burns — because of facial oedema).

Upper limbs

The upper limbs should be elevated on pillows with the shoulder in abduction and slight flexion, the elbows and wrists in extension, and the hands with MCP joints in flexion, IP joints in extension, and thumb in palmar abduction. The joints of the hand are held in position by static splints.

Lower limbs

The lower limbs are rested with the hip joints in extension and slight abduction, knees in extension and ankles in 90-degree dorsiflexion (in a foot drop splint). Elevation is obtained by raising the end of the bed, not by placing pillows under the legs, which would put the hips into flexion.

4

Splinting

Splints may be static or dynamic.

Static splints

Static splints are used when it is essential to maintain a certain joint position until movement can start or to maintain a satisfactory resting position between exercises. These are designed and made to individual requirements using thermoplastics and modified as the patient recovers, such as after passive stretching. Splinting may be required at night only to prevent soft-tissue tightening whilst the patient is asleep. Nearly all patients will require hand-resting splints and foot-drop splints.

Dynamic splints

Dynamic splints can permit controlled movement of various joints. For example, an MCP extension splint to all four fingers allows some flexion of the fingers, thus allowing damaged extensor tendons to move in a limited range but not to be overstretched.

With a dynamic finger MCP joint flexion and thumb abduction splint (Figure 4.5), wrist extension is maintained and leather loops are positioned over the proximal phalanges of each finger and pulled volarly by elastic traction. The thumb is pulled into abduction to widen the first web space.

With a flexor glove wrist extension is maintained, and straps pass from the fingers to the volar aspect of the splint, thus performing passive composite flexion of the fingers (Figure 4.6).

A collar may be necessary to maintain the neck position because the skin over the anterior aspect of the neck contracts very readily, pulling the lower jaw down to the chest. A soft material may be adequate for daytime and a firmer one used at night (Figure 4.7).

General points for splinting

- The position has to be effective, but is not necessarily the position of function.
- Joints must not be included unnecessarily in splints.
- Tight encircling must be avoided. Splints must be bandaged on evenly.

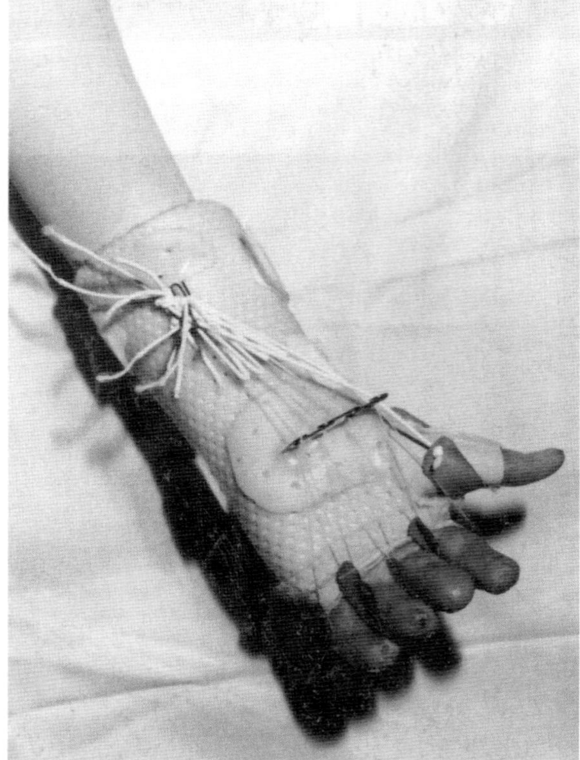

Figure 4.5 Dynamic finger MCP joint flexion and thumb abduction splint.

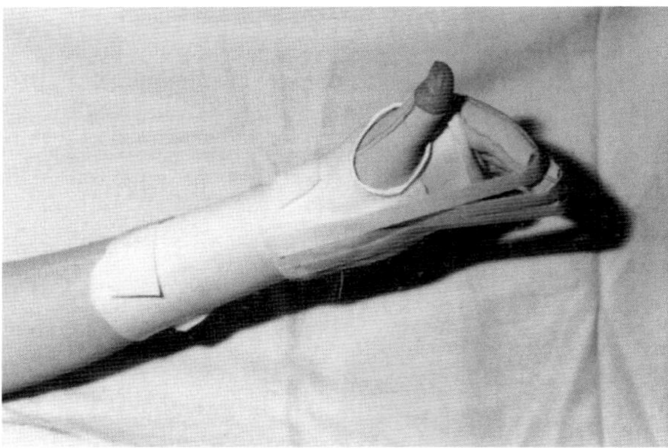

Figure 4.6 Flexor glove.

- Grafts and flaps must not be subjected to pressure from the splint material.
- Bony prominences must be avoided where possible or require corresponding padding within the splint.
- Nerve compression must be avoided.

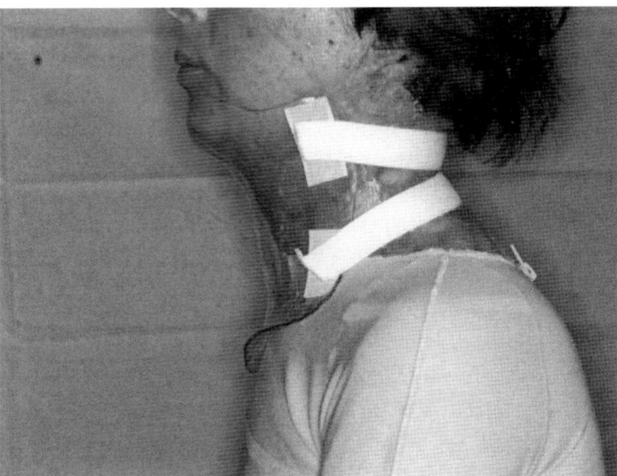

Figure 4.7 Rigid collar to maintain soft-tissue length following deep dermal burns to the neck and chest.

- Correction and prevention of deformity is essential but so too is muscular activity. Therefore, intermittent and dynamic splinting must be used where possible.

Exercises

Every joint should, where possible, be moved through full range of movement each day. An active exercise programme must be devised to achieve this. Assisted active exercises or passive movements are necessary for the damaged limbs and free active exercise for undamaged areas. If the patient is sedated and unable to perform exercises, passive movements must be carried out at regular intervals. Movement should be performed frequently to reduce oedema and resultant joint stiffness.

During bathing, the patient is immersed in water and, where possible, physiotherapy should be incorporated. All joints should be moved individually through full range and composite movements carried out, either actively or passively, with respect to exposed tendons and any other associated injuries: for example, fractures. The exercise programme can be started on the day of the burn and must take place daily.

Exercise can be very painful. Where possible, treatment should be timetabled to coincide with the patient's medication; alternatively Entonox may be utilised. The physiotherapist may take the opportunity to mobilise restricted joints whilst the patient is under anaesthetic in the operating theatre. This is an ideal forum because the surgeon will be able to assess the need for release of scar tissue if this is causing the limited range. The range of movement gained during treatment will be controlled by the patient's tolerance level of pain and the limitations of movement of the burnt tissues.

The physiotherapist may perform passive movements through the dressings or the hand bags. If movement is restricted by the adherence of the dressings, then treatment can be carried out whilst the dressings are down. Therefore good communication and cooperation are essential between the therapists and the nursing staff.

Once the patient is alert enough and the intravenous drips and lines are minimal, he or she can be allowed to sit out of bed and may attempt standing. A tilt table may be used to bring the patient gradually into the vertical position. Once the patient is able to stand, walking is commenced. The use of a pulpit frame or Zimmer walking frame may be necessary.

As soon as possible, the patient must be encouraged to be independent in self-care and activities of daily living.

Muscle strengthening

Where joints can be moved, the patient must work the muscles for each joint through full range at least twice a day. Muscles working over joints, which are fixed, can be worked isometrically. The use of small weights, graded rubber exercise bands and springs can increase muscle strength. An exercise programme can be devised for the patient to carry out during the day.

As soon as possible, the patient should be up and about and following an exercise/activity programme. Where possible, an exercise circuit in the physiotherapy gym should be commenced.

Regaining maximum function

Function is the ability to perform activities of daily living at home, work and leisure. An individual circuit is worked out which involves free exercise and equipment work. Goals should be set, such as so many minutes on an exercise bike, so many repetitions without rest on skipping, jumping a height, or reaching a grip strength by a given time (in weeks). This programme continues and is progressed as the patient improves, with modifications following grafting. Trips to the hospital shop and then to neighbouring shops and pubs may be included so that the patient starts to feel like a member of society again. A home visit may be carried out to assess the patient's mobility and level of independence. Discharge home is arranged as soon as the patient and relatives are ready.

Outpatient physiotherapy

Some patients may require continuation of dressings once discharged from hospital and will attend the burns outpatient clinic. The physiotherapist should be present to assess the range of movement, the healing process and scar formation. Contractures must be prevented by regular passive stretching, and mobility of scar tissue is maintained by techniques of scar management (see later). The patient can continue with the rehabilitation programme at the same time, which may involve continuing gym work. When all the wounds have fully healed and the grafts are stable, the patient is assessed and measured for pressure garments (see later).

As a member of an outreach team, the physiotherapist may visit patients near to or at their home. This concept of the burns care team travelling to different sites to treat the burns patient has been piloted and proven to be of value. These outreach teams are essential for continuity of care and have the following functions:

- enabling patient discharge with support in or near the patient's home
- education of the local general hospital-based nurses and therapists and of community rehabilitation teams
- offering an accessible expert resource for the local hospital and community health professionals, patients and their families (British Burns Association 2006, p. 40).

> **Clinical note**
>
> Smaller burns may be treated by physiotherapy on an outpatient basis. Active exercise is just as important for small burns as for larger ones so that scar tissue is kept mobile and prevented from causing adhesions or contracting.

Return to active lifestyle

From the start the patient's independence is encouraged, and the entire multidisciplinary team dealing with the patient work together to encourage, sympathise and cajole. The physiotherapist has sometimes to push the patient hard, particularly where likelihood of contractures or loss of function is high, as with burns to the hands, axillae, chest, feet and anterior aspect of the neck.

Many patients with a burn injury find the transfer from hospitalisation to life in the community challenging and exhibit a whole range of problems at different times in the recovery process. Sometimes it helps to have patients meet people who have recovered from severe injuries, and self-help groups can provide invaluable long-term support. Return to work is obviously dependent on the nature of work and type of injury but generally the patient should return, even if there are interruptions for release operations, follow-up appointments and pressure garment refits. Family, friends and employers have, therefore, to play a part in the restoration of a full active lifestyle.

Children

The treatment of children follows the same principles as for adults. The physiotherapist will need to teach the family how to perform exercises and stretches. The family must encourage the child to be as independent as possible (e.g. feeding). The patient will be reviewed on a regular basis during the years of growth until reaching adulthood.

INTRODUCTION TO PLASTIC SURGERY

The term 'plastic surgery' was introduced in the early nineteenth century. It describes the technique of moulding tissues. The work is largely reconstructive following trauma, excision of diseased tissue or correction of a congenital deformity. Burns are usually managed by the plastic surgeon in the acute phase and then in the correction of resultant deformities (Morgan and Wright 1986).

This section discusses the use and management of skin grafts and flaps.

Definition

Skin grafts consist of slices of skin removed from one part of the body (the donor area) and applied to a raw surface in another part (the recipient site).

Skin grafts

Skin grafts may be used for any part of the body in areas where there has been damage by burns, lacerated wounds, ulceration, pressure sores, skin cancers or healed contracted scars. A graft is used only when the recipient site is vascular (i.e. in soft-tissue injuries). Types include split-skin grafts and full-thickness grafts.

Split-skin grafts

Split-skin (Thiersch) grafts consist of a very thin layer of epidermis, or a thicker layer, up to the whole epidermis and part dermis. These grafts are transferred without blood supply.

This type of graft can be taken from several parts of the body, the most common being the volar aspect of the thigh and the medial aspect of the upper arm.

The graft may be applied to the recipient site in strips or large sheets. If the recipient site is large and the split skin is smaller, the skin can be meshed to increase the area of coverage. The graft is passed through an instrument that shreds the skin at intervals to give an even meshwork (Figure 4.8).

Any skin that has been cut in excess of requirements can be stored at a temperature of 4° C and remains viable for later use for up to 21 days. The graft is wrapped in gauze moistened with saline and placed in a sterile closed container within the refrigerator (McGregor 1989).

The recipient site

Split-skin grafts are applied to raw surfaces or granulating wounds. The area must be as flat as possible and bleeding stopped. The graft is cut to size and applied raw surface down. It may be sutured, stapled or glued in place. Petroleum jelly gauze and crêpe bandages are applied.

Where it is necessary to hold the graft in contact with the recipient site, such as in a concave defect, the graft will be dressed with either a pressure or a 'tie-over' dressing. Sutures applied to the edges of the graft are left long enough to be tied over the top of the cotton wool pressure dressing, thus holding the graft down on to the bed.

For the first 48 hours nutrition is obtained from free tissue fluid of the recipient site. Capillaries grow into the graft and vascularisation is generally established after 48 hours. This is a critical time because movement of the graft destroys the capillary buds and the graft does not 'take'. Reasons for failure of a graft may be a haematoma under the graft or 'tenting' where the graft has contracted and lifted the central area off the recipient bed.

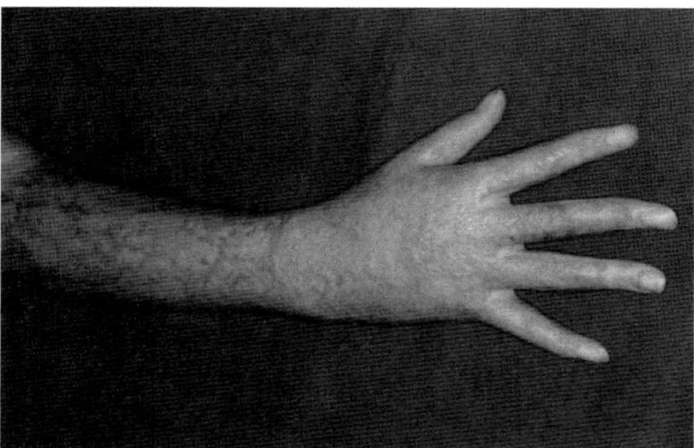

Figure 4.8 Dorsum of hand with meshed split skin 8 weeks after grafting. Note the mesh pattern in the skin surface.

The dressings are taken down after 24 hours to look for formation of a haematoma or a seroma. Grafts to the lower leg are redressed with double crêpe bandage and Tubigrip. These patients can then commence physiotherapy and mobilise.

The donor site

Donor sites are healed in 9–14 days, depending on the thickness of skin removed. A donor area used for full-thickness skin has to be covered by a split-skin graft or closed primarily.

The donor area for a split-skin graft is dressed with petroleum jelly gauze and crêpe bandage and left undisturbed for 14 days. If attempts are made to remove the dressing too early, the area bleeds and is very painful as the regenerating epithelium is torn away.

Once healed, the donor area is managed with moisturising cream and massage, and if necessary protected with sun block.

Full-thickness grafts

A 'full thickness' (Wolfe) graft includes the skin down to but excluding superficial fascia. This type of graft has little tendency to contract and has an appearance similar to normal skin. Because of this, these grafts are commonly used on the face or the hand (Figure 4.9).

The donor site will not heal spontaneously and will require direct closure by suture or coverage with a split-skin graft. Common donor sites are behind the ear (post-auricular) for the face, as there is a good colour match, and the upper arm, as closure is easy.

The management of full-thickness grafts is the same as for split-skin grafts. Scar management is still necessary, although the graft should not contract as much.

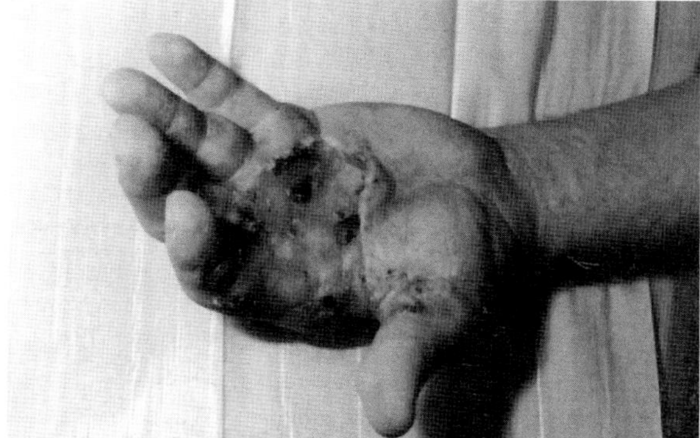

Figure 4.9 Full-thickness skin graft to the palm following fasciectomy, 2 weeks after grafting.

Physiotherapy following skin grafting

General principles

Range of movement of the surrounding joints is maintained by exercises. If the patient is on bed rest, a regime of bed maintenance exercises is implemented. Once the graft is stable, the patient is instructed in active range-of-motion exercises to the joints affected by the graft. This is best carried out with the dressing removed.

The circulation to the graft should not be impaired by this activity and the therapist should observe the colour of the graft. Where the grafted area is 'squeezed' or folded, as it is in the palm of the hand on full flexion of the fingers, the circulation is intermittently occluded. The same occurs when a graft is put on excessive stretch and it will blanch. The graft should be allowed to 'pink up' in between each movement as the circulation re-establishes in the tissues. The area should not be rested with any stretching or folds to the grafted area; nor should the graft be rested upon, as this may compromise the capillary flow to the new skin.

After about 14 days, the graft begins to contract and there is a danger that it will become adherent to underlying tissues. The physiotherapist must be aware of this and practise scar management techniques to maintain range of movement and soft-tissue length.

Scar management

The complications that arise from scar formation are:

- adherence of graft to underlying tissues
- contracting scar tissue
- reduced range of movement
- hard immobile tissues
- red raised areas
- discomfort of tight skin
- persistent itching.

The objectives of physiotherapy are therefore to:

- mobilise soft tissues
- increase range of movement — passive and active
- prevent further contraction of the scar
- reduce redness and flatten raised areas
- reduce pain and discomfort
- lengthen soft tissues.

Treatment techniques

Passive stretches

Where there is restricted range of movement caused by tight scar tissue, the physiotherapist performs passive movement at the end of range to create a stretch to the scar. The amount of force applied will be controlled by the pain tolerance of the patient, the 'give' of the tissues under stretch and the circulation to the area. The physiotherapist must observe the colour changes of the scar carefully; when at full stretch it will blanch and this can be used as a guide to the effectiveness of the treatment. When the scar tissue does not respond to repeated treatments or the contraction increases, the tissues will require surgical release to regain the range of movement.

Massage

Once the graft is stable and the edges fully healed, massage can be commenced. A moisturising cream can be applied during this process. The massage should initially be carried out at the edges of the graft with small movements and superficial pressure. Gradually work more centrally as the graft matures. It is important to avoid pressure and sliding over the skin, as this will cause blistering of the graft. The aim is to soften and mobilise the grafted tissue to enable freedom of movement, improve nutrition and therefore restore function.

Pressure garments

These garments are made to measure and constructed from elasticated material (Figure 4.10). They are worn for nearly 24 hours a day and removed for washing and cream massage of the scars. They are used to reduce hypertrophic scarring, which is excessive formation of collagen resulting in thick, rope-like, uneven scars, which both limit function and look unsightly. They also assist in flattening raised areas and reducing the redness of skin grafts. Pressure by an elasticated garment worn almost continuously for up to 2 years reduces this scarring.

The individual requires reassessment on a regular basis for adjustments to the garment size and shape as the person either grows or puts on weight.

The garments may be manufactured by staff on the hospital site or can be ordered from specialist suppliers.

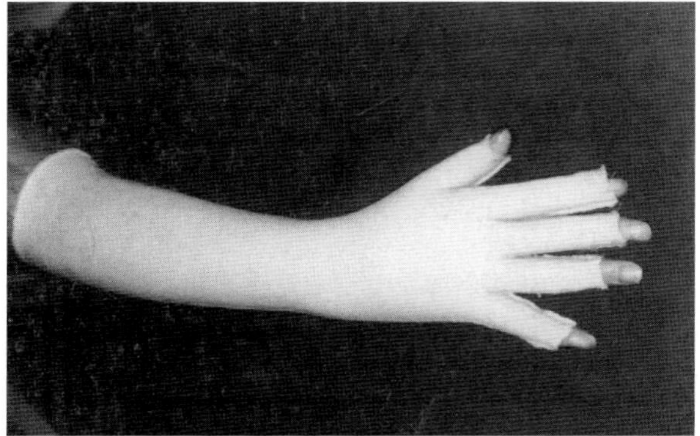

Figure 4.10 The same arm as in Figure 4.8 wearing a pressure garment.

The patient is provided with sleeves, tights, vests or gloves, depending on the area affected. If the garment is fitted over a concave area — for example, a glove over the palm of the hand — silicone can be moulded to fit in the space in order to apply pressure.

There are various products available to apply extra pressure to areas of concavity or persistent raised scarring. These include silastic elastomer, silastic foam, Otoform and silicone gel sheets or liquid. Some require a pressure garment to hold them in place.

Silicone causes the following changes to the scar:

- The scar becomes softer and smoother.
- Colour changes from red to pink.
- Scar thickness is reduced.

It is thought the silicone product hydrates the stratum corneum and releases some silicone fluid into the scar.

The silicone is introduced to the patient gradually in order to build up a tolerance level. Thus it is applied for a short time initially and the length of time it is worn is gradually increased. The pressure garments, silicone material and skin must be washed and thoroughly dried on a regular basis, and careful instructions provided for the patient and relative.

Splintage

Thermoplastic splints are used to prevent contractures of the graft and to prevent joint deformities developing. The splint may only be required at night while the patient sleeps. This may be necessary for several months until the graft has matured and become softer and more malleable, with less risk of contracting. The initial splint is worn over dressings and remoulded to gain conformity with the area as the dressings are reduced.

Soft splintage may also be used where there is a tendency for the graft to contract as a result of function. For example, grafting on the volar aspect of a finger would contract with repetitive finger flexion. The splint may be a cylindrical pressure garment or a Neoprene™ tube with a double layer of material on the dorsum. The tension in the material maintains the finger IP joints in extension when the hand is relaxed, thus preventing shortening of soft tissues.

Flaps

Definition

A flap consists of a transfer of tissue that relies on a functioning arterial and venous circulation.

Flaps may be attached to the blood supply throughout the transfer process; the part that remains attached is the pedicle or base. A flap that is detached temporarily in order to transfer the tissue is called a *free flap*. As flaps have their own blood supply they can be used to cover avascular defects: for example, open joints, exposed bone, cartilage or tendon. They may consist of:

- full-thickness skin — a cutaneous flap
- skin and fascia — a fasciocutaneous flap
- muscle and skin — a myocutaneous flap
- bone, muscle and skin — an osteomyocutaneous flap.

Complications of flaps include arterial insufficiency due to spasm or thrombosis, and venous thrombosis. Either will cause the flap to necrose if the anastomosis is not revised as soon as possible.

Common types of flap

- *Local flap.* This is a flap transferred from a site adjacent to the defect. It is used where the skin is pliable or loose and direct closure of the donor site is possible.
- *Transposition flap.* A square of skin is raised and moved to an adjacent defect, leaving a triangular defect which requires a split skin graft to cover.
- *Rotation flap.* A semi-circle of skin is raised and rotated to cover a triangular defect. There is no secondary defect to be grafted.
- *VY advancement flap.* This is the transfer of a V shape of skin; it is moved towards the defect, leaving a Y-shaped closure. It is commonly used to cover fingertip injuries.
- *Distant flap.* This is used to cover an area not adjacent to the flap. For example, a defect on the hand may be covered by a flap raised from the groin. The donor area is covered with a split-skin graft or closed directly. The hand remains attached to the groin by the pedicle (through which pass the artery and vein). This remains intact for 3 weeks, after which the pedicle is divided.
- *Myocutaneous flap.* The skin and the underlying muscle are harvested to cover the recipient site. A common example of this is the latissimus dorsi muscle used in the reconstruction of the breast.
- *Osteomyocutaneous flap.* This may be taken from the forearm and used for maxillofacial reconstruction. The donor site is covered with a split-skin graft and a protective plaster of Paris applied for 4–6 weeks. The wrist and hand require mobilising, as would a fractured radius.

Free flaps

With a free flap the skin and underlying tissues are raised, together with the artery and vein, and detached from the body. The vessels are then anastomosed to the vessels of the recipient area. These operations are performed with the use of a microscope — hence the term 'microsurgery'.

As mentioned above, these free flap transfers can involve bone and muscle as well as skin. The free flap should be elevated postoperatively, but not in high elevation, and care must be taken to eliminate any pressure applied to the vessels proximal to the flap.

Physiotherapy following flap transfer

The respiratory system

Breathing exercises with huffing or coughing to clear the lung fields may be necessary, especially after a long time under anaesthetic when microsurgery is performed. The patient may well return to the intensive care unit following such procedures. The treatment of these patients as a whole is as for any other surgical patient on the unit.

Exercises

If the patient is sedated, the physiotherapist will carry out passive movements to all joints. Care must be taken when moving the areas adjacent to and involving the flap. The flap must not be compressed for any length of time; nor must the vessels to the flap be kinked or stretched.

Any splints that are required for positioning joints or immobilising parts must be constructed in such a way as to avoid compression of the flap or the vessels proximal to the flap.

When a pedicle flap has been used and the patient's arm or leg is attached to another part of the body, stiffness of the joints of that limb will develop. The physiotherapist must assist the patient to move the affected joints as much as possible with respect to the circulation of the flap.

Scar management

The same principles apply as for skin grafts. The flap may well be bulky and raised because of the fat layer, and this will not respond to pressure therapy. An operation may be performed some months later to debulk such a flap. A flap involving muscle tissue will reduce in size over time as the muscle fibres atrophy.

CASE STUDY — BURNS

A 22-year-old man caught in a house fire sustained burns to his face, back, arms, legs, buttocks, hands and feet, and was admitted to the regional burns unit. The burns were partial-thickness and the total percentage area of burns was 35 per cent. Approximately 4 per cent of these burns were full-thickness. The man had no previous medical history.

4

FIRST OPERATION

On admission to the burns unit the patient underwent surgery for debridement of burns and escharotomies to both hands. See Table 4.2 for the initial assessment.

SECOND OPERATION

One week later further surgery was carried out, consisting of debridement and grafting to both arms. The patient developed a chest infection with oxygen saturation levels of 96 per cent and 60 per cent O_2 via face mask. See Table 4.3 for the new assessment.

OPERATION THREE

Two weeks later the man returned to the operating theatre for grafting to upper limbs, application of skin grafts to raw areas, and left-hand PIP joints K-wired in extension. See Table 4.4 for the new assessment.

COMPLICATIONS

Over a period of 4–8 weeks after the burning incident the patient developed reduced range of movement at the right elbow joint, which was painful. Heterotopic ossification of the elbow joint was confirmed with an MRI scan. The exercise regimen for the elbow was limited to active movements within the limits of pain. A night splint was worn to hold the elbow in extension to maintain soft-tissue length on the anterior aspect of the elbow joint.

Bone exposed at the tip of the left index finger was corrected by terminalisation of the index finger at the level of the DIP joint.

The web space of the left thumb began to contract, thus limiting abduction of the thumb and therefore reducing function of the left hand. Passive stretches of the thumb into palmar abduction and active abduction exercises were carried out by the physiotherapist and the family to achieve the desired range of movement. A 'C' splint was fitted to the first web space and the patient instructed to wear it between treatment and at night.

PROGRESSION

At 1 month the patient commenced standing between two physiotherapists. This was carried out twice daily and progressed to walking once the patient had acquired standing balance. The distance walked was gradually increased, as the patient was able. A stair assessment was carried out and followed with a home visit, as the patient lived in the vicinity of the burns unit.

At 10 weeks the patient was discharged from the unit with follow-up appointments at the burns dressing clinic. These appointments took place three times a week and involved 1 hour of physiotherapy in the rehabilitation room.

Once areas of grafting had healed and the condition of the skin allowed, the patient was assessed

Table 4.2 Case study: assessment 1

Problems	Active needs	Treatment plan
Potential for decreased ROM in affected joints due to burn	Increased ROM in all affected joints until fully healed Maintain full active movement of unaffected joints	Passive exercises while patient sedated, progress to active Twice daily
Swelling due to burn	Prevent swelling until healed	Elevate affected areas, especially hands and feet
Pain	Reduce pain to a tolerable level to allow exercises	Liaise with nursing staff on pain control
Potential deformity or contracture of joints	Prevent contractures and deformities while scar tissue forms and matures	Hand-resting splints and foot-drop splints Passive and active exercises twice daily
Potential respiratory problems due to smoke inhalation	Prevent respiratory problems and maintain clear airway	Breathing exercises and coughing 2–3 times daily Encourage fluid intake

ROM = range of movement.

Table 4.3 Case study: assessment 2

Problems	Active needs	Treatment plan
Respiratory problems due to anaesthetic and previous smoke inhalation	Improve O_2 saturation levels to 98 per cent with oxygen at 35 per cent via face mask	Breathing exercises and coughing 2–3 times daily Encourage fluid intake
Potential for reduced ROM in joints due to the immobilisation of joints adjacent to grafts	Increase ROM in all affected joints until fully healed	Active and passive exercises once the grafts are stable Twice daily

Table 4.4 Case study: assessment 3

Problems	Active needs	Treatment plan
Potential respiratory problems due to anaesthetic	Prevent respiratory problems and maintain clear airway	Breathing exercises and coughing 2–3 times daily Encourage fluid intake
Pain due to surgery	Reduce pain to a tolerable level	Liaise with nursing staff on pain control
Potential for decreased ROM in joints due to the immobilisation of joints adjacent to grafts	Increase ROM in all affected joints until fully healed	Active and passive exercises once the grafts are stable Twice daily
Decreased ROM of wired joints	Increase ROM of PIP joints when wires removed after 5 weeks	Passive flexion of each joint and active exercises, 10-hourly Dynamic splintage if necessary

for the provision of pressure garments. These were manufactured by the senior therapy assistant, who then fitted the garments and instructed the patient on how to use them. The left glove was converted into a flexor glove to combine the pressure therapy with passive flexion of the fingers. This garment was worn for intervals of approximately 30 minutes followed by active flexion and extension exercises of the fingers. In between sessions with the flexor glove the patient wore a glove and a dynamic MCP joint flexion splint. Gradually the range of flexion improved at the MCP and PIP joints of the left hand and function increased.

Over a period of several weeks the patient attended the rehabilitation room for intensive treatment to return to function. Activities included balance work, cycling, dressing, writing, playing cards and therapeutic putty exercises. The treatment was adapted as progress was made and the pressure garments were reviewed at regular intervals as the scar tissue matured.

DISCUSSION

The recovery period following such extensive burns is a long and arduous one; it requires a great deal of cooperation and commitment from all members of the multidisciplinary team, which includes the patient and relatives. In order for the patient to regain as much function as possible, clear objectives must be set out at the beginning and all members must be included in the decision-making process. It is essential once the patient is discharged from the hospital that the burns care continues on an intensive level with the involvement of specialists, and that the patient complies with the treatment plan and its execution.

4

FURTHER READING

Glassey N 2004 Physiotherapy for Burns and Plastic Reconstruction of the Hand. Whurr: London
Leveridge A (ed.) 1991 Therapy for the Burns Patient. Chapman & Hall: London
Morgan B, Wright M 1986 Essentials of Plastic and Reconstructive Surgery. Faber & Faber: London
Settle ADJ 1986 Burns — the First Five Days. Smith & Nephew Pharmaceuticals: London

REFERENCES

British Burns Association (BBA) 2001 National Burn Care Review. BBA: London
British Burns Association (BBA) 2006 National Burn Care Review. BBA: London
CSP (Chartered Society of Physiotherapy) Therapy Standards Working Group 2000 Standards for Burns. CSP: London
Glassey N 2004 Physiotherapy for Burns and Plastic Reconstruction of the Hand. Whurr: London
Herndon DN 2002 Total Burn Care, 2nd edn. WB Saunders: London
Leveridge A (ed.) 1991 Therapy for the Burns Patient. Chapman & Hall: London
McGregor IA 1989 Fundamental Techniques of Plastic Surgery. Churchill Livingstone: Edinburgh
Morgan B, Wright M 1986 Essentials of Plastic and Reconstructive Surgery. Faber & Faber: London
Muir IFK, Barclay TL 1962 Treatment of burn shock. In: Burns and their Treatment. Lloyd Luke: London
Settle JAD (ed.) 1996 Principles and Practice of Burns Management. Churchill Livingstone: Edinburgh
Wachtel TL, Berry CC, Wachtel EE, Frank HA 2000 The inter-rater reliability of estimating the size of burns from various burn area chart drawings. Burns 26(2): 156–170

Chapter 5

Physiotherapy in women's health

Gill Brook, Yvonne Coldron, Georgina Evans, Georgie Gulliford, Jeanette Haslam, Ruth Hawkes, Judith Lee, Alison Lewis, Melanie Lewis, Daphne Sidney, Ros Thomas, Jacquelyne Todd, Kathleen Vits and Pauline Walsh

CHAPTER CONTENTS

INTRODUCTION

This chapter offers an overview of the role of the physiotherapist in women's health. Some of the expert contributors are members of the Association of Chartered Physiotherapists in Women's Health (ACPWH), a recognised clinical interest group of the Chartered Society of Physiotherapy (CSP). Originally known as the Obstetric Physiotherapists Association, it was formed in 1948 and is one of the oldest such organisations.

Weblink

Association of Chartered Physiotherapists in Women's Health (ACPWH), c/o CSP, 14 Bedford Row, London WC1R 4ED:
www.acpwh.org.uk

The ACPWH forms a representative body that can be consulted, and will act in the professional interest of the physiotherapist working in women's health and in the specific field of continence. By promoting relevant post-registration courses and workshops it encourages and provides means by which the physiotherapist may improve specialist therapeutic skills and understanding of the specialty. A journal is published twice a year and there is an annual conference. In order to nurture interest in this field amongst student physiotherapists there is a student award, which provides funding to attend the annual conference. There is a lack of evidence for many of the interventions used in women's health physiotherapy and, to encourage research, support may be offered in the form of a small bursary. There is, in addition, a research officer who works closely with the CSP and other relevant funding bodies, to set the future agenda for research.

The women's health physiotherapist is a vital member of the multiprofessional team, so there is a need to foster mutual understanding between the members of the obstetric and gynaecological healthcare team and their professional bodies. The association continues to seek new alliances with other organisations and maintains strong ties with the Royal College of Midwives, the Association for Continence Advice and the Continence Foundation.

Health promotion is also an important aspect of this specialty and this can take the form of leading classes, advising individuals or couples, and providing a support group for an identified clientele. There is an abundance of ACPWH literature to accompany health education, and communication with other local organisations (e.g. branches of the National Childbirth Trust) can be invaluable.

Since 1999, ACPWH has been a member of the International Organization of Physical Therapists in Women's Health (IOPTWH), an official subgroup of the World Confederation for Physical Therapy (WCPT). The organisation's mission is to provide a means by which WCPT members having a common interest in the physical therapy problems and concerns of women may meet, confer and promote these interests. Its membership in 2006 was 15 countries.

> **Weblink**
>
> International Organization of Physical Therapists in Women's Health (IOPTWH):
> www.ioptwh.org

The scope of practice of the physiotherapist is forever altering and the field of women's health is no exception. For example, knowledge and understanding of the assessment and treatment of incontinence has advanced considerably, and includes the male sufferer. Similarly, the needs of the partner through pregnancy, childbirth and gynaecological procedures are now recognised and must be included in any advice or treatment protocol. Cultural differences, sexuality and religious beliefs must also be considered.

ANATOMY AND PHYSIOLOGY

A physiotherapist needs to know about female anatomy and physiology in order to appreciate the difficulties that pregnancy may bring.

Bones and joints of the pelvis

The pelvis is multi-purpose, being protective of the pelvic contents, supportive of the trunk and able to transfer weight to the legs in walking and ischial tuberosities in sitting. The joints of the pelvis (Figure 5.1) are held together by some of the strongest ligaments in the body, which become more lax in pregnancy due to the increased levels of oestrogen, progesterone and relaxin (Ostgaard 1997). There is frequently separation of the pubic symphysis up to 1 cm during pregnancy and labour (Jain and Sternberg 2005).

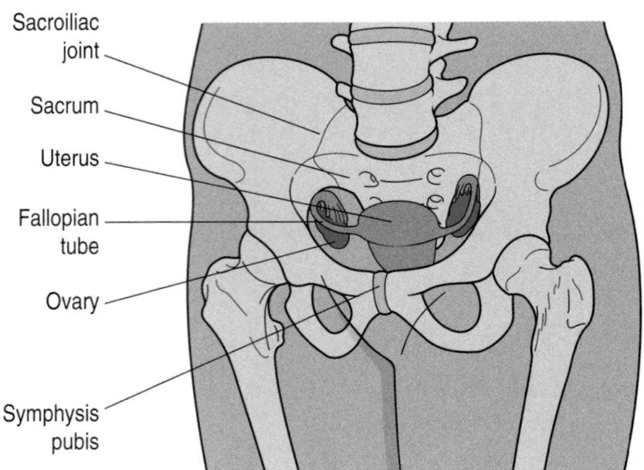

Figure 5.1 True and false pelvis: female reproductive organs.

The pelvic brim or inlet divides the pelvis into the 'false' pelvis above and the 'true' pelvis below. The pelvic outlet at the base of the pelvis is comprised of the pubic arch, ischial spines, sacrotuberous ligaments and the coccyx (Haslam 2004a).

The gynaecoid pelvis is ideal in that it has a well-rounded inlet and symmetrical orderly outlet. Other pelvic shapes can make a vaginal delivery problematical; for example, it has been shown that a narrow suprapubic arch predisposes to prolonged labour and postpartum anal incontinence (Frudlinger et al. 2002).

Muscles

The abdominal muscles — rectus abdominis, the internal and external abdominal obliques, and transversus abdominis — form a muscular 'four-way stretch' elastic support for the abdominal contents (Figure 5.2). The obliques and transversus abdominis insert into an aponeurosis joining in the midline at the linea alba. The recti abdominis attach to the xiphoid process and lower ribs above and to the pubis below, and run in sheaths formed by the aponeurosis on either side of the linea alba. These sheaths are deficient posteriorly in their lower portion.

Towards the end of pregnancy the growing uterus stretches the abdominal muscles and can cause the recti to be separated in midline by several finger widths as the connective tissue forming the linea alba also becomes lax (Sapsford et al. 1998). This can persist into the postnatal period (Barton 2004a).

The main function of the recti is to flex the lumbar spine (Sapsford et al. 2001), whilst the obliques, interlaced

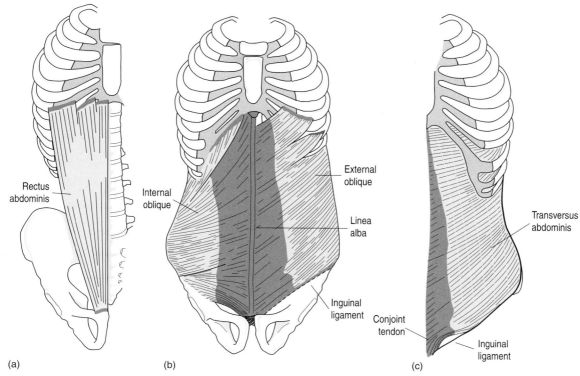

Figure 5.2 (a) Right rectus abdominis. (b) Right internal oblique and left external oblique muscles. (c) Left transversus abdominis. (Reproduced from Palastanga et al. 2002, with permission.)

diagonally in midline deep to the recti, produce side-flexion and rotation of the spine. Transversus abdominis, the deepest muscle, has horizontal fibres, which provide considerable postural support for the abdominal contents and help maintain intra-abdominal pressure, along with the pelvic floor muscles (Cresswell et al. 1992).

The pelvic floor muscles (Figure 5.3) form an elastic sling at the pelvic outlet to support the pelvic and abdominal contents. The pelvic floor comprises four layers. The deepest is the viscerofascial layer, important for both organ support and muscle attachment. The next layer is muscular; it is part of the supportive mechanism and assists with the sphincteric control of the bladder and bowel. This layer is formed by the levator ani muscles — comprising pubococcygeus (sometimes known as the pubovisceral muscle) and ileococcygeus — and ischiococcygeus. The next layer is a dense triangular membrane lying anteriorly, known as the perineal membrane; it is of importance for connection of the urethra, vagina and perineal body to the ischiopubic rami (DeLancey 2001). The most superficial external genital muscles — ischiocavernosus, bulbocavernosus and the transverse perineal muscles — have a sexual function in assisting a woman to achieve orgasm. The external anal sphincter is important for anal control and lies posteriorly and inferior

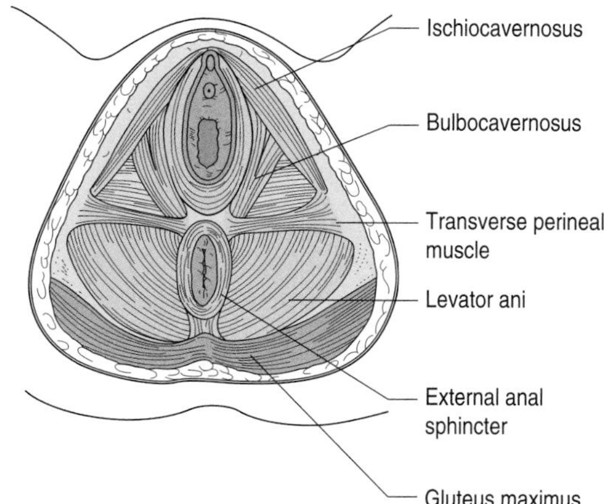

Figure 5.3 Pelvic floor muscles.

to the other parts of the pelvic floor. Contraction of the pelvic floor muscles (PFM) results in a cranioventral lift movement that has been observed by real-time ultrasound (Dietz et al. 1998). It has always been believed that the pudendal nerve, from the sacral nerve root S2–4, supplies all of the pelvic floor muscles. However, Barber et al. (2002) have suggested that, although the pudendal nerve supplies the urethral sphincter and the external genital muscles, the levator ani has a distinctive separate nerve supply from S3–5, which has been named the 'nerve to levator ani'; this theory is in some dispute.

Pregnancy and childbirth are major contributory factors to pelvic floor muscle dysfunction (Freeman 2002). It has been shown that those women who suffer urinary incontinence in pregnancy are twice as likely to suffer with it 15 years after childbirth (Dolan et al. 2003). The act of vaginal delivery has also been shown to increase the likelihood of future urinary and faecal disorders, but caesarean section may not be fully protective (MacArthur et al. 2006). It is also thought that there is a possible genetic collagen factor, as it has been found that having a mother or older sister suffering from urinary incontinence is a predictive factor for a woman developing symptoms (Hannestad et al. 2004).

The pelvic floor muscles are composed of approximately two-thirds slow oxidative (tonic) fibres and one-third fast glycolytic (phasic) fibres (Gilpin et al. 1989).

Organs of reproduction

The uterus — a hollow, pear-shaped organ — comprises the fundus, body, isthmus and cervix, and weighs about 50 grams (g) in its normal state. Together with the ovaries, it is suspended in connective tissue and peritoneum inside the true pelvis. The broad ligament (a double fold of peritoneum) extends from the lateral walls of the uterus to the side walls of the pelvis, dividing the pelvic cavity into two compartments — the anterior, containing the bladder, and the posterior, containing the rectum. The ovaries lie in the broad ligament on each side of the uterus. Just behind and slightly above are the trumpet-shaped open ends of the contractile fallopian tubes. Their tentacle-like fringes (fimbriae) catch the ovum when it erupts from the ovary at ovulation. The free ovum is propelled along the fallopian tube to the uterus by a peristaltic wave and by the cilia lining the tube walls. On fertilisation, the ovum is embedded in the endometrium lining the uterus. If fertilisation has not occurred, the lining is shed (menstruation).

The uterus has a remarkable capacity to grow as the fetus develops during pregnancy, and able to accommodate the baby (in 1 litre of amniotic fluid within a membranous sac) and placenta, which attaches it to the uterine wall.

THE PHYSIOLOGY OF PREGNANCY

Following fertilisation of the ovum, the first sign of pregnancy is amenorrhoea (cessation of menstruation). As pregnancy progresses, the uterus grows, its muscle fibres lengthening and thickening, and weight increasing from 50 g to 1000 g at term. By 12 weeks it has enlarged to become an abdominal organ. Gestational dates can be determined by the level of the uterus, which continues to rise until the latter weeks of pregnancy. Coordinated contraction of the uterus may be felt by the woman from about 20 weeks (Braxton Hicks contractions). These contractions assist in blood flow through the placental site, and in development of the lower uterine segment. The cervix gradually increases in size with an increase in collagen content, hypertrophy of external muscle fibres and increase in vascularity (McNabb 1997), and becomes slightly softer in consistency. A mucous plug acts as a barrier to infection.

The disc-shaped placenta grows during pregnancy and has the major responsibility of maintaining the fetal circulation in order to facilitate blood gas exchange, nutrition and excretion, and act as a barrier to noxious substances. It also produces progestogens and oestrogens.

The fetus grows and develops within the amniotic sac and is nurtured by the placenta via the umbilical cord. Its heartbeat can be detected at about 10 weeks with Sonicaid ultrasonic equipment, and movements may be felt by primigravidae (women pregnant for the first time) at 18–20 weeks; multigravidae (women who have experienced a previous pregnancy) may notice movement at 16–18 weeks.

Pregnancy is governed and controlled by hormones, which affect various systems. Some are of particular relevance to the physiotherapist:

- Progesterone decreases smooth muscle tone, initiates sensitivity to CO_2 in the respiratory centre, and causes an increase in maternal temperature, breast development, and storage of fat deposits for milk production.
- Oestrogen influences uterine and breast growth and development, prepares prime receptor sites for relaxin (e.g. pelvic joints), and causes increased water retention. An unwanted effect is that of increased vaginal glycogen, predisposing to thrush.
- In target areas relaxin replaces collagen with a modified form which has greater pliability and extensibility. It has a softening effect on connective tissue (pelvic floor and abdominal fascia), increasing extensibility in those structures. It also inhibits myometrial activity up to 28 weeks' gestation.

Pregnancy lasts on average 40 weeks and is divided into three trimesters (periods of approximately 3 months). During this time many changes occur in the body owing to the growth of the fetus, the changes effected by the above hormones, weight gain and subsequent postural alterations.

Physiotherapists treating pregnant women should be conversant with these changes and consider them during assessment and treatment, or when planning or taking classes. Likewise, they should have an understanding of the complications that might arise during pregnancy — such as placenta praevia (a low-lying placenta) or high blood pressure.

Chapter coverage

Within this text attention will be paid to the changes and complications of most relevance to the physiotherapist dealing with women during pregnancy and the postnatal period. Further reading is advised (see the end of the chapter).

MUSCULOSKELETAL CHANGES DURING PREGNANCY

Postural changes

The overall equilibrium of the spine and pelvis alters as pregnancy progresses but there is still confusion as to the exact nature of any associated postural adaptation. With weight gain, increased blood volume and ventral growth of the fetus, the centre of gravity no longer falls over the feet and the woman may need to lean backwards to gain equilibrium (Abitol 1997), resulting in disorganisation of spinal curves. Reported postures include a reduction in lumbar lordosis (Moore et al. 1990), an increase in both lumbar lordosis and thoracic kyphosis (Bullock-Saxton 1991) or a flattening of the thoracolumbar spinal curve (Gilleard et al. 2002). These differences imply that there are individual variations with no 'normal' posture in pregnancy, and it might be that antenatal lumbopelvic posture is an accentuation of the woman's normal posture pre- pregnancy. However, there will still be compensatory changes to posture in the thoracic and cervical spines, and this, combined with the extra weight of the breasts, may result in posterior displacement of the shoulders and thoracic spine and an increase of the cervical lordosis. Postural changes may still be present 12 weeks postnatally (Bullock-Saxton 1991).

Articular and connective tissue changes

Altered levels of relaxin, oestrogen and progesterone during pregnancy result in a change to collagen metabolism, and increased connective tissue pliability and extensibility. Therefore, ligamentous tissues are predisposed to laxity with resultant reduced passive joint stability. The symphysis pubis and sacroiliac joints are particularly affected to allow for passage of the baby. This ligamentous laxity may continue for 6 months postpartum (Foti et al. 2000).

Biomechanical changes of the joints of the spine and pelvis may involve an increase in sacral promontory, an increase in the lumbosacral angle, a forward rotatory movement of the innominate bones, and downward and forward rotation of the symphysis pubis (Borg-Stein et al. 2005). The normal pubic symphyseal gap of 4–5 mm shows an average increase of 3 mm during pregnancy (Abramson et al. 1934). Pelvic joint loosening begins around 10 weeks with maximum loosening near term. Joints should return to normal at 4–12 weeks postpartum (Snow and Neubert 1997). The sacrococcygeal joint also loosens. By the last trimester, the hip abductors and extensors, and the ankle plantar flexors increase their net power during gait (Foti et al. 2000) and there is an increase in load on the hip joints of 2.8 times the normal value when standing and working in front of a worktop (Paul et al. 1996).

As the uterus rises in the abdomen, the rib cage is forced laterally and the diameter of the chest may increase by 10–15 cm (Barton 2004b).

Neuromuscular changes

Abdominal and pelvic muscles contribute to spinal and pelvic stability via active tension exerted on the passive ligamentous and fascial stability structures. During pregnancy the enlarged uterus results in elongation of the abdominal muscles and separation of the linea alba (Boissonnault and Blaschak 1988). Passive joint instability (as seen in pregnancy) alters afferent input from joint mechanoreceptors and probably affects motor neurone recruitment. A decrease in muscle stiffness and thus active stability of a joint may result from alteration of muscle spindle regulation (Bullock-Saxton 1998) and this is applicable particularly to muscles around the pelvic girdle. These changes may lead to poor recruitment of the muscles responsible for pelvic girdle stability (particularly gluteus medius and maximus) and result in decreased tension of these muscles during walking, perhaps resulting in pelvic girdle pain (PGP).

Rectus abdominis

As pregnancy progresses, rectus abdominis elongates (Gilleard and Brown 1996) and becomes wider and thinner (Coldron 2006). In many women the disproportion between width and thickness remains even at 12 months postpartum (Coldron 2006). Although the consequences of this are unknown, the strength of gross muscle flexion has been shown to be impaired at 24 weeks postpartum (Potter et al. 1997b).

As the fetus grows anteriorly, the aponeurosis of the linea alba becomes wider and thinner via hormonally mediated changes, the two bellies of rectus abdominis curving round the abdominal wall (Haslam 2004b). This divarication of the linea alba during the third trimester is normally about 2–4 cm (20–40 mm) wide and 2–5 cm (20–50 mm) long, though it can split and become a diastasis, i.e. an inter-recti distance (IRD) of > 27 mm at the umbilicus (Rath et al. 1996). The IRD at the umbilical level normally resolves to about 20 mm by 8 weeks postpartum when it reaches a plateau, though in a minority of women a diastasis may persist (Coldron 2006).

Lateral abdominal muscles

There is very little information on the effect of pregnancy on the three lateral abdominal muscles (transversus abdominis, internal and external obliques). However, research on normal subjects has identified the importance of transversus abdominis as the prime stabiliser of the trunk (Hodges 1999). Decreased stabilisation of the pelvis happens in late pregnancy and poor stability persists at 8 weeks postpartum (Gilleard and Brown 1996).

Pelvic floor muscles

During pregnancy there is stretching to the pelvic floor, and trauma/tearing during labour and vaginal delivery. It is now thought that the function and recruitment of transversus abdominis and the pelvic floor musculature are closely associated, with voluntary activity in the deep abdominal muscles resulting in increased pelvic floor muscle activity (Sapsford and Hodges 2001). There is an association between pelvic floor muscle dysfunction and pregnancy-related lumbopelvic pain (Pool-Goudzwaard et al. 2005).

LABOUR, BIRTH AND THE PUERPERIUM

Definition

Labour is defined as the process by which the products of conception are expelled from the uterus after the 24th week of gestation.

Monitoring

Uterine activity, the progress of labour and fetal condition are monitored regularly throughout labour, by abdominal palpation, by vaginal assessment and by listening to the fetal heart rate. The latter may be done intermittently (e.g. by Pinard fetal stethoscope) or by continuous electronic monitoring (through the abdomen or via a clip electrode attached to the presenting part of the baby, with a printout on a cardiotocograph machine). Information is recorded on a partogram (progress chart), which will show any deviation from a 'normal' labour.

The mother's temperature, pulse, respiration, blood pressure, state of hydration, bladder fullness and psychological state are monitored regularly.

Onset of labour

The exact 'trigger' for labour is unknown, but there are biochemical events resulting in a fall in progesterone and a rise in oestradiol, prostaglandins and oxytocin. Signs are a 'show' of the mucous plug, rupture of membranes and regular uterine contractions.

Stages of labour

First stage

This is from commencement of established labour to full dilatation of the cervix, averaging 12 hours in a primigravid woman (one having her first baby). Contraction and retraction of the myometrial fibres of the uterus achieve effacement and dilatation of the cervix. The contractions increase in intensity, duration and frequency, pulling the uterus forwards into line with the pelvic inlet and birth canal and driving the presenting part downwards.

The cervix must be fully dilated (10 cm) before pushing commences. Transition (the final part of this first stage) can be very difficult as the woman may experience mood swings, overwhelming pain, intense fatigue and a strong desire to push.

Second stage

This is the expulsive stage, from full dilatation to the birth of the baby — averaging 1–2 hours in the primigravid. The fetal head must adapt to the various segments of the pelvis. The head engages in the transverse position, flexes and rotates as it strikes the pelvic floor, passes under the pubic arch, extending as it distends both the perineum and introitus maximally, and is 'crowned' and delivered with the face towards the anus. The position of the umbilical cord is checked. The head rotates back again as the anterior shoulder is born, followed by the second shoulder and the body. The cord is clamped and cut.

The mother assists expulsive contractions of the uterus with short pushes, and the adoption of comfortable gravity-aided positions to facilitate delivery (Russell 1982; Gardosi et al. 1989; Caldeyro-Barcia 1997). She may be asked to pant at the crowning of the head, as the baby is being delivered.

Episiotomy

During delivery, a woman's perineum can stretch and remain intact, but it may tear. A third- or fourth-degree tear (involving the anal sphincter and mucosa respectively) may have serious implications, even faecal incontinence (Sultan et al. 1994; Kamm 1994). An episiotomy (cut) may be deemed necessary to avoid excessive trauma, to hasten the birth or to prepare for an instrumental delivery. A mediolateral incision is performed to avoid tearing into the anus.

Instrumental delivery

Delay in the second stage, or fetal or maternal distress, might be an indication for instrumental delivery, by vacuum extraction or forceps.

- With vacuum extraction (e.g. Ventouse, Kiwi Omni-Cup) a suction cap is applied to the fetal scalp and traction is used with contractions.
- With forceps delivery, metal blades cradle each side of the fetal head. Traction is applied steadily during contractions. A choice of forceps allows lift out or rotation as required.

Third stage

This is the shortest stage of labour, lasting up to 30 minutes and commencing after the birth of the baby. The uterus contracts and shears the placenta off its wall, pushing it down through the vagina. The process may be aided by an injection of Syntocinon at delivery and cord traction. The placenta and membranes will be examined for completeness on delivery. On occasion, part or all of the placenta and/or membranes may be retained, requiring manual removal.

Caesarean section

This is a surgical procedure performed electively, or as an emergency, before or during labour. The baby is removed through the abdominal wall by a transverse incision through the lower uterine segment (LSCS). A vertical incision in the upper segment may be necessary but can increase morbidity. Epidural anaesthesia or spinal block is commonly used instead of a general anaesthetic, reducing the risk of aspiration of acid stomach contents into the mother's lungs (Mendelson's syndrome).

Indications for caesarean section include fetal or maternal distress, prolonged or obstructed labour, and malpresentation of the fetus or placenta.

Induction

Labour can be induced when the continuation of pregnancy is considered disadvantageous. Common indications are post-maturity (overdue), pre-eclampsia (associated with high blood pressure), diabetes, intrauterine growth retardation and antepartum haemorrhage.

Induction may be performed by 'stretch and sweep' (when a midwife or doctor attempts, during digital vaginal examination, to stretch the cervix gently and separate the membranes from the walls of the cervix), the insertion of vaginal prostaglandins (to 'ripen' the cervix), artificial rupture of membranes, oxytocin infusion, or a combination of some or all of these.

Pain relief

Henderson and Jones (1997) describe labour pain as being unique and isolating. Pain and the perception of pain will vary from individual to individual and from labour to labour.

Pain in the first stage is experienced mainly in the abdomen and lower back, becoming more intense as the contractions increase in strength and length. It is due to dilatation of the cervix, contraction and distension of the uterine muscle, and pressure of the uterus on other areas.

In the second stage a sharp, burning pain is caused by distension and dilatation of the birth canal (vagina) and perineum.

A woman, possibly using pain management techniques taught at antenatal classes, may be able to cope with the pain she experiences. However, many will request additional analgesia.

Drugs

Entonox

This mixture of 50 per cent nitrous oxide and 50 per cent oxygen is inhaled and administered by the woman via a mask or mouthpiece. There are no known adverse effects to her or the fetus. It may be particularly useful in the later part of the first stage and during the second stage. The analgesic effect is delayed, so inhalation from the start of a contraction is required.

Pethidine and diamorphine

These opioid drugs are readily available and easily administered by intramuscular injection. Possible disadvantages include nausea and vomiting, and neonatal respiratory depression, which may be corrected by administration of naloxone.

Epidural

An epidural is a local anaesthetic introduced into the lumbar epidural space, reducing or eradicating the pain of uterine contractions (Howell and Chalmers 1992) without affecting uterine activity. Although it is an invasive procedure administered by an anaesthetist, it has been found to be not only effective, but safe (Thorp and Breedlove 1996) with a low risk of complication (Paech et al. 1998). Potential disadvantages include reduced mobility for the mother, prolonged second

5

stage with higher risk of a forceps delivery, vasodilatation in the lower limbs necessitating an intravenous infusion, and urine retention. Headaches (due to dural puncture at the time of administration), infection and neural damage might follow delivery. Although women may report backache as a consequence of epidural, the occurrence of new-onset chronic back pain has not been supported (MacArthur et al. 1995). Epidural may be advised when operative delivery is suspected (e.g. with multiple births). It can also be an advantage for women with high blood pressure, as its administration reduces blood pressure.

Transcutaneous electrical nerve stimulation

TENS (or TNS) can be used in labour. A low-frequency high-intensity current of 2–10 Hz is thought to increase the production of endorphins and encephalins. This is applied throughout labour, and a high-frequency low-intensity current at 100–200 Hz which activates the pain-gate mechanism (Melzack and Wall 1982) is used during the more intense contractions. A special two-channel battery-operated obstetric machine enables the woman to change from one frequency to the other by depression of a button. The current is introduced via four electrodes placed over the nerve roots to the uterus (T10–L2) and the pelvic floor and perineum (S2–S4). The two channels enable individual control of each pair of electrodes.

TENS is easy to apply and non-invasive, with no known side-effects to mother or baby. It allows mobility and affords the woman some control of her analgesia. It cannot be used in water, and may on occasion interfere with the cardiograph tracings. Randomised controlled trials (RCTs) have provided no compelling evidence for TENS having any analgesic effect during labour (Carroll et al. 1997), though a reduction in use of narcotics has been reported (Bortoluzzi 1989).

Alternative methods of pain control

These include the use of water (birthing pool), hypnotherapy, acupuncture, aromatherapy and reflexology.

The puerperium

Puerperium describes the first 6 weeks after childbirth. Some body systems return to their non-pregnant state and other changes are initiated (e.g. lactation). Within this period the uterus involutes (returns to its pre-pregnant size and position). As the site of the placenta heals and the endometrium regenerates, the woman experiences a discharge (lochia), initially bloody, for up to 8 weeks.

Potential complications during this period that might involve the women's health physiotherapist include perineal or wound swelling or bruising, musculoskeletal problems, urinary incontinence, faecal incontinence and constipation (see also the section on postnatal physiotherapy).

PHYSIOTHERAPY IN THE CHILDBEARING YEAR

The women's health physiotherapist works as part of the multidisciplinary team caring for the pregnant woman, along with obstetricians, GPs, midwives, health visitors, occupational therapists, social workers or other physiotherapists. Contact with the pregnant woman may be in the community, health centre, leisure centre or physiotherapy department.

The role of the women's health physiotherapist is to:

- educate the pregnant woman for pregnancy, labour and beyond (see the section on antenatal classes)
- advise on safe and appropriate exercise (see the section on exercise and pregnancy)
- identify, assess and treat musculoskeletal problems (dealt with in this section).

Pelvic floor dysfunction

See the section on urogenital dysfunction. During pregnancy, physiotherapists may consider it prudent to limit their intervention to advice.

Pregnancy-related lumbopelvic pain

Lumbopelvic pain is common during pregnancy, with a prevalence described variously as ranging from 50 per cent to 70 per cent (Mantle et al. 1977; Fast et al. 1987; Berg et al. 1988; Ostgaard et al.1991; Wu et al. 2004; Mogren and Pohjanen 2005; Gutke et al. 2006), and it may be of spinal and/or pelvic girdle origin (Ostgaard et al. 1996; Stuge et al. 2003; Wu et al. 2004; Vleeming et al. 2004; Mogren & Pohjanen 2005; Gutke et al. 2006). Pain of spinal origin is normally referred to as low back pain (LBP). Pregnancy-related PGP is a global term that encompasses symphysis pubis dysfunction, diastasis symphysis pubis and sacroiliac joint pain. Lumbopelvic pain is often regarded as 'a normal part of pregnancy' but, without appropriate treatment, a minor episode may develop into a chronic problem. A third of women report severe back pain that interferes with daily life and compromises their ability to work (Ostgaard et al. 1991; Mens et al. 1996). Most backache resolves in the first few weeks postpartum, but for some may continue for 18 months (Ostgaard and Andersson 1992) or may present postpartum for the first time (Russell and Reynolds 1997). Some patients may experience a relapse around menstruation and in a subsequent pregnancy (Mens et al. 1996).

The anatomical origins of pregnancy-related lumbopelvic pain vary and are difficult to determine and diagnose (Nilsson-Wikmar et al. 1999). Common conditions include unilateral sacroiliac dysfunction, symphysis pubis dysfunction, minor lumbar disc herniation, lumbar zygapophyseal joint problems, thoracic spine pain and coccydynia. Women describe pain variously as occurring in the low back, sacral, posterior thigh and leg, anterior thigh, pubic, groin and hip areas. These may occur simultaneously or separately, antenatally, during delivery or postnatally (Heiberg and Aarseth 1997). There is often associated cervical, thoracic or coccygeal pain. Sciatic pain is common and may be of lumbar origin or from sacroiliac joint involvement because the L5 and S1 components of the lumbosacral plexus run immediately anterior to the sacroiliac joints. Several studies have differentiated between pregnancy-related LBP and PGP (Ostgaard et al. 1994; Ostgaard et al. 1996; Ostgaard 1997; Noren et al. 2002; Vleeming et al. 2004; Bastiaanssen et al. 2005; Gutke et al. 2006). It is important that both the lumbar spine and pelvic girdle are examined in order to determine the origin of symptoms and plan appropriate management.

Causes of lumbopelvic pain appear to be multifactorial and may include postural adaptations, fatigue, increased joint mobility, increased collagen volume causing pressure on pain-sensitive structures, weight gain, and pressure from the growing fetus (Haslam 2004b). The main risk factors are a history of previous lumbopelvic pain and/or previous trauma to the pelvis, and possibly high workload and multiparity (Berg et al. 1988; Ostgaard and Andersson 1991; Kristiansson et al. 1996a; Larsen et al. 1999; Vleeming et al. 2004). Other risk factors may include PGP in a previous pregnancy (Larsen et al. 1999), poor workplace ergonomics and awkward working conditions (Larsen et al. 1999), abdominal sagittal and transverse diameters and a naturally large lumbar lordosis (Ostgaard et al. 1993), and decreased fitness level before pregnancy (Ostgaard et al. 1993).

Reported musculoskeletal factors contributing to pregnancy-related PGP include the pelvic girdle joints moving asymmetrically (Damen et al. 2001), symphyseal laxity (Bjorklund et al. 1999) and ligamentous strain and muscle weakness (Mens et al. 1996). PGP is probably caused by a combination of these factors plus altered activity in the spinal (Sihvonen et al. 1998), abdominal, pelvic girdle, hip (Pool-Goudzwaard et al. 1998) and pelvic floor muscles (Pool-Goudzwaard et al. 2005), leading to abnormal pelvic girdle biomechanics and stability. However, a small number of women might have non-biomechanical but hormonally induced pain in the pelvic girdle.

Symphysis pubis dysfunction

Symphysis pubis dysfunction (SPD) relates to pain in the region of the symphysis pubis joint, whereas diastasis symphysis pubis (DSP) is a true separation of the symphysis pubis joint; diagnosis of the latter is made radiologically. The definition of DSP is symphyseal separation of more than 10 mm and/or vertical shift of more than 5 mm (Hagen 1974). The amount of symphyseal separation does not always correlate with symptoms (Snow and Neubert 1997) and not all symptomatic patients have an increased gap. SPD or DSP may occur antenatally, during delivery or postnatally, and might cause severe social difficulties (Fry 1999).

Pain distribution may be in the groin, medial and anterior thigh, perineum, coccyx, and one or both sacroiliac joints (Fry 1999; Coldron 2005). Severity and irritability vary from mild to severe and may be different from day to day. Common physical signs are pain on abduction of the thighs, a shuffling or waddling gait, severe symphyseal tenderness, inability to weight-bear unilaterally, and pain on turning in bed, lifting a light weight, getting up from a chair and using stairs (Fry 1999; Hansen et al. 1999). Minor trauma such as stepping down from a kerb may cause severe symphysis pubis pain. A forward rotation and oblique slip of the innominate caused by overactivity in the adductor muscles of the thigh may contribute to SPD (Röst 1999). With poor use of the glutei and lack of force closure of the pelvis, disruption of the self-locking mechanism of the pelvis may occur.

Proposed non-musculoskeletal factors for PGP include an increased level of the enzyme hyaluronidase (Schwartz et al. 1985), oral contraceptives (Wreje et al. 1997) — although this is disputed by Bjorklund et al. (2000b), and genetic susceptibility (MacLennan and MacLennan 1997). The contribution of relaxin to pregnancy-related lumbopelvic pain is controversial, with some evidence showing an association between relaxin and PGP (MacLennan et al. 1986b; Kristiansson et al. 1996b) but with other evidence showing no association (Albert et al. 1997; Bjorklund et al. 2000a). Relaxin levels are at their highest during labour but fall to almost non-pregnant levels by three days postpartum (MacLennan et al. 1986a), suggesting that other reasons must be contributory, as many women experience postpartum lumbopelvic pain.

Conclusive association between new-onset postpartum backache and epidural analgesia has not been demonstrated (Breen et al. 1994; Russell et al. 1996; Macarthur et al. 1997; Howell et al. 2002; Loughnan et al. 2002), though its masking effect on pain may lead to women adopting unsuitable positions in labour (MacArthur et al. 1990).

Management of lumbopelvic pain and dysfunction

It is important to acknowledge that pregnancy-related lumbopelvic pain and dysfunction is a common, recognised condition, better managed with prompt identification and assessment and appropriate treatment. It is known that, if left untreated, this condition may last more than 2 years (Albert et al. 2001).

Advice, posture, education and general exercise

Antenatal education on posture and back pain by a physiotherapist has been shown to reduce back and pelvic pain, reduce sick leave and continue to benefit women in the postnatal period (Noren et al. 1997). Antenatal advice should cover adopting comfortable resting positions, how best to move out of bed, chair or car, postures in walking and standing, and lifting and handling. In addition, postnatal advice includes positions for breast-feeding, nappy changing, bathing and handling the growing baby.

Treatment of articular dysfunctions/movement restriction of the spine and pelvic girdle

There is some evidence that pregnancy-related lumbopelvic pain may respond to manual therapy (Daly et al. 1991; Diakow et al. 1991; McIntyre and Broadhurst 1996), and accurate assessment of the spine and pelvic girdle is imperative to enable treatment to be targeted at the correct structures. Providing severity and irritability have been properly assessed, many manual therapy techniques in use in the non-pregnant population can be used and adapted for women with pregnancy-related lumbo-pelvic pain. Many techniques can be adapted to the side-lying position.

Management depends upon whether there are movement restrictions caused by a true articular restriction, or those where the joint is held in an abnormal position by the imbalance or altered recruitment of the muscles (Lee and Vleeming 2000). Lee (1999) recommends that articular restrictions be treated first with mobilisation or manipulation techniques, followed by treatment of myofascial structures using muscle energy techniques (MET). Other techniques for treating myofascial dysfunctions include trigger point massage, strain/counterstrain, positional release, and soft tissue manipulation techniques or taping to offload overactive muscles. Unilateral or bilateral muscles that may be overactive with PGP are the hip adductors, psoas, erector spinae and quadratus lumborum. Tightness may be palpated in the posterior fibres of the pubococcygeus.

With SPD, special attention should be paid to overactive pelvic adductors, underactive abductors, unilateral displacement of one innominate bone (Röst 1999), and poor pelvic girdle and spinal stabilising muscle function. Advice regarding unilateral weight-bearing activities and hip abduction should be given. Crutches, or in the most severe cases a wheelchair, may be required.

The use of a sacroiliac/trochanteric belt for sacroiliac and symphysis pubis instability both antenatally and postnatally may stabilise the pelvic girdle joints (Damen et al. 2002; Mens et al. 2006) and substitute the work of the internal oblique muscle (Snijders et al. 1998), but its effect on pain is equivocal (Depledge et al. 2005). However, a belt should be tried if the active straight leg raising test is positive. A large tubular bandage for the abdomen, or maternity belt, may give added support.

Liaison with midwives is essential. Women should be aware of the masking effect of epidural and spinal anaesthesia in relation to excessive abduction of the hips during labour and delivery. If possible, they should adopt the most comfortable position during labour (for example, left side-lying, or kneeling upright with support). They should be discouraged from placing their feet on attendants' hips and care should be taken if lithotomy is required (ACPWH 2007a). Suturing should take place in the most comfortable position for the mother.

Muscle re-education

Abdominal, spinal and pelvic girdle muscle recruitment needs to be retrained to stabilise an unstable spinal segment or pelvic girdle joint. Specific spinal and pelvic girdle stabilising programmes have been shown to be effective in reducing pain antenatally (Elden et al. 2005) and postnatally (Stuge et al. 2004a; Stuge et al. 2004b; Stuge et al. 2006).

Rehabilitation exercises antenatally and postnatally should concentrate initially on correct recruitment of both pelvic girdle stabilising muscles (gluteus medius and maximus) and core lumbopelvic stabilising muscles (transversus abdominis, lumbar multifidus, pelvic floor muscles). Poor recruitment and decreased strength of hip adductors and flexors has been shown to be a factor in pregnancy-related PGP (Mens et al. 2002), and altered recruitment of gluteus maximus has been shown in patients with sacroiliac joint pain. No studies of gluteus medius in pregnancy-related PGP have been undertaken, but the waddling gait of these patients is a common sign and is probably due to poor gluteus medius control. Therefore, it is proposed that the main muscles to be targeted in women with PGP are the core stability muscles as described above, plus the hip abductors, adductors, flexors and extensors. Consideration of the balance between adductors and abductors should be given due to their function in providing stability across the symphysis pubis (Lee 1999). Exercises for global stabilising muscles such as the oblique abdominals, erector spinae, latissimus dorsi and iliopsoas should follow, though possibly only postnatally. Once core stability has been gained, the woman should be encouraged to increase her strength, and general aerobic and cardiovascular fitness, particularly postnatally.

Rehabilitation exercises need to be functional, as many women cannot regularly attend a physiotherapy department owing to family commitments.

Pain management

There is increasing evidence that acupuncture is effective in relieving antenatal lumbopelvic pain (Wedenberg et al. 2000; Ternov et al. 2001; Guerreiro da Silva et al. 2004; Kvorning et al. 2004; Elden et al. 2005; Lund et al. 2006), though caution must be taken to avoid acupuncture points that might provoke abortion.

TENS may be used postnatally, but the use of TENS antenatally is controversial. A recent statement (ACPWH 2007b) declares that although it is of lower risk to the fetus than strong medication, careful consideration of the appropriate use of TENS must be given.

Management of diastasis rectus abdominis (DRA)

The consequences of a persistent DRA are not known but it is possible that the mechanical advantage of the two RA bellies is compromised and thus could affect muscle strength and potentially result in lumbopelvic pain. It is advisable for physiotherapists to examine the postnatal gap between the recti manually at the level of the umbilicus and assess the IRD. The IRD should resolve to approximately 20 mm by 8 weeks postpartum (Coldron 2006), which approximates to 1–2 finger widths. If there appears to be a persistent DRA (> 3 finger widths), advice regarding exercise should be given, including initial training of the deep abdominal muscles (transversus abdominis) (Sheppard 1996; Potter et al. 1997a) and avoidance of strong trunk-curling exercises to prevent herniation of abdominal contents.

Rib flare

Costal margin pain along the anterior surface of the lower ribs (possibly related to pressure from the ascending uterus and commonly called 'rib flare') may be accompanied by thoracic spinal and lateral chest pain. This may be relieved by side-flexion manœuvres away from the pain, and manual therapy techniques.

Nerve compression syndromes

Fluid retention may occur during the third trimester, which can lead to a variety of nerve compression syndromes. These include carpal tunnel syndrome (CTS), brachial plexus compression, meralgia paraesthetica (compression of the lateral cutaneous nerve of the thigh as it passes under the inguinal ligament, presenting as tingling and burning in the outer thigh) and posterior tibial nerve compression. These entrapments normally resolve postpartum. Wrist splints and ice are useful for CTS. Postural advice can be used for brachial plexus compression. Ice and elevation may help posterior tibial nerve compression (Barton 2004b).

EXERCISE AND PREGNANCY

General issues

Physiological, emotional, social and psychological issues influence physical fitness in pregnancy. The physiotherapist must be sensitive towards these, and be aware of other issues such as language, ethnic cultures, equal opportunities and women with special needs. The therapist's approach to the pregnant woman should be holistic, flexible, individual, and — where available — evidence-based.

Many women now incorporate regular exercise into their lifestyle and wish to continue during their pregnancy. A significant minority of women decide to take up exercise for the first time when they become pregnant.

The research available suggests that mild to moderate exercise is beneficial to the healthy pregnant woman (Clapp 2000) and is not harmful to the fetus (Riemann et al. 2000; Clapp et al. 2000; ACOG 2002; Arena and Maffulli 2002). Moderate intensity is defined as being able to talk easily, whilst increasing the heart rate to a maximum 140 beats per minute. Choice of exercise must be influenced by the physiological changes which will occur (Artal et al. 2003). For example, plasma volume increases before red cell volume, leading to a decreased ability to provide oxygen in response to demand. Also, increased demand causes raised respiratory rates, cardiac output values increase during pregnancy for the same activity (over the non-pregnant woman), and there is a loss of cardiac reserve. Strenuous activity might compromise the mother's health and that of the fetus.

Benefits and contraindications

Potential *benefits* of exercise include:

- maintenance of cardiovascular fitness
- maintenance of healthy weight range
- improvement of body awareness, posture, coordination and balance
- improvement in circulation
- increase in endurance and stamina
- provision of social interaction with exercise, enhancing feelings of social and emotional well-being

- possible reduction in problems during labour and delivery
- potentially shorter labour
- possible prevention of gestational diabetes
- reduction in minor complaints of pregnancy
- more rapid postnatal recovery.

Contraindications to exercise include:

- cardiovascular, respiratory, renal or thyroid disease
- diabetes (type 1, if poorly controlled)
- history of miscarriage, premature labour, fetal growth restriction, cervical incompetence
- hypertension, vaginal bleeding, reduced fetal movement, anaemia, breech presentation, placenta praevia (ACOG 2002).

Advice

The advice given to regular and non-regular exercisers will differ.

Regular exercisers

- Consult your doctor or midwife before beginning exercise.
- Exercise at a moderate level most days for 30 minutes or more (ACOG 2002; Hefferman 2000).
- Discontinue contact sports and activities that carry a high risk of falling or abdominal trauma. Avoid scuba diving (ACOG 2002).
- Self-regulate both the level of intensity and duration of exercise, aiming to keep core temperature below 38 degrees C.
- Aim for low-impact activity.
- Wear suitably supportive footwear to reduce musculoskeletal stresses.
- Maintain adequate fluid intake to prevent dehydration, and avoid exercise during hot and humid weather, or with pyrexia.
- Warm up and cool down for at least 5 minutes.
- Do not use developmental stretching (because of the effects of relaxin).
- Seek professional advice on specific exercises (e.g. for the pelvic floor muscles).
- Avoid ballistic exercise, low squats, crossover steps and rapid changes of direction.
- Do not exercise in the supine position after 16 weeks' gestation, to avoid aortocaval compression.
- Eat to appetite without calorific restriction.
- Work towards cross-training to avoid over-training, and stop exercise before fatigue sets in.

Non-regular exercisers

In addition to the above, women not used to regular exercise should be advised on the following:

- Do not start an exercise programme until > 13 weeks' gestation.
- Consider beginning with non-weight-bearing exercises such as aquanatal.
- Progress from simple and basic levels of exercise, increasing exercise tolerance gradually, under the supervision of a suitably qualified professional.

When to stop

All women should stop exercising immediately and seek advice from a doctor if they experience:

- abdominal pain
- per vaginum (PV — from the vagina) bleeding
- shortness of breath, dizziness, faintness, persistent severe headache, palpitations or tachycardia
- PGP which may also lead to difficulty in walking.

Most women will naturally reduce the amount of exercise they take during pregnancy as their weight increases, and as they fatigue and become breathless more rapidly.

Types of exercise

General categories

- *Leisure sports.* Provided the contraindications have been noted and the woman is familiar with her chosen activity, it is safe to continue pursuing leisure sports. These may include brisk walking, swimming, jogging, hiking, rowing and dancing. The pace adopted should be sufficient to cause aerobic changes. If pelvic pain is a problem, avoid the kicking motion of the legs during breast stroke swimming.
- *Low-impact aerobics* (or equivalent classes). The emphasis is on maintaining fitness levels.
- *Pilates or yoga* (modified for pregnancy). These cater for the non-aerobic elements of fitness — flexibility, control of breathing and relaxation.
- *Back care classes.* Core stability exercises may be taught, sometimes using a Swiss ball.
- *Gym work.* The pregnant woman may have access to a static bicycle, treadmill or cross-trainer, all of which encourage aerobic activity. Technique is especially important when strength-training. Women should use light weights, with submaximal lifts, aiming to use both upper and lower body muscle groups in a variety of exercises. Weights, sets and repetitions should be decreased further as pregnancy progresses (Avery et al. 1999).

Aquanatal classes

Aquanatal classes — that is, exercise classes in water designed specifically for pregnant and postnatal women — have grown in popularity in the UK in recent years. Pregnant women find exercise and relaxation in water enjoyable and beneficial, largely because of the feeling of weightlessness and the reduced jarring of the joints. It has been suggested that a woman submerged up to the level of the xiphisternum will experience only 28 per cent of her body weight (Harrison and Bulstrode 1987). Women in aquanatal classes notice that they get relief from aches and pains, feel they have more energy after the class, and sleep better. Another important benefit is the absence of post-exercise muscle soreness because, during immersion, all muscle work is concentric (Newham 1988). Other significant advantages are less obvious to the women themselves. Exercise in water helps to tone the respiratory muscles; the leg movements of swimming and exercise in water aid venous return; and the diuretic effect of immersion is helpful to a pregnant woman troubled by fluid-retention as immersion for 20–40 minutes results in a loss of 300–400 ml of fluid (Katz et al. 1991).

Women must be screened for contraindications and for any musculoskeletal problem of which the teacher should be aware (ACPWH 2004). Exercises can be amended for someone with a back, pelvic girdle, neck or other orthopaedic problem. Pregnant women with sacroiliac or symphysis pubis discomfort should be advised to modify their breast stroke leg movements and take small rather than wide steps sideways. All women should take short backward steps to avoid an increase in lumbar lordosis. Exercises that will overstretch the already compromised abdominal muscles should be excluded. Conversely, squatting, which is difficult on land and thought by some to be damaging, is safe in water as virtually no weight goes through the knee joints.

The aim of the class is to help maintain, not improve, a woman's level of fitness. Exercises must be safe and carefully chosen, and each included for a reason. Water exercises should be considered in their own right and not taken unchanged from exercise classes on land (Evans 2002). It is necessary to warm up in the water before starting aerobic and strengthening exercises. Buoyancy can be used to assist movement and to make the exercises easier, or to resist movement and allow muscle-strengthening. Pelvic floor muscle exercises should be included before, during or at the end of the class. Good posture should be taught at the beginning of the class, and participants reminded to maintain it throughout. If the water is warm enough, a relaxation session is an excellent way to end.

Antenatal classes

The Department of Health National Institute for Health and Clinical Excellence (NICE) guidelines (NICE 2003) recommend that all pregnant women should receive appropriate antenatal advice and information about childbirth.

The provision of high-quality and accessible antenatal education and advice for all pregnant women is important in order to prevent pelvic floor disorders. The most common of these is urinary incontinence, which is a major clinical problem that can have a profound impact on quality of life (Laycock et al. 2001). It affects about 10–30 per cent of women aged 15–64 years, with a much higher incidence among pregnant women, estimated at between 20 and 67 per cent (Hannestad et al. 2000; Mørkved et al. 2003). Lower urinary tract symptoms are so common in early pregnancy that they are often considered to be normal (Cutner and Cardozo 1990). Norwegian studies have reported an incidence of 42 per cent during pregnancy and symptoms persisting at 8 weeks for 38 per cent of all women (Mørkved and Bø 1999).

It is well documented and acknowledged by clinicians that low back and PGP in pregnancy is also common, incidence ranging from 50 to 70 per cent (Mantle et al. 1977; Fast et al. 1987; Berg et al. 1988; Ostgaard et al. 1991; Wu et al. 2004; Mogren and Pohjanen 2005; Gutke et al. 2006). Increasingly, there is theoretical evidence of coexisting low back and/or PGP with pelvic floor dysfunction, commonly urinary incontinence (Pool-Goudzwaard 2003; Lee and Lee 2004).

These figures highlight the need for a prevention and treatment strategy for these women in the perinatal period. By active involvement in antenatal care, women's health physiotherapists are well placed to provide advice and instruction to prevent and alleviate the physical stresses of pregnancy and childbirth and encourage a healthy lifestyle.

Midwives, physiotherapists and health visitors typically work together to provide antenatal education in the form of classes and group activity, though health visitors are more usually involved in postnatal groups. The sessions take many different formats, and vary in number and timing to suit the needs of each patient group. The challenge is to provide high-quality advice and information at a convenient time in a location that is accessible and in a format that is appropriate to the woman's needs and those of her partner, if appropriate.

Best practice would be to offer advice on safe exercise in pregnancy and on back care and pelvic floor early in pregnancy. 'Early bird' groups are held around 16 weeks of pregnancy when the physiotherapist's role is to discuss the changes in pregnancy, how these will affect the working woman, and how to adapt to the changes. One of the most important topics is to encourage a healthy lifestyle that includes regular safe exercise, walking being the simplest. Also care of the back should be addressed, to alleviate backache and prevent long-term problems. Women's work activities will be discussed and advice given on seating, lifting and so on. The structure and function of the pelvic floor muscles and the importance of pelvic floor muscle exercises to prevent long-term continence problems will be explained. Transversus abdominis activation will be taught, its role in providing stability to the lower back explained, and the importance of bringing activation of these muscles into everyday functional activities discussed.

The majority of the classes are held later in pregnancy from about 30 weeks onwards, commonly as a 4–6-week course held during the day or evening, or as a weekend course. Pregnant women only or couples may attend. The classes may be for first-time mothers or for women who have had previous pregnancies. Commonly they include a mixture of both. In some large hospitals there will be specific classes for twin pregnancies and elective caesarean deliveries. Attendees of these groups will benefit from meeting other women in a similar situation.

The physiotherapy content may have to be prioritised to fit into one 2-hour session, and drop-in sessions work well, especially for teenage and ethnic groups.

Classes may be held in the hospital, in local health centres or in other community settings.

The physiotherapy input to the later antenatal classes may include:

- the benefits of safe exercise in pregnancy
- postural advice on standing, sitting and lying
- the practice of transversus abdominis and pelvic floor muscle exercises, relating these to functional activities
- advice on back care and prevention of long-term problems
- advice on how to access physiotherapy services for musculoskeletal problems
- exercises and advice for the circulation
- coping strategies for labour, which include relaxation, positions of comfort and breathing awareness
- advice on early postnatal exercises and return to fitness.

In most cases the midwives will discuss labour, feeding and baby care.

There is a constant need to evaluate the classes to confirm that they are meeting the expectations of women and to ascertain whether all women have an equal opportunity to attend a class of their choice.

Postnatal physiotherapy

The role of the physiotherapist in the days, weeks and sometimes even months following the birth includes advice for the new mother on how to regain and perhaps improve her former level of fitness through appropriate exercise and education. Also included are the assessment and treatment of specific physical problems, emotional support and health education. Contact with the new mother may be in the postnatal ward, in the outpatients' physiotherapy department, or in community-based postnatal groups.

Although it might be considered the ideal for every woman to be advised by a women's health physiotherapist postnatally, this is becoming increasingly uncommon. Many women will not be seen by a physiotherapist, but should be given appropriate advice and literature.

Physiotherapy intervention may be limited to some or all of the following.

Caesarean section

Education during antenatal classes may help to prepare the mother for a caesarean. Postnatally, the physiotherapist should be aware of the reasons for the caesarean and offer emotional support and advice when required. Bed exercises and mobility, followed by early ambulation, reduce the risk of respiratory problems, back pain or deep venous thrombosis (DVT). Wound haematomas may respond well to ultrasound or pulsed electromagnetic energy (PEME). Abdominal and pelvic floor muscle exercises and optimal feeding postures should be taught.

Painful perineum

A prolonged or difficult delivery, episiotomy or an extended tear may result in a bruised, painful and oedematous perineum. Physiotherapeutic interventions might include ice packs, PEME, ultrasound, pelvic floor muscle exercises (to increase blood supply and aid healing), advice on supported defaecation, and the use of pillows under each buttock when sitting to prevent pressure on the wound. Scar tissue may cause longer-term pain or psychosexual problems.

Incontinence

Urinary urgency and incontinence can occur after delivery, particularly after a prolonged second stage, episiotomy, instrumental delivery, or delivery of a large baby. Training in pelvic floor muscle exercises by a physiotherapist postnatally, incorporating strategies to improve compliance, has been shown to reduce the incidence and severity of urinary incontinence (Chiarelli and Cockburn 2002), and the effect of postnatal pelvic floor muscle training on the prevention and treatment of stress urinary incontinence has been shown still to be present 1 year after delivery (Mørkved and Bø 2000). Persistent pelvic floor dysfunction should always be assessed and treated (see the section on urogenital dysfunction).

Incontinence of stool can also occur, and has been found to be more prevalent among women who experienced a third-degree tear (partial or complete disruption of the anal sphincter) or fourth-degree tear (complete disruption of the external and internal anal sphincter and epithelium) during delivery (Eason et al. 2002). See also the section on anorectal dysfunction.

Musculoskeletal problems

See the earlier section on musculoskeletal problems in the childbearing year.

Postnatal groups

Many new mothers find difficulty adjusting to, and caring for, a baby during the first few weeks. Extreme fatigue may result. Physiotherapists are well placed to motivate women, encouraging them to attend postnatal groups, support groups, relaxation or exercise classes. Input from a team of health professionals provides education and information on a wide range of topics relevant to the new mother.

Physiotherapists may lead a low-impact aerobics or Pilates exercise class, teach baby massage, or hold discussion/support groups. Stress-free physical activity is associated with a reduced likelihood of developing postnatal depression (Koltyn and Schultes 1997). Physiotherapists may detect new or previously undisclosed symptoms, and should be instrumental in referring the sufferer to an appropriate health professional. Postnatal groups promote a positive outlook, reinforcing healthy living for life.

UROGENITAL DYSFUNCTION

Problems relating to the female urinary and genital tracts are common and often complex. Increasingly, physiotherapy is the first line of treatment. The problems encountered most frequently are bladder dysfunction and genitourinary prolapse.

Bladder dysfunction

Most common is urinary incontinence, which may occur at any time in a woman's life but rises in incidence with age. A study of women aged 50–74 found that some leakage of urine was reported by 47 per cent, and regularly by 31 per cent (Holtedahl and Hunskaar 1998); other authors report similar findings. Six categories of incontinence are described: stress (SUI, USI), overactive bladder (OB, OAB), mixed, overflow, neurogenic detrusor overactivity and functional incontinence, and it is important to distinguish between these.

Stress urinary incontinence

Definition

The International Continence Society (ICS 2002) defines stress urinary incontinence as the complaint of involuntary leakage on effort or exertion, or on sneezing or coughing. Urodynamic stress incontinence (USI) is now the preferred term, replacing the original 'genuine stress incontinence'. USI is noted during filling cystometry and is defined as the involuntary leakage of urine during increased intra-abdominal pressure in the absence of a detrusor contraction.

This is the most common type of incontinence and may coexist with overactive bladder. It is associated with urethral hypermobility and/or an incompetent sphincter (closure) mechanism. The urethra has to remain closed and sealed, except during voluntary bladder emptying. Continence is maintained by urethral closure pressure, which must remain higher than detrusor (bladder muscle) pressure, both at rest and on physical exertion. Physical effort causes a sudden rise in intra-abdominal pressure, which is transmitted to the bladder. When pressure in the bladder rises above that of the urethra, there will be an involuntary escape of urine. The pelvic floor muscles contribute significantly to the continence mechanism, providing about one-third of urethral closure pressure (Raz and Kaufman 1977; Rud et al. 1980).

Overactive bladder

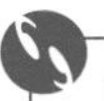

Definition

Overactive bladder is a urodynamic observation characterised by involuntary detrusor contractions during the filling phase, which may be spontaneous or provoked. Urge incontinence (the symptom) is the complaint of involuntary leakage accompanied or immediately preceded by urgency: that is, a sudden compelling desire to pass urine, which is difficult to defer (ICS 2002).

This form of leakage occurs when the detrusor contracts inappropriately as the bladder fills. The literature describes detrusor inhibition mediated by peripheral reflexes, which originate in the pelvic floor, perineum and urethra. Laycock (1998) suggests that activation of the dermatomes and myotomes from S2 to S4 — for example, a rapid contraction of the pelvic floor or standing on 'tip-toe' — may have an inhibitory effect on the detrusor, and so suppress inappropriate detrusor activity, leading to a decrease in urgency.

5

Overflow incontinence

Overflow incontinence

This was originally termed 'retention with overflow' and may be acute or chronic.

In hypotonic ('floppy') bladders, the normal response to the increase in pressure that occurs during filling may be absent, and the detrusor fails to contract. Retention is associated with outflow obstruction (e.g. in men with prostate disease), neuropathy, low spinal cord lesions, radical pelvic surgery and multiple sclerosis, or it may be secondary to drug therapy (especially with psychotropic drugs). Incontinence sometimes, but not always, occurs with retention.

Neurogenic detrusor overactivity

Definition

This term replaces 'hyperreflexia' (ICS 2002) and describes bladder dysfunction of neurological origin.

Neurogenic detrusor overactivity occurs in the presence of a suprasacral cord lesion where the bladder is isolated from cortical control (e.g. cerebrovascular incident, tumour, spinal cord injury or multiple sclerosis). One of the earliest symptoms of multiple sclerosis may be urinary urgency and it is important that physiotherapists are aware of this.

Functional incontinence

Definition

Functional incontinence includes all cases where there is involuntary loss of urine resulting from a deficit in ability to perform toileting functions secondary to physical or mental limitations (Mantle 2004).

Genital prolapse

Pelvic organ prolapse is the descent of one or more of:

- the anterior/posterior vaginal wall (known as cystocele and rectocele respectively)
- the top of the vagina (cervix, uterus)
- the vault (cuff) after hysterectomy.

Symptoms include the feeling of a lump ('something coming down'), low backache, heaviness and dragging sensation, or the need to replace the prolapse digitally in order to defaecate or pass urine. It can occur with other lower urinary tract dysfunction and may mask incontinence.

Prolapse occurs when the fibromuscular supports of the pelvic organs fail. Fifty per cent of parous women (those who have had children) have some degree of genital prolapse but only 10–20 per cent are symptomatic. Severity increases with age (Sultan et al. 1996). Norton (1990) reports a link between joint hypermobility, the presence of striae ('stretch marks') and prolapse, features which are present in other connective tissue disorders. It is suggested that some women exhibit an immature collagen type and that total collagen content may be reduced significantly (Jackson et al. 1995), leading to genital prolapse.

A trained pelvic floor will contract reflexly in response to a sudden rise in intra-abdominal pressure, thereby limiting downward movement of the organs and reducing the risk of damage to their supports. A voluntary contraction, performed before such episodes (e.g. coughing, lifting), will afford protection and should become a life-long habit.

Factors contributing to urogenital dysfunction

It is widely accepted that urogenital problems are associated with vaginal delivery (Wilson et al. 1996; Toozs-Hobson 1998). For many women, childbirth is probably the most significant factor contributing to the development of symptoms. Allen et al. (1990) suggest that a woman's first vaginal delivery causes muscle, fascial and nerve damage, and it is likely that further damage will occur with future deliveries. Chiarelli and Campbell (1997) suggest that forceps delivery increases this risk. There are other reported risk factors: pregnancy itself, straining at stool, heavy lifting, inappropriate exercise, chronic cough, obesity, pelvic surgery, hormonal status and ageing.

Pelvic floor muscle exercises

Women with stress incontinence, stress with urge incontinence, and urge incontinence and/or genital prolapse may all benefit from specialist physiotherapy.

The pelvic floor muscles have a significant role to play in the continence and organ support mechanisms; they contribute to urethral closure pressure and provide tonic inhibition to the bladder. They are capable of a brisk forceful contraction to counteract a rapid rise in intra-abdominal pressure or to suppress a sudden compelling need to void.

Key point

Recent guidance from the National Institute for Health and Clinical Excellence (NICE 2006) states that the first line treatment for women with stress or mixed urinary incontinence should, following digital assessment of the muscle contraction, be a trial of supervised pelvic floor muscle training of at least 3 month's duration.

Bump et al. (1991) state that all women presenting with pelvic floor dysfunction should undergo a digital vaginal examination to ensure correct muscle action. Their research demonstrated that fewer than 50 per cent of women were able to perform an optimal or correct pelvic floor contraction when given verbal or written instruction only, and that the feedback provided by digital examination is the only way to ensure appropriate pelvic floor muscle activity.

Teaching pelvic floor muscle exercises

Many widely differing exercise protocols are described in the literature and, unfortunately, no standardised outcome measures have been employed to allow evaluation. It is generally accepted, however, that certain principles are fundamental to success.

Clinical note

- To exercise the pelvic floor muscles, imagine that you are trying to stop yourself from passing wind, and at the same time trying to stop your flow of urine in mid-stream. The feeling is one of 'squeeze and lift', closing and drawing up the back and front passages. Continue the lift for as long as you can (up to 10 seconds). Release and rest for several seconds.
- Repeat as many times as you can (up to a maximum of 10 repetitions at a time). This will help to increase the endurance of your pelvic floor muscles.
- It is important to do this without tightening your buttocks, holding your breath or squeezing your legs together. You may feel your lower abdomen working at the same time, in the area just above your pubic bone.
- It is also important that the muscles are able to react quickly to stop leakage with coughs, sneezes etc. Practise tightening hard and fast, then relaxing immediately.
- Both these exercises can be practised anywhere, at any time and in any position, but not while emptying your bladder.

Principles of exercise: specificity, overload and maintenance

Gilpin et al. (1989) demonstrated that the pelvic floor exhibits 65 per cent type 1 fibres and 35 incontinence type 2, although these proportions vary depending on the subject's age, parity and hormonal status, and on the pelvic floor muscle site that is sampled. An exercise regime should include work for both fibre types specifically.

Type 1 fibres exhibit tonic activity and are engaged at lower levels of work and during a submaximal sustained contraction. Type 2 fibres are recruited during maximal pelvic floor activity, producing a brisk forceful contraction but fatiguing rapidly. Overload is developed by increasing the exercise frequency and duration appropriately as muscle function improves. Maintenance of improved function requires that exercises be continued for life.

Although sometimes suggested as an exercise, interrupting the flow of urine mid-stream is strongly discouraged since it may contribute to incomplete emptying and infection.

The pelvic floor as a synergist

Traditionally, pelvic floor muscle exercise has been taught in isolation from other trunk muscles. Although further studies are needed, there is some evidence that the pelvic floor forms part of the functional unit of local spinal stabilisation, acting in synergy with transversus abdominis and other segmental stabilisers (Sapsford et al. 1997; Richardson et al. 1999). Appropriate training of transversus abdominis, therefore, may facilitate re-education of the pelvic floor.

Adjuncts to exercise

The principal aim of physiotherapy is to strengthen the pelvic floor muscles, and the basis of treatment is an individualised exercise regimen that is progressed appropriately. Bø (1995) suggests that a successful outcome depends on 5–6 months of exercise, plus contact with the therapist. Other modalities may complement this programme, and might include biofeedback, neuromuscular electrical stimulation (NMES) and behavioural modification.

Biofeedback

Biofeedback may be via electromyography, a pressure sensor or real-time ultrasound. The woman receives immediate visual information regarding her pelvic floor activity and is able to modify/increase her effort accordingly. This can provide high levels of motivation. Because of the many variables involved, biofeedback does not measure muscle strength but simply monitors a trend.

Electrical stimulation

NMES is not an alternative to voluntary exercise, but an additional means of strengthening and improving the function of a weakened pelvic floor. Detrusor inhibition may be achieved by targeting the sensory afferent fibres of the pudendal nerve, using a frequency of 5–10 Hz. Higher frequencies of 30–50 Hz will reinforce cortical awareness and stimulate the type 2 fibres to produce a contraction.

Behavioural modification

Many women experience urinary frequency. Pressure from a prolapse, urgency or the belief that keeping the bladder empty of urine will prevent involuntary leakage may all be contributing factors. Bladder training aims gradually to increase both the amount of urine passed and the intervals between voiding. Normal bladder capacity is 350–500 ml, and this capacity can be sustained only if the muscular bladder remains compliant. Allowing it to fill to normal volumes will maintain its elasticity.

> ***Clinical note***
>
> Bladder dysfunction is not confined to women. LUTS are present in up to 30 per cent of men aged over 50, who have not undergone surgery (Chute et al. 1993). Physiotherapy intervention for male problems does not feature significantly in the literature but help is often sought from physiotherapists who specialise in continence management. Dorey (1998, 2000) discusses the subject in some detail and provides relevant references for further reading.

ANORECTAL DYSFUNCTION

The physiotherapist seeing patients with urogenital dysfunction might also treat anorectal dysfunctions such as faecal incontinence and constipation.

Faecal incontinence

The problem

Faecal incontinence affects 1 per cent or more of community-dwelling adults (Nelson et al. 1995; Perry et al. 2002) and over 10 per cent of those in residential care for the elderly (Tobin and Brocklehurst 1986). It can have a negative impact on quality of life (Madoff et al. 2004). Causes are similar to those listed under urogenital dysfunction, the most common being obstetric trauma.

> ***Definition***
>
> Leakage is described as *passive* (patient not aware) or *urge* (patient is aware of a need to defaecate, but is unable to control it).

Arguably of greatest significance is the consistency of stool. If this is liquid or very soft, then it is far more difficult to contain. Ideally, the referring doctor will have addressed this issue before the patient attends for physiotherapy.

Anal sphincters

The internal anal sphincter comprises smooth muscle, and provides 80–85 per cent of resting pressure. The external anal sphincter (EAS) is under voluntary control, and contracts in response to rectal distension to allow the individual to defer defaecation until an appropriate time.

Puborectalis

Puborectalis, part of the levator ani, also contributes to the continence mechanism, by forming an acute angle at the top of the anal canal (anorectal angle) to prevent the escape of rectal contents.

Physiotherapy intervention

As in urogenital dysfunction, muscle re-education may be indicated — exercises to improve the function of puborectalis and the EAS, with or without biofeedback. Electrical stimulation may also be used. Enck (1993), in a review, reported a cure or improvement rate of 79 per cent with biofeedback. Fynes et al. (1999) suggested the addition of electrical stimulation was more beneficial than exercises and biofeedback alone, but Mahony et al. (2004) found no enhanced symptomatic outcome from the addition of electrical stimulation to intra-anal electromyographic biofeedback.

As in all aspects of physiotherapy, appropriate advice should be given: for example, as regards diet and deferment (for urge incontinence). Interestingly, Norton et al. (2003), in a study of 171 patients with faecal incontinence, concluded that neither pelvic floor muscle exercise nor biofeedback was superior to standard care supplemented by advice and education.

Constipation

The problem

Constipation has been reported to affect between 2 and 34 per cent of adults, and a literature review (D'Hoore and Penninckx 2003) has suggested that obstructed defaecation (see below) specifically affects 7 per cent.

> ***Definition***
>
> Constipation may be defined as infrequent bowel motions (fewer than three times a week) or the need to strain at defaecation. It may be subdivided into slow-transit and obstructed defaecation.

Slow-transit defaecation

This may be idiopathic, but can be a result of the avoidance or postponement of defaecation by an individual amongst other causes. It has been claimed (Gattuso and Kamm 1993) that up to 50 per cent of patients with severe idiopathic constipation may have a history of childhood bereavement or of emotional, sexual or physical abuse.

Obstructed defaecation

This presents as an urge to defaecate, but an inability to empty fully. It may be associated with a failure to relax puborectalis (pelvic floor dyssynergia) or the EAS, or a lack of pelvic floor support (and resulting descent of the perineum) during defaecation (Markwell and Sapsford 1995). Causes are many, including obstetric trauma, pelvic surgery and prolonged straining. As with slow transit, authors have suggested an association with sexual abuse (Leroi et al. 1996). Obstructed defaecation may be found in combination with slow transit (Hutchinson et al. 1993).

Physiotherapy intervention

The physiotherapist is more commonly involved in the treatment of obstructed defaecation. The aim of treatment is to teach effective defaecation without straining (Markwell and Sapsford 1995) and should include correct positioning on the toilet, relaxation of puborectalis and the EAS, and optimum abdominal muscle action with an expulsive effort. Biofeedback might also be used, and a review of the literature undertaken by Bassotti et al. (2004) concluded that, although controlled trials were few and open to criticism, two-thirds of patients with obstructed defaecation due to pelvic floor dyssynergia should benefit from biofeedback.

If there is evidence of perineal descent or a rectocele, women might be advised to offer manual support to the perineum or digital support to the posterior vaginal wall, respectively, to facilitate bowel emptying.

As there is an increase in colonic transit following meals, patients can be encouraged to attempt defaecation at these times.

GYNAECOLOGICAL SURGERY

Operations

Major gynaecological surgery may be necessary for many reasons, including the removal of benign or malignant tumours, urogynaecological conditions (if they fail to respond to physiotherapy), and the treatment of problems related to fertility or ectopic pregnancy. The physiotherapist should be aware of the indication for surgery and the social and emotional implications for the woman and her family.

A list of procedures undertaken is prohibitively long for this text, but those more commonly encountered by the physiotherapist include:

- hysterectomy (removal of the womb), which can be undertaken vaginally or abdominally
- tension-free vaginal tape, e.g. TVT/TOT (transobturator tape)/TVT-O (transvaginal tension-free vaginal tape-obturator) (for stress urinary incontinence) (NICE 2003)
- Burch colposuspension (for stress urinary incontinence)
- anterior or posterior repair (for genital prolapse)
- salpingectomy (removal of a fallopian tube, often for an ectopic pregnancy)
- vulvectomy (removal of the vulva, for benign or malignant disease).

Physiotherapy

5

The physiotherapist working on the gynaecological ward is in a unique position to be able not only to prepare women for surgery, but also to provide health education for future life. Ergonomic advice for home and work, sports and leisure, postural care, abdominal and pelvic floor exercise and relaxation should be provided, preferably pre-operatively, and ideally before admission to hospital. This will give the patient an opportunity to organise changes at home. A group setting is good use of the therapist's time and gives a forum for peer support and discussion.

The physiotherapist must know each woman's history so as to be aware of any special needs (e.g. a diagnosis of malignancy). Special attention should be given to the psychosocial and psychosexual effects of gynaecological surgery on the patient and her family. Referral to other professional groups — for example, a Macmillan nurse or social worker — may be appropriate.

Pre-operative assessment will give the physiotherapist an opportunity to instigate treatment for problems such as urogenital or anorectal dysfunction and musculoskeletal problems.

Pre-operative care

This can include:

- assessment of risk factors (e.g. respiratory conditions, current medication etc.)
- identification of urogenital or anorectal dysfunction
- identification of musculoskeletal problems
- exercises and strategies to promote postoperative mobility and comfort
- postoperative recovery plan, both before and after discharge from hospital
- relaxation.

Postoperative care

The presence of an intravenous infusion, urinary catheter (suprapubic or urethral), patient-controlled analgesia and vaginal pack should be noted. The physiotherapist must be aware of the findings at surgery, and their potential physical and psychological impact on the patient. There may be concerns about relationships or resuming sexual activity, and referral to the relevant professional may be appropriate (Sacco Ezzell 1999).

Respiratory function
Patients may be instructed in appropriate respiratory techniques and wound support when coughing, especially women who have undergone surgery for prolapse. Those with predisposing factors to postoperative respiratory complications, those undergoing extensive and invasive surgery, and those who are already debilitated are at increased risk of postoperative chest problems (Webber and Pryor 1998).

Circulation
Patients considered at risk of developing DVT are fitted with anti-embolus stockings and prophylactic anticoagulant therapy is administered. Ankle and quadriceps exercises will help prepare for mobilisation postoperatively and therefore reduce the risk of DVT (Webber and Pryor 1998).

Mobility, comfort and posture
The patient should be taught correct movement patterns for bed mobility, transfer from bed to chair, movement from sitting to standing, and positions of comfort on the bed and in a chair. This will reduce strain on the operation site and facilitate mobility. Reassurance that correct movement patterns can do no harm to the wound, along with good analgesic cover, will contribute to early mobilisation.

Urination and defaecation
The patient should sit on the toilet or commode with feet supported. When defaecating in the early postoperative period, she may feel more confident and comfortable if supporting her wound with hands placed over a folded towel (or perineal pad following vaginal surgery).

Abdominal exercises
Contractions of transversus abdominis should be taught to maintain the musculature of the abdominal wall. Pelvic tilting and knee rolling might ease LBP and painful flatus. Abdominal massage applied in a clockwise direction can also help the latter. These exercises and self-help strategies may be commenced as soon as the woman feels ready (e.g. the first or second day after surgery). Early mobilisation will also help to relieve these postoperative discomforts.

Pelvic floor muscle exercises and advice
The physiotherapist should confirm with the consultant any local policy for commencement of pelvic floor muscle exercises. (Jarvis et al. 2005). Women who have undergone surgery for prolapse and/or incontinence may already have poor connective tissue. If returning to a lifestyle that may have contributed to the necessity for surgery, they should be given appropriate advice — correct lifting techniques, avoidance of standing for long periods, awareness of the role of the pelvic floor and its interaction with transversus abdominis. Outpatient follow-up might be beneficial.

Going home
Women are generally anxious to return to full activity. Consideration must be given to the surgery undergone when advice is sought concerning progression of physical activity (e.g. work and sports). Discharge from hospital may be as early as 3 days following some surgery, though it can be considerably longer. Convalescence is usually for 1–2 months with a gradual increase in physical activity, but heavy lifting should be avoided for at least 2 months (Chamberlain 1995).

Relaxation
If time allows, the physiotherapist may teach relaxation to help the patient cope with the anxieties of hospitalisation and any future stresses.

PELVIC PAIN

Acute and chronic pain

Pelvic pain in women has many varied sources, diagnoses and outcomes. It can be acute or chronic. Acute pain usually has an easily identifiable cause, such as dyspareunia (pain on sexual intercourse) caused by scar tissue following childbirth. Appropriate treatment will alleviate it.

When pain has lasted more than 6 months it is termed chronic. Although it may still have a well-defined cause (e.g. endometriosis), it can involve a much more complex interplay between biomechanical, behavioural, emotional and sociocultural influences, all of which need to be taken into account in the treatment. This has led to clinicians involved in treating this group of women advocating a multidisciplinary integrated approach (Steege et al. 1998).

Prevalence

The annual prevalence of chronic pelvic pain has been estimated at between 24.4 cases per 1000 women (Davies et al. 1992) and 38.3 per 1000 (Zondervan et al. 1999). It has been estimated that the economic burden to the National Health Service is £158 million, with indirect costs of a further £24 million (Davies et al. 1992).

Pelvic pain has traditionally been ascribed (from a gynaecological view) to endometriosis, pelvic inflammatory disease, adhesions secondary to infection or surgery, and — more recently — pelvic venous congestion. The most important non-gynaecological cause is irritable bowel syndrome. Other causes include ilio-inguinal nerve entrapment, levator ani syndrome, coccydynia, interstitial cystitis, vulval vestibulitis/vulvodynia and musculoskeletal dysfunction.

Two studies have shown that between 28 and 61 per cent of patients involved never receive a diagnosis (Zondervan et al. 1999; Mathias et al. 1996). This is highly significant for all health professionals working with this group of patients, as sufferers often feel that their pain has not been validated and will not be taken seriously until they have a diagnosis (Grace 1995). This may result in a fruitless round of clinicians.

Role of the physiotherapist

The role of the physiotherapist in the management of women with chronic pelvic pain is to decrease the pain, increase function and treat existing (and help prevent future) musculoskeletal dysfunction.

Following a detailed musculoskeletal examination, including assessment of the pelvic floor muscles, the treatment modalities used to achieve this may include the measures listed in Table 5.1.

The modalities chosen will vary according to the needs of the patient and the experience of the clinician involved. Close liaison with other members of the multidisciplinary team is essential to maximise the benefit of treatment.

Table 5.1 Treatment modalities for pelvic pain

- Muscle imbalance work
- Muscle energy techniques
- Core stability exercises
- Pelvic floor rehabilitation
- Electrical stimulation
- Soft-tissue mobilisations
- Joint manipulation
- Breathing and relaxation techniques
- Heat/cold therapy
- Hydrotherapy
- Biofeedback and alternative therapies

MENOPAUSE

Menopause is the cessation of menstruation and marks the end of a woman's reproductive years. It has significant implications for a woman's health and quality of life, and so is of great relevance to the physiotherapist.

Menopause in the context of a woman's life

Average life expectancy has risen significantly in the last 150 years, but the age at which menopause occurs has remained remarkably constant at 50¾ years.
A British woman can expect to enjoy about 30 years of postmenopausal life (Belsey 1999). Biochemical and metabolic changes following menopause may cause distressing symptoms that adversely affect quality of life.

Oestrogens are the group of female hormones produced by the ovary. Oestrogen receptors are present in many tissues, and normal physiological function is dependent on the presence of this steroid. The perimenopause describes the period during which ovarian function declines. The menstrual cycle becomes erratic and a woman may seek help for symptoms of oestrogen depletion.

Vasomotor effects

Examples are hot flushes and night sweats. The cause of this vasomotor instability is complex and unclear (Bachmann 2001), and severity varies widely between individuals.

Musculoskeletal and articular effects

Osteoporosis, characterised by low bone mass, is one of the most clinically significant sequelae of oestrogen deficiency.

Articular changes may occur due to a decrease in the collagen content of ligaments and articular soft tissues (Whitehead and Godfree 1992). Muscular changes are attributed to an overall reduction in muscle mass, with a decrease in both strength and endurance of muscle tissue. These changes result in an increased risk of falls and injury, which may require physiotherapy.

Cardiovascular disease

Cardiovascular disease (CVD) is the biggest killer of postmenopausal women in Western society. It had generally been accepted that postmenopausal oestrogen replacement conferred protection against CVD, greatly reducing the risk (Mendelsohn and Karas 1999). However, this postulation is now questioned (Burger and Teede 2001), with suggestions that oestrogen may actually *increase* the risk of cardiovascular events. The conflicting evidence that has emerged during the last 5 years requires that robust RCTs be performed so that women may be advised appropriately.

Cognitive function

Oestrogen lack is thought to be involved in alteration of neurotransmitters in the brain (Genazzani et al. 1998), with a consequent decline in cognitive function and increased incidence of dementia. These changes will have implications for the woman, her family and health professionals, including the physiotherapist who may be involved in her care.

Urogenital oestrogen deficiency syndrome

Oestrogen receptors are present in the urogenital tract and the pelvic floor (Smith et al. 1990) and the ageing woman may experience vaginal dryness, soreness, infection and dyspareunia (pain on intercourse). Genital prolapse and urinary symptoms, including incontinence, frequency, urgency and voiding difficulties, are common (Samsioe 1998). The physiotherapist has an important role to play in the conservative management of these problems (see the section above on urogenital dysfunction).

BREAST CANCER

Breast cancer is the most common cancer affecting women in the United Kingdom, with an average of 1 in 9 being diagnosed. Around 41 000 new cases of breast cancer are recorded yearly and it causes over 12 000 deaths annually. The highest incidence of breast cancer is found in North America, with 99.4 women per 100 000 affected; the lowest incidence is in China, with 11.77 per 100 000. The Egyptians first documented breast cancer in 2650 BC and up until 1999 it was the primary cause of cancer death in women (Office for National Statistics 2004).

The risk factors for breast cancer are shown in Table 5.2.

Initial diagnosis is made by mammography and ultrasound scan, followed by needle aspiration or biopsy to establish the extent and stage of the disease and its hormonal (oestrogen and progesterone) status. There are four stages of breast cancer, I–III potentially being curable (Table 5.3).

Table 5.2 Risk factors for breast cancer

- *Gender* – predominately a female disease
- *Age* – risk increases with age
- *Hormonal factors* – uninterrupted menstrual cycles; early menarche/late menopause
- *Reproductive history* – no children or delay; lack of breast-feeding
- *Exogenous hormones* – contraceptive pill/hormone replacement therapy (HRT)
- *Family or personal history* of breast cancer
- *Other factors* – postmenopausal obesity, lack of physical activity, excessive alcohol consumption, exposure to ionising radiation, a fatty diet, higher socioeconomic status

(Clavel-Chapelon 2002; van den Brandt et al. 2000; Dixon 2001.)

Table 5.3 Stages of breast cancer

Stage I	Tumour up to 2 cm No lymph nodes affected No evidence of spread beyond the breast
Stage II	Tumour between 2 cm and 5 cm and/or Lymph nodes in armpit affected No evidence of spread beyond armpit
Stage III	Tumour more than 5 cm Lymph nodes in armpit affected No evidence of spread beyond armpit
Stage IV	Tumour of any size Lymph nodes in armpit often affected Cancer has spread to other parts of body

The majority of patients will undergo surgery to remove the cancer, although management depends on the stage of the disease. Many women choose breast-sparing surgery such as wide local excision or lumpectomy, which removes the breast lump and the surrounding tissue. The scars are normally small and the cosmetic appearance of the breast is good with obvious psychological benefit. However, if the cancer is large or below the nipple a mastectomy is more appropriate. For some patients primary breast reconstruction is achieved at the same time as the mastectomy, although it is usual to delay this until treatment has been completed. During surgery, axillary lymph nodes are excised to assess whether the cancer has spread beyond the breast. Historically all the axillary lymph nodes were removed; however, newer techniques of sampling lymph nodes and sentinel node biopsy are now in use, which may reduce the incidence of lymphoedema (see below).

Adjuvant therapies

- *Radiotherapy* is frequently given following breast surgery, particularly after breast-sparing operations; its main aim is to irradiate any cancer cells that may remain in the area.
- *Chemotherapy* is mainly used as an adjuvant therapy for pre-menopausal women and when the cancer has spread to the axillary lymph nodes. Chemotherapy may also be given as neo-adjuvant therapy to shrink the tumour, thereby facilitating more conservative surgery. Women who have oestrogen-sensitive tumours also receive some form of hormonal therapy, e.g tamoxifen or anastrozole to block the cancer-promoting effect of oestrogen. There are a number of

ongoing trials to establish the best regimes and therapies for pre- and postmenopausal women (Wishart et al. 2002).

Role of the physiotherapist

Physiotherapists have an important role in the rehabilitation of breast cancer patients. Their problem-solving approach and anatomical and physiological knowledge of the shoulder complex makes them the ideal healthcare professional to encourage patients. Through rehabilitation, physiotherapists promote independence and a return to normal activities, ultimately improving quality of life. Exercise groups on a ward level can work well postoperatively, with patients offering each other peer support.

Pre-operative care

This can include:

- full assessment of any existing musculoskeletal shoulder or neck problems that may affect postoperative outcomes
- identification of any risk factors
- information and advice, including a leaflet on postoperative exercise routines
- strategies to prevent the occurrence of lymphoedema (1 in 4 breast cancer patients will suffer with this). Ideally, circumferential measurements could be taken as a baseline recording.

Postoperative care

Immediately after surgery patients usually have at least one drain in place that remains in situ for 3–7 days. Any form of cancer diagnosis is distressing and the physiotherapist must be aware of the psychological impact and resultant altered body image that can occur with the loss of a breast.

- *Postoperative exercise*. Daily general upper limb mobility exercises need to be encouraged. Specific shoulder exercises are taught to prevent stiffness. Some hospitals limit shoulder mobility to 90 degrees until the drains are removed. The evidence for and against this is limited; however, there is some support for the belief that physiotherapy aids recovery of shoulder mobility after breast cancer (Schultz et al. 1997; Clodius 2001; Box et al. 2002).
- *Pain*. It is usual for patients to experience postoperative pain and this is relieved by medication. However, some patients can go on to suffer from chronic pain, which may be far more complex due to biomechanical, behavioural, emotional and sociocultural influences. Physiotherapy modalities such as TENS, muscle imbalance work, soft-tissue and joint mobilisations, relaxation techniques and alternative and cognitive therapies can all help.
- *Prevention of lymphoedema*. This will be covered in the lymphoedema section below, but patients are encouraged to moisturise the arm and breast area daily with an emollient cream and to avoid any invasive medical interventions such as venepuncture or blood pressure measurements on the affected limb.
- *Cording/axillary web syndrome*. Tender cord-like structures, thought to be a result of lymphangitis or lymphatic thrombosis, may arise from the chest wall to the axilla, sometimes extending down the arm itself. These cords restrict movement and cause significant pain. Physiotherapists need to mobilise them gently with soft tissue massage, and encourage passive and active physiological movements to initiate their dispersal.
- *Scarring*. Surgical scars may become adhered to underlying structures, i.e. fascia, resulting in tightness and discomfort in the axilla and chest wall regions. Patients should be encouraged to massage scars, once healed, to improve tissue pliability.
- *Postural advice*. Removal of the breast tissue causes weight imbalance and as a consequence patients tend to protract their shoulder. If this is not corrected, the pectoral muscles will shorten and tighten, leading to muscle imbalance and pain.
- *Numbness*. During axillary surgery the cutaneous nerves are incised, resulting in sensory loss in the axilla, lateral chest wall and upper arm. It is not uncommon for patients to experience pain and paraesthesia as sensory recovery occurs.
- *Radiotherapy treatment*. Prior to radiotherapy it is imperative that patients have good shoulder mobility to facilitate radiotherapy positioning. Post-radiotherapy patients should be encouraged to continue their shoulder mobility exercises, as treatment can cause delayed-onset stiffness.
- *Return to function*. All patients are encouraged to lead an active and normal life after having breast surgery. Care is always needed to prevent lymphoedema but patients should not be discouraged from activities of daily living that could improve quality of life.

LYMPHOEDEMA

The condition

Definition

Lymphoedema is chronic and progressive swelling caused by a low-output failure of the lymphatic system, resulting in the development of a high-protein oedema in the tissues (Földi et al. 2003).

Lymphoedema is a form of chronic oedema, which is a persistent swelling due to the excess accumulation of fluid in the tissues (British Lymphology Society 2001). In addition to lymphoedema, chronic venous insufficiency and dependency can result in chronic oedema. Provided there is no indication for medical intervention, a combination of physical therapies, as used in the treatment of lymphoedema, may be beneficial.

Lymphoedema is classified as primary or secondary in origin.

5

Classification of lymphoedema

- *Primary lymphoedema* – lymphoedema due to a congenital lymphatic dysplasia
- *Secondary lymphoedema* – lymphoedema due to anatomical obliteration of part of the lymphatic system due to an extrinsic process (e.g. surgery or repeated infections) or as a consequence of functional deficiency (e.g. paralysis) (ISL 2003).

In the Western world, cancer or its treatment is a common cause of lymphoedema. Surgical removal of part of the lymphatic system, or fibrotic changes subsequent to surgery or radiotherapy, result in a partial obstruction in lymphatic drainage and the development of lymphoedema in the affected limb and associated part of the trunk. The time of onset varies and in some cases can be many years after the initial cancer treatment (Stanton et al. 1996).

Prevalence and incidence of cancer-related lymphoedema

Recent evidence suggests a crude prevalence for chronic oedema of 1.3 per 1000 (Moffat et al. 2003). Evidence around incidence is available for people with breast cancer-related lymphoedema and is estimated to be around 25 per cent of the population receiving treatment (Pain and Purushotham 2000). Evidence around the incidence of lower limb and midline lymphoedema is limited, although there are indications that the risk of lymphoedema is at least equal to that for breast cancer patients (Keeley 2000).

Recent evidence has indicated that the number of people in the United Kingdom with a non-cancer-related lymphoedema is greater than the number of those with a cancer-related lymphoedema by a ratio of 3:1 (Moffat et al. 2003). The prevalence of lymphoedema increases with age (5.4 per 1000 over 65 years).

The onset of lymphoedema is often marked by intermittent swelling and paraesthesia (Piller 1999). Initially, the oedema is soft and pitting and reduces on elevation (Keeley 2000). With time and recurrent skin infections, fibrotic changes occur in both the skin and subcutis, with a progressive swelling and distortion of shape. The skin and tissues become thickened with enhanced skin folds and increased adiposity, and the swelling becomes largely non-pitting. The size of the limb increases and is sometimes accompanied by a distortion in shape. Movement becomes restricted as the limb becomes increasingly heavy and uncomfortable.

Women with lymphoedema are predisposed to recurrent attacks of acute inflammatory episodes (AIE), often referred to as cellulitis (Browse et al. 2003). These apparent skin infections are recognised by signs and symptoms that include acute pain, swelling, anorexia, fevers, vomiting and rigors.

The psychosocial impact of living with lymphoedema can be profound, resulting in negative feelings such as embarrassment, loss of self-esteem and increased feelings of anxiety and depression. Patients also experience impaired physical mobility and pain (Tobin et al. 1993; Woods et al. 1995; Williams et al. 2004).

Although no curative treatment is available, a combination of physical therapies is used to control and reduce the complications associated with lymphoedema. Patient education is a primary aim of any treatment programme. Assessment and treatment are provided by specialist trained physiotherapists and nurses. A treatment plan is agreed and negotiated with the patient following a comprehensive assessment of needs. Ongoing reviews are usually required to monitor progress and to provide a new supply of compression garments.

Role of the physiotherapist

Treatment is based around four key areas (Földi et al. 2003; Jenns 2000):

- skin care
- compression/support
- exercise
- lymphatic massage.

Skin care

This involves the daily application of emollient cream and the provision of information and advice on skin care to minimise the risk of AIE. Advice includes protection of the skin from cuts, insect bites and burns (e.g. when sewing, gardening or sunbathing). Whenever possible, medical interventions such as venepuncture or taking blood pressure should be undertaken on the unaffected side, to minimise any potential risk.

Compression garments

These are used to limit and control swelling in the limbs. In breast cancer, a glove, sleeve or combined glove and sleeve may be used, depending on the extent of the swelling. Garments are usually worn during the day, especially for exercise and when working. In some cases a bandaging system described as multilayer lymphoedema bandaging (MLLB) is used in combination with lymphatic massage to reverse complications such as severe swelling or distorted limb shape, prior to the introduction of compression garments (Badger et al. 2000). Pneumatic compression therapy (e.g. Flotron) is a traditional method of treatment, but there is concern that continued use will increase the risk of midline swelling (Boris and Lasinski 1989; Casley-Smith and Casley-Smith 1997).

Dynamic exercise

This is beneficial, as lymphatic drainage is enhanced by the effect of the muscle pump, particularly when a compression garment is worn. Gentle stretching exercises also help to maintain or improve range of movement and to facilitate good posture (Harris et al. 2001). Excessive exercise can increase the lymphatic load and result in further swelling, so patients are warned to introduce any new activity gradually and with caution.

Lymphatic massage

Manual lymphatic drainage (MLD) is characterised by the pressure and sequence of the technique, designed to stimulate drainage through the functioning lymphatics. This is usually the only method of care available to treat midline oedema (i.e. face, trunk). A simplified method is shown to the patient for self-treatment (Williams et al. 2002).

PSYCHOSEXUAL ISSUES

Sexual activity and enjoyment is essentially a psychophysical act, which can be affected by obstetric and gynaecological problems, and by emotions. The use of the term 'psychosexual' is important, as any sexual relationship involves whole people with previous experiences and feelings, attached to anatomical sexual parts.

Physiotherapists usually feel they must be 'doing' something to treat their patients. However, unless they are also able to listen and acknowledge the real problem, change will not occur. The physiotherapist may be the first person the patient trusts enough to share this problem. The women's health physiotherapist is one of the few professionals who may include a vaginal examination as part of her assessment. This is a very intimate procedure and a time of self-awareness for the patient. In psychosexual counselling it is referred to as the 'moment of truth' and should be approached with sensitivity and care. This may be the occasion when past feelings come to light: for example, previous sexual abuse.

Childbirth is said to be the greatest emotional crisis in a woman's life and she can find it very traumatic. Some women take time to come to terms with the experience and the consequent changes to their body caused by pregnancy and birth, which may affect their sexual activity in the short or long term. The perineum can feel painful for some time after an episiotomy or tear, and intercourse may be difficult and therefore avoided. This pain and a perceived change in body image may affect any close relationship. The physiotherapist and other health professionals must encourage the woman to talk about her labour and about any feelings of disappointment or loss of control, particularly how the experience made her feel.

A woman who suffers from faecal and urinary incontinence is embarrassed and often unable to speak to anyone about the problem. She is afraid that she smells, she feels dirty and is ashamed that she leaks, and so may avoid having intercourse or close contact with her partner. This can have a devastating effect on the relationship.

Concern about a change in body image can occur after breast and gynaecological surgery, particularly for malignancy. Some women grieve for the loss of their uterus. To them, it is an intrinsic part of being a woman and its removal feels like a bereavement.

During the menopause, many changes take place, both physical and emotional. Women may suffer from loss of libido (sex drive), and vaginal tissues can become dry and cause pain during intercourse. Dyspareunia can also be the result of a surgical procedure, or acute or chronic pelvic pain, as well as after childbirth.

Feelings play a large part in psychosexual problems and the physiotherapist must be prepared to listen to patients who choose to share these feelings. If the patient feels she needs further help, the physiotherapist should know what options are available for referral. It is also very important that the therapist knows whom to go to for a debriefing, as experienced support might be required with these sometimes complex issues.

FURTHER READING

Physiotherapy in women's health

Association of Chartered Physiotherapists in Women's Health: www.acpwh.org.uk

Mantle J, Haslam J, Barton S (eds) 2004 Physiotherapy in Obstetrics and Gynaecology, 2nd edn. Butterworth–Heinemann: Oxford

Sapsford R, Bullock-Saxton J, Markwell S 1998 Women's Health: A Textbook for Physiotherapists. WB Saunders: London

Pregnancy and Childbirth

Fraser DM, Cooper MA (eds) 2003 Myles' Textbook for Midwives, 14th edn. Churchill Livingstone: Edinburgh

Antenatal Classes, Advice and Exercise

Brayshaw E 2003 Exercises for Pregnancy and Childbirth: A Guide for Educators. Books for Midwives: Oxford

Brayshaw E, Wright P 1994 Teaching Physical Skills for the Childbearing Year. Books for Midwives: Hale

Nolan M 2000 Antenatal Education. A Dynamic Approach. Baillière Tindall: London

Schott J, Priest J 2002 Leading Antenatal Classes: A Practical Guide. Books for Midwives Press: Oxford

Breast Cancer

Weblink

www.breastcancercare.org
www.cancerresearchuk.org

Lymphoedema

Twycross R, Jenns K, Todd J (eds) 2000 Lymphoedema. Radcliffe Medical: Oxford

Psychosexual Issues

Weblink

Institute of Psychosexual Medicine: www.ipm.org.uk

Skrine RL 1997 Blocks and Freedoms in Sexual Life. Radcliffe Medical: Oxford

Skrine RL, Montford H (eds) 2001 Psychosexual Medicine: An Introduction. Edward Arnold: London

REFERENCES

Abitol MM 1997 Quadrupedalism, bipedalism, and human pregnancy. In: Vleeming A, Mooney V, Dorman T (eds) Movement, Stability and Low Back Pain. Churchill Livingstone: Edinburgh

Abramson D, Roberts SM, Wilson PD 1934 Relaxation of the pelvic joints in pregnancy. Surg Gynaecol Obstet 58: 595–613

ACOG (American College of Obstetricians and Gynecologists) 2002 Exercise during pregnancy and the postpartum period. Obstet Gynecol 99: 171–173

ACPWH (Association of Chartered Physiotherapists in Women's Health) 2004 Aquanatal guidelines. Available from ACPWH, Chartered Society of Physiotherapy, 14 Bedford Row, London WC1R 4ED or via www.acpwh.org.uk

ACPWH 2007a Pregnancy-related pelvic girdle pain. www.acpwh.org.uk

ACPWH 2007b ACPWH guidance on the safe use of transcutaneous electrical nerve stimulation (TENS) for musculoskeletal pain during pregnancy. www.acpwh.org.uk

Albert H, Godskesen M, Westergaard JG et al. 1997 Circulating levels of relaxin are normal in pregnant women with pelvic pain. Eur J Obstet Gynecol Reprod Biol 74: 19–22

Albert H, Godskesen M, Westergaard J 2001 Prognosis in four syndromes of pregnancy-related pelvic pain. Acta Obstet Gynecol Scand 80: 505–510

Allen RE, Hosker GL, Smith AR, Warrell DW 1990 Pelvic floor damage and childbirth: a neurophysiological study. Br J Obstet Gynaecol 97: 770–779

Arena B, Maffulli N 2002 Exercise in pregnancy: how safe is it? Sports Med Arthrosc 10(1): 15–22

Artal R, O'Toole M 2003 Guidelines of the American College of Obstetricians and Gynecologists for exercises during pregnancy and the postpartum period. Br J Sports Med 37: 6–12

Avery ND, Stocking KD, Tranmer JE et al. 1999 Foetal responses to maternal strength conditioning exercises in late gestation. Can J Appl Physiol 24(4): 362–376

Bachmann G 2001 Physiological aspects of natural and surgical menopause. J Reprod Med 46(3 Suppl): 307–315

Badger CMA, Peacock JL, Mortimer PS 2000 A randomized controlled parallel group clinical trial comparing multilayer bandaging followed by hosiery versus hosiery alone in the treatment of patients with lymphedema of the limb. Cancer 88(12): 2832–2837

Barber MD, Bremer RE, Thor KB et al. 2002 Innervation of the female levator ani muscles. Am J Obstet Gynecol 187: 64–71

Barton S 2004a The postnatal period. In: Mantle J, Haslam J, Barton S (eds) Physiotherapy in Obstetrics and Gynaecology, 2nd edn. Butterworth–Heinemann: London, pp 205–247

Barton S 2004b Relieving the discomforts of pregnancy. In: Mantle J, Haslam J, Barton S (eds) Physiotherapy in Obstetrics and Gynaecology, 2nd edn. Butterworth–Heinemann: London, pp 141–164

Bassotti G, Chistolini F, Sietchiping-Nzepa F et al. 2004 Biofeedback for pelvic floor dysfunction in constipation. BMJ 328(7436): 393–396

Bastiaanssen JM, de Bie RA, Bastiaenen CH et al. 2005 A historical perspective on pregnancy-related low back and/or pelvic girdle pain. Eur J Obstet Gynecol Reprod Biol 120: 3–14

Belsey J 1999 Evidence-based review of tibolone and oestrogen-based hormone replacement therapy. J Br Meno Soc 5(Suppl 1): 33–35

Berg G, Hammar M, Moller-Nielsen J 1988 Low back pain during pregnancy. Obstet Gynaecol 71: 71–75

Bjorklund K, Nordstrom ML, Bergstrom S 1999 Sonographic assessment of symphyseal joint distention during pregnancy and post partum with special reference to pelvic pain. Acta Obstet Gynecol Scand 78: 125–130

Bjorklund K, Bergstrom S, Nordstrom ML et al. 2000a Symphyseal distention in relation to serum relaxin levels and pelvic pain in pregnancy. Acta Obstet Gynecol Scand 79: 269–275

Bjorklund K, Nordstrom ML, Odlind V 2000b Combined oral contraceptives do not increase the risk of back and pelvic pain during pregnancy or after delivery. Acta Obstet Gynecol Scand 79: 979–983

Bø K 1995 Pelvic floor muscle exercise for the treatment of stress urinary incontinence: an exercise physiology perspective. Int Urogynecol J 6: 282–291

Boissonnault JS, Blaschak MJ 1988 Incidence of diastasis recti abdominis during the childbearing year. Phys Ther 86: 1082–1086

Borg-Stein J, Dugan SA, Gruber J 2005 Musculoskeletal aspects of pregnancy. Am J Phys Med Rehabil 84: 180–192

Boris M, Lasinski B 1989 The risk of genital oedema after external pump compression for lower limb lymphoedema. Lymphology 31: 15–20

Bortoluzzi G 1989 Transcutaneous electrical nerve stimulation in labour: practicability and effectiveness in a public hospital labour ward. Aust J Physiother 35: 81–87

Box RC, Reul-Hirche HM, Bullock-Saxton JE et al. 2002 Shoulder movement after breast cancer surgery: results of a randomised controlled study of post operative physiotherapy. Breast Cancer Res Treat 75: 35–50

Breen TW, Ransil BJ, Groves PA, Oriol NE 1994 Factors associated with back pain after childbirth. Anesthesiology 81(1): 29–34

British Lymphology Society 2001 Clinical Definitions. www.lymphoedema.org/bls

Browse N, Burnand K, Mortimer P 2003 Diseases of the Lymphatics. Edward Arnold: London

Bullock-Saxton JE 1991 Changes in posture associated with pregnancy and the early postnatal period measured in standing. Physiother Theory Pract 7: 103–109

Bullock-Saxton JE 1998 Musculoskeletal changes associated with the perinatal period. In: Sapsford R, Bullock-Saxton J, Markwell S (eds) Women's Health: A Textbook for Physiotherapists. WB Sanders: London, pp. 134–161

Bump R, Hurt WG, Fantl A, Wyman J 1991 Assessment of Kegel pelvic muscle exercise performance after brief verbal instruction. Am J Obstet Gynecol 165: 322–329

Burger H, Teede H 2001 Cardiovascular disease. Maturitas 40: 1–3

Caldeyro-Barcia R 1997 The influence of maternal position on time of spontaneous rupture of membranes, progress of labour, and foetal head compression. Birth Fam J 6: 7–15

Carroll D, Tramèr M, McQuay H et al. 1997 Transcutaneous electrical nerve stimulation in labour pain: a systematic review. BJOG 104(2): 169–175

Casley-Smith JR, Casley-Smith JR 1997 Modern Treatment for Lymphoedema, 5th edn. Terrance: Adelaide, pp. 288–301

Chamberkain G 1995 Gynaecology by Ten Teachers. Edward Arnold: London, p. 282

Chiarelli P, Campbell E 1997 Incontinence during pregnancy: prevalence and opportunities for continence promotion. Aust NZ J Obstet Gynaecol 37(1): 66–73

Chiarelli P, Cockburn J 2002 Promoting urinary continence in women after delivery: randomised controlled trial. BMJ 324(7348): 1241–1243

Chute CG, Panser LA, Girman CJ et al. 1993 The prevalence of prostatism: a population-based survey of urinary symptoms. J Urol 150: 85–89

Clapp JF 2000 Exercise during pregnancy: a clinical update. Clin Sports Med 19(2): 273–286

Clapp JF, Kim H, Burciu B, Lopez B 2000 Beginning regular exercise in early pregnancy: effect on foetoplacental growth. Am J Obstet Gynecol 183: 1484–1488

Clavel-Chapelon F 2002 Differential effects of reproductive factors on the risk of pre- and postmenopausal breast cancer. Results from a large cohort of French women. Br J Cancer 86(5): 723–727

Clodius L 2001 Minimizing Secondary Arm Lymphedema From Axillary Dissection: Lymphology 34: 106–110

Coldron Y 2005 Mind the gap — symphysis pubis dysfunction revisited. J Assoc Chart Physiother Wom Health 96: 3–15

Coldron Y 2006 Characteristics of recutus abdominis during the first postnatal year. In: Characteristics of Abdominal and paraspinal Muscles in Postnatal Women. St George's, University of London (unpublished PhD thesis), pp. 185–225

Cresswell AG, Grundstrom H, Thortensson A 1992 Observations on intra-abdominal pressure and patterns of abdominal intramuscular activity in man. Acta Physiol Scand 144: 409–418

Cutner A, Cardozo L 1990 Urinary incontinence: clinical findings. Practitioner 234: 1018–1024

Daly JM, Frame PS, Rapoza PA 1991 Sacroiliac subluxation: a common, treatable cause of low-back pain in pregnancy. Fam Pract Res J 11: 149–159

Damen L, Buyruk HM, Guler-Uysal F et al. 2001 Pelvic pain during pregnancy is associated with asymmetric laxity of the sacroiliac joints. Acta Obstet Gynecol Scand 80: 1019–1024

Damen L, Spoor CW, Snijders CJ et al. 2002 Does a pelvic belt influence sacroiliac joint laxity? Clin Biomech 17: 495–498

Davies L, Gangar KF, Drummond M et al. 1992 The economic burden of intractable gynaecological pain. J Obstet Gynaecol 12(Suppl 2): S54–56

De Lancey JLO 2001 Anatomy. In: Cardozo L, Staskin D (eds) Textbook of Female Urology and Urogynaecology. Isis Medical Media: London, pp. 112–124

Depledge J, McNair PJ, Keal-Smith C et al. 2005 Management of symphysis pubis dysfunction during pregnancy using exercise and pelvic support belts. Phys Ther 85: 1290–1300

D'Hoore A, Penninckx F 2003 Obstructed defecation. Colorectal Dis 5(4): 280–287

5

Diakow PR, Gadsby TA, Gadsby JB et al. 1991 Back pain during pregnancy and labor. J Manipulative Physiol Ther 14: 116–118

Dietz HP, Clarke B, Wilson PD 1998 A new method for quantifying levator activity and teaching pelvic floor muscle exercises. Neurourol Urodyn 17(4): 436–437

Dixon JM 2001 Hormone replacement therapy and the breast. BMJ 323(7326): 1381–1382

Dolan LM, Hosker GL, Mallett VT et al. 2003 Stress incontinence and pelvic floor neurophysiology 15 years after the first delivery. BJOG 110(12): 1107–1114

Dorey G 1998 Physiotherapy for male continence problems. Physiotherapy 85: 556–663

Dorey G 2000 Physiotherapy for the relief of male lower urinary tract symptoms. Physiotherapy 86: 413–426

Eason E, Labrecque M, Marcoux S, Mondor M 2002 Anal incontinence after childbirth. CMAJ 166(3): 326–330

Elden H, Ladfors L, Olsen MF et al. 2005 Effects of acupuncture and stabilising exercises as adjunct to standard treatment in pregnant women with pelvic girdle pain: randomised single blind controlled trial. BMJ 330: 761

Enck P 1993 Biofeedback training in disorded defecation: a critical review. Digest Dis Sci 38: 1953–1960

Evans GM 2002 Aquanatal exercise. In: Campion MR, Pattmann J (eds) Hydrotherapy: Principles and Practice, 2nd edn. Butterworth–Heinemann: Oxford

Fast A, Shapiro D, Ducommun EJ 1987 Low back pain in pregnancy. Spine 12: 368–371

Földi E, Földi M, Kubik S (eds) 2003 Textbook of Lymphology. Urban & Fischer: Munich

Foti T, Davids JR, Bagley A 2000 A biomechanical analysis of gait during pregnancy. J Bone Joint Surg Am 82: 625–632

Freeman RM 2002 The effect of pregnancy on the lower urinary tract and pelvic floor. In: MacLean AB, Cardozo L (eds) Incontinence in Women. RCOG: London, pp. 331–345

Frudlinger A, Halligan S, Spencer JAD et al. 2002 Influence of the suprapubic arch angle on anal sphincter trauma and anal incontinence following childbirth. BJOG 109: 1207–1212

Fry D 1999 Perinatal symphysis pubis dysfunction: a review of the literature. J Assoc Chart Physiother Wom Health 85: 11–18

Fynes MM, Marshall K, Cassidy M et al. 1999 A prospective, randomized study comparing the effect of augmented biofeedback with sensory biofeedback alone on fecal incontinence after obstetric trauma. Dis Colon Rectum 42: 753–761

Gardosi J, Sylvester SB, Lynch C 1989 Alternative positions in the second stage of labour: a randomised controlled trial. Br J Obstet Gynaecol 96B: 1290

Gattuso J, Kamm M 1993 The management of constipation in adults. Aliment Pharmacol Ther 7: 487–500

Genazzani AR, Bernadi F, Stomati M et al. 1998 Sex steroids and the brain. J Br Meno Soc 5(Suppl 1): 11–12

Gilleard WL, Brown JMM 1996 Structure and function of the abdominal muscles during pregnancy and the immediate post birth period. Phys Ther 7: 750–762

Gilleard WL, Crosbie J, Smith R 2002 Static trunk posture in sitting and standing during pregnancy and early postpartum. Arch Phys Med Rehabil 83: 1739–1744

Gilpin SA, Gosling JA, Smith ARB et al. 1989 The pathogenesis of genitourinary prolapse and stress incontinence of urine: a histological and histochemical study. Br J Obstet Gynaecol 96: 15–23

Grace VM 1995 Problems of communication, diagnosis, and treatment experienced by women using the New Zealand health services for chronic pelvic pain: a quantitative analysis. Health Care Women Int 16(6): 521–535

Guerreiro da Silva JB, Nakamura MU, Cordeiro JA et al. 2004 Acupuncture for low back pain in pregnancy — a prospective, quasi-randomised, controlled study. Acupunct Med 22: 60–67

Gutke A, Ostgaard HC, Oberg B 2006 Pelvic girdle pain and lumbar pain in pregnancy: a cohort study of the consequences in terms of health and functioning. Spine 31: E149–E155

Hagen R 1974 Pelvic girdle relaxation from an orthopaedic point of view. Acta Orthop Scand 45: 550–563

Hannestad YS, Rortveit G, Sandvik H et al. 2000 A community-based epidemiological survey of female urinary incontinence: the Norwegian EPINCONT study. Epidemiology of Incontinence in the County of Nord-Trondelag. J Clin Epidemiol 53: 1150–1157

Hannestad YS, Lie RT, Rortveit G, Hunskaar S 2004 Familial risk of urinary incontinence in women: population based cross sectional study. BMJ 329: 889–891

Hansen A, Jensen DV, Wormslev M et al. 1999 Symptom-giving pelvic girdle relaxation in pregnancy. II: Symptoms and clinical signs. Acta Obstet Gynecol Scand 78: 111–115

Harris SR, Hugi MR, Olivotto IA et al. 2001 Clinical practice guidelines for the care and treatment of breast cancer: 11. Lymphedema. CMAJ 164(2): 191–199

Harrison R, Bulstrode F 1987 Percentage weight bearing during partial immersion in a hydrotherapy pool. Physiother Pract 3: 60–63

Haslam J 2004a Anatomy. In: Mantle J, Haslam J, Barton S (eds) Physiotherapy in Obstetrics and Gynaecology, 2nd edn. Butterworth–Heinemann: London, pp. 1–25

Haslam J 2004b Physiology of pregnancy. In: Mantle J, Haslam J, Barton S (eds) Physiotherapy in Obstetrics and Gynaecology, 2nd edn. Butterworth–Heinemann: London, pp. 27–52

Hefferman AE 2000 Exercise and pregnancy in primary care. Nurse Pract 25(3): 42, 49, 53–56

Heiberg E, Aarseth SP 1997 Epidemiology of pelvic pain and low back pain in pregnant women. In: Vleeming A et al. (eds) Movement, Stability and Low Back Pain. Churchill Livingstone: Edinburgh, pp. 405–410

Henderson C, Jones K (eds) 1997 Essential Midwifery. Mosby: London

Hodges PW 1999 Is there a role for transversus abdominis in lumbo-pelvic stability? Manual Ther 4(2): 74–86

Holtedahl K, Hunskaar S 1998 Prevalence, 1-year incidence and factors associated with urinary incontinence: a population based study of women 50–74 years of age in primary care. Maturitas 28(3): 205–211

Howell CJ, Chalmers I 1992 A review of prospectively controlled comparisons of epidural with non-epidural forms of pain relief during labour. Int J Obstet Anesth 1: 93

Howell CJ, Dean T, Lucking L et al. 2002 Randomised study of long term outcome after epidural versus non-epidural analgesia during labour. BMJ 325: 357

Hutchinson R, Notghi A, Mostafa AB et al. 1993 Audit of transit abnormality in chronic idiopathic constipation. Gut 34(Supp 4): W49

ICS (International Continence Society) 2002 Standardisation of Terminology in Lower Urinary Tract Function. ICS: London

ISL (International Society of Lymphology) 2003 The diagnosis and treatment of peripheral lymphedema. Lymphology 36(2): 84–91

Jackson S, Avery N, Eckford S et al. 1995 Connective tissue analysis in genitourinary prolapse. Neurourol Urodynam 14: 412–414

Jain N, Sternberg LB 2005 Symphyseal separation. Obstet Gynecol 105: 1229–1232

Jarvis SK, Hallam TK, Lujic S et al. 2005 Peri-operative physiotherapy improves outcomes for women undergoing incontinence and or prolapse surgery: results of a randomised controlled trial. Aust NZ J Obstet Gynaecol 45(4): 300–303

Jenns K 2000 Management strategies. In: Twycross R, Jenns K, Todd J (eds) Lymphoedema. Radcliffe Medical: Oxford, pp. 98–117

Kamm MA 1994 Obstetric damage and fecal incontinence. Lancet 344: 730–733

Katz VL, McMurray RG, Cefalo RC 1991 Aquatic exercise during pregnancy. In: Mittelmark RA, Wiswell RA, Drinkwater BL (eds) Exercise in Pregnancy, 2nd edn. Williams & Wilkins: Baltimore, pp. 271–278

Keeley V 2000 Classification of lymphoedema. In: Twycross R, Jenns K, Todd J (eds) Lymphoedema. Radcliffe Medical: Oxford, pp. 22–44

Koltyn KF, Schultes SS 1997 Psychological effects of an aerobic exercise session and a rest session following pregnancy. J Sports Med Phys Fitness 37(4): 287–291

Kristiansson P, Svardsudd K, von Schoultz B 1996a Back pain during pregnancy: a prospective study. Spine 21: 702–709

Kristiansson P, Svardsudd K, von Schoultz B 1996b Serum relaxin, symphyseal pain, and back pain during pregnancy. Am J Obstet Gynecol 175: 1342–1347

Kvorning N, Holmberg C, Grennert L et al. 2004 Acupuncture relieves pelvic and low-back pain in late pregnancy. Acta Obstet Gynecol Scand 83: 246–250

Larsen EC, Wilken-Jensen C, Hansen A et al. 1999 Symptom-giving pelvic girdle relaxation in pregnancy. I: Prevalence and risk factors. Acta Obstet Gynecol Scand 78: 105–110

Laycock J 1998 An update on the management of female urinary incontinence. J Assoc Chart Physiother Wom Health 83: 3–5

Laycock J et al. 2001 Clinical Guidelines for the Physiotherapy Management of Females aged 16–65 with Stress Urinary Incontinence. London: CSP

Lee D 1999 Biomechanics of the lumbo-pelvic-hip complex. 5 In: The Pelvic Girdle, 2nd edn. Churchill Livingstone: Edinburgh, pp. 43–72

Lee D, Lee LJ 2004 Stress urinary incontinence, a consequence of failed load transfer through the pelvis? Presented 5th World Interdisciplinary Congress in Low Back Pain and Pelvic Pain: www.dianelee.ca

Lee D, Vleeming A 2000 Current concepts on pelvic impairment. In: Singer KP (ed.) Proceedings of the 7th Scientific Conference of the IFOMT in Conjunction with the MPAA International Federation of Orthopaedic Manipulative Therapists: Perth, pp. 465–491

Leroi AM, Bernier C, Watier A et al. 1996 Prevalence of sexual abuse among patients with functional disorders of the lower gastrointestinal tract. Int J Colorectal Dis 10(4): 200–206

Loughnan BA, Carli F, Romney M et al. 2002 Epidural analgesia and backache: a randomized controlled comparison with intramuscular meperidine for analgesia during labour. Br J Anaesth 89: 466–472

Lund I, Lundeberg T, Lonnberg L et al. 2006 Decrease of pregnant women's pelvic pain after acupuncture: a randomized controlled single-blind study. Acta Obstet Gynecol Scand 85: 12–19

MacArthur C, Lewis M, Knox BJ, Crawford JS 1990 Epidural anaesthesia and long-term backache after childbirth. BMJ 301: 9–12

MacArthur A, MacArthur C, Weeks S 1995 Epidural anaesthesia and low back pain after delivery: prospective cohort study. BMJ 311: 1336–1339

MacArthur AJ, MacArthur C, Weeks SK 1997 Is epidural anesthesia in labor associated with chronic low back pain? A prospective cohort study. Anesth Analg 85: 1066–1070

MacArthur C, Glazener CM, Wilson PD et al. 2006 Persistent urinary incontinence and delivery mode history: a six-year longitudinal study. BJOG 113(2): 218–224

MacLennan AH, Nicolson R, Green RC 1986a Serum relaxin in pregnancy. Lancet 2: 241–243

MacLennan AH, Nicolson R, Green RC et al. 1986b Serum relaxin and pelvic pain of pregnancy. Lancet 2: 243–245

MacLennan AH, MacLennan SC 1997 Symptom-giving pelvic girdle relaxation of pregnancy, postnatal pelvic joint syndrome and dysplasia of the hip. Acta Obstet Gynecol Scand 76: 760–764

Madoff R, Parker SC, Madhulika GV, Lowry AC 2004 Faecal incontinence in adults. Lancet 364: 621–632

Mahony RT, Malone PA, Nalty J et al. 2004 Randomized clinical trial of intra-anal electromyographic biofeedback physiotherapy with intra-anal electromyographic biofeedback augmented with electrical stimulation of the anal sphincter in the early treatment of postpartum fecal incontinence. Am J Obstet Gynecol 191(3): 885–890

Mantle J 2004 Urinary function and dysfunction. In: Mantle J, Haslam J, Barton S (eds) Physiotherapy in Obstetrics and Gynaecology, 2nd edn. Butterworth–Heinemann: Oxford, p. 348

Mantle MJ, Greenwood RM, Currey HLF 1977 Backache in pregnancy. Rheumatol Rehabil 16: 95–101

5

Markwell SJ, Sapsford RR 1995 Physiotherapy management of obstructed defaecation. Aust J Physiother 41: 279–283

Mathias SD, Kuppermann M, Liberman RF et al. 1996 Chronic pelvic pain: prevalence, health-related quality of life, and economic correlates. Obstet Gynecol 87: 321–327

McIntyre IN, Broadhurst NA 1996 Effective treatment of low back pain in pregnancy. Aust Fam Physician 25: S65–S67

McNabb M 1997 Maternal and foetal physiological responses to pregnancy. In: Sweet BR (ed.) Mayes Midwifery, 12th edn. Baillière Tindall: London, pp. 123–147

Melzack R, Wall P 1982 The Challenge of Pain. Penguin: Harmondsworth

Mendelsohn ME, Karas RH 1999 The protective effects of oestrogen on the cardiovascular system. N Engl J Med 340: 1801–1811

Mens JM, Vleeming A, Stoeckart R et al. 1996 Understanding peripartum pelvic pain. Spine 21: 1363–1370

Mens JM, Vleeming A, Snijders CJ et al. 2002 Reliability and validity of hip adduction strength to measure disease severity in posterior pelvic pain since pregnancy. Spine 27: 1674–1679

Mens JM, Damen L, Snijders CJ et al. 2006 The mechanical effect of a pelvic belt in patients with pregnancy-related pelvic pain. Clin Biomech 21: 122–127

Moffat CJ et al. 2003 Lymphoedema: an underestimated health problem. Q J Med 96: 731–738

Mogren IM, Pohjanen AI 2005 Low back pain and pelvic pain during pregnancy: prevalence and risk factors. Spine 30: 983–991

Moore K, Dumas GA, Reid JG 1990 Postural changes associated with pregnancy and their relationship with low-back pain. Clin Biomech 5: 169–174

Mørkved S, Bø K 1999 Prevalence of urinary incontinence during pregnancy and post partum. Int Urogynecol J Pelvic Floor Dysfunct 10(6): 394–398

Mørkved S, Bø K 2000 Effect of postpartum pelvic floor muscle training in prevention and treatment of urinary incontinence: a one year follow up. Br J Obstet Gynaecol 107: 1022–1028

Mørkved S, Bø K, Schei B et al. 2003 Pelvic floor muscle training during pregnancy to prevent urinary incontinence: a single-blind randomized controlled trial. Obstet Gynecol 101(2): 313–319

Nelson R, Norton N, Cautley E, Furner S 1995 Community-based prevalence of anal incontinence. JAMA 274: 559–561

Newham DJ 1988 The consequences of eccentric contraction and their relationship to delayed onset of muscle pain. Eur J Appl Physiol 57: 3353–3359

NICE (National Institute for Health and Clinical Excellence) 2003 Final Appraisal Determination: Tension-free Vaginal Tape (Gynecare TVT) for Stress Incontinence. Accessed 24 June 2006: www.nice.org.uk

NICE 2003 Antenatal care: Routine Care for the Healthy Pregnant Woman. NICE Clinical Guideline 6. NICE: London, www.nice.org.uk

NICE 2006 Urinary incontinence; the management of urinary incontinence in women. NICE: London, www.nice.org.uk

Nilsson-Wikmar L, Harms-Ringdahl K 1999 Back pain in women post-partum is not a unitary concept. Physiother Res Int 4(3): 201–213

Noren L, Ostgaard S, Nielson TF, Ostgaard HC 1997 Reduction of sick leave for lumbar back and posterior pain in pregnancy. Spine 22: 2157–2160

Noren L, Ostgaard S, Johansson G et al. 2002 Lumbar back and posterior pelvic pain during pregnancy: a 3-year follow-up. Eur Spine J 11: 267–271

Norton C, Chelvanayagam S, Wilson-Barnett J et al. 2003 Randomized controlled trial of biofeedback for fecal incontinence. Gastroenterology 125(5): 1320–1329

Norton P 1990 Genitourinary prolapse: relationship with joint mobility. Neurourol Urodynam 9: 321–322

Office for National Statistics 2004 Mortality Statistics: Cause. England and Wales. Stationery Office: London

Ostgaard HC 1997 Lumbar back and posterior pelvic pain in pregnancy. In: Vleeming A et al. (eds) Movement, Stability and Low Back Pain. Churchill Livingstone: Edinburgh, pp. 411–420

Ostgaard HC, Andersson GB 1991 Previous back pain and risk of developing back pain in a future pregnancy. Spine 16: 432–436

Ostgaard HC, Andersson GBJ 1992 Postpartum low back pain. Spine 17: 53–55

Ostgaard HC, Andersson GB, Karlsson K 1991 Prevalence of back pain in pregnancy. Spine 16: 549–552

Ostgaard HC, Andersson GBJ, Schuttz AB, Miller JA 1993 Influence of some biomechanical factors on low back pain in pregnancy. Spine 18: 61–65

Ostgaard HC, Zetherstrom G, Roos-Hansson E et al. 1994 Reduction of back and posterior pelvic pain in pregnancy. Spine 19: 894–900

Ostgaard HC, Roos-Hansson E, Zetherstrom G 1996 Regression of back and posterior pelvic pain after pregnancy. Spine 21: 2777–2780

Paech MJ, Godkin R, Webster S 1998 Complications of obstetric epidural analgesia and anaesthesia: a prospective analysis of 10,995 cases. Int J Obstet Anesth 7(4): 280–281

Pain SJ, Purushotham AD 2000 Lymphoedema following surgery for breast cancer. Br J Breast Surg 87: 1128–1141

Palastanga N, Field D, Soames R 2002 Anatomy and Human Movement, 4th edn. Butterworth–Heinemann: Oxford

Paul JA, Salle H, Frings-Dresen MH 1996 Effect of posture on hip joint moment during pregnancy, while performing a standing task. Clin Biomech 11: 111–115

Perry S, Shaw C, McGrother C et al. 2002 Prevalence of faecal incontinence in adults aged 40 years or more living in the community. Gut 50: 480–484

Piller NB 1999 Gaining an accurate assessment of the stages of lymphedema subsequent to cancer: the role of objective and subjective information in when to make measurements and their optimal use. Eur J Lymphol 7(25): 1–9

Pool-Goudzwaard A 2003 Biomechanics of the sacro iliac joints and pelvic floor. PhD thesis. Ch 8. Relation between low back and pelvic pain, pelvic floor activity and pelvic floor disorders

Pool-Goudzwaard AL, Vleeming A, Stoeckart R et al. 1998 Insufficient lumbopelvic stability: a clinical, anatomical and biomechanical approach to 'a-specific' low back pain. Man Ther 3: 12–20

Pool-Goudzwaard AL, Slieker ten Hove MC, Vierhout ME et al. 2005 Relations between pregnancy-related low back pain, pelvic floor activity and pelvic floor dysfunction. Int Urogynecol J Pelvic Floor Dysfunct 16: 468–474

Potter HM, Downey JL, Jones ST 1997a Effect of an intense training programme for the deep antero-lateral abdominal muscles on rectus abdominis diastasis: a single case study. In: Proceedings of the 10th Biennial Conference of the Manipulative Physiotherapists Association of Australia (MPAA) Manipulative Physiotherapists Association of Australia. Victoria, pp 153–155

Potter HM, Randall HF, Strauss GR 1997b Effect of pregnancy and motherhood on trunk muscle strength: an examination of isokinetic trunk strength at 24 weeks postpartum. In: Proceedings of the 10th Biennial Conference of the Manipulative Physiotherapists Association of Australia (MPAA) Manipulative Physiotherapists Association of Australia. Victoria, pp 151–152

Rath AM, Attali P, Dumas JL et al. 1996 The abdominal linea alba: an anatomo-radiologic and biomechanical study. Surg Radiol Anat 18: 281–288

Raz S, Kaufman JJ 1977 Carbon dioxide urethral pressure profile in female incontinence. J Urol 117: 765–769

Richardson C, Jull G, Hodges P, Hides J 1999 Therapeutic Exercise for Spinal Segmental Stabilization in Low Back Pain. Churchill Livingstone: Edinburgh, p. 95

Riemann MK, Kanstrup Hansen IL 2000 Effects on the foetus of exercise in pregnancy (review). Scand J Med Sci Sports 10(1): 12–19

Röst C 1999 Bekkenpijn Tijden En Na De Zwangerschap Een Programma ter Voorkoming van Chronische Bekkeninstabiliteit. Elsevier/De Tijdstroom: Maarssen

Rud T, Anderson KE, Asmusson M et al. 1980 Factors maintaining the intraurethral pressure in women. Invest Urol 17: 343–347

Russell JGB 1982 The rationale of primitive delivery positions. Br J Obstet Gynaecol 89: 712

Russell R, Dundas R, Reynolds F 1996 Long term backache after childbirth: prospective search for causative factors. BMJ 312: 1384–1388

Russell R, Reynolds F 1997 Back pain, pregnancy and childbirth. BMJ 314: 1062

Sacco Ezzell P 1999 Managing the effects of gynaecological cancer treatment on quality of life and sexuality. Soc Gynaecol Nurs Oncol 8(3): 23–26

Samsioe G 1998 Urogenital ageing: a forgotten problem. Meno Rev 3(1): 5–6

Sapsford RR, Hodges PW 2001 Contraction of the pelvic floor muscles during abdominal manoeuvres. Arch Phys Med Rehabil 82: 1081–1088

Sapsford RR, Hodges PW, Richardson CA 1997 Activation of the abdominal muscles is a normal response to contraction of the pelvic floor muscles. International Continence Society Conference, Japan (abstract)

Sapsford RR, Bullock-Saxton J, Markwell S 1998 Women's Health: A Textbook for Physiotherapists. WB Saunders: London

Sapsford RR, Hodges PW, Richardson CA et al. 2001 Co-activation of the abdominal muscles and pelvic floor muscles during voluntary exercises. Neurourol Urodynam 20: 31–42

Schultz I, Barholm M, Grondal S 1997 Delayed shoulder exercises in reducing seroma frequency after modified radical mastectomy. Ann Surg Oncol 4(4): 293–297

Schwartz Z, Katz Z, Lancet M 1985 Management of puerperal separation of the symphysis pubis. Int J Gynaecol Obstet 23: 125–128

Sheppard S 1996 The role of transversus abdominis in post partum correction of gross divarication recti. Man Ther 1: 214–216

Sihvonen T, Huttunen M, Makkonen M et al. 1998 Functional changes in back muscle activity correlate with pain intensity and prediction of low back pain during pregnancy. Arch Phys Med Rehabil 79: 1210–1212

Smith P, Heimer G, Norgren A et al. 1990 Steroid hormone receptors in pelvic muscles and ligaments in women. Gynecol Obstet Invest 30: 27–30

Snijders CJ, Ribbers MTLM, de Bakker HV et al. 1998 EMG recordings of abdominal and back muscles in various standing postures: validation of a biomechanical model on sacroiliac joint. J Electromyogr Kinesiol 8: 205–214

Snow RE, Neubert AG 1997 Peripartum pubic symphysis separation: a case series and review of the literature. CME Review 7: 438–443

Stanton AWB, Levick JR, Mortimer PS 1996 Current puzzles presented by post mastectomy oedema (breast cancer related lymphoedema). Vasc Med 1: 213–225

Steege JF, Metzger DA, Levy BS (eds) 1998 Chronic Pelvic Pain: An Integrated Approach. WB Saunders: Philadelphia

Stuge B, Hilde G, Vollestad N 2003 Physical therapy for pregnancy-related low back and pelvic pain: a systematic review. Acta Obstet Gynecol Scand 82: 983–990

Stuge B, Laerum E, Kirkesola G et al. 2004a The efficacy of a treatment program focusing on specific stabilizing exercises for pelvic girdle pain after pregnancy: a randomized controlled trial. Spine 29: 351–359

Stuge B, Veierod MB, Laerum E et al. 2004b The efficacy of a treatment program focusing on specific stabilizing exercises for pelvic girdle pain after pregnancy: a two-year follow-up of a randomized clinical trial. Spine 29: E197–E203

Stuge B, Holm I, Vollestad N 2006 To treat or not to treat postpartum pelvic girdle pain with stabilizing exercises? ManTher 11(4): 337–343: epub 9 Jan 2006

Sultan AH, Kamm MA, Hudson CM, Bartram CI 1994 Third degree obstetric and sphincter tears: risk factors and outcomes of primary repair. BMJ 308: 887

Sultan AH, Monga AK, Stanton SL 1996 The pelvic floor sequelae of childbirth. Br J Hosp Med 55: 575–579

5

Ternov NK, Grennert L, Aberg A et al. 2001 Acupuncture for lower back and pelvic pain in late pregnancy: a retrospective report on 167 consecutive cases. Pain Med 2: 204–207

Thorp JA, Breedlove G 1996 Epidural analgesia in labor: an evaluation of risks and benefits. Birth 23(2): 63–83

Tobin GW, Brocklehurst JC 1986 Faecal incontinence in residential homes for the elderly: prevalence, aetiology and management. Age Ageing 15(1): 41–46

Tobin MB, Lacey HJ, Meyer L, Mortimer P 1993 The psychological morbidity of breast cancer related arm swelling. Cancer 72: 3248–3252

Toozs-Hobson P 1998 Pelvic floor ultrasonography: the current state of ultrasound imaging of the pelvic floor in relation to urogynaecology and childbirth. J Assoc Chart Physiother Wom Health 84: 18–22

van den Brandt A, Spiegelman D et al. 2000 Pooled analysis of prospective cohort studies on height, weight, and breast cancer risk. Am J Epidemiol 152(6): 514–527

Vleeming A, Albert H, Ostgaard HC et al. 2004 European guidelines on the diagnosis and treatment of pelvic girdle pain. www.backpaineurope.org

Webber BA, Pryor JA 1998 Physiotherapy for Respiratory and Cardiac Problems. Churchill Livingstone: Edinburgh, pp. 295–305

Wedenberg K, Moen B, Norling A 2000 A prospective randomized study comparing acupuncture with physiotherapy for low-back and pelvic pain in pregnancy. Acta Obstet Gynecol Scand 79: 331–335

Whitehead M, Godfree V 1992 Consequences of oestrogen deficiency. In: Hormone Replacement Therapy: Your Questions Answered. Churchill Livingstone: Edinburgh, pp. 13–36

Williams AF, Vadgama A, Franks PJ, Mortimer PS 2002 A randomized controlled crossover study of manual lymphatic drainage therapy in women with breast cancer-related lymphoedema. Eur J Cancer Care 11: 254–261

Williams AF, Moffatt CJ, Franks PJ 2004 A phenomenal study of the lived experiences of people with lymphoedema. Int J Palliat Care 10(6): 279–296

Wilson PD, Herbison RM, Herbison GP 1996 Obstetric practice and the prevalence of urinary incontinence three months after delivery. Br J Obstet Gynaecol 103: 154–161

Wishart GC, Gaston M, Poultsidis AA, Purushotham AD 2002 Hormone receptor status in primary breast cancer — time for a consensus? Eur J Cancer 38(9): 1201–1203

Woods M, Tobin MB, Mortimer P 1995 The psychosocial morbidity of breast cancer patients with lymphoedema. Cancer Nursing 18(6): 467–471

Wreje U, Isacsson D, Aberg H 1997 Oral contraceptives and back pain in women in a Swedish community. Int J Epidemiol 26: 71–74

Wu WH, Meijer OG, Uegaki K et al. 2004 Pregnancy-related pelvic girdle pain (PPP), I: Terminology, clinical presentation, and prevalence. Eur Spine J 13(7): 575–589

Zondervan KT, Yudkin PL, Vessey MP et al. 1999 Prevalence and incidence of chronic pelvic pain in primary care: evidence from a national general practice database. Br J Obstet Gynaecol 106: 1149–1155

Chapter **6**

Biomechanics

Jim Richards

CHAPTER CONTENTS

INTRODUCTION

This chapter will give you an introduction to clinical gait analysis, definitions and detailed descriptions of the movement and force patterns found during walking, and the mathematical basis of how muscle force and power may be calculated. More information about clinical biomechanics is available in the textbook *Biomechanics in Clinic and Research: An interactive teaching and learning course* (Richards 2008).

Clinical gait analysis

In 1953, Saunders and co-workers referred to the major determinants in normal gait and applied these to the assessment of pathological gait. Inman (1966, 1967) and Murray (1967) both published detailed analyses of the kinematics and conservation of energy during human locomotion, and these are resources to which we still frequently refer. Inman et al. (1981) later published *Human Walking*, a comprehensive textbook on human locomotion.

Brand and Crowninshield (1981) highlighted the distinction between the use of biomechanical techniques to 'diagnose' or 'evaluate' clinical problems. The authors stated: 'Evaluate, in contrast to diagnose, means to place a value on something. Many medical tests are of this variety and instead of distinguishing diseases, help determine the severity of the disease or evaluate one parameter of the disease. Biomechanical tests at present are of this variety.' Brand and Crowninshield also gave a guide of six criteria for tools used in patient evaluation:

1. The measured parameter(s) must correlate well with the patient's functional capacity.
2. The measured parameter must not be directly observable and semi-quantifiable by the physician or therapist.
3. The measured parameters must clearly distinguish between normal and abnormal.

4. The measurement technique must not significantly alter the performance of the evaluated activity.
5. The measurement must be accurate and reproducible.
6. The results must be communicated in a form which is readily identifiable.

Brand and Crowninshield stated: 'It is clear to us that most methods of assessing gait do not meet all of these criteria. We believe that it is for this reason that they are not widely used.'

Advances in biomechanical assessment in the last 25 years have been considerable. The description of normal gait in terms of movement and forces about joints is now commonplace. The relationship between normal gait patterns and normal function is also well supported in both scientific papers and textbooks (Bruckner 1998; Rose and Gamble 1994; Perry 1992). This allows deviations in gait patterns to be studied in relation to changes in function in subjects with particular pathologies. It is possible for a clinician or physician to study gait subjectively, but the value and repeatability of this type of assessment is questionable owing to poor inter- and intra-tester reliability (Pomeroy et al. 2003). It is impossible for one individual to study simultaneously, by observation alone, the movement pattern of all the main joints involved in an activity like walking. Studying movement patterns using objective motion analysis allows information to be gathered simultaneously with known accuracy and reliability. In this way changes in movement patterns due to intervention by physical therapists and surgeons may be assessed unequivocally.

Most motion analysis systems now report on the joint kinematics for the individual recorded, and also contain information for the mean for normal on the same graph, allowing a direct comparison of the individual's movement pattern in relation to a predefined normal.

Weblink

Such information is also available on the Internet at sites such as
www.biomechanicsonline.com

Patrick (1991) reviewed the use of movement analysis laboratory investigations in assisting decision-making for the physician and clinician. Patrick concluded that the reasons for the use of such facilities not being widespread were due to:

- the time of analysis being considerable
- bioengineers designing systems and presenting results for researchers and not clinicians
- a lack of understanding by physicians and clinicians of applied mechanics and its relevance to assessment of treatment outcome.

Since 1991 the movement analysis laboratory has become more widely accepted by physicians, and the time needed for analysis is ever decreasing, resulting in new laboratories appearing in the clinical setting. Winter (1993) reviewed techniques of gait analysis; this was a reply to the criticisms from Brand and Crowninshield. Winter provided evidence to show that clinical gait assessments can give a valuable contribution to: diagnostic information to assist surgeons in planning orthopaedic procedures; planning of rehabilitation; and the assessment of prosthetic devices. Winter also demonstrated the use of a generalised strategy and diagnostic checklist developed for all pathologies. This checklist did not focus on a particular pathology, but rather targeted gait problems that may be common to many pathologies. Winter demonstrated the use of such a checklist using five case studies: knee arthroplasty, below-knee amputation; cerebral palsy hemiplegia; above-knee amputation; and patellectomy. The paper concluded by stating that assessment of pathological gait is not an easy task, and can require considerable expense in equipment, software and specialised personnel. Winter also stressed the need for a database of normal data for children, adult and elderly subjects.

A common argument against movement analysis laboratories has been cost. The cost of movement analysis equipment and its potential use in the clinical setting has been reported (Bell et al. 1996). A broader question indeed could be put with regard to any clinical assessment or treatment that requires the use of technology. One example of this is the relative cost of radiography to that of movement analysis equipment, which in comparison is modest. Gage (1994) claimed that gait analysis costs are comparable with MRI or CT scans. Gage also stated that the use of movement analysis, as a detailed form of assessment, may have wider cost benefits and improve clinical services more than first realised.

Bell et al. (1995) highlighted the use of an holistic approach to motion analysis including muscle performance and joint range of motion, as well as kinematic and kinetic parameters of gait. This holistic approach may be applied to many pathologies to give a detailed assessment of pathology and the subsequent effects of treatment.

Many of the techniques of collection and analysing human locomotion have been applied to clinical practice. This has led to more detailed clinical assessment of therapeutic and surgical intervention, which is becoming increasingly important in the age of evidence-based practice.

The development of equipment

Instrumented walk mat systems

Spatial parameters can be measured in a variety of simple ways. These include putting ink pads on the soles of the subjects' shoes and asking them to walk on paper (Rafferty and Bell 1995), and using marker pens attached to shoes (Gerny 1983). Although very cheap, these systems can require awkward and time-consuming analysis. Temporal parameters can be measured by timing how long it takes an individual to walk a set distance and then counting the number of steps it took to cover that distance. At best, this will only give average velocity and cadence, and will give no value to the symmetry of these parameters. This technique is extremely susceptible to human error.

In the last two decades of the 20th century, advances in computer technology led to the development of a number of instrumented walk mat systems. These allow fast collection of temporal and spatial gait data. Using a computer also allows easier, less time-consuming analysis. These systems include: Durie and Farley (1980), Arenson et al. (1983), Hirokawa and Matsumura (1987), Crouse et al. (1987) and Al-Majali et al. (1993).

Walk mat systems are now commercially available that do not require any modifications to footwear. These offer far less interference with the gait cycle. One such system is the GAITRite™ system, which uses pressure sensor arrays to determine the foot positions (Figure 6.1).

Movement analysis

In the late 19th century the first motion picture cameras recorded patterns of locomotion in both humans and animals. In 1877, Muybridge demonstrated, using photographs, that when a horse is moving at a fast trot there is a moment when all of the animal's hooves are off the ground; in 1887 he published his findings in *Animal Locomotion*. Muybridge later used 24 cameras to study the movement patterns of a running man and in 1901 published *The Human Figure in Motion*.

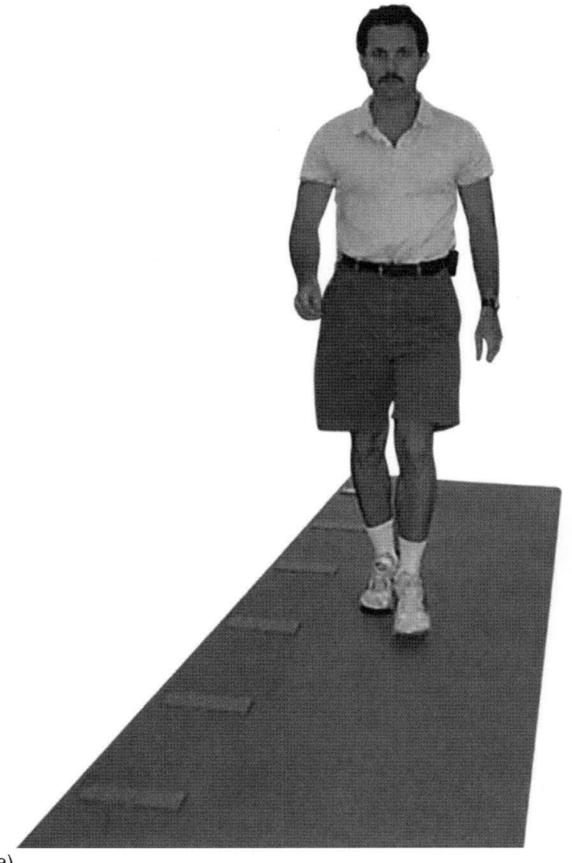

(a)

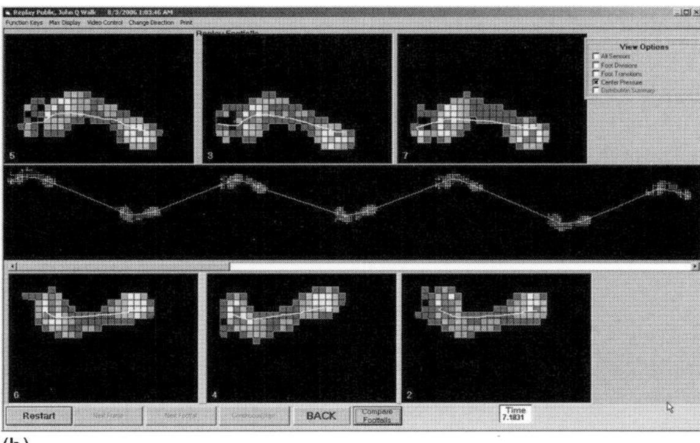

(b)

Figure 6.1 GAITRiteTM system and typical output from GAITRiteTM.

Marey, a French physiologist, used a photographic rifle to photograph movement of animals in 1873, and in 1882 and 1885 to record displacements in human gait, producing the first stick figure of a runner.

In the second half of the 20th century many systems capable of automated and semi-automated computer-aided motion analysis were developed. One of the first to become commercially available was the Ariel Performance Analysis System, which required the operator to identify manually the location of each marker used for each frame. Since then, the problems of automatic marker identification have been at the forefront of the development of computer-aided motion analysis. In 1974 SELSPOT came on the market, which allowed automatic tracking of active light-emitting diode (LED) markers. Later Watsmart and Optotrak used a similar technique. VICON, a television camera-based system, became commercially available in 1982. Since then, many systems based on television camera technology have been developed; these include the Motion Analysis Corporation system, Elite, and ProReflex by Qualisys (Figure 6.2).

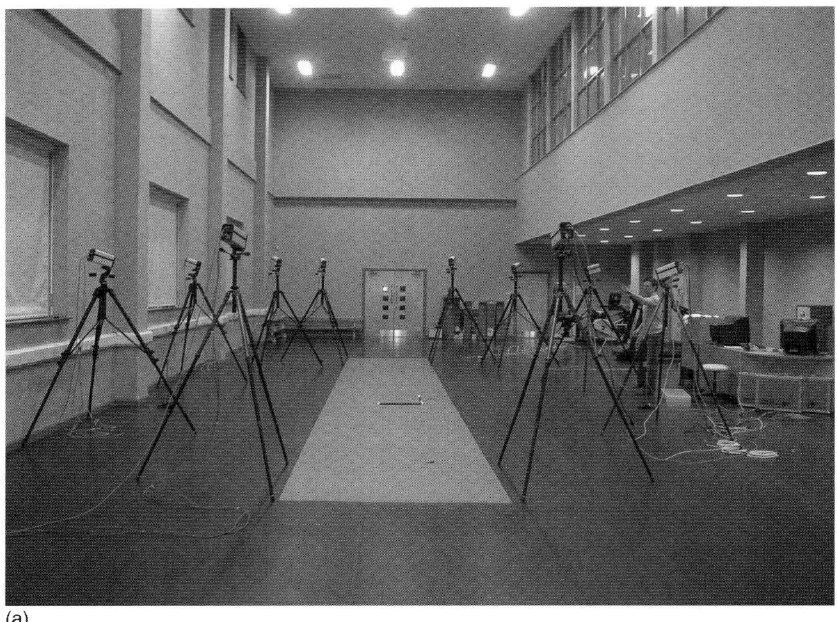

(a)

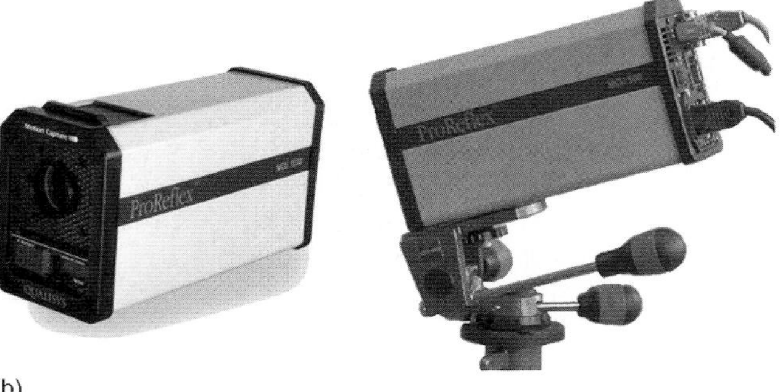

(b)

Figure 6.2 (a) UCLan's Movement Analysis Laboratory in the Faculty of Health. (b) Qualisys ProReflex CCD camera.

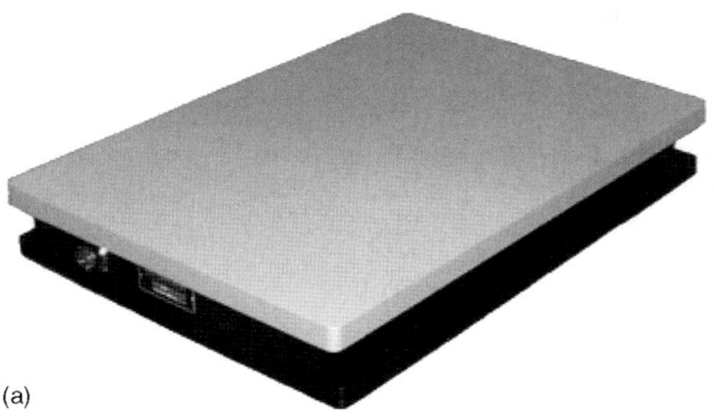

(a)

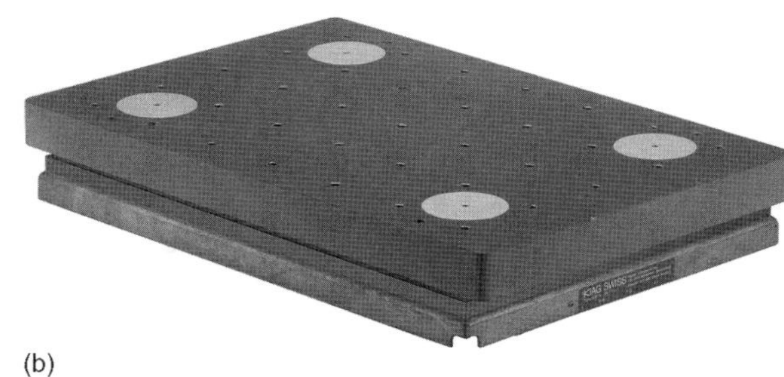

(b)

Figure 6.3 (a) AMTI force platform. (b) Kistler force platform.

Force analysis

Force platforms are devices which measure the ground reaction forces acting beneath the feet. They are considered to be a basic but fundamentally important tool for gait analysis. The first force measurements date back as far as the late 19th century, when Marey used a wooden frame on rubber supports. Elftman (1938) used a similar method with a platform on springs. However, it was not until the advancement of computers and electronic technology that the readings could be accurately measured. In 1965, Peterson and co-workers developed one of the first strain-gauge force platforms. A plethora of publications now exists on the applications of such devices in both clinical research and sports.

Since 1965 force platforms have undergone considerable development by three internationally accepted manufacturers: Kistler Instruments, AMTI and the Bertec Corporation. Advances have been in the form of greater accuracy of the platforms (reducing crosstalk), increased sensitivity (increasing the natural frequency) and portability of the platforms (Figure 6.3).

KINEMATICS

The gait cycle

For normal walking, the obvious division is the length of time that the foot is in contact with the ground and the period when it is not. These are known as 'stance phase' (approximately 60 per cent of the gait cycle) and 'swing phase' (approximately 40 per cent of the gait cycle) respectively.

Definition

The *stance phase* can be subdivided into: heel strike, foot flat, mid-stance, heel off and toe off. The *swing phase* can be subdivided into: early swing, mid-swing and late swing.

Spatial and temporal parameters of gait

The simplest way to look at walking patterns is by studying distances and times for which the foot is in contact with the ground.

Spatial parameters

The spatial parameters of foot contact during gait are (Figure 6.4):

- *step length* — the distance between two consecutive heel strikes
- *stride length* — the distance between two consecutive heel strikes by the same leg
- *foot angle or angle of gait* — the angle of foot orientation away from the line of progression
- *base width or base of gait* — the medial lateral distance between the centre of each heel during gait

Temporal parameters

Temporal parameters are (Figure 6.5):

- *step time* — the time between two consecutive heel strikes
- *stride time* — the time between two consecutive heel strikes by the same leg: one complete gait cycle
- *single support* — the time over which the body is supported by only one leg
- *double support* — the time over which the body is supported by both legs

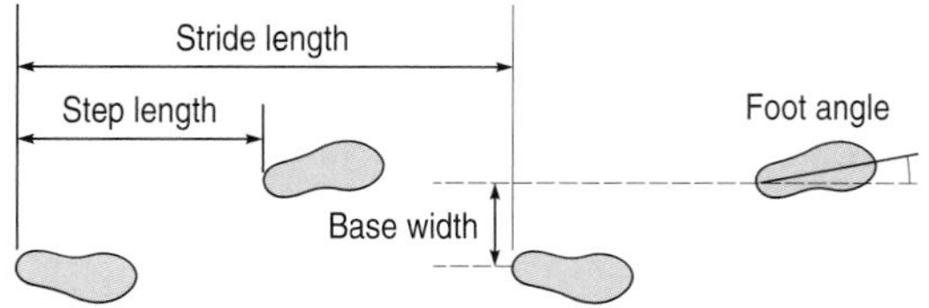

Figure 6.4 Spatial parameters.

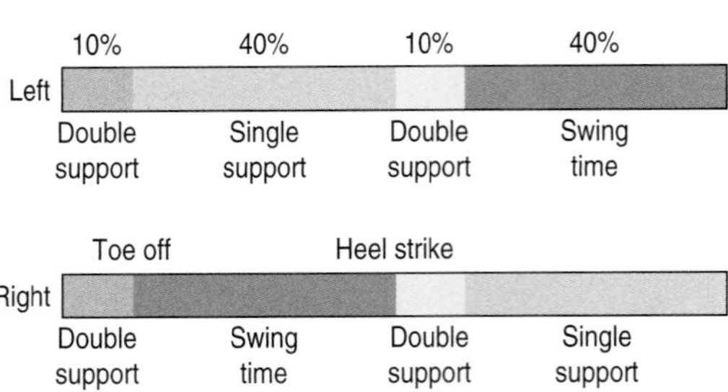

Figure 6.5 Temporal parameters.

6

- *swing time* — the time taken for the leg to swing through while the body is in single support on the other leg
- *total support* — the total time a foot is in contact with the ground during one complete gait cycle.

Two other parameters may easily be calculated using this information: *cadence* and *velocity*. The cadence is the number of steps taken in a given time, usually steps per minute. Velocity may be calculated using the formula below:

$$\text{Cadence (steps/min)} = \frac{\text{number of steps}}{\text{time (min)}}$$

$$\text{Velocity (m/s)} = \frac{\text{step length (m)} \times \text{cadence (steps/min)}}{60 \text{ (number of seconds in 1 min)}}$$

Symmetry can also be found by dividing the value of a parameter found for the left over that of the right:

$$\text{Symmetry of step length} = \frac{\text{step length for the left}}{\text{step length for the right}}$$

These parameters, although simple, can be a very useful means of assessing treatment outcome. It must be noted, however, that they may not always be appropriate for some more complex pathological gait patterns (Wall et al. 1987).

Analysis of joint motion

Calculation of segment angles and joint angles

Normal movement patterns during gait

Human walking allows a smooth and efficient progression of the body's centre of mass (Inman 1967). To achieve this, there are a number of different movements of the joints in the lower limb. The correct functioning of the movement patterns of these joints allows a smooth and energy-efficient progression of the body. The relationship between the movements of the joints of the lower limb is critical. If there is any deviation in the coordination of these patterns, the energy cost of walking may increase, and also the shock absorption at impact and propulsion may not be as effective.

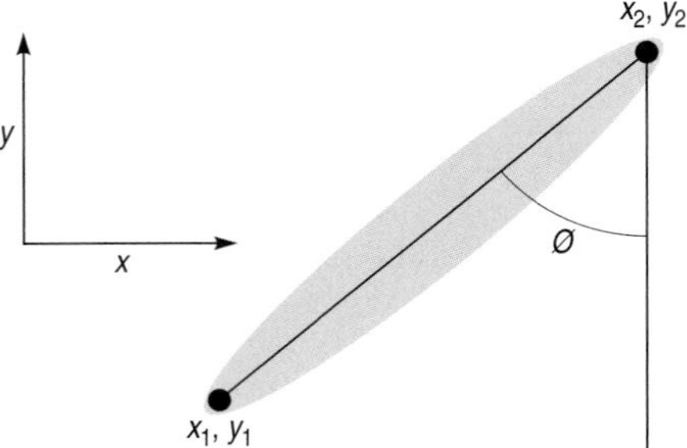

Figure 6.6 The segment angle.

Definition

Segment angle is defined as the angle of the body segment away from the vertical axis (Figure 6.6). The segment angles can be calculated by knowing the coordinates of the proximal and distal ends of a body segment in a particular plane. The angle can then be found by trigonometry.

$$\text{Tan } \theta = \frac{x_2 - x_1}{y_2 - y_1}$$

Joint motion patterns commonly reported include: ankle plantar flexion/dorsiflexion, foot rotation, knee flexion/extension, knee valgus/varus, knee rotation, hip flexion/extension, hip abduction/adduction, hip rotation, pelvic tilt, pelvic obliquity and pelvic rotation. Although all these movement patterns are of interest, only major movement patterns of the lower limb are covered here. These include:

- plantar flexion and dorsiflexion of the ankle joint
- knee flexion/extension
- hip flexion/extension
- motion of the pelvis in the coronal plane
- motion of the pelvis in the transverse plane.

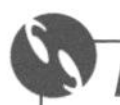

Definition

Joint angle is defined as the angle between the line of the proximal and distal segments of a joint. The example shown in Figure 6.7 is the knee joint angle, which is usually defined such that full extension is zero degrees and an increase in flexion is positive. This may be calculated by the equation shown below:

$$\text{Tan } \phi = \frac{x_2 - x_1}{y_2 - y_1} \quad \text{Tan } \beta = \frac{x_2 - x_3}{y_3 - y_2}$$

$$\text{Joint angle } \Theta = \pm\beta \pm \phi$$

However, care must be taken as the formula changes depending on which quadrant the body segments are acting in. This may result in the segment angles needing to be added or subtracted to find the true joint angle.

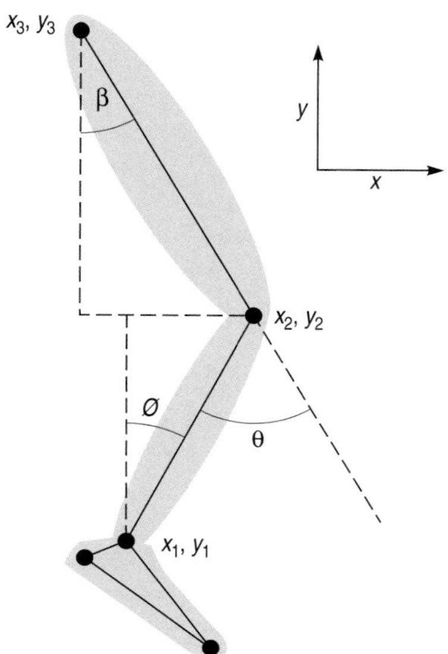

Figure 6.7 Joint angle definitions.

Motion of the ankle joint

The movement about the ankle joint is of great importance, as it allows shock absorption at heel strike and progression of the body forwards during the stance phase, as well as being vital in the 'push off' or propulsive stage immediately before the toe leaves the ground. During the swing phase, the motion of the ankle joint allows foot clearance, which can be lacking in some pathological gait patterns and is generally known as 'drop foot'.

The range of motion that occurs in walking varies between 20 degrees and 40 degrees, with an average value of 30 degrees. However, this does not tell us how the motion of the ankle varies throughout gait. During gait the ankle has four phases of motion (Figure 6.8):

- *Phase 1*. At initial contact, or heel strike, the ankle joint is in a neutral position; it then plantar-flexes to between 3 and 5 degrees until foot flat has been achieved (Figure 6.9). This is sometimes referred to as 'first rocker' or 'first segment', which refers to the foot pivoting about the heel or calcaneus. During this period the dorsiflexor muscles in the anterior compartment of the foot and ankle are acting eccentrically, controlling the plantar flexion of the foot. This gives the effect of a shock absorber and aids smooth weight acceptance to the lower limb.
- *Phase 2*. At the position of foot flat the ankle begins to dorsiflex. The foot becomes stationary and the tibia becomes the moving segment, with dorsiflexion reaching a maximum of 10 degrees as the tibia moves over the ankle joint (Figure 6.10). The time from foot flat to heel lift is referred to as 'second rocker' or 'second segment', which refers to the pivot of the motion now being at the ankle joint with the foot firmly planted on the ground. During this time the plantar flexor muscles are acting eccentrically to control the movement of the tibia forwards.
- *Phase 3*. The heel then begins to lift at the beginning of double support, causing a rapid ankle plantar flexion reaching an average value of 20 degrees at the end of the stance phase at toe off (Figure 6.11). The ankle plantar-flexes at a rate of 250 degrees/s. This rapid movement is associated with power production. During this propulsive phase of the gait cycle the plantar flexor muscles in the posterior compartment of the foot and ankle concentrically contract, pushing the foot into plantar flexion and

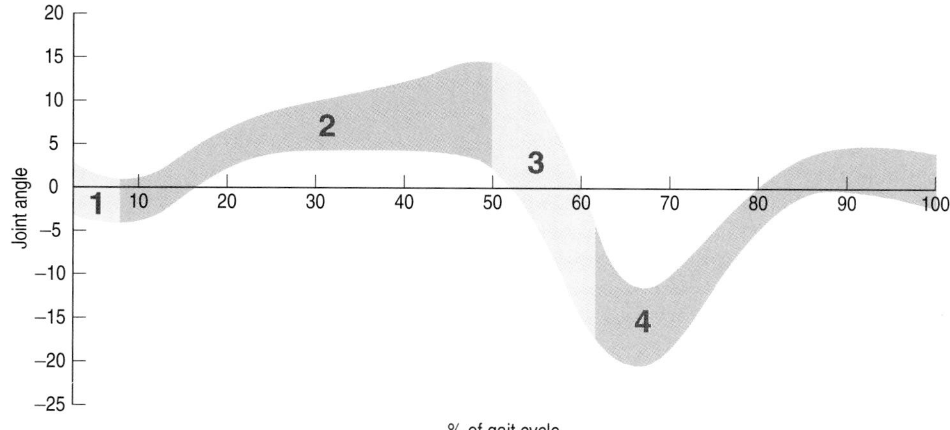

Figure 6.8 Ankle plantar/dorsiflexion.

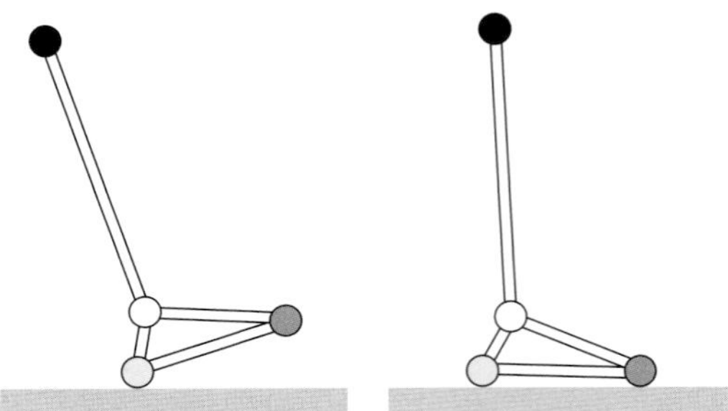

Figure 6.9 Motion of the ankle joint phase 1.

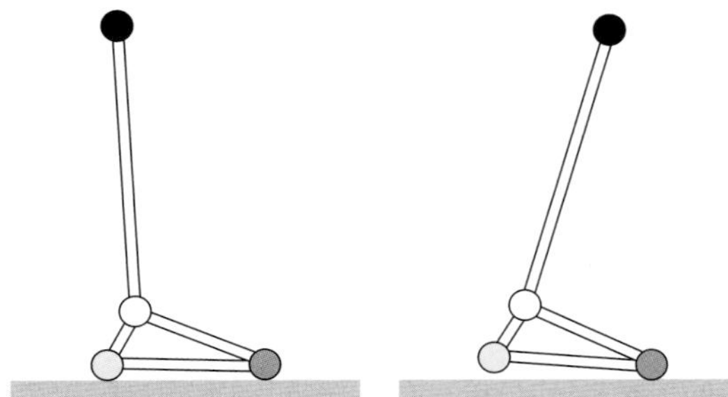

Figure 6.10 Motion of the ankle joint phase 2.

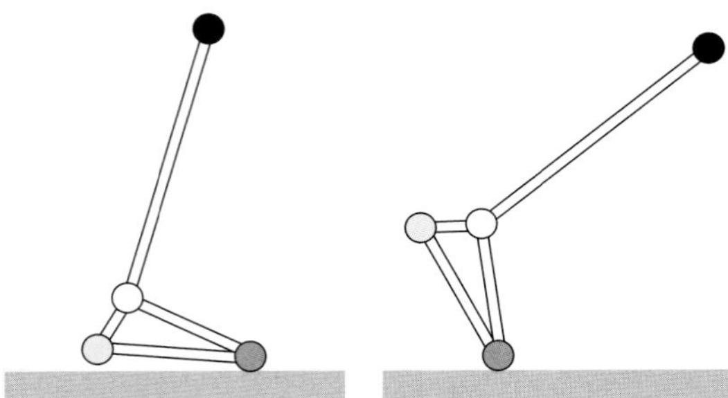

Figure 6.11 Motion of the ankle joint phase 3.

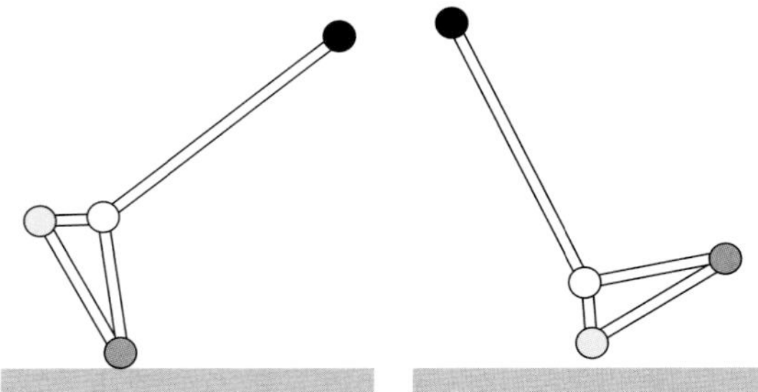

Figure 6.12 Motion of the ankle joint phase 4.

propelling the body forwards. This is referred to as 'third rocker' or 'third segment' as the pivot point is now under the metatarsal heads.

- *Phase 4*. During the swing phase the ankle rapidly dorsiflexes (150 degrees/s) to allow the clearance of the foot from the ground (Figure 6.12). A neutral position (0 degrees) is reached by mid-swing, which is maintained during the rest of the swing phase until the second heel strike. This is referred to as the 'fourth segment'. It has been recorded that there is sometimes a 3–5 degree dorsiflexion during the swing phase. During this phase the ankle dorsiflexors concentrically contract to provide foot clearance from the ground and prepare for the next foot strike.

Motion of the knee joint

During gait the knee joint moves in the sagittal, transverse and coronal planes. However, the majority of the motion of the knee joint is in the sagittal plane, which involves the flexion and extension of the knee joint. The flexion and extension of the knee joint is cyclic, and varies between 0 and 70 degrees, although there is some variation in the exact amount of peak flexion occurring. These differences may be related to differences in walking speed, subject individuality, and the landmarks selected to designate limb segment alignments. There are five phases (Figure 6.13):

- *Heel strike*. At heel strike, or initial contact, the knee should be flexed (Figure 6.14). However, people's knee posture can vary between slight hyperextension (−2 degrees) to 10 degrees of flexion, with a mean value of 5 degrees.
- *Phase 1*. After the initial contact there is a flexion of the knee joint to about 20 degrees when the knee is flexed under maximum weight-bearing load (Figure 6.15). The knee joint flexes to absorb the loading at a rate of 150–200 degrees/s. This occurs at the same time as the ankle joint plantar-flexes, with a net effect to act as a shock absorber during the loading of the lower limb. During this time the knee extensors are acting eccentrically.
- *Phase 2*. After this first peak of knee flexion the knee joint extends at a rate of 80–100 degrees/s to almost full extension (Figure 6.16). This is concerned with a smooth movement of the body over the stance limb.
- *Phase 3*. The knee then begins its second flexion, which coincides with heel lift (Figure 6.17). During this second flexion the lower limb is in the propulsive phase of the gait cycle. The knee undergoes a rapid flexion in preparation for swing phase, sometimes referred to as pre-swing.
- *Phase 4*. Toe off occurs when knee flexion is approximately 40 degrees, at which time the knee is flexing at a rate of 300–350 degrees/s (Figure 6.18). This

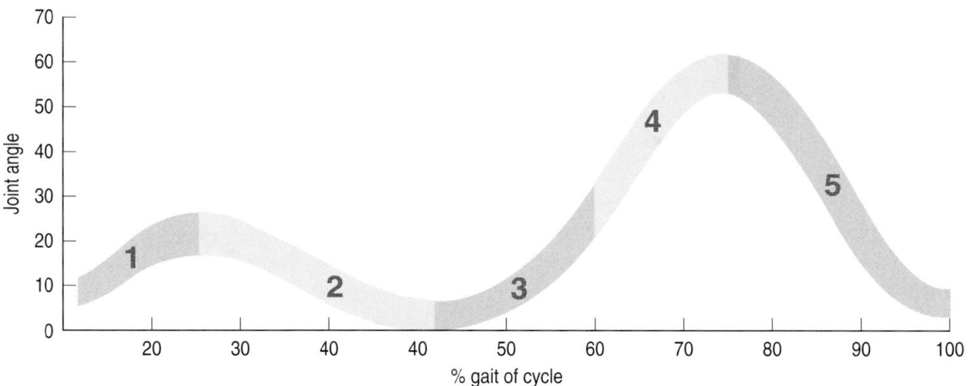

Figure 6.13 Knee flexion/extension.

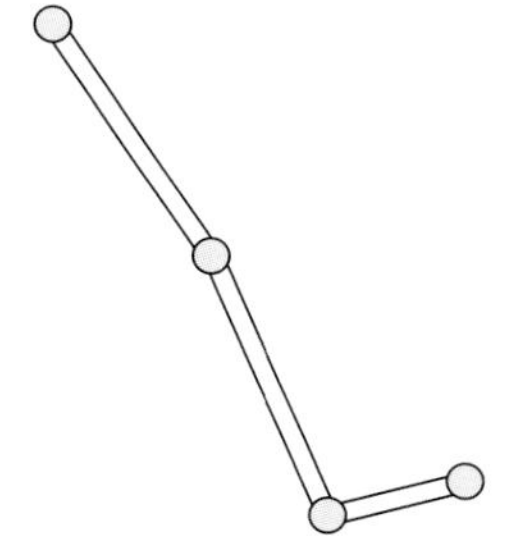

Figure 6.14 Motion of the knee joint – heel strike.

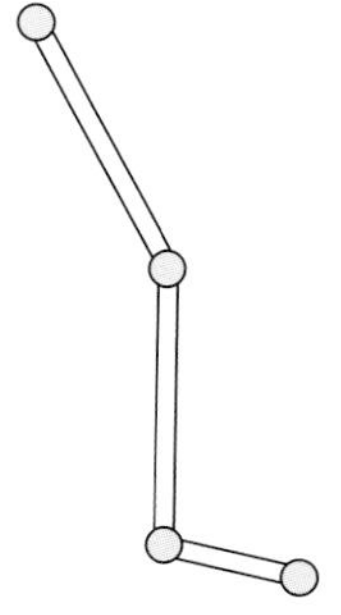

Figure 6.15 Motion of the knee joint – phase 1.

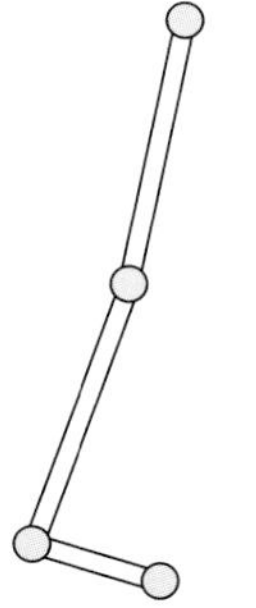

Figure 6.16 Motion of the knee joint – phase 2.

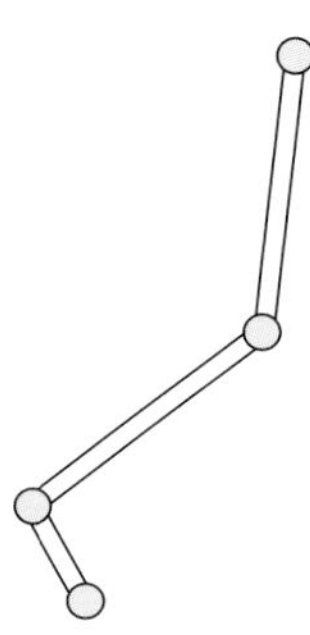

Figure 6.17 Motion of the knee joint – phase 3.

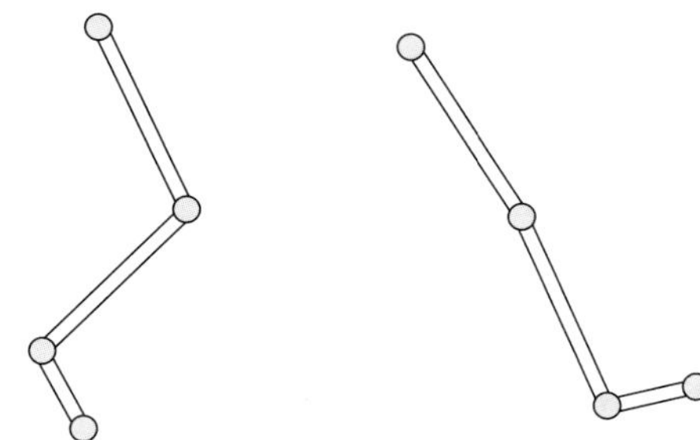

Figure 6.18 Motion of the knee joint – phase 4 and 5.

flexion, coupled with ankle dorsiflexion, allows the toe to clear the ground. During initial to mid-swing the knee continues to flex to a maximum of 65–70 degrees.

- *Phase 5*. During late swing, the knee undergoes a rapid extension, 350–400 degrees/s to prepare for the second heel strike (Figure 6.18).

Motion of the hip joint in the sagittal plane

During walking the leg flexes forward at the hip joint to take a step and then extends until push off. This motion

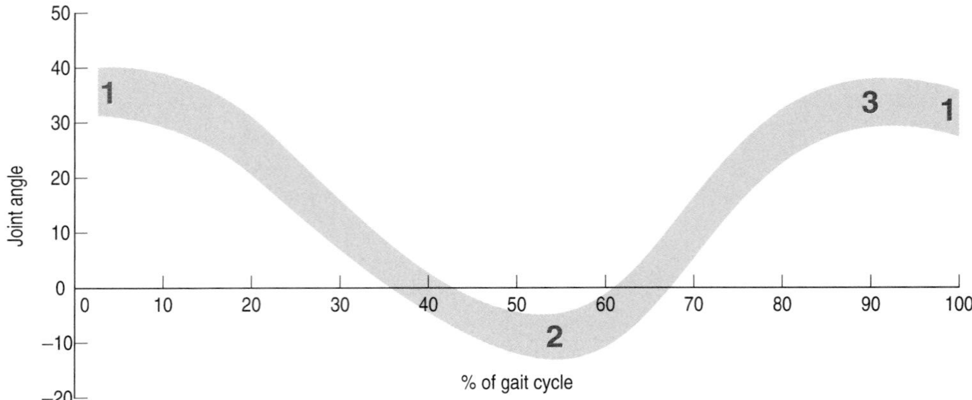

Figure 6.19 Hip flexion/extension.

forms an arc starting at initial contact and finishing at toe off.

The motion of the hip joint is quite simple. The pattern may be described as follows (Figure 6.19). Maximum hip flexion occurs during terminal swing (3); this is followed by a slight (movement towards) extension before initial contact (1) (Figure 6.20). After initial contact (1) the hip then extends as the body moves over the limb at a rate of 150 degrees/s. Maximum hip extension occurs just after opposite foot strike (2) (Figure 6.21); weight is then transferred to the forward limb and the trailing limb begins to flex at the hip. This is the pre-swing period. The toe leaves the ground at 60 per cent of the gait cycle and the hip flexes rapidly at a rate of 200 degrees/s. This can be seen from the slope of the angle against time plot below, to progress the limb forward and prepare for the next initial contact (1).

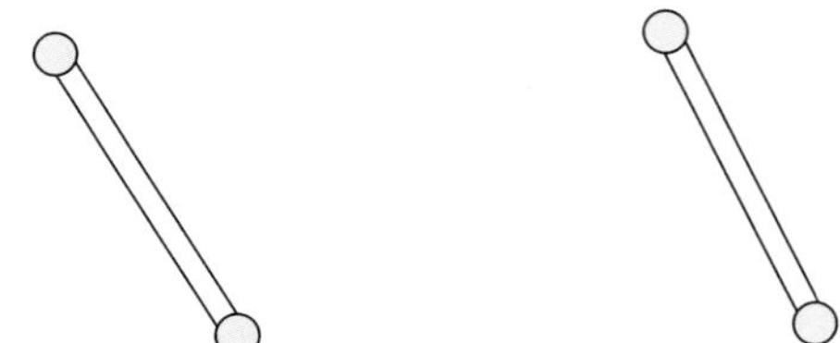

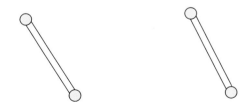

Figure 6.20 Motion of the hip joint at point 3 and 1.

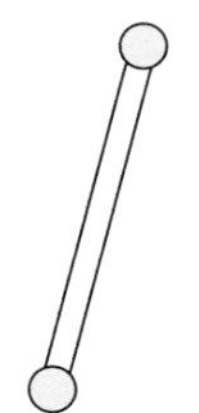

Figure 6.21 Motion of the hip joint 2.

Motion of the pelvis in the coronal plane (pelvic obliquity)

During the early stance phase the contralateral side of the pelvis drops downwards in the coronal plane (Figure 6.22). In order for foot clearance to be achieved, the knee undergoes rapid flexion. In normal gait the peak pelvic obliquity (drop down) occurs just after opposite toe off, which corresponds to the early stance phase on the weight-bearing limb.

Pelvic obliquity serves three purposes: to aid shock absorption, to allow limb length adjustments, and to reduce the vertical excursions of the body (improving efficiency).

To illustrate these points we consider an above-knee amputee gait (with a fixed knee joint). The pelvic obliquity does not always follow the normal pattern, as normal control of the knee joint has been lost. Hitching up the contralateral side of the pelvis often ensures foot clearance. In this way pelvic obliquity can be used to shorten the effective limb length when required. However, this increases energy expenditure as it increases the excursion of the vertical body.

Motion of the pelvis in the transverse plane (pelvic rotation)

During normal level walking the pelvis rotates about a vertical axis alternately to the left and to the right (Figure 6.23). This rotation is usually about 4 degrees on each side of this central axis, the peak internal rotation occurring at foot strike and the maximal external rotation at opposite foot strike. This rotation effectively lengthens the limb by increasing the step length and prevents excessive drop of the body, making the walking pattern more efficient. Pelvic rotation has the effect of smoothing the vertical excursion of the body and reducing the impact at foot strike.

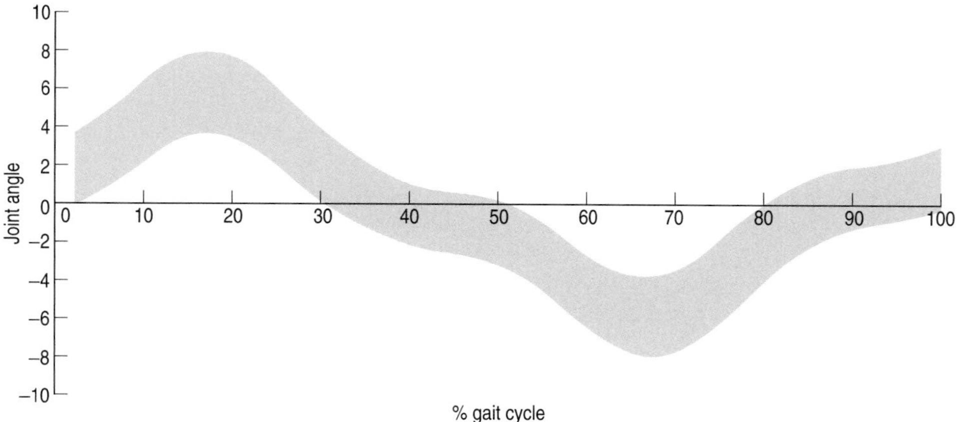

Figure 6.22 Pelvic obliquity.

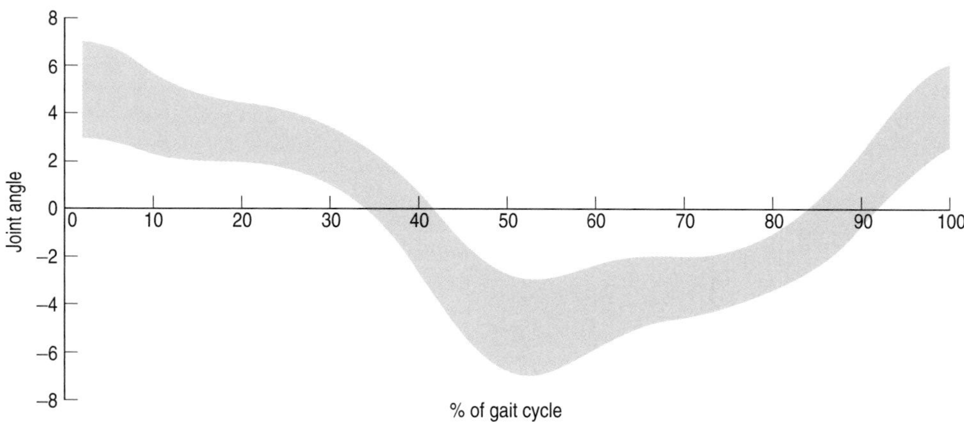

Figure 6.23 Pelvic rotation.

Linear Motion

Terminology

s = displacement
v = final velocity
u = initial velocity
a = acceleration
t = time

Definitions

Displacement. The average velocity multiplied by time. The average velocity may be found by adding the initial and final velocities and dividing by two:

Average velocity = {1/2} (u + v)

Velocity. The rate of change of displacement: that is, the distance covered in a particular time:

Velocity = change in displacement/time

Acceleration. The rate of change of velocity: that is, the change in velocity over a given time:

Acceleration = change in velocity/time

TEST YOURSELF

From the displacement data shown in Figure 6.24 and Table 6.1, the linear velocity and acceleration of the hand may be found. The data was collected at 10 readings per second. Calculate the velocity and acceleration of the hand and plot the displacement, velocity and acceleration on graph paper.

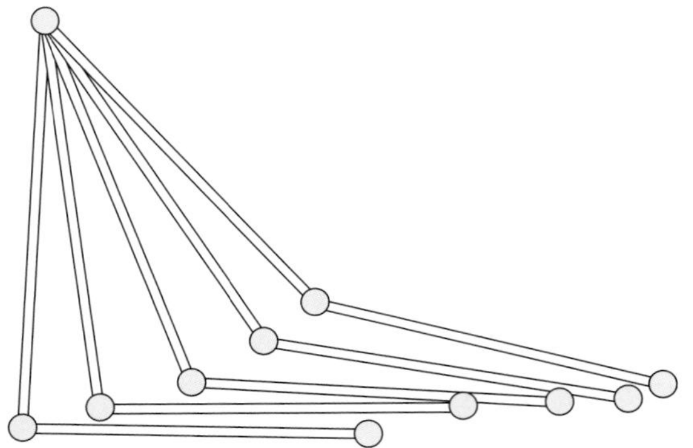

Figure 6.24 Motion of the upper limb during reaching.

Table 6.1 Data for the 'Test yourself' task

Time	Displacement	Velocity	Acceleration
0	0.003973		
0.1	0.005293		
0.2	0.007077		
0.3	0.028080		
0.4	0.089244		
0.5	0.171660		
0.6	0.235259		
0.7	0.267247		
0.8	0.281803		
0.9	0.289150		
1.0	0.291820		

Linear displacement graph

This graph is drawn from knowing how the linear position of the hand varies over time. The graph in Figure 6.25 shows how the hand starts at a position zero and moves forwards in a reaching motion. The gradient of the curve indicates the velocity at which the hand is moving throughout the task.

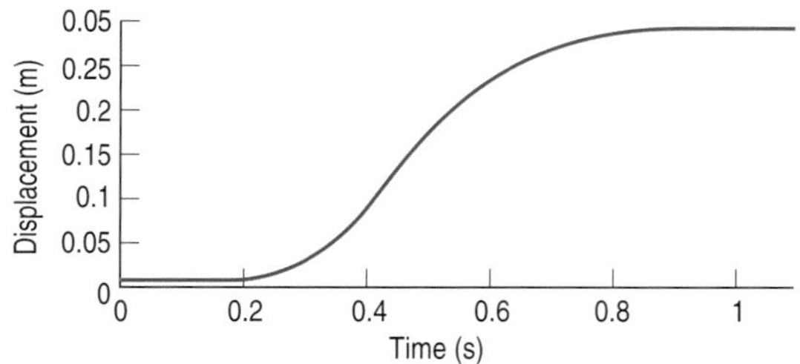

Figure 6.25 Linear displacement of the hand.

Linear velocity graph

The velocity graph is found by measuring the change in the linear displacement over each successive time interval. The linear velocity graph for the hand during reaching shows a bell-shaped curve (Figure 6.26). Initially the velocity of the hand is zero; the hand then accelerates to its maximum velocity at approximately the mid-point of the reaching movement. The hand now decelerates, as the hand gets closer to its target; this takes slightly longer than the acceleration phase to ensure accuracy of hand position.

Linear acceleration graph

The acceleration graph is found by measuring the change in the linear velocity over each successive time interval. The graph in Figure 6.27 shows an initial acceleration peak early in the movement. The acceleration then decreases to zero as the hand reaches its maximum velocity. The hand then goes into a deceleration phase as the hand reaches its target. The peak deceleration is lower than the acceleration phase, but it lasts for a longer period of time, as shown with the velocity curve; again this is to ensure accuracy of positioning of the hand at the target.

The difference between displacement, velocity and acceleration graphs

The information presented above for displacement, velocity and acceleration comes from exactly the same

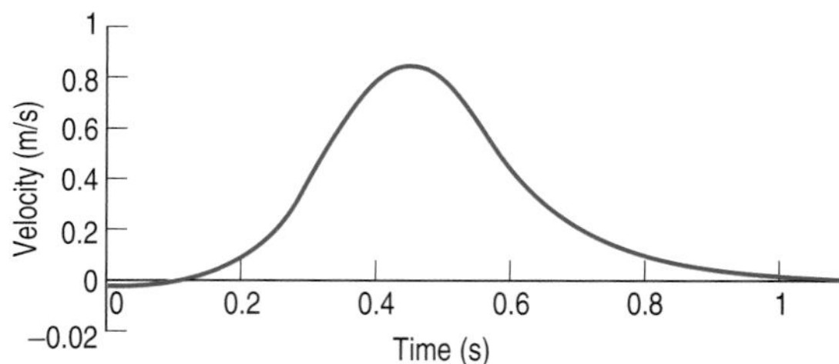

Figure 6.26 Linear velocity of the hand.

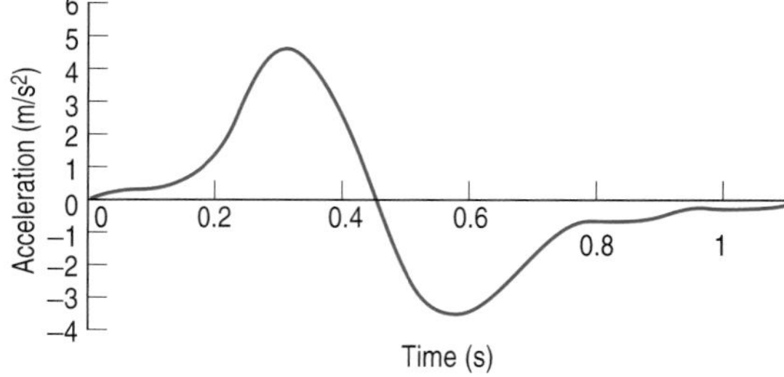

Figure 6.27 Linear acceleration of the hand.

original numbers. However, it is important to realise that each of these graphs gives us different information about the movement strategy. The process of finding velocity from displacement and acceleration from velocity is called *differentiation*.

Angular Motion

Definitions

Angular displacement (θ). This can be measured in two ways: either in degrees or in radians. There are 360 degrees in a full circle, or 2π radians. Pi (π) is the ratio of the circumference of a circle to its diameter (a ratio that is for all circles) and is very close to 3.1416. So 1 radian is approximately 57.3 degrees.
Angular velocity (ω). The change in angle over time.

$$\omega = \frac{\text{Change in } \theta}{\text{Time}}$$

Angular velocity can be expressed in degrees/s or radians/s.
Angular acceleration (α). The change in angular velocity over time.

$$\alpha = \frac{\text{Change in } \omega}{\text{Time}}$$

Angular acceleration can be written in degree/s^2 or radians/s^2.

TEST YOURSELF

From the data in Table 6.2, calculate the knee angular velocity and angular acceleration. Plot the angular displacement, velocity and acceleration on graph paper.

Table 6.2 Data for the 'Test yourself' task

Time	Displacement (degrees)	Velocity (degrees/s)	Acceleration (degrees/s²)
0	6		
0.1	18		
0.2	24		
0.3	20		
0.4	12		
0.5	25		
0.6	50		
0.7	65		
0.8	55		
0.9	27		
1.0	6		

Knee angular displacement

The description of the angle against time graph can be found in 'Normal movement patterns during gait' above. This graph is drawn from knowing how the angle between the femoral and tibial segments varies over time (Figure 6.28).

Knee angular velocity

The velocity graph is found by measuring the change in the angular displacement over each successive time interval. This graph (Figure 6.29) shows the speed of movement into flexion or extension during walking. This tells us more about how the movement is achieved. A flexing angular velocity is defined as being positive, and extension angular velocity as negative. These graphs have been used to determine the performance of the joint and to determine functional deficits in different pathologies (Richards 2003).

Knee angular acceleration

The acceleration graph (Figure 6.30) is found by measuring the change in the angular velocity over each successive time interval. It shows the smoothness of movement and can give information about control of the movement.

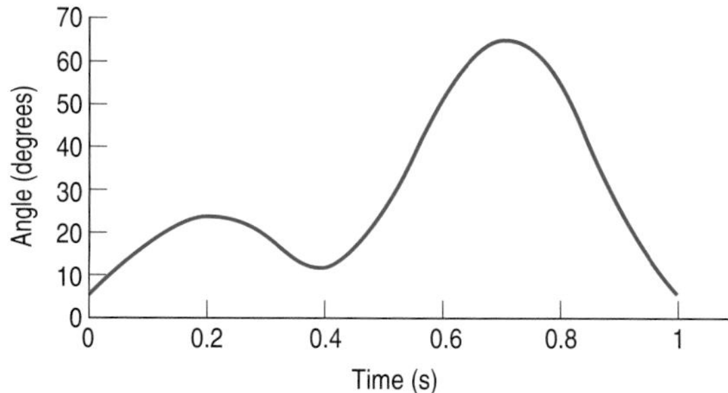

Figure 6.28 Knee angular displacement.

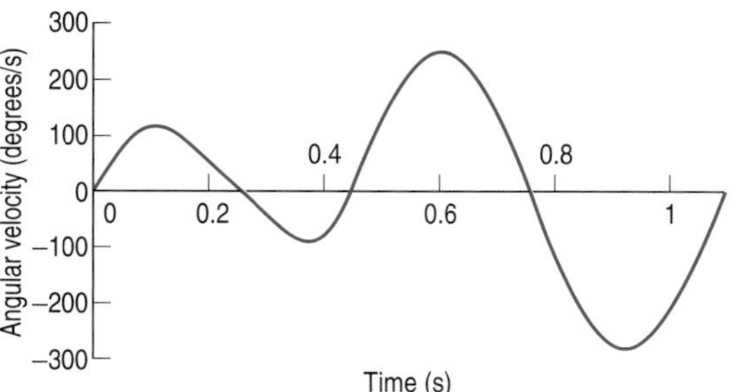

Figure 6.29 Knee angular velocity.

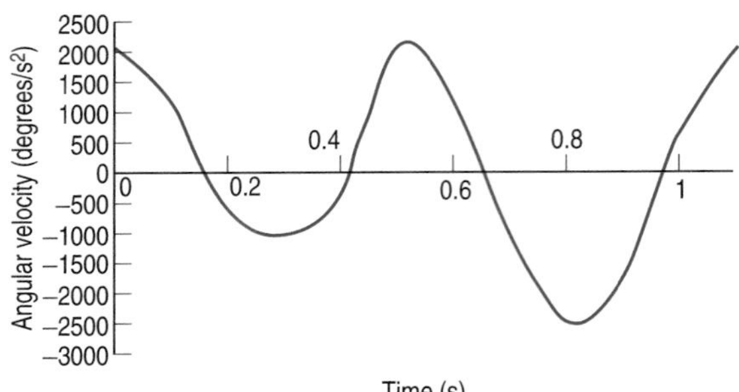

Figure 6.30 Knee angular acceleration.

6

Solutions to the 'Test yourself' tasks

The solutions are shown in Tables 6.3 and 6.4.

Table 6.3 Answer to the 'Test yourself' task — motion of the upper limb during reaching

Time	Displacement	Velocity	Acceleration
0	0.003973	0	0
0.1	0.005293	0.0132	0.132
0.2	0.007077	0.01784	0.0464
0.3	0.028080	0.21003	1.9219
0.4	0.089244	0.61164	4.0161
0.5	0.171660	0.82416	2.1252
0.6	0.235259	0.63599	−1.8817
0.7	0.267247	0.31988	-3.1611
0.8	0.281803	0.14556	−1.7432
0.9	0.289150	0.07347	−0.7209
1.0	0.291820	0.02670	−0.4677

Table 6.4 Answer to the 'Test yourself' task — motion of the knee during walking

Time	Displacement (degrees)	Velocity (degrees/s)	Acceleration (degrees/s^2)
0	6	0	2100
0.1	18	120	1200
0.2	24	60	-600
0.3	20	-40	-1000
0.4	12	-80	-400
0.5	25	130	2100
0.6	50	250	1200
0.7	65	150	-1000
0.8	55	-100	-2500
0.9	27	-280	-1800
1.0	6	-210	700

BASIC KINETICS: NEWTON'S LAWS

Forces

Forces make things move, stop things moving, or make things change shape. They can either push or pull. Force is a *vector*, which simply means it has both direction and magnitude. All forces thus have two characteristics, magnitude and direction, and both need to be stated in order to describe the force fully.

In *statics* we apply the fundamental concepts of mechanics, forces and moments to the analysis of objects. A good place to start is with the laws formulated by Sir Isaac Newton. In 1687 Newton published three simple laws, which together enshrine the fundamental principles of mechanics.

Newton's first law

If an object is at rest, it will stay at rest. If it is moving with a constant speed in a straight line, it will continue to do so, as long as no external force acts on it. In other words, if an object is not experiencing the action of an external force, it will either keep moving or not move at all (Figure 6.31).

This law expresses the concept of *inertia*. The inertia of a body can be described as being its reluctance to start moving, or to stop moving once it has started.

Why not perpetual motion?

Why does a car slow down when rolling on a flat road? The answer is that there are a number of external forces that need to be considered, such as wind resistance and friction in the bearings of the wheels and axle. This means we have to be careful to consider *all* the forces that are acting on an object in order to find out how it is going to move.

Newton's second law

The rate of change of velocity is directly proportional to the applied external force acting on the body and takes place in the direction of the force (Figure 6.32). Therefore forces can cause either an acceleration or a deceleration of an object. *Acceleration* is usually defined as being positive and *deceleration* as being negative.

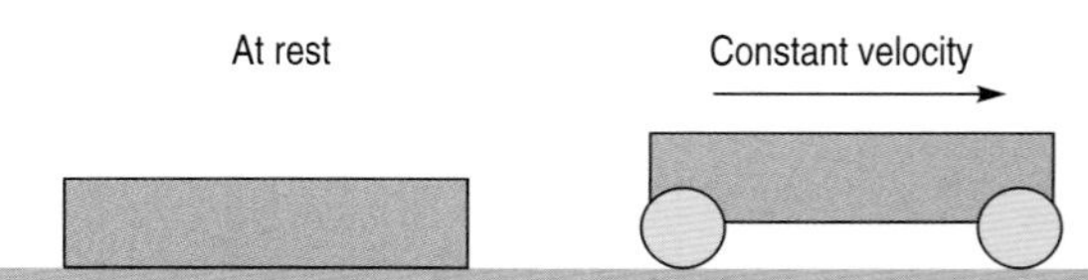

Figure 6.31 Newton's first law.

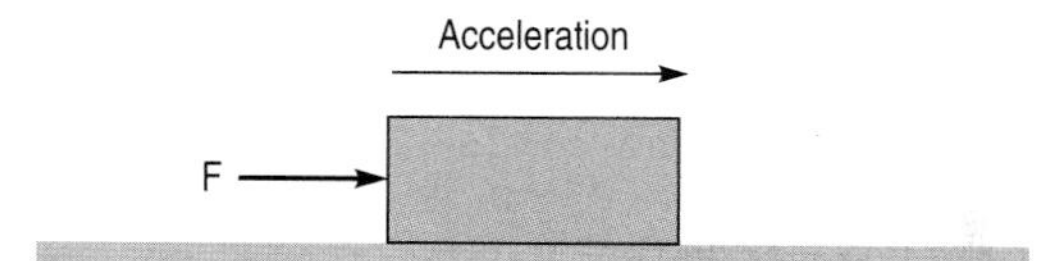

Figure 6.32 Acceleration of an object with a constant force.

If F is the applied force (in Newtons), m is the mass of the body (kg) and a is the acceleration of the body (m/s^2), then $F = ma$. Therefore 1 N is that force which produces an acceleration of 1 m/s^2 when it acts on a mass of 1 kg.

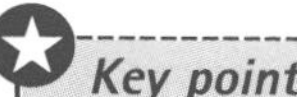

Key point

In the SI system of units, forces are measured in Newtons (N).

Newton's third law

If the box shown in Figure 6.33 exerts a force on the table top (*action*), then the table will exert an equal and opposite force on the box (*reaction*). This does not mean the forces cancel each other out, because they act on two different objects.

The action of a force on the ground receives an equal and opposite reaction force. This is known as a *ground reaction force* (GRF).

Mass and weight

Mass

Mass is the amount of matter an object contains. This will not change unless the physical properties of the object are changed, wherever the object is moved.

Weight

Weight is a force. This depends on both the mass of the object and the acceleration acting on it. Weight is often interpreted as being the force acting beneath our feet (i.e. scales measure this force, although they never use the correct units which are Newtons).

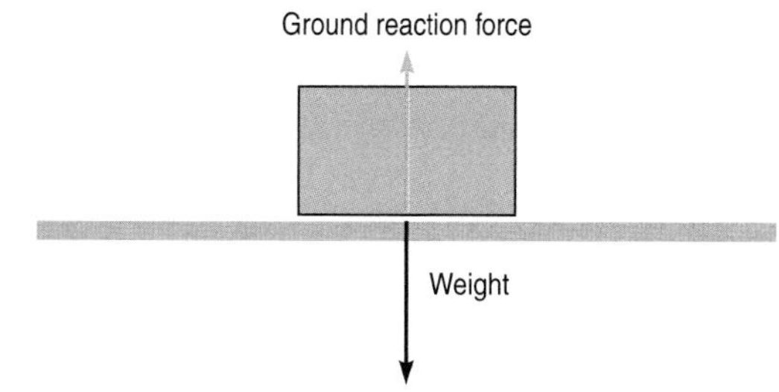

Figure 6.33 Newton's third law.

Therefore a good way to lose weight is to stand in a lift and press the down button. You will lose weight (the GRF will reduce) as the lift accelerates downwards. Unfortunately, when the lift comes to a stop, you will gain weight again as the lift decelerates downwards.

Another example of the difference between mass and weight is to consider astronauts. When they are in space they are weightless, but this does not mean they have gone on an amazing diet, only that there is no acceleration acting on them. Therefore weight watchers should really be called mass watchers.

Acceleration due to gravity

Wherever you are on planet Earth, there is acceleration due to gravity acting on you. This does vary a small amount but the value is generally close to 9.81 m/s^2. For the purposes of rough calculations, this is often rounded up to 10 m/s^2. It is acceptable to use 10 m/s^2 for the biomechanics covered in this book. However, for the best possible accuracy the figure of 9.81 m/s^2 should be used.

Static equilibrium

The concept of static equilibrium is of great importance in biomechanics, as it allows us to calculate forces that are unknown.

Newton's first law tells us that there is no resultant force acting if the body is at rest — i.e. the forces balance. Therefore if an object is at rest, the sum of the forces on the object, in any direction, must be zero. So when we resolve in a horizontal and vertical direction the resultant force must be zero.

Free-body analysis

Free-body analysis is a technique of looking at and simplifying a problem. The example below considers someone pulling a box along the ground with a piece of string at an angle to the horizontal (Figure 6.34a). We now break down what force must be acting on the box and form a simplified picture of just the box. The forces acting are the tension in the string, the frictional force, the weight of the box and the GRF (Figure 6.34b).

Worked example

With reference to Figure 6.35, find the horizontal acceleration and the GRF.

Horizontal forces

Horizontal force in string = 10 cos 30° = 8.66
Therefore 8.66 − 2.66 = mass × acceleration
$6 = 4 \times a$
1.5 m/s = a

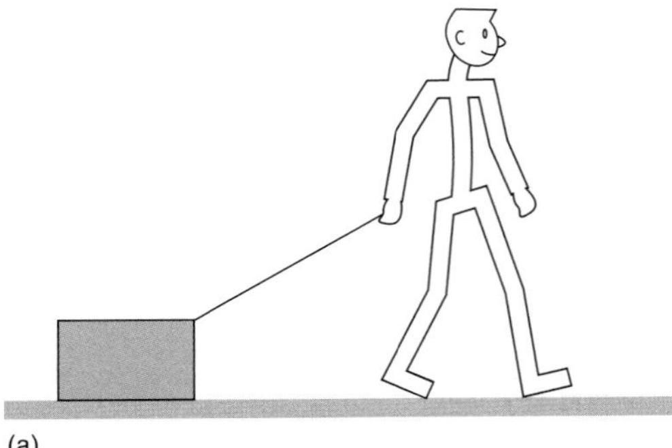

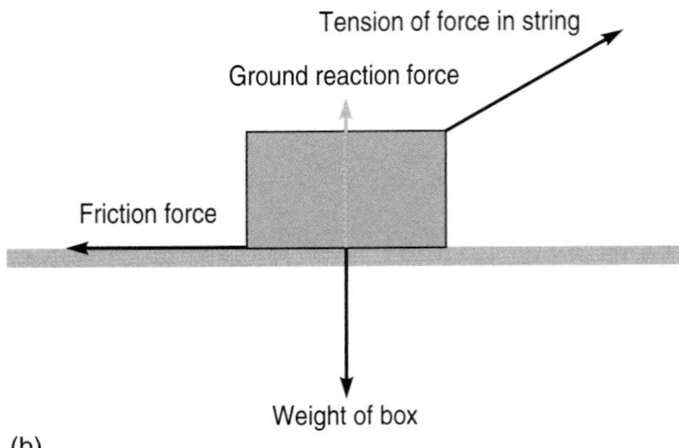

Figure 6.34 Free-body analysis.

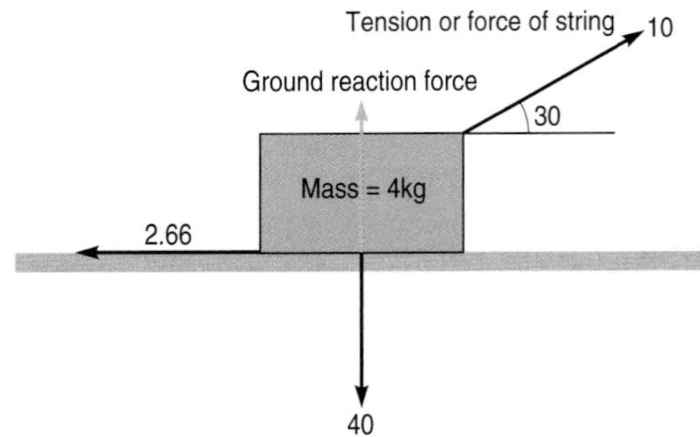

Figure 6.35 Worked example of Newton's laws.

Vertical forces

Vertical force in string $= 10 \sin 30° = 5$

$\text{GRF} + 5 - 40 = 0$

$\text{GRF} = 40 - 5 = 35\,\text{N}$

KINETICS IN BODILY MOVEMENTS

Ground reaction forces

Definition

A ground reaction force is the force that acts on a body as a result of the body resting on the ground or hitting the ground.

If someone stands on a floor without moving, that person is exerting a force (the person's weight) on the floor, but the floor exerts an equal and opposite reaction force on the person. That is an example of the simplest GRF, but it never happens as easily as that as in real life humans do not balance perfectly because of sway.

When standing, we naturally sway backwards and forwards (anterior–posterior, Figure 6.36) and from side to side (medial–lateral, Figure 6.37). As we rock like that, horizontal forces come into play in addition to the vertical force (Figure 6.38). The *centre of pressure* (CoP) is the point at which the force is acting beneath the feet. The CoP moves forwards, backwards and side to side between the two feet (Figure 6.39).

Force platforms

Force platforms are devices that measure and record GRFs and their point of application at the centre of pressure (Figure 6.40).

A GRF is made up of three forces acting in three directions at the centre of pressure: vertical, anterior–posterior and mediolateral. At each corner of the force platform there is a load cell or transducer. These measure the forces in the three directions at each corner. To find the total force acting in an anterior–posterior direction, for example, all the anterior–posterior forces measured by the load cells will be added to give the total force in that direction.

Ground reaction forces during the gait cycle

Vertical force component

The vertical component of the GRF can be split into four sections (Figure 6.41).

- *Heel strike to first peak.* This is where the foot strikes the ground and the body decelerates downwards, transferring the loading from the back foot to the front foot during initial double support. The first peak should be in the order of 1.2 times the person's bodyweight.
- *First peak to trough.* The knee extends, so raising the body. As the body approaches its highest point, it is slowing down (decelerating the body) in its upward motion. This reduces the vertical GRF. This has the same effect as going over a hump-backed bridge in a car; as you reach the top of the hump you feel very light, because the contact force between you and the seat is reduced. The trough should be in the order of 0.7 times the person's bodyweight.
- *Trough to second peak.* The centre of mass now falls as the heel lifts and the foot is pushed down and back into the ground by the action of muscles in the posterior compartment of the ankle joint.

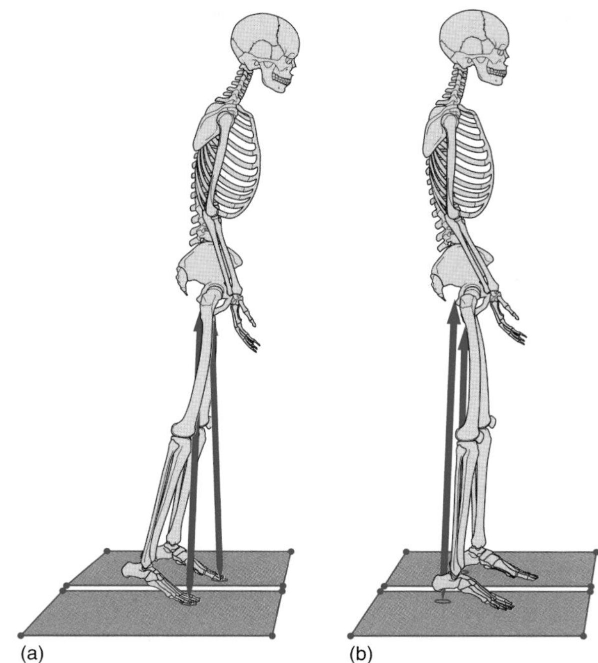

Figure 6.36 Postural sway in the anterior posterior direction.

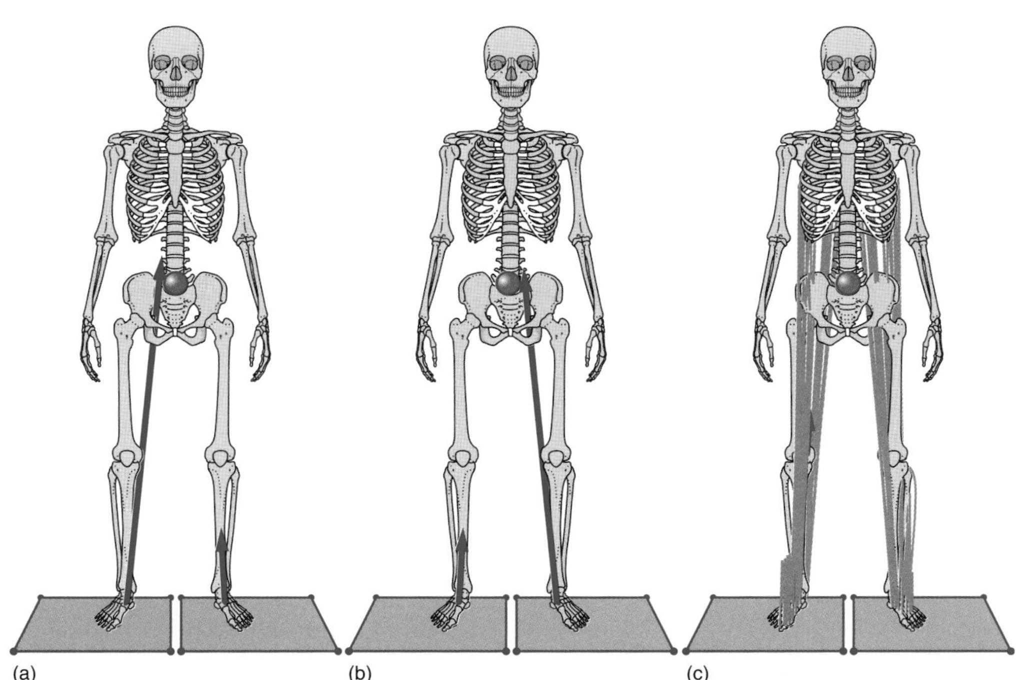

Figure 6.37 Postural sway in the medial lateral direction.

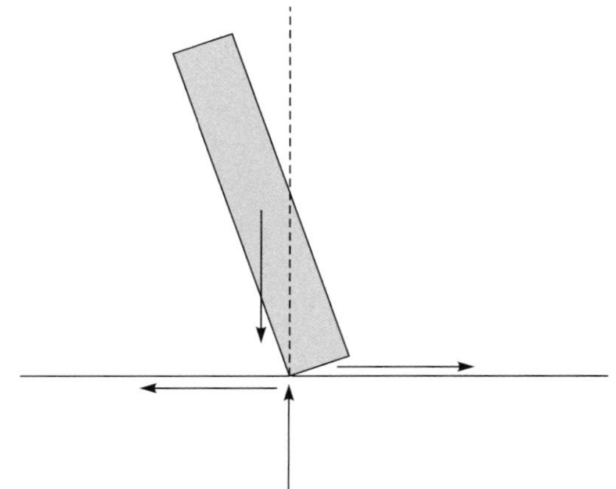

Figure 6.38 Postural sway during balance.

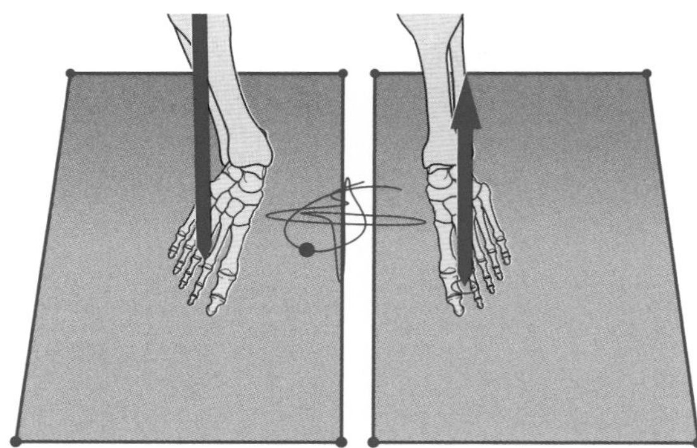

Figure 6.39 Movement of the centre of pressure during postural sway.

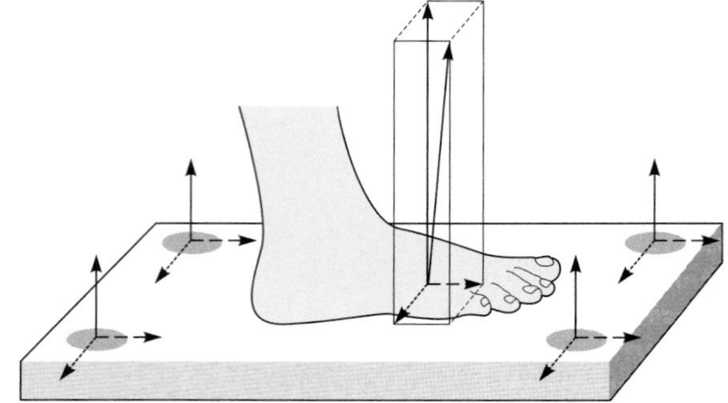

Figure 6.40 A force platform.

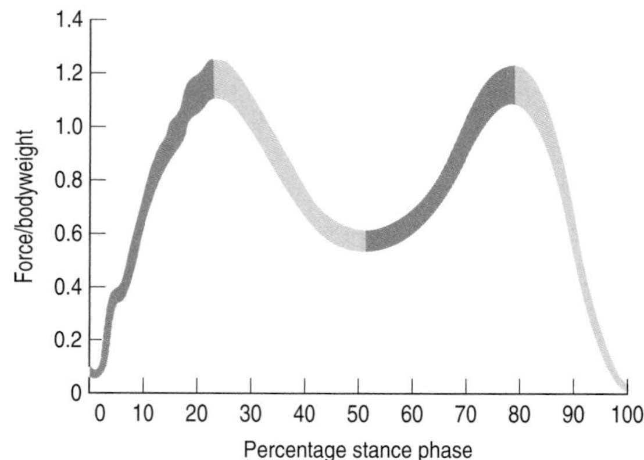

Figure 6.41 Vertical force during normal walking.

Both the deceleration downward and propulsion from the foot–ankle complex cause the second peak. The second peak should be in the order of 1.2 times the person's bodyweight.

- *Second peak to toe off*. The foot is unloaded as the load is transferred to the opposite foot.

Anterior–posterior force component

The anterior–posterior component may also be split into four sections (Figure 6.42).

- *Clawback*. Clawback is an initial anterior force, which is not always present during walking. This is caused by the swinging limb hitting the ground with a backwards velocity, thus causing an anterior reaction force as it decelerates. Clawback is often exaggerated during marching as the swing limb is driven back to meet the ground.
- *Heel strike to posterior peak*. After the initial clawback (if present) the heel is in contact with the ground and the body decelerates, causing a posterior shear force. Imagine you are walking on a thick carpet, loading your front foot, and suddenly you are transported to an ice rink — your leg would slide forwards. This is because the frictional force between the ice and your foot is very low, whereas the carpet can provide a much larger posterior reaction force that stops your leg from slipping forwards. The posterior peak should be in the order of 0.2 times the person's bodyweight.
- *Posterior peak to crossover*. The posterior component reduces as the body begins to move over the stance limb, reducing the horizontal component of the resultant GRF.
- *Crossover to anterior peak*. The heel lifts and the foot is pushed down and back into the ground by the action of muscles in the posterior compartment of the ankle joint. This has the effect of produ-cing an anterior component of the GRF, which propels the body forwards. The anterior peak should be in the order of 0.2 times the person's bodyweight.
- *Anterior peak to toe off*. This is now the period of terminal double support where the force is being transferred to the front foot. The anterior force therefore reduces.

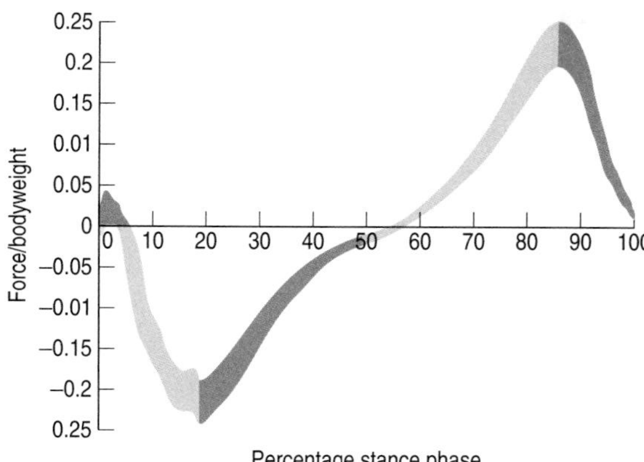

Figure 6.42 Force in the anterior–posterior direction during normal walking.

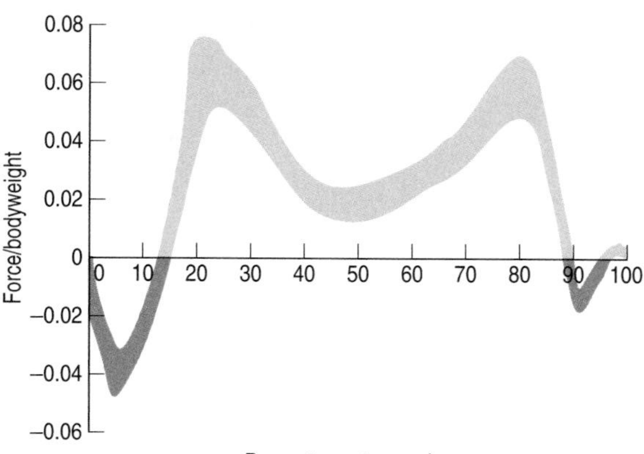

Figure 6.43 Force in the mediolateral direction during normal walking.

Mediolateral force component

The mediolateral component may be split into two main sections (Figure 6.43). Initially at heel strike there is a lateral thrust during loading; during this time the foot is working as a mobile adaptor. After the initial loading, the forces push in a medial direction as the body moves over the stance limb. Small lateral forces are often seen during the final push-off stage.

The mediolateral forces are the most variable of the three components, and can easily be affected by footwear and foot orthotics. Normal maximum medial force is between 0.05 and 0.1 times the person's bodyweight. The maximum lateral force should be less than the maximum medial force.

How to study the measurements taken from these graphs

For each of these measurements the percentage difference can be studied between the left and right sides, and between the subject tested and non-pathological data. This will not only identify what differences are present in the walking patterns, but also how big the differences are.

Pedotti diagrams

The interaction of the vertical and anterior–posterior forces described above may be shown with a Pedotti diagram. This demonstrates the magnitude of the resultant GRF.

Pedotti diagrams rely on the information provided by force platforms. To construct a Pedotti diagram we need to know the vertical and horizontal forces and the positions of the forces beneath the foot in the plane of interest for each moment in time.

As a subject walks, the forces during the stance phase move forward from under the heel to the toe, so the position of the force moves from posterior to anterior. As we have seen in the previous section, the vertical and horizontal GRFs are continually changing during the stance phase, so changing the direction and magnitude of the resultant GRF (Figure 6.44).

Figure 6.45 shows the vertical, horizontal and resultant GRF components being drawn at heel off. The CoP has moved forwards from the heel to the forefoot and the new vertical, horizontal and resultant GRF components are drawn from the new position. This process is repeated throughout the stance phase, producing a butterfly-like diagram.

TEST YOURSELF

Use the data in Figure 6.46 and Table 6.5 to plot a Pedotti diagram on graph paper.

Video vector generators

The video vector generator is a piece of equipment that combines the information from a force platform with a video image. The resultant force can be superimposed on top of the video information, giving a picture of the action of the GRFs (Figure 6.47). This uses the same information as displayed in the Pedotti diagram, but also allows the action of the forces to be seen with respect to the joints of the lower limb. This information may be used to identify biomechanical pathologies and monitor gross changes due to treatment.

Definition

A moment (M) is defined as the magnitude of force F (how hard you push) multiplied by the perpendicular distance d of the force away from the pivot. So $M = Fd$ (Figure 6.48).

6

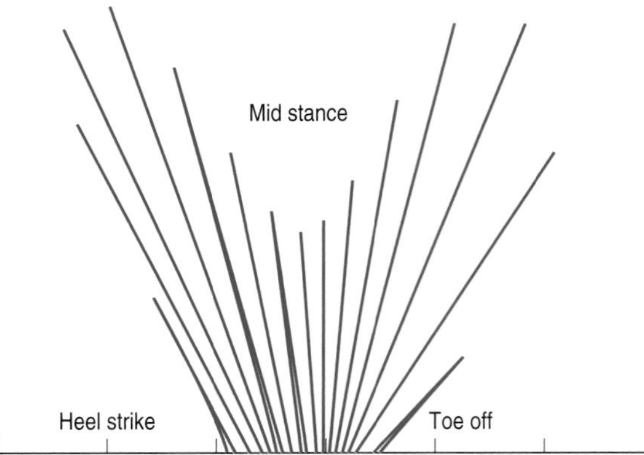

Figure 6.44 Pedotti diagram during normal walking.

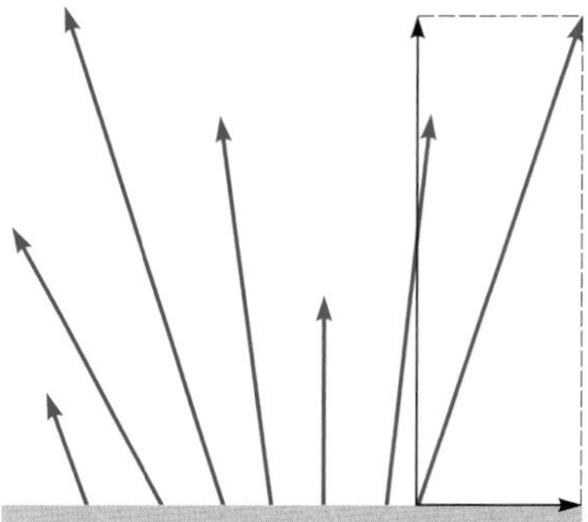

Figure 6.45 Vertical, horizontal and resultant GRFs at heel off.

INVERSE DYNAMICS: MOMENTS

When a force acts on a body some distance away from its pivoting point, a turning effect is set up. Consider opening and closing a door, whereby you are creating sufficient force to turn the door on its hinges. The force required to do this action multiplied by the distance away from the hinges is referred to as the *moment* (also sometimes called torque).

Now consider the see-saw in Figure 6.49a. It is clear that the see-saw will not balance. However, if the 1000 N force is moved so it is half the distance away from the pivot (point of rotation), as in Figure 6.49b, it will balance. This is explained below.

To solve problems with moments we have to consider the action of each force in turn. To do this we consider whether it will rotate the object (in this case a see-saw) in a clockwise or anticlockwise direction. If it is in a clockwise direction it is considered to be in a positive direction, and if anticlockwise it is considered to be in a negative direction (these are arbitrary choices).

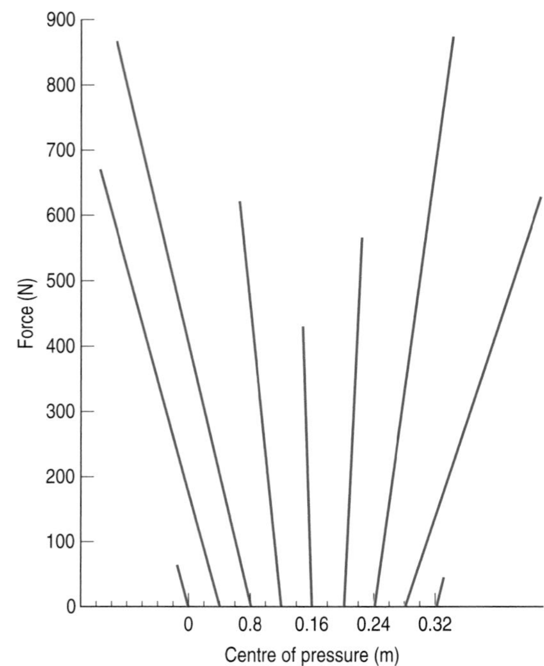

Figure 6.46 Data for the 'Test Yourself' Task.

Table 6.5 Data for the 'Test yourself' task

Position (m)	Anterior–posterior force (N)	Vertical force (N)
0	-8	66
0.04	-155	678
0.08	-180	878
0.12	-54	622
0.16	-13	457
0.2	26	564
0.24	106	889
0.28	180	626
0.32	10	16

Therefore the 1000 N force will try to turn the seesaw clockwise and the 500 N force will try to turn the seesaw anticlockwise.

If the see-saw balances then the sum of the clockwise turning effects and anticlockwise turning effects must be zero. If we say that anticlockwise moments are negative and clockwise ones are positive, then:

$$\text{Sum of the moments} = -(1000 \times 1) + (500 \times 2)$$
$$\text{Sum of the moments} = -(1000) + (1000) = 0$$

That is, if the sum of the moments on the see-saw is zero then the see-saw will balance.

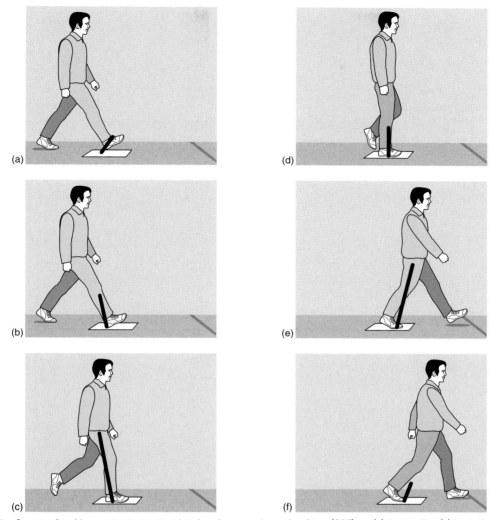

Figure 6.47 Output of a video vector generator, showing the ground reaction force (GRF) at: (a) heel strike; (b) just after heel strike; (c) at foot flat; (d) at mid-stance; (e) at heel off; and (f) just before toe off.

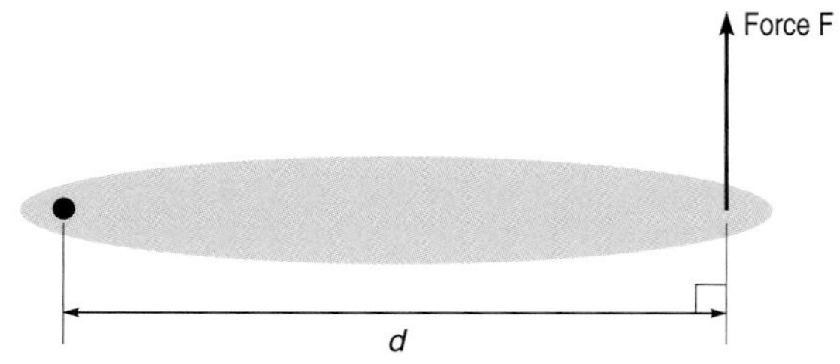

Figure 6.48 The moment of a force.

Although there seems to be little effect when we consider the see-saw vertically, we have a mass on each side, giving a total force of $500 + 1000 = 1500$ N downwards. From Newton's third law we know that there must be an equal and opposite reaction at the pivot of 1500 N acting up on to the pivot of the see-saw (Figure 6.49c).

CALCULATION OF MOMENTS ABOUT JOINTS

These values can be calculated in the same way as finding moments acting on a see-saw, as in the preceding section. Therefore all we need to know is the forces acting about a joint and the distances at which they act from the joint.

However, forces seldom act at 90 degrees to body segments. Therefore we invariably need first to *resolve* the forces. There are two methods we can use:

6

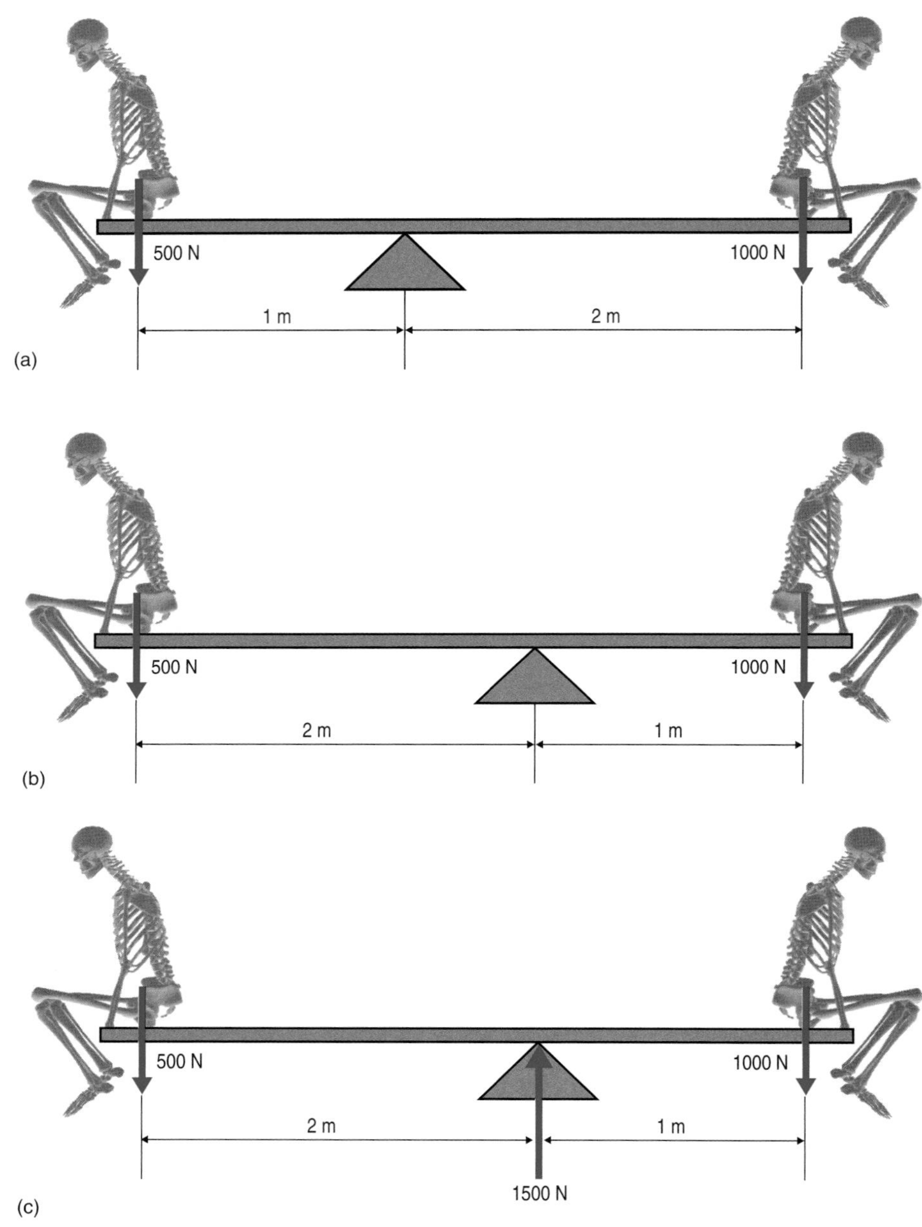

Figure 6.49 (a) Unbalanced seesaw. (b) Balanced seesaw. (c) Pivot reaction force.

- method 1 — the component of force at 90 degrees to the body segment
- method 2 — the horizontal and vertical components of the force relative to the ground.

Students' note

This author's preference is to use the component of force at 90 degrees to the body segment for *upper limb and upper body* (trunk) problems, and the horizontal and vertical components of the force relative to the ground for *lower limb* problems which involve GRFs.

Calculation of moments in the upper limb using method 1

Figure 6.50 shows the weight of the forearm acting straight down. This will produce an extending moment about the elbow.

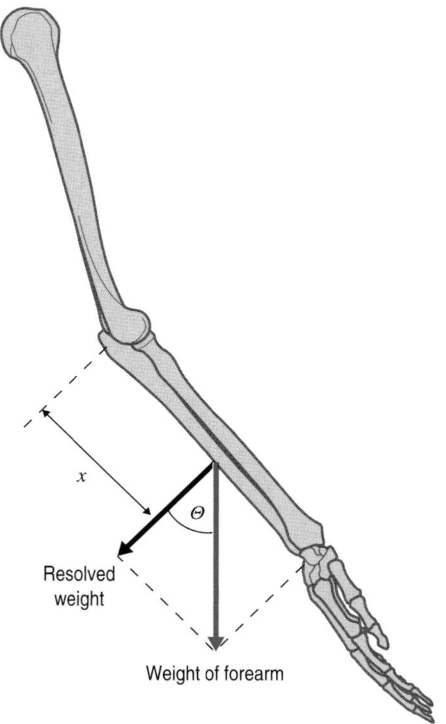

Figure 6.50 Moments in the upper limb using method 1.

Resolving the force

The weight of the forearm is not acting perpendicular to the forearm, so we cannot use it to find the moment. However, if we find the component of the weight acting perpendicular to the forearm then we can find the moment.

Component acting perpendicular to the forearm = weight of the forearm $\times$ cos Θ

Moments about the elbow

The component of the weight is acting a perpendicular distance of x away from the elbow. Therefore:

Moment about the elbow = weight of the forearm $\times$ cos $\Theta \times x$

Calculation of moments in the lower limb using method 2

Figure 6.51 shows the resultant GRF seen at foot flat in a normal subject. The resultant force can be broken up into two separate components: one in the vertical direction and the other in the horizontal direction.

If we consider the moments about the knee, we need to find out the effects of both the vertical and horizontal components of the resultant GRF.

Resolving the forces

Vertical component = resultant $\times$ sin Θ
Horizontal component = resultant $\times$ cos Θ

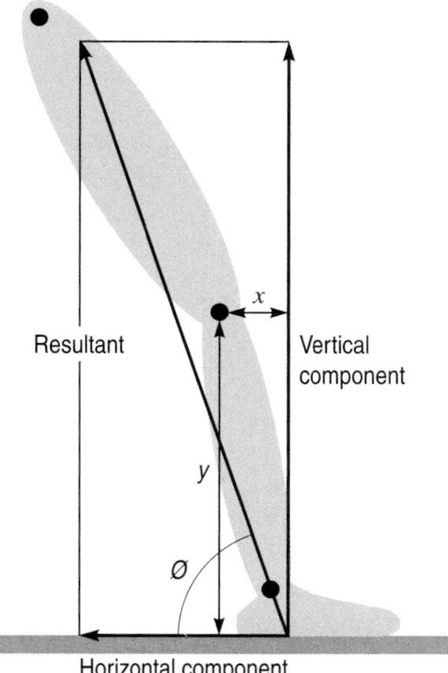

Figure 6.51 Moments in the lower limb using method 2.

Moments about the knee

To find the moment about the knee we are going to consider each of these forces separately:

- The horizontal force (resultant × cos Θ) is passing a perpendicular distance y below the knee. This force will try to turn the knee in a clockwise direction.
- The vertical force (resultant × sin Θ) is passing a perpendicular distance x in front of the knee. This force will try to turn the knee in an anticlockwise direction.

If we say all moments going clockwise are positive and those going anticlockwise are negative, then moments about the knee may be written:

$$\text{Moment about the knee} = \text{resultant} \times \cos \Theta \times y - \text{resultant} \times \sin \Theta \times x$$

CALCULATION OF MUSCLE AND JOINT FORCES

Students without a maths background should not become too worried as this section uses exactly the same principles dealt with in previous sections.

Muscle forces may be considered in the same way as balancing forces on a see-saw, and joint forces may be considered in the same way as the force at the pivot in the middle of the see-saw.

Muscle forces

One way to calculate the moment due to a force inclined at an angle is to break the force up into two perpendicular components. This is usually necessary in biomechanics calculations where the muscle acts at an angle to a body segment, as in the example in Figure 6.52. The muscle force has components along and perpendicular to the axis of the arm.

- The *rotary component* is the force that tries to turn the body segment around the proximal joint (e.g. flexing or extending the elbow joint), and balances the external moments acting on the body segment.

$$\text{Rotary component} = \text{muscle force} \times \sin A$$

- The *stabilising component* is the force that acts along the body segment (e.g. the forearm) forcing into, or pulling out of, the joint.

$$\text{Stabilising component} = \text{muscle force} \times \cos A$$

The first of these component forces acts through the pivot and has zero moment; the second will produce a moment about the proximal joint.

Joint forces

To find the joint force we first need to think back to the see-saw, where the force at the pivot was equal to the sum of the two forces acting downwards. We shall adopt the same technique here (Figure 6.53).

First we need to find all the forces acting in a vertical direction (including the vertical component of the muscle force). The only force we will not know is the vertical force at the joint. The sum of all these forces must be zero.

Then we need to find all the forces acting in a horizontal direction (including the horizontal component of the muscle force). The only force we will not know is the horizontal force at the joint. The sum of all these forces must also be zero.

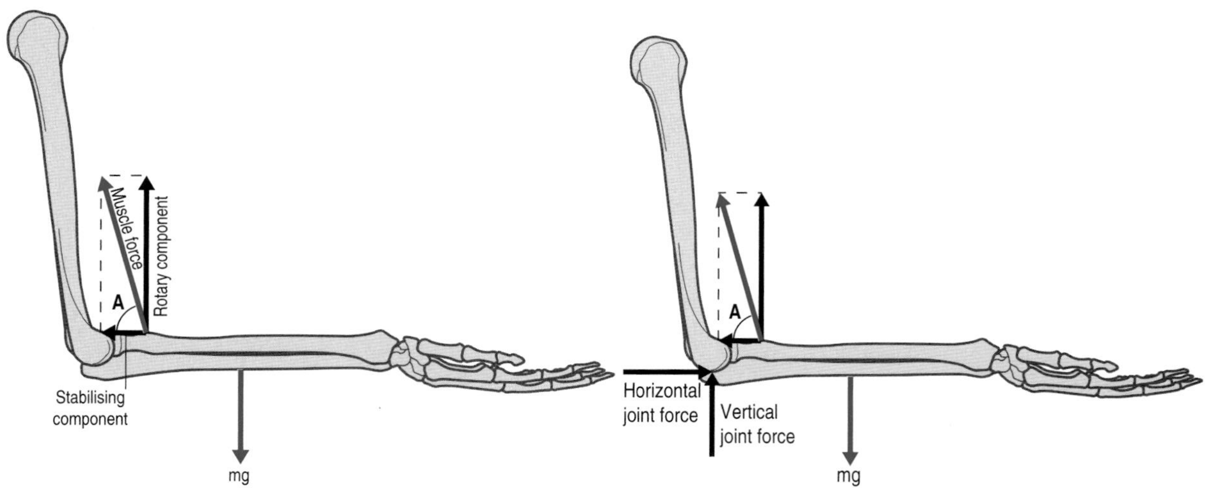

Figure 6.52 Components of muscle force.

Figure 6.53 Components of joint force.

Worked example 1: calculation of muscle and joint forces in the upper limb

Consider the tuning moments about the elbow joint while holding a pint of beer (Figure 6.54). Assume that the weight of a pint of beer is 7 N and the weight of the forearm and hand is 25 N. The distance d_1 from the elbow joint to the centre of mass of the forearm and hand is 0.15 m, and the distance d_2 from the elbow joint to the beer is 0.4 m.

Finding the moment about the elbow joint

Moment = force × perpendicular distance

Therefore:

Moments about the elbow joint
$= (\text{weight of forearm} \times d_1)$
$+ (\text{weight of beer} \times d_2)$

Moments about the elbow joint
$= (25 \times 0.15) + (7 \times 0.4)$

Moments about the elbow joint
$= 3.75 + 2.28 = 6.55\,\text{Nm}$

Finding the force in the muscle

Assume that the muscle is inclined to the forearm at 80 degrees (angle A) and the muscle insertion point is 0.04 m away from the elbow joint (Figure 6.55).

The muscle must provide an equal and opposite moment to support the weight of the arm and the weight of the beer. However, the muscle is inclined to the forearm, so the muscle force needs to be resolved in order to be perpendicular to the distance from the elbow joint.

If the muscle force is given the symbol m_f so the vertical component (or rotary component) of it will be $m_f \sin 80°$.

As the muscle produces an equal and opposite moment, the clockwise component must equal the anticlockwise component, i.e. the muscle must provide an equal and opposite moment to:

Moments about the elbow joint = 6.55 Nm

Therefore:

$m_f \sin 80\ °0.04 = 6.55$
$m_f = 6.55/(\sin 80° \times 0.04)$
$m_f = 166.3\,\text{N}$

Finding the joint force (Figure 6.55)

Vertical forces

In the problem above the vertical forces include: $m_f \sin 80°$ (163.75 N), weight of beer (7 N), weight of the forearm (25 N) and the vertical joint force.

If the force is acting up we will call it positive; if it is acting down we will call it negative. Therefore:

$163.75 - 7 - 25 - \text{vertical joint force} = 0$
$163.75 - 7 - 25 = \text{vertical joint force}$
$131.75\,\text{N} = \text{vertical joint force}$

Horizontal forces

The horizontal forces in this problem are easier; the only forces which will have a horizontal component are the muscle force and the joint force:

$m_f \cos 80°(28.9\ \text{N})$ and the horizontal joint force

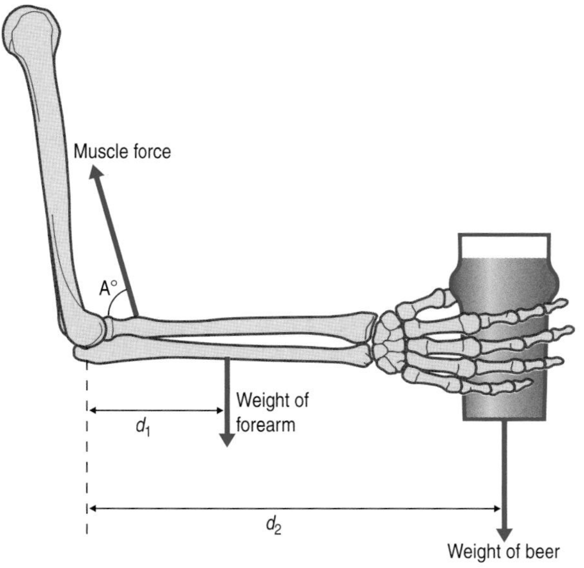

Figure 6.54 Schematic for worked example 1.

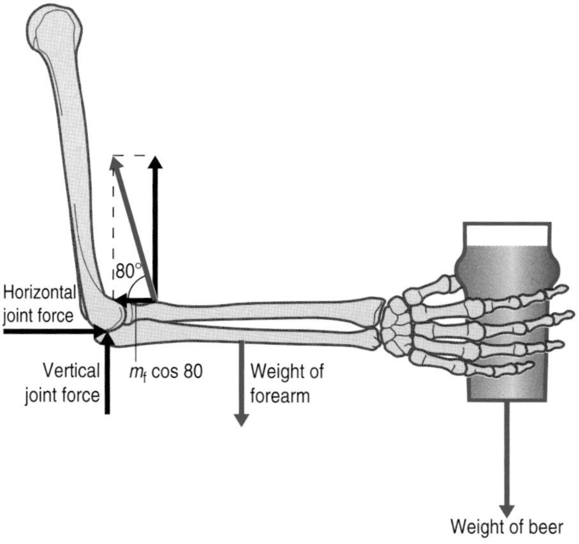

Figure 6.55 Resolving the horizontal and vertical forces.

If the force is acting to the right we will call it positive; if it is acting to the left we will call it negative:

Horizontal joint force − 28.9 = 0
Horizontal force = 28.9 N

Resultant joint force

There is one last step. What we want to find is the total effect on the joint, or the resultant joint force. This can simply be found by using Pythagoras:

6

$131.75^2 + 28.9^2 = R_2$
$134.9 = R =$ resultant joint force

Worked Example 2: Calculation of moments in the lower limb

Figure 6.56 shows the GRF acting at heel strike. The point of application of the GRF and the position of the ankle, knee and hip joints are known. We wish to calculate the moments produced by the GRF about (i) the ankle joint, (ii) the knee joint, and (iii) the hip joint. The GRF, 950 N, is acting at 82 degrees to the horizontal.

Resolving

Horizontal GRF = 950 × cos 82
Vertical GRF = 950 × sin 82

Horizontal GRF = 132.2 N
Vertical GRF = 940.75 N

Once the vertical and horizontal forces have been found, we can now consider the action of each component about each joint separately.

Moments about the ankle

The vertical component of the GRF acts straight through the joint; therefore this will not produce a moment.

The horizontal component acts to the right and below the ankle (Figure 6.57).

Moment about the ankle =
940.75 × 0 + 132.2 × 0.1 = 13.2 Nm

Moments about the knee (Figure 6.58)

The vertical component of the GRF acts in front of the knee joint.

The horizontal component acts to the right and below the knee.

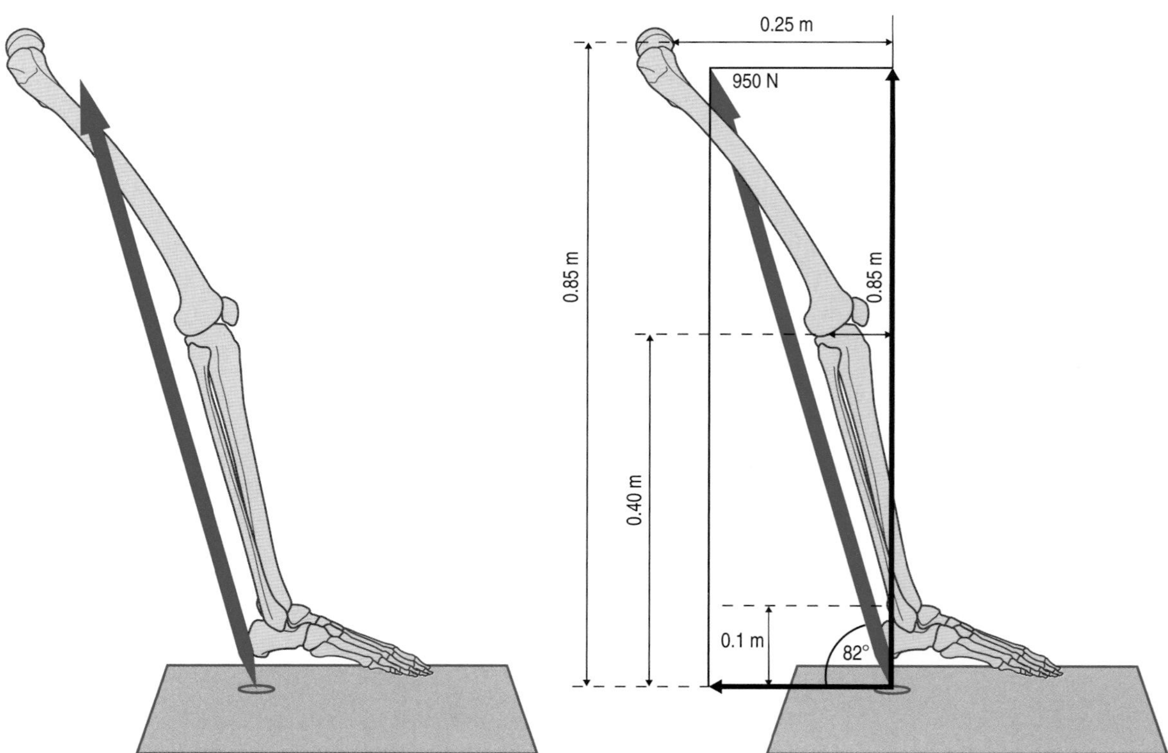

Figure 6.56 Joint moments in the lower limb during walking.

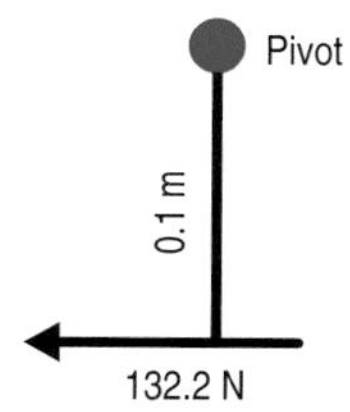

Figure 6.57 Moments about the ankle.

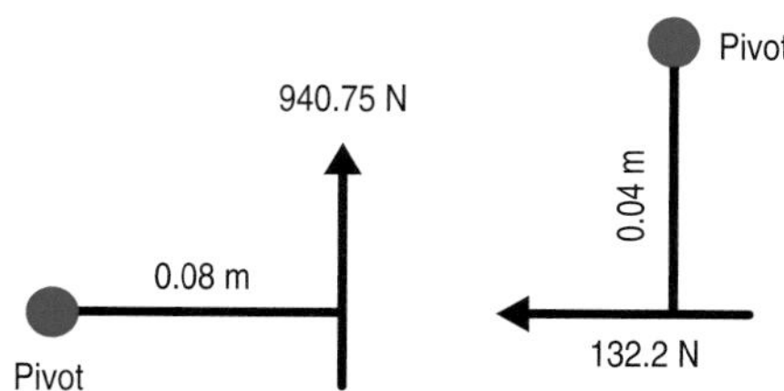

Figure 6.58 Moments about the knee.

Moment about the knee =

$$940.75 \times 0.08 + 132.2 \times 0.4 = 22.38 \text{ Nm}$$

Moments about the hip (Figure 6.59)

The vertical component of the GRF acts in front of the hip joint.

The horizontal component acts to the right and below the hip.

$$M_{hip} = -940.75 \times 0.25 + 132.2 \times 0.85 = -122.82 \text{ Nm}$$

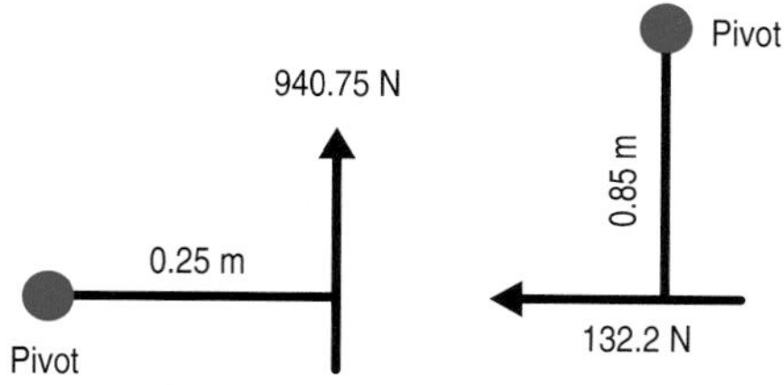

Figure 6.59 Moments about the hip.

So what are the effects of these moments on the muscles?

- The moment about the ankle joint is a plantarflexing moment; therefore the muscles in the anterior compartment of the ankle joint must be active (dorsiflexors).
- The moment about the knee joint is a flexing moment; therefore the muscles in the anterior compartment of the knee joint must be active (knee extensors).
- The moment about the hip joint is a flexing moment; therefore the muscles in the posterior compartment of the hip joint must be active (hip extensors).

Worked example 3: calculation of muscle and joint forces on the base of the spine

A person lifts a weight of 600 N, as shown in Figure 6.60a.

- Mass of trunk = 52.5 kg
- Mass of head = 8.5 kg
- Mass of upper arms = 5.8 kg
- Mass of forearm = 3.4 kg.

(i) If the centre of mass of the trunk, arms and head is a horizontal distance of 0.2 m from L5–S1 (the base of the spine) and the weights being lifted are a horizontal distance of 0.42 m from L5–S1, find the moment about L5–S1.
(ii) If this moment were supported entirely by the muscle E acting 0.07 m away from L5–S1, what would be the force in the muscle?
(iii) Find the resultant force at L5–S1 if the force E is acting at 40 degrees to the vertical.

Solution

(i) $M = 600 \times 0.42 + 702 \times 0.2 = 392.4$ Nm.
(ii) 392.4 Nm = E × 0.07
392.4/0.07 = E
5606 N = E
(iii) Force E is acting at an angle to vertical and horizontal, so we find the vertical and horizontal component by resolving:
$E_v = 5606 \times \cos 40 = 4294$ N
$E_h = 5606 \times \sin 40 = 3603$ N
Total force vertical = 4294 + 600 + 702 = 5596 N
Total force horizontal = 3603 N
Resultant = sq root $(5596^2 + 3603^2)$
Resultant = 6655 N.

MOMENTS ABOUT THE ANKLE, KNEE AND HIP JOINTS DURING NORMAL WALKING

We have previously considered the movements and GRFs during the gait cycle. We will now consider the effects of the position of the GRF in relation to the ankle, knee and hip joints.

Typical ankle moments during normal gait

At heel strike the GRF passes very close to the ankle joint centre, thereby producing a very small moment. In some cases this will be behind the ankle joint, giving rise to a plantar flexion moment. After heel strike the

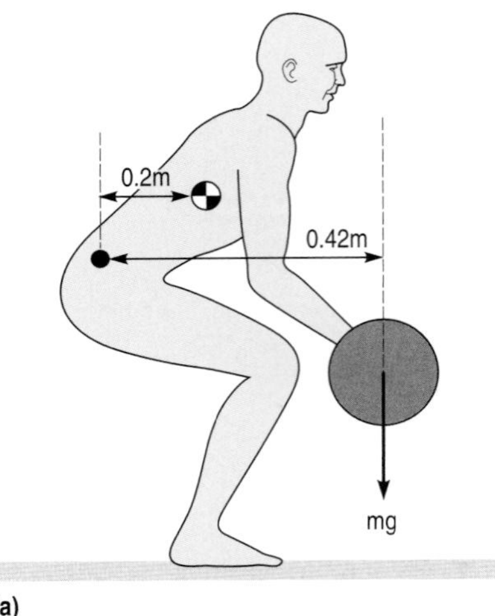

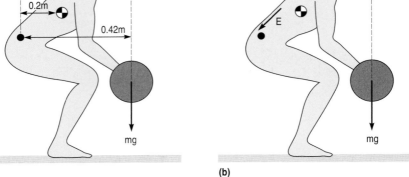

Figure 6.60 Muscle and joint forces on the spine.

GRF moves in front of the ankle joint, producing a dorsiflexion moment. This increases as the force moves under the metatarsal heads and the force increases during push off (Figure 6.61).

Typical knee moments during normal gait

At heel strike the GRF initially passes anterior to the knee joint, giving rise to an extension moment. The GRF then quickly passes behind the knee joint, causing a flexion moment. After mid-stance the force passes in front of the knee again until toe off. During swing phase the knee also has significant moments due to the acceleration and deceleration of the foot and tibia (Figure 6.62).

Typical hip moments during normal gait

At heel strike the GRF passes quite far anterior to the hip joint, producing a peak flexion moment. After heel strike the GRF still passes anterior to the hip; however, the distance from the force to the hip is much reduced. After mid-stance the force passes posterior to the hip, giving rise to an extension moment. As with the knee, there are significant moments during swing phase due to the acceleration and deceleration of the lower limb (Figure 6.63).

LINEAR WORK, ENERGY AND POWER

Linear work

Definition

Work is a product of a force applied to a body and the displacement of the body in the direction of the applied force (Figure 6.64).

Work = force × displacement ($W = Fs$)

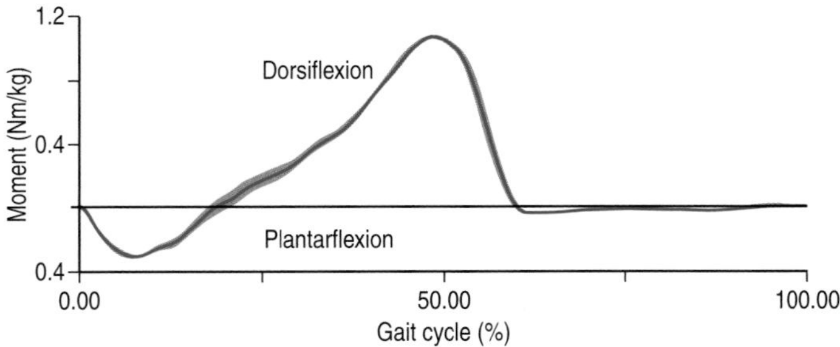

Figure 6.61 Typical ankle moments during normal gait.

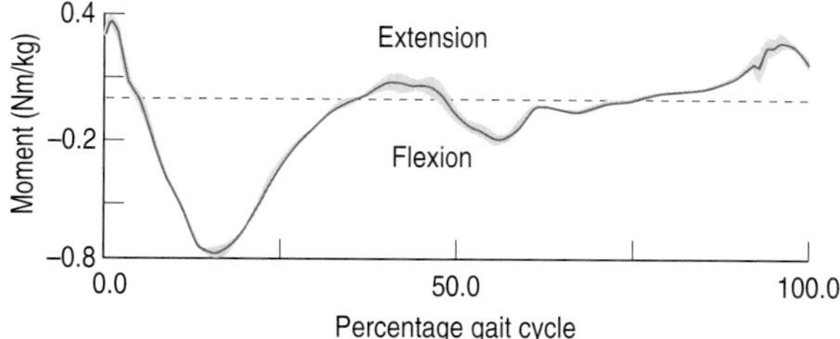

Figure 6.62 Typical knee moments during normal gait.

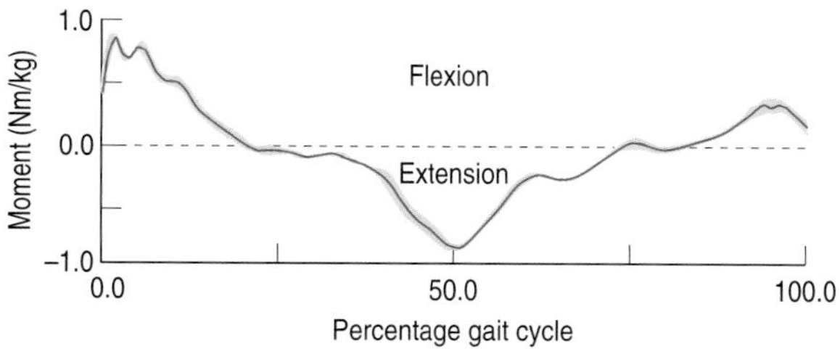

Figure 6.63 Typical hip moments during normal gait.

Linear work does not refer to muscular or mental effort. Work is basically a force overcoming a resistance and moving an object through a distance. If, for example, an object is lifted from the floor to the top of a table, work is done in overcoming the downward force due to gravity. On the other hand, if a constantly acting force does not produce motion, no work is performed.

> ***Key points***
>
> - Holding a book steadily at arm's length does not involve any work, irrespective of the effort required, because there is no movement of the applied force.
> - The units of work are Newtons × metres, or *joules* (J).

Linear power

Power is the *rate* of performing work or transferring energy. So power measures how quickly the work is done.

Suppose a person pushes a box from one end of the room to the other in 10 seconds, then pushes the box back to its original position in 5 seconds. In each trip across the room, the force applied and the distance the box is moved are the same, so the work done in each case is the same. But the second time the box is pushed across the room, the person has to produce more power than in the first trip because the same amount of work is done in 5 seconds rather than ten.

Power = work done/time taken

> ***Key point***
>
> The units of power are joules per second (J/s) or *watts* (W).

Linear energy

While work is done on a body, there is a transfer of energy to the body, and so work can be said to be 'energy in transit'.

> ***Key point***
>
> Energy has the same units as work (*joules*), as the work done produces a change in energy.

Energy is the capacity of matter to perform work as the result of its motion or its position in relation to forces acting on it. Energy related to position is known as *potential energy*, and energy associated with motion is known as *kinetic energy*. A swinging pendulum has maximum potential energy at the terminal points; at all intermediate positions it has both kinetic and potential energy in varying proportions.

Conservation of energy

Energy can be transformed but it cannot be created or destroyed. In the process of transformation either kinetic or potential energy may be lost or gained, but the sum total of the two always remains the same.

Potential energy

This is stored energy possessed by a system as a result of the relative positions of the components of that

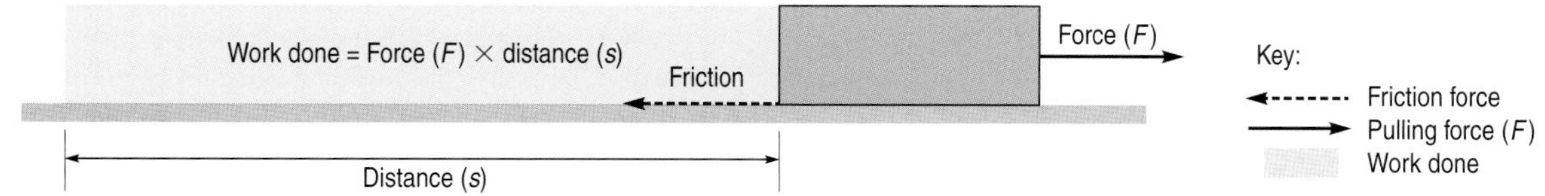

Figure 6.64 Linear work.

system. For example, if a ball is held above the ground, the system comprising the ball and the earth has a certain amount of potential energy; lifting the ball higher increases the amount of potential energy the system possesses. This is expressed mathematically as $PE = mgh$ (mass times gravity times height).

Work is needed to lift the ball up, giving the system potential energy. It takes effort to lift a ball off the ground. The amount of potential energy a system possesses is equal to the work done on the system.

6

Potential energy also can be transformed into other forms of energy. For example, when a ball is held above the ground and released, the potential energy is transformed into kinetic energy.

Kinetic energy

This is energy possessed by an object, resulting from the motion of that object. The magnitude of the kinetic energy depends on both the mass and the speed of the object according to the equation $KE = \{1/2\}\ mv^2$.

Angular work and power

Angular work

Work (w) = force (F) × distance moved (s)

The distance the force is moved is not in a straight line, as with linear work, but in an arc. To find the angular work, the length of the arc must first be found.

The length of the arc is affected by the radius of the arc and the angle moved through:

$$\text{Length of an arc (s)} = \text{radius (r)} \times \text{angular displacement } (\Theta)$$

$$\text{Length of an arc (s)} = r\Theta$$

Note: The angular displacement must be measured in radians (rads):

$1 \text{ radian} = 57.3°$
$\text{Work} = Fs$
$\text{Angular work} = Fr\Theta$

However:

$\text{Force} \times r = \text{Moment } (M)$

Therefore:

$\text{Work} = \text{Moment } (M) \times \Theta$

Angular power

$$\text{Power} = \frac{\text{Work done}}{\text{Time taken}}$$

$$\text{Power} = \frac{\text{Force } \Theta \times \text{r}}{t}$$

Or:

$$\text{Power} = \frac{\text{Moment}(M) \times t}{\text{Time taken}}$$

$$\text{Power} = \frac{M \times \Theta}{t}$$

However:

$\Theta/t = \omega$ (angular velocity)

so:

$\text{Power} = M\omega$
ω is in radian/s (rad/s)

JOINT POWER DURING NORMAL WALKING

The results covered in this section are found by multiplying the joint moments (M) and joint angular velocities (ω). Positive values show power generation; negative values show power absorption. It is also beneficial to consider whether muscle action is either concentric or eccentric. Concentric activity is associated with power development, whereas eccentric activity is associated with power absorption. These graphs can be hard to interpret; however, they become easier if you consider whether the moments are trying to flex or extend and what movements are occurring at each time. The examples below consider the power absorption and generation of the ankle, knee and hip joints during walking. Power absorption, eccentric activity, is shown as negative and power generation, concentric activity, is positive.

Ankle power

If the ankle has a dorsiflexion velocity and the moment is dorsiflexing about the ankle joint, then the posterior muscles must be working eccentrically and absorbing power. If the ankle has a plantar flexion velocity and a dorsiflexion moment, then the posterior muscles must be working concentrically and therefore generating power.

At heel strike there is a plantar flexion moment and angular velocity; therefore at heel strike there is eccentric power absorption from the dorsiflexors. This is followed by an eccentric power absorption by the plantar flexors as the body moves forwards over the foot. During push off there is a dorsiflexion moment and a plantar flexion velocity; therefore power is generated by concentric activity of the plantar flexors (Figure 6.65).

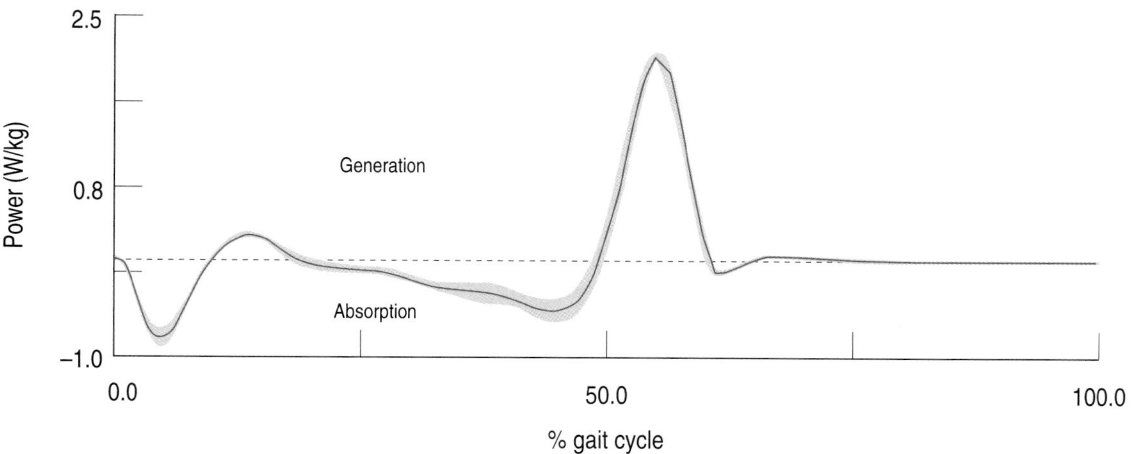

Figure 6.65 Typical ankle power during normal gait.

Knee power

At heel strike the knee shows power generation; this is due to the GRF being in front of the knee and therefore producing an extension moment while the knee is flexing. This initial power generation or concentric contraction of the hamstrings ensures that the knee does indeed flex at heel strike, rather than moving into a hyperextended position. After this point the GRF falls behind the knee, creating a flexion moment whilst the knee is flexing; therefore the quadriceps will be working eccentrically to act as a shock absorber. The knee then shows power generation at approximately 20 per cent of the gait cycle. At this point the GRF is behind the knee and therefore this relates to the quadriceps acting concentrically and pulling the femur over the tibia. As the knee extends the GRF passes through the knee joint, producing no moment, and therefore little or no power is generated or absorbed. It is interesting to note the involvement of the knee during push off at 50–60 per cent of the gait cycle. During this time the GRF falls behind the knee, creating a flexion moment, but at this time the knee is flexing and therefore power is being absorbed and not generated. The knee thus has little or no involvement in the power production during push off (Figure 6.66).

Hip power

At heel strike the hip shows power absorption at heel strike; this is due to the hip having a small period of flexion velocity coupled with a flexion moment. The hip then extends to start to move the body over the stance limb whilst the moment is still trying to flex the hip; this is achieved by power generation by the hip extensors. At approximately 25 per cent of the gait cycle the moment passes behind the hip, changing from a flexion moment to an extension moment; however, the hip is still extending. This relates to power absorption, or eccentric control of the hip flexors as the body moves over the stance limb. After 50 per cent of the gait cycle the hip reaches its maximum extended position; after this point there is a rapid power generation during push off. This power generation is due to the GRF creating an extension moment while the hip changes from a flexing angular velocity to an extending angular velocity, and therefore contributes to power production during push off (Figure 6.67).

STRENGTH TESTING AND TRAINING

So far in this chapter we have been looking at moments, muscle forces and joint forces. There is another way in which we often talk about muscle and joint performance, and that is strength. But what exactly is strength? The dictionary tells us that strength is the capacity for exertion or endurance or the power to resist force, but a better way of thinking about muscle strength is the amount of force a particular muscle or muscle group can produce. However, when evaluating muscle strength, the measures we can take do not directly measure actual strength of the muscle or muscle group. What is usually recorded is the effective moment being produced by the muscle. This is because muscle forces are hard to measure, requiring information about the position of muscle, position of the body segment, muscle insertion points and the line of pull of the muscle, all

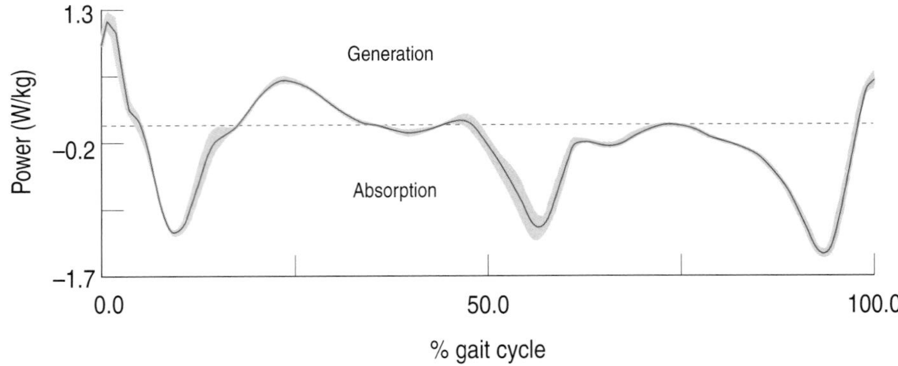

Figure 6.66 Typical knee power during normal gait.

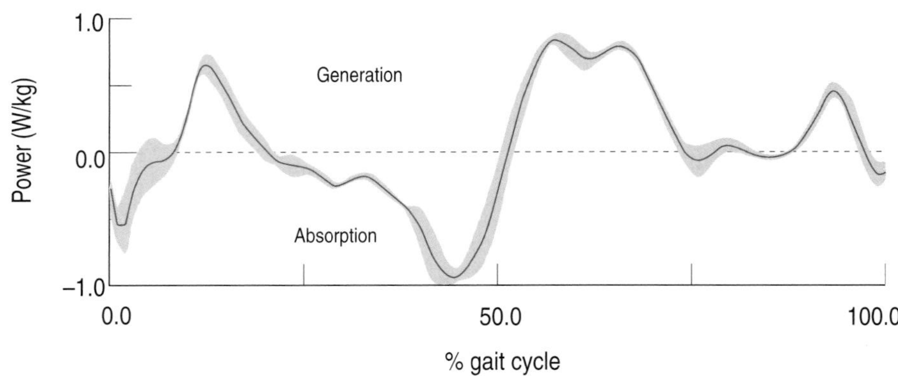

Figure 6.67 Typical hip power during normal gait.

of which will be constantly changing during dynamic activities.

Most measures taken in the clinical setting do not go as far as to estimating actual muscle forces. However, there are a number of methods of indirect evaluation. Indirect evaluation of the force produced by a muscle can be influenced by a number of factors. The follow section will consider the different permutations of these factors when considering upper limb muscle strength.

These factors include:

- the body segment inclination
- the position and size of the applied load
- muscle insertion points
- angle of muscle pull
- type of contraction
- speed of contraction.

Changing the effective moment caused by the body segment inclination

The inclination of body segments can have a very large effect on joint moments. The effect of the weight of the forearm in the three positions shown is very different (Figure 6.68). The maximum moment about the elbow is when the forearm is level; when the forearm is inclined either up or down, the moment reduces; and when the forearm in vertical, there will be no moment about the elbow at all, as the entire weight of the segment will be acting through the joint. It is also important to note the direction of the 'stabilising' component that acts along the forearm. When the forearm is angled down, the component acting along the forearm will try to pull the forearm away from the upper arm, whereas with the forearm angled up the forearm is pushed into the upper arm; this will have

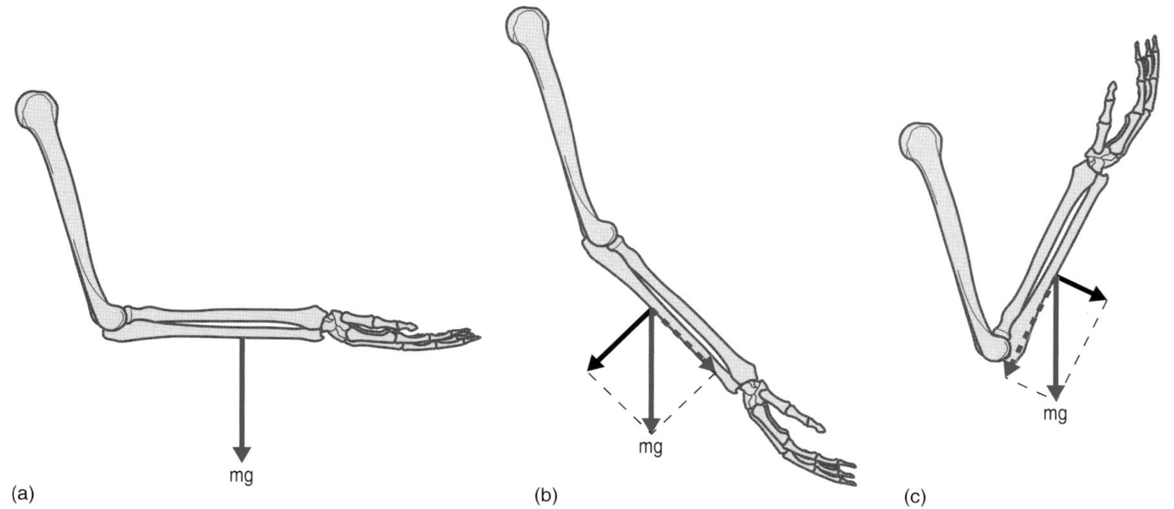

Figure 6.68 (a) Forearm horizontal. (b) Forearm angled down. (c) Forearm angled up.

the effect of reducing and increasing the joint force at the elbow respectively.

The position and size of the applied load

The position and size of the load applied have an important effect on the moment about the elbow, and will in turn have a significant effect on the muscle and joint forces. When assessing muscle strength both these factors should be measured and taken into account. If you position a load at the end of a subject's arm to see if he or she can support it, the moment will depend on the size of the load and the subject's limb length (Figure 6.69).

Both the size of the load and the subject's limb length need to be considered when assessing an individual's muscle performance or strength. For example, if two individuals of different heights and therefore different tibial (shank) lengths conducted the same leg raise activity with the same loads, the shorter of the two would in fact use less muscle force (strength) to lift the same load, assuming the muscle insertion points were not significantly different.

Muscle insertion points

Different muscles will have different insertion points. The position of these insertion points will have a large effect on the muscle force required to support a given turning moment. Two examples are shown in Figure 6.70. In Figure 6.70a the muscle insertion point is close to the elbow joint, while in Figure 6.70b the muscle insertion point is much further away.

For a particular load there will be a larger force in the muscle if its insertion point is close to the joint. Conversely, if there is a maximum force that a muscle group can cope with, then larger loads will be able to be carried with the insertion point further away from the joint.

This leads us to an interesting point when we consider weight lifters. Is a weight lifter able to lift the larger load because he or she can support larger muscle forces, or is this due to a difference in the muscle insertion points? If the latter is the case, are we actually assessing something different from *strength* (the force in the muscle) with the task?

The effect of the angle of muscle pull

As the body segment moves relative to the ground, so the angle of the muscle moves relative to the body segment. Consider different inclinations of the body segment, but instead of thinking about the moment due to the weight, think about the line of action of the force in relation to the forearm. The maximum moment that the muscle can produce is when the elbow is at 90 degrees, as this makes an approximately 90 degree angle between the muscle and the body segment, and therefore produces the greatest rotary component from the muscle force. As the elbow joint is moved away from this position, either flexed or extended, the moment that the muscle can produce is reduced as the rotary component of the muscle force acting at 90 degrees to the forearm is reduced. When the forearm is vertical with the elbow fully extended, the muscle

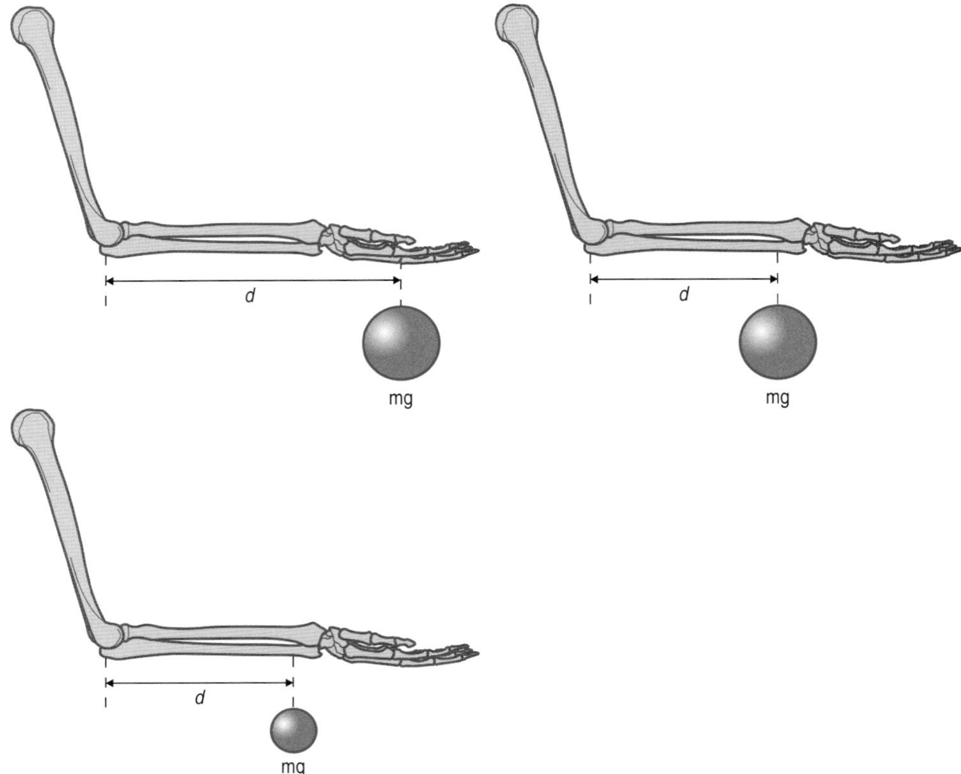

Figure 6.69 Position and size of the applied load.

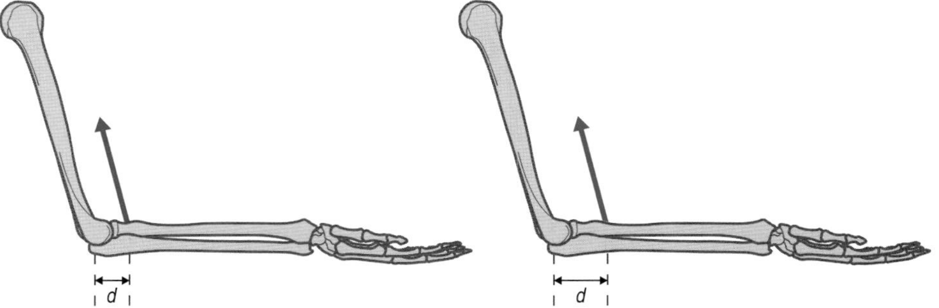

Figure 6.70 (a) Muscle insertion point close. (b) Muscle insertion point further away.

would find it much harder to produce a moment as the rotary component will be at its smallest. It is also interesting to note the direction of the 'stabilising' component of the muscle force when the elbow is flexed. This appears to be pulling the forearm away from the joint and will not provide a compressive stabilising force into the joint; however, in this position the rotary component will be providing a compressive force into the joint. In reality we will also have a co-contraction from the extensor muscles to stabilize the elbow joint (Figure 6.71).

Type of muscle contraction

The type of muscle contraction affects the resistance that can be controlled, held or overcome. The three types of muscle contraction are isometric, concentric and eccentric. Isometric contractions are stabilising

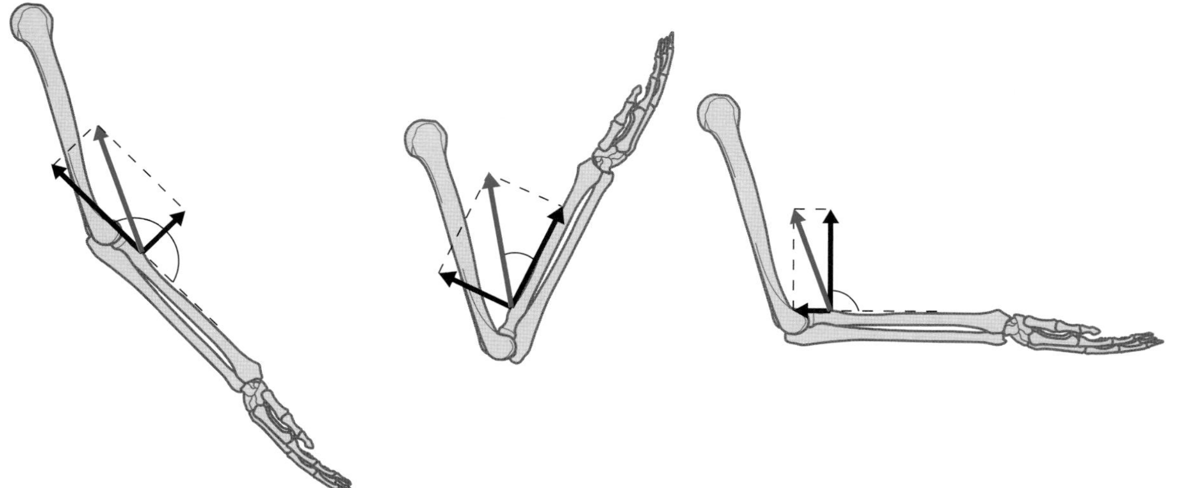

Figure 6.71 Effect of the angle of muscle pull.

contractions where the muscle length remains virtually constant. Concentric contractions are where the muscle shortens during the activity. These are generally the weakest muscle contractions, requiring more motor unit recruitment than isometric and eccentric for a particular load. Eccentric contractions are where the muscle lengthens during the activity. These are generally the strongest muscle contractions, requiring less recruitment than isometric and concentric for a particular load.

The effect of the speed of contraction

There are three ways of classifying speed during exercises: isotonic, isokinetic and isometric.

- *Isotonic* is when a constant load is applied but the angular velocity of the movement may change; this allows an infinite variation in the rate of contraction of a muscle. Although this is closest to real-life muscle and joint function, the change in speed continually affects the amount of force that a muscle can produce and makes the exact muscle function quite hard to assess.
- *Isokinetic* is when the velocity or angular velocity of the movement is kept constant but the load may be varied; this setting of the speed of working helps improve our assessment of muscle performance, but the speed or velocity of the joints is restricted to only one set speed at any one time.
- *Isometric* relates to the force varying but the joint is held in a static position; therefore muscle length remains the same as no movement occurs. This tells us what static moment may be supported; however, this does not necessarily relate to the moments that can be produced or supported dynamically.

Methods of objective assessment

One method of improving the measurements of force taken in clinical assessment uses a device called a myometer; this can be attached to different body segments using a sling. One example is the Nottingham Mecmesin Myometer, a force gauge which has been used to asses the muscle strength component of the constant score to evaluate shoulder function (Figure 6.72). It does, however, have the drawback of assessing isometrics and not dynamic tasks, and care must still be taken in the position of the sling on the body segments to ensure repeatable and useful measurements.

Another method uses an isokinetics dynamometer, which allows for a standardised assessment by controlling or presetting the angular velocity and measuring the resistance that can be produced by an individual.

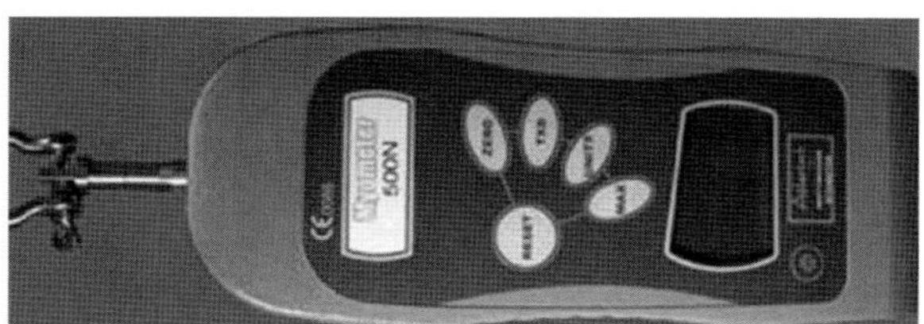

Figure 6.72 Nottingham Mecmesin myometer.

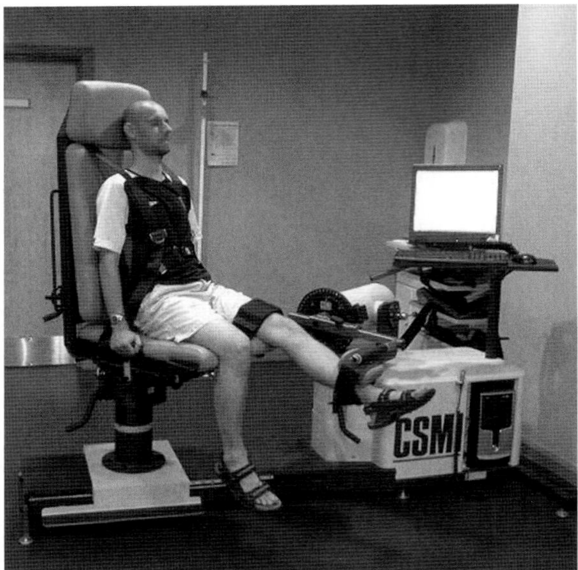

Figure 6.73 Isokinetic machine.

6

In controlling the angular velocity and measuring the resistance, the muscle power produced becomes very easy to find. Isokinetics also allow concentric, eccentric and isometric moments (commonly referred to as torque in isokinetics) and concentric and eccentric power to be found separately. Many isokinetic machines are also capable of isotonic assessment, isotonic referring to constant load or torque throughout the range of motion. Isotonic testing is a simulation of free weights, although isokinetic machines also have the ability to allow for the weight of the segment through the range of motion being tested, therefore giving a true representation of the torque and power provided by the muscles (Figure 6.73).

CONCLUSION

This chapter highlights some of the background theory and methods necessary for the analysis and interpretation of the assessment of movement, forces, moments, strength and power. It should help the reader to understand the movement patterns of individuals who are pain- and pathology-free and to become familiar with some of the techniques used in the clinical research literature. All these techniques may be applied to the assessment of pathologies and conditions that affect movement to enable objective assessment and monitoring of recovery through treatment and rehabilitation programmes.

REFERENCES

Al-Majali M, Solomonidis SE, Spence W et al. 1993 Design specification of a walk mat system for the measurement of temporal and distance parameters of gait. Gait Posture 1: 119–120

Arenson JS, Ishai G, Bar A 1983 A system for monitoring the position and time of feet contact during walking. J Med Eng Technol 7(6): 280–284

Bell F, Ghasemi M, Rafferty D et al. 1995 An holistic approach to gait analysis. Glasgow Caledonian University's CRC. Gait Posture 3: 185

Bell F, Shaw L, Rafferty D et al. 1996 Movement analysis technology in clinical practice. Phys Ther Rev 1: 13–22

Brand RA, Crowninshield RD 1981 Locomotion studies: caves to computers (abstract). J Biomech 14: 497

Bruckner J 1998 The Gait Workbook: a Practical Guide to Clinical Gait Analysis. SLACK: Thorofare, NJ

Crouse J, Wall JC, Marble AE 1987 Measurement of temporal and spatial parameters of gait using a microcomputer based system. J Biomed Eng 9(1): 64–68

Durie ND, Farley RL 1980 An apparatus for step length measurement. J Biomed Eng 2(1): 38–40

Elftman H 1938 Forces and energy changes in the leg during walking. Am J Physiol 125: 339–356

Gage JR 1994 The role of gait analysis in the treatment of cerebral palsy. J Pediatr Orthoped 4: 701–702

Gerny K 1983 A clinical method of quantitative gait analysis. Phys Ther 63: 1125–1126

Hirokawa S, Matsumura K 1987 Gait analysis using a measuring walkway for temporal and distance factors. Med Biol Eng Comput 25: 577–582

Inman VT 1966 Human locomotion. Can Med Assoc J 94: 1047–1054

Inman VT 1967 Conservation of energy in ambulation. Arch Phys Med Rehab 48: 484–488

Inman VT, Ralston HJ, Todd F 1981 Human Walking. Williams & Wilkins: Baltimore

Marey EJ 1873 Animal Mechanism: A Treatise on Terrestrial and Aerial Locomotion. Appleton: New York (republished as vol. XI of the International Scientific Series)

Murray MP 1967 Gait as a total pattern of movement. Am J Phys Med 40: 290–333

Muybridge E 1887 Animal locomotion. In: Brown LS (ed.) 1957 Animals in Motion. Dover: New York

Muybridge E 1901 The Human Figure in Motion. Chapman & Hall: London

Patrick J 1991 Gait laboratory investigations to assist decision making. Br J Hosp Med 45: 35–37

Perry J 1992 Gait Analysis: Normal and Pathological Function. SLACK: Thorofare, NJ

Peterson WA, Brookhart JM, Stone SA 1965 A strain-gage platform for force measurements. J Appl Physiol 20: 1095–1097

Pomeroy VM, Pramanik A, Sykes L et al. 2003 Agreement between physiotherapists on quality of movement rated via videotape. Clin Rehabil 17(3): 264–272

Rafferty D, Bell F 1995 Gait analysis — a semiautomated approach. Gait and Posture 3(3): 184

Richards J 2008 Biomechanics in Clinic and Research: An Interactive Teaching and Learning Course. Churchill Livingstone: Edinburgh

Richards JD, Pramanik A, Sykes L, Pomeroy VM 2003 A comparison of knee kinematic characteristics of stroke patients and age-matched healthy volunteers. Clin Rehabil 7(5): 565–571

Rose J, Gamble JG 1994 Human Walking. Williams & Wilkins: Baltimore

Saunders JBDM, Inman VT, Eberhart HS 1953 The major determinants in normal and pathological gait. J Bone Joint Surg 35A: 543–558

Wall JC, Charteris J, Turnbull G 1987 Two steps equals one stride equals what? Clin Biomech 2: 119–125

Winter DA 1993 Knowledge base for diagnostic gait assessments. Med Prog Technol 19(2): 61–81

Chapter 7

Osteoporosis

Kirsty Carne

CHAPTER CONTENTS

INTRODUCTION

Physiotherapists encounter osteoporosis in a wide range of clinical situations. This chapter provides important background physiology, aetiology, diagnostic procedures and other essential information that physiotherapists need to manage and treat this increasingly common condition effectively.

Bone is an amazing tissue. It is alive and has the unique ability to remodel itself. It can change its density and internal architecture according to whether we exercise more or exercise less, as it is stressed by muscles and tendons, and as our diet and health status changes.

Osteoporosis is very closely linked with the natural ageing process of human beings, but until quite recent times very little has been done to recognise it as an actual disease process and to investigate ways of treating it. Examination of medieval skeletons from a site in England found evidence of very similar age-related bone loss at the femur (Mays et al. 1998), despite the huge differences in lifestyle between the way we lived then and the way we live now. Populations are on the increase and we can now expect to live well into old age, unlike our medieval ancestors. We also expect to have a much better quality of life, and greater independence during our later years. This means that osteoporosis will be an enormous problem for the modern world, and has huge implications in terms of both personal suffering and the costs to health services of treating such a condition.

Definition

At the Consensus Development Conference for the World Health Organization (CDC 1991), osteoporosis was defined as 'a progressive skeletal disorder, characterised by low bone mass and microarchitectural deterioration of bone tissue, leading to a consequent increase in bone fragility and susceptibility to fracture'.

Brittle bone disease

Note that osteoporosis is not the same as brittle bone disease (osteogenesis imperfecta), which is a genetic condition. If you require more information about brittle bone disease, write to Brittle Bone Society, 30 Guthrie Street, Dundee DD1 5BS (telephone 01382 204446), or visit www.brittlebone.org. There is a Freephone helpline on 08000 282459 – for advice only.

Throughout childhood and our early adult years, many different aspects of skeletal growth occur. Longitudinal growth of bone ceases and each individual's peak bone size is eventually achieved. During the end of a person's third decade of life the peak bone mineral density (BMD) is also realised. These factors combine to give our skeletons the dimensions, flexibility and strength that we require to be able to function as active human beings. Skeletal growth does not then cease altogether; bone is living tissue and needs to renew itself constantly to maintain an optimal level of health. It is this process of renewal or *bone turnover* that is the important factor in osteoporosis. The action of osteogenic cells, specifically osteoclasts and osteoblasts, is key to the potential maintenance or loss of BMD.

Weblink

- National Osteoporosis Society: www.nos.org.uk
- For general enquiries: National Osteoporosis Society, Camerton, Bath BA2 0PJ
- Telephone: 0845 130 3076 or 01761 471771

The National Osteoporosis Society (NOS) is based in the United Kingdom. It campaigns to ensure that all people with or at risk of osteoporosis receive appropriate information and treatment to enable them to avoid fractures and enjoy a better quality of life. The NOS provides information and support for people with osteoporosis and for their carers by promoting education for the public and health professionals, by lobbying government and health organisations, and by encouraging fundraising for support services and research into osteoporosis prevention and treatment.

The society offers membership packages for both lay people and health professionals. There are quarterly magazines containing the latest information about and research into osteoporosis. The society also provides a medical helpline service run by nurses who are specialists in osteoporosis for health professionals and lay members alike, whether they are members or not.

The society has a large network of patient support groups around the UK. These are run by volunteers and provide an opportunity for people with osteoporosis to get together and learn about other peoples' experiences, and to hear outside speakers on a number of topics.

The society produces a wide range of publications, ranging from information booklets about all aspects of the disease, to position statements for health professionals providing guidance on certain issues. The NOS is independent of any drug company and all information is evidence-based.

PHYSIOLOGY OF BONE TURNOVER

The skeleton comprises two types of bone:

- *Cortical bone* is found mainly in the shafts of long bones and the surfaces of flat bones. Approximately 80–90 per cent of the skeleton is made up of cortical bone.
- *Trabecular or cancellous bone* forms the internal part of flat bones, and is also found at the ends of long bones.

These two types of bone are subject to different types of force. Trabecular bone is designed mainly to resist compression, whereas cortical bone needs to withstand twisting and bending forces as well as compression. Bone turnover or remodelling occurs throughout the skeleton at random, scattered sites. The process of remodelling takes place on the surfaces of these different bone structures, which means that the rate of remodelling in trabecular bone is significantly higher than that of cortical bone because trabecular bone has a much greater surface area.

Osteoclasts are the bone cells that are responsible for *resorption* of bone. They position themselves on the bone surface at any selected site for remodelling and absorb the old bone, creating a cavity. Following a short interval, the osteoblasts then position themselves in the newly formed cavity. These are the bone-forming cells and their main function is the formation and mineralisation of osteoid, the protein component of bone. The osteoblasts are also responsible for the regulation of some of the growth factors that are found in the protein-based bone matrix, and it is because of this fact that the osteoblasts are the cells that are generally considered to govern bone metabolism.

Key point

Although a fair amount is known about the progress of these cells, what prompts the osteoclasts to move into position at the sites that need remodelling, and causes the osteoblasts to follow behind, is still largely unclear.

Both osteoclasts and osteoblasts, like many other cells in the body, have a reasonably short life. New ones are constantly being produced and the old ones die by a process called *apoptosis*. Oestrogens and bisphosphonates (a group of non-hormonal drugs used for the prevention and treatment of osteoporosis) can promote apoptosis in the osteoclasts and inhibit this process in osteoblasts. Glucocorticoids, however, can have the opposite effect; they inhibit apoptosis in the osteoclasts, and promote the death of the osteoblast cells (Weinstein and Manolagas 2000).

The process of bone remodelling is slow, and gets even slower as we age (Figure 7.1). One complete cycle of turnover, including a resting phase, can take 3–6 months in an adult, and to replace the entire skeleton would take anything from 7 to 10 years; in children this can be completed in just 2–3 years. During this cycle any changes in bone shape and amount are barely noticeable. It is because this process is so slow that patients with osteoporosis are generally not monitored by bone density scans more frequently than two-yearly (apart from in exceptional cases).

Ordinarily, bone remodelling aims to replace exactly the same amount of bone as it takes away. When functioning correctly this is a balanced cycle (Figure 7.2a). It is when this cycle becomes unbalanced that problems occur. When the osteoclasts experience increased activity or the osteoblasts have reduced activity, there will be a deficit in bone; more bone will be absorbed than made, leading to a loss of BMD and, potentially, osteoporosis (Figure 7.2b). As bone density decreases, the structure of the bone starts to lose some of its rigidity and strength (Figure 7.3).

Bone density is not the only component of bone strength. Other factors such as bone quality are equally important but are very difficult to measure. As there is a strong inverse correlation between bone density and fracture risk, with a two- to three-fold increase in the incidence of fracture for each standard deviation reduction in BMD (see the later section on the diagnosis of osteoporosis) (Marshall et al. 1996), and BMD is measurable, it is the BMD that is usually used to diagnose and monitor patients.

Loss of BMD is heavily influenced by age. Studies looking at bone density levels during a lifetime period show that bone mass is steadily built up throughout childhood and the early adult years (Figure 7.4). Men achieve a higher peak bone mass than women because they generally have a larger bone structure, but both sexes achieve their peak and then maintain that level until their early to mid-forties. After that point, natural age-related loss of BMD starts to occur, and this happens because the osteoclasts and osteoblasts are no longer working at quite the same rates. Several other factors such as oestrogen deficiency will also affect loss of BMD.

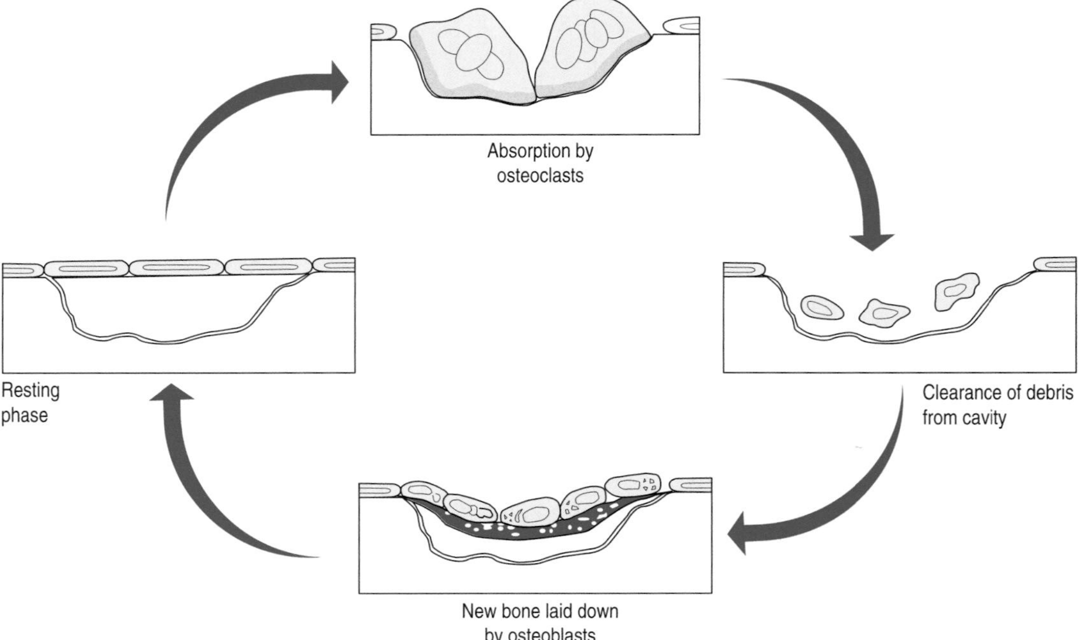

Figure 7.1 The cycle of bone turnover.

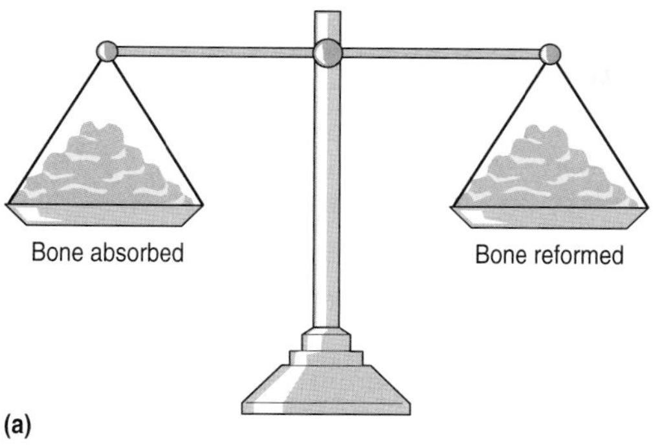

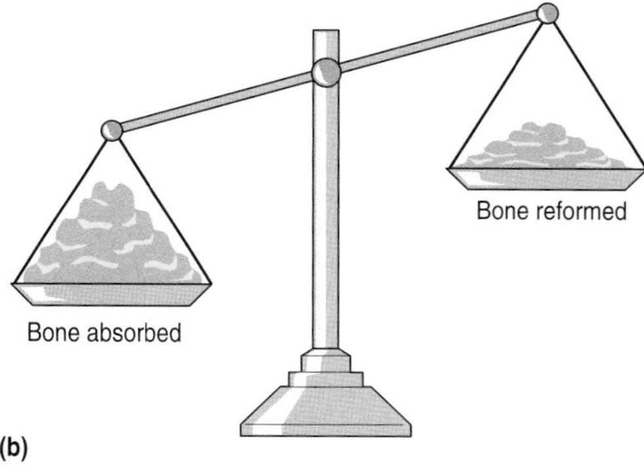

Figure 7.2 Bone remodelling: (a) normal – osteoblast activity matches osteoclast activity; (b) osteoporosis – osteoclast activity exceeds osteoblast activity.

THE EXTENT OF THE PROBLEM

Osteoporosis is an enormous problem and has huge implications in terms of both personal suffering and the cost to the National Health Service. The combined cost of hospital and social care in the UK for patients with a hip fracture amounts to more than £1.73 billion per year (Torgerson et al. 2001). The cost of treating all osteoporotic fractures in post-menopausal women has been predicted to rise to more than £2.1 billion by 2020 (Burge 2001). Osteoporosis is often referred to as a 'silent' condition. This is because having a low bone density is not a disorder that one can feel in any way. Many people do not know there is a problem until they sustain a fracture. This, combined with either a lack of awareness of the condition or a general assumption that osteoporosis affects only elderly people, means that prevention is a huge challenge, and at present we may only be tackling the tip of the iceberg.

Key point

One in two women and one in five men will suffer a fracture after the age of 50 (Van Staa et al. 2001).

Key point

Life expectancy is increasing. The UK 2001 Census showed that one-third of the population (nearly 20 million people) were aged 50 or over. By 2020 this is predicted to have increased to 25 million (Shaw 2004). This will have massive implications for health services as the rates of age-related illnesses increase.

AN ANALYSIS OF RISK FACTORS

Refer to Table 7.1.

Age

Many factors combine with ageing to contribute to the increasing rates of osteoporosis and associated fractures around the world. Factors directly linked to older age — such as reduced mobility and increased risk of falling — have a direct impact on the number of hip fractures. The increase in incidence of hip fracture correlates directly with increasing age, and for women from the age of 50 the risk is approximately twice that for men.

Lifestyle

New technology leading to changes in lifestyle — such as the invention of the motor car — mean that people no longer walk very far and often get very little physical exercise. Westernised diets with a heavy emphasis on convenience foods have had an enormous impact on the incidence of osteoporosis. This has led to less healthy diets, with people often not achieving recommended calcium levels for healthy bone, alongside other issues such as the consumption of fat, which brings about more health problems. Other elements of advanced technology — such as the increasing numbers of women who have oophorectomies (removal of the ovaries), often at the time of a hysterectomy, leaving them with reduced natural levels of oestrogen — increases the number of post-menopausal women who are at risk of low bone density.

Key point

There is some evidence to suggest that people are gradually growing taller when information from the last century is studied. This leads to an increase in the length of the hip axis, which may again increase a person's risk of hip fracture (Dennison and Cooper 2001).

7

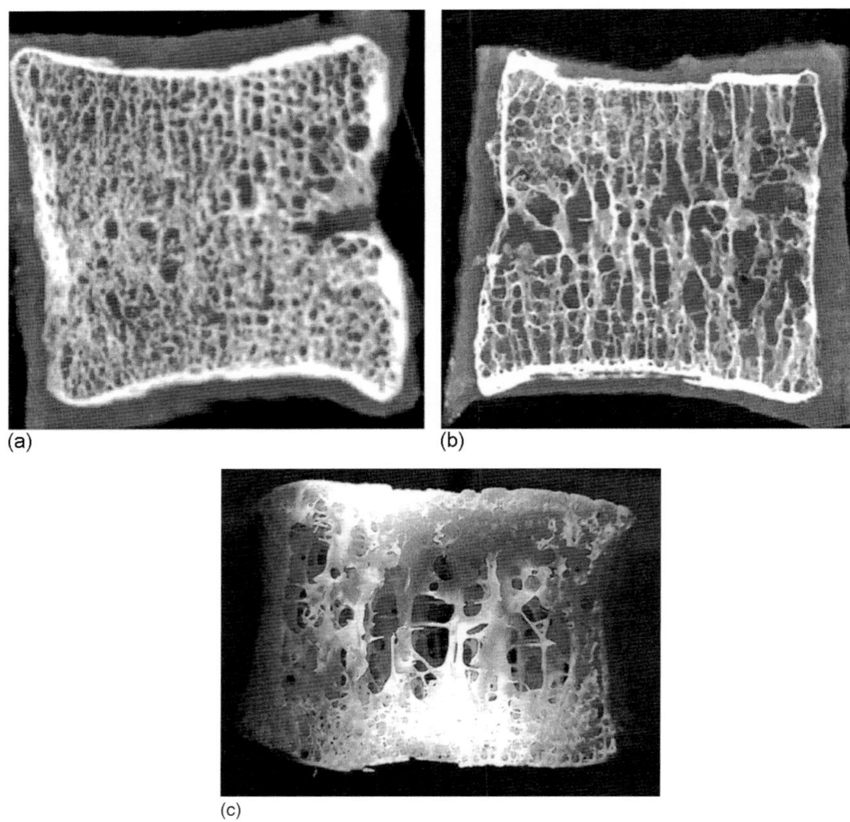

Figure 7.3 (a) Cross-section of a vertebra showing normal bone density. (b) Cross-section through an osteoporotic vertebra. (c) Lateral view of an osteoporotic vertebra.

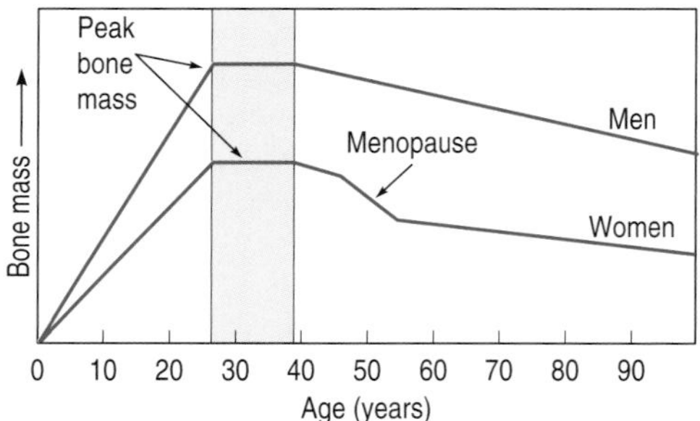

Figure 7.4 Bone mass throughout life.

Hormonal changes

Loss of oestrogen

Women run a much higher risk of developing osteoporosis than men. Not only is their peak bone density lower, but bone loss is faster owing to a decrease in the level of the hormone oestrogen. As women go through their menopause they suddenly experience a much more dramatic rate of loss of their BMD: approximately 4 per cent per year in the 5–10 years after the menopause. This then slows to a more gradual rate of loss similar to that of men: approximately 1 per cent per year (Cummings et al. 1985).

Oestrogen is known to have some 'protective' effect on bone, but exactly what that role is remains unclear. It is thought that the osteoclast and osteoblast cells may contain oestrogen receptors, although only at a very low concentration. This means that a change in oestrogen level will affect the rate of bone remodelling. A low oestrogen level results in loss of BMD or has a detrimental effect on peak bone mass obtained, through increased osteoclast activity, and simply through an increase in the rate of bone turnover.

Currently a woman's life expectancy in the UK is around 80 years, meaning many women may well spend 30 or more years of their life in a post-menopausal state with a depleted oestrogen level. In view of the fact that life expectancy is increasing, this figure is set to rise

Table 7.1 Major osteoporosis risk factors in men and women

Risk factors for women

Lack of oestrogen, caused by:

- Early menopause (before the age of 45)
- Early hysterectomy (before the age of 45), particularly when both ovaries are removed by oophorectomy
- Missing periods for 6 months or more (excluding pregnancy) as a result of over-exercising or over-dieting

Risk factors for men

- Low levels of testosterone (hypogonadism)

Risk factors for men and women

- Long-term use of high-dose corticosteroid tablets (for conditions such as rheumatoid arthritis and asthma)
- Close family history of osteoporosis (maternal or paternal), particularly with history of a maternal hip fracture
- Medical conditions such as Cushing's syndrome, liver and thyroid problems
- Malabsorption problems (coeliac disease, Crohn's disease, intestinal diseases or gastric surgery)
- Long-term immobility
- Heavy alcohol consumption and smoking
- Poor diet
- Low bodyweight in proportion to height

dramatically. This, combined with natural age-related loss, which is also continuing for longer, could obviously have a very negative effect on bone density.

Increasing numbers of women will also find themselves experiencing premature ovarian failure for reasons other than a natural menopause. For some women, having a hysterectomy, even without oophorectomy, can induce spontaneous ovarian failure, and as treatments advance for other medical conditions, such as chemotherapy and radiotherapy for cancers, women can again experience premature ovarian failure.

Younger women, and even young girls, may also be at risk. The media bombards us with images of the stereotypical 'perfect' woman who is incredibly thin, and many women and young girls are finding themselves under pressure to conform to this ideal. Eating disorders such as anorexia nervosa and bulimia can in severe cases not only leave the sufferer malnourished in terms of minerals such as calcium, but can also lead to a decline in body function and production of hormones such as oestrogen — causing menstruation to cease. Over-exercising can also have this effect (Keay et al. 1997).

It is believed that the low energy availability caused by too little dietary energy intake in comparison to the energy used affects the hypothalamus, pituitary and thyroid glands and the amount of the hormones they produce. Amenorrhoea (absence of periods) for 6 months or more may have long-term implications for a woman's BMD, particularly if this is occurring during her younger years whilst she is still building her bone density.

Male osteoporosis

The single osteoporosis risk factor that is particular to men is hypogonadism, or low levels of the hormone testosterone. This can occur for a number of reasons, such as disorders of the testes or pituitary gland, damage to or removal of the testes, chemotherapy and radiotherapy, and alcohol abuse (Figure 7.5).

Why hypogonadism causes loss of BMD is not entirely clear. It is believed that testosterone has a direct effect on BMD, acting on the androgen receptors in osteoblasts, and therefore influencing the remodelling of bone. It is also thought that oestrogen has an influence here. As already mentioned, osteoclasts and osteoblasts are known to be receptive to oestrogen. A small amount of testosterone in men is converted into oestrogen naturally. Therefore oestrogen deficiency may well be a contributory factor in male osteoporosis (Riggs et al. 1998; Center et al. 1999).

Although osteoporosis is far more common in women than in men, male osteoporosis should not be ignored. About 30 per cent of all hip fractures are in men (Pande and Francis 2001). On the basis of current trends, hip fracture rates in the UK may increase from approximately 46 000 in 1985 to 117 000 in 2016 (Dennison et al. 2005), so the problem is going to increase. It has also been suggested that vertebral deformity in older men may be as common as it is in women, with a more severe degree of deformity (O'Neill et al. 1993).

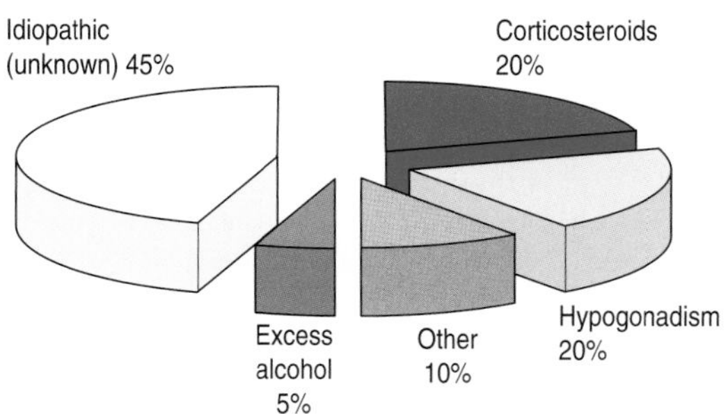

Figure 7.5 Causes of male osteoporosis.

7

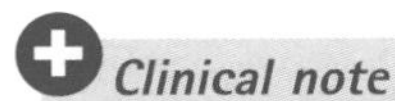

Clinical note

All of the remaining risk factors to be considered in this chapter apply to both men and women.

Corticosteroid use

The influence of corticosteroid treatments on a person's bone density can be dramatic. Corticosteroids interfere with the natural lifespan of the osteogenic cells. They shorten the life of the osteoblasts and lengthen the life of the osteoclasts, which then means that the remodelling process becomes unbalanced with more bone being resorbed than built, so causing a loss in BMD. Corticosteroids can also slow the rate of remodelling generally.

Moderate to high doses of oral corticosteroids taken long-term will affect a person's bone density. It is also now becoming clear that other methods of administering corticosteroids, such as by means of inhalers, can still cause bone density loss (Israel et al. 2001), although this does seem to be related to dose and duration of treatment. The comparative effect of different methods of corticosteroid delivery is difficult to measure, as many patients who use inhalers, for example, may have periods of more severe illness that require short durations of oral medication. Obviously most people are prescribed this sort of treatment for major illnesses or conditions that could be life-threatening, and in this case omitting to take them is not an option. However, in view of the fact that about 40 per cent of patients on high-dose or long-term corticosteroid treatments may experience fractures, it is important that the professionals managing such cases should be aware of the risk.

Genetics

Osteoporosis is a hereditary condition. As much as 75 per cent of the population variance in BMD amongst age- and sex-matched individuals can be attributed to genetic or inherited factors (Gueguen et al. 1995). Parental history of fracture (particularly a family history of a hip fracture after the age of 50) increases an individual's risk of experiencing a fracture (Kanis et al. 2004). It is thought that a woman whose mother broke her hip has nearly double the risk of having a fracture herself (Cummings et al. 1995).

Many women follow the same pattern as their mother with the timing of their menopause. This means that early menopause, a risk factor for osteoporosis, can possibly run in families. Also other factors such as a small body frame can be inherited from one's parents. This is known to be a contributory risk factor for developing osteoporosis. Since these factors cannot be changed, awareness of osteoporosis is crucial to enable people to modify their lifestyle.

Other medical conditions

Conditions such as coeliac disease, Crohn's disease and those requiring major gastric surgery will have important implications for the person's ability to absorb essential minerals and vitamins from food. Without nutrients our bodies do not continue to function at an optimum level. Without general good health and the correct amounts of calcium and vitamin D, alongside other minerals such as magnesium and boron, our bones will no longer be able to remain healthy and maintain BMD by balanced remodelling.

Disorders of the thyroid and parathyroid glands are also quite common, and can lead to a low bone density. The thyroid gland in the neck produces thyroid hormone (thyroxine), which is responsible for controlling many of the bodily functions. Hyperthyroidism occurs when the thyroid gland becomes overactive, and the excess of thyroxine that is produced causes the rate of remodelling and loss of BMD to increase. Hypothyroidism (an underactive thyroid) is not a risk factor for osteoporosis unless the thyroxine medication that is given as replacement is not monitored to prevent the level becoming too high.

Hyperparathyroidism is another condition that impacts upon bone health. The parathyroid glands are situated in the neck just behind the thyroid gland. Parathyroid hormone produced by the parathyroid gland has an important role in regulating the level of calcium in the blood. If the blood calcium falls too low, then the parathyroid gland increases the level of parathyroid hormone. This then releases calcium from the bones and also allows the gut to absorb more calcium from the food, which in turn then increases the blood calcium level again. People suffering from hyperparathyroidism are producing too much parathyroid hormone and are therefore continually leaching calcium from their bones.

Diseases or disorders of the liver have an impact on bone density. The liver is responsible for filtering and processing digestive products, neutralising toxins, secreting bile and many other metabolic processes. If the liver becomes diseased or damaged in any way it will not be able to perform these functions properly, which in turn has a negative effect on bone density as the body is not receiving the correct amounts of nutrients or metabolism is increased greatly.

Immobility

This has particular relevance to physiotherapists. People become immobile for many reasons, some temporary and some permanent. When the body is no longer exercised in any way bone density decreases. Bone health is maintained partly by the regular stresses and load-bearing that it was designed to receive. Studies in astronauts and of the effect of weightlessness on bone density have shown that approximately 1 per cent of the skeleton is lost during each month spent in a zero-gravity environment (Holick 1998). Studies into the effect of acute immobilisation have suggested a bone loss of 1–2 per cent per month (Shackelford et al. 2004), although this is thought to stabilise after 6 months. Remobilisation can cause the bone density to improve again, but obviously some people are permanently unable to mobilise and are then at a very high risk of fracture, particularly if they have a fall.

Smoking and alcohol consumption

Smoking is believed to cause reduced BMD by increasing bone resorption. This is possibly due to a reduction in the production, and acceleration of the degradation, of oestrogen. Excessive amounts of alcohol, too, cause a reduction in BMD, but this time through decreased bone formation.

Key point

Studies in this area are limited, but many have linked both smoking and heavy drinking with increased risk of fracture (Kanis et al. 2005; Kanis et al. 2004).

Apart from the obvious detrimental effects to health in general, smoking is also associated with premature menopause. Overton and Davies (1999) reported that women who smoke tend to have their menopause approximately 2 years earlier than they would have done otherwise. This means that female smokers experience 2 extra years of depleted oestrogen levels, which is associated with a reduction in BMD.

Smoking and excessive alcohol consumption will also affect a person's lifestyle. Smoking is known to be an appetite suppressant, and alcohol abuse often leads to a poor diet. This is associated with low nutrient intake, which contributes to poor health and, more specifically, poor bone health and loss of density.

The WHO risk assessment tool

The World Health Organization (WHO) is currently working on developing an osteoporosis risk assessment tool. The aim is to provide health professionals at all levels, but particularly those in primary care, with a way of accurately assessing an individual's risk of fracture in the next 10 years.

Currently diagnosis of osteoporosis and decisions about treatments are usually based on the measurement of BMD by dual energy X-ray absorptiometry (DXA) scan. There is a distinct correlation between having a low bone density measurement and having an increased risk of fracture. This method of measuring bone quantity does not, however, take into account bone quality, which will also influence an individual's risk of fracture.

As bone quality is difficult to measure unless invasive techniques are used, the WHO is working on devising a system of looking at other clinical risk factors that influence a person's risk of fracture independently of bone density measurement. Factors such as age, previous fragility fracture, smoking, alcohol intake, steroid use, family history and secondary osteoporosis (osteoporosis due to other known factors or conditions) are all seen as clinical risk factors that make an independent contribution to a person's risk of fracture. The more risk factors a person has, the greater their risk of fracture becomes.

The WHO is aiming to give each one of the clinical risk factors some sort of weighting or score to allow healthcare professionals to calculate a person's risk of fracture over the next 10 years. This may help to identify those people who would then benefit from also having a bone density scan as well, and ultimately those who would need treatment to reduce their risk of fracture. Work on this risk assessment tool is still ongoing and a target date for completion has not yet been established.

Public awareness

Public awareness of the risk factors discussed in this section is an extremely important issue. If people are armed with the knowledge that they could be at risk of having low bone density or of developing osteoporosis in the future, then they can seek advice, diagnosis and treatment from their doctor, and make changes towards a bone-healthy lifestyle to maximise the bone density that they do have.

COMMON SITES OF FRACTURES RELATED TO OSTEOPOROSIS

The three most common sites of fracture for people with osteoporosis are:

- the wrist
- the spine
- the hip.

These parts of the skeleton are predominantly made up of cancellous bone. In Britain, fracture rates for women for hip, spine and distal forearm are 14 per cent, 11 per cent and 13 per cent respectively; for men they are 3 per cent, 2 per cent and 2 per cent (Dennison and Cooper 1996). This translates into over 60 000 hip fractures, 50 000 wrist fractures and 120 000 spinal fractures being seen in the UK each year (Van Staa et al. 2001; Keene et al. 1993).

Wrist fractures

7

Fractures of the distal forearm (Colles' fracture) tend to happen to women most commonly during the perimenopausal period. In white women the incidence of Colles' fractures increases between the ages of 40 and 65, and then stabilises. In men, however, the incidence remains constant between the ages of 20 and 80. Wrist fractures are nearly always the consequence of falling on to an outstretched hand.

There is an increase of these fractures during the winter months, but this seems to be due to falls outside on icy ground rather than for any other reason. Wrist fractures do not continue to increase with age, and this is probably due to the fact that our neuromuscular coordination decreases with age, so we are less likely to put out a hand to break a fall as we get older, and instead land straight on to the hip.

Spinal fractures

It is believed that only one-third of people with spinal fractures caused by osteoporosis come to medical attention (Cooper et al. 1993), and as few as 13 per cent of patients who have had a moderate to severe vertebral fracture in the thoracic region receive a diagnosis when they have a chest X-ray as part of their normal medical care (Gehlbach et al. 2000). Therefore the estimated figures for these fractures are much lower than the number of fractures in reality.

Fractures of the vertebrae can happen spontaneously and silently (no symptoms), often leaving victims unaware of their presence until they discover that they have been gradually losing height or developing a kyphosis and wonder what has caused it. Alternatively fractures can occur very obviously when a person makes a specific movement or has a fall, in which case the injury may cause intense pain.

The vertebrae that are most commonly involved tend to correspond with the weakest regions in the spine: T8, T12 and L1. With the loss of strength caused by reduced BMD, the vertebrae crush down into themselves. Although the bones still heal, they are unable to reform their original cubic shape and they remain in a shortened, squashed shape, causing the spine to shorten. They can also fracture irregularly to form a wedge shape, and these fractures are the cause of a kyphosis. They are often referred to as 'crush' and 'wedge' fractures (Figure 7.6).

Unlike wrist fractures, spinal fractures do seem to increase with age, particularly in women. True figures, however, are very difficult to obtain, as so few of these fractures are actually reported. Firstly, as already stated, many are silent and are simply not known about. Secondly, there is nothing that can be done other than giving pain relief for these fractures, so many people who have experienced one do not seek medical attention for any further fractures. Studies have shown that once a person has experienced one such vertebral deformity, he or she is then at 7–10 times greater risk of suffering further deformities.

Hip fractures

Key point

In 1990 there were an estimated 1.66 million hip fractures worldwide. As long ago as 1993, hip fractures accounted for over 20 per cent of orthopaedic bed occupancy in the United Kingdom (Cryer et al. 1996). Hip fractures are significantly more common in women than in men, and they are specifically associated with the very elderly.

Although hip fractures tend to happen much later in life than wrist or spinal fractures, they represent the most serious consequence of osteoporosis. They are associated with considerable mortality and morbidity (subsequent illness/complications) (Cooper et al. 1993). A study by Baudoin and colleagues in 1996 showed that hip fractures are associated with a 20 per cent mortality rate within the first year, and there is also a greater risk of functional impairment and institutionalisation. Hip fractures may require surgery or hospitalisation, and all require a long period of recovery and rehabilitation. Physiotherapists play a key role in rehabilitating people after femoral neck fractures.

Hip fractures most commonly occur following a fall from standing height. It is also not unusual for people to say that they heard the bone break before the fall, indicating that the fracture caused the fall, and not the fall the fracture. The risk of falls also increases with age. Reduced neuromuscular coordination, reduced muscle tone, strength and balance, poorer eyesight, and general greater frailty all combine to increase the likelihood of someone falling.

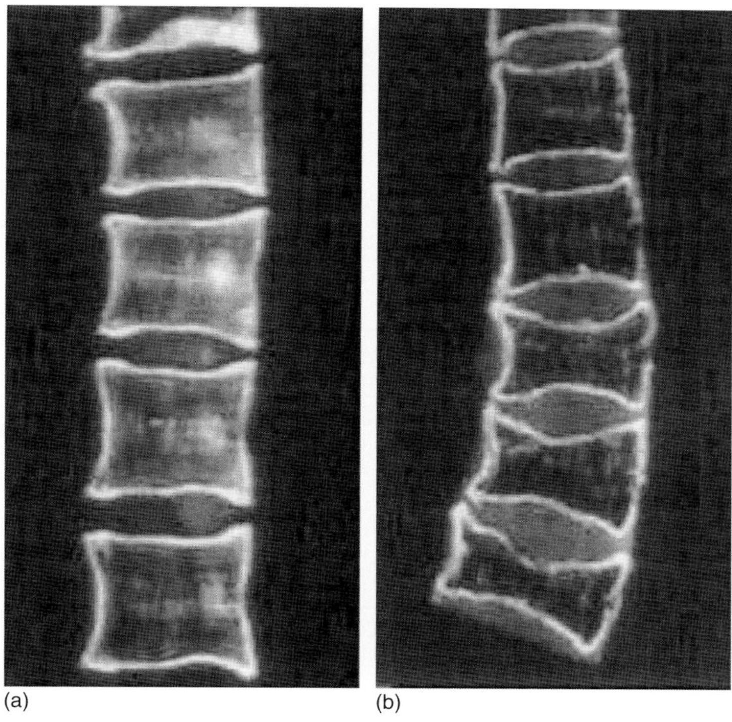

Figure 7.6 (a) Appearance of normal vertebrae on X-ray. (b) Osteoporotic vertebral column showing biconcave shape and compression fractures.

> **Other types of fracture**
>
> The three types of fracture considered in this section, although the most common, are not the only fractures that can occur in someone with osteoporosis. The disease can affect any bone anywhere in the skeleton, so fractures at other sites are possible.

SYMPTOMS AND CLINICAL FEATURES

Silent onset

Osteoporosis is a silent condition, often giving no indication of its presence. One cannot feel changes in bone density, and without knowledge of the risk factors the first thing to alert the individual to a problem may be a fracture, by which point there has already been significant loss of BMD. The fact that people do not suffer problems with pain in the early stages of the condition is a good thing, but the lack of any early warning signs often means ignorance of bone ill-health until osteoporosis is established and fractures are occurring.

Having a low bone density per se does not cause pain. Although pain is very much a feature of osteoporosis, it does not occur until fractures happen. Obviously the pain from any recent fracture can be extremely acute for some people, often causing temporary immobility and requiring strong analgesia. For some people, this pain then subsides as the fracture heals and they have no further problems. For others, permanent discomfort (often from nerve or muscle involvement) rising to intense, chronic pain can remain. The control of this pain then becomes the key clinical feature of that person's osteoporosis management.

Complications

Although the process of healing continues as normal in someone with osteoporosis, the fractures that people experience can then cause many associated problems as well as pain. Vertebral fractures are often the main culprit. Multiple vertebral fractures can eventually lead to kyphosis, a curvature of the top of the spine often referred to as a 'dowager's hump'. They can also cause considerable loss of height. These two factors combined can cause immense problems. A dramatic change in body image, with enormous difficulty in finding clothes to fit, has a huge psychological impact, causing social isolation and depression.

Spinal curvature and height loss lead in turn to reduced space for the internal organs. This tends to involve the lungs, stomach, bladder and bowel in particular. People can find themselves feeling more short of breath, as the lungs do not have the room to fill to capacity and expand properly. They will also feel easily full after small portions of food and often lose their appetite, which can quickly lead to poor nutrition, particularly in the elderly. Similarly, people can find themselves needing to pass urine more frequently, and having trouble with bloating and bowel function as these organs also become squashed into a smaller space. As these organs struggle to function owing to the lack of room many people with osteoporosis develop a distended abdomen. The skeleton provides a vertical barrier confining the internal organs, so the only possible extra space to be found is by horizontal expansion at the lower abdominal area.

Investigations and diagnosis

Osteoporosis is sometimes diagnosed purely on the strength of a person's medical history or even physical appearance. Significant height loss, kyphosis, a history of low-trauma fractures and the presence of other risk factors may be enough for a doctor to diagnose osteoporosis in some patients.

Advanced technology has brought about sophisticated scanning methods that enable the measurement of bone density in people who are at high risk of the disease. Three types of scan are commonly used in the UK to examine BMD in detail:

- hip and spine DXA
- peripheral DXA and single energy X-ray absorptiometry (SXA)
- ultrasound (diagnostic, not therapeutic).

The WHO scoring system

The WHO has developed a definition of osteoporosis based on the scoring system of the DXA scan (which is discussed below). The system is now used to diagnose the condition more accurately.

These scores are expressed in 'standard deviations' (SDs) away from the normal range (Figure 7.7). The T-score, which compares the individual's BMD to that of the young adult mean, is the score that is used for diagnosis, monitoring and treatment decisions. The Z-score is where the individual's BMD is compared to the age-matched mean. This is helpful to assess the BMD of an older person.

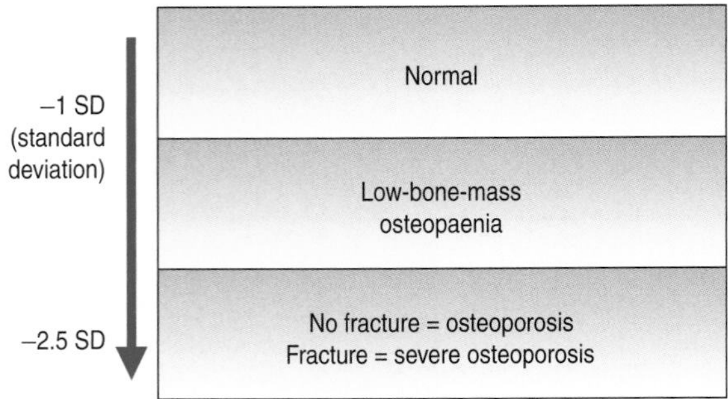

Figure 7.7 The WHO definition of T-scores (WHO 1994).

DXA (dual energy X-ray absorptiometry) scans

The hip and spine DXA scan

This is very much considered to be the 'gold standard' in osteoporosis scanning. For the patient it is a very simple procedure, and is low-risk in terms of the amount of radiation emitted. It is a quick procedure, taking only a few minutes.

The patient lies on the scanner's bed and does not even have to undress, except to remove any metal items (Figure 7.8). The arm of the scanner then passes over the lower spine and non-dominant hip, producing the scan image and measurements on a screen in front of the radiographer. The scan result is sent to the radiologist for interpretation.

The peripheral scan

These are either DXA or SXA. They may be performed on either the distal forearm or the calcaneus. Owing to the varying amounts of trabecular and cortical bone in these sites at different positions, these scans are not able to diagnose osteoporosis as easily as the hip and spine DXA.

Forearm scanning can use the same scoring system, if positioned correctly, and can either indicate a person's need for treatment (T-score at −2.5 SD) or indicate the need for a hip and spine DXA if the T-score is between −1 and −2.5 SD. The distal forearm is not sufficiently sensitive to be able to monitor changes in BMD with treatments and time (National Osteoporosis Society 2001). The calcaneus is a site that could potentially be used to monitor change because, unlike the distal forearm, it is mainly trabecular bone. However, the threshold score of −2.5 SD is not applicable to the heel and adjustments to those scores need to be made. It is not yet clear whether those adjustments would be appropriate for different makes of scanner.

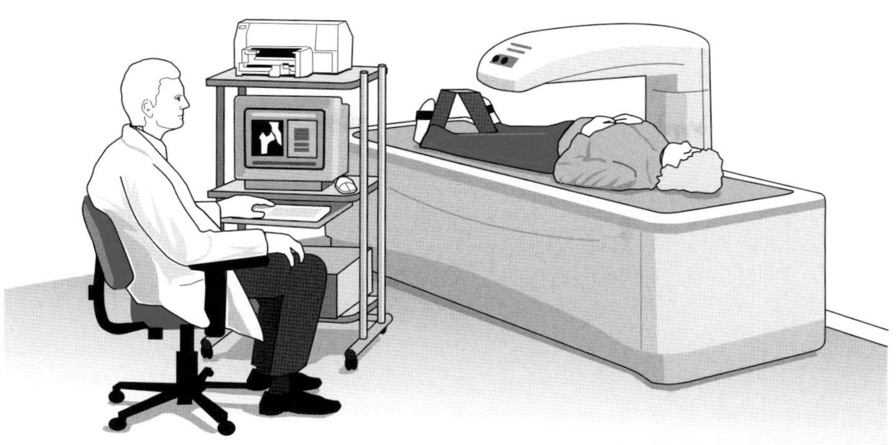

Figure 7.8 A bone density scan in progress.

Ultrasound scans

These scans use the calcaneus. There is no ionising radiation involved, and the machines themselves are often easily portable (unlike the hip and spine DXA). They are also considerably cheaper than other scanners.

Ultrasound cannot diagnose osteoporosis, as it does not measure bone mineral content or density directly. However, a low result from an ultrasound scan is recognised as an independent risk factor for future osteoporotic hip fracture. Ultrasound also cannot yet (in most cases) be used to monitor bone loss and response to treatment in an individual patient.

> ***Key point***
>
> This method of scanning was designed to look at post-menopausal women, so its use in children, younger women and men is not recommended for clinical purposes.

Ultrasound scanners need to be operated by properly trained personnel in the right conditions to achieve accurate results.

Other methods of measuring bone density

It is worth remembering that other methods of scanning may be used to diagnose osteoporosis, directly or indirectly. Computerised tomography (CT) may be used, although this is not common. Plain X-rays are, however, very commonly used. Often a patient may have an X-ray to investigate back pain or an unrelated problem, and a degree of bone density loss will be noted. This is not an entirely reliable way of diagnosing reduction in BMD, as the development process of the X-ray film can sometimes give the appearance of low BMD, which is open to misinterpretation.

Urine testing to measure breakdown products (biochemical markers) produced during the bone remodelling process is being researched. Although this is currently available in some specialist centres, and even available in kit form from supermarkets (to be sent away for analysis), it is not a process that has yet reached its full potential. In the future this could be a much cheaper and simpler form of monitoring a person's response to a treatment. Using repeat scanning every few years as a method of monitoring a person's progress is much less common these days. Many specialists feel that a bone density measurement gives only limited information when trying to predict a person's risk of fracture, and believe they are not necessary if that patient is settled on a treatment without further fractures.

PREVENTATIVE MEASURES

Certain lifestyle factors, such as diet and exercise, have an influence on bone density and bone health in general. If positive population-wide lifestyle changes could be made to increase peak bone mass, this would be a step in the right direction towards reducing the incidence of osteoporosis.

7

Diet

Diet plays a major role in bone health. The protein component of bone, the osteoid, needs to be mineralised to give the bone its hardness and strength. The key mineral required in this process is calcium. Calcium is freely available in our diets with many rich food sources available.

The human body contains over a kilogram of calcium, almost all of which is in our skeleton; the remaining 1 per cent is found in the blood stream and other body fluids. To maintain this level, calcium-rich foods such as dairy products, green leafy vegetables, bony fish, cereal products and dried fruit, to name just a few, need to be included in the diet. Some people, however, are not able to obtain everything that they require from their diet alone and will use a calcium supplement to top this level up. The National Osteoporosis Society recommends that someone who has a diagnosis of osteoporosis, and is taking a treatment as well, may need to boost calcium intake to 1200 mg per day, and many people will find this amount difficult to achieve from dietary sources alone.

Calcium, however, is only one part of a bone-friendly diet. Humans need to have a healthy, balanced diet that includes all of the major food groups, in order to provide the essential vitamins and minerals, and the right balance of acid and alkali, required to function properly. A balanced diet should give more than adequate amounts of all the other nutrients that we require, such as boron, copper, zinc, magnesium, manganese, potassium, vitamins B6, C and K, and essential fatty acids.

Of course, there are also elements of our diet that can cause the potential deterioration of bone health. Several things can inhibit our natural ability to absorb calcium. These include caffeine, excess sodium (salt), excess protein and even phosphate, which is a preservative used in some carbonated (fizzy) drinks. There is also much scientific discussion over the possible detrimental effects of a diet that is too acidic or alkaline. The key to all of these issues is to have a balanced diet without excess.

Key point

Diet is not merely an issue for adults. It is essential that children and young adults have a healthy, balanced diet too. It is during these early years that bone density is built and bone health firmly established. A good diet with all the important nutrients will ensure that person's peak bone mass is as high as possible.

Phytoestrogens are very weak plant oestrogens that are similar to one type of human oestradiol. Isoflavones and ligans are types of phytoestrogens that are found in soya products, grains, cereals and linseed. These are of great interest to scientists and researchers, as it seems that populations who consume diets rich in these phytoestrogens have much lower rates of certain cancers and diseases such as osteoporosis. Their use in the diet or in supplement form to prevent bone density loss, however, is still not proven and further research does need to be done.

Exercise

Exercise has two important roles in the prevention of fractures. Firstly, it is shown to aid bone density; secondly, it tones and strengthens muscles, thereby ensuring good balance, coordination and skeletal support.

Bone is designed to bear certain stresses and loads, and appears to be at its healthiest when this functional 'use' is maintained (Lanyon 1996). A meta-analysis (overall review) of several studies looking into the effect of exercise on bone mass showed a prevention, or reversal, of bone loss of almost 1 per cent per year (Wolff et al. 1999). However, studies looking at the effect of exercise are only relatively short-term, so we do not know what the long-term effect will be. Increases in BMD may possibly plateau unless the intensity of exercise is continually increased, which is not really feasible. Maintenance of exercise will help maintenance of BMD.

Weight-bearing exercise is important when considering osteoporosis prevention. High-impact exercise such as jogging will target the hips and spine, and resistance exercises like weight lifting can target specific areas such as the wrist. Loading the skeleton with physical weights or bodyweight stimulates the osteogenic cells, giving rise to a maintenance or possible increase in BMD. A greater load provides greater stimulation. Bodyweight is multiplied during high-impact exercise (a jump where you leave the ground and then land again, compared to a step where a foot always remains on the floor, for example), and this is why exercises such as jogging and aerobics have more effect than brisk walking.

Obviously, exercise needs to be appropriate and safe, and high-impact exercise is not suitable for everyone. Many people are not used to doing any regular exercise and would need to start very gently and carefully. Something like walking may be appropriate, despite the fact that it does not give as effective results on BMD; however, a non-threatening form of exercise such as walking may well mean that a person does some exercise instead of none at all, giving other health benefits as well. Also, many people will have other medical conditions to take into account, such as arthritis or myalgic encephalopathy (ME), which may restrict activity.

People who have established osteoporosis with fractures and those who have very low bone density obviously need to approach exercise with care. Bone-loading and impact exercises and some stretches — such as an extreme forward flexion, for example — could be dangerous for them by possibly causing further fractures. People in this situation need to do gentle muscle-toning and strength-building exercises instead.

Key point

There are still exercise groups that are safe for such people to go to if they wish. Organisations such as Extend run classes involving movement to music for the over-sixties and for people with disabilities at any age.

The important features of these lifestyle factors are that they do not have to involve any major cost, and they can be addressed in the privacy of a person's own home. No major adjustment to a person's daily routine needs to be made, unless he or she chooses to join an exercise class or gym. They will, however, not only provide extra help for the health of a person's bones; they will also benefit overall general health and fitness too.

TREATMENT OF OSTEOPOROSIS

Drugs and supplements

There are a wide variety of medications available for the prevention and treatment of osteoporosis, and fortunately further research and increased technology in pharmacology mean that new developments in the management of this disease are frequently occurring.

There are three commonly used types of medication for osteoporosis prevention and treatment in the UK. These are the bisphosphonates, strontium ranelate and raloxifene (a selective oestrogen receptor modulator or 'SERM'). The majority of people requiring treatment will be able to use one of these drugs, but some will not for various reasons. There are several other types of treatment available, which a specialist may consider.

Although many of the drug treatments are licensed for the prevention of osteoporosis as well as for treatment, they are in practice not often prescribed for prevention these days. The treatments all aim specifically to reduce the individual's risk of fracture and so treatment is very much targeted at those with a diagnosis of osteoporosis who are considered to have a high risk of fracture. It is only in specific circumstances relating to certain risk factors for osteoporosis (such as corticosteroid users) that the treatments are prescribed as a preventative therapy.

The bisphosphonates

This is a family of non-hormonal drugs specifically for the treatment of osteoporosis. The most common drugs within this family are alendronate (Fosamax and alendronic acid), risedronate (Actonel), ibandronate (Bonviva) and cyclical etidronate (Didronel PMO).

These drugs are anti-resorptive and work by directly inhibiting the osteoclasts, whilst allowing the osteoblasts to continue working. This will slow or stop the loss of BMD that is occurring, and possibly encourage a slight increase. The main aim of these drugs is to reduce the person's risk of fracture. It is thought that they do this by also affecting the structure (and therefore strength) of the bone.

People taking bisphosphonates must follow very strict instructions for their safe and effective administration. The drugs must be taken on an empty stomach whilst in an upright position and must be accompanied by a glass of plain tap water. The various brands differ slightly in their instructions and are available as daily, weekly or monthly preparations. These drugs can be associated with a degree of gastric irritation so the instructions do need to be followed accurately. Ibandronate is also now available as a quarterly intravenous injection for those people who cannot manage the oral regimes.

The bisphosphonates are licensed for the prevention and treatment of osteoporosis in post-menopausal women. Fosamax is also licensed for use in men. They have been shown to be effective in reducing fractures of the spine, hip and other non-vertebral sites. They are also licensed for the prevention of corticosteroid-induced osteoporosis. Specialists will sometimes use these drugs outside of their licences on younger people or on men. For any drug to become legally licensed for use, it has to undergo trials to prove its safety and efficacy. The easiest, most readily available group of people to study with osteoporosis is post-menopausal women. This does not mean, however, that these medications will not work on other groups, such as men and pre-menopausal women; they just have not yet been studied in large trials (except for Fosamax).

Another bisphosphonate called pamidronate is sometimes used for the treatment of osteoporosis. It is not actually licensed for this use; it was developed for a different condition called Paget's disease, but again some specialists will choose to use it in their patients. This drug is given in the form of an intravenous drip as a day case in hospital on an intermittent basis.

Finally, there is not yet a great deal known about the long-term use of the bisphosphonates. We do not really know what the optimum duration of treatment is or how long they may continue to offer protection to the bones, even after the treatment regimen has ceased. Furthermore, a newer and potentially more potent bisphosphonate is being trialled; it is called zolendronic acid, and the manufacturers hope it will be suitable for being given as a once-a-year injection.

Strontium ranelate

Strontium ranelate (Protelos) is a newer drug treatment for osteoporosis. Other drug treatments for osteoporosis work by suppressing the action of the osteoclasts, which break down bone, or by stimulating the action of the osteoblasts, which build bone. Strontium ranelate is the first treatment that works by performing both these functions. It is licensed for post-menopausal women, to reduce the risk of fracture in the hip and spine.

Similar to the bisphosphonates, strontium ranelate needs to be taken on an empty stomach, but instead of being in the form of a tablet, strontium ranelate is given as a sachet of powder that is mixed with water into a drink. Unlike the bisphosphonates, strontium ranelate does not cause gastric irritation, so is often quite a useful alternative to that family. It does, however, carry a slight increase in the risk of venous thromboembolism (VTE). Again we do not yet know about the long-term implications of this treatment.

Selective oestrogen receptor modulators

SERMs are a different type of drug. Raloxifene (Evista) is the first of these drugs to be designed and licensed as a treatment for osteoporosis, but others are currently being trialled. Again this is licensed for post-menopausal women, and it works by acting as an oestrogen agonist in bone and an oestrogen antagonist in areas like the breast and uterus.

Evista is not a hormone replacement, so will not have any of the other effects that hormone replacement therapy (HRT) has. It too carries an increased risk of VTE. Evista has been shown to reduce the risk of vertebral fractures, but no effects have been noted so far on non-vertebral sites. Evista is very convenient and easy to take at any time of the day and there are no food restrictions.

Teriparatide

Teriparatide (Forteo) is a very different type of drug treatment for osteoporosis. Rather than having an anti-resorptive effect, this has an anabolic effect on bone, stimulating the osteoblasts and causing an increase in bone density. Teriparatide is based on parathyroid hormone and is licensed for post-menopausal women to reduce the risk of vertebral fractures.

In the UK teriparatide is only rarely used. The National Institute for Health and Clinical Excellence (NICE) has produced guidelines for doctors on the treatment of osteoporosis in those people who have already had a fracture. These guidelines recommend very strict restrictions on the prescribing of teriparatide. They state that patients need to be over 65, have had three or more vertebral fractures, have very low T scores or have other risk factors as well. In comparison to the other osteoporosis drug treatments, teriparatide is very expensive, and this is part of the reason for it being less commonly used.

Teriparatide is given as an 18-month course of treatment in the form of a daily injection which the patient is taught to administer. After the 18-month course has finished, patients will need to return to one of the other osteoporosis treatments to try to maintain the increase in bone density that the teriparatide has hopefully produced.

Calcium and vitamin D

All the clinical trials looking at osteoporosis treatments and their efficacy have ensured that the correct amount of calcium is being used as well. In some cases, however, calcium and vitamin D supplements are used as a treatment on their own.

Vitamin D is required to metabolise calcium and we normally get most of what we need from sunshine. Elderly people, in particular, are often unable to go out and about and may very well be deficient in this vitamin. Studies have shown that, although regular supplementation in the frail elderly nursing home population may reduce the risk of non-vertebral fractures, routine supplementation in the independent-living elderly population does not reduce the risk of fracture (Cameron and Kurrle 2005).

Given the fact that calcium and vitamin D supplements have very few side-effects, other than some constipation with calcium, they are often a good treatment option for those people who cannot tolerate other treatments.

Hormone replacement therapy (HRT)

HRT, like the bisphosphonates, has an anti-resorptive therapy effect on bone and works by stimulating the oestrogen receptors on the bone cells. HRT used to be very commonly used in women for the prevention and treatment of osteoporosis, but is now rarely used in post-menopausal women due to the potential health risks that are associated with long-term use. These include an increase in the risk of breast cancer, heart disease, stroke and VTE. Although HRT is known to be beneficial to bone, these risks seem to increase with both age and duration of use.

HRT may still be used for bone protection in the younger woman and continued up until the natural age of the menopause (around 50). This group includes those women who have had an early or premature menopause, or young women with very low hormone levels due to anorexia nervosa and other such conditions.

Hip protectors

Hip protectors are an external hip protection system that aims to reduce the risk of a hip fracture, should the wearer fall. They comprise of two hip-protecting shells, made of polypropylene, integrated into a pair of stretchy, cotton-mix pants. The shells disperse the impact of a fall into the soft tissue and muscles around the pelvis. Various research projects have been completed into the acceptability and safety of hip protectors; studies are ongoing and so far have not been conclusive about their effectiveness. One of the main problems with hip protectors is that they are not easy to put on and take off. This means that the people who would benefit most from wearing them tend to not wear them when they are most vulnerable, such as at night. Hip protectors are not available on prescription and have to be purchased.

REFERENCES

Baudoin C, Fardellone P et al. 1996 Clinical outcomes and mortality after hip fracture: a 2-year follow-up study. Bone 18(3 Suppl): 149S–157S

Burge RT 2001 The cost of osteoporotic fractures in the UK: Projections for 2000–2020. J Med Econ 4: 51–62

Cameron ID, Kurrle S 2005 Prevention of low-trauma fractures in older people: results of the RECORD calcium and vitamin D study. Lancet 366: 543

CDC (Consensus Development Conference) 1991 Prophylaxis and treatment of osteoporosis. Am J Med 90: 107–110

Census 2001: National Report for England and Wales. 2002. National Statistics

Center JR, Nguyen TV, Sambrook PN, Eisman JA 1999 Hormonal and biochemical parameters in the determination of osteoporosis in elderly men. J Clin Endocrinol Metab 84: 3626–3635

Cooper C, Atkinson EJ, Jacobsen SJ et al. 1993 Population based study of survival after osteoporotic fractures. Am J Epidemiol 137: 1001–1007

Cryer PC, Davidson L, Styles CP, Langley JD 1996 Descriptive epidemiology of injury in the south east: identifying priorities for action. Public Health 110(6): 331–338

Cummings SR, Kelsey JL, Nevitt MC et al. 1985 Epidemiology of osteoporosis and osteoporotic fractures. Epidemiol Rev 7: 178–208

Cummings SR, Nevitt MC, Browner WS et al. 1995 Risk factors for hip fracture in white women. N Engl J Med 332: 767–773

Dennison E, Cooper C 1996 The epidemiology of osteoporosis. Br J Clin Pract 50: 33–36

Dennison E, Cooper C 2001 Epidemiology of Osteoporotic Fractures: Effective Management of Osteoporosis. Aesculapius Medical: London

Dennison E, Cole Z, Cooper C 2005 Diagnosis and epidemiology of osteoporosis. Curr Opin Rheumatol 17: 456–461

Gehlbach SH, Bigelow C, Heimisdottir M et al. 2000 Recognition of vertebral fracture in a clinical setting. Osteoporos Int 11: 577–582

Gueguen R, Jouanny P, Guillemin F et al. 1995 Segregation analysis and variance components analysis of bone mineral density in healthy families. J Bone Min Res 12: 2017–2022

Holick MF 1998 Perspective on the impact of weightlessness on calcium and bone metabolism. Bone 22(Suppl 5): 105s–111s

Israel E, Banerjee T, Fitzmaurice G et al. 2001 Effects of inhaled glucocorticoids on bone density in premenopausal women. N Engl J Med 345: 941–947

Kanis JA, Johansson H, Oden A et al. 2004 A family history of fracture and fracture risk: a meta-analysis. Bone 35: 1029–1037

Kanis JA, Johnell O, Oden A et al. 2004 Smoking and fracture risk: a meta-analysis. Osteoporos Int 16: 155–162

Kanis JA, Johansson H, Johnell O et al. 2005 Alcohol intake as a risk factor for fracture. Osteoporos Int 16: 737–742

Keay N, Fogelman I et al. 1997 Bone mineral density in professional female dancers. Br J Sports Med 31(2): 143–147

Keene GS, Parker MJ, Pryor GA 1993 Mortality and morbidity after hip fractures. BMJ 307: 1248–1250

Lanyon LE 1996 Using functional loading to influence bone mass and architecture: objectives, mechanisms and relationship with estrogen of the mechanically adaptive process in bone. Bone 18: S37–S43

Marshall D, Johnell O, Wedel H 1996 Meta-analysis of how well measures of bone mineral density predict occurrence of osteoporotic fractures. BMJ 312: 1254–1259

Mays S, Less B, Stevenson JC 1998 Age-dependent bone loss in the femur in a medieval population. Int J Osteoarchaeol 8: 97–106

National Osteoporosis Society 2001 Position Statement on the Use of Peripheral X-ray Absorptiometry in the Management of Osteoporosis. NOS: Bath

O'Neill TW, Varlow J, Cooper C et al. 1993 Differences in vertebral deformity indices between three European populations. J Bone Min Res 8(Suppl 1): S149

Overton C, Davies M 1999 Factors which Determine the Age of the Menopause: Handbook of the British Menopause Society. BMS: London

Pande I, Francis RM 2001 Osteoporosis in men. Best Pract Res Clin Rheumatol 15: 415–427

Riggs BL, Khosla S et al. 1998 A unitary model for involutional osteoporosis: estrogen deficiency causes both type I and type II osteoporosis in postmenopausal women and contributes to bone loss in aging men. J Bone Miner Res 13: 763–773

Shackelford LC, LeBlanc AD, Driscoll TB et al. 2004 Resistance exercise as a countermeasure to disuse-induced bone loss. J Appl Physiol 97: 119–129

Shaw C 2004 Interim 2003-based national population projections for the United Kingdom and constituent countries. Government Actuary Department: London

Torgerson D, Iglesias C, Reid DM 2001 The economics of fracture prevention. In: Barlow DH, Francis RM, Miles A (eds) The Effective Management of Osteoporosis. Aesculapius Medical: London, pp. 111–121.

Van Staa TP, Dennison EM, Leufkens HG, Cooper C 2001 Epidemiology of fractures in England and Wales. Bone 29: 517–522

Weinstein RS, Manolagas SC 2000 Apoptosis and osteoporosis. Am J Med 108: 153–154

WHO (World Health Organization) 1994 Assessment of Fracture Risk and its Application to Screening for Postmenopausal Osteoporosis. WHO technical report series 843. WHO: Geneva

Wolff I, Van Croonenborg JJ, Kemper HCG et al. 1999 The effect of exercise training programs on bone mass: a meta-analysis of published controlled trials in pre- and post-menopausal women. Osteopor Int 9: 1–12

Chapter **8**

Physiotherapy in thoracic surgery

Anne Dyson

CHAPTER CONTENTS

ANATOMY OF THE THORAX

The skeleton of the thorax is an osteocartilagenous framework within which lie the principal organs of respiration, the heart, major blood vessels and the oesophagus. It is conical in shape, narrow apically, broad at its base and longer posteriorly. The bony structure consists of 12 thoracic vertebrae, 12 pairs of ribs and the sternum (Figure 8.1).

The musculature of the thoracic cage is in two layers. The outer layer consists of latissimus dorsi and trapezius, the inner layer of the rhomboids and serratus anterior muscles. Anteriorly the chest wall is covered by pectoralis major and minor. The intercostal muscles run obliquely between the ribs. The diaphragm forms the lower border of the thorax. It is convex upwards showing two cupolae, the right being slightly higher than the left. It is made up of muscle fibres peripherally and is tendinous centrally.

The lungs

The two lungs are basically very similar (Figure 8.2). The right lung is made up of three lobes and the left of two lobes. The lingular segment of the left lung corresponds to the middle lobe on the right. Each lobe is divided into segments.

The thoracic cage is lined by the pleura. There are two layers, the parietal and visceral, which are continuous with each other and enclose the pleural space. The parietal pleura is the outer layer and lines the thoracic cavity. The visceral pleura covers the surface of the lung, entering into the fissures and covering the interlobar surfaces. The two layers are lubricated by a thin layer of pleural fluid lying within the pleural space, which in health contains no other structure.

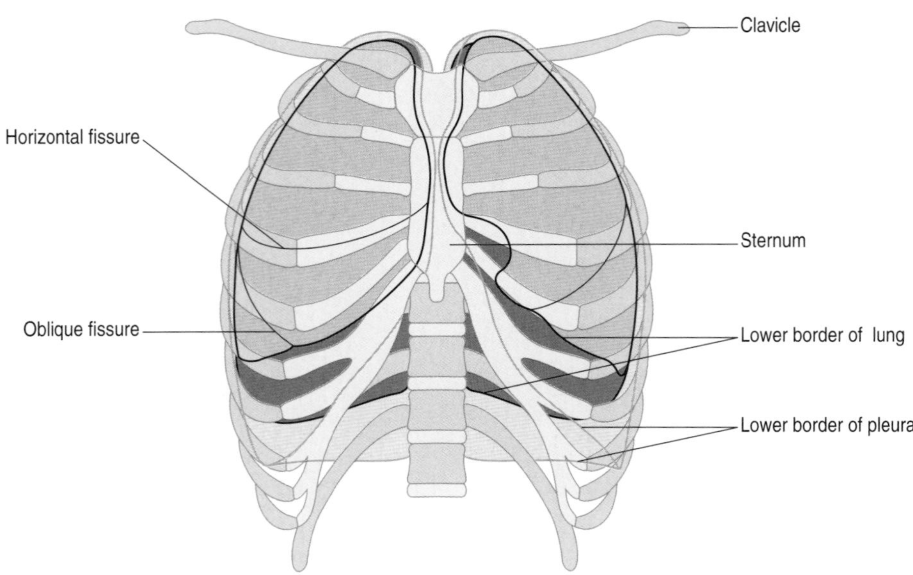

Figure 8.1 Anatomy of the thorax. (Reproduced from Jacob 2001, with permission.)

The oesophagus

The oesophagus is a muscular tube stretching from the pharynx to the stomach. It is composed of mucosa and circular and longitudinal muscle layers. The oesophagus enters the stomach below the diaphragm at approximately the level of the eleventh thoracic vertebra.

THORACIC SURGERY

Indications for surgery

Tumour

The most common reason for pulmonary and oesophageal resection is a malignant tumour (carcinoma). A small percentage of tumours can be benign.

Incidence of lung and oesophageal cancer

Lung cancer is the most common form of cancer in the world and the second most common form in the UK, after breast cancer. In 2003 there were 37 100 new cases of lung cancer diagnosed in the UK. This represents around 70 cases per 100 000 population. The male to female ratio is 3:2.

Oesophageal cancer is the ninth most common form of cancer in the UK. There were 7600 new cases diagnosed in the UK in 2003 (Cancer Research UK).

There are two histological types of lung cancer (WHO):

- *non-small-cell*: squamous-cell type 45–60 per cent; adenocarcinoma 11–28 per cent; large-cell type fewer than 1 per cent
- *small-cell*: 35 per cent.

Non-small-cell tumours are treated by resection if possible, if the tumour can be safely removed with clear margins and if metastatic disease is not in evidence. Small-cell cancer is virtually always widespread at diagnosis so surgery is usually not an option.

Malignant tumours of the oesophagus are generally adenocarcinoma, especially in the lower end. They may have arisen in the cardia of the stomach and spread proximally. In the middle and upper oesophagus squamous carcinomas predominate.

Benign tumours of the oesophagus and lungs are rare.

Pneumothorax

This is a collection of air in the pleural cavity. It usually occurs spontaneously and is due to rupture of the visceral pleura of an otherwise healthy lung. Pneumothorax is more common in men than women and more usual in the under-forties.

Patients with chronic obstructive pulmonary disease (COPD) can rupture a bulla, resulting in a pneumothorax. Other much rarer causes include tumour, abscess and tuberculosis (TB). Traumatic pneumothoraces can occur with blunt trauma to the chest wall, such as following a car accident or heavy fall, or from a penetrating chest wound, i.e. stabbing or gunshot. Iatrogenic (medical in

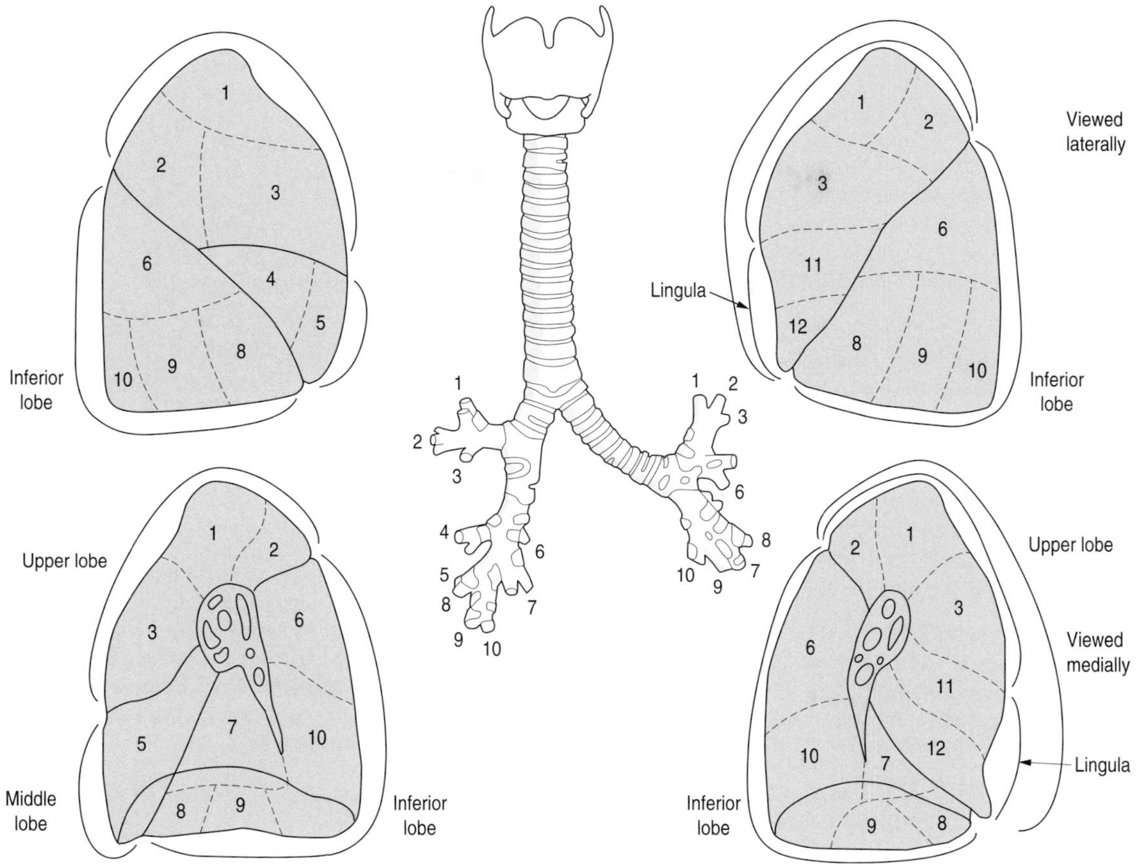

Figure 8.2 Anatomy of the lungs. Bronchopulmonary segments: 1 = apical, 2 = posterior, 3 = anterior, 4 = lateral, 5 = medial, 6 = apical basal, 7 = medial basal, 8 = anterior basal, 9 = lateral basal, 10 = posterior basal, 11 = superior, 12 = inferior. (Reproduced from Palastanga et al. 2002, with permission.)

origin) pneumothoraces can occur following intravenous line insertion, pacemaker insertion or in ventilated patients on high levels of positive end expiratory pressure (PEEP).

Empyema

Empyema is a collection of pus in the pleural cavity. The cause is commonly pneumonia, lung carcinoma or abscess, bronchiectasis or more rarely TB. It can occur in patients with septicaemia or osteomyelitis of the spine or ribs. Most empyemas are located basally but they can occur between two lobes.

Bronchiectasis

Bronchiectasis is a chronic lung condition in which abnormal dilation of the bronchi occurs, associated with obstruction and infection. Patients present with excessive production of purulent secretions, which become chronically infected. Bronchiectasis is generally managed medically with a physiotherapy regime and antibiotics. In some severe cases where the condition is localised to one area of the lung, lobectomy can offer some relief of symptoms.

Oesophageal perforation

Trauma and perforation to the oesophagus may result from the accidental swallowing of a foreign body (such as a dental plate). The oesophagus can rupture in cases of severe vomiting, especially if the patient tries to suppress the vomiting action. Iatrogenic perforation can occur following oesophagoscopy or surgery associated with the pharynx.

Preoperative investigations

Patients are assessed pre-operatively in order to establish the nature of the lesion, and whether they are fit for operation. The following investigations are commonly performed.

8

Chest X-ray

A standard chest X-ray is carried out on all patients to establish pre-operative lung status.

CT scan

In patients with cancer a CT scan is done universally. The scan will locate the lesion accurately and show if there is invasion into surrounding structures, which determines operability. The presence of metastases in distant organs is a contraindication to surgery.

Bronchoscopy/oesophagoscopy

This will establish the site of the lesion and allow biopsy or bronchial washings to be sent for histology. It can be carried out under sedation or general anaesthetic.

Pulmonary function tests (PFTs)

Respiratory function tests will help the surgeon decide whether the patient can withstand lung resection. It will also provide the anaesthetist with valuable information to assess suitability for general anaesthesia.

Arterial blood gases (ABGs)

Blood gases may be analysed routinely at some hospitals or in high-risk patients, such as those with a pre-existing lung condition.

Types of thoracic incision

Posterolateral thoracotomy

This incision is most commonly used for operations on the lung (Figure 8.3). It is a curved incision, which starts at the level of the third thoracic vertebra and follows the vertebral border of the scapula and the line of the rib extending forwards to the anterior angle or costal margin. An incision through the bed of the fifth or sixth rib is used for pneumonectomy or lobectomy.

The muscles cut are trapezius, latissimus dorsi, rhomboids, serratus anterior and the corresponding intercostal. A small piece of rib, approximately 1 cm, may be removed to allow easier retraction and avoid a painful fracture.

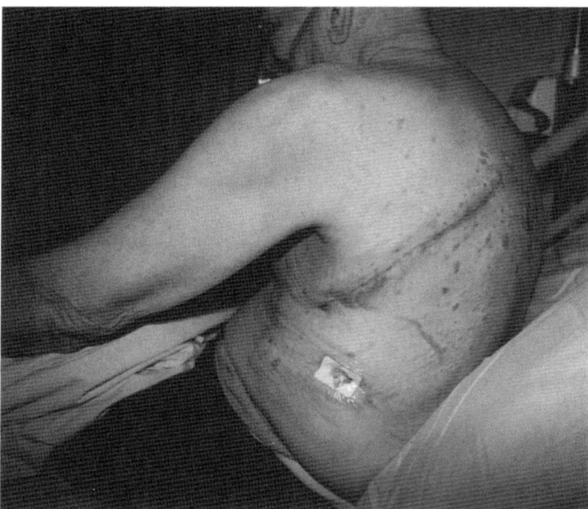

Figure 8.3 The incision for a posterolateral thoracotomy.

Anterolateral thoracotomy

This incision is used primarily for cardiac surgery but can be used to perform pleurectomy.

The incision starts at the level of the fifth costal cartilage. At the sternal edge it follows the rib line below the breast to the posterior axillary line. The muscles cut are pectoralis major and minor, serratus anterior, and the corresponding intercostal (Figure 8.4).

Median sternotomy

This incision is used for lung volume reduction surgery and bilateral pleurectomy. It is a vertical incision that involves splitting the sternum.

The incision extends from just above the suprasternal notch to a point about 3 cm below the xiphisternum. No muscle is cut, except the aponeuroses of pectoralis major (Figure 8.4c).

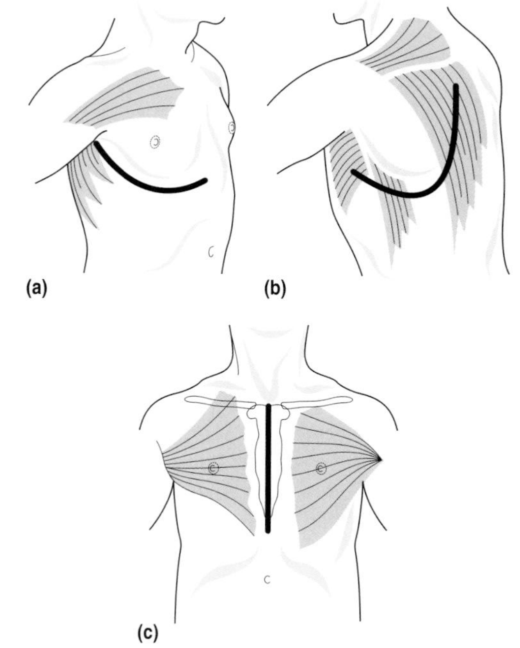

Figure 8.4 Sternotomy. Common incisions: (a) anterolateral thoracotomy; (b) posterolateral thoracotomy; (c) median sternotomy.

Left thoracolaparotomy

This incision is used for surgery on the lower oesophagus and stomach. The thoracotomy incision follows the curve of the seventh rib and extends anteriorly over the costal margin towards the umbilicus. The muscles involved are latissimus dorsi, serratus anterior, the corresponding intercostal muscles and the abdominal muscles.

> **Video-assisted thoracoscopic incisions**
>
> This relatively new technique aims to carry out conventional thoracic operations through several very small (1–2 cm) incisions, as opposed to a posterolateral thoracotomy. Instead of the surgeon seeing inside the patient directly, an endoscope with video camera attachment is introduced into the chest through one of the small incisions and the surgeon sees the image produced on television monitors in theatre. Specialised instruments are inserted via the other incisions so the operation can be completed. Advantages are reduced pain and less impact on respiratory mechanics in the postoperative period, and much smaller scars.

If an oesophageal tumour is involving the middle third of the oesophagus, surgical access may be easier through a right thoracotomy and a separate abdominal incision. If the tumour is in the upper third, then a cervical incision will also be required.

OPERATIONS ON THE LUNG

Figure 8.5 shows resection margins in lung surgery.

Pneumonectomy

Extrapericardial pneumonectomy is carried out for tumours involving a main bronchus. The whole lung is removed and the resulting cavity will fill with protein-rich fluid and fibrin over a period of weeks.

Lateral shift of the mediastinum, upward shift of the diaphragm, and reduction of the intercostal spacing on the operated side reduce the size of the cavity.

Intrapericardial pneumonectomy is a more radical procedure involving the removal of part of the pericardium. This is required when the tumour growth involves the pericardium.

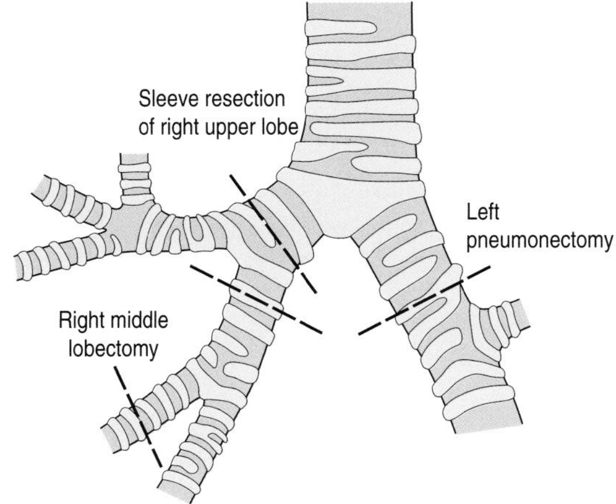

Figure 8.5 Resection margins in lung surgery.

Lobectomy

This means removal of a complete lobe with its lobar bronchus. On the right side, two lobes can be removed together: the upper and middle or middle and lower. Removal of the upper lobe on the right can sometimes include a section of right main bronchus; this is known as a 'sleeve resection'.

8

Segmental resection

A segment of a lobe, along with its segmental artery and bronchus, is removed.

Wedge resection

This is a small local resection of lung tissue.

Lung volume-reduction surgery (LVRS)

LVRS is a procedure designed to improve respiratory function in patients with severe bullous emphysema. These patients present with hyperinflated lungs and a flattened diaphragm. By excising the bullous tissue and shaping the remaining lung, expansion of the healthy lung and doming of the diaphragm can be achieved. This will result in improved respiratory mechanics and symptomatic relief of dyspnoea (breathlessness). Patients should undergo a period of pulmonary rehabilitation pre-operatively to maximise their respiratory function.

Complications of pulmonary surgery

The major complications of pulmonary surgery are listed in Table 8.1.

OPERATIONS ON THE PLEURA

Pleurectomy

Recurrent pneumothoraces will require surgical treatment. In young patients this is usually on the second or third occasion. In a small number of patients, bilateral pleurectomy will be required. In the older patient presenting with pneumothorax as a complication of COPD, surgery may be required on the first occasion.

The procedure involves removing the parietal layer of pleura from the chest wall in the area adjacent to the lung injury. This leaves a raw area to which the

Table 8.1 Complications of pulmonary surgery

Respiratory
- Sputum retention ± infection
- Atelectasis/lobar collapse
- Persistent air leak/pneumothorax
- Bronchopleural fistula (breakdown of the bronchus from which the lung tissue has been resected, more likely to occur following pneumonectomy and generally occurs about 8–10 days after surgery)
- Pleural effusion
- Surgical emphysema
- Respiratory failure

Circulatory
- Haemorrhage
- Cardiac arrhythmia: atrial fibrillation will occur in approximately 30% of lung resection patients
- Deep vein thrombosis
- Pulmonary embolus
- Myocardial infarction

Wound
- Infection
- Chronic wound pain
- Failure to heal

Neurological
- Stroke
- Recurrent laryngeal nerve (RLN) damage (the RLN supplies the vocal chords and trauma during surgery will impair the patient's ability to cough)
- Phrenic nerve damage, resulting in paralysis of the hemidiaphragm

Loss of joint range
- Loss of shoulder range on operated side
- Postural changes

lung becomes adherent and thus unable to 'collapse' again. At the same time any bullous lung tissue can be either ligated or excised.

Decortication

Decortication is carried out following chronic empyema. The procedure involves the removal of the thickened, fibrous layer of visceral pleura from the surface of the lung. This allows the lung to re-expand into the space previously occupied by the empyema.

OPERATIONS ON THE OESOPHAGUS

Oesophageal resection

Tumours in the lower third of the oesophagus are resected via a left thoracolaparotomy. The upper third of the stomach is removed, along with the oesophagus from about 10 cm above the tumour margins. The remaining stomach is passed through the hiatus of the diaphragm into the posterior pleural cavity and a circular anastamosis is created between the distal oesophagus and tip of the gastric tube.

Tumours in the middle third are more easily dealt with via a right thoracotomy and separate laparotomy. This is known as an Ivor–Lewis procedure. The stomach is passed into the right pleural cavity and the anastamosis constructed above the level of the aortic arch.

Tumours of the upper third will require resection of virtually all the oesophagus and the anastamosis will be made via an incision in the neck. The stomach is placed as with the previous procedures.

Repair of oesophageal perforations

Oesophageal perforations are treated surgically by direct repair. The site of the perforation will decide the nature of the operation. Some perforations can be treated conservatively and allow natural healing of the perforation without operative intervention.

Complications of oesophageal surgery

All the complications of pulmonary surgery apply to oesophageal operations. In addition there may be chylothorax, a pleural effusion resulting from the severing of the thoracic chyle duct. The effusion, when drained, will appear milky and on testing contains fat-staining globules. Occasionally surgical repair will be required but usually an intercostal drain (see below) will suffice until the leak stops.

There may also be anastamosis breakdown, usually due to a variable degree of gastric tube necrosis.

INTERCOSTAL DRAINS

Key point

When thoracotomy has been performed and the pleura opened, it is necessary to insert chest drains. These will commonly be referred to as intercostal drains.

Most patients will require two intercostal drains, one sited in the apex of the pleural cavity to drain air and allow the lung to re-expand, and a second drain in the basal area to drain postoperative bleeding. Patients undergoing pneumonectomy need only a single drain.

The drainage tubes are introduced through stab incisions, in an intercostal space below the level of the thoracotomy and positioned within the chest before closure. They are secured with a purse-string suture, which will allow a tight seal to be achieved whilst the drain is in situ and on its removal. The apical drain is generally sited anteriorly and the basal posteriorly. It is always wise to check this in the operation notes.

The drainage tube passes from inside the pleural cavity down to a bottle containing sterile water, and attaches to a tube that continues to below the level of the water (Figure 8.6). Above water level is a second tube that is open to the atmosphere. This maintains atmospheric pressure within the bottle. Known as an 'underwater sealed drain', it provides a simple one-way valve allowing air and blood to drain from the pleural cavity. Suction can be applied to the short tube to reduce the pressure in the bottle to below atmospheric and therefore encourage the evacuation of air and blood.

On free drainage the fluid level in the tubing will rise and fall. On inspiration the negative pressure in the thorax pulls water up the tube, and on expiration there is less negative pressure in the thorax and the water level falls. If the level ceases to swing, then either the lung is fully expanded or the drain is blocked. There will be no swing if the drain is connected to suction.

Drainage bottles must be kept below the level of insertion to prevent the siphoning of fluid back into the pleural cavity (Figure 8.7).

Amount and type of drainage

The amount of drainage is measured on a calibrated scale on the side of the bottle. Initially this will be bloodstained but it progresses to serous fluid and then stops. Air drainage can be seen as bubbles in the water, especially after coughing. Persistent air leaks are the result of a hole in the lung tissue or at the resection site. Bubbling may continue for many days and an apical

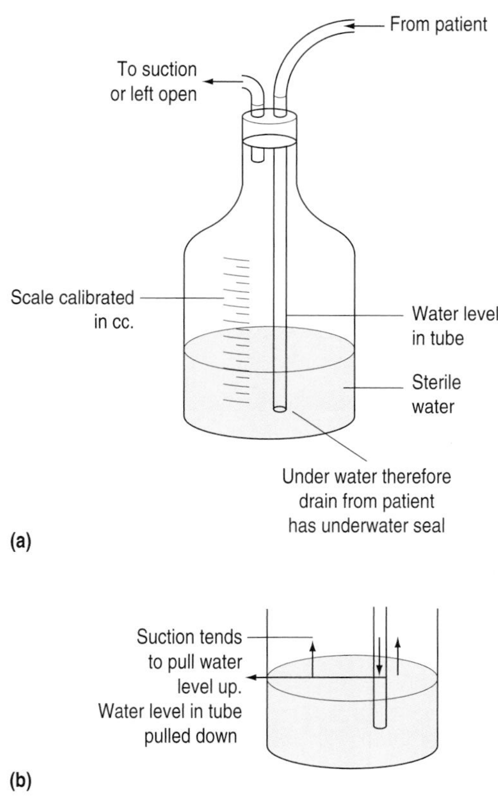

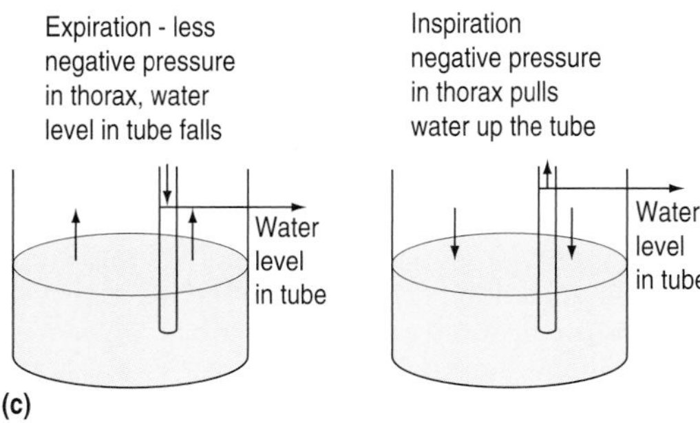

Figure 8.6 Effects of suction on water level: (a) the drainage bottle; (b) the effect of suction on water level; (c) the effect of the patient's breathing.

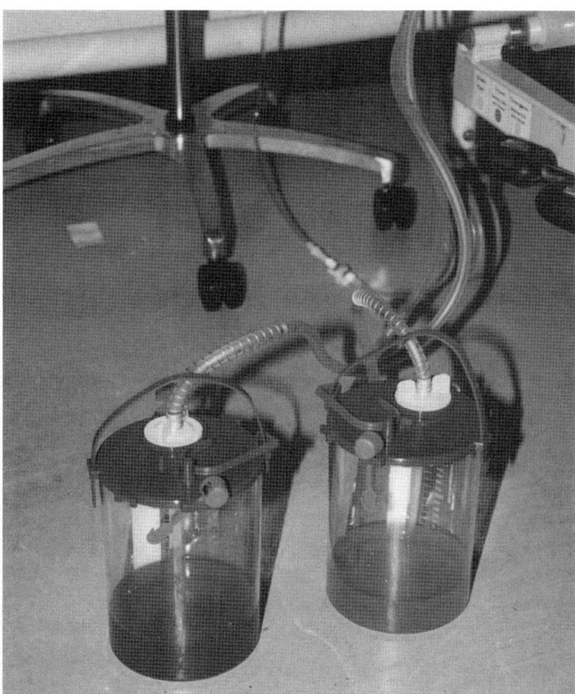

Figure 8.7 Underwater seal drainage in use.

8

drain cannot be removed until this stops. The basal drain will be taken out 24–48 hours postoperatively, the apical drain after 48–72 hours unless there is continued drainage.

PAIN CONTROL IN THORACIC SURGERY

> **Quotation**
>
> 'For all the happiness man can gain is not in pleasure but rest from pain.' (John Dryden, 1631–1700)

Postoperative pain relief is not solely for the relief of an unpleasant sensation. Disturbances of pulmonary function are common after any form of intrathoracic operation. A decrease in functional residual capacity (FRC) with minimal change in closing volume leads to atelectasis (Sabanathan et al. 1990). Patients also experience an inability to cough effectively, thus becoming prone to sputum retention leading to infection and arterial hypoxaemia (Ali et al. 1974). Pain from the incision site and drains can be severe for up to 3 days (Kaplan et al. 1975) and abnormal patterns of breathing due to pain will only worsen these problems.

Good postoperative pain control is essential in order to carry out effective physiotherapy. This can be delivered in several ways; epidural anaesthesia, paravertebral block, patient-controlled analgesia (PCA), transcutaneous nerve stimulation (TENS) and oral analgesia are the most commonly used.

Epidural anaesthesia (Figure 8.8)

An epidural provides delivery of a local anaesthetic agent such as bupivicaine and an opiate such as fentanyl directly into the small space just outside the dura mater — the 'epidural space'. The local agent will provide dermatomal relief over the incision site and the opiate a more central effect.

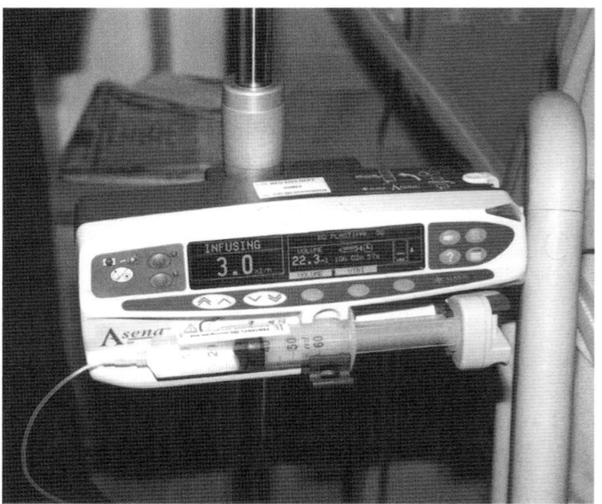

Figure 8.8 An epidural used to provide pain relief after surgery.

Epidurals can provide profound analgesia in considerably smaller doses of opiate drug than if used systemically (Chaney 1995). This will minimise the unwanted side-effect of respiratory depression commonly seen in opiate use. Lui et al. (1995) demonstrated improved analgesia with physiotherapy in thoracotomy patients using bupivicaine epidurals. An epidural will be inserted by an anaesthetist before the operation begins.

Paravertebral block

If it is not possible to insert an epidural, continuous delivery of a local anaesthetic agent can be achieved using a paravertebral catheter positioned in the paravertebral groove. This can provide safe and effective pain relief after thoracotomy (Inderbitzi et al. 1992). The catheter will be sited by the surgeon prior to closure of the chest.

Patient-controlled analgesia (PCA)

PCA allows the administration of small doses of intravenous opioids on demand by the patient. The patient must be awake, be cooperative and have had adequate instruction pre-operatively on how to use the system. The dose delivered is dependent upon patient weight. A 'lock-out' interval is set to allow time for the opiate to work, and this will also prevent overdosing.

Transcutaneous nerve stimulation

TENS can be useful if it is initiated postoperatively to relieve referred shoulder pain. The phrenic nerve supplies the diaphragm and if it is irritated during operation patients can experience ipsilateral referred shoulder pain (Scawn et al. 2001). TENS can also be of benefit in patients with persistent wound pain when an epidural or paravertebral has been removed.

Oral analgesia

Epidurals, paravertebrals and PCAs will continue, on average, for 72 hours, but analgesia will still be required for many days. The pain experience is individual and oral analgesia required will vary from patient to patient. Simple analgesia such as paracetamol or ibuprofen may be adequate, but some patients require stronger medication such as dihydrocodeine or diclofenac. Oral medication can be prescribed on a regular basis or 'as required' (p.r.n.).

Most hospitals will have a specialist nurse for pain control. The nurse will be very helpful in the care of patients with severe pain that is difficult to control on standard analgesia.

THE PHYSIOTHERAPIST AND THORACIC SURGERY

Clinical note

Chest physiotherapy has a place in the prevention as well as the treatment of postoperative pulmonary complications.

Preoperative care

The provision of preoperative chest physiotherapy is not routine, but it has been shown to be of benefit in high-risk patients. For example, Nagasaki et al. (1982) demonstrated that pre-operative physiotherapy for elderly patients and those with COPD reduced postoperative pulmonary morbidity.

Patients with pre-existing COPD are prone to increased bronchial secretions (Massard and Wihlm 1998) and may require chest clearance prior to surgery. Physiotherapy may be requested by the patient's medical team following bronchoscopic findings (i.e. sputum retention).

The pre-operative care may vary from simple education in postoperative techniques to more intensive chest clearance.

Key point

Communication is of great importance in the successful treatment of thoracic patients. The physiotherapist must communicate with nursing and medical staff in order to monitor the patient's progress. Medical notes and chest X-rays should be monitored on a daily basis. Effective communication skills will result in improved patient compliance and make treatment more effective.

Postoperative care

Postoperative complications commonly present as a restrictive pattern with reduced inspiratory capacity, reduced vital capacity (VC) and reduced functional residual capacity (FRC) (Craig 1981). There are changes in defence mechanisms due to anaesthesia and reduced cough effort (Scuderi and Olsen 1989) that can lead to retention of secretions.

Key point

The provision of chest physiotherapy after thoracic surgery is fairly routine in the UK, even though there has been little research specifically on the subject.

Postoperative physiotherapy aims to minimise the risk of non-infectious and infectious pulmonary complications (Scuderi and Olsen 1989), the most common being atelectasis and pneumonia. Other problems frequently encountered are loss of joint range in the shoulder on the incision side and reduced mobility. So the main aims of physiotherapy are:

- patient education
- maximisation of lung volume
- prevention of sputum retention
- sputum clearance
- maintenance of shoulder range of movement
- early mobilisation.

Patient assessment

The initial assessment of the patient leads to identification of specific problems. Without an accurate assessment an appropriate treatment plan cannot be initiated (Pryor et al. 1998). Re-assessment is then an ongoing process to judge the effectiveness of treatment, to identify new problems and to modify a treatment plan. Table 8.2 lists what the initial patient assessment should include.

8

Table 8.2 The Initial Patient Assessment Notes
Database: obtained from medical notes
■ Pre-operative information: PFTs/ABGs
■ Surgical procedure and incision
■ Concise relevant history of present condition
■ Relevant past medical history, including previous surgery
■ Social history
■ Drug history, with specific note of respiratory medicines, e.g. inhalers
Subjective: information the patient gives you
■ Ask open-ended questions: how do you feel?
■ Ask about pain control: can the patient cough?
Objective: information based on examination of the patient and tests carried out
■ CVS: blood pressure, heart rate and rhythm
■ Oxygen delivery system and F_iO_2
■ Blood gases or O_2 saturation
■ Respiratory rate
■ CXR
■ Method of pain control
■ Number and type of drains
■ Auscultation
■ Ability to cough
■ Range of movement of shoulder on incision side

ABGs, arterial blood gases; CVS, cardiovascular status; CXR, chest X-ray; F_iO_2, fraction of inspired oxygen; PFTs, pulmonary function tests.

Following assessment, the problems identified will commonly include:

- reduced lung volume
- retention of secretions
- increased work of breathing
- poor breathing control/pattern
- ineffective cough
- pain.

MODALITIES OF PHYSIOTHERAPY

From the initial assessment and problem identification a treatment plan can be formulated.

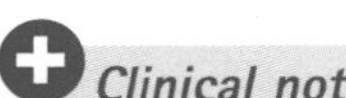

Clinical note

A particular treatment modality can be used to address more than one problem. For example, the active cycle of breathing technique (ACBT – see below) will be effective in treating reduced lung volume and sputum retention.

The amount of chest physiotherapy required will vary from patient to patient. The patient's individual requirements will primarily dictate how often and for how long treatment is needed. Consultant preference and hospital protocols may also influence this (Stiller et al. 1992).

Breathing exercises

The active cycle of breathing technique (ABCT)

The ACBT used in sitting may be sufficient to maintain effective airway clearance (Pryor and Webber 1998). ACBT consists of cycles of breathing control and thoracic expansion exercises followed by the forced expiratory technique (FET) (Figure 8.9). The thoracic expansion exercises can be combined with inspiratory hold and vibrations. In patients with reduced breath sounds, atelectasis and/or sputum retention, positioning in conjunction with ACBT may be indicated.

The whole cycle should be repeated 2–3 times or until the patient becomes non-productive. In early post-operative patients, fatigue may be an issue and treatment should be terminated at this point.

The thoracic expansions should be slow deep breaths in through the nose and then sighing out through the mouth. The end-inspiratory hold can improve air flow to poorly ventilated regions (Hough 2001); the breath hold should be encouraged at the height of the inspiratory effort for 2–3 seconds.

Patients should be encouraged to carry out at least two full cycles every waking hour in order to maintain improvements gained in lung function.

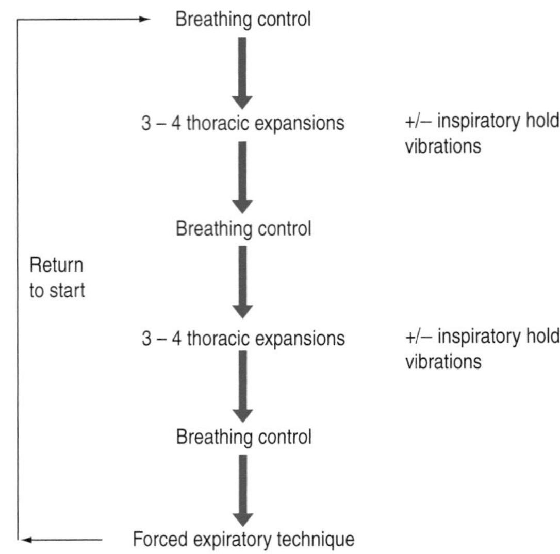

Figure 8.9 The active cycle of breathing technique (ACBT). (Adapted from Pryor and Webber et al. 1998.)

Forced expiration technique (FET)

FET is used to help in the clearance of excess bronchial secretions.

The forced expiratory technique

The technique was defined by Pryor and Webber in 1979. FET is one or two forced expirations from mid-lung to low-lung volumes (Partridge et al. 1989).

An effective FET should sound like a forced sigh. It is dependent on:

- mouth open
- glottis open
- abdominal wall contracted
- chest wall contracted.

Crackles may be heard if secretions are present.

FET performed to low lung volumes will aid removal of peripherally situated secretions. High lung volumes will clear secretions from proximal airways (Pryor and Webber 1998).

Supported cough

A cough is created by forced expiration against a closed glottis. This causes a rise in intrathoracic pressure. As the glottis opens there is rapid, outward airflow and shearing of secretions from the airway walls.

Improved coughing and FET can be achieved if the wound is supported (Figure 8.10). This can be done by the physiotherapist during treatment sessions or by

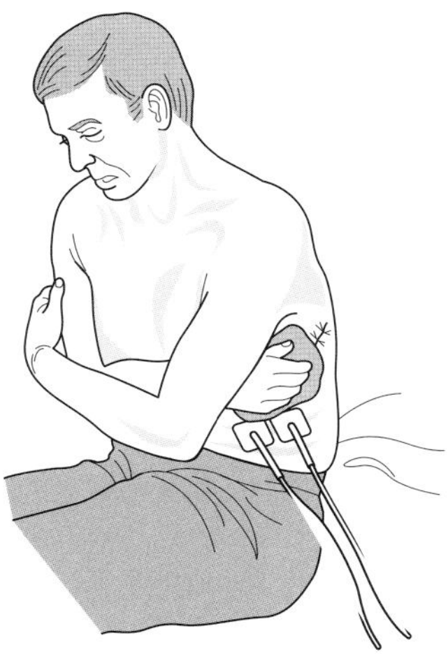

Figure 8.10 Coughing: patient supporting wound.

the patient. The arm on the unoperated side is placed across the front of the thorax and over the incision and drain sites. Firm overpressure is applied during coughing/FET. A towel, folded lengthways, passed around the back of the patient and pulled across the front of the thorax can also be useful to support coughing.

Positioning

Key point

The major function of positioning postoperatively is to improve FRC. A good sitting position either in or out of bed, as opposed to slumped in the bed, can achieve this (Jenkins et al. 1988).

There are recognised positions for segmental drainage (Thoracic Society 1950) and these may be utilised if there is a segmental or lobar-specific problem. It is much more likely, however, that modified positions only will be required, especially in view of the changed anatomy of the area.

Positioning can also be used to improve gas exchange. Improvement in oxygenation can be achieved in side-lying with the affected lung uppermost; the ventilation/perfusion match is improved, resulting in increased oxygen uptake (Winslow et al. 1990).

Pneumonectomy patients should *not* be positioned on their unoperated side. This can result in bronchopleural fistula due to space fluid washing over the bronchial stump. Patients undergoing intrapericardial pneumonectomy should be treated in sitting for the first 4 days unless advised otherwise by the medical team.

Early mobilisation

Mobilisation should commence as soon as is safely possible, as FRC is maximally improved in standing (Jenkins et al. 1988). Dull et al. (1983) proposed that early mobilisation in uncomplicated patients could render breathing exercises unnecessary. Patients must be cardiovascularly stable and not requiring high concentrations of oxygen before mobilisation can begin. If intercostal drains are on suction, mobility will be restricted to standing and spot-marching at the bedside. Some anaesthetic departments restrict mobility when an epidural is in situ, owing to the risk of profound hypotension on mobilising. Hospital protocols should be noted.

Shoulder exercises

8

The shoulder on the operated side should be checked for range of movement. The patient should practise elevation and abduction of the shoulder at least three times a day. Auto-assisted exercises may be necessary to begin with. Any limitation of range should be more formally assessed and treated.

Adjuncts to physiotherapy

Physiotherapy is a 'hands on' practice. There are several adjuncts that can be used to augment the basic breathing exercise regimen.

Incentive spirometer (Figures 8.11 and 8.12)

Incentive spirometry is a feedback system to encourage patients to take a deep breath and produce a sustained maximal inspiration in order to open atelectatic areas of lung (Su et al. 1991). It is cheap to provide, non-invasive and, when taught well, needs minimal supervision.

Bastin et al. (1997) deduced that deterioration in incentive spirometer performance could be used as a warning of pulmonary deterioration.

Mini-tracheostomy

Sputum retention is a frequent complication in patients recovering from thoracic surgery (Busch et al. 1994). It can be a result of sputum tenacity or a weak ineffective cough. Mini-tracheostomy can be an invaluable tool in the postoperative patient to aid removal of secretions in conjunction with a physiotherapy regimen.

Quidaciolu et al. (1994) concluded that mini-tracheostomy was safe and effective in reducing respiratory morbidity in high-risk patients following pulmonary surgery.

Heated humidification

Pulmonary secretions can become tenacious following surgery. This may be due to anaesthesia, infection or

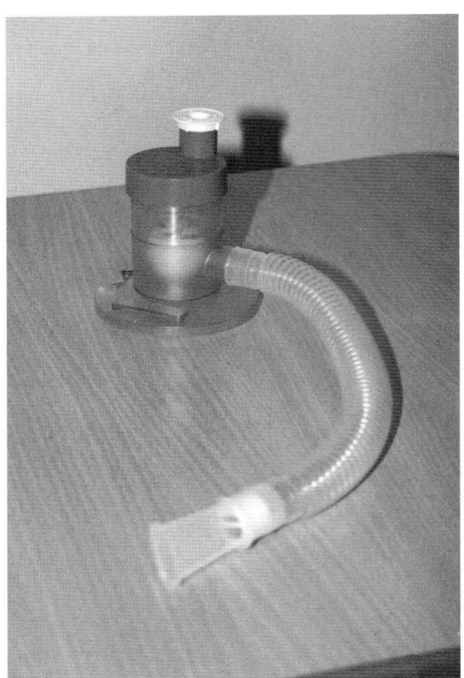

Figure 8.11 The incentive spirometer.

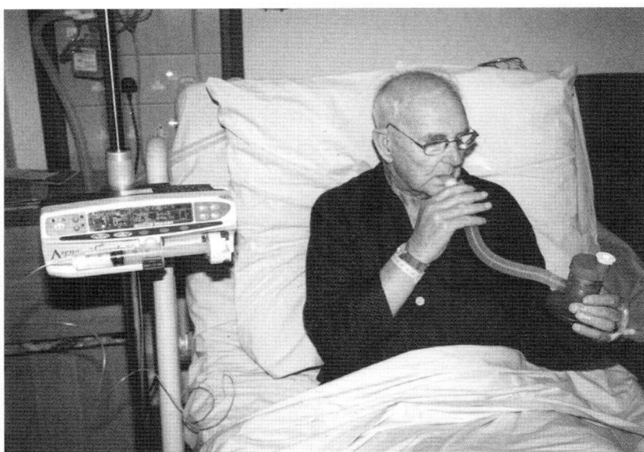

Figure 8.12 The incentive spirometer in use.

dehydration — especially in oesophageal patients who are 'nil by mouth'. Improving humidification to the airways by heating the oxygen/air delivery can help in mucous clearance.

Continuous positive airways pressure (CPAP)

Patients with poor ABGs and reduced lung volume can be supported by the use of CPAP. It can be used continuously or intermittently. When used continuously, it must be humidified.

CPAP is effective in improving FRC and arterial oxygen in patients with acute respiratory failure. It can also reduce the work of breathing (Keilty et al. 1992). Care must be taken in thoracic patients because of the anastamosis, and medical opinion should be sought.

Intermittent positive pressure breathing (IPPB)

There is little literature to support the use of IPPB, but with good teaching and in the right patient it can be effective. It is of particular use in patients who have loss of lung volume and are tiring. It works to improve lung volume and reduces the work of breathing.

Extreme care must be used when considering IPPB on lung resection patients , as the anastamosis may be vulnerable to positive pressure. The physiotherapist should discuss the use of IPPB with the patient's medical team.

DISCHARGE

Patients will reach discharge from treatment at varying points in their recovery. A low-risk patient with no postoperative complications may need only 3–4 days of physiotherapy. High-risk patients and those experiencing pulmonary complications will need considerably more. FRC and VC can be regained, even in lung resection patients. The time for full recovery of FRC is about 2 weeks; for VC it can be in excess of 3 weeks (Craig 1981). Once discharged, the patient should be advised to continue with regular breathing exercises and to increase mobility gradually.

ACKNOWLEDGEMENTS

The author and editor would like to thank Mr Richard Page (consultant thoracic surgeon), Mary Kilcoyne (physiotherapist) and all physiotherapy staff at the Cardiothoracic Centre, Liverpool, along with Jo Sharp (lecturer) at the University of Liverpool.

FURTHER READING

Hough A 2001 Physiotherapy in Respiratory Care, 3rd edn. Nelson Thornes: London

Pryor A, Webber J, Barbara A et al. 1998 Physiotherapy for Respiratory and Cardiac Problems. Churchill Livingstone: Edinburgh

REFERENCES

Ali J, Weisel RD, Layug AB et al. 1974 Consequences of postoperative alterations in respiratory mechanics. Am J Surg 128: 376–382

Bastin R, Moraine J-J, Bardocsky G et al. 1997 Incentive spirometry performance: a reliable indicator of pulmonary function in the early postoperative period after lobectomy? Chest 111: 559–563

Busch E, Verazin G, Antkowiak VG et al. 1994 Pulmonary complications in patients undergoing thoracotomy for lung carcinoma. Chest 105: 760–766

Chaney MA 1995 Side-effects of intrathecal and epidural opioids. Can J Anaesth 42: 891–903

Craig D 1981 Postoperative recovery of pulmonary function. Anaesth Analg 60(1): 46–52

Dull JL, Dull WL 1983 Are maximal inspiratory breathing exercises or incentive spirometry better than early mobilisation after cardiopulmonary bypass? Phys Ther 63: 655–659

Hough A 2001 Physiotherapy in Respiratory Care, 3rd edn. Nelson Thornes: London

Inderbitzi R, Fleveckiger K, Ris HB 1992 Pain relief and respiratory mechanics during continuous intrapleural bupivicaine administration after thoracotomy. Thorac Cardiovasc Surg 40(2): 87–89

Jacob S 2001 Atlas of Human Anatomy. Churchill Livingstone: Edinburgh

Jenkins SC, Soutar SA, Moxham J 1988 The effects of posture on lung volumes in normal subjects and in pre- and post-coronary artery surgery. Physiotherapy 74: 492–496

Kaplan JA, Miller ED, Gallagher EG 1975 Postoperative analgesia for thoracotomy patients. Anaesth Analg 54: 773

Keilty SE, Bott J 1992 Continuous positive airways pressure. Physiotherapy 78(2): 90–92

Lui S, Angel JM, Owens BD et al. 1995 Effects of epidural bupivicaine after thoracotomy. Reg Anaesth 20: 303–310

Massard G, Wihlm JM 1998 Postoperative atelectasis. Chest Surg Clin N Am 8: 281–290

Nagasaki F, Flehinger BJ, Martini N 1982 Complications of surgery in the treatment of carcinoma of the lung. Chest 82(1): 25–29

Palastanga M, Field D, Soames R 2002 Anatomy and Human Movement, 4th edn. Butterworth–Heinemann: Oxford

Partridge C, Pryor J, Webber B 1989 Characteristics of the forced expiratory technique. Physiotherapy 75(3): 193–194

Pryor A, Webber J et al. 1998 Physiotherapy for Respiratory and Cardiac Problems. Churchill Livingstone: Edinburgh

Quidaciolu F, Gausone F, Pastorino G et al. 1994 Use of mini-tracheostomy in high risk pulmonary resection surgery: results of a comparative study. Minerva Chir 49: 315–318

Sabanathan S, Eng J, Mearns AJ 1990 Alterations in respiratory mechanics following thoracotomy. J R Coll Surg Edinb 35(3): 144–150

Scawn ND, Pennefather SH, Soorae A et al. 2001 Ipsilateral shoulder pain after thoracotomy with epidural and the influence of phrenic nerve infiltration with lidocaine. Anesth Analg 93: 260–264

Scuderi J, Olsen GN 1989 Respiratory therapy in the management of post operative complications. Respiratory Care 34: 281–290

Stiller KR, Munday RM 1992 Chest physiotherapy for the surgical patient. Br J Surg 79: 745–749

Su M, Chiang CD, Huang WL et al. 1991 A new device of incentive spirometry. Zhonghua Yi Xue Za Zhi (Taibei) 48(4): 274–277

Thoracic Society 1950 The nomenclature of broncho-pulmonary anatomy. Thorax 5: 222–228

Winslow EH, Clark AP, White KM et al. 1990 Effects of a lateral turn on mixed venous oxygen saturation and heart rate. Heart Lung 19: 551–561

Chapter 9

Cardiac disease

Jonathan P. Moore

CHAPTER CONTENTS

INTRODUCTION

Diseases of the heart and circulation (cardiovascular disease or CVD) claim more lives worldwide than any other condition. Although death rates have been falling in the United Kingdom since the early 1970s, just over 216 000 people died from CVD in the UK in 2004. This figure represents more than 1 in every 3 deaths (38 per cent). The primary aim of this chapter is to provide an introduction to the diseases and disorders of the heart. An overview of the healthy heart is included. However, readers requiring more detail should refer to texts in the suggested further reading list at the end of this chapter.

Key point

In clinical terms, cardiovascular diseases may be divided into those that affect the heart and those that affect the circulation. These are referred to as cardiac and vascular disease respectively.

STRUCTURE AND NORMAL FUNCTIONING OF THE HEART

The heart is basically a muscular pump that provides the driving pressure for blood flow through the various blood vessels. Each day, the average heart will fill and empty around 100 000 times and pump around 7500 L (5000 gallons) of blood.

Anatomy of the heart

The heart is found in the mediastinum between the two lungs and lies posterior to the sternum and superior to the diaphragm (Figure 9.1). The apex of the heart projects to the left of the midline and can be felt pulsating with each heartbeat. Weighing between 200 and 425 grams

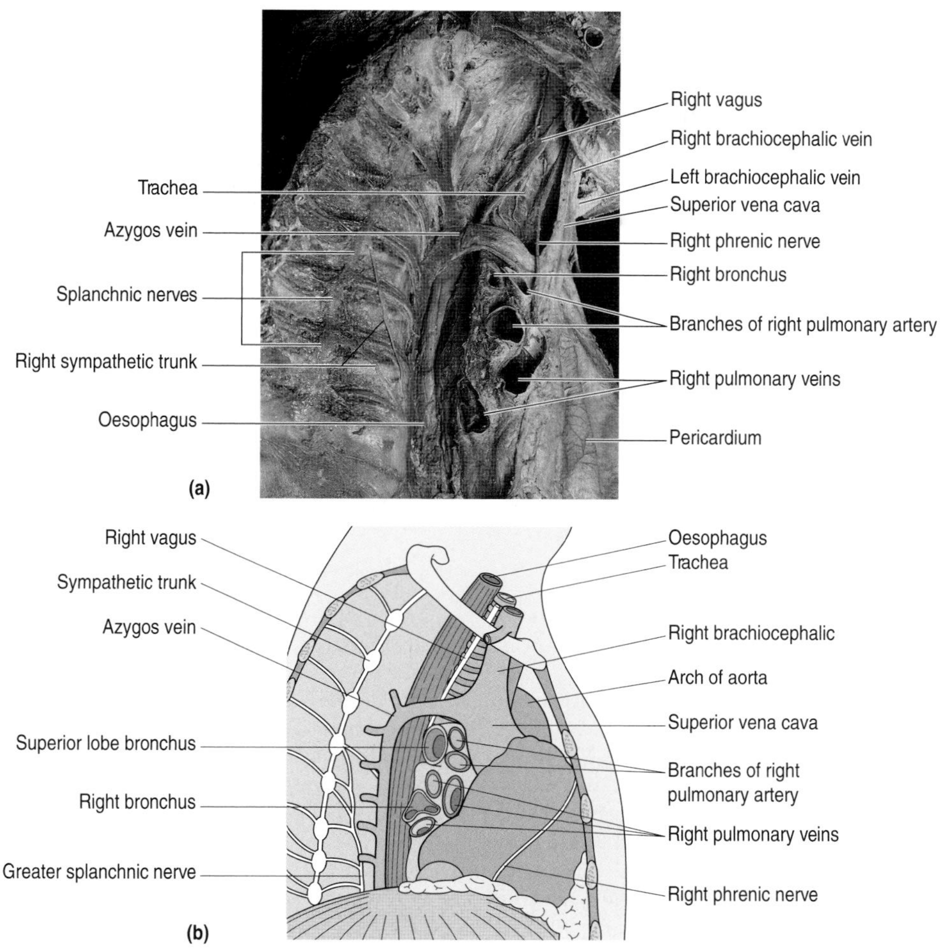

Figure 9.1 Position of the heart and associated structures in the mediastinum. (Reproduced from Jacob S 2001 Atlas of Human Anatomy. Churchill Livingstone: Edinburgh, with permission.)

when it is filled with blood, the heart is a little larger than the size of a clenched fist. The superficial anatomy of the heart is shown in Figure 9.2. A pair of thin-walled *atria* lie behind and above a pair of thicker-walled *ventricles*. The atria act as receiving chambers for blood entering the heart and the more muscular ventricles pump blood out of the heart. Both atria and both ventricles lie side by side and the portions of the walls that separate them are called the *interatrial and interventricular septums*.

Although anatomically the heart is a single organ, the left and right sides are functionally distinct pumps separated by the septum. Consequently each pump consists of an atrium and a ventricle. The right heart receives deoxygenated blood from the great veins and distributes it into the low-pressure pulmonary circulation, where it gives up carbon dioxide and takes up oxygen. Oxygen-enriched blood returns via the pulmonary veins to the left heart, which pumps it around the systemic circuit.

Structure of the heart wall

A membranous sac called the *pericardium* encloses the heart. This consists of two principal portions that are separated by a fluid-filled space called the *pericardial cavity*. An outer pericardial layer surrounds the origins of the great blood vessels and is attached by ligaments to the spinal column and diaphragm so that the heart is relatively fixed in the mediastinum. This layer, referred to as the *parietal pericardium*, is composed of tough fibrous connective tissue lined with a more delicate serous membrane that secretes a small amount of fluid into

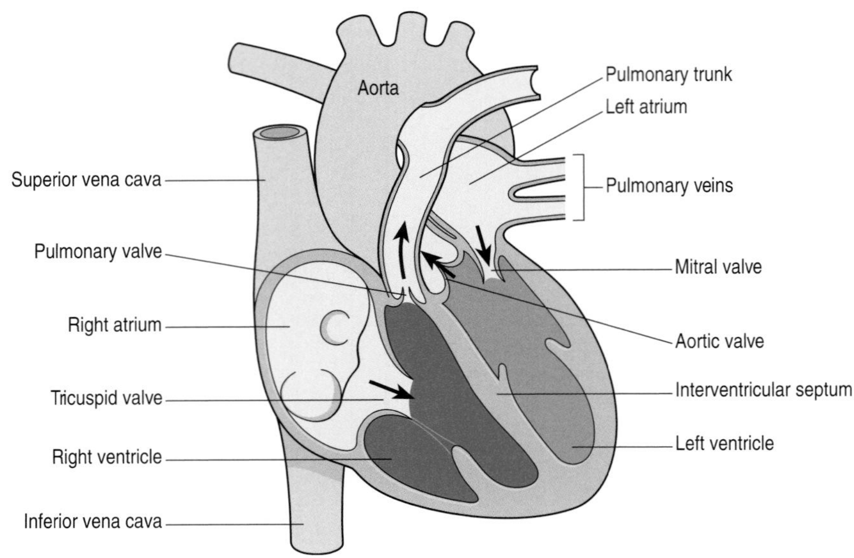

Figure 9.2 The structure of the heart.

the pericardial cavity. The fibrous connective tissue of the parietal pericardium serves to protect the heart from excessive expansion due to overfilling with blood, whereas the pericardial fluid serves as a lubricant to allow friction-free movement of the heart within the pericardium as it contracts and relaxes.

The second inner pericardial portion, the *visceral pericardium*, adheres tightly to the surface of the heart. Also known as the *epicardium*, this represents the most superficial of three layers that comprise the heart wall. Underneath the epicardium is the *myocardium*, which is the predominant layer. The myocardium is the contractile element of the heart and is composed of specialised striated muscle fibres called *cardiac muscle*. The innermost layer, the *endocardium*, which comes into direct contact with the blood, lines all four heart chambers and covers the heart valves.

Generation of the heartbeat

Alternating contractions and relaxation of the myocardium facilitate the pumping action of the heart, commonly referred to as the 'heartbeat'. Like skeletal muscle, the myocardium contracts (i.e. shortens and thickens) when it becomes electrically stimulated, or depolarised. Unlike skeletal muscle contraction, however, myocardial depolarisation is initiated within the heart muscle itself (i.e. myocardial cells show an inherent or intrinsic rhythm that is independent of any extrinsic nerve supply). However, autonomic nerves that carry impulses to the heart, and chemical messengers in the blood, are also capable of influencing the rate of heart muscle depolarisation.

Although every individual myocardial cell is potentially capable of initiating its contraction, the heart possesses a specialised excitatory and conductive system that controls cardiac contraction (Figure 9.3). The cardiac action potential begins in a group of cells referred to as the *sinoatrial* (SA) *node*. This small mass of specialised cells is located close to the point of entry of the great veins into the right atrium and is often referred to as the 'pacemaker node'. This region establishes its

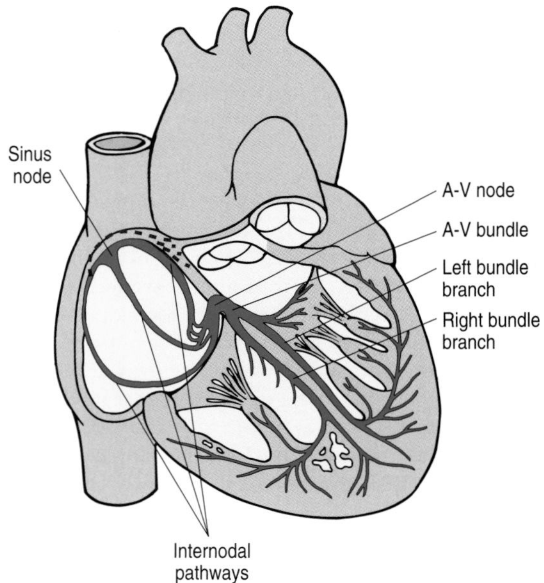

Figure 9.3 The sinus node and the Purkinje system of the heart. (Reproduced from Guyton and Hall 2005, with permission.)

dominance because its cycle of electrical depolarisation and repolarisation is more rapid than in other regions.

An electrical impulse emitted by the SA node disperses through the myocardium of the right atrium and then the left, leading to excitation and contraction of atrial muscle fibres as a single unit.

Since the atria are almost entirely separated from the ventricles by a band of connective tissue that does not conduct impulses, a conductive path from atria to ventricles is needed from a second group of specialised cells located at the base of the interatrial septum. This second area of the conductive system is called the *atrioventricular* (AV) *node*, and it consists of a narrow bundle of fibres through which conduction is relatively slow. Consequently, the impulse originating in the SA node is delayed for about one-tenth of a second at the AV node. This ensures that the atria have time to contract before ventricular muscle is excited.

The depolarisation wave emerging from the AV node is quickly transmitted over a bundle of modified myocardial fibres — the *atrioventricular* (AV) *bundle* (also known as the 'bundle of His') — in the interventricular septum.

The bundle of His splits to form left and right bundle branches that carry the depolarisation wave at around 1 metre per second to the apex of the ventricles. The electrical impulse spreads out very quickly (at 3–5 m/s) from the base of the heart through an extensive network of branching fibres, called the *Purkinje fibres*. Consequently, the ventricular contraction radiates from the apex, forcing blood upwards out of the heart and into the large arteries.

Key point

The action potential of cardiac muscle is 100 times longer than that of skeletal muscle. The refractory period of cardiac muscle is also longer, preventing summation of repetitive stimuli and sustained cardiac contractions. Consequently, cardiac contractions consist of relatively brief twitches.

The electrocardiogram

Electrical activity arising from the sequential electrical depolarisation and repolarisation of the heart muscle is transmitted through the tissues by body fluids, which are rich in electrolytes that are good conductors of electricity. Voltage differences (around 1 mV) between pairs of electrodes (leads) placed on the skin surface on each side of the heart can be amplified and recorded as an electrocardiogram (ECG) trace.

The appearance of the ECG trace depends on the position of the electrodes with respect to the electrical activity of the heart. Standardised limb leads I, II or III or chest leads are used for this purpose.

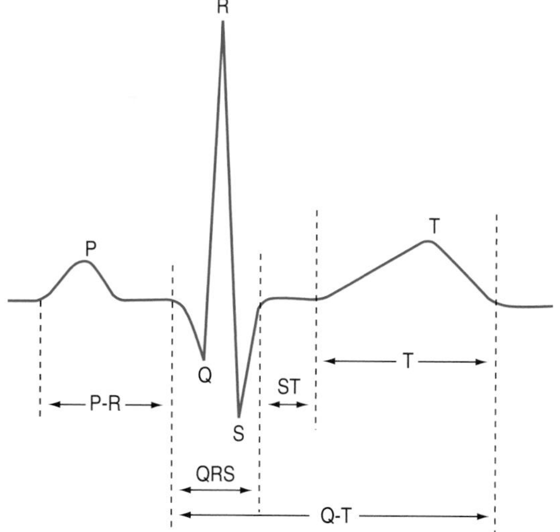

Figure 9.4 Configuration of a typical electrocardiogram (ECG). The P-wave signifies atrial depolarisation, the QRS complex signifies onset of ventricular depolarisation, and the T-wave signifies ventricular repolarisation. (Reproduced from Berne and Levy 2000, with permission.)

A typical ECG trace is shown in Figure 9.4. The *P-wave* corresponds to atrial depolarisation, the *QRS complex* occurs as the impulse travels through the ventricles, and finally the *T-wave* corresponds to repolarisation of the ventricles.

Atrial repolarisation occurs during ventricular depolarisation and is masked by the QRS complex. The *P–R interval* is due to the delay in transmission through the AV node. *The ECG thus gives information about the normal and abnormal function of the ventricular myocardium.*

Regulation of heart rhythm

The rate at which the SA node discharges electrical impulses is referred to as *sinus rhythm*. SA nodal discharge frequency is influenced by cardiac autonomic nerves, metabolic factors and respiratory activity, and sinus rhythm may increase or decrease depending upon a variety of physiological conditions that bring about changes in these factors. For example, during exercise, emotional excitement or fever, sinus rhythm will temporarily increase, and a heart rate in excess of 200 beats per minute is possible. This speeding up of heart rate is referred to as *sinus tachycardia*, and it is stimulated by increased activity in sympathetic nerves supplying the SA node and an increase in the circulating levels of the adrenal medullary catecholamines, *adrenaline* and *noradrenaline* (epinephrine and norepinephrine).

A reduction of sinus rhythm, referred to as *sinus bradycardia*, is caused by parasympathetic stimulation via the vagus nerve; it is common under less stressful conditions and during sleep. Sinus rhythm during peaceful resting usually falls to give a resting heart rate of around 60–70 beats per minute. In certain physically fit individuals sinus rhythm can be slow enough to produce a heart rate of 40–50 beats per minute. Sinus rhythm is also affected by a variety of pathological conditions, and abnormal heart rhythms may be symptomatic of underlying cardiac disease. Examples of ECGs of sinus rhythms are shown in Figure 9.5.

The heart valves

Two pairs of valves, the *atrioventricular* (AV) and *semilunar valves*, cover the inlets and outlets of both ventricles (Figures 9.6 and 9.7). Each valve consists of two or three flexible flaps, or cusps, of a yellowish-brown connective membrane.

9

The AV valves — the *bicuspid mitral valve* on the left and the *tricuspid valve* on the right — lie between the atria and the ventricles and ensure that blood cannot move backwards into the atria during ventricular contraction.

The AV valves are planted in a ring of fibrous tissue that is continuous with that which separates the atria from the ventricles. Figure 9.8 shows a set of tendons, the *chordae tendineae*, that attach the free edges of each cusp of an AV valve to papillary muscles in the ventricles and prevent them from being pushed into the atria during systole.

At the ventricular outlets, the tricuspid *semilunar valves* — the *pulmonary valve* on the low-pressure pulmonary circuit and the *aortic valve* on the high-pressure systemic circuit — ensure that blood cannot flow back into the ventricles during ventricular relaxation. Unlike the AV valves, the semilunar valves are not supported by chordae tendineae.

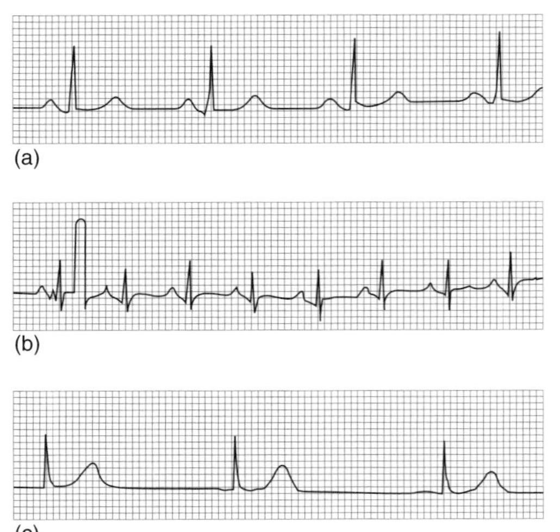

Figure 9.5 Sinus rhythms: (a) normal sinus rhythm; (b) sinus tachycardia; (c) sinus bradycardia. (Reproduced from Berne and Levy 2000, with permission.)

Key point

Sequential opening and closing of the heart valves in response to pressure changes within the heart chambers is vital in the prevention of backflow of blood from the ventricles to the atria during contraction, and from the aorta and pulmonary arteries into the ventricles during relaxation. Consequently, blood normally flows in one direction only through the heart during each heartbeat.

Circulation through the heart

Figure 9.9 summarises the flow of blood through the heart chambers and great vessels.

Deoxygenated venous blood is carried to the right atrium via the *superior and inferior vena cavae*. This blood continues its passage through the tricuspid valve into the right ventricle, which propels it via the pulmonary valve into the pulmonary trunk and on to the left and right *pulmonary arteries*. As it passes through the pulmonary circulation, the blood comes into contact with inhaled air, picks up oxygen and gives up carbon dioxide.

Oxygenated blood is returned to the left atrium through *pulmonary veins*, from where it flows to the left ventricle via the mitral valve, and into the *aorta* through the aortic valve.

Passage of blood from the left ventricle through the aorta and tissues of the body requires a considerable amount of driving force. Therefore, the left ventricle has the thickest walls of the four heart chambers, as it has to generate the greatest pressure to propel blood.

The cardiac cycle

Alternating contraction and relaxation of the myocardium allows the heart to pump blood from the veins to the arteries, and the combined events of one contraction and the subsequent relaxation is known as the *cardiac cycle*. In a resting individual with a heart rate of around 70 beats per minute each cardiac cycle lasts approximately 0.8 seconds.

The contraction phase, known as *systole*, lasts around 0.3 seconds. The relaxation phase, known as *diastole*, lasts longer (around 0.5 seconds) and it is during this period that the heart chambers fill with returning blood. Each cycle is initiated by spontaneous generation of an action potential in the SA node. Figure 9.10 shows the relationship between the electrical events and mechanical events during the cardiac cycle.

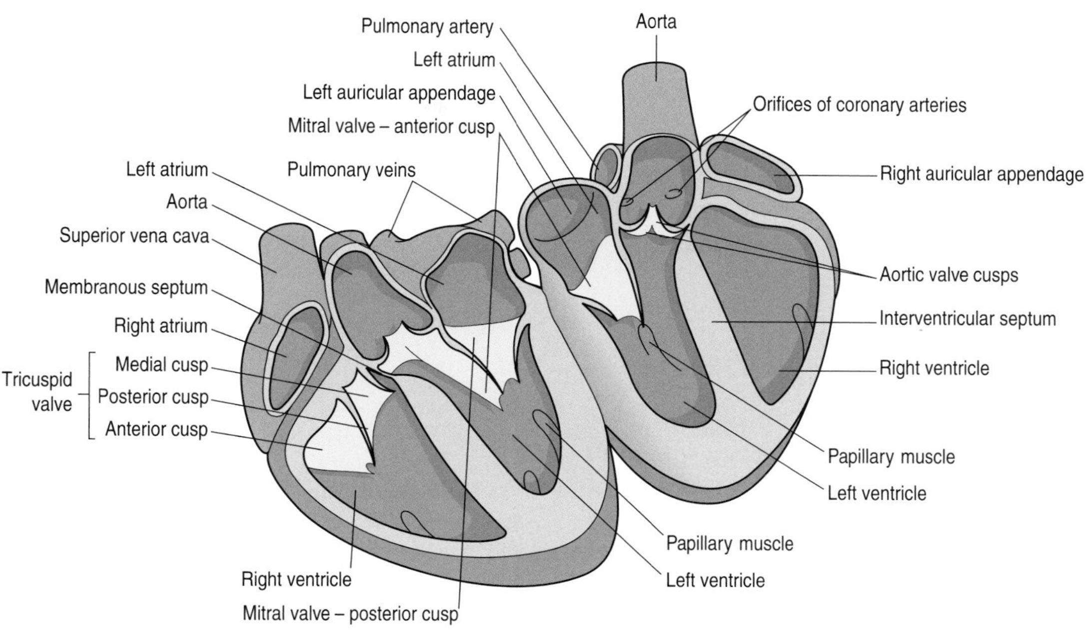

Figure 9.6 Section through the heart showing the anatomical relationships of the cardiac valves. (Reproduced from Berne and Levy 2000, with permission.)

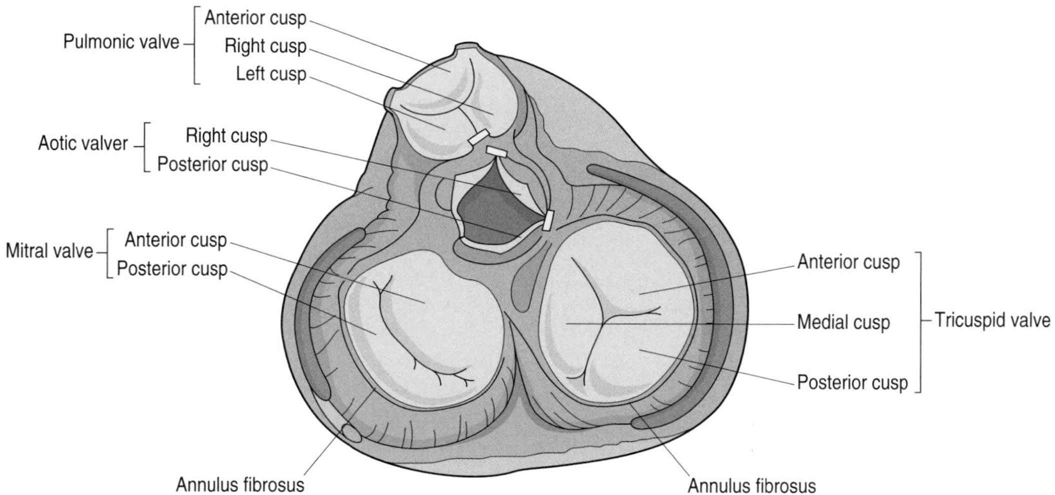

Figure 9.7 Four cardiac valves viewed from the base of the heart. (Reproduced from Berne and Levy 2000, with permission.)

Atrial systole, which coincides with the P-wave of the ECG and precedes ventricular systole, forces blood from the atria into the still-relaxed ventricles. The volume of blood (around 130 mL) present in each ventricle at the end of diastole is called the *ventricular end-diastolic volume* (EDV).

Ventricular contraction starts at the peak of the R-wave of the ECG (Figure 9.4) and forces blood from the right and left ventricles into the pulmonary artery and aorta respectively. The volume of blood (around 50–60 mL) remaining in each ventricle at the end of ventricular contraction is the ventricular end-systolic volume (ESV).

The amount of blood expelled from one ventricle during a single heartbeat (EDV minus ESV) is called the *stroke volume* and is about 70 mL in a resting human. The proportion of blood ejected during systole is called the *ejection fraction* (i.e. SV divided by EDV) and is normally around 60 per cent.

The ability of the ventricles to fill with blood under low pressure and to squeeze this into the pulmonary and systemic circulations against high arterial pressures

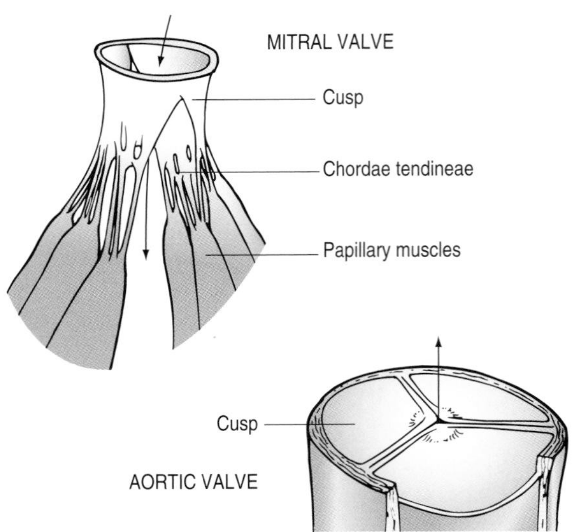

Figure 9.8 Mitral and aortic valves. (Reproduced from Guyton and Hall 2005, with permission.)

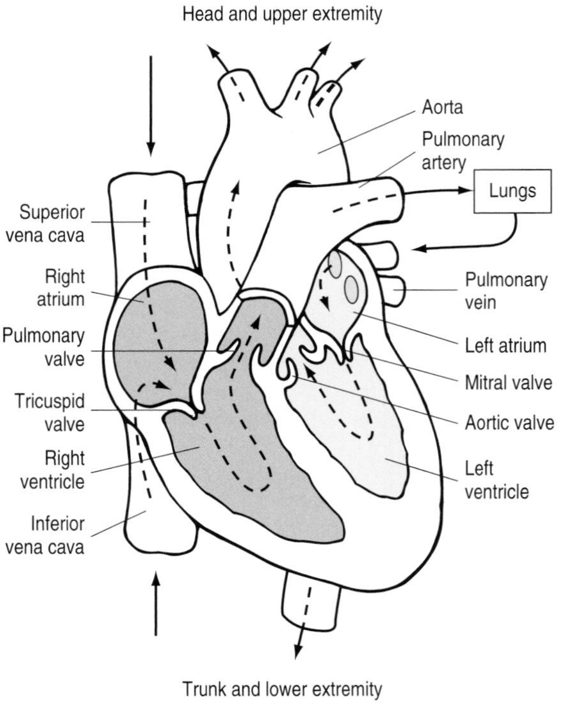

Figure 9.9 Direction of blood flow through the heart chambers. (Reproduced from Guyton and Hall 2005, with permission.)

is critically dependent on the precise operation of the AV and semilunar valves. If ventricular relaxation is taken arbitrarily to be the start of the cycle, at this point in time the pressures in the atria are higher than those in the ventricles. Consequently, the AV valves are open and venous blood is able to flow via the atria into the ventricles. This is known as the *ventricular filling phase* of the cardiac cycle. At the same time the pulmonary arterial and aortic pressures are greater than the ventricular pressures. The aortic and pulmonary valves are therefore closed and there is no outflow of blood from either ventricle.

The volume of blood in the ventricles increases during this passive ventricular filling and the ventricular pressures begin to rise. Ventricular filling continues as long as AV valves remain open (i.e. while the atrial pressures exceed those in the ventricles).

Atrial pressures are elevated further by atrial contraction (denoted by *a* in the atrial pressure curve of Figure 9.10). This ensures that more blood is forced into the ventricles through the still-open valves. Atrial contraction contributes the final 20 per cent of the blood filling the ventricles at the end of ventricular diastole.

With the onset of ventricular contraction, the ventricular pressure exceeds that of the atria and the AV valves snap shut. Closure of the AV valves prevents movement of blood in either direction between atria and ventricles. At the time of AV valve closure, both the aortic and pulmonary valves are still closed and each ventricle is in effect a sealed container. This phase of ventricular contraction is referred to as *isovolumetric ventricular systole* because there is no outlet for the blood contained within the ventricles and the intraventricular volumes remain unchanged, even though the ventricles are contracting.

Compression of blood contained within the ventricles contributes to a rapid increase in ventricular pressures. At the same time, bulging of the AV valves backwards towards the atria causes an elevation in atrial pressure referred to as the *c-wave.* As soon as the ventricular pressures exceed those in the great arteries, the semilunar valves are forced open and blood is now able to flow into the pulmonary and systemic circulations. This is the *ejection phase of ventricular systole*, which consists of a period of rapid ejection, followed by a period of rather slower emptying. Rapid ejection is characterised by increasing ventricular and arterial pressures as blood flows from the ventricles into the pulmonary and systemic circulations.

Throughout this phase of the cycle the semilunar valves remain closed and the blood leaving the ventricles is not being replaced by venous blood that is filling the atria. The combination of a reduction in ventricular volume and the onset of ventricular relaxation, however, rapidly results in ventricular pressures falling below those in the pulmonary artery and aorta. Consequently, the semilunar valves snap shut, preventing reflux of blood from the arterial system into the ventricles during diastole. Immediately before the aortic valve closes, there is a brief period of backward flow; this is followed

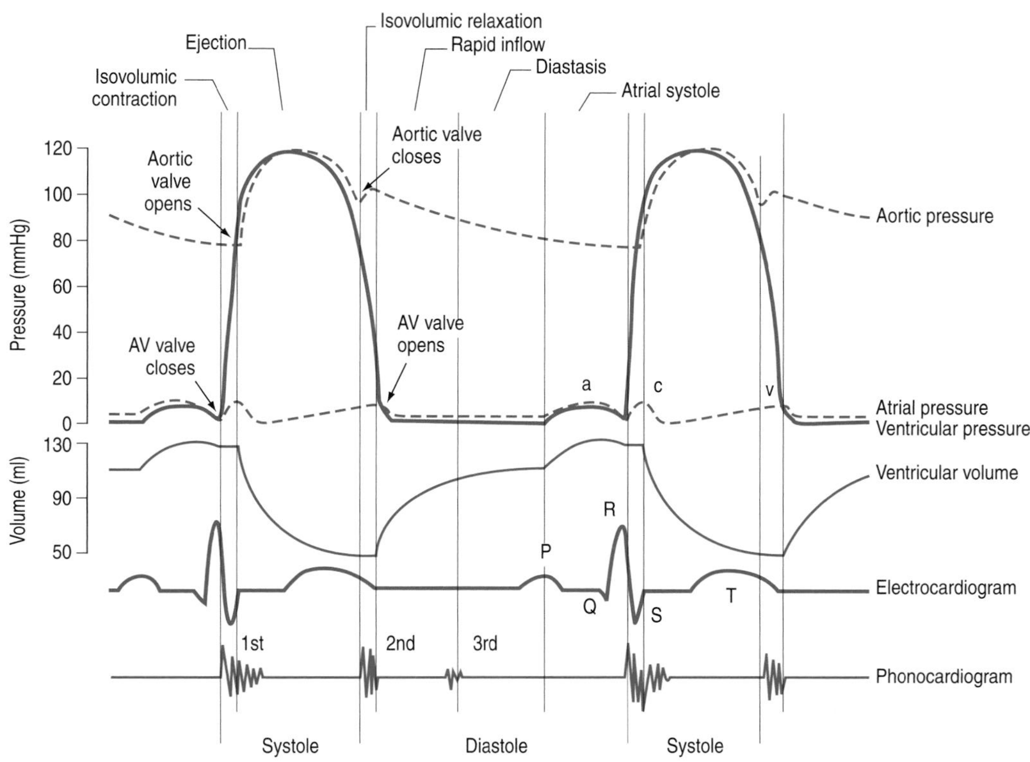

Figure 9.10 Events of the cardiac cycle for the left heart, showing changes in atrial pressure, ventricular pressure, aortic pressure, ventricular volume, the ECG and heart sounds (phonocardiogram). (Reproduced from Guyton and Hall 2005, with permission.)

by a brief surge in aortic pressure once the valve has closed. These aortic pressure changes are apparent as the 'notch' on a pressure trace recorded in a large systemic artery.

Once the semilunar valves have closed, another brief period during which all the heart valves are simultaneously closed ensues. During this isovolumetric relaxation phase, in which no blood can enter or leave the ventricles, relaxation of the ventricular myocardium accounts for a rapid decline of intraventricular pressures. Soon these fall below those pressures in the atria which have been filling with venous blood whilst the ventricles have been contracting, resulting in the *v pressure wave* in the atrial pressure curve of Figure 9.10. The mitral and tricuspid valves open and blood flows from the atria into the ventricles.

This restoration of the filling phase of ventricular diastole represents the completion of one complete cardiac cycle.

Normal heart sounds

The rhythmic closure of the heart valves during each cardiac cycle may be detected at the chest wall with a stethoscope, or by a technique known as phonocardiography that uses a low-frequency microphone connected to an amplifier and recording device.

Normally, closure of the mitral and tricuspid valves is characterised by a low, slightly prolonged 'lub' sound that identifies the onset of ventricular systole. This is referred to as the *first heart sound*. A *second heart sound*, a sharper, higher-pitched 'dup', identifies closure of the semilunar valves and the end of systole. Occasionally, a *third heart sound*, soft and low-pitched, is audible in normal hearts. This coincides with early diastole and is thought to be produced by vibrations of the ventricular wall.

Key point

Abnormal heart sounds — *heart murmurs* — may indicate the presence of a serious heart problem. These soft swishing or hissing sounds indicate that blood may be leaking through an imperfectly closing valve.

The coronary circulation

The heart muscle, like every other organ or tissue of the body, needs oxygen-rich blood to survive. Blood is

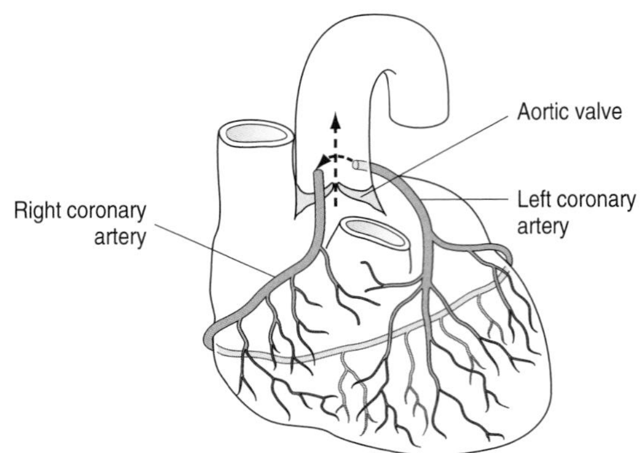

Figure 9.11 The coronary circulation. (Reproduced from Guyton and Hall 2005, with permission.)

supplied to the myocardium by its own special vascular system, called the *coronary circulation*.

Figure 9.11 shows how two main coronary arteries branch off from the aorta and divide into smaller arteries that supply the myocardial capillary network with oxygen-rich blood. The right coronary artery supplies blood mainly to the right side of the heart. The left coronary artery, which branches into the left anterior descending artery and the circumflex artery, supplies blood to the left side of the heart.

Veins accompany all the major arterial branches of the coronary circulation. Most eventually drain into the large *coronary sinus*, which lies on the AV groove on the posterior surface of the heart and opens into the right atrium.

The coronary arteries are composed of three layers. The outer layer, the *tunica adventitia*, is a loose fibrous tissue sheath that serves to anchor the blood vessel to the myocardium. A thick and elastic middle layer, the *tunica media*, is composed of smooth muscle that provides the mechanical strength of the blood vessel. Furthermore, contraction and relaxation of this muscular layer alters the radius of the coronary arteries — known as 'vasoconstriction' and 'vasodilatation' respectively — and changes the vascular resistance to coronary blood flow. The inner layer of the artery, the *tunica intima*, is made of a smooth layer of endothelial cells overlying a thin layer of connective tissue.

Key point

At rest, around 225 mL per minute of blood flows through the coronary circulation, which accounts for about 4–5 per cent of the output of the left ventricle.

An important feature of coronary blood flow is that it is intermittent. During systole, the external pressure exerted by the contracting myocardium compresses the coronary vessels — known as 'extravascular compression' — which impedes the free flow of blood through the coronary circulation. This is despite the fact that there is a high pressure driving blood out of the aortic root and into the coronary arteries during ventricular systole. Consequently, flow to the myocardium is at its peak during early diastole when the mechanical compression of the coronary vessels is minimal.

Figure 9.12 shows the pattern of coronary blood flow in the left and right coronary arteries. The differences in flow may be attributed to the fact that the left ventricle has a greater muscle mass, and therefore larger blood supply, and the fact that myocardial contraction — and therefore coronary artery compression — is greatest in the walls of the left ventricle.

Despite the compression of coronary blood vessels that occurs during each cardiac cycle, coronary perfusion and myocardial metabolism are closely matched. Indeed, during maximal cardiac work the coronary blood flow can increase from a resting level of around 75 mL per minute to as much as 300–400 mL per minute for each 100 g of heart tissue. This increase in flow, known as 'hyperaemia', is mediated largely by local metabolic vasodilatation and takes place despite a

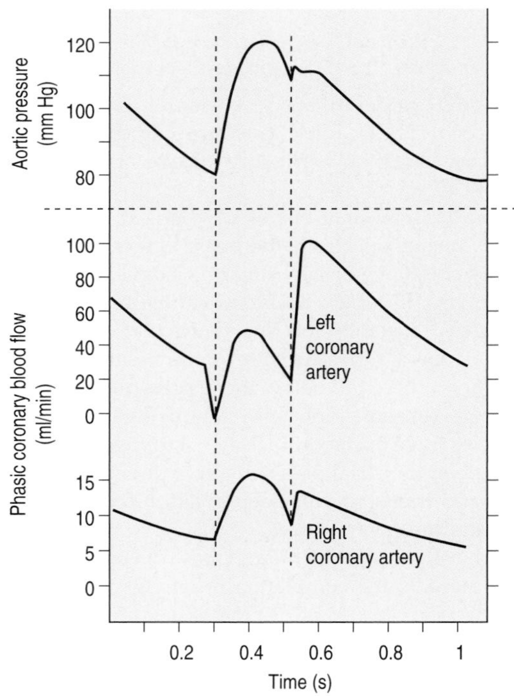

Figure 9.12 Comparison of phasic coronary blood flow in the left and right coronary arteries. (Reproduced from Berne and Levy 2000, with permission.)

reduction in the duration of diastole at high heart rates.

The precise nature of metabolic vasodilatation is largely unclear, but it is generally accepted that a decrease in the ratio of oxygen supply to oxygen demand releases some vasodilator substance(s) from the myocardium into the interstitial fluid, where it can relax the coronary resistance vessels. Among the substances implicated are CO_2, O_2, hydrogen ions (liberated from dissociation of lactic acid produced by myocardial tissue), potassium ions and adenosine.

Normal cardiac function

The primary physiological function of the heart is to pump blood to vital organs and tissues to meet their metabolic requirements (i.e. delivery of oxygen and nutrients and removal of metabolic by-products). The volume of blood pumped out of the heart each minute, the *cardiac output*, is a measure of the total blood flow through the lungs and around the body and is the product of heart rate and stroke volume.

$$\text{Cardiac output (litres per minute)} = \text{stroke volume (mL)} \times \text{heart rate (beats/min)}$$

Cardiac output is closely matched to the fluctuating demands of the body's organs and tissues for blood flow. Under steady-state conditions, the cardiac output of the right heart equals that of the left heart — i.e. flows in the pulmonary and systemic circulations are equal. In an adult human at rest, the cardiac output is between 4 and 7 L per minute. Normally this figure decreases during sleep, and is raised following a heavy meal or under conditions of stress. During periods of strenuous physical activity, cardiac output may be raised by as much as six-fold.

Since it is the product of heart rate and stroke volume, cardiac output is altered by changes in one or both of these variables. The influence of autonomic and humoral factors on heart rate, via the pacemaker cells of the SA node, has already been briefly discussed. Stroke volume is also influenced by autonomic and humoral factors, which alter the force of myocardial contraction. However, as stroke volume is equal to the end-diastolic volume minus the end-systolic volume, factors that influence these volumes also affect the stroke volume.

Myocardial muscle is similar to skeletal muscle in that it can generate a more forceful contraction when it has been prestretched or preloaded. This phenomenon is summarised by the *Frank–Starling relationship*, which states that the greater the degree of tension in myocardial fibres at the end of diastole, the more forceful the subsequent myocardial contraction. The degree of tension in myocardial fibres at the end of diastole is determined by the end-diastolic volume, a phenomenon known as *preload*. Common examples of alterations to preload may be observed under conditions when the amount of blood returning to the heart, the *venous return*, is changing. This may occur during postural changes and in the transition from relative inactivity to moderate exercise. For example, if there is a transient increase in the venous return, the end-diastolic volume and therefore preload will be increased, resulting in a more forceful myocardial contraction.

Another determinant of stroke volume is the resistive forces in the circulation that oppose ventricular ejection. The term *afterload* describes this resistance and an increase in this factor usually results in a transient reduction in stroke volume. However, stroke volume is normally able to recover within one or two heartbeats; reflex mechanisms ensure an unchanged venous return and this, combined with the increased end-systolic volume, results in ventricular distension and an increased preload. This produces a greater force of myocardial contraction and a more complete emptying of the ventricles, returning the stroke volume to normal. This feedback mechanism is known as *intrinsic regulation of myocardial contractility*.

Sympathetic nerve activity and circulating levels of various hormones, such as catecholamines, are also responsible for increasing the force of myocardial contraction. This extrinsic mechanism is particularly important when there has been an increase in heart rate — during exercise, for example — which reduces the time available for ventricular filling. Under these conditions an increase in venous return plus increased sympathetic activity increase the force of contraction so that the ejection fraction increases.

Figure 9.13 summarises the four factors that determine cardiac output.

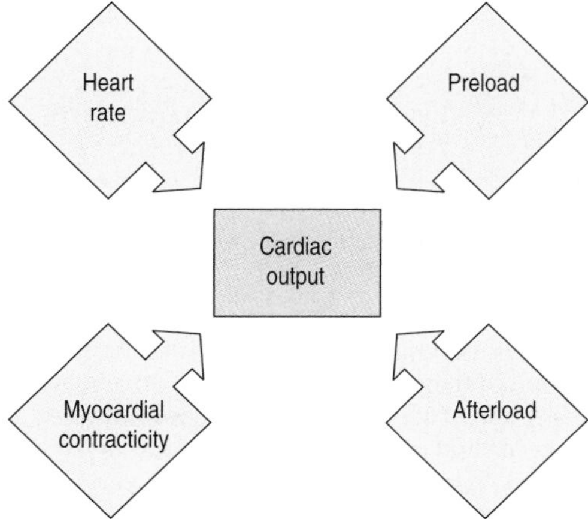

Figure 9.13 Factors that determine cardiac output.

HEART FAILURE

Definition

An abnormal pumping action is a principal component of almost all forms of heart disease. Consequently, heart failure may be defined as the pathological state arising from some cardiac abnormality that is responsible for the heart's inability to pump enough blood to satisfy the demands of the body.

Introduction

The causes of heart failure are numerous because many conditions and diseases affect the heart, its valves and its blood supply. In most cases, the common denominator is severe myocardial damage leading to an extra workload being imposed on the heart. Current British Heart Foundation statistics for the UK indicate that around 675 000 people have definite heart failure (and a further 235 000 have probable heart failure).

This reduced capability to pump blood is often associated with a reduction in the *ejection fraction* that is accompanied by cardiac enlargement. There is a resultant fall in cardiac output and perception of a low blood pressure by neurohumoral reflexes. This results in a range of compensatory responses, including systemic vasoconstriction and blood volume expansion. The aim of these is to maintain perfusion to critical organs, notably the brain and the heart, which cannot survive a prolonged reduction in blood flow.

Whilst these compensations aid survival, they may become maladaptive over time and lead to further pump dysfunction. For example, the peripheral vasoconstriction that serves to maintain perfusion acutely causes an increase in afterload, which when sustained becomes detrimental by exacerbating pump dysfunction.

Key point

Heart failure may be acute or chronic. Acute failure may be caused by toxic quantities of drugs or by certain pathologies, such as sudden coronary artery occlusion. Chronic heart failure may occur in conditions such as hypertension or ischaemic heart disease (IHD).

In the early stages of heart failure there may be no obvious circulatory impairment, though the heart may be dilated and enlarged on a chest X-ray. As the syndrome develops, the symptoms are related predominantly to the retention of fluid and vascular congestion — oedema — throughout the body. Congestion can vary from the most minimal of symptoms to a sudden abnormal accumulation of fluid in the lungs. The term 'congestive heart failure' is often used to describe the clinical syndrome that results from central heart failure and the compensatory response of the peripheral organs and circulation.

Signs and symptoms of heart failure

Fluid retention leading to vascular congestion is a prominent feature of early and untreated heart failure. A major cause of vascular congestion is an alteration in the person's ability to excrete sodium and water. Although the exact nature of these changes is unclear, it may be in some way related to a fall in renal blood flow.

It is well established that renin, a hormone released by the kidneys under conditions of decreased renal flow, initiates a sequence of events (involving angiotensin and aldosterone) that promotes the retention of salt and water. Accumulation of salt and water in the extracellular fluid can lead to clinical oedema. Whilst the person is in the upright position the fluid may gather around the ankles and feet, and in severe cases this peripheral oedema may extend to the lower legs, thighs and groin. Whilst the person is lying down, fluid may accumulate in the back and around the abdomen, and is referred to as *ascites*.

Heart disease most frequently affects the left ventricle in some way or another. If the left ventricle fails to pump blood adequately around the systemic arteries, a rise in left ventricular end-diastolic pressure will cause an elevation of left atrial pressure that is transmitted to the pulmonary veins. The 'back pressure' resulting from an increase in pulmonary venous pressure can cause congestion of the pulmonary circulation and reduce the amount of space available in the lungs for air. Pulmonary congestion also tends to reduce lung compliance.

In extreme cases, pulmonary capillary pressure may reach a point at which there is transudation of fluid from the vascular space to the pulmonary interstitium and eventually the alveoli. Accumulation of fluid in the alveoli, referred to as *pulmonary oedema*, can result in breathing difficulties, and respiratory distress is the most dramatic symptom of pulmonary congestion. Less severe symptoms of pulmonary congestion include breathlessness (dyspnoea) during exercise, whilst lying flat at rest or when asleep (paroxysmal nocturnal dyspnoea). The combination of left ventricular failure and pulmonary congestion is often called *left heart failure*.

Increased pulmonary venous pressure in left heart failure can also cause an increase in pulmonary arterial pressure, known as *pulmonary hypertension*. This often contributes to the development of right ventricular failure.

Under conditions of an elevated pulmonary arterial pressure, the right ventricular end-diastolic pressure becomes increased and is transmitted to the right atrium, causing back pressure in the veins all over the body. People with right heart failure often develop clinical signs of peripheral oedema, congestion of the liver and high pressure in the veins.

Key point

Other causes of pulmonary hypertension, which are independent of left heart failure, include tricuspid valve disease and cor pulmonale, the latter a condition that develops secondary to lung disease.

Detection and treatment of heart failure

Detection

Throughout the various stages of heart failure it is rare for there to be any evidence that blood flow is insufficient to provide adequate tissue perfusion. One exception is the shock state that occurs in acute and severe cardiac failure and in which there is acute inadequacy of flow to some critical tissues.

In the early stages of heart failure the inadequacy of the heart may become apparent only under stressful situations. Symptoms such as fatigue and weakness are generally related to poor perfusion of active muscles during exercise following a decline of cardiac output. Difficulty in breathing during exertion may also occur, but pulmonary oedema is not usually present. Other manifestations of a reduced cardiac performance and low output state include sinus tachycardia, light-headedness or fainting (syncope), mental confusion and cool pallid skin.

In moderate congestive heart failure, there is marked limitation of physical activity. Signs and symptoms may also become apparent at rest. Should the condition become severe, there will be increasing manifestations of left and right heart failure and the patient will become more disabled. Ultimately heart failure may become totally disabling, with severe respiratory distress and the inability to lie flat and to exercise. When such circumstances are prolonged, general ill-health may develop, with various secondary effects such as malnutrition or diarrhoea.

A degree of heart failure, from mild to severe, may occur following acute and severe cardiac damage (e.g. acute myocardial infarction). This can result in a rapidly lethal shock-like state characterised in most cases by low blood pressure, a weak, rapid pulse, and cold sweaty skin. This is referred to as *cardiogenic shock* and it may or may not be accompanied by other symptoms of cardiac failure — peripheral oedema and pulmonary congestion — depending on the duration and severity of the shock state.

Treatment

Treatment of people with heart failure is generally aimed at:

- increasing the pumping function of the heart
- reducing the volume of blood that must be pumped
- reducing fluid retention
- controlling the vascular tone.

Digitalis drugs (also known as cardiac glycosides) increase the force of myocardial contraction without increasing heart rate, and for many years these were the cornerstones of drug treatment for heart failure. One of these, digoxin, is still very useful in patients with arrhythmias that can lead to heart failure, but it is not often prescribed now for people with a normal rhythm. However, it retains a place in the treatment of heart failure in certain patients.

Blood volume reduction is achieved through the use of diuretics, which increase the amount of water excreted in the urine. This is a very effective way to reduce the amount of blood that must be pumped by the heart and to relieve any vascular congestion caused by heart failure. However, diuretic therapy sometimes causes excessive potassium loss through the urine. Low potassium can trigger abnormal heart rhythms, especially in those taking digitalis. The imbalance may be corrected by using potassium supplements or a potassium-sparing antidiuretic.

Another group of drugs used to treat heart failure are vasodilators, which reverse the narrowing of blood vessels. This results in a reduction in resistive load, which is of major benefit to the heart as it reduces the amount of work that it must perform to pump the blood around the circulation. Several classes of drug are prescribed for their vasodilator effect: nitrates, angiotensin-converting enzyme (ACE) inhibitors, calcium-channel blockers, and sympatholytics.

Diagnosing heart disease

Electrocardiography, which was discussed earlier in the chapter, provides information on the passage of the cardiac action potential through the myocardium and is commonly used to detect heart rhythm disorders. Another common non-invasive diagnostic test during the initial evaluation of heart disease is a chest X-ray to determine if there is any cardiac enlargement.

In recent years, echocardiography, which produces an ultrasound picture of the heart and valves, has been more commonly used to provide a diagnosis of cardiac enlargement. By determining cardiac volumes during the cardiac cycle, echocardiography also provides an indication of the degree of myocardial dysfunction.

Cardiac catheterisation is an invasive procedure that enables a number of other tests to be performed. Catheterisation requires a fine tube to be introduced through a vein in the arm or the femoral artery in the groin. The tube is advanced under X-ray guidance to the heart chambers. Once in place, the catheter may be used in a number of ways. A radio-opaque contrast medium may be injected through the catheter and its progress through the heart chambers followed by X-ray cinematography. This technique, known as angiocardiography, shows the movement of the heart walls, valve defects and the extent of coronary artery occlusion by establishing where and by how much the arteries are narrowed. The catheter may also be used to measure the rate of blood flow and blood pressures within the heart during the cardiac cycle. From the results of these tests it is possible to gain an idea of how well or poorly the heart is pumping.

Sometimes small pieces of heart muscle (biopsies) are also taken during the cardiac catheterisation for laboratory study. Such heart muscle biopsies are helpful in the evaluation of possible infections of the heart, as well as certain metabolic abnormalities of the heart.

DISTURBANCES OF HEART RHYTHM

> **Key point**
>
> The normal heartbeat is initiated by the pacemaking sinoatrial node and then passes along the conducting pathways so that the heart beats with a regular rhythm. If the conduction system fails, the heartbeat may be abnormal – either tachycardic, bradycardic or irregular.

Arrhythmias

The general term for an irregular heartbeat is *arrhythmia*, although the term *dysrhythmia* is also used. Occasional arrhythmias, such as an extra beat or skipped beat, can take place in a healthy heart and may be of minimal consequence. However, abnormal heart rhythms may also occur if there is a birth defect, coronary heart disease and other less common heart disorder. Various systemic conditions, including hyperthyroidism, and certain drugs, caffeine for example, can disturb the heart rhythm.

A common manifestation of disordered heart rhythm is an uncomfortable awareness of a very rapid heartbeat, referred to as *palpitation*. However, exercise or anxiety is another possible cause of this.

Prolonged or chronic arrhythmias often lead to severe pump dysfunction and a reduction in cardiac output that lowers blood pressure and affects perfusion of vital organs like the brain and heart. Consequently, arrhythmias may also be associated with shortness of breath, light-headedness, fatigue, blackout or syncope, and in extreme cases, sudden cardiac death. The presence of an arrhythmia usually represents a lack of normal communication between the atrial and ventricular conduction systems.

Atrial flutter and fibrillation

Atrial flutter is a term used to describe regular atrial activity so rapid — between 240 and 400 contractions per minute — that the conduction of impulses to the ventricles may be impaired so that only every other or every third impulse excites ventricular activity and a detectable pulse. This is characterised by the absence of a normal P-wave on the ECG and overall the pulse is around 150 beats per minute. Because the atria are electrically isolated from the ventricles except for the conduction system, the atria can enter tachycardia without the ventricle being affected.

Atrial fibrillation (AF) describes a common form of arrhythmia in which the atria beat rapidly and incompletely in a chaotic and irregular manner. Atrial fibrillation may be transient or persistent, and may contribute to ineffective pumping of blood by the heart. Figure 9.14 shows the ECG during atrial fibrillation.

Development of blood clots within the atrial walls is a complication of atrial fibrillation. If a formed clot fragments and passes into the circulation, it may precipitate a stroke or a pulmonary embolism.

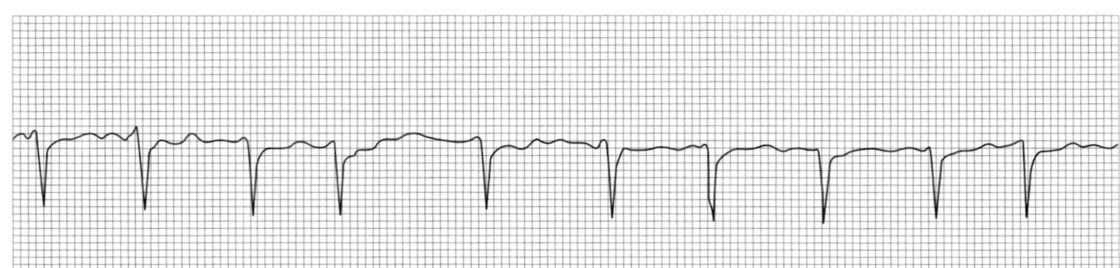

Figure 9.14 Atrial fibrillation. (Reproduced from Berne and Levy 2000, with permission.)

Ventricular tachycardia and fibrillation

Ventricular tachycardia (VT) is a dysrhythmia characterised by a heart rate typically greater than 120 beats per minute and wide QRS complexes on the ECG (Figure 9.15). If a run of tachycardia lasts less than 30 seconds, it is referred to as *unsustained VT*; a longer duration is considered *sustained VT*. VT is commonly associated with coronary heart disease and contributes to interference with normal cardiac filling and ejection. Consequently, prolonged VT may result in congestive failure, whereas severe and acute VT leads to the development of a shock state.

Ventricular fibrillation (VF) is a pulseless arrhythmia with irregular and chaotic electrical activity and ventricular contraction (Figure 9.16).

Consequences and treatment of arrhythmia

Fibrillating atria and/or ventricles lose the ability to function as a pump relatively quickly. During ventricular fibrillation in particular, a sudden loss of cardiac output, with subsequent lowering of tissue perfusion (hypoperfusion), creates global tissue ischaemia. The cells of the brain and myocardium are most susceptible to infarction.

Clinical note

If treated in time, many atrial and ventricular arrhythmias can be converted into normal rhythm by applying an electrical shock that resets and restores the normal rhythm to the heart. This is referred to as *cardioversion* or *defibrillation* (Figure 9.17).

Drug treatments for arrhythmia include beta-blockers, calcium-channel blockers, digitalis drugs and quinidine.

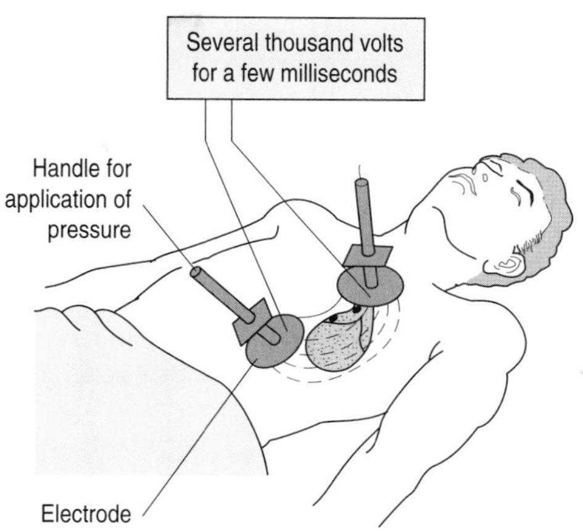

Figure 9.17 Application of electrical current to the chest to stop ventricular fibrillation. (Reproduced from Berne and Levy 2000, with permission.)

These anti-arrhythmic drugs work by altering the conduction rate of the cardiac action potential through the myocardium. In patients who have had a life-threatening arrhythmia, or those with risk factors for such arrhythmias, an implantable cardioverter-defibrillator (ICD) can deliver a small internal shock directly to the heart when an abnormal rhythm is detected. This returns the heart to a normal rhythm.

Heart block

Occasionally, malfunction of the conduction system results in the cardiac action potential impulse becoming delayed or interrupted. This results in a *bradycardia* or heart block. Also known as *atrioventricular* (AV) *block*, heart block is a condition characterised by a lack of synchronisation between atrial and ventricular contractions. This situation

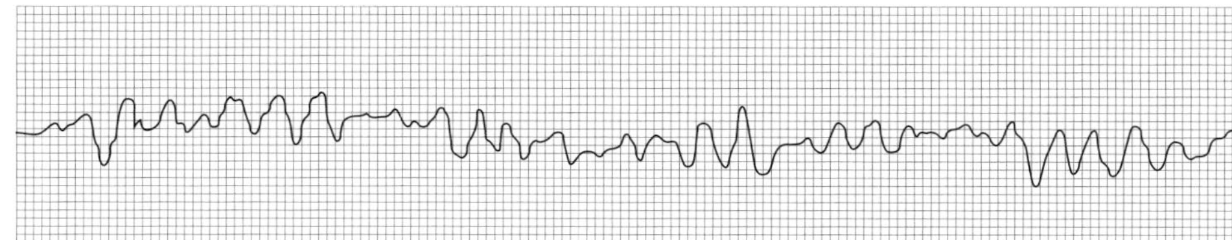

Figure 9.15 Ventricular tachycardia. (Reproduced from Berne and Levy 2000, with permission.)

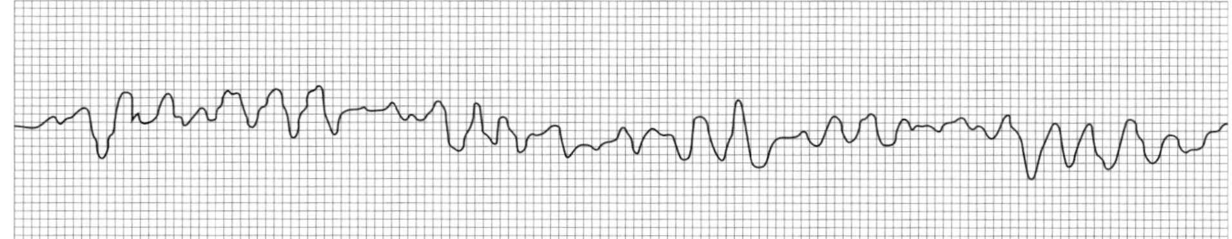

Figure 9.16 Ventricular fibrillation. (Reproduced from Berne and Levy 2000, with permission.)

can be diagnosed on an ECG and is classified according to the severity of impairment. In *first-degree heart block* the conduction time from the atria to the ventricles is prolonged; this is characterised by a longer than normal (> 0.2 seconds) interval between the P-wave and QRS complex on an ECG (Figure 9.18a).

Electrophysiological studies have shown that first-degree heart block may be due to conduction delay in the AV node, in the His–Purkinje system, or both. This condition does not normally result in clinical manifestation. Certain drugs used in the treatment of other heart conditions such as digitalis can cause first-degree heart block.

In *second-degree heart block* some action potentials that have travelled normally from the SA node to the AV node fail to induce ventricular contractions and a QRS complex on the ECG (Figure 9.18b). This results in missing or 'dropped' heartbeats. Since the conduction system below the AV node divides into two major branches, blockage of impulse transmission in either of these is termed *right- or left-bundle block*.

Third-degree (complete) heart block occurs when the cardiac action potential does not pass from the atria to the ventricles. In this situation, atrial contraction usually continues at a normal or higher than normal rate (Figure 9.18c). Ventricular contraction is established at a rate independent of atrial contraction. Consequently, there is total dissociation of atrial and ventricular contraction, and third-degree heart block is characterised on the ECG by an abnormal relationship between the P and the QRS waves. If ventricular contraction is established at a rate close to normal, this condition may be without consequence to the circulation. However, if ventricular contraction is slower than normal, some degree of heart failure may ensue.

Complete heart block is often associated with heart disease or is a side-effect of drug toxicity. Other causes of heart block include congenital abnormalities of the conduction system or trauma caused during heart surgery. In these circumstances a pacemaker may be necessary to monitor the heart's rhythm and take over control if it becomes too slow.

PERICARDIAL DISEASE

> **Clinical note**
> Pericardial disease may occur as an isolated process or as a manifestation of disease elsewhere in the body.

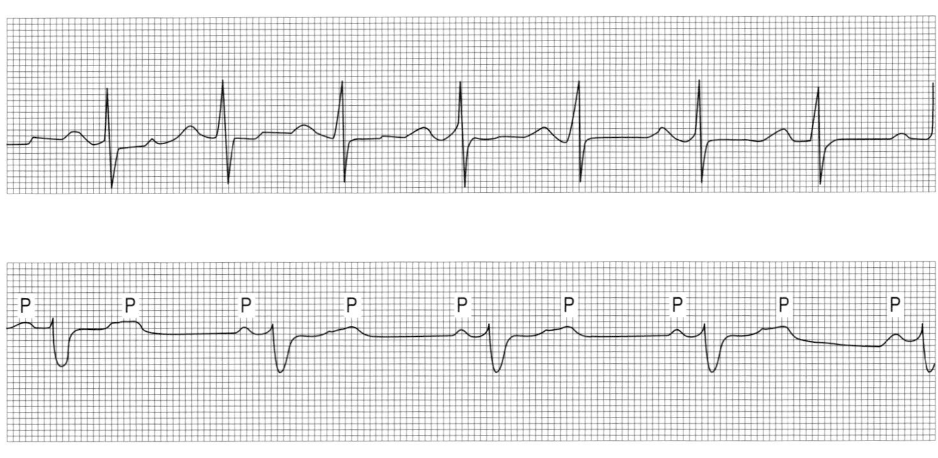

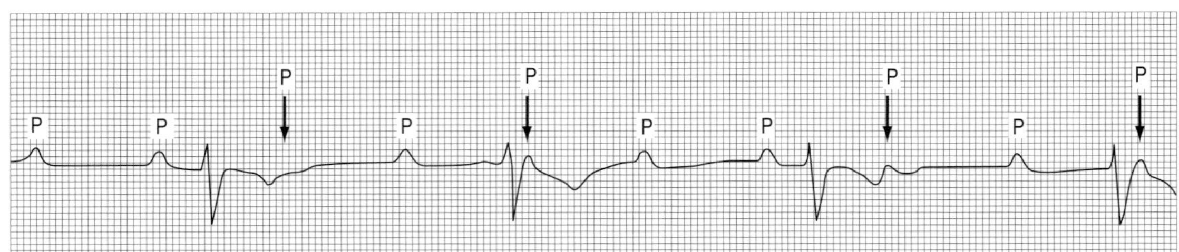

Figure 9.18 Heart block: (a) first-degree; (b) second-degree; (c) third-degree. (Reproduced from Berne and Levy 2000, with permission.)

Most commonly, pericardial disease involves inflammation of the pericardium — *pericarditis* — which is caused by a rubbing together of the visceral and parietal layers. Sometimes an outpouring of the pericardial contents (fluid, blood, pus, gas) — a pericardial effusion or hydropericardium — develops. The presence of excessive amounts of fluid in the pericardial space may be determined by abnormal findings on a chest X-ray or echocardiogram. Accumulation of large amounts of fluid can lead to an increase in the pressure within the pericardial sac and impaired diastolic filling of the ventricles. On rare occasions this can lead to cardiac tamponade, a form of heart failure that causes a fatal shock-like state.

Pericarditis has a number of causes. The pericardium may become inflamed due to an infection (bacterial, viral, fungal or protozoal) or as the result of a chemical or metabolic disturbance. Pericarditis can also develop during myocardial infarction and certain inflammatory or autoimmune diseases. In some cases pericarditis may have an idiopathic (unknown or non-specific) origin. Carcinoma, connective tissue disease and specific injury to the pericardium are also potential causes of pericardial disease. In constrictive pericarditis, thickening and fibrosis of the pericardium restrict diastolic expansion of the heart.

The most common symptom of pericarditis is chest pain, although it may exist without pain. A characteristic sound, called 'friction rub', can be heard on the left sternal border during examination with a stethoscope. Sometimes a person may get some relief from the pain by adopting a certain position: for example, sitting up. There will also be symptoms related to the cause of the pericarditis (e.g. fever).

Treatment for pericarditis usually involves administering aspirin or other NSAIDs. If there is evidence of cardiac tamponade, a needle is inserted just under the xiphoid process to drain excess fluid. This is referred to a 'pericardiocentesis'. Sometimes treatment may involve surgical removal of thickened pericardium from around the heart, which permits normal filling and expansion of the ventricles and restores adequate cardiac output to the organs.

MYOCARDIAL DISEASE

Key point

Conditions that affect the myocardium and decrease the pumping ability of the heart are recognised as a major cause of morbidity and mortality worldwide.

Clinically, a number of diseases can cause damage to myocardial tissue. For example, certain infections may occasionally affect the heart muscle to cause an inflammation known as *myocarditis*. Infections that can cause myocarditis include the Coxsackie A and B viruses, the influenza virus, the diphtheria bacterium, the parasite *Trypanosoma* and rheumatic fever. A number of systemic disorders can also affect the heart muscle; these include rheumatic disease, acromegaly, thyrotoxicosis and myxoedema. Alcoholism and drug toxicity can also be a cause of myocarditis.

Myocarditis is a condition that can affect people of any age but young adults seem to be most susceptible. The patient usually experiences chest pains and there may be symptoms of heart failure and an abnormal ECG. Treatment includes rest and drug therapy to treat the cause. The majority of people who develop myocarditis recover after several weeks without permanent damage to the heart.

About 120 000 people in the UK have cardiomyopathy, and no disease is responsible for more sudden deaths in the under-25s. Although it may be distinguished in general clinical terms from other forms of heart disease, cardiomyopathy is often misdiagnosed or is not detected at all.

In general, the signs and symptoms of cardiomyopathy are similar to those of heart failure. The clinical and pathological features of cardiomyopathies are sufficiently different, however, for them to be divided into three main classes: dilated, hypertrophic obstructive, and restrictive.

Definition

Cardiomyopathy is the term used to describe a syndrome of non-inflammatory heart muscle damage, or changes that affect the heart's pumping performance (*myo* relates to muscles, and *pathy* refers to damage). Although other forms of heart disease (e.g. coronary heart disease) can eventually lead to cardiomyopathy, the term is generally reserved for myocardial changes that are independent of other forms of heart disease. Some clinicians use the terms 'primary' and 'secondary' to distinguish between the causes. Currently four separate and distinct conditions of cardiomyopathy are recognised.

Dilated cardiomyopathy (DCM)

Also known as *congestive cardiomyopathy*, DCM is most notable for an enlarged heart that contracts poorly. Stretching, or dilatation, of the heart walls causes them to become thin and flabby so that the heart becomes weak and is unable to pump as well as it should. This is indicated by a reduction in the ejection fraction.

DCM is not a common condition; it affects 35 in every 100 000 of the population, and twice as many men as women. Most cases of DCM are idiopathic (unknown cause). However, one known cause of DCM is myocarditis, possibly because of severe damage to the heart during the initial infection, or because the virus triggers an autoimmune reaction. In 20–40 per cent of all cases there will be a family history of DCM, although the specific genetics are still not fully understood. Other causes of DCM are believed to be excessive alcohol consumption and exposure to toxic compounds.

Uncommonly, women in mid- to late pregnancy, or soon after delivery, can develop DCM. This is termed *peripartum cardiomyopathy* and occurs in approximately one in 10 000 pregnancies. Some of these cases of DCM may be due to one of the other causes outlined above, but coincidence makes the disease first become obvious during pregnancy, probably because of the extra demands placed on the heart. In around half the cases of genuine peripartum cardiomyopathy the condition resolves within 6–8 weeks of the delivery, but may recur in subsequent pregnancy. The cause of the occurrence or recurrence of peripartum cardiomyopathy is unknown. Women who have not completely recovered are advised to avoid further pregnancies.

DCM occurs with a spectrum of severity and outcomes. Depending on the cause and the degree of irreversible damage to the heart muscle following the acute illness, about one-third of patients have persistent very poor heart function, one-third improve but are left with some heart dysfunction, and one-third recover completely. It is difficult to predict into which category an individual patient will fall, so frequent cardiology follow-up is extremely important. Patients who do have irreversible damage and persistent poor function may go on to require a heart transplant. Sudden death as a culmination of chronic low-output heart failure is a feature of DCM.

Hypertrophic cardiomyopathy (HCM)

The most notable sign of hypertrophic cardiomyopathy, also known as *hypertrophic obstructive cardiomyopathy* (HOCM), is an excessive thickening of the heart muscle. This wall thickening (hypertrophy) can result in problems with obstruction to outward flow and problems with relaxation of the ventricles, and can thereby affect the ability of the heart to fill.

The distribution of hypertrophy is variable. The left ventricle is almost always affected and in some individuals the muscle of the right ventricle also thickens. Typically, the septum is thicker than the free wall of the left ventricle, the left ventricular volume is reduced, and the diastolic pressure is raised.

It is important to note that heart muscle may also hypertrophy in normal individuals as a result of prolonged athletic training. In these athletic cases, the thickened muscle is healthy and usually contracts well and ejects most of the blood from the heart. In hypertrophic cardiomyopathy, however, the muscle is often stiff and relaxes poorly, requiring higher pressures than normal to expand with the inflow of blood. Ventricular end-diastolic volumes are therefore reduced and this will limit the amount of blood that can be ejected with the next contraction.

Typical presentations include dyspnoea and arrhythmia, but tragically sudden death is sometimes the first indication that something was wrong with the heart muscle. Although the incidence of sudden death is relatively rare (less than 1 per cent), it is common in young people with HCM in whom a keen interest in sport has exacerbated the condition. Risk factors for sudden death include episodes of sinus tachycardia, passing out and a family history of sudden death.

It is estimated that 1 in 500 people have HCM. The precise cause is unclear, although there is evidence for a familial connection in the majority of cases. In other cases of HCM there is either no evidence of inheritance or there is insufficient information about the individual's family to assess inheritance.

Restrictive cardiomyopathy (RCM)

The hallmark feature of RCM is ventricles with normal or near-normal ventricular pumping function but abnormal filling due to fibrosis or scarring of the myocardium. Because a stiff rigid ventricle has difficulty in filling, damming of blood behind one or both AV valves ensues, and the atria become distended and enlarged. The ventricles remain normal or near-normal in size.

RCM is notable for increased work of breathing, often associated with a respiratory illness such as a cold, bronchitis or pneumonia. Other symptoms are those of left and right heart failure, including systemic and pulmonary congestion.

RCM is a very rare form of cardiomyopathy, accounting for around 5 per cent of patients with cardiomyopathy. It may be idiopathic or may be secondary to another systemic disease. Endomyocardial fibrosis is common in tropical Africa. One cause of RCM in the UK is deposition of abnormal protein in the myocardium and endocardium. This condition is called amyloidosis. Other causes include scleroderma and sarcoidosis.

The prognosis for sufferers of DCM depends upon the underlying cause but is generally poor.

Arrhythmogenic right ventricular cardiomyopathy (ARVC)

The hallmark feature of ARVC is the replacement of heart muscle by fibrous and fatty tissue that may result in abnormal electrical activity and rhythm disturbances, and in some cases problems with heart contraction.

The distribution of fibrous and fatty tissue is patchy and predominately affects the right ventricle, resulting initially in wall thickening. Later loss of cardiac muscle can result in dilatation and a thinner heart wall. It used to be thought that only the right ventricle was affected but it is now recognised that the left side of the heart, as well as the atria, may become affected if the disease progresses.

Rhythm disturbances are a primary sign of ARVC and symptoms may include palpitation, light-headedness, fatigue, and blackout or fainting. Less common symptoms are those of right heart failure, including systemic and pulmonary congestion. Features of left heart failure may occur late in the disease, if at all.

This disease has been recognised only recently and it is very difficult to determine how many people are affected. Currently, estimates are that it affects between 1 in 3000 and 1 in 10 000 people. The precise cause is unknown. One theory under investigation is that expression of an abnormal gene or genes may result in heart muscle cell damage and loss. The damaged or lost cells are replaced by fibrous and fatty tissues and the resulting disorganised structure of myocardium leads to abnormal electrical activity.

Detection and treatment of cardiomyopathies

Key point

Signs and symptoms of congestive heart failure – such as rapid breathing, abnormal heart rhythms, abnormal lung and heart sounds and an enlarged liver – are common in patients with a cardiomyopathy. However, their absence does not rule out the diagnosis.

Although there is a long list of possible causes of cardiomyopathy, few of them are directly treatable and most therapy is aimed at treating the secondary effects on the heart.

Treatment is usually with drugs and is aimed at minimising symptoms and preventing the development of complications and progression of the disease. A combination of drugs used to treat heart failure may be prescribed. These include ACE inhibitors, beta-blockers, digoxin and diuretics. Patients with RCM are at high risk for blood clots within the heart, particularly the enlarged upper chambers, so use of an anticoagulant such as heparin is vital. Rhythm problems may be treated using anti-arrhythmic drugs, although in some cases ablation (removal of a small area of abnormal heart tissue) or implantation of a pacemaker or ICD may be necessary.

Some patients with cardiomyopathies do not respond to medical treatment and deteriorate to such an extent that their quality of life is very poor. At this stage the individual may be referred to a specialist hospital where an assessment will be made to see if heart transplantation is appropriate.

VALVED DISEASE AND ENDOCARDITIS

There are two ways in which a diseased or damaged valve can affect the flow of blood through the heart. If a valve becomes constricted or narrowed, the forward flow of blood is accelerated and turbulent, a condition called *valvular stenosis*. Alternatively, deformation of a valve may result in its incomplete opening and closure, allowing backward flow of blood, called *regurgitation*, during myocardial contraction. This situation is referred to as *valvular incompetence* or *insufficiency*.

Stenosis and incompetence interfere with normal flow of blood through the heart. In a case of stenosis, the heart must contract more forcefully to pump blood through the narrowed valve. With incompetence, the heart also has to work harder to pump the increased volume of blood forwards; however, some of this energy will be wasted as blood is going backwards also.

Key point

Stenosis and regurgitation often occur simultaneously in advanced disease. The heart becomes dilated in order to accommodate the greater than normal blood volume.

There are several causes of valvular disease; these include congenital abnormalities, and acquired diseases such as bacterial endocarditis or rheumatic fever. In bacterial endocarditis, an infection becomes established on the endothelial lining of the heart chambers. Endocarditis may be acute or severe, or it may be chronic, often referred to as 'subacute endocarditis'. The endothelium becomes inflamed and frequently the location of the inflammation is at the line of valve closure. It may erode the valve structure, or it may produce nodules with the ulcerative surface of active infection. Subsequent fibrosis and scarring of the valves and chordae tendineae often results in deformity of one or more of the heart valves, which may cause valve malfunction.

Rheumatic fever is another example of an inflammatory condition that can cause endocarditis and valve malfunction. This involves a delayed hypersensitivity reaction in susceptible individuals, usually children and young adolescents, following an untreated streptococcal throat infection. The severity and incidence of the acute phase of rheumatic fever is decreasing, owing to improved social conditions and rapid and effective treatment or prevention of streptococcal infections.

9

However, rheumatic fever is still a major cause of death from heart disease in 5–24-year-olds of less developed countries of the third world. It is common for cardiac surgeons to perform operations to repair valves in middle-aged or older persons that were damaged years ago by the disease in childhood or young adulthood. Valve defects are also associated with a number of other diseases, including ankylosing spondylitis, rheumatoid arthritis and systemic lupus erythematosus (SLE).

Abnormalities of the mitral valve apparatus are the most common valve defects caused by disease. Mitral stenosis is more common in women than men and the most frequent cause is rheumatic endocarditis. Scarring or fusion of the valve cusps, so that the valve opening becomes funnel-shaped, causes mitral stenosis, and calcification of the valve in middle age makes it more narrow and non-compliant. Mitral regurgitation is the most common lesion of rheumatic heart disease. Changes in the chordae tendineae and papillary muscle of one or both cusps, or dilatation of the valve ring, cause the valve to remain open during systole. Incomplete valve closure permits backflow of blood from the left ventricle to the left atrium during systole. Mitral stenosis and incompetence often coexist, but one or the other may be functionally predominant.

The tricuspid valve is subject to defects less frequently than either the mitral or aortic valves. These deformities almost always exist with mitral and aortic lesions and occur in approximately 10 per cent of patients with chronic rheumatic heart disease. Pulmonary valve deformities are the most rare complication of rheumatic endocarditis.

Detection and treatment of valve disease

The symptoms of valvular heart disease depend on which valve is affected and on the severity of the deformation. People with mild valvular heart disease may have few symptoms, although heart murmurs are a common feature. A murmur during ventricular diastole generally indicates an abnormal flow into the ventricle that is typical of a mitral stenosis. A murmur during ventricular systole, however, indicates an abnormal flow of blood back into the left atrium. This latter murmur is typical of mitral regurgitation. The presence of aortic stenosis may lead to a marked left ventricular hypertrophy. Over time there may be atrial dilatation and ventricular hypertrophy that is typical of congestive heart failure, and increasing strain on the heart can cause tiredness or breathlessness on exercise. If the obstruction is severe, the onset of congestive heart failure may be relatively rapid.

Medical treatment for valvular heart disease involves medication to relieve the symptoms of heart failure and will depend on the severity of the condition. If the obstruction or leaking of valves is severe, then medicines alone may not be enough to maintain an adequate cardiac function. In these cases some form of remedial surgery is the only option to repair a defective valve or valves and prevent further damage to the heart muscle.

One relatively common procedure is valvuloplasty. This is carried out during cardiac catheterisation. A catheter with a small inflatable balloon at its tip is inserted into a vein in the groin and passed through to the orifice of the damaged valve. The balloon is gently inflated so that the deformed valve is stretched and widened. This is commonly used in the treatment of mitral stenosis. If a valve is damaged beyond repair it can be replaced with either an artificial valve made of stainless steel, or a valve from a deceased human or animal (usually pig) donor. The advantage a donor valve has over an artificial valve is the absence of clotting, which occurs occasionally using an artificial valve.

CORONARY HEART DISEASE

Definition

Coronary heart disease (CHD) describes a number of interdependent syndromes that are manifestations of a poor supply of oxygen-rich blood to the heart muscle. The main examples of CHD are angina pectoris (chest pain), and acute myocardial infarction (heart attack).

Although death rates have been falling since the early 1970s, CHD causes over 105 000 deaths in the UK each year: approximately 21 per cent of deaths in men and 15 per cent of deaths in women. Furthermore, illness and disability arising from CHD in older age groups is increasing. Around 1.3 million people in the UK have had a heart attack, and around 2 million suffer from angina. Thus, in addition to the human cost, CHD has major economic consequences. It is estimated that in the UK the combined CHD cost to the healthcare system and production losses from death and illness in those of working age represent a total of £10 000 million annually.

Pathogenesis

The pathological basis of CHD is partial or complete obstruction of one or more of the main coronary arteries. Under these conditions blood flow through the artery is decreased. Typically this results in an inadequate supply of oxygen and other nutrients to the heart muscle. The state in which the myocardial energy requirements exceed the energy supply is referred to as *myocardial ischaemia* (from the Greek *iskho*, to keep back, and *haima*, blood). Consequently, the term *ischaemic heart disease* (IHD) may be used as a more precise alternative to CHD.

Initially, the ischaemia may be mild or transient. Under conditions requiring an increase in the myocardial oxygen supply — for example, during physical or emotional stress — the blood flow through a blocked or restricted artery may be insufficient to deliver the required amount of oxygen. Under these conditions the person often experiences chest pain that is symptomatic of an angina attack. With repeated angina attacks, or greater degrees of coronary blockage, or following a very sudden decrease in coronary blood supply, any area of myocardial tissue that is cut off from its oxygen supply for more than a few minutes will usually be irreversibly damaged and may even die. A region of dead cells is known as an *infarct*. The myocardial contractility of the affected area is severely compromised and this may precipitate abrupt loss of cardiac function, or cardiac arrest. It is estimated that around 275 000 people have a heart attack each year in the UK and that about 2.1 million people have or have had angina.

Coronary atherosclerosis

Progressive changes to the wall and the inner lining of the coronary arteries are significant precursors of the syndromes of CHD. Known collectively as *coronary atherosclerosis* (*athero* is Greek for porridge, and *sclerosis* is hardening) or coronary artery disease, these changes include proliferation, or thickening, of the coronary arterial intima, and excessive deposition of fatty tissue, fibrous cellular debris and calcium salts in the endothelium. These deposits, referred to as *atherosclerotic plaques* or lesions, generally begin forming in childhood and clinical manifestations appear in middle to late adulthood.

Thickening of the intimal layer reduces the elasticity of the arterial walls, whereas plaques encroach into the lumen of the artery. The left coronary artery is more commonly affected than the right, and eventually this 'hardening' and 'narrowing' of the coronary vessels impedes blood flow to the left ventricle, apex, interventricular septum and anterior surface of the atria; chronic occlusive syndromes of CHD may ensue.

However, it is worth noting that while coronary artery disease is responsible for almost all cases of CHD, many more individuals have plaques than those who have CHD. Furthermore, not all mechanisms that trigger coronary artery disease are the same as those that lead to CHD. For example, signs of CHD might never appear in an individual with a lesion of the left coronary artery, provided the area of heart muscle supplied by the artery is adequately supplied with oxygenated blood (e.g. from an alternative coronary artery circuit).

Plaque formation

The earliest lesions of the coronary arteries, fatty lipid streaks, may be found in children as young as 10 years of age. However, these areas of yellow discoloration may not be a precursor to atherosclerotic plaques in all cases. An advanced lesion, the fibrous atherosclerotic plaque, generally appears during early adulthood and progresses with age. Fibrous plaques are white in appearance and it is these that can increase in size, leading to progressive arterial obstruction. Plaques can be complicated by ulceration, haemorrhage, thrombosis and calcification.

The pathogenesis underlying coronary artery disease is complex and incompletely understood. It is generally accepted, however, that there are three important components to consider in relation to advanced coronary atherosclerotic lesions:

- endothelial injury
- lipid infiltration
- platelet–fibrin deposition.

Potential causes of injury to the delicate lining of the coronary arteries include mechanical trauma caused by:

- the coronary arterial pressure pulse
- repeated compression of the arteries during heart contractions.

Another possible source of endothelial injury is believed to be chronic exposure to a high level of cholesterol-carrying lipoproteins, referred to as *hyperlipidaemia* or *hypercholesterolaemia*. This is supported by a strong association between a high level of lipoproteins in the circulation and coronary atherosclerosis in human populations and experimental animals. Other potential causes of endothelial damage include immunological injury to the endothelium and exposure to certain vasoactive substances.

Lipid infiltration is an important feature of plaque formation inside the lumen of the coronary arteries. According to one hypothesis, white blood cells migrate into damaged arterial endothelium and become macrophages that accumulate lipid. In addition, macrophages synthesise and secrete a number of growth factors that are believed to stimulate thickening of the smooth muscle and connective tissue layers of the coronary arterial wall. The instability of cholesterol-rich low-density lipoproteins (LDLs) and LDL receptors on arterial walls has also been implicated in the lipid infiltration stage of plaque formation. As the plaques accumulate fat, they enlarge and the arterial lumen becomes progressively occluded.

Activation of the blood-clotting system is an additional complication that can be seen, and the third and final stage of plaque formation involves the deposition of fibrous cellular debris and calcium salts in the plaques.

Several factors relating to the formation of advanced lesions may contribute to the involvement of thrombosis in coronary atherosclerosis. Cracks and fissures that appear in the advanced lesion may act as sites for platelet attachment and formation. Damage to the endothelium may be sufficient to cause a low-grade inflammation that leads to adherence of platelets and the formation of microthrombi (minute clots) in the vessel lining. A reduction of blood flow at the site of a lesion may activate clotting. Activation of the blood-clotting system results in the formation of microthrombi consisting of cellular debris and calcium salts. These may become incorporated into existing advanced atherosclerotic plaques, from which unstable thrombi frequently break away. Alternatively. a clot may become lodged in a coronary artery, a process described as a *coronary thrombosis*, causing severe occlusion that results in an *acute myocardial infarction* (MI).

Although the precise stages of plaque formation are unclear, it is obvious that a number of synergistic processes are involved. Endothelial injury promotes:

- macrophage emigration and proliferation in the intima
- accumulation of lipid, principally in the form of free cholesterol within the cell and surrounding connective tissue
- formation of platelet fibrinogen thrombi.

Growth factors released by platelets, macrophages and other formed elements stimulate proliferation of smooth muscle cells in the artery walls and formation of large amounts of connective tissue, including collagen and elastic fibres.

Key point

It is unclear whether plaques are reversible. Experimental evidence from studies in animal models and human femoral arteries suggests that lesions may undergo reversal. The extent to which it is possible to reduce advanced obstructive lesions in human coronary arteries is not yet understood.

Hypercholesterolaemia

It is widely acknowledged that individuals with elevated levels of total serum cholesterol (> 5.2 mmol/L) have a higher than normal risk of developing plaques. However, it is the ratio of low-density lipoprotein (LDL) cholesterol to high-density lipoprotein (HDL) cholesterol, rather than the total serum cholesterol, which is thought to be the best indicator of the risk of developing coronary artery diseases.

LDL cholesterol is composed of about 20 per cent protein and 80 per cent lipid (around half of which is cholesterol), and this represents the main carrier of cholesterol to the tissues. Under most conditions it is incorporation of LDL cholesterol into plaques that determines whether or not the plaque progresses. Consequently, this type of cholesterol is considered 'bad'. On the other hand, HDL cholesterol, which is being transported away from tissues to the liver, is considered 'good'. HDL cholesterol is around 50 per cent protein and 5 per cent lipid, of which around two-fifths is cholesterol.

There is accumulating experimental evidence to suggest that some defect of LDL receptors prevents the specific uptake of cholesterol into cells by receptor-mediated endocytosis, resulting in elevated levels of circulating cholesterol. It appears that this defect is inherited, although the influence of environmental factors cannot be ruled out. For example, it is reported that dietary fatty acids influence the relative proportions of LDL and HDL in the blood; unsaturated fatty acids increase the proportion of HDL, while saturated fatty acids increase the proportion of LDL. It is also believed that cigarette smoking is associated with a reduction in plasma HDL, whereas exercise causes an elevation of HDL. Finally, oestrogens cause an increase of HDL and a reduction of both total cholesterol and LDL. This may explain why the incidence of CHD is lower in pre-menopausal than post-menopausal women.

Symptoms of coronary heart disease

An angina attack is characterised by the sensation of severe pain and heaviness or tightness behind the sternum. Pain radiating to the arms, neck, jaw, back or stomach is also common. One of the more common causes of angina is physical activity, particularly after a large meal. However, sufferers can also have an attack during other forms of stress, or even whilst resting or asleep. Symptoms usually fade within 10–15 minutes, and an angina attack is also known as a transient ischaemic attack (TIA).

Myocardial infarction (MI) is a continuous process. Interruption of the myocardial blood supply is the first stage and the outstanding clinical feature is a heavy pain in the chest. This pain may also spread to the arms, neck, jaw, face, back or stomach, and in some cases may be mistaken for indigestion. There may also be sweating, nausea or vomiting, and often there is a shortness of breath and an impending sense of doom. The affected person may look ill and pale, and as the damaged heart may then lack the strength to circulate an adequate volume of blood, fainting (syncope) can occur.

The important difference between myocardial infarction and angina is that the MI pain lasts for a much longer period, at least 15–30 minutes, and sometimes for several hours or perhaps a day. A heart attack may also be complicated by the appearance of one or more cardiac arrhythmias.

The severity of the symptoms of MI varies. Often there is severe pain and collapse, but sometimes a heart attack is 'silent' and produces very little or trivial discomfort. Signs of silent heart attack often remain undiscovered until the sufferer has a routine physical examination or undergoes a medical investigation for other symptoms.

Diagnosis of coronary heart disease

As the symptoms of angina often occur during exertion, a resting ECG may be normal. Therefore a patient may be asked to perform a stress test on an exercise bicycle or treadmill. Even then, some cases will show only transient changes with exercise.

Another test is a radionuclide scan, which is useful for people who cannot exercise, and for females, in whom it is sometimes difficult to make an accurate diagnosis with an exercise ECG. A very small amount of thallium, a radioisotope of potassium, is injected into the blood. A large camera, positioned close to the chest, picks up the gamma rays emitted by the isotope. This shows which parts of the heart muscle are short of blood and measures how severe the condition is. Another common test for angina is cardiac angiography.

Diagnosis of MI may be confirmed by an elevation of cardiac enzymes in the blood, which indicates leakage from damaged heart muscle cells, or by ECG, which in most cases shows distinct abnormalities.

Treatment of coronary heart disease

Drug treatments

Inhaled amyl nitrate or sublingual (under the tongue) glyceryl trinitrate (GTN) are good examples of drugs that can help to dilate the coronary vessels temporarily, as well as reduce the resistive load on the heart. Taken regularly, beta-blockers can help reduce the frequency of angina attacks by reducing the work of the heart so that it needs less oxygen, blood and nutrients. Beta-blockers are not usually suitable for people with asthma or bronchitis, and calcium-channel blockers may be used as an alternative. Potassium-channel activators are a new type of drug given to relieve angina. They have a similar effect to nitrates as they relax the walls of the coronary arteries and therefore improve blood flow. Unlike nitrates, however, they do not appear to become less effective with continued use. Nitrates and beta-blockers are often used together from the start of treatment. If they do not control the angina, a calcium-channel blocker may be used as well.

Clinical note

There are a number of alternative treatments for CHD and the one selected will depend upon the nature and the severity of the symptoms. One or more from a range of medications may be administered, with the aim of increasing the coronary blood supply and reducing the myocardial workload.

Surgery

If the symptoms of angina cannot be stabilised using drug therapy alone, the sufferer may require varying degrees of surgical intervention.

Coronary angioplasty is often used in cases where obstructive lesions are relatively isolated and incomplete. A small balloon is gently inflated so that it squashes the fatty tissue responsible for the narrowing and widens the artery. Coronary angioplasty is usually successful, but it can sometimes lead to a blockage of the artery; this will need immediate surgery. Sometimes the artery will become narrow again over the 4–6 months after the coronary angioplasty. The angioplasty can be repeated if necessary. Increasingly, specialists who carry out angioplasty place a short tube of stainless steel mesh, called a stent, inside the artery. The stent helps to hold the vessel open, reducing the chances of the artery narrowing again.

Revascularisation techniques, involving the use of a laser to drill small holes in the myocardium that allow blood to gain muscular access, are used in patients for whom angina cannot be eliminated by angioplasty. In cases where there is a more severe blockage in two or all three main coronary arteries, a more complicated surgical procedure — a *coronary artery bypass graft* (CABG) — may be necessary (see Figure 9.21).

Complications and sequelae of a heart attack

Complications of a heart attack include abnormal heart rhythms, heart failure, cardiogenic shock and pericarditis. Around 20 per cent of heart attack victims die before they reach hospital and most of these deaths are attributed to ventricular fibrillation. Therefore the sooner paramedics or an attending physician can monitor the ECG, the greater the chance of survival. Aspirin, a drug that helps to improve the anti-clotting effect of any subsequent treatments, is also administered as early as possible. Ideally, the patient should receive a thrombolytic drug, such as streptokinase or tissue plasminogen activator, within 90 minutes of the heart attack. Thrombolytics help to dissolve the clot that is blocking the artery and prevent the formation of any further clots. These drugs can be given later, but are less effective as time goes by.

A number of additional medications, such as anticoagulants, beta-blockers or anti-arrhythmic drugs, may be administered to prevent further heart attacks. Diuretics or ACE inhibitors may be given to relieve heart failure and the associated breathlessness. The patient may also be prescribed other drugs used to relieve the symptoms of angina, and drugs that lower serum cholesterol.

The amount of myocardial damage after a heart attack is often relatively small, with the result that there is enough good muscle left for the heart to carry on its work satisfactorily. The area of the heart muscle that was damaged does not regenerate so the infarction is replaced by fibrous scar tissue; this takes from a few days to a few weeks. Within 2–3 months the hearts of many heart attack patients are functioning just as well as they were before the attack. These individuals do, however, have an increased potential for subsequent myocardial infarction. If a large area of tissue is involved there may be residual evidence of heart failure or other cardiac malfunction with the result that the pumping action of the heart is not as good as before. This can lead to symptoms of varying degrees associated with heart failure. Also, some people continue to experience angina symptoms because there is still narrowing of the coronary arteries.

Risk factors for coronary heart disease

A number of factors are identified as increasing the risk of an individual developing CHD. These are:

- hypercholesterolaemia
- physical inactivity
- blood pressure > 140/90 mmHg (hypertension)
- tobacco smoking
- obesity.

Since the occurrence of CHD is undoubtedly due to many independent and interdependent influences, it is difficult to distinguish any one of these major risk factors over another. It is clear, however, that the coexistence of two or more risk factors can greatly increase the risk of developing CHD.

There is evidence that hypercholesterolaemia and hypertension may be inherited. Consequently, the inherited nature of these factors may make them less susceptible to modification. Furthermore, familial (genetic) predisposition to CHD, whilst it is acknowledged, is not well understood. Research is ongoing with the aim of identifying rogue genes that contribute to CHD. However, it is worth noting that reducing human health to the activity of human genes ignores the fact that the surrounding environment in which those genes are operating has a profound influence upon the ways in which the effects are manifested.

Finally, a number of secondary factors — such as predisposition to develop thrombosis, metabolic disorders such as diabetes mellitus, and rarely oral contraceptives — increase the risk of CHD in susceptible persons.

Healthcare professionals recommend a number of lifestyle changes to reduce the risk of CHD. These include eating a healthy diet, increasing levels of physical activity, stopping smoking, and maintaining weight within normal limits. However, whilst there is impressive evidence from a wide range of sources supporting the effectiveness of these measures, much of this is circumstantial and not all of the recommendations have been shown to be as effective as expected or predicted.

Lowering high serum levels of cholesterol has a great impact on heart disease, particularly in people with familial hypercholesterolaemia. It has been estimated that reducing the intake of saturated fat by 10 per cent is linked with a reduction of 20–30 per cent of deaths from CHD. However, conclusive evidence for this is yet to be presented.

Key point

It is reported that within a few years of stopping smoking, a risk factor for heart disease is attainable that is nearly equal to that of people who have never smoked.

Regular daily physical activity, such as brisk walking, swimming or cycling, can help improve serum cholesterol levels. Physical activity increases the level of HDL cholesterol (the protective cholesterol), but does not affect LDL cholesterol.

It is also reported that people at risk of CHD benefit from treatment with statin drugs to lower blood cholesterol levels, with the suggestion that use of statins reduces the risk of being hospitalised because of worsening angina and reduces heart attacks by around one-third.

SUDDEN CARDIAC DEATH

Definition

Sudden cardiac death (SCD) is an unexpected death arising from cardiac arrest, often brought on by exercise or some form of strenuous physical activity. It occurs instantaneously or shortly after the first symptoms appear. Although heart disease or some other cardiac abnormality is a common cause of SCD, no definitive cause of death can be found in about 1 in every 20 cases. This is referred to sudden arrhythmic death syndrome (SADS), and although it is rare it is most commonly found in apparently fit and healthy adolescents and young adults.

Cardiac arrest occurs when the heart abruptly and without warning stops pumping blood to the rest of the body. All known heart diseases can lead to cardiac arrest and sudden death, but the most common underlying reason for a person to die suddenly from cardiac arrest is CHD. Other factors that can cause cardiac arrest include respiratory arrest, electrocution, drowning, choking or trauma.

Cardiac arrest can also occur without any known cause. One in 20 of all cases of sudden cardiac death in people aged under 65 years is unexplained, with no cardiac abnormalities ever found. Researchers feel that many people who have died suddenly may have inherited an undiagnosed tendency to an abnormal heart rhythm.

Simple clinical methods can be used to investigate and possibly identify some of the causes of unexplained sudden cardiac death in the population. These include resting or exercise ECG testing, 24-hour monitoring of ECG, and in some cases MRI screening to exclude certain forms of cardiomyopathy.

CONGENITAL HEART DISEASE

Types of malformation

Fetal heart development is a complicated process that can sometimes go wrong. There are many different kinds of cardiac malformation and these are referred to as 'congenital abnormalities' or defects. Most occur because part of the heart, its valves or the adjoining vessels is missing or improperly formed. Other defects may arise from disturbance of the heart rhythm or if the pumping action of the heart does not work properly.

Most congenital heart defects have little effect before birth because the fetal circulation is adapted so that oxygenation of the blood is accomplished across the placenta. After birth, however, specific defects impair the normal circulation of blood through the heart, lungs and great vessels. Some infants are born with only one isolated abnormality, while others have two or more.

In around a half of cases the defect is relatively minor and repairs itself without treatment. These are referred to as 'asymptomatic defects'. The remaining half have major defects, which are repaired by medical or surgical procedures with varying degrees of success. Death is common in the most severe malformations.

Congenital heart defects may be categorised as *cyanotic* or *non-cyanotic*:

- In the cyanotic types the lungs are partially or completely bypassed, and poorly oxygenated blood finds it way into the systemic circulation. This results in a bluish colouring of the skin, nail beds and lips (cyanosis comes from the Greek *cyan* for blue).
- In non-cyanotic defects, oxygenated blood is shunted from the left heart to the right side. This may increase the preload in the right heart and may also cause blood that has already been oxygenated to pass into the pulmonary circulation.

In severe non-cyanotic varieties of congenital heart disease, the infant may experience symptoms of congestive heart failure, a higher than normal risk of respiratory infection, and poor growth.

Fetal circulation

Two shunts, the foramen ovale between the right and left atria, and the ductus arteriosus between the pulmonary artery and the first segment of the aortic arch, create a short-circuit in the fetal circulation so that most blood does not pass through the lungs. These organs do, however, receive enough blood to ensure their adequate development. Normally, functional closure of the foramen ovule and ductus arteriosus occurs spontaneously within a few hours of being exposed to atmospheric oxygen at birth. However, closure of either structure is sometimes delayed or does not occur at all, and some mixing of oxygenated and deoxygenated blood occurs.

Patent ductus arteriosus

Patent or *persistent ductus arteriosus* (PDA) describes the condition in which the ductus arteriosus remains open, or patent, following birth (Figure 9.19). While this condition is much more common in premature babies, it may also occur in term infants. If it is small, the PDA may be asymptomatic, although it might be detected as a heart murmur.

Closure of a PDA in premature babies and young infants may be induced using a drug called indometacin; alternatively, a surgical intervention may be required in older infants and children. In cases when

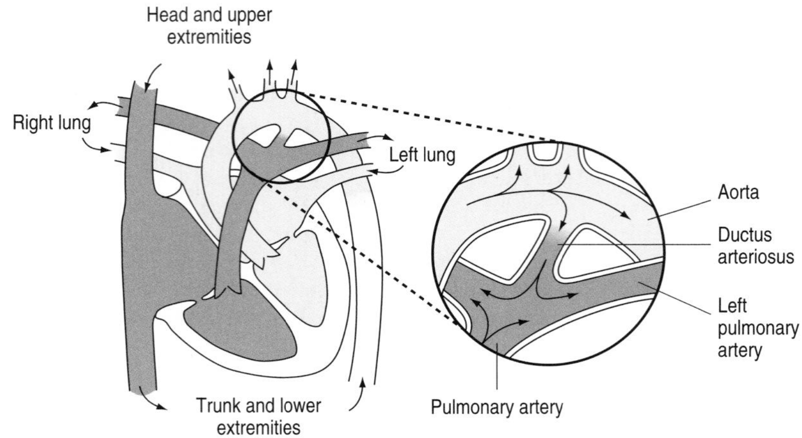

Figure 9.19 Patent ductus arteriosus. (Reproduced from Guyton and Hall 2005, with permission.)

an infant is born with another cardiac abnormality, doctors may try to delay closure of the ductus by administering prostaglandins, until corrective surgery or a heart transplant can be performed. Alone, this defect is often not too serious, and in some malformations of the heart is actually necessary for continued life.

Congenital valve abnormalities

Abnormal development within the womb often leads to infants being born with heart valves that are not well formed. The most common congenital valve defect is *pulmonary stenosis*, which is caused by thickening of the valve cusps and narrowing of the orifice. In some cases the valves are completely closed, a condition known as *atresia*.

Mild stenosis is usually compatible with normal activities and a normal life. More severe narrowing or complete atresia is often associated with the development of other heart abnormalities before or after birth.

Another problem of congenitally faulty valves is valvular incompetence. For example, a small percentage of the population (less than 2 per cent) are born with fusion of the aortic valve, which is usually bicuspid rather than tricuspid. The valve is often obstructed and incompetent. Tricuspid atresia is an example of a valve defect that coexists with another congenital deformity; the pulmonary artery and valve also tend to be underdeveloped since a less than optimal volume of blood leaves the right ventricle.

Treatment of congenital valve defects depends upon the severity of the defect and whether or not the person has any symptoms. Surgery is sometimes required early in life. On the other hand, people may have a normal life expectancy.

Septal defects

Septal defects are a common example of non-cyanotic congenital heart disease. Holes of variable size in the interatrial, atrioventricular or interventricular septum enable blood to be shunted between the left and right sides of the heart.

A large right-to-left shunt at the level of the atria is a physiological condition in the fetus and atrial septal defects (ASDs) are commonly located in the area prenatally occupied by the foramen ovale. *Septum primum* refers to a hole in the portion of the septum below the site of the foramen ovale, whereas *septum secundum* refers to a hole above this site. Secundum ASDs, which are the most common, are usually isolated, but may be related to other cardiac lesions (such as mitral, pulmonary, tricuspid or aortic atresia). In extreme cases, virtually no septum may exist between the atrial chambers.

Ventricular septal defects (VSDs) represent around 30 per cent of all heart abnormalities' they may be isolated or be part of a complex or multiple heart defect. A large proportion of these are relatively small and close spontaneously within the first year of life; this is not usually associated with serious disability. Larger, more severe defects allow a significant amount of blood to be shunted from the left to the right heart and infants with these defects normally present with manifestations of congestive heart failure at 2–8 weeks of life. Because many septal defects close spontaneously, they may be monitored for a short period before surgical closure is undertaken. Survival rates from surgery exceed 90 per cent and survivors have a normal life expectancy and normal exercise tolerance.

Abnormalities of the great vessels

In complex forms of congenital heart disease, the origins of the aorta and pulmonary artery are malformed. For example, in a cyanotic condition known as *transposition of the great arteries*, the outflow tracts of the ventricles are reversed so that venous blood is pumped around the systemic circulation and oxygenated blood is circulated through the lungs. In some cases both the aorta and pulmonary artery may originate from the same ventricle; survival of infants born with this form of defect is dependent upon the coexistence of a patent ductus arteriosus or septal defect that allows oxygenated blood to enter the aorta. When there is no such shunt, it may be created surgically.

In *truncus arteriosus*, the aorta and pulmonary arteries arise from a common 'trunk', and blood from both ventricles mixes together as it all exits the heart through a single valve. *Coarctation of the aorta* is a common abnormality that involves a narrowing of the aortic wall just distal to the origin of the left subclavian artery. Consequently, there is a reduction in blood flow to the lower half of the body and an increase in upper body blood pressure. Cutting out the constriction and stitching the normal ends together can repair this defect.

Anomalous pulmonary venous return

One or more of the pulmonary veins may connect either directly or indirectly to the right atrium, instead of the left. This is referred to as *anomalous pulmonary venous return* and is an example of a non-cyanotic congenital defect. Partial forms of anomalous pulmonary venous return, in which only one or two pulmonary veins are connected abnormally, may have few symptoms of vascular congestion, although surgical correction may be performed. Infants born with total anomalous pulmonary venous return (TAPR) usually develop problems related to cardiac failure within the first few weeks or months and thus require cardiac surgery.

Heart chamber abnormalities

Abnormalities of the heart chambers may be serious and potentially life-threatening. One of the most complex cardiac defects seen in a neonate is severe underdevelopment, or hypoplasia, of one or more heart chambers. In *hypoplastic left heart syndrome* (HLHS) an infant may be born with a reduction in left ventricular/left atrial size, and the mitral and aortic valves are either very small or completely atretic. The initial part of the aorta is also very small, often only a few millimetres in diameter. This results in a situation where the left side of the heart is completely unable to support the circulation needed by the body's organs, though the right side of the heart is typically developed normally. Under these conditions, and provided that the ductus arteriosus remains patent, the right ventricle may be capable of performing a dual pumping role, distributing blood both to the lungs and out to the body. Children with HLHS rarely survive more than 2 or 3 days from their birth and cardiac transplantation can be considered.

Tetralogy of fallot

This condition, which is a classic example of a cyanotic form of congenital heart disease, takes its name from the French physician who first described it. It is a relatively uncommon malformation consisting of a VSD, pulmonary valve stenosis, right ventricular hypertrophy and a shift of the aorta from the left to the right side so that it receives blood from both sides of the heart (Figure 9.20). A child born with this congenital disease can survive beyond infancy, but few survive to adulthood without surgery.

Causes of congenital heart disease

In most cases, the precise cause of a congenital heart defect is unknown. Certain chronic illnesses, such as diabetes and SLE, may increase the risk of giving birth to an infant with a congenital heart defect. However, this does not imply that women with diabetes or epilepsy cannot have healthy children; they do, however,

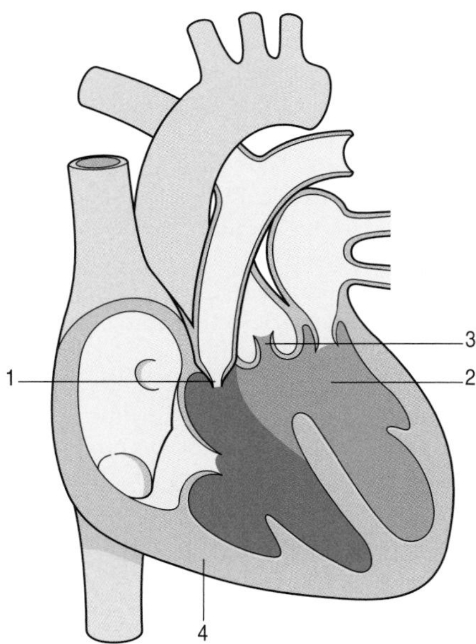

Figure 9.20 Tetralogy of Fallot. (1) = pulmonary stenosis; (2) = ventricular septal defect; (3) = dextra-position of aorta; (4) = hypotrophy of right ventricle. (Reproduced from Guyton and Hall 2005, with permission.)

need to be carefully monitored during their pregnancies. Acute illness, such as the viral infection rubella, during pregnancy can also cause abnormalities before birth or interfere with an infant's heart as it develops. Finally, drugs taken in pregnancy, such as some of those prescribed for epilepsy, illegal drugs, or alcohol, are also known to cause certain heart defects. Smoking is also thought to be a contributing factor.

In some cases, a genetic factor has been identified. This may be the result of a single mutant gene or it may be associated with a chromosomal abnormality. Down's syndrome is the most common example of chromosomal abnormality associated with congenital heart defects. Although the search for the causes of congenital heart diseases continues, it is generally accepted that in most cases it is probably caused by a variety of factors. Any inherited factor is usually unmasked only if it occurs together with an appropriate environmental hazard. The risk of a sibling of a child with congenital heart disease being similarly affected is 2–4 per cent. The precise recurrence can vary for individual congenital cardiovascular defects. Between 2 and 5 babies in every 100 born to women with a defect have a similar abnormality. The risk is obviously greater in the unlikely event that the father also has a heart defect.

Detection and treatment of congenital defects

Some abnormalities are diagnosed in utero (within the womb). Amniocentesis is an established method by which fetal chromosomes may be tested for abnormalities associated with congenital heart disease. A hollow needle introduced via the mother's abdomen into the womb is used to collect a small amount of amniotic fluid in order to study cells shed by the fetus. There is a small risk to the fetus with this test; about 1 in every 100 babies aborts after amniocentesis. A non-invasive ultrasound test, called a fetal echocardiogram, performed at about 16–20 weeks of pregnancy, is becoming increasingly effective at detecting some heart defects.

The presence of a congenital defect is not always detected at birth. Some are detected for the first time in older children when a heart murmur is heard. Furthermore, some defects do not become apparent or symptomatic until later in adult life. For example, a malformed bicuspid aortic valve may initially function near to normal, but can calcify and become stenotic and require replacement in middle age.

Some isolated defects, such as an atrial septal defect, a small ventricular septal defect, and patent ductus arteriosus, are not severe and the patient may live a normal life because the shunt is not great. However, there is an increased predisposition to respiratory infections and endocarditis with these abnormalities. Other more complex defects are survivable, but right heart failure eventually occurs. Modern heart surgery has advanced so much in recent years that it is now standard practice to operate on tiny babies. Severe defects such as hypoplastic left heart syndrome are generally not survivable and cardiac transplantation can be considered.

HEART SURGERY

Surgical treatment of heart disease may require the surgeon to make an incision into one or more of the heart chambers; this is referred to as 'open-heart surgery'. Such a procedure is made possible by the use of a cardiopulmonary bypass device, which maintains circulation and oxygenation outside of the patient's body so that beating of the heart may be temporarily suspended. This means that the surgeon has a dry and motionless heart on which to work.

The most common open-heart procedures are those for correction of congenital heart defects, to repair diseased valves, and in the treatment of severe CHD. Cardiopulmonary bypass also enables surgery to repair damage to the great vessels that transport blood to and from the heart.

Other cardiac surgery can be performed without opening the heart. The main advantages of these over open-heart procedures is that not all require cardiopulmonary bypass and they are less invasive, and consequently may be less traumatic.

Repair of diseased valves

For many years congenital and acquired disease of the heart valves was corrected using open-heart surgery. In the case of the mitral valve, an incision made into the wall of the left atrium gave access to the damaged valve. Replacement of the tricuspid valve, although less common than mitral valve surgery, may also be performed in open-heart procedures. Defects of the pulmonary valve can usually be repaired without opening the heart. The valve may be approached through the pulmonary artery and cut in three places to create a valve with three cusps. In older children and adults, pulmonary valvuloplasty represents a less invasive alternative to surgery. In the case of a malfunctioning aortic valve, the severity of the damage and whether or not the valve must be replaced will dictate whether a bypass is required.

Repair of congenital heart defects

Most congenital malformations can be repaired surgically and fall into two categories. The first consists of those that require cardiopulmonary bypass, such as intracardiac abnormalities. For example, an incision into the heart enables the tissue on each side of a small septal defect to be sutured together; larger septal defects may require a patch of material to close the opening. The second category consists of procedures that do not need a bypass, such as ligation of a patent ductus arteriosus or removal of an aortic constriction.

Coronary artery bypass graft (CABG)

The aim of the operation is to restore adequate blood flow to the myocardium beyond severe atherosclerotic obstructions of the coronary arteries. Cardiopulmonary bypass is used to support the circulation in most operations to replace these diseased arteries. Narrowed sections of the main coronary arteries are bypassed by grafting a blood vessel between the aorta and a point in the artery beyond the narrowed or blocked area (Figure 9.21). Multiple grafts are often used for multiple atheromatous lesions. For many years a section of vein removed from the leg was used for this, but increasingly the two internal mammary arteries (arteries that run down the inside of the chest wall) are also used. The internal mammary arteries are less likely than vein grafts to narrow over time. However, since there are only two internal mammary arteries many patients have a mixture of vein grafts and an internal mammary graft.

The principal uses of CABGs may be to relieve angina that is resistant to other forms of treatment and/or to prolong a person's life.

Heart transplantation

In many cases of irreversible heart damage (by long-lasting disease or viral infection) that cannot be treated by any other medical or surgical means, heart transplantation is the only option. This procedure, which involves removing the diseased organ and replacing it with a healthy human heart, was first attempted in 1967 by surgeons in Cape Town, South Africa. On that pioneering occasion the recipient survived for 18 days before succumbing to a pulmonary infection caused in part by immunosuppressive medication required to reduce the chance of donor organ rejection. Since then, however, long-term survival rates have improved and around 300 transplants are performed in the UK each year. A smaller number of combined heart and lung transplants are also performed each year in patients with lung disease, or heart disease that has caused secondary damage to the lungs. The number of available donor organs limits the number of transplants that may be attempted. Experimental artificial hearts have also been implanted, but these require an external power supply and long-term survival rates are unknown.

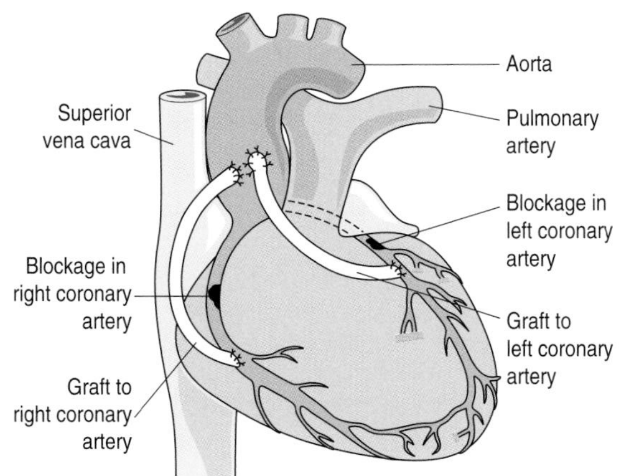

Figure 9.21 Coronary artery bypass.

Perhaps the major factor affecting long-term survival in recipients of donor organs is the risk of rejection. Human beings have evolved a complex immune system that recognises and attacks foreign materials that enter the body. Unfortunately, this system cannot differentiate between disease-causing pathogens and the cells of a life-saving transplant. Consequently, even before a transplant may be attempted, a number of tests must be undertaken to determine the compatibility of the tissue types of the potential recipient and the donor. This is referred to as 'histocompatibility', and the principles of tissue typing are similar to those for red blood cell typing. Unfortunately, a number of very sick patients may never have the opportunity to receive a donor heart, as they die before a compatible organ becomes available.

If a compatible heart is found and transplanted, immunosuppressive drugs, such as azathioprine, cortisone, prednisolone and ciclosporin, must be administered in the weeks and months following the operation to reduce the chance of acute transplant rejection. Unfortunately, this means that the patient has a greater risk of developing a postoperative infection. Another complication of chronic immunosuppression is the higher risk of skin cancer and lymph gland tumours. Consequently, the regimen of immunosuppressants must be carefully monitored and after some months the dosage can often be reduced.

Acute rejection of the heart is rare after 6 months, although the body may continue to attack the coronary arteries of the donor heart, and symptoms of coronary heart disease may become a problem after several years.

Aside from the risk of rejection, recovery from heart transplantation is similar to that from other forms of cardiac surgery, although the patient may have been weaker than most before the procedure. Because the transplanted heart has no nerve supply, it will respond much more slowly to the demands of physical activity. However, most people who have undergone transplants are eventually able to undertake a normally active life.

The outlook for those people fortunate enough to receive a heart transplant is good. Between 85 and 90 per cent of recipients survive for at least 1 year after the operation; 75 per cent are still alive after 5 years; and 50–60 per cent live for a further 5 years.

FURTHER READING

Allender S, Peto V, Scarborough P et al. 2006 Coronary Heart Disease Statistics. British Heart Foundation: London

Berne RM, Levy MN 2001 Cardiovascular Physiology, 8th edn. Mosby: London

Guyton AC, Hall JE 2005 Textbook of Medical Physiology, 11th edn. WB Saunders: London

Jacob S 2001 Atlas of Human Anatomy. Churchill Livingstone: Edinburgh

Julian DG, Camm AJ, Fox KM et al. 1996 Disease of the Heart, 2nd edn. WB Saunders: London

Levick JR 2003 An Introduction to Cardiovascular Physiology, 3rd edn. Arnold: London

Rang HP, Dale MM, Ritter JM, Moore P 2003 Pharmacology, 5th edn. Churchill Livingstone: Edinburgh

Zipes DP, Libby P, Bono RO, Braunwald E 2005 Braunwald's Heart Disease: A Textbook of Cardiovascular Medicine, 7th edn. WB Saunders: London

Chapter 10

Management of respiratory diseases

Stephanie Enright

CHAPTER CONTENTS

INTRODUCTION

Students' note

Other relevant information, such as the active cycle of breathing technique (ACBT) and basic respiratory anatomy and physiology of the lungs, can be found in Chapter 8, Physiotherapy in Thoracic Surgery.

Diseases of the respiratory system are a major cause of illness worldwide and are an increasingly important cause of mortality and morbidity (Rimington et al. 2001). In the UK they are the most common reason for consulting a general practitioner, and result in more days lost from work than any other type of illness (Yelin et al. 2006).

Respiratory diseases can be broadly divided into obstructive and restrictive types, although most patients have elements of both:

1. *Obstructive diseases* include conditions in which there is a resistance to airflow either through reversible factors such as bronchospasm or inflammation, or through irreversible factors such as airway fibrosis or loss of elastic recoil owing to damage to the airways and the alveoli.
2. *Restrictive disorders* are characterised by reduced lung compliance leading to the loss of lung volume, which may be caused by disease affecting the lungs, pleura, chest wall or neuromuscular mechanisms. These diseases are therefore different from the obstruc-tive diseases in their pure form, although mixed restrictive and obstructive conditions can occur.

Obstructive diseases are by far the most common and are secondary only to heart disease as a major cause of disability (Prescott et al. 2003). Therefore their pathophysiology and treatment will be discussed initially in some detail. These diseases include:

- chronic bronchitis
- emphysema
- chronic bronchitis and emphysema together
- asthma
- bronchiectasis
- cystic fibrosis.

Next, as the changing pattern of respiratory disease has resulted in opportunistic pneumonias, which are a common presentation in patients with acquired immune deficiency syndrome (AIDS), the restrictive disorders and their management will then be considered. They are:

- pneumonia
- pleurisy
- pleural effusion
- pneumothorax
- acute respiratory distress syndrome (ARDS)
- fibrosing alveolitis.

Finally, there are other lung disorders that fit into neither of the first two categories but need to be included owing to their prevalence within the community or hospital environment. They are:

- lung abscess
- pulmonary tuberculosis
- bronchial and lung tumors
- respiratory failure.

CHRONIC OBSTRUCTIVE PULMONARY DISEASE: BASIC ISSUES

Chronic obstructive pulmonary disease (COPD) is an ill-defined term that is often applied to patients who have a combination of chronic bronchitis and emphysema, which frequently occur together (and may also include asthma). In the majority of cases, chronic bronchitis is the major cause of obstruction, but in some cases emphysema is predominant. There are many patients who report shortness of breath increasing in severity over several years and, on examination, are found to have a chronic cough, an overinflated chest and poor exercise tolerance. It is often difficult to assess clinically to what extent these patients have chronic bronchitis or emphysema or a mixture of both.

Patients may also present with a more episodic form of disease, which is a characteristic of an asthmatic component. Therefore, 'chronic obstructive pulmonary disease' is a convenient term that encompasses one or all of these pathological components.

> ***Key point***
> Chronic bronchitis and emphysema often coexist in COPD; the disease is progressive and is characterised by acute exacerbations. It is not usually diagnosed until irreversible damage has occurred.

It is difficult to determine the exact prevalence of COPD. However, figures from general practice suggest that 5 per cent of men and 2 per cent of women will be diagnosed as suffering from COPD, although in the population as a whole it is estimated that 11 per cent of men and 8 per cent of women have evidence of obstructed airways when specifically tested by spirometry (Joint Health Surveys Unit 1996). COPD is projected to be the fifth major cause of death worldwide by 2010 (Office for National Statistics 1997).

The survival rate for COPD varies between 5 and 30 years, but eventually cardiac and ventilatory failure will occur. Avoidance of the precipitating factors listed below will tend to improve the prognosis:

- stopping smoking
- control of atmospheric pollution
- prompt treatment of all acute infections
- maintenance of good general health.

Since COPD is characterised by obstruction, the greater the obstruction, the lower the chance of survival (Pearson and Calverley 1995). Obstruction to flow is measured by FEV_1, which stands for *forced expiratory volume in one second*; together with age, FEV_1 is the most important determinant of survival (Table 10.1).

CHRONIC BRONCHITIS

> ***Definition***
> Chronic bronchitis is a chronic or recurrent increase in the volume of mucus secretion sufficient to cause expectoration when this is not due to localised bronchopulmonary disease. In the definition of this disease, chronic/recurrent is further defined as a daily cough with sputum for at least 3 months of the year for at least 2 consecutive years and airways obstruction that does not change markedly over periods of several months (West 1995). Chronic bronchitis is a clinical diagnosis (unlike the definition of emphysema).

Aetiology of chronic bronchitis

This is more common in middle to late adult life and in men more than women (Clarke 1991), although recent

Table 10.1 The relationship between age, FEV_1 and survival

Age	FEV_1	3-year survival probability
< 60	$> 50\%$ of expected	90%
>60	$> 50\%$ of expected	80%
> 60	40–50% of expected	75%
> 60	30–40% of expected	60%

data suggest that mortality is now rising faster in women (Dransfield et al. 2006).

Cigarette smoking is the chief culprit and, although in the UK over 20 per cent of the adult population continue to smoke (DOH 1997), only 15–20 per cent of smokers develop COPD. The reason for this is probably genetic (Silverman et al. 2000), although the number of cigarettes smoked does have an effect on the progression of the disease.

Exposure to Risk: Pack-Years

Rather than simply recording a patient's current smoking habits, a much better indicator of any potential deterioration in lung function is an assessment of pack-years, which is the number of packs (20 cigarettes per pack) smoked daily multiplied by the number of years of smoking. For example, someone aged 60 years who has smoked five cigarettes per day (0.25 of a pack) since the age of 15 has a lifetime exposure equal to $0.25 \times 45 = 11$ pack-years. Another person of the same age who smoked 30 cigarettes per day (1.5 packs) between the ages of 15 and 25, gave up till age 40 and since then has smoked one pack per day, has a lifetime exposure of $(1.5 \times 10) + (1 \times 20) = 35$ pack-years.

Atmospheric pollution (e.g. industrial smoke, smog and coal dust) will also predispose to the development of the disease, which is therefore more common in urban than in rural areas. It is more prevalent in socioeconomic groups 4 and 5 (Yelin et al. 2006) and is costly in terms of working days lost annually in Britain.

Pathology of chronic bronchitis

The hallmark is hypertrophy and an increase in number of mucous glands in the large bronchi with evidence of inflammatory changes in the small airways (Thurlbeck 1976). Some irritative substance stimulates overactivity of the mucus-secreting glands and the goblet cells in the bronchi and in the bronchioles, which causes secretion of excess mucus. This mucus coats the walls of the airways and tends to clog the bronchioles, which is functionally more important (West 1995). The cells increase in size and their ducts become dilated and may occupy as much as two-thirds of the wall thickness (West 1995). The airways become narrowed and show inflammatory changes, which results in mucosal oedema, thus further decreasing the diameter of the airways. The ciliary action is also inhibited.

Airflow limitation in COPD is more closely related to the dimensions of the distal (small) airways than proximal (large) airways (Hasegawa et al. 2006), and this narrowing of the lumen of the airways is further emphasised during expiration by the normal shortening and narrowing of the airways. Consequently, the airways obstruction is enhanced during expiration, with resulting trapping of air in the alveoli. The lungs gradually lose their elasticity as the disease progresses. They will gradually become permanently distended, which eventually may cause extensive rupture of the alveolar walls. After repeated exacerbations due to infection there is widespread damage to the bronchioles and the alveoli, with fibrosis and kinking occurring as well as compensatory overdistension of the surviving alveoli. This is closely allied to and contributory to the development of emphysema (Hogg 2004).

Clinical features of chronic bronchitis

The most important clinical features are cough, sputum, wheeze and dyspnoea.

Cough

10

The patient will complain of a cough for many years, initially intermittent and gradually becoming continuous. Fog, damp or infection increases it. The patient may also complain of bouts of coughing occasionally on lying down or in the morning. The cough and sputum production are not associated with either mortality or disability, and are reversible in most smokers once they stop smoking. The cough is caused either by irritation of airway nerve receptors due to the release of compounds from inflammatory cells or by the presence of increased mucous production.

Sputum

This is mucoid and tenacious, usually becoming mucopurulent during an infective exacerbation.

Wheeze

Wheezing is a symptom described by as many as 80 per cent of patients with COPD. It is a characteristic feature of COPD, although it is also reported in many other acute and chronic respiratory diseases. Caused by the sound generated by turbulent airflow through the narrowed conducting airways, it may be worse in the mornings or may be related to weather changes.

Dyspnoea (shortness of breath)

This occurs in patients with COPD and, together with the energy-requiring consequences of chronic infection and inflammation, leads to increased work of breathing (Donahoe et al. 1989). The patient becomes progressively more short of breath as the disease progresses.

Other signs and symptoms

Exercise intolerance

Owing to abnormalities of respiratory function, patients with COPD ventilate excessively and ineffectively at all work levels compared with subjects with normal lung function (O'Donnell 2006). This limits exercise performance. Limitation of exercise tolerance is, however, determined not only by pulmonary function but also by many other factors — including motivation, muscle mass and nutritional status (Decramer et al. 2005). Of equal importance is the impact these symptoms have on the patient's quality of life, activities of daily living and recreational activities. Patients should also be assessed for the impact that these symptoms have on:

- ability to work
- psychological well-being
- sexual function.

Deformity

These patients often develop a barrel chest due to hyperinflation and use of accessory muscles of respiration. The thoracic movements are gradually diminished and paradoxical indrawing in the intercostal spaces may develop.

10

Cyanosis

This is a blue coloration of the skin caused by the presence of desaturated haemoglobin due to reduced gaseous exchange. Cyanosis is also related to the development of complications, such as poor cardiac output due to ventricular failure leading to increased peripheral oxygen extraction. Cyanosis may also be due to an increase in red blood cells (polycythaemia) in response to chronic hypoxaemia.

Cor pulmonale

This may occur in the later stages of COPD. The impaired gas exchange in COPD caused by the disruption of ventilation and perfusion and the resulting hypoxia leads to widespread hypoxic pulmonary vasoconstriction. This causes an increase in pulmonary vascular resistance, resulting in pulmonary hypertension (Vender 1994). The increase in the pressure within the pulmonary artery will create a resistance, which the right ventricle must overcome. This eventually leads to hypertrophy and dilatation, a condition known as 'cor pulmonale'.

Right heart failure leads to an increased pressure in the peripheral tissues, resulting in the development of peripheral oedema. The combination of renal hypoxia and the increase in blood viscosity from polycythaemia increases the systemic blood pressure (BP) and eventually leads to left heart failure. The development of pulmonary oedema, which exacerbates the hypoxia and low cardiac output in patients with COPD, leads to a terminal stage of the disease. The mechanism of this cycle is illustrated in Figure 10.1.

Lung function

There is reduction of FEV_1 and the *forced vital capacity* (FVC) is grossly reduced. The residual volume (RV) will be increased at the expense of the vital capacity (VC) because of air trapping and the inability of the expiratory muscles to decrease the volume of the thoracic cavity. The expiratory flow–volume curve is grossly abnormal in severe disease; after a brief interval of moderately high flow, flow is strikingly reduced as the airways collapse, and flow limitation by dynamic compression occurs. A scooped-out appearance is often seen.

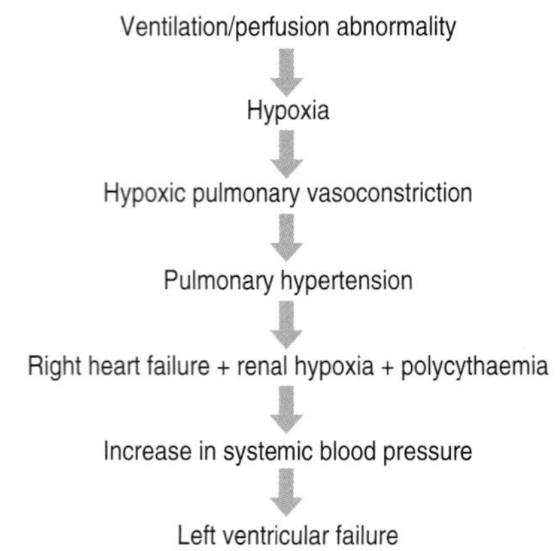

Figure 10.1 Mechanism of development of cor pulmonale and congestive heart failure in COPD.

Blood gases

Ventilation/perfusion mismatch is inevitable in COPD and leads to a low arterial oxygen pressure (PaO_2) with or without retention of carbon dioxide (CO_2). As the disease becomes severe, the arterial carbon dioxide pressure ($PaCO_2$) may rise, and there is some evidence that the sensitivity of the respiratory centre to CO_2 is reduced (Fleetham et al. 1980), which may leave the respiratory stimulus dependent upon the hypoxic drive. However, more recent evidence suggests that the administration of high levels of oxygen (> 70 per cent) in patients with COPD may increase hypercapnia owing to the reversal of pre-existing regional pulmonary hypoxic vasoconstriction, resulting in greater dead space (Crossley et al. 1997).

Auscultation signs

There will be inspiratory and expiratory wheeze with added coarse crepitations. The breath sounds are vesicular with prolonged expiration.

X-ray signs

No characteristic abnormality is seen in the early stages of the disease. If there is significant airways obstruction there may be signs of chest overexpansion (flattening of the diaphragm) and an enlarged retrosternal airspace.

EMPHYSEMA

Incidence of this condition is probably highest in England when compared to the rest of Europe, especially in the major centres of industry — although often there is a family history of the disease and it is more common in males (Corda et al. 2006).

Definition

Emphysema is a condition of the lung characterised by permanent dilatation of the air spaces distal to the terminal bronchioles with destruction of the walls of these airways. It is nearly always associated with chronic bronchitis and it is difficult to distinguish the two conditions during life.

Causes and types of emphysema

Causes and predisposing factors

Congenital or primary emphysema may be caused by alpha$_1$-antitrypsin deficiency. This is a rare inheri-ted condition, which affects one person in 4000 and results in the complete absence of one of the key antiprotease systems in the lung (Corda et al. 2006). The consequence is the early development of COPD, especially if the patient is already a smoker (Senn et al. 2005). Although alpha$_1$-antitrypsin deficiency is responsible for less than 1 per cent of cases of COPD, its hereditary nature means that it is worth diagnosing. It should, therefore, be considered in any young COPD patient.

Emphysema may be secondary to other factors, such as:

- obstructive airways disease — e.g. asthma, cystic fibrosis, chronic bronchitis
- occupational lung diseases — e.g. pneumoconiosis
- compensatory to contraction of one section of the lung — e.g. fibrous collapse or removal, when the remaining lung expands to fill the space.

Types of emphysema

Definition

Centrilobular (centri-acinar) emphysema tends to affect the respiratory bronchioles, with most of the alveoli remaining normal. *Panlobular* (panacinar) emphysema results in widespread destruction of most alveoli, as well as respiratory bronchioles.

Emphysema is usually of the panacinar (panlobular) type. In centrilobular emphysema the upper zones of the lung are usually affected. This causes gross disturbance of the ventilation/perfusion relationship since there is a relatively well-preserved blood supply to the alveoli, but the amount of oxygen reaching the capillary is decreased owing to the damage to airways proximal to the alveoli. Panacinar emphysema predominantly affects the lower lobes and lower lobe involvement is more common in individuals with alpha$_1$-antitrypsin deficiency (Stavngaard et al. 2006). This has a less drastic effect on the ventilation/perfusion relationship, since the blood supply in the damaged areas is decreased in proportion to the decreased ventilation in those areas.

Pathology of emphysema

Smoking causes the clustering of pulmonary alveolar macrophages (which are the major defence cells of the respiratory tract) around the terminal bronchioles. These macrophages are abnormal in smokers and release proteolytic enzymes, which destroy lung tissue locally. Polymorphonuclear leucocytes, necessary to combat infection in the lung, release an enzyme that also destroys lung tissue. The defence mechanism against the unwanted action of these enzymes lies in the serum alpha$_1$-antitrypsin, which is normally present in the airway lining fluids. Oxidants released by both cigarette smoke and the leucocytes tend to inactivate the antiproteolytic action of the alpha$_1$-antitrypsin, thus causing destruction of lung tissue, as seen in centrilobular emphysema (Stavngaard et al. 2006).

Subsequently, the walls of the airways become weak and inelastic owing to the damage from repeated infections. They tend to act as a one-way valve since the walls collapse on expiration. This causes air trapping and consequent increase in the intra-alveolar pressure during expiration. The alveolar septa break down and form bullae (Figure 10.2).

During expiration, the pressure from the trapped air in the bullae may compress adjacent healthy tissue, thus causing occlusion and trapping of air in that tissue. The capillaries around the alveolar walls become stretched, causing the lumen to decrease and atrophy to occur. This causes an alteration in the ventilation/perfusion relationship, owing to the loss of surface area for gaseous exchange and the decrease in blood supply resulting from damage to the pulmonary capillary network.

Clinical features of emphysema

Progressive dyspnoea

Shortness of breath occurs initially on exertion, but as the disease progresses it will gradually occur after less and less activity and finally at rest. This disabling breathlessness is what prevents the patient from working and gradually transforms the patient's state into one of severe exercise intolerance and disability (Folgering and von Herwaarden 1994).

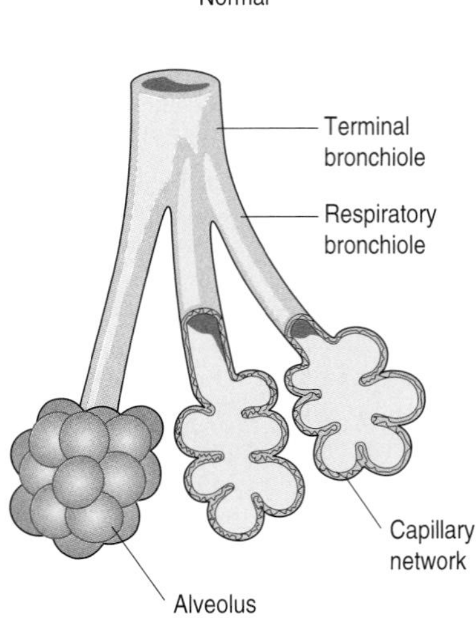

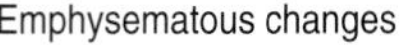

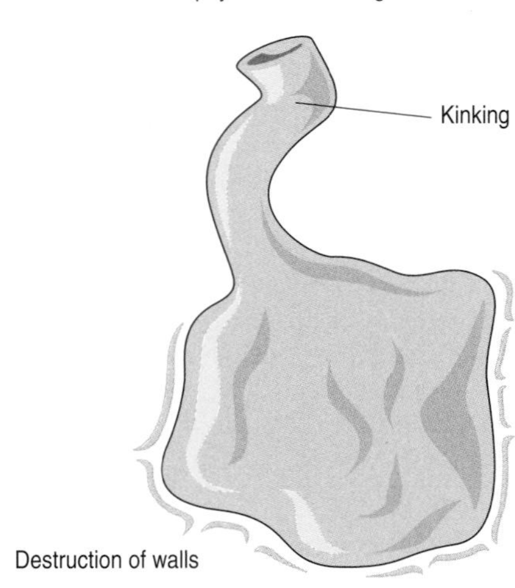

Figure 10.2 Emphysematous changes in the lung.

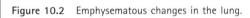

Respiratory pattern

The patient has a 'fishlike' inspiratory gasp, which is followed by prolonged, forced expiration usually against 'pursed lips'. The latter creates back-pressure, which tends to prevent airways shutdown during expiration. Owing to increased intrathoracic pressure the jugular veins fill on expiration. A 'flick' or 'bounce' of the abdominal muscles may be seen on expiration as the outward flow of air is suddenly checked by the obstruction of the airways (Figure 10.3).

Cough with sputum

This will be present if the disease is associated with chronic bronchitis or if there is infection.

Chest shape

The chest becomes barrel-shaped and fixed in inspiration, with widening of the intercostal spaces. There may also be indrawing of the lower intercostal spaces and supraclavicular fossa on inspiration. This is associated with the difficulty of ventilating stiff lungs through narrowed airways. The ribs are elevated by the accessory muscles of respiration and there is loss of thoracic mobility.

Poor posture

There may be a thoracic kyphosis plus elevated and protracted shoulder girdles.

Polycythaemia

This may develop in response to prolonged decrease in PaO_2 owing to the ventilation/perfusion imbalance.

Cor pulmonale

This occurs in the advanced stages of the disease.

Lung function

The FEV_1/FVC ratio is usually below 70 per cent. RV is increased and lung volume may exceed the predicted total lung capacity (TLC) (Decramer 1989).

Examination

The percussion note will be normal or hyper-resonant due to air trapping. Auscultation will reveal decreased breath sounds and prolonged expiration. The chest X-ray shows low flat diaphragms and hyperinflation.

Prognosis of emphysema

The patients become progressively more disabled, with death ultimately occurring from respiratory failure. Complications of the disease are pneumothorax due to rupture of an emphysematous bulla, and congestive cardiac failure.

COMBINED CHRONIC BRONCHITIS AND EMPHYSEMA

Within the spectrum of COPD, two extremes of clinical presentation are recognised: type A and type B. At one time these were classified as either 'pink puffers' (type A) or 'blue bloaters' (type B) to correlate with the relative amounts of emphysema and chronic bronchitis respectively (Figure 10.4). Whilst these definitions

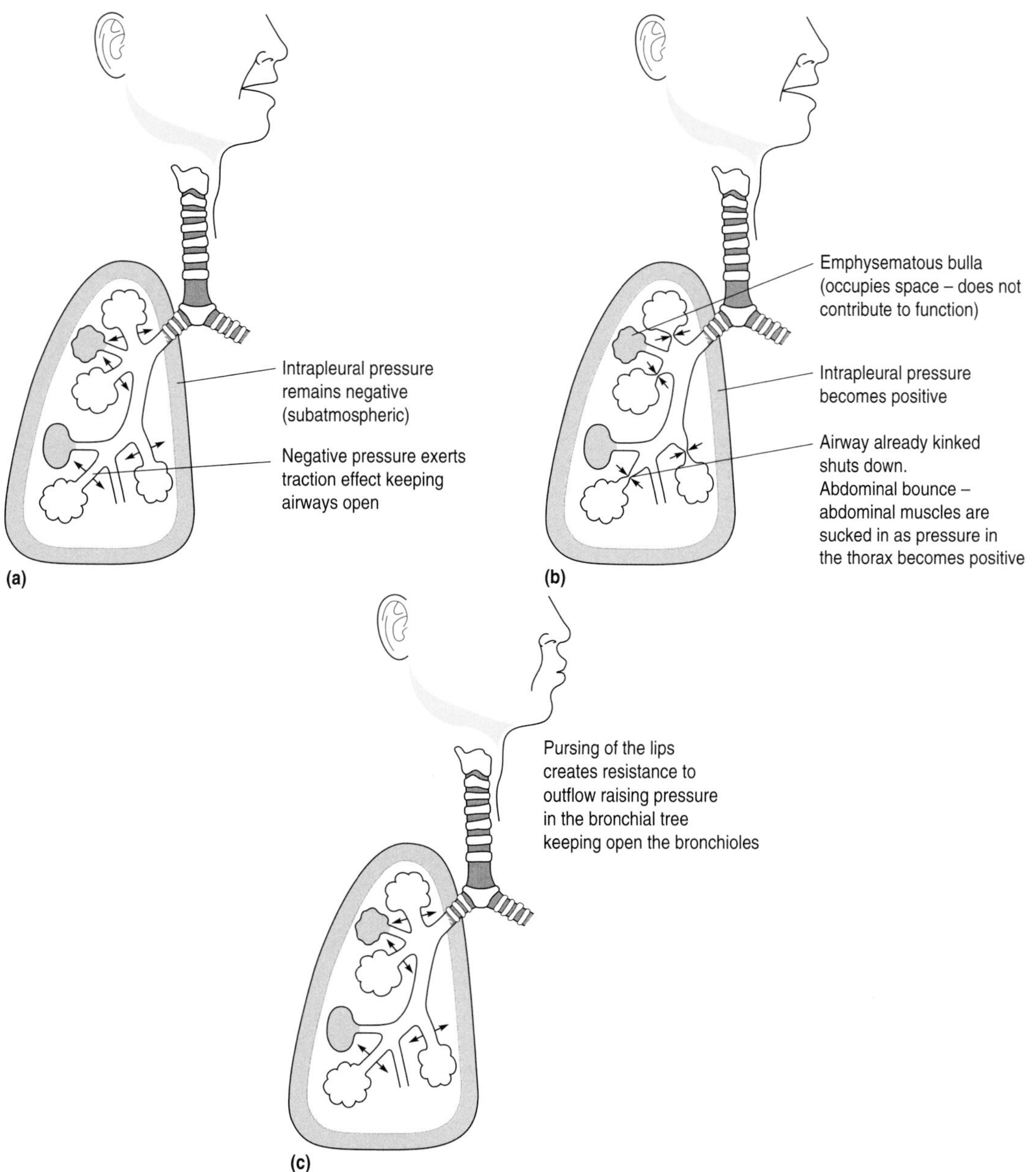

Figure 10.3 End of expiration: (a) normal; (b) in emphysema; (c) pursed-lip breathing.

are oversimplistic, it is worth remembering that patients can present in dramatically different ways (Kesten and Chapman 1993).

Blue bloaters

Patients with this syndrome often show the following symptoms:

- obesity
- comparatively mild dyspnoea
- copious sputum, which may become infected
- low PaO_2 and high $PaCO_2$ ($PaO_2 > 8$ kPa; $PaCO_2 > 6.5$ kPa) because they tend to hypoventilate
- central cyanosis with cor pulmonale
- peripheral oedema
- an increased residual volume but normal TLC.

10

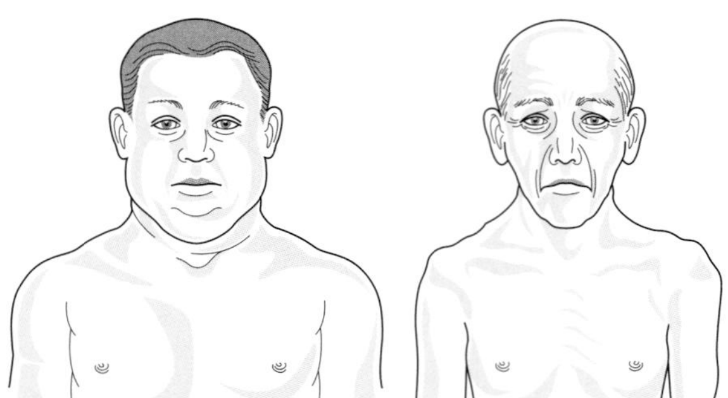

Figure 10.4 Blue bloater and pink puffer.

Pink puffers

Patients with this syndrome often show the following symptoms:

- an anxious expression
- general thinness
- severe breathlessness
- little or no sputum production
- relatively normal PaO_2 and $PaCO_2$ (PaO_2 < 8 kPa; $PaCO_2$ normal/low) due to hyperventilation early on in the disease
- central cyanosis and the development of cor pulmonale in the later stages of the disease
- generally no peripheral oedema until the late stages of the disease
- an increased TLC due to hyperventilation.

10

MEDICAL TREATMENT OF COPD

Principles of treatment

1. *Decrease the bronchial irritation to a minimum.* The patient should be advised to stop smoking and avoid dusty, smoky, damp or foggy atmospheres. Occupation or housing conditions may need to be changed.
2. *Control infections.* All infections should be treated promptly, as each exacerbation will cause further damage to the airways. The patient should have a supply of antibiotics at home and receive a vaccination against influenza each winter. The main affecting organisms are *Streptococcus pneumoniae* and *Haemophilus influenzae,* which are usually sensitive to amoxicillin or trimethoprim.
3. *Control bronchospasm.* Although bronchospasm is not a prominent feature of this disease, drugs (e.g. salbutamol) may be given to relieve the airways obstruction as much as is possible.
4. *Control/decrease the amount of sputum.* Patients with chronic bronchitis may present with excessive bronchial secretions and are usually able to eliminate this by themselves. However, during an episode when secretions may become difficult to eliminate, physiotherapy techniques, including humidification, positioning and manual techniques, may aid expectoration and reduce airflow obstruction in the short term (Cochrane et al. 1977).
5. *Oxygen therapy.* Oxygen must be prescribed and should be given with great care, especially if a normal pH indicates a chronic compensated respiratory acidosis (renal conservation of bicarbonate ions (HCO_3) to maintain pH within 7.35–7.45). In this instance HCO_3 is raised above 24 mmol/L whilst the PaO_2 is low and the $PaCO_2$ is raised. Controlled oxygen may be given via a Ventimask (or equivalent) with careful monitoring of blood gas levels.
6. *Long-term oxygen therapy* (LTOT). As respiratory function deteriorates, the level of oxygen in the blood falls, leading to an increase in pulmonary hypoxic vasoconstriction and a deterioration in cardiac function. In 1981, the Medical Research Working Party examined the effects of supplementary low concentrations of oxygen (24 per cent) for 15 hours a day in COPD and found that it reduced 3-year mortality from 66 per cent to 45 per cent. The British Thoracic Society guidelines (1997) suggest that patients who have a PaO_2 of less than 7.3 kPa, with or without hypercapnia, and a FEV_1 of less than 1.5 L, should receive LTOT. This therapy should be considered also for patients with a PaO_2 between 7.3 and 8.0 kPa and evidence of pulmonary hypertension, peripheral oedema or nocturnal hypoxia.

Medications

Drugs used in the treatment of respiratory disease broadly fall into two categories: relievers and preventers.

- The *relievers* are used to reduce bronchospasm and include the beta$_2$-agonists (which may be short- or long-acting), the anticholinergics and the xanthene derivatives.
- The *preventers* may be used to prevent bronchial hyperreactivity and reduce bronchial mucosal inflammatory reactions; they include the corticosteroids.

Beta$_2$ (β_2)-agonists

Beta-agonists such as salbutamol (Ventolin) and terbutaline (Bricanyl) work by stimulating beta$_2$-receptors, which are widespread throughout the respiratory system. These stimulate adenylate cyclase, which leads to bronchodilation. Beta-receptors are also found in other tissues, including the heart, although these are of the $beta_1$ subtype.

Even though modern bronchodilators are designed to be $beta_2$-selective, they may still cause an increase in heart rate and other side-effects, which include fine tremor, tachycardia, and hypokalaemia (low potassium) after high doses. Inhaled therapy is therefore preferred to oral, as the former limits the amount of drug that finds its way into the general circulation. The long-acting beta-agonist agents, salmeterol and formoterol, offer a more favourable dose regimen, and respiratory physicians are adding a long-acting beta-agonist for patients who have not responded fully to short-acting beta-agonists and an anticholinergic used together.

Anticholinergics

Anticholinergic bronchodilators work by preventing bronchoconstriction, mediated by the parasympathetic nervous system. Two agents are currently available, ipratropium bromide and oxitropium bromide. Most studies suggest that these agents are at least as potent as beta-agonists when used alone in COPD (Tashkin et al. 1986). A short-acting bronchodilator ($beta_2$-agonist or anticholinergic) used 'as required' is recommended as initial therapy in the British Thoracic Society guidelines (BTS 1997).

Xanthene derivatives

The precise mode of action of the xanthene derivatives, such as theophylline and aminophylline, remains somewhat uncertain, although they are moderately powerful bronchodilators. They have, however, been shown to improve symptoms in COPD by increasing the contractual ability of the diaphragm (Murciano et al. 1989).

Corticosteroids

The role of inhaled steroids (beclometasone, budesonide) in COPD will vary from patient to patient. Steroids work by reducing inflammation and reducing bronchial hyperactivity. Trials have shown that about 10–20 per cent of COPD patients will improve significantly following a short course of high-dose oral steroids (Gross 1995).

The most serious limitation to oral steroid therapy is the risk of long-term side-effects, which include osteoporosis, adrenal suppression, muscle wasting, poor immune response and impaired healing. However, a positive response to corticosteroids justifies the administration of regular inhaled steroids.

Drug delivery systems

The objective of inhaled therapy in COPD is to maximise the quantity of drug that reaches its site of action while minimising side-effects from unintended systemic absorption. Most metered-dose inhalers (which are later described in detail for asthmatic patients) are designed to deliver particles of between 0.5 and 10 microns (micrometres). Unfortunately, poor inhaler technique tends to mean that only a relatively small proportion of the drug actually reaches its site of action. It is therefore imperative that a good inhaler technique be adopted (as described for patients with asthma).

In acute exacerbations, when conventional inhalers have proved inadequate, nebulisers may be used to deliver a therapeutic dose of a drug as an aerosol within a fairly short period of time, usually 5–10 minutes (BTS 1997). The type of nebuliser for home use consists of a compressor or pump, a chamber and a mask or mouthpiece. The compressor blows air into the chamber, where it is forced through a drug solution and past a series of baffles. The solution is converted into a fine mist, which is then inhaled by the patient through the mask or the mouthpiece.

PHYSIOTHERAPY TECHNIQUES IN COPD

General aims of treatment

The general aims are:

- to relieve any bronchospasm, facilitate the removal of secretions and optimise gaseous exchange
- to improve the pattern of breathing, breathing control and the control of dyspnoea
- to teach local relaxation, improve posture and help allay fear and anxiety
- to increase knowledge of the patient's lung condition and control of the symptoms
- to improve exercise tolerance and ensure a long-term commitment to exercise
- to give advice about self-management in activities of daily living.

The treatment given must be appropriate to the stage of the disease and the patient's general health.

Treatment in the early stages

Key point

The most important themes are clearing the airways of secretions, establishing a correct breathing pattern, improving or maintaining exercise capacity, and patient education in self-management.

Removal of secretions

The active cycle of breathing technique

The ACBT is a cycle of breathing control, thoracic expansion exercises and the forced expiratory technique (FET) that has been shown to be effective in the clearance of bronchial secretions (Prior and Webber 1979; Wilson et al. 1995) and the improvement of lung function (Webber et al. 1986).

Thoracic expansion exercises are deep breathing exercises (three or four), which may be combined with a 3-second hold on inspiration (unless the patient is very breathless, in which case this may not be tolerated). This increase in lung volume allows air to flow via collateral channels (e.g. the pores of Kohn) and may assist in mobilising the secretions as air is able to get behind them. The increase in lung volume during the inspiratory phase of the cycle may also be achieved by the patient performing a 'sniff' manœuvre at the end of a deep inspiration. Manual techniques — for example, shaking, vibrations or chest clapping — may further aid in removal of secretions.

The FET manœuvre is a combination of one or two forced expirations (huffs) against an open glottis (as opposed to a cough, which is a forced expiration against a closed glottis). An essential part of the FET manœuvre is a pause for some breathing control, which prevents an increase in airflow obstruction.

Postural drainage/positioning

This may also aid sputum removal and may be combined with the ACBT. The optimum position for effectiveness must be established with each individual, although postural drainage for the lower lobe segments may be difficult as some patients may not tolerate the head-down position or even lying flat. The ACBT alone may be effective for many patients in the seated position (Cecins et al. 1999) and changes in position should be used to optimise gaseous exchange. In the lateral position, the lower lung is always better ventilated regardless of the side on which the subject is lying, although there still remains a bias in favour of the right side due to its larger size when compared to the left lung (Svanberg 1957). Perfusion is also preferential to the lower lung in the lateral position (West 1995), although if pathology exists within the lowermost lung, gaseous exchange may be compromised due to the presence of pulmonary hypoxic vasoconstriction which cannot be overcome by gravity (Chang et al. 1993).

Humidification

If the secretions are very thick and tenacious, the patient may be given humidification via a nebuliser. Inhalations with pine oil added to near-boiling water may also be given prior to treatments to remove excessive bronchial secretions.

Improving the breathing pattern

The patient is taught how to relax the shoulder girdle in a supported, posturally correct position such as crook half-lying. Breathing control is taught following clearance of secretions. If the patient is breathless, respiratory control is regained starting with short respiratory phases and allowing the rate to slow as the patient's breathing pattern improves.

Increasing/maintaining exercise tolerance

The patient may be treated as an inpatient or as an outpatient, in a health centre or at home by a community physiotherapist. It is important to see the patient regularly. Advice should be given on taking regular exercise: for example, a short walk every day. If possible, the patient should be offered participation in a multidisciplinary comprehensive programme of pulmonary rehabilitation.

Definition

The National Institutes of Health in the USA define pulmonary rehabilitation as 'a multidimensional continuum of services directed to persons with pulmonary disease and their families, usually an interdisciplinary team of specialists, with the goal of achieving and maintaining the individual's maximum level of independence and functioning in the community' (American Thoracic Society 1995).

There is unequivocal evidence to suggest that pulmonary rehabilitation improves both exercise capacity and health-related quality of life (Lacasse et al. 1996; Guell et al. 2006). In essence, the components of a pulmonary rehabilitation programme include aerobic exercise training, education about the background of the disease, smoking cessation, compliance with medication, nutritional support and energy-conserving strategies for activities of daily living. Pulmonary rehabilitation programmes may also include psychosocial support with regard to advice on benefits, sexual function and anxiety management.

Inspiratory muscle training

The potential for fatigue of the ventilatory muscles is now recognised as an important component of ventilatory limitation in patients with COPD (Moxham 1990; Green and Moxham 1993). Fatigue may be due to a combination of:

- increased mechanical load on the respiratory muscles
- reduced muscle strength
- reduced energy supply to the respiratory muscles (Roussos and Zakynthinos 1996).

It has also been established that respiratory muscle weakness, which may be a predisposition to muscle fatigue, is present in patients with COPD (Clanton and Diaz 1995; Polkey et al. 1995). It therefore follows that training techniques, which might specifically target the respiratory muscles, may prove beneficial in patients with COPD who may develop respiratory muscle weakness due to a loss of muscle mass.

Many studies have been performed to examine the benefits of inspiratory muscle training (IMT), particularly in patients with COPD (Smith et al. 1992). Despite this intensive investigation, IMT has failed to become part of routine clinical practice. In part this has been due to the paucity of controlled clinical trials, but more importantly it stems from the nature of the training adopted. In general the trials were confounded by the nature of their training methodology in which the frequency, duration and intensity of training were less than that required to achieve a true training response (Smith et al. 1992). Therefore the training methodology employed during IMT should follow the same principles that are applied to other skeletal muscles in terms of the frequency, duration and intensity of the training.

Training methodologies should also control for the lung volume at which the training takes place; otherwise the patient may alter the lung volume at which the training is performed in order to cope with the resistive load more easily (Goldstein et al. 1993). However, recent studies that have incorporated these principles during training at 80 per cent of maximum inspiratory pressure (MIP) have shown evidence of muscle fatigue (Chatwin et al. 2000), which indicates that an appropriate training response has been applied. By using an appropriate training methodology, increase in exercise capacity in moderately trained (Chatham et al. 1999) and highly trained subjects has been achieved (Enright et al. 2000). In addition to these improvements, associated increases in lung function and diaphragm thickness have been observed in healthy subjects and in adult patients with cystic fibrosis (Enright et al. 2004; Enright et al. 2006).

Treatment in the later stages

It is imperative that patients with COPD are able to maintain as much independence and maximum function as is possible through support from the hospital or community healthcare team. During acute exacerbations, the ACBT may be continued to assist clearance of secretions. Breathing control should be emphasised so that the patient can walk or climb stairs with confidence. Relaxation positions should be taught for regaining breathing control after activity has made the patient breathless. If the patient becomes very disabled, a walking frame may help to retain some degree of independence, as the arms are fixed and accessory muscles of inspiration may be used.

Non-invasive positive-pressure ventilation (NIPPV)

Tracheal intubation and mechanical ventilation providing intermittent positive-pressure ventilation (IPPV) is used in intensive care or high-dependency units to manage patients with deteriorating respiratory failure. However, tracheal intubation may result in complications, which include tracheal injury and infection. Furthermore, some patients find it difficult to stop using IPPV, resulting in a prolonged stay in intensive care.

NIPPV is therefore indicated for the delivery of intermittent positive pressure and may be applied via the nose or mouth using a silicone mask attached to a bedside ventilator. Unlike IPPV, NIPPV can be administered on a general ward for patients in respiratory failure (Sinuff et al. 2000). The ventilator is programmed to supplement the patient's own respiratory effort, and if required, oxygen therapy may be given in conjunction with NIPPV. NIPPV can be used during an acute exacerbation and has been shown to improve quality of life and arterial blood gas pressures (Meecham-Jones et al. 1995) and to reduce mortality in patients with COPD (Brochard et al. 1995).

Physiotherapy will be required for short spells but frequently throughout the day and sometimes at night. Intermittent positive pressure breathing (IPPB) may also be given using a mask if the patient is too drowsy to use a mouthpiece. Postural drainage may be necessary, if tolerated, together with rigorous shaking applied during the expiratory phase of the ventilator. Patients should be positioned appropriately in order to facilitate gaseous exchange.

Suction via an airway or the nose may have to be used as a last resort to remove secretions if the patient is unable to cough spontaneously. If $PaCO_2$ is high and PaO_2 is low, the patient should not be given a high concentration of oxygen. Two litres of oxygen through a nebuliser with the IPPB respirator driven off air gives a 25 per cent oxygen-to-air mix, which is generally suitable. Drugs such as mucolytic agents or bronchodilators may be provided through the nebuliser attached to the ventilator. The patient should be encouraged to sip drinks because dehydration makes the secretions viscid.

As the patient recovers, treatment should be directed towards that given in the 'early' stages, with special emphasis on a daily maintenance programme of regular exercise, sputum clearance and breathing exercises.

Terminal care

The main theme is to keep the patient as comfortable as possible. Treatment needs to be short and frequent. Non-invasive nasal ventilation may be provided for home use. Inhalations may be used to loosen and liquefy secretions. Suction may be necessary and the GP may provide medication for the patient if the person is being managed at home.

ASTHMA

Definition

Asthma is a clinical syndrome characterised by attacks of wheezing and breathlessness due to narrowing of the intrapulmonary airways. The severity of the narrowing varies over short periods and is reversible either spontaneously or as a result of treatment (Hargreave et al. 1990).

Types of asthma

It has been common practice to divide asthma into *extrinsic* and *intrinsic* forms. There is a degree of overlap, and many asthmatics, particularly adults, do not fall clearly into either group.

10

Extrinsic asthma

Extrinsic (atopic) asthma occurs in the younger age groups and is caused by identifiable trigger factors, such as specific allergens. Patients are usually sensitive to different factors (e.g. pollen, house dust mites, feathers, fur, dust, pollution and, occasionally, food, drugs and exercise) and have a family history of similar sensitivities Atopic subjects show an immediate skin reaction, elicited by pricking the skin through a drop of antigenic extract. Exposure to the precipitating factor causes a mucosal inflammatory allergic reaction. This type of asthma tends to be episodic. House dust mites provide the most common positive skin test in Britain, being positive in 80 per cent of children with severe asthma. Extrinsic asthma is common in young people and is associated with a family history of asthma, hay fever and eczema, although new evidence suggests that the presence of more than one of these factors is also associated with the development of asthma in later life (Porsbjerg et al. 2006).

Intrinsic asthma

Intrinsic (non-atopic) asthma tends to occur in the older patient as a chronic condition. This type of asthma is precipitated by, or associated with, chronic bronchitis, strenuous exercise, stress or anxiety. Respiratory infections are also a common factor in precipitating acute attacks; the majority of these are viral in origin (Nicholson et al. 1993), so antibiotics are inappropriate in their treatment.

Aetiology and prevalence of asthma

The condition can occur at any age but is most common in children, especially boys (ratio of about three to two). Approximately 10 per cent of children under 10 years of age in the UK have bouts of coughing and wheezing related to narrowing of the airways. Asthma accounts for more absences from school than any other chronic disease, although days lost from school may be underestimated owing to the underdiagnosis and undertreatment of childhood asthma (Speight 1983).

Childhood asthma generally remits after puberty but it may return in later life. Asthma that starts in middle age is more common in women than men and remission in this age group is rare.

The majority of cases of asthma are mild, although the course of the disease is unpredictable. The mortality rate is unacceptably high and has shown a slow rise since the 1960s to around 2000 deaths per year in England and Wales.

The rise in the prevalence of asthma has continued since 1988 but had been shown to decline by 2003 (Burr et al. 2006). This decline in asthma prevalence is thought to be due to better disease management, as more children are now using inhaled corticosteroids as a preventive treatment (Burr et al. 2006). However, despite the rise in the use of corticosteroids, undertreatment and inadequate appreciation of the severity of asthma by patients and doctors are important factors in determining mortality, with up to 86 per cent of asthma deaths being preventable (British Thoracic Association 1982). Those most at risk are patients who underestimate their symptoms. About 15–20 per cent of asthmatics do not notice moderate changes in their airflow obstruction (Rubinfeld and Pain 1976) and may quickly deteriorate until they suddenly present with severe asthma (Kikuchi et al. 1994). Patients with inadequately controlled severe persistent asthma are at a particularly high risk of exacerbations, hospitalisation and death, and often have severely impaired quality of life (Peters et al. 2006).

Pathology of asthma

In all types of asthma an underlying problem seems to be abnormal reactivity of the airways; that is, they narrow excessively in response to stimuli which would not affect normal subjects (Bone 1996). The main pathological changes occurring during an asthmatic attack are:

- spasm of the smooth muscle in the walls of the bronchi and bronchioles (bronchoconstriction)
- oedema of the mucous membrane of the bronchi and bronchioles
- excessive mucus production and mucus plugging.

These changes result in airways obstruction. The bronchial walls become infiltrated with eosinophils and there is thickening of the epithelial basement membrane.

At the end of an attack these changes are almost totally reversible, but if attacks occur frequently then long-standing changes will occur. Such changes are:

- hypertrophy of the smooth bronchial muscle, which increases the effect of bronchial spasm during an attack
- permanent thickening of the mucous membrane with an increase in the number of goblet cells and mucous glands
- overdistension of the alveoli due to trapping of air
- atelectasis of alveoli when a bronchiole, already narrowed, becomes blocked by mucus plugs.

Where the predominant factor precipitating asthma is an allergic reaction, there is antigen-mediated bronchoconstriction. This means that the antigen (allergen or precipitating factor) binds to two IgE molecules (immunoglobulin antibodies) on the membranes of mast cells present in the bronchial lining. This binding releases mediators that act on receptor sites on smooth muscle cells, causing changes in intracellular cyclic adenosine monophosphate (AMP) levels, which in turn result in muscular contraction. The mediators histamine, neutrophil chemotactic factor (NCF-A), platelet activating factor (PAF) and eosinophil chemotactic factor (ECF-A) are stored in granules within the mast cells as preformed mediators. This antigen–antibody reaction is part of the body's immune response, and previous exposure to the antigen results in greater bronchoconstriction.

Clinical features of asthma

Extrinsic asthma

In extrinsic asthma the onset is often sudden and paroxysmal, frequently at night. An attack starts with chest tightness, dryness or irritation in the upper respiratory tract. Attacks tend to be episodic, often occurring several times a year. Their duration varies from a few seconds to many months and the severity may be anything from mild wheezing to great distress. The most predominant features are summarised below.

Wheeze and dyspnoea

Dyspnoea may be intense and chiefly occurs on expiration, which becomes a conscious exhausting effort with a short gasping inspiration. Wheezing is always present on expiration but may also occur on inspiration in severe asthma.

Cough

At the initial stage of an attack the cough may be unproductive and 'barking' in nature. It causes an increase in bronchospasm and dyspnoea. As the attack subsides, the cough becomes productive of casts or plugs of sputum. Such plugs — made up of yellow viscid mucus and desquamated epithelial cells and eosinophils — are often coughed up during acute attacks, which may produce a marked relief of symptoms. Particularly in children, a cough may be the only presenting symptom of asthma (Corraco et al. 1979).

Posture

The patient will prefer to sit upright with the shoulder girdle fixed (by grasping a table or bed) to assist the accessory muscles of respiration. The chest is hyperinflated.

Pulse

This is rapid and there may be an increased drop in blood pressure during inspiration (> 10 mmHg) owing to an exaggeration in intrathoracic pressure swings due to severe airways obstruction (pulsus paradoxus). However, pulsus paradoxus may be absent even in very severe attacks of asthma. When it is present, the measurement is easily performed with a sphygmomanometer and provides a guide to progress and response to treatment (Pearson et al. 1993).

10

Electrocardiogram (ECG)

This will show a tachycardia and may show signs of right ventricular strain or the development of a large P-wave (P pulmonale). These abnormalities will return to normal as the attack subsides.

Cyanosis

This may occur at a very late stage in the progression of the disease due to worsening hypoxaemia (low PaO_2) if this is not corrected with adequate oxygen therapy.

Blood gases

Analysis of blood gases provides important information to help the management of severe asthma. The usual finding is of a low arterial PaO_2 (hypoxaemia) due to ventilation/perfusion mismatch, and a low $PaCO_2$ (hypocapnia) due to the effects of hyperventilation. Later in the disease process, the $PaCO_2$ may be found to be high because the hyperventilation fails to compensate for the fact that there are many underventilated alveoli distal to the blocked bronchioles. When the $PaCO_2$ is found to be increasing and the pH is low, this is a danger sign that the patient may be becoming tired and is likely to need assisted ventilation if immediate improvement cannot be achieved (British Thoracic Society 1997).

Breath sounds

These are vesicular, with evidence of a prolonged expiration and high-pitched wheeze. Crackles may also be heard if sputum is present. During severe attacks with worsening obstruction, the breath sounds may be diminished and occasionally become inaudible (silent chest) due to diminished airflow.

Percussion note

The note may be hyper-resonant if the patient is hyperinflated.

Chest X-ray

Radiography is not usually helpful in the management of asthma. It usually shows only overinflation, although it may be useful to demonstrate a pneumothorax if this is suspected.

Lung function

FEV_1 and FVC drop during a severe attack, with little sign of reversibility (Figure 10.5). However, if FEV_1 is measured before and after giving bronchodilators and there is a 15 per cent increase in FEV_1, this amounts to significant reversibility. The FEV_1 may be less than 30 per cent of FVC. TLC, FRC and RV may be increased due to overinflation of the lungs. Recovery is associated with a reduction in these lung volumes. Recordings of the peak expiratory flow rate (PEFR) for a week at home will often make the diagnosis of asthma obvious (Prior and Cochrane 1980). PEFR dips in the morning, especially during the recovery phase (Figure 10.6). If the dip is severe (less than 33 per cent of predicted), then respiratory arrest may occur (British Thoracic Society 1997). In a severe attack, the PEFR may drop below 100 litres/minute.

> **Clinical note**
>
> No abnormality should be detectable between attacks, although children with severe asthma may develop a pigeon chest or have a persistent, low-pitched wheeze with a productive cough.

Intrinsic (chronic) asthma

This is less paroxysmal in character than extrinsic asthma and is often associated with chronic bronchitis.

Clinical features are similar to those described above for extrinsic asthma, but wheeze and dyspnoea tend to be continuous and worse in the morning, cough produces mucoid sputum, respiratory infections occur with increasing frequency, and X-rays may show emphysematous changes.

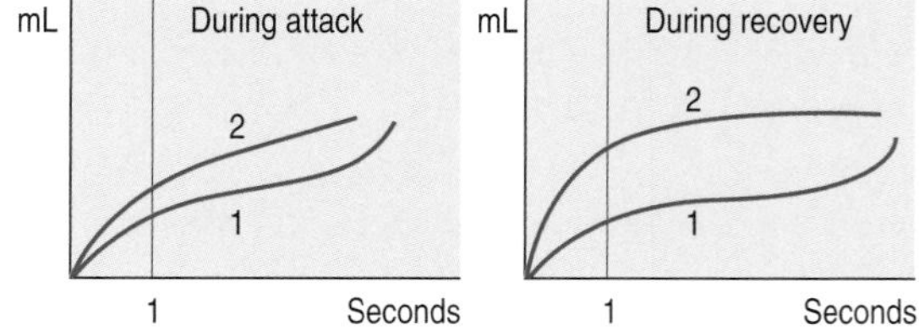

Figure 10.5 Asthma: FEV_1 and FVC reversibility during an attack and recovery. 1 = before bronchodilator; 2 = after bronchodilator.

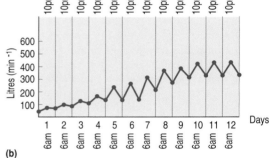

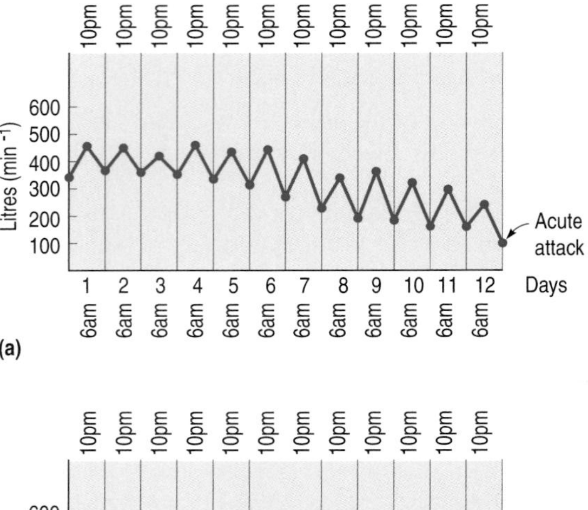

Figure 10.6 Dipping charts in asthma. (a) Recording of peak flow at home showing deterioration before onset of acute attack. Intervention when there is a chart like this can prevent the attack. (b) During recovery there is still diurnal variation. These patients are at risk and should have long-term monitoring.

Acute severe asthma

As asthma is by nature a paroxysmal condition, acute attacks that are resistant to bronchodilators may occur. Such attacks are potentially life-threatening, so prompt and effective treatment is imperative. In general, clinical criteria are most helpful, as is a person's own recognition that his or her asthma symptoms are worsening. Table 10.2 lists warning signs of an acute severe attack.

Table 10.2 Warning signs of an attack of acute severe asthma

Early warning signs	Signs of increasing severity
■ Increase in symptoms	■ Dyspnoea at rest
■ Sleep disturbance	■ Peak flow below 100 L/min
■ Increase in bronchodilator use	■ Deteriorating blood gases
■ Fall in peak flow	■ Pulsus paradoxus
■ Decrease in exercise tolerance	■ Tachycardia

MEDICAL TREATMENT OF ASTHMA

Oxygen therapy

Unlike patients with long-standing COPD, patients with asthma may tolerate higher levels of oxygen to correct hypoxaemia. During an acute episode it is essential that oxygen therapy be titrated according to the level of PaO_2. It may be evident on clinical examination, however, that the asthmatic patient also has evidence of COPD. In this situation examination of the blood gases will reveal whether the patient has a chronic compensated respiratory acidosis where the use of controlled oxygen will be required.

Medications

Suitable drugs are discussed in the earlier section on the management of patients with COPD. Their use is included here particularly with regard to the treatment of asthma.

Beta$_2$ (β_2)-agonists

The side-effects of salbutamol (Ventolin) and terbutaline (Bricanyl) include fine tremor, tachycardia, and hypokalaemia (low potassium) after high doses.

Corticosteroids

In a small proportion of asthmatic people, long-term oral corticosteriods (e.g. beclometasone and budesonide) will be necessary. In circumstances when an attack supervenes very rapidly, a short course of oral steroids (prednisolone) is required. It cannot be emphasised enough that this approach is safe and certainly much safer than a poorly controlled attack of asthma. There have been suggestions that the adverse effects associated with long-term steroids, such as osteoporosis, might be less common in asthma but this has been shown to be untrue (Adinoff and Hollester 1983). The introduction of inhaled corticosteroids in 1972 radically changed the management of asthma, as side-effects from oral steroids were prevented.

Leukotriene antagonists

Oral inhibitors of leukotriene action may help to reduce the inflammatory component of asthma (Israel et al. 1993).

> **Mucolytic agents and asthma**
>
> There is no evidence that mucolytic agents are effective in the treatment of acute or chronic asthma (Rudolf et al. 1978).

Other agents

Other types of medication that may be useful include:

- anticholinergic agents
- long-acting beta$_2$-agonists
- theophylline
- salmeterol.

Delivery of medication

Metered-dose inhalers

It is good practice to use inhaled therapy for asthma. This keeps the dose down and reduces side-effects.

Beta$_2$-agonists, anticholinergic agents and corticosteroids are frequently prescribed in metered-dose inhalers (MDIs). The particles leaving an MDI do so with considerable velocity and, even with a perfect technique of inhalation, only about 10 per cent of the dose reaches the respiratory tract; the remainder is deposited in the mouth or swallowed (Davies 1973). The MDI does have the advantage of being small and portable and familiar to many asthmatics. The MDI can also be used with a spacer, which virtually removes oropharangeal deposition, thereby increasing lung deposition to 20–30 per cent (O'Callahan et al. 1997).

Breath-activated devices (Figure 10.7) are primed before actuation and the MDI is triggered by inspiratory airflow. The airflow required is low and the triggering of the device is quiet enough not to disturb the inspiration. Beta$_2$-agonists, anticholinergic agents and corticosteroids can be prescribed in this form of inhaler.

There are various *dry powder systems* (Figure 10.8):

- The Diskhaler contains four or eight doses in one disc. Each dose is sealed to prevent problems with humidity.
- The Turbohaler is a multidose dry powder system that requires an inspiratory airflow of only 60 L/minute. Patients therefore tend to find this system easy to use.
- The Disk/Accuhaler is a dry powder multidose system used for the delivery of salmeterol and fluticasone propionate.
- With Rotocaps each dose of medication is loaded into the inhaler prior to use and so the inhaler needs to be stored in a dry place. Rotocaps absorb moisture and the particles can become too large to inhale.

Nebulisers

If asthma symptoms become severe, inspiratory airflow may become limited to such an extent that the contents of an MDI cannot be inhaled adequately. With a nebuliser, a high-velocity jet of air or oxygen sucks liquid up a tube and the liquid is broken into tiny particles that

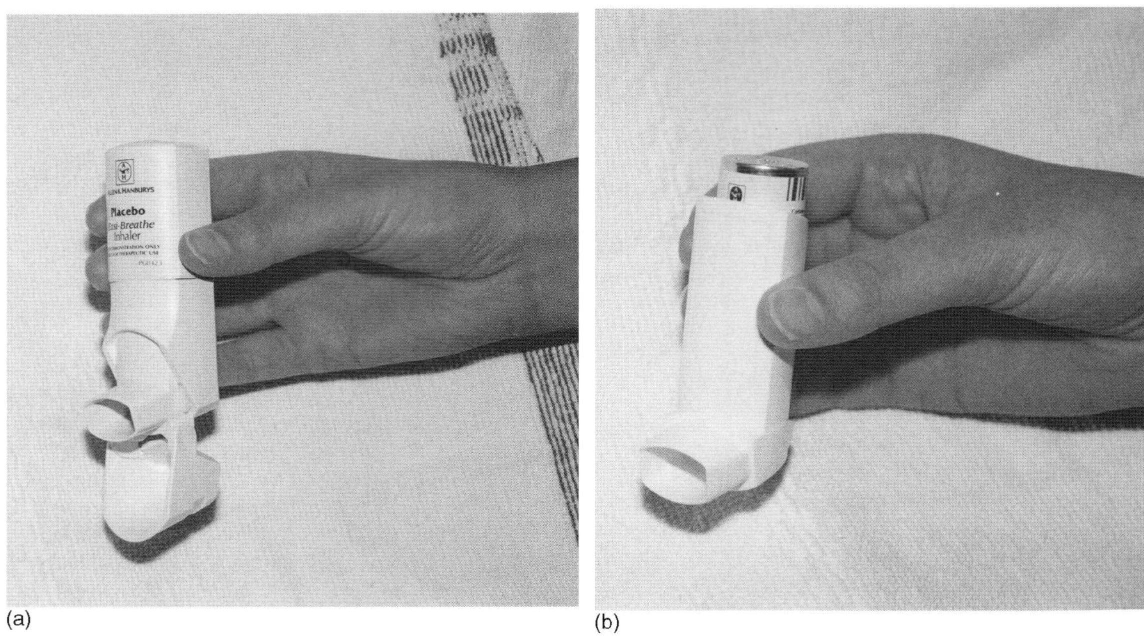

(a) (b)

Figure 10.7 Breath-activated metered-dose inhalers. (Courtesy of Melanie Reardon and Joanne Kenyon.)

are inhaled and deposited in the lungs (Rees et al. 1982) (Figure 10.9). Ultrasonic nebulisers may also be used to deliver medication, although currently there is insufficient data to verify their advantage over other nebulisers in the management of patients with asthma and COPD (Brocklebank et al. 2001).

Guidelines for drug therapy

The British Thoracic Society (1997) has introduced guidelines on the drug management of asthma. Steps 1 to 3 below apply to the treatment of less severe asthma, and relate to the attempt to control symptoms. Steps 4 and 5 apply to the treatment of more severe asthma, when it may not be possible to abolish symptoms. Stepping down and up this treatment ladder is recommended to match therapy to the person's current need.

- *Step 1*: Inhaled short-acting beta$_2$-agonists p.r.n. (when required), but not more than once daily. If needed more than once daily, move on to step 2. No prophylaxis (preventers such as inhaled corticosteroids).
- *Step 2*: Inhaled short-acting beta$_2$-agonists p.r.n. Regular low-dose inhaled steroids, such as 100–400 micrograms of beclometasone twice daily, or budesonide daily via a large-volume spacer.
- *Step 3*: Inhaled short-acting beta$_2$-agonists p.r.n. Regular high-dose inhaled steroids, such as 800–2000 micrograms of beclometasone, or budesonide daily via a large-volume spacer. In a very small number of patients who experience side-effects with high-dose inhaled steroids, either the long-acting inhaled beta$_2$-agonists option is used *or* a sustained-release theophylline may be added to step 2 medication.
- *Step 4*: Inhaled short-acting beta$_2$-agonists p.r.n. Regular high-dose inhaled steroids, such as 800–2000 micrograms of beclometasone, or budesonide daily via a large-volume spacer. Add in long-acting inhaled beta$_2$-agonists *or* sustained-release theophylline or high-dose inhaled bronchodilators.
- *Step 5*: Inhaled short-acting beta$_2$-agonists p.r.n. Regular high-dose inhaled steroids, such as 800–2000 micrograms of beclometasone, or budesonide daily via a large-volume spacer. Add in one or more long-acting bronchodilator as in step 4 *plus* regular oral prednisolone as a single daily dose.

Management between attacks

The environment

This comprises identifying and removing the cause, if known. For example, a patient may have to avoid certain foods and damp. The home environment should be cleaned regularly, bedding vacuumed frequently, and synthetic fibres used in place of feathers for pillows and quilts. Gortex mattress covers are not inexpensive but are impervious to mites and their faecal particles. It may also be of benefit to avoid certain domestic animals, although getting rid of a loved family pet may

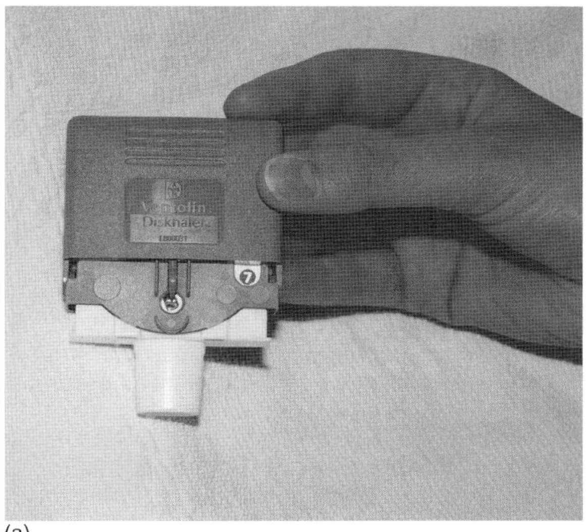

(a)

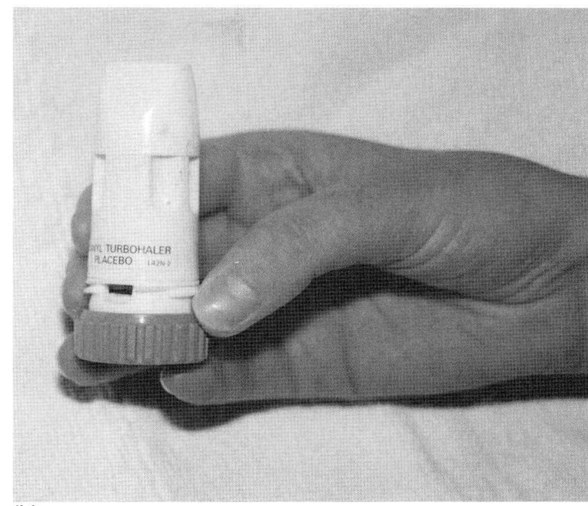

(b)

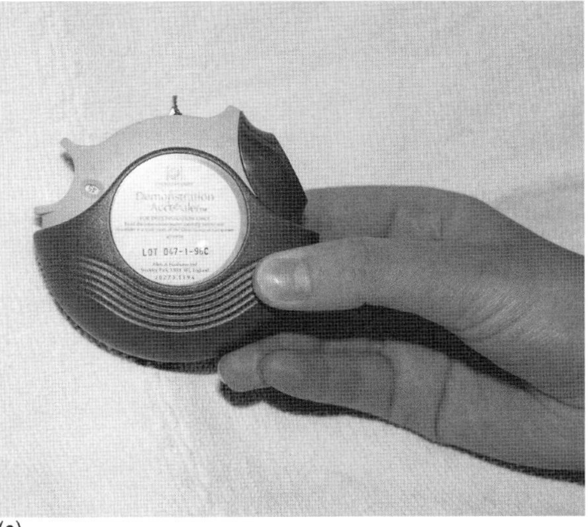

(c)

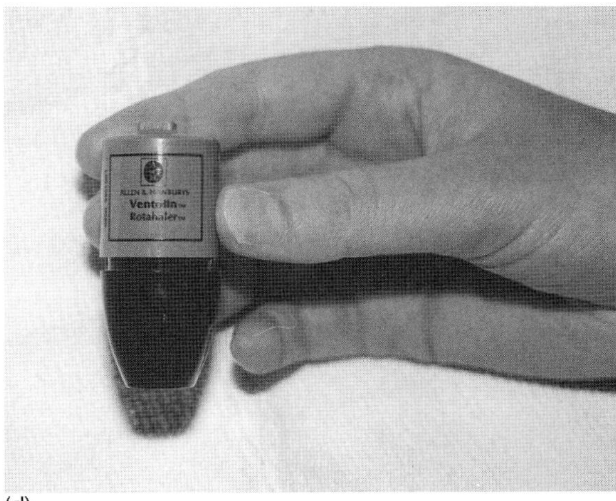

(d)

Figure 10.8 Dry powder systems. (a) Diskhaler; (b) Turbohaler; (c) Disk/Accuhaler; (d) Rotocaps. (Courtesy of Melanie Reardon and Joanne Kenyon.)

provoke emotional problems in children, which can make their asthma worse. Desensitisation may be possible by injection of mild doses of the allergen, which will have been identified by a skin test, although avoidance of these allergens altogether may be difficult.

Measurement of peak flow

Measurement of peak flow can be useful so that variability of lung function is clearly seen and treatment is titrated accordingly. The patient may then alter medication in order to control his or her symptoms. This is based upon the extent to which the peak flow deteriorates (60 per cent, 40 per cent or 30 per cent of the patient's expected value). An example of a peak flow action plan, which will be kept by the patient for reference and which is based on the British Thoracic Society (1997) guidelines, is shown in Table 10.3.

Inhaler technique

When drugs are administered by aerosol/inhaler, it is important that the patient be taught how to use the device correctly. The use of various inhaler devices

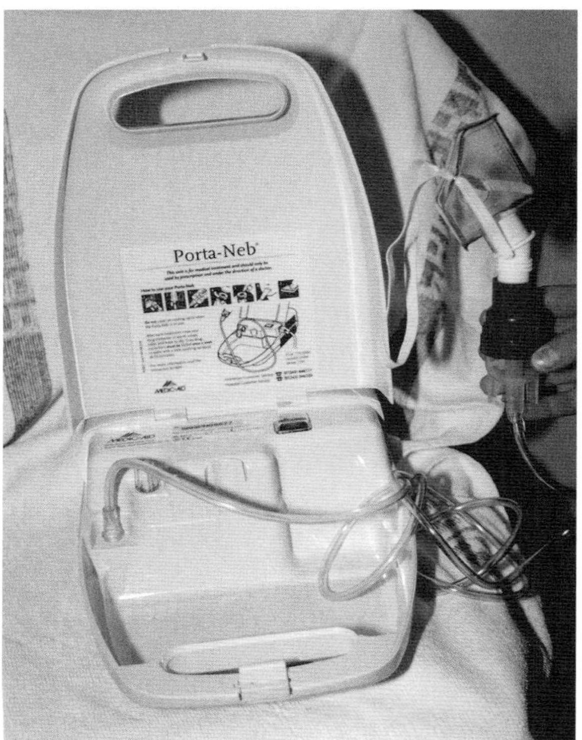

Figure 10.9 Portable nebuliser.

requires some skill on the part of the patient and teaching the correct method of use is an essential part of the prescription of such treatment. Failure to master an MDI occurs in many patients of all ages. The technique for an MDI in which the drug is suspended in a propellant is as follows.

1. *Shake the inhaler.* This disperses the drug uniformly throughout the propellant.
2. *Hold the inhaler upright and direct into the mouth.* If it is not held upright, the metering chamber will not fill correctly.
3. *Start inspiration and press the activating mechanism.* The drug will be effective only if it is breathed in during inspiration. Although there is some controversy regarding the lung volume at which the actuation should occur (Newman et al. 1981), it is simpler to teach the person to discharge the inhaler at the beginning of inspiration.
4. *Breathe in slowly through the mouth.* The flow rate of inspiration should be slow (Newman et al. 1982). This helps to reduce impaction on the pharynx and allow for further penetration of the drug into the bronchial tree, since flow is laminar rather than turbulent.
5. *Hold the breath at maximum inspiration for 5–10 seconds.* This allows particles of the drug to settle on the airway walls. Ideally, the breath should be held for 10 seconds.
6. *Relax and allow easy expiration.* Patients need to be aware of when their inhaler is getting close to empty and should be instructed to shake their inhaler in order to gauge this. Another method is to place the inhaler in water. If it floats symmetrically upright then it is close to empty. It is always good advice to instruct the patient to have two inhalers at home, to avoid being caught out in an exacerbation without adequate relief.

PHYSIOTHERAPY TECHNIQUES IN ASTHMA

General aims of treatment

The principal aims are:

- to relieve any bronchospasm and to facilitate the removal of secretions
- to improve breathing control and the control of dyspnoea during attacks

Table 10.3 Peak flow action plan

Daily medication	Seretide (purple inhaler) **1 suck every morning and evening**
As-needed medication	Salbutamol (blue inhaler) **2 puffs as needed**
Best peak flow reading when well	390 L/min
If unwell with cough, wheeze, breathlessness or tight chest or peak flow 310 L/min or below	Continue daily medication(s) as above Commence salbutamol (blue) **4 puffs every 4 hours** Record peak flow readings every 4 hours before taking blue inhaler
If peak flow falls to 230 L/min	Commence oral steroids **8 tablets once a day** for 3 days See your doctor within 24 hours of commencing oral steroids
If the action plan does not help relieve your child's symptoms for 4 hours or peak flow reading falls to 150 L/min, then you must seek urgent medical attention.	

- to teach local relaxation, improve posture and help allay fear and anxiety
- to increase knowledge of the lung condition and control of symptoms
- to improve exercise tolerance and ensure a long-term commitment to exercise
- to give advice about self-management.

The management of asthmatic patients should include maintenance of a good general fitness, and a vital part of asthma management is to educate the patient.

Patient education

All asthmatic patients and their close relatives should be aware of how to manage their asthma, and the physiotherapist is integral is the education process. Prevention of infection is important. The patient should have plenty of fresh air, avoid smoky atmospheres and keep away from people with infections such as bronchitis and influenza. Stress or anxiety must be minimised, as these can precipitate an attack.

Patients must know what therapy to take and how to take it and where they should go to seek further help. All this should be carefully planned beforehand and incorporated into a written action plan and self-management strategy (Amado and Portnoy 2006) that guides patients to increase treatment when their asthma becomes more severe and to reduce treatment when it gets better (Table 10.3).

Acute attacks

Treatment during acute exacerbations will involve the physiotherapist in aiding removal of excessive bronchial secretions using the ACBT (see above), with the addition of postural drainage, if tolerated. Percussion and shakings should be applied sensitively, as they may increase bronchospasm. Breathing control and the adoption of relaxed positions may be necessary.

Pulmonary rehabilitation

Pulmonary rehabilitation has largely been confined to patients with COPD, but there is now a recognition that other patient groups may benefit. The principles are the same as those previously described for patients with COPD but with some additional considerations.

Patients with asthma are younger but very commonly have a fear and inhibition of exercise (Cochrane et al. 1990) and therefore can benefit from improved cardiorespiratory fitness (Patessio et al. 1993). Also, unlike patients with COPD, individuals with asthma usually show a greater variability in airflow obstruction, and are more susceptible to exercise-induced exacerbations (EIEs). Consideration needs to be given to the prevention of exacerbations (such as by the self-administration of beta$_2$-agonists prior to exercise), although certain forms of exercise — for example, swimming — are less likely to cause an EIE than others. In addition to whole-body programmes, inspiratory muscle training may also be incorporated into the exercise programme (as described previously for COPD patients).

Removal of secretions

Some patients, especially children, have constant excessive secretions and may require sputum clearance techniques such as the ACBT on a daily basis. It may be essential to teach a forced expiration technique for clearing secretions without increasing bronchospasm.

Relaxation

If the patient is able to practise relaxation it may be possible to ward off an attack when there has been exposure to an allergen. The onset of an attack is often preceded by a 'tickle' in the throat or a sensation of tightness in the chest. Relaxation and breathing control in an appropriate position may prevent an attack developing. 'Appropriate position' depends on where the patient is and may have to be against a wall or the back of a chair.

Breathing control

Encouraging a longer expiratory phase is helpful, but neither inspiration nor expiration should be forced. This may be helped by counting (e.g. 'in 1–2, out 1-2-3') and by manual pressure just under the xiphisternum to encourage diaphragmatic excretion. The patient must breathe at a rate and rhythm that suits him or her. Children may be taught to breathe to a nursery rhyme.

BRONCHIECTASIS

Definition

Bronchiectasis is a condition that is characterised by the permanent dilatation of the bronchi associated with destruction of elastic and muscular components of their walls, usually due to acute or chronic infection (Rosen 2006).

The most common cause of bronchiectasis is damage to the bronchial tree after infection. Bronchiectasis may also complicate bronchial obstruction or a more widespread disorder (e.g. cystic fibrosis) (Cole 1995).

Types and prevalence of bronchiectasis

The condition most commonly affects the lower lobes, the lingula and then the middle lobe. It tends to involve the left lung more than the right, although 50 per cent of cases are bilateral. The upper lobes are least affected since they drain most efficiently with the assistance of gravity. There are broadly two types of disease.

Congenital bronchiectasis

This is very rare and occurs in Kartagener's syndrome ('immotile cilia' syndrome), where there is a congenital microtubular abnormality of the cilia that prevents normal cilial beating. It is characterised by bronchiectasis, sinusitis, dextrocardia and complete visceral transposition. There may also be associated male infertility.

Acquired bronchiectasis

Bronchial obstruction and bacterial infection are the principal factors responsible for this disease. Obstruction of a bronchus, which may be due to a tumour or foreign body, will cause collapse of the lung tissue supplied by that bronchus. Bronchiectasis may also occur following an infection, which causes the production of sticky sputum leading to obstruction of multiple small bronchi. Classically, this is associated with whooping cough, TB, measles and pneumonia in childhood, when the airways are smaller and therefore more easily 'plug' with sputum. Very occasionally, bronchiectasis may occur as a late complication of TB, which has affected the right middle lobe and caused that segment to collapse. It may also occur following lung abscess and pneumonia and be associated with immune defects in patients with hypogammaglobulinaemia. Allergic bronchopulmonary aspergillosis, which is associated with an autoimmune response, can cause formation of mucus plugs resulting in bronchiectasis of the medium-sized bronchi.

Prevalence

The prevalence of bronchiectasis following a childhood infection is decreasing since these infections are now treated with antibiotics, but the condition may occur in individuals with an underlying disorder that predisposes them to chronic or recurrent infection. This includes cystic fibrosis, immunodeficiency, human immunodeficiency (HIV) infection and primary ciliary dyskinesia (Rosen 2006).

Pathology of bronchiectasis

Bronchial obstruction may be localised (due perhaps to an inhaled foreign body such as a peanut or broken tooth or obstruction due to a tumour or enlarged gland) or generalised (e.g. pneumonia that is slow to resolve owing to whooping cough or measles).

The bronchial obstruction will cause absorption of the air from the lung tissue distal to the obstruction and this area will therefore shrink and collapse. This causes a traction force to be exerted upon the more proximal airways, which will distort and dilate them. If the obstruction can be cleared and the lung re-expanded quickly, then the dilatation is reversible. Secretions may collect distal to the obstruction if it is not relieved quickly and these easily become infected. This causes inflammation of the bronchial wall with destruction of the elastic and muscular tissue. These infections occur repeatedly, with the walls becoming weaker and weaker. They will eventually dilate owing to the negative intrapleural pressure. As the disease advances, the bronchi become grossly dilated and pockets containing pus are formed. The elastic and muscle tissue is destroyed and the mucous lining is replaced by granulation tissue with loss of cilia. Therefore, the mucociliary transport mechanism is disrupted and passage of mucus out of the lungs is thus hindered (Figure 10.10).

Several types of obstruction are recognised pathologically: tubular, fusiform or sacular. The arterial vessels within the bronchial walls anastomose with the pulmonary capillaries and this results in the common feature of haemoptysis.

Clinical features of bronchiectasis

Key point

Although symptoms often begin in childhood, diagnosis is not usually made until adult life.

Cough and sputum

Patients complain of persistent cough with purulent sputum since childhood. Initially, it is present only following colds or influenza, but if the disease is allowed to progress in severity the affected segments continually accumulate purulent secretions, resulting in cough and sputum production. The sputum is usually green, often foul-smelling and present in fairly large volume. The breath is fetid. The cough is particularly troublesome on a change of position and on rising first thing in the morning.

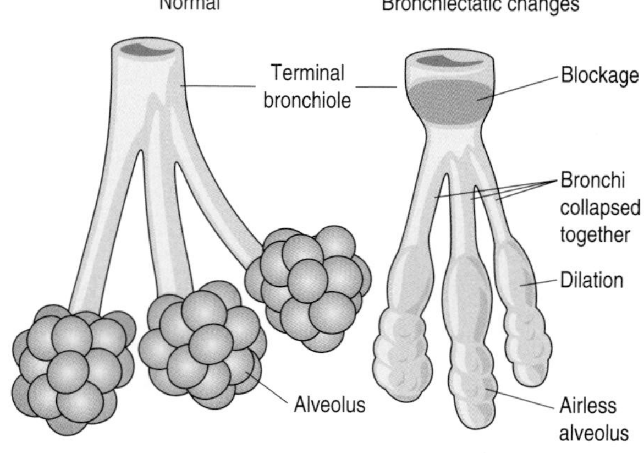

Figure 10.10 Changes of bronchiectasis.

Initially, the sputum culture will isolate *Haemophilus influenzae* and/or *Staphylococcus*. In the later stages of the disease *Pseudomonas aeruginosa* and *Klebsiella* may be isolated.

Dyspnoea

Shortness of breath is noticeable only if disease is particularly severe and widespread. If the bronchiectasis is localised, other well-ventilated and perfused alveoli should maintain blood gases at a reasonable level, although bronchospasm may be a feature, particularly during an exacerbation.

Haemoptysis

This occurs quite commonly, usually in association with an acute infection. It can be life-threatening if severe and may require surgical resection of the affected lung tissue.

Recurrent pneumonia

Characteristically this will affect the same sites and is a common feature.

Chronic sinusitis

This occurs in approximately 70 per cent of patients.

General ill-health

Patients may suffer pyrexia, night sweats, anorexia, malaise, weight loss, lassitude and joint pains.

Clubbing

In about 50 per cent of patients fingers and toes become clubbed. The first sign of clubbing is loss of the angle between the nail and the nail bed. This is followed by curvature of the nail, and an increase in the soft tissue of the ends of the fingers, forming so-called 'drumstick' fingers.

Thoracic mobility

This gradually decreases, as do shoulder girdle movements.

Radiography

Initially, the X-ray will be normal but the patient gradually develops an increase in the bronchovascular markings and sometimes shows multiple cysts with fluid levels (Armstrong et al. 1995). Bronchography is used for accurate localisation of the area affected and will reveal dilated bronchi. A CT scan will show bronchial wall thickening and dilatation of the bronchi and cysts.

Prognosis of bronchiectasis

The vast majority of these patients can lead normal lives with a nearly normal life expectancy, provided medical care is adequate. Possible complications, however, are:

- recurrent haemoptysis (common)
- pneumonia (common)
- pleurisy and empyema
- abscess formation (in lung/cerebrum) (rare)
- emphysema (rare)
- respiratory failure
- right ventricular failure (commonly develops after years of pulmonary sepsis and arterial hypoxaemia if there is widespread bronchiectasis)
- systemic amyloidosis (rare).

Management of bronchiectasis

Principles of treatment

The anatomical picture makes very little difference to the treatment of the disease.

- Relieve the obstruction before permanent damage occurs (recognition of either localised obstruction or appropriate treatment for whooping cough or measles).
- Control infection. Antibiotics are given prophylactically in all but very mild cases. The dosage of the antibiotics should be altered if an acute infection occurs. Intravenous treatment is indicated for severe infections (Currie 1997). Inhaled (delivered by a nebuliser) or continuous oral therapy may be used for chronic sepsis and more resistant pathogens (e.g. *Staph. aureus* and *P. aeruginosa*).
- Promote good health with a good diet and fresh air.
- Maintain and improve exercise tolerance, as some patients with bronchiectasis become deconditioned owing to fatigue and shortness of breath.
- Inhaled steroids may be used in order to reduce inflammation and reduce the volume of sputum produced (Elborn et al. 1992).
- Surgery to remove the area of affected lung may be indicated in young patients with localised disease, although there is conflicting evidence regarding the efficacy of surgery when compared to conservative treatment (Corless and Warburton 2000).

Physiotherapy

Aims of treatment

The principal aims of physiotherapy in bronchiectasis are:

- to remove secretions and clear lung fields
- to teach an appropriate sputum clearance regimen
- to educate the patient in the pathology and management of the condition
- to promote good general health and maintain or improve exercise tolerance
- to teach the patient how to fit in home treatment within his or her lifestyle.

Clearing secretions

Postural drainage may be indicated, if tolerated, for patients with excessive bronchial secretions. The position must be accurate for the areas of lung affected. Accuracy is judged by production of sputum and by identification of the affected areas on a chest X-ray. This minimises the danger of secretion overspill into the least affected side, which could cause spread of the disease or pneumonia. Percussion, shaking and vibrations with the ACBT are also necessary and must be accurately applied over the affected area of the lungs.

The patient may be taught the FET. A flutter or positive expiratory pressure (PEP) valve may be used to facilitate the movement of peripheral mucus plugs and pus into the trachea, from where they are cleared by coughing. The patient must perform a combination of these treatments 2–3 times daily. It is important to ensure that the patient has disposable sputum pots and polythene or paper bags to dispose of the infected sputum without the risk of reinfection or endangering other members of the family. Should the patient develop a cold or influenza, antibiotics must be readily available, together with physiotherapy, so that infection and secretions can be cleared promptly.

Maintaining exercise tolerance

Mobility of the thorax, good posture and good general health are achieved by the patient performing a daily exercise programme. This is comprised of general deep breathing, maintenance of good posture and aerobic exercise such as brisk walking. The patient may also attend a pulmonary rehabilitation session, as this has been shown to be effective in increasing exercise capacity in patients with bronchectasis (Bradley and Moran 2006). The patient should also be encouraged to partake in sports such as jogging, walking, cycling, tennis or swimming.

CYSTIC FIBROSIS

Definition

Cystic fibrosis (CF) is a hereditary disorder of exocrine glands, with a high sodium chloride content in sweat and pancreatic insufficiency, resulting in malabsorption. There is hypertrophy and hyperplasia of mucus-secreting glands, resulting in excessive mucus production in the lining of bronchi, which predisposes the patient to chronic bronchopulmonary infection.

Cystic fibrosis is the most common hereditary disorder, being transmitted by a recessive gene estimated to be present in 1 in 20 in the UK. It is the most common life-shortening autosomal recessive disorder in the Caucasian population. The disease is caused by mutations in a single gene on the long arm of chromosome 7 that encodes the cystic fibrosis transmembrane conductance regulator (CFTR) (Mansoura 1998).

Pathology of cystic fibrosis

Mutations in the CFTR gene result in defective chloride transport, which is accompanied by decreased transport of sodium and water in the epithelial cells in the respiratory, hepatobiliary, gastrointestinal and reproductive tracts and in the pancreas (Quinton 1990). This results in dehydration and hence an increase in the viscosity of secretions that are associated with luminal obstruction and scarring of various exocrine ducts (Oppenheimer and Esterly 1975). Other than in the respiratory system, the resultant clinical manifestations include pancreatic insufficiency, diabetes mellitus, azoospermia in affected men, and evidence of biochemical liver abnormality in up to 80 per cent of children (Ling et al. 1999).

The primary causes of morbidity and mortality in patients with CF, however, are bronchiectasis and obstructive pulmonary disease; the latter accounts for over 90 per cent of deaths. Infants with CF have persistent endobronchial bacterial infections (Abman et al. 1991), which are associated with an intense inflammatory response that damages the airway and impairs local host defence mechanisms (Konstan and Berger 1993). Continuous inflammation, coupled with thickened pulmonary secretions, leads to airways obstruction and hyperinflation (Davis et al. 1996). Hyperinflation becomes a marked feature of the disorder, leading to altered pulmonary mechanics that cause the inspiratory muscles, particularly the diaphragm, to be foreshortened prior to contraction. In such cases, even a small change in breathing pattern (Bellemare and Grassino 1982) or an increase in ventilatory requirement induced by exercise could be enough to induce inspiratory muscle fatigue (Levine and Guillen 1987).

Pulmonary changes

- *Excessive mucus.* There is excess mucus production, especially in the small bronchi and bronchioles. These respiratory passages are structurally normal at birth but become blocked by mucus plugs. Lung disease in CF is also characterised by impaired mucociliary clearance of secretions.
- *Viscid mucus.* The abnormality in the mucous glands results in production of mucus with a reduced water content, so that the secretions produced are very viscid and stick to the bronchial walls.
- *Infection.* The accumulated mucus provides a medium for growth of bacteria and so the secretions become

infected and purulent. This leads to irritation of the bronchial wall tissue, which then becomes inflamed.

- *Bronchiectasis.* Inflammation leads to weakening of the bronchial walls and dilatation occurs as in bronchiectasis.
- *Lack of development of lung tissue.* Mucus and inflammation resulting in airway obliteration inhibit the development of normal lung tissue.

Other pathological changes

Fibrosis of the pancreas causes digestive malfunction and may lead to development of diabetes. Intestinal obstruction may occur owing to gallstones or faecal impaction. In newborn babies, there is intestinal obstruction — known as 'meconium ileus' because there is excess meconium (a greenish-black viscid discharge from the bowel of newborn babies), which plugs the small intestine necessitating an emergency operation. Right ventricular hypertrophy occurs owing to pulmonary congestion, which develops as fibrosis, and thickening of the pulmonary arterial walls takes place.

Prognosis of cystic fibrosis

With early diagnosis and good management, the life expectancy of patients with CF is increasing and survival may be to the fourth or fifth decade (Elborn et al. 1991). The majority, however, die before 40 years of age from respiratory failure related to pulmonary infection. In addition to the relentless progression of lung disease, acute exacerbations of chronic infection adversely affect the nutritional status of these patients. During the terminal phase of their life many patients with CF enter into a vicious circle of repeated respiratory exacerbations with evidence of a deterioration in lung function measurements and declining bodyweight (Elborn et al. 1993). This evidence strongly suggests that the systemic consequences of infection and inflammation are in part responsible for weight loss in patients with CF. Chronic infection may also cause anorexia due to physical factors such as increased mucus production and the anorectic effects of cytokines.

Thus, in patients with CF there may be reduced energy intake, reduced nutrient absorption due to maldigestion, and an increase in energy expenditure resulting from abnormal pulmonary function and sepsis (Bell et al. 1996).

Clinical features of cystic fibrosis

Children

At birth the infant is normal, but symptoms of organ dysfunction can appear soon after. The presenting features vary widely:

- *Meconium ileus.* This may present in approximately 10 per cent of infants and is caused by the abnormally viscid nature of the meconium giving rise to obstruction of the terminal ileum.
- *Failure to thrive and gain weight.* This results from chronic malnutrition.
- *Cough producing copious, often purulent, sputum.* Recurrent *Staph. aureus* infections are common and *Pseudomonas* and *Burkholderia capacia* colonise the respiratory tract.
- *Dyspnoea.* This is particularly evident during an exacerbation.
- *Wheezing.* This is due to airway obstruction caused by inflammation and bronchospasm.
- *High level of sodium in sweat.* Sweat sodium and chloride concentrations are elevated (sweat sodium > 7 mmol/L) in children under 10 years of age. The test is reliable in older children and adults and is a reliable diagnostic sign.
- *Frequent, foul-smelling stools.* This is because of malabsorption and steatorrhoea (fat in the stools) due to secondary dysfunction of the exocrine pancreas.

10

Adolescents and adults

- *Progressive breathlessness.* This may be associated with infective exacerbations and increasing disease severity.
- *Reduced FEV_1 and deteriorating blood gases.* Pulmonary function tests deteriorate as chronic airways obstruction develops. As the disease progresses, ventilation/perfusion imbalance occurs leading to hypoxaemia and pulmonary hypertension.
- *Continued wheezing and productive cough.* This is associated with purulent sputum from which may be cultured strains of *Pseudomonas*, *Staphylococcus* or *Burkholderia capacia*.
- *Haemoptysis.* This occurs secondary to bronchiectasis.
- *Chest X-ray.* This will show hyperinflation and bronchial wall thickening, particularly in the upper zones and bronchiectasis.
- *Finger clubbing.* This is associated with bronchiectasis.
- *Delayed puberty.* This may affect both male and female patients. Most women have normal or near-normal fertility, although pregnancy may be inadvisable if pulmonary function is less than 60 per cent of expected.
- *Infertility in males.* This occurs owing to blockage of the vas deferens, which is either absent or blocked; affected males can still produce sperm.
- *Lung function tests* (LFTs). There is reduction of the FEV_1/FVC ratio and the FVC is grossly reduced. The RV will be increased at the expense of the VC because of air trapping and the inability of the

expiratory muscles to decrease the volume of the thoracic cavity.

- *Blood gases*. Ventilation/perfusion mismatch is inevitable in CF and leads to a low PaO_2 with or without CO_2 retention. As the disease becomes severe, the arterial $PaCO_2$ may rise and a diffusion abnormality will also be apparent.
- *Auscultation*. There will be inspiratory and expiratory wheeze with added coarse crepitations.
- *X-ray*. No characteristic abnormality is seen in the early stages of the disease. If there is significant airways obstruction, there may be signs of chest overexpansion (flattening of the diaphragm) and an enlarged retrosternal airspace.

Complications

- *Haemoptysis*. This is usually mild but occasionally frank haemoptysis may occur.
- *Spontaneous pneumothorax*. This may occur due to rupture of emphysematous bullae.
- *Osteoporosis*. There has been a recent recognition of the high prevalence of low bone mineral density leading to osteoporosis and an increased susceptibility to fractures (Haworth et al. 1999).
- *Liver disease*. This usually presents as biliary cirrhosis and may be associated with portal hypertension and oesophageal varices.
- *Diabetes mellitus*. This results from progressive fibrosis damaging the exocrine glands that produce insulin.
- *Deformity*. These patients often develop a barrel chest due to hyperinflation with use of accessory muscles of respiration. There may be evidence of a poor posture, including kyphosis and lordosis and associated musculoskeletal pain.
- *Cor pulmonale*. This may occur in the later stages of the disease.

Social-psychological problems

The disease carries with it some unfortunate social and psychological problems. Coughing and spitting are antisocial, so people, in avoiding the patient, are unwittingly unkind. The parents may feel guilty as they are carrying the gene. They have to spend a lot of time with the patient, which creates resentment in siblings. The patient, on reaching adolescence, may become resentful of treatment and the increasing inability to participate in a full social life. Clearly, this is only a brief mention of the total picture, of which the physiotherapist must be aware.

Terminal features

The terminal features include respiratory failure, cyanosis, cor pulmonale and severe nutritional depletion (accelerated loss of lean body mass and fat mass).

MANAGEMENT OF CYSTIC FIBROSIS

General principles

Paediatric and adult patients with CF should receive care from a specialist CF centre. A low-fat, high-calorie diet is recommended, supplemented with vitamins. In addition to maintaining or improving dietary status, treatment of CF is directed towards the correction of organ dysfunction (Davis 1996), including pancreatic enzyme replacement and reversal of secondary nutritional and vitamin deficiencies (Ramsey et al. 1992), although the majority of treatment is directed towards the management of abnormalities of pulmonary function. This includes clearance of lower airway secretions (Zach and Oberwaldner 1989), treatment of persistent pulmonary infections (Turpin and Knowles 1993) and the alleviation of the symptoms of pulmonary dysfunction, especially breathlessness.

Owing to abnormalities of pulmonary function, patients with CF ventilate excessively and ineffectively at all work levels compared with subjects with normal lung function (Cerny et al. 1982). This results in loss of functional status because aerobic exercise in CF is limited by both cardiovascular and pulmonary mechanisms. Thus, maintenance of exercise capacity in patients with CF is imperative.

Medications

Antibiotics

Antibiotics are essential and the patient will be prescribed one form or another for life. There is much evidence that aggressive intravenous antibiotic therapy in children with CF has resulted in a significantly improved survival rate (Turpin and Knowles 1993). More recent investigations suggest that the use of prophylactic antibiotics is associated with a reduced requirement for additional courses of oral antibiotics and fewer hospital admissions in the first 2 years of life, although no effect on infant lung function has been identified (Smyth and Walters 2000). In older patients with CF, who are chronically infected with *Pseudomonas* species, no differences in lung function or mortality rate were identified between two groups of 30 patients who were given either elective or symptomatic antibiotic therapy over a 3-year period (Elborn et al. 2000).

Bronchodilators

These may be useful when there is airways obstruction that is reversible. During an acute exacerbation, a nebuliser may be used at home.

Oxygen therapy

Oxygen therapy may be appropriate in the terminal stages when there is persistent hypoxaemia.

Mucolytic agents

Because lung disease in CF is characterised by impaired mucociliary clearance, recurrent bronchial infections and inflammation, methods that may enhance the removal of retained bronchial secretions may act to lessen the destructive inflammatory process in the airways (Solomon et al. 1996).

Nebulised hypertonic saline has been shown to increase mucociliary clearance immediately after administration. This may have a long-term beneficial effect, although the effect on PFTs, quality of life and frequency of exacerbations remains unclear (Wark and McDonald 2000).

Recombinant human deoxyribonuclease (rhDNase) is currently used to treat pulmonary disease in patients with CF by facilitating protein breakdown in pulmonary secretions, thereby aiding expectoration (Christopher et al. 1999). When compared to nebulised saline, evidence suggests that rhDNase may improve FEV_1 by $>$ 200 mL in 37 per cent of patients, as compared to only 3 per cent of patients after saline when tested over a maximum of three 4-week assessment periods (Bollert et al. 1999). Also when compared to other mucolytic agents, in the short term (6 months) rhDNase has been shown to reduce the risk of respiratory exacerbations (Christopher et al. 1999), although randomised controlled trials to date have been of insufficient duration to answer important questions about long-term outcomes (Kearney and Wallace 2000). In addition to this, a large interindividual variability in response to rhDNase treatment has been documented and the benefits have been found to be unpredictable in around 50 per cent of patients (Cobos et al. 2000).

Physiotherapy

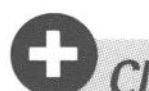

Clinical note

Daily physiotherapy for life is an essential part of the treatment of the pulmonary features of cystic fibrosis, and currently airways clearance is recommended as soon as the diagnosis is made. The treatment approach should be adapted to changes in the patient's lifestyle as he or she matures and as the disease progresses.

The aims of physiotherapy are:

- to reduce bronchospasm and to clear the lung fields
- to encourage activities for maintaining physical fitness/increasing exercise tolerance
- to train postural awareness and relaxation
- to educate the patient in self-management.

Clearing lung fields

This is the cornerstone of management of patients with CF, because the primary causes of morbidity and mortality are bronchiectasis and obstructive pulmonary disease, the latter accounting for over 90 per cent of deaths. It is important that the parents and the rest of the family are involved in the treatment of the child at a young age so that physiotherapy can become an accepted routine.

Chest clearance techniques in the infant include the use of postural drainage, percussion and shaking. The optimal position is usually sitting in the upright position, as the infant will spend a lot of time in supine lying. Prior to these techniques it is useful to have an active game with a child so that he or she laughs, producing deeper respiration and then becoming breathless. This is required twice a day, every day, even when the patient is apparently well, as there is some evidence that inflammation and infection exist during infancy (Konstan et al. 1994).

10

Key point

During exacerbations, or when the child has an upper respiratory tract infection, these treatment sessions may have to be increased up to as much as six times a day.

A baby may be positioned on a pillow on the knee of either the physiotherapist or parent. The physiotherapist has to identify the most effective position for each individual patient and relate the treatment to the home situation. As the child grows, there comes a stage where it may be necessary to position for drainage using cushions if secretions are evident in the lower zones. A tipping frame that supports the patient totally is more comfortable for draining the anterior and lateral segments of the lower lobes, and the middle lobe or lingula. Adolescents and adult patients may have blocks made so that their own bed may be tipped.

In addition to postural drainage and manual techniques, the use of a positive expiratory pressure (PEP) mask and the Flutter device can be used to facilitate the clearance of secretions by enhancing expiratory airflow (Freitag et al. 1989). Infants tend to swallow their secretions and for children under 3 years and babies the sputum needs to be cleared with a tissue. Disposal of infected sputum should be discussed with parents, relatives or patient, as it is essential to avoid reinfection.

Some form of humidification is useful to reduce the viscosity of the mucus, and may be applied using a mouthpiece and nebuliser. Ultrasonic nebulisers have been shown to be preferred by CF patients (Thomas et al. 1991). For babies and children, a mask may be necessary. Saline solution may be used as a mucolytic agent. For home use, patients may have an electric compressor with a nebuliser.

As soon as the patient is old enough, he or she should be encouraged to become involved in the treatment. The person should also be encouraged to expectorate the secretions and not to swallow the sputum, as this may cause an exacerbation of abdominal symptoms. During exacerbations of infection, patients may be admitted to hospital where intensive physiotherapy is essential.

A community physiotherapist should visit the patient's home at regular intervals and will become very well known to the involved family. The patient has to attend regular follow-up clinics to be seen by a chest specialist, as well as being taken care of by the GP. It is also essential that the patient is seen regularly by the physiotherapist, so that treatment can be updated and problems discussed.

Maintenance of physical fitness/increasing exercise tolerance

Aerobic fitness in both children and young adults with CF can be improved by aerobic exercise training (Kaplan et al. 1991). Higher levels of aerobic fitness in patients with CF have been shown to be associated with a significantly improved length of survival (Nixon et al. 1992). Exercise has also been shown to decrease breathlessness (O'Neill et al. 1987) and improve quality of life (de Jong et al. 1997), and also makes an important contribution to sputum expectoration (Sahl et al. 1989).

Parents of an infant with CF should be encouraged to treat the child as normally as possible so that the child joins in physical activities at school and with friends at weekends. It is helpful for the parents to meet the child's teachers so that they know it is important to encourage the child to participate fully in school life.

Adult patients may benefit from regular swimming or short sessions of jogging and, if possible, should be encouraged to attend the hospital or clinic when clinically stable to have their baseline exercise capacity measured. This will allow the physiotherapist to recommend a level of exercise that will provide an appropriate training effect. It is also important to establish the goals of an exercise programme and to tailor the programme to the patient's level of fitness and disease severity.

Terminal stages

The advanced stages of CF are characterised by repeated exacerbations, reduced mobility and eventually respiratory failure. As the blood gases deteriorate and the $PaCO_2$ begins to rise as a result of ventilatory failure, NIPPV will be indicated. This is a distressing time for the patient, the family and the multidisciplinary team, as the patient becomes very ill and recognises that death is imminent. The family will require a great deal of emotional support from the multidisciplinary team.

The principal theme is to keep the patient as comfortable as possible, which usually means sedation using morphine or one of its derivatives to relieve the sensation of breathlessness and reduce anxiety. It is inappropriate to discontinue contact with the physiotherapist, even though active treatment is no longer effective. The aim in the terminal stages of the disease is positioning of the patient in high side-lying or forward lean-sitting to make the person as comfortable as possible and to assist with the clearance of secretions from the upper airways if these become uncomfortable and distressing. Nasopharyngeal suction is not indicated in the terminal stages of the disease.

Surgery

The maintenance of mobility is essential for those patients who are waiting for lung transplantation, if this is indicated. Although exercise tolerance at this stage of the illness may be restricted, the physiotherapist should maintain muscle strength and cardiovascular function. Postoperatively, rehabilitation should be extensive in order to maximise function and quality of life.

RESTRICTIVE PULMONARY DISEASES

Pneumonia

Definition

Pneumonia is an acute inflammation of the lung tissue — the alveoli and adjacent airways.

Classification

Pneumonia may be classified in many ways, for example:

- according to its anatomical distribution (e.g. lobar, which is confined to one lobe, or bronchopneumonia, which is a more widespread, patchy infection)
- according to its microbiological cause.

In clinical terms it may also be defined:

- according to where the infection is acquired (i.e. in the community or in hospital)
- according to whether the patient is immunocompromised (e.g. by AIDS).

All of these factors may determine the outcome of the disease, the likely causative factors and the clinical features of the disease.

Community-acquired pneumonia

Infection is acquired through the inhalation of droplets containing the specific micro-organism, and the individual is unable to overcome the infection through the natural pulmonary defence mechanism.

Community-acquired pneumonia is a common pulmonary disease and may be responsible for over one million hospital admissions a year in the UK. Specific microbiological causes do, however, tend to affect different age groups:

- *Streptococcus pneumoniae* pneumonia is the most prevalent community-acquired pneumonia and affects all age groups.
- *Mycoplasma pneumoniae* pneumonia usually occurs in adolescents and young adults.
- Influenza, parainfluenza, measles and adenovirus pneumonias are more common in children and the elderly.
- Chickenpox pneumonia occurs in adults.
- Respiratory syncytial virus (RSV) is an important cause of morbidity and mortality in children under 2 years of age.
- *Legionella pneumophila* infection (Legionnaire's disease) may occur in all age groups but is more common in men than women. It thrives in warm water and frequently contaminates badly maintained air-conditioning systems.
- *Haemophilus influenzae* may produce bronchopneumonia in those with pre-existing pulmonary disease (e.g. chronic bronchitis). It is therefore more common in the elderly.
- *Staphylococcus pyogenes, Klebsiella pneumoniae* and *Mycoplasma pneumoniae* infections are rare in healthy individuals but may commonly complicate viral pneumonia.

Predisposing factors

These are: winter or springtime, overcrowded circumstances where bacteria and viruses are easily transmitted, alcoholism, smoking (cigarette smoke and alcohol depress ciliary function and phagocytosis), atmospheric pollution, lower socioeconomic groups and pre-existing respiratory disease. The disease may also occur secondary to impaired consciousness and malnutrition.

Pathological changes

The invading organism causes inflammation in the bronchioles and alveoli. The exudates spread into neighbouring alveoli to provide a medium for rapid spread of bacteria. The alveoli become filled with red blood cells, leucocytes, macrophages and fibrin (red hepatisation) and there is congestion throughout the lobe. The overlying pleural surface is inflamed and a pleural effusion may develop. Resolution occurs when the leucocytes engulf the bacteria and macrophages clear the debris by phagocytosis (grey hepatisation).

In lobular or bronchopneumonia the inflammation is scattered irregularly in the lungs, whereas in lobar pneumonia the inflammation is spread throughout but contained within one entire lobe.

Without treatment, resolution occurs by liquefaction of the consolidation, which is then expelled by coughing.

Clinical features

The onset may be sudden (lobar pneumonia) or gradual (bronchopneumonia or lobular pneumonia) and is associated with malaise, pyrexia (temperature often $> 40\,^{\circ}C$), rigors, vomiting, confusion due to hypoxaemia (especially in the elderly), and tachycardia.

- *Cough*. This is dry at first, but after a few days purulent sputum is produced.
- *Breathlessness*. Blood passing through the affected alveolar membranes is inadequately oxygenated so that the PaO_2 falls. Hyperventilation cannot compensate for this hypoxaemia because blood passing through the normal lung tissue is almost saturated. The inflammation that occurs makes the lung stiff and compliance is reduced, with the result that the effort of breathing is increased. Respiration therefore becomes rapid and shallow.
- *Pain*. If inflammation spreads to the pleura, there is a sharp pain aggravated by taking a deep breath or by coughing.
- *X-ray*. Consolidation can be seen as an opacity, especially in lobar pneumonia. There may also be evidence of a pleural effusion.
- *Auscultation*. Bronchial breathing can be heard (especially in lobar pneumonia) because the consolidated lung tissue conducts the sounds of air movement in the trachea. Whispering pectoriloquy and increased vocal resonance can be heard. Wheeze may be evident if bronchospasm is present.

Investigations

- *Haematology*. This may reveal a raised white blood cell count.
- *Biochemistry*. Arterial blood gases should be measured to reveal the extent of arterial hypoxaemia.
- *Microbiology*. Sputum should be sent for Gram staining to identify the causative organism (e.g. *Strep. pneumoniae*) and to identify which antimicrobial agents are sensitive to the organism.

- *Pleural aspiration for culture.* This should be considered if the pneumonia is complicated by a pleural effusion.

Prognosis

The outcome depends on predisposing factors, the virulence of the bacteria, and the age and general fitness of the patient. Improvement starts within 3–4 days of the patient having antibiotics, and within 10 days the sputum should be less in quantity and mucoid in nature — by which time the patient begins to feel better. In an otherwise fit person, the X-ray should be clear in 6 weeks.

Generally, lobar pneumonia resolves and patients recover, particularly those who are generally fit and are between the ages of 20 and 50 years. Bronchopneumonia is more serious, is often secondary to other problems, and may be the terminal illness in patients who are elderly. The disease may be fatal in the very young because the secretions readily block the narrow, underdeveloped airways.

Management

- Antibiotics are given to control infection. Specimens of sputum should be sent for culture and sensitivity as soon as possible to confirm or alter antibiotic therapy.
- Adequate fluids must be taken to ensure fluid balance.
- Analgesics are given to relieve pleuritic pain.
- Oxygen therapy may be necessary and blood gases should be monitored regularly.
- Bed rest at home may be sufficient, but an acutely ill patient should be admitted to hospital.

Complications

Possible complications of pneumonia are:

- spread to other lung areas
- delayed resolution — due to the wrong antibiotic being given, poor compliance with medication, or bronchial obstruction (e.g. due to carcinoma)
- pleural disease resulting in pleural effusion or empyema — this will require an intercostal tube and drainage (possibly surgical drainage), along with antibiotics if an empyema is evident
- lung abscess — this will cause a swinging pyrexia and will require antibiotics
- cardiac failure
- septicaemia
- pneumococcal meningitis
- pneumothorax — this is particularly associated with *Staph. aureus* pneumonia and will require intercostal tube drainage
- deconditioning due to malaise.

Physiotherapy in pneumonia

Physiotherapy is indicated when the inflammation has begun to resolve. The aims of treatment are:

- to reduce bronchospasm (if present) and to clear lung fields of secretions
- to gain full re-expansion of the lungs
- to regain exercise tolerance and fitness.

Clearing lung fields

Humidification may be necessary to moisten secretions. The method will vary according to the severity of the illness and may be by steam inhalation, nebuliser or IPPB. Clapping, shaking and breathing exercises may all be necessary in a postural drainage position appropriate to the area of the lung affected. Sometimes suction is required for the very ill patient who cannot cough or expectorate. If there is an underlying bronchospasm, then a bronchodilator may be given.

Re-expansion of the lungs

Positioning should be used to increase ventilation to the affected area.

Exercise tolerance and fitness

As soon as possible, the patient should be mobilised and start walking short distances which are progressively increased in length.

Pleurisy

Definition

Pleurisy is a process whereby inflammation occurs on the visceral and parietal pleura which come into direct contact with each other to cause pain.

Aetiology and pathological changes

This condition is common in town dwellers where there is dust and grit in the atmosphere. It may also be secondary to TB or lobar pneumonia. Infection or irritation of the pleura causes inflammation and vascular congestion. A fibrinous exudate is formed within the pleural cavity and the pleural surfaces are roughened. The inflammation may resolve or develop into a pleural effusion (see below), depending upon any underlying conditions. When resolution occurs, fibrin laid down within the exudate tends to form adhesions between the two layers of the pleura.

The causes of pleurisy are:

- viral infection, which is the most common cause
- pulmonary infarction
- bronchial carcinoma
- pneumonia

- autoimmune rheumatic diseases (e.g. SLE, rheumatoid arthritis).

Clinical features

- *Pleuritic pain*. This is due to stretching of the inflamed pleura. The pain is sharp (knife-like), severe and related to movement of the chest (e.g. deep inspiration or coughing). It is usually well localised to the area of the chest under which the pleural irritation lies. Irritation of the diaphragmatic pleura, however, causes pain sensation via the phrenic nerve and this is often referred to the tip of the shoulder.
- *Pleural rub*. There is a creaking or grating sound heard through a stethoscope on both inspiration and expiration. It is localised to the affected area. This disappears if an effusion develops.
- *Cough*. Coughing may be present if respiratory infection is the cause.
- *X-ray*. The diaphragm may be raised on the affected side.
- *Other clinical signs*. Tachycardia and pyrexia may be present, depending on associated conditions.

Investigations and treatment

Haematology shows a high white cell count if infection is present. Identification and treatment of any underlying conditions are essential. Analgesics are given to relieve pain, and possibly sedative linctus to reduce coughing. Rest is important to allow the inflammation to subside and to minimise the pain.

Physiotherapy in pleurisy

Physiotherapy is usually inappropriate in the early stages. During the recovery stage, however, the aims are:

- to regain full thoracic expansion
- to minimise adhesion formation between the pleural layers
- to mobilise the thorax.

Thoracic expansion is regained by teaching the patient localised expansion exercises with manual resistance over the affected area both to guide rib movement and to relieve pain. General deep breathing exercises and mobility exercises, such as sitting with trunk bending side to side, are important to regain mobility of the thorax and thoracic spine.

Pleural effusion

Definition

Pleural effusion is an excessive accumulation of fluid in the pleural cavity.

Aetiology

Pleural effusion is often secondary to conditions such as:

- malignancy of the lungs or bronchi
- pneumonia
- TB
- pulmonary infarction
- bronchiectasis
- lung abscess
- blockage of lymph vessels
- rupture of blood vessels
- left ventricular failure.

Pathological changes

Fluid accumulates in the pleural cavity, the composition of which varies according to the underlying cause. The fluid may be reabsorbed naturally or removed by surgical intervention. As the pleural layers come together, they may become adherent owing to organisation of fibrin if the fluid contains plasma proteins.

Fluid may accumulate in the pleural cavity as transudate or exudate. *Transudate* occurs when there is an increased pulmonary capillary pressure (as in congestive cardiac failure) or a decreased osmotic pressure (as in hypoproteinaemia associated with malnutrition) across the pleural membrane. *Exudate* occurs when there is inflammation resulting in increased permeability of capillaries and visceral pleura, together with impaired lymphatic reabsorption (as in pneumonia or malignancy).

Exudate is cloudy with a high protein content, in contrast to transudate, which is clear with a low protein content. Consequently, exudate tends to become consolidated, whereas transudate can be reabsorbed if the underlying condition is treated.

Clinical features

- *Breathlessness*. The pressure of fluid reduces lung expansion.
- *Cyanosis*. This may be present in a large effusion.
- *Pyrexia*. This is usually associated with infection.
- *Lethargy*. The person complains of a lack of energy.
- *Pain*. The person complains of pain.
- *Thorax*. Thoracic expansion is restricted on the affected side.

Investigations and treatment

A fluid level can be identified on X-ray. There is a stony dullness on percussion over the fluid. Breath sounds are absent over the effusion (> 500 mL of fluid), although bronchial breathing may be heard just above the effusion. Small effusions (220–500 mL) are revealed by chest radiography.

If the fluid does not become reabsorbed naturally, then it should be aspirated (drained surgically). Oxygen therapy may be necessary.

Physiotherapy in pleural effusion

The aims of physiotherapy are:

- to prevent the formation of disabling adhesions between the two layers of pleura
- to obtain full expansion of the affected lung
- to increase ventilation of the lungs
- to increase exercise tolerance following immobility.

The treatment must be modified to take into account any underlying condition. Following aspiration, breathing exercises should be given to encourage localised expansion of the affected side. The patient is encouraged to practise these exercises, possibly with the aid of a belt.

If patients have difficulty in localising the expansion, it may be helpful for them to lie on the unaffected side over a firm pillow to help stretch the affected side. Breathing exercises may also be practised in this position several times a day. When the patient has regained lung expansion, the treatment programme should be expanded to include mobilisation of the patient and to increase exercise tolerance.

Some malignant pleural effusions may require a pleurodesis — the insertion of a powder such as tetracycline into the pleural cavity

Empyema

Definition

Empyema is a collection of pus in the pleural cavity.

Aetiology

The condition of empyema usually arises secondary to pre-existing lung disease, such as bacterial pneumonia, TB, lung abscess or bronchiectasis. The most common cause is direct spread of infection into the pleural space in a patient with pneumonia caused by *Strep. pneumoniae*. It may also arise as a result of a stab wound or as a complication of thoracic surgery.

Pathological changes

Infected material enters the pleural cavity. Both layers of pleura become covered in thick inflammatory exudate within which fibrous tissue is laid down. As this fibrous tissue contracts, it acts as a physical barrier to lung expansion. The pressure of the fibrous tissue on the pus may cause rupture of the pleura and lung tissue, and the pus may then be coughed up. Alternatively, an abscess may form. Healing occurs when the pus has been surgically removed or the infection has been overcome by the patient's natural antibodies, assisted by antibiotics. The layers of the pleura come together and adhesion formation may take place, restricting lung movement.

Clinical features

These include:

- pyrexia
- lassitude and loss of weight
- tachycardia
- dyspnoea
- pleuritic pain, severe at first then decreasing in severity
- diminished thoracic movements.

There may be a history of pneumonia or other associated condition.

Investigations and treatment

On X-ray the empyema can be seen as a D-shaped shadow, the straight line of the D being on the lung surface. Pleural aspiration or tap will confirm the diagnosis, as the sample is often thick and purulent, and may be foul-smelling. Pleural fluid cytology will reveal an exudate with pus cells and organisms.

Antibiotics are given to combat infection. Aspiration through a needle inserted into the cavity may remove sufficient pus to relieve the condition, but continuous underwater drainage may be necessary. Rib resection may be indicated if the effusion is very thick or loculated.

If the condition results in fibrosis of the pleura that severely limits lung expansion, then a rib resection may be performed and the pleura stripped off the lung (decortication).

The prognosis depends on the cause, but untreated infection can make the patient very ill from toxins absorbed into the blood stream (toxaemia).

Physiotherapy in empyema

The aims are:

- to minimise adhesion formation within the pleura
- to regain full lung expansion
- to clear the lung fields
- to maintain good posture and thoracic mobility
- to improve exercise tolerance.

If the patient has a chest drainage tube inserted, the physiotherapy is similar to that following a thoracotomy. Good posture should be encouraged whenever physiotherapy is being given. The tendency is for the patient to protect the affected side, by side-flexing to that side. Therefore, the patient should be taught to take weight evenly on both buttocks, to keep the shoulders level and to practise stretching to the opposite side from the lesion as well as stretching backwards.

Breathing exercises to expand the lung on the affected side need to be carried out three or four times daily. Postural drainage may be indicated to clear the lungs if secretions are accumulating.

As the patient recovers, general leg, arm and trunk exercises should be taught. Walking should begin as soon as possible with breathing control practised over progressively longer distances, and with going down (then up) stairs incorporated. As the patient regains lung expansion, the treatment programme should be expanded to increase exercise tolerance.

Pneumothorax

Definition

Air collects between the visceral and parietal pleura. Air in the pleural space will allow the lung to move away from the chest wall and the lung will partially deflate.

There are two types of pneumothorax: spontaneous (which may be secondary to an underlying disease) and traumatic.

Spontaneous pneumothorax

This can occur at any age but is most common in young men (a ratio of 6:1 young men to old men) who are otherwise apparently healthy. It may also be associated with emphysema and chronic bronchitis in men over 50 years of age, or result from other underlying disease or be associated with mechanical ventilation. These spontaneous causes may be summarised as:

- airflow limitation due to asthma or bullous emphysema
- positive pressure ventilation, particularly with the use of PEEP
- infections (e.g. staphylococcal pneumonia, TB)
- cystic fibrosis
- Marfan's syndrome.

Traumatic pneumothorax

A traumatic pneumothorax may be caused by:

- penetrating injury to the chest (e.g. by stab wound or a bullet)
- non-penetrating injury to the chest wall (e.g. impact of a road traffic accident involving the chest)
- during the insertion of an intravenous (e.g. subclavian) line
- during surgery to the chest wall
- during pleural aspiration or biopsy.

When the chest wall remains intact, the condition is termed a *closed pneumothorax*, but if the chest wall is opened following the trauma the term used is *open pneumothorax*. In the presence of an open wound, emergency treatment involves the application of a large dressing pad over the chest wall.

Pathological changes

As air escapes into the pleural cavity and reduces the subatmospheric pressure (i.e. less negative), the lung collapses. The hole in the pleura closes, the air becomes absorbed and the lung gradually re-expands. Sometimes this does not happen and the hole in the pleura becomes like a valve. Air then enters the pleural cavity on inspiration but cannot escape during expiration. The lung remains collapsed and, as air accumulates in the pleural cavity and the pressure increases, there is displacement of the heart together with compression of the other lung and great vessels. This is termed a *tension pneumothorax* and has to be treated as an emergency by needle aspiration and thereafter by insertion of a drain connected to an underwater seal.

Clinical features

The onset is often sudden with severe chest pain and progressive breathlessness. There is diminished chest movement unilaterally, and an absence of breath sounds often over the apex of the affected side.

Other clinical features may be related to the underlying pathology (e.g. emphysema). In a patient with known lung disease a pneumothorax should always be considered if the patient becomes more breathless for no apparent reason.

Subcutaneous emphysema may develop at the time of the pleural air leak or following the insertion of an intercostal drain, when air may track into the subcutaneous tissues. Subcutaneous air results in a crackling sensation on palpation.

Investigations and treatment

The chest X-ray shows absence of lung markings and the edge of the collapsed lung can be seen. This will confirm the diagnosis. Inspiratory and expiratory X-rays will help define the visceral pleura where there is a small pneumothorax.

A small pneumothorax requires no treatment, apart from a few days bed rest until it resolves. A large pneumothorax (i.e. more than 25 per cent of the pleural space is filled with air) is treated by needle aspiration or by an intercostal drain that connects the pleural cavity to a drainage bottle, creating an underwater seal. The drain is removed when there are no more bubbles in the drainage bottle — indicating that the pleural cavity is free of air.

Surgery is indicated for a recurrent pneumothorax. Pleurodesis comprises the insertion of a powder into the pleural cavity. This acts as an irritant to the pleural surfaces, causing them to adhere to each other. Pleurectomy is the removal of the parietal pleura from the chest wall, leaving a raw surface to which the visceral layer sticks. A hole in the visceral pleura may have to be stitched.

Physiotherapy in pneumothorax

A patient who has an underwater drainage system requires expansion breathing exercises to re-expand the lung. Also, full-range shoulder movements are necessary to maintain shoulder, shoulder girdle and thoracic mobility. This treatment is generally given 3–4 times daily until the drain is removed.

Following pleurodesis, expansion breathing exercises are essential to ensure that when the adhesions form between the layers of the pleura the lung is fully expanded. The patient must be taught to practise expansion breathing exercises so that thoracic mobility is maintained; otherwise there may be sharp pleuritic pain if the intrapleural adhesions become too contracted. If the lung does not re-expand within 36 hours, then a second operation is required. Physiotherapy after a pleurectomy follows the same principles as for any thoracotomy.

Acute respiratory distress syndrome (ARDS)

A catastrophic event can, either directly or indirectly, cause damage to the pulmonary epithelium or the alveolar capillary membrane. ARDS is, therefore, the respiratory manifestation of a systemic condition, which appears within 12–48 hours after the initial triggering event.

> ***Definition***
>
> The acute respiratory distress syndrome (ARDS) is a severe and acute form of respiratory failure precipitated by a wide range of catastrophic events – including shock, septicaemia, major trauma, or aspiration or inhalation of noxious substances (Bernard et al. 1994).

Examples of triggering events are: pulmonary aspiration, severe burns with or without inhalation injury, disseminated intravascular coagulation (a coagulation defect due to clotting abnormalities), cardiopulmonary bypass, severe trauma, massive blood transfusion, near-drowning, pre-eclampsia, septicaemia, amniotic fluid embolism (substances entering the maternal circulation usually following a vigorous labour), pancreatitis, and fat embolism resulting from fracture of (long) bones.

Pathological changes

Activated neutrophils are thought to release a number of vasoactive mediators that damage the integrity of the alveolar membrane. As a result of increased endothelial permeability within the alveolar–capillary membrane, fluid moves from the pulmonary capillaries into the gas exchange areas of the lung. This results in alveolar oedema and extravasation of inflammatory cells. The pulmonary oedema is therefore said to be non-cardiogenic because there is normal hydrostatic pressure in the pulmonary vasculature (unlike in left ventricular failure, when this is raised). As this acute phase progresses, there is increasing congestion in the capillaries. The loss of functioning alveoli results in severe hypoxaemia and respiratory failure.

Clinical features

The defining features of ARDS are:

- severe refractory (resistant to treatment) hypoxaemia
- the presence of pulmonary oedema with normal hydrostatic pressure in the pulmonary vasculature
- the appearance of diffuse bilateral pulmonary infiltrates on chest X-ray
- a falling pulmonary compliance (< 50 mL/cmH_2O).

Increasing breathlessness is evident; left untreated, it may lead to acute tachypnoea (> 20 breaths per minute). There is evidence of the appearance of diffuse bilateral pulmonary infiltrates on chest X-ray, and widespread wheezes and crackles on auscultation. Despite oxygen, the disease usually progresses to a state of severe respiratory failure, which requires the support of mechanical ventilation. The lungs become progressively stiffer and adequate oxygenation and ventilation becomes more difficult.

Investigations and treatment

On blood gas analysis the PaO_2 is reduced to critical levels. If this is not corrected, the $PaCO_2$ may begin to rise.

Any underlying pathological cause is treated. Adequate ventilatory support will be necessary, and this may include high inspired oxygen, IPPV and the application of PEEP to restore adequate function by allowing for the recruitment of hypoventilated alveoli. This will result in an improved PaO_2. High levels of oxygen may be used initially to reduce a dangerous hypoxaemia, but since oxygen is toxic at high concentrations (causing further damage to the alveolar membrane), this should be reduced to a level that will give an adequate PaO_2. Although the application of PEEP in this condition has been standard practice for over two decades, overdistension of lung tissue may result in barotrauma and volutrauma with the development of pneumothorax and subcutaneous emphysema (Montgomery et al. 1985).

Complications

Nosocomial pneumonitis is a common complication in patients with ARDS on prolonged mechanical ventilation and is directly related to oropharyngeal colonisation of Gram-negative bacilli — the stomach being one of the possible reservoirs of these micro-organisms (Driks et al. 1987). The loss of mucosal integrity and clearance mechanisms is a predisposing factor that leads to secondary infection and may contribute to worsening gas exchange.

Hence, adequate removal of retained bronchial secretions using chest physiotherapy techniques is an integral part of the management of these patients.

Prognosis

A substantial number of studies have now confirmed that the primary cause of death in patients with ARDS is not the inability to oxygenate arterial blood adequately, but rather the result of the development of multiple organ dysfunction and failure (MOF) due to poor tissue oxygen extraction and altered tissue blood flow (Montgomery et al. 1985; Fowler et al. 1990). These manifestations are associated with a high mortality rate. Approximately 30–60 per cent of patients with ARDS die, despite increasing awareness of the mechanisms of acute injury and the introduction of novel forms of therapy and support (Bernard et al. 1994).

Physiotherapy in ARDS

The aims of physiotherapy are:

- removal of retained secretions
- passive/active movements.

Chest physiotherapy involves four principal manœuvres: positioning to enhance removal of secretions and to improve gas exchange; manual hyperinflation; endotracheal suctioning; and manual techniques (which include shaking and vibrations).

Passive and active exercises need to be performed regularly whilst the patient's mobility remains restricted during the critical stages of disease, in order to maintain the mobility of joints and the extensibility of the soft tissues (e.g. the muscles, tendons and ligaments).

Fibrosing alveolitis

Definition

In fibrosing alveolitis the alveolar walls become thickened, with an increase in type II pneumocytes and macrophages. As the disease progresses, the alveolar walls fibrose and fibrosis spreads to the lung parenchyma.

The aetiology of fibrosing alveolitis is unknown (in most cases), although sometimes there is evidence of a pre-existing specific disease. These may be autoimmune (e.g. rheumatoid arthritis, systemic sclerosis) or gastrointestinal (e.g. chronic active hepatitis, ulcerative colitis).

Clinical features

- *Dyspnoea.* There is an insidious onset of breathlessness, often accompanied either by a dry unproductive cough or by a little clear sputum.
- *Auscultation.* A typical feature is mid- to late inspiratory crackles, which are said to be 'metallic' in nature.
- *Finger clubbing.* As the disease progresses, most patients develop gross finger clubbing.
- *Cyanosis.* This is due to impaired gas exchange.

Investigations and treatment

Blood gases reveal a progressive hypoxaemia with hypercapnia evident late in the disease. The chest X-ray will first show a ground-glass appearance, mainly in the lower zones; as the disease progresses, this becomes discrete and nodular. Transbronchial or open lung biopsy shows interstitial and alveolar fibrosis. LFTs reveal a restrictive deficit with reduced gas transfer factor.

10

Chronic forms of fibrosing alveolitis are treated with high doses of oral corticosteroids. Other immunosuppressive drugs (e.g. cyclophosphamide) are sometimes used if the alveolitis is associated with an autoimmune disease. Long-term oxygen therapy (LTOT) should be considered to correct hypoxaemia that leads to pulmonary hypertension and the development of cor pulmonale. Heart–lung transplantation may be considered in younger patients.

The median survival time of patients with fibrosing alveolitis is less than 5 years, although some patients may live for much longer. In general, the earlier the onset of the disease, the worse the prognosis.

Physiotherapy in fibrosing alveolitis

Physiotherapy should be directed at teaching breathing control and maintaining exercise tolerance as the patient becomes deconditioned due to fatigue and shortness of breath.

OTHER PULMONARY DISEASES

Lung abscess

Definition

A lung abscess is a localised formation of pus, usually surrounded by a fibrous capsule, within lung tissue.

Antibiotics and improved anesthesia have reduced the incidence of lung abscess and the condition tends now to occur secondary to bronchial carcinoma, particularly in patients who are over 40 years.

Aetiology

A variety of bacteria may enter the lungs by one of the following routes:

- through the air passages due to bronchopneumonia or following inhalation of a foreign body
- through the open chest wall following a wound from a knife stab or bullet
- from the blood stream
- due to bronchial carcinoma — an abscess forms where secretions accumulate distal to the tumour.

Pathological changes

The invading organisms cause inflammation of the lung tissue. At the centre of the area there is necrosis of lung tissue with liquefaction and suppuration. The area becomes distended and fibroblasts lay down fibrous tissue around the area until there is complete encapsulation. The capsule contracts and the abscess bursts, resulting in the production of foul-smelling sputum. Sometimes the pus drains into the pleura, causing empyema, and if drainage spills into adjacent lung tissue there is a danger of bronchiectasis. Toxins from the pus can be absorbed into the blood stream and there is then a danger of septicaemia. Healing occurs with the formation of a fibrous scar.

Clinical features

There is malaise, fever, cough and dyspnoea. The cough is at first irritable and unproductive but later is productive of foul-smelling sputum accompanied by a bad taste in the mouth. The cough may be painful if the pleura are inflamed. Haemoptysis and halitosis are further features.

Finger clubbing may become evident if the abscess becomes chronic.

Investigations and treatment

Blood analysis may reveal an increased white cell count. Cultures of sputum or lung aspirate will reveal the organism. A chest X-ray will show an area of cavitation within the lung tissue, which may contain an air-fluid level.

Most lung abscesses will respond to large intravenous doses of antibiotics to which the organism is sensitive. Drainage of the abscess may be necessary via needle aspiration or a thoracotomy. If there is an endobronchial obstruction caused by a foreign body, removal is essential.

Physiotherapy for a lung abscess

The site of the abscess is ascertained on the X-ray and the patient is positioned accurately for 10–15 minutes every 4 hours. Shaking is applied to the chest wall and breathing exercises are taught to regain breath control after coughing. Deep inspiration should not be encouraged because the increase in negative pressure may move the pus through healthy lung tissue.

It is important to adjust the patient's position to obtain maximum effective drainage and to ensure that precautions are taken to avoid any danger of cross-infection.

Pulmonary tuberculosis (TB)

Definition

In pulmonary tuberculosis the bacillus *Mycobacterium tuberculosis* causes irritation of the mucous lining in the bronchioles or alveoli and inflammatory changes take place.

In 1882, Robert Koch isolated the tubercle bacillus, of which there are two types, one human and the other bovine. Since then the disease has been controlled by inoculation, mass radiography, drugs and pasteurised milk.

Key point

The lungs are not the only tissues to be affected by TB. Types of TB other than pulmonary are: acute miliary (the blood is affected, with spread of the disease to spleen, liver, kidneys, meninges and lymph nodes); surgical TB; bone or joint TB; lupus vulgaris (the skin is affected); and TB adenoma (the lymph nodes are affected).

Aetiology and prevalence

Mycobacterium tuberculosis is spread by droplets during coughing and sneezing, so that a person can be infected from a patient's sputum.

TB is common worldwide, though its incidence has increased in Britain in recent years. The disease is still very common in Africa and Asia. In Europe the age group most frequently affected is middle age, but it also often occurs in elderly men. In Britain, the disease occurs mainly in the immigrant population from Ireland, Asia and the West Indies.

Predisposing factors are the environment, poor hygiene, overcrowding, lower socioeconomic groups, malnutrition, smoking and alcoholism. Other factors are diseases such as diabetes mellitus, congenital heart-disorder, leukaemia, Hodgkin's disease, long-term corticosteroids or immunosuppressive drugs.

Pathological changes

The bacilli are ingested by leucocytes and then absorbed by macrophages. More leucocytes form a barrier around this collection of cells and the complete mass is known as a 'tuberculous follicle'. The centre of the area undergoes necrosis and becomes soft and cheesy in consistency, the process being known as 'caseation'. This material may be moved into a bronchus and coughed up, leaving a cavity behind. Fibroblasts lay down a capsule around the tubercle in which calcium salts become deposited and healing takes place.

Cavity formation and calcification are the features of TB, with the calcified lesion remaining a potential source of infection. The bacillus may be reactivated and cause *postprimary pulmonary TB*. The danger then is that the disease may spread to other areas of the lungs, including the pleura, and through the blood stream to other parts of the body.

Clinical features

These are:

- malaise, lassitude and irritability
- loss of appetite and loss of weight
- pyrexia and tachycardia
- night sweats
- productive cough — the bacillus can be cultured from the sputum
- haemoptysis
- diminished respiratory movements with possibly some dyspnoea
- pain if there is pleural involvement.

Investigations

The chest X-ray shows cavity formation and calcification. In children these clinical features may be present to a mild degree and the disease can pass undetected. Other investigations are as follows:

- *Haematology*. The full blood count may show anaemia.
- *Immunology*. The Mantoux test is usually strongly positive in postprimary pulmonary TB, but is frequently negative in miliary TB.
- *Microbiology*. Sputum culture will show tubercle bacilli after 4–5 weeks of the primary infection. Bacilli may be cultured from the bone marrow in patients with miliary TB.
- *Diagnostic imaging*. In postprimary TB the chest X-ray may demonstrate a pleural effusion or pneumonia. A soft spreading apical shadowing is strongly suggestive of TB. In miliary TB there is widespread shadowing (i.e. small nodules 2–3 cm diameter).

Prevention

Vaccination with BCG (bacille Calmette–Guérin) greatly reduces the incidence of the disease and is currently offered to schoolchildren at 12–13 years of age. The vaccination may also be offered to people who might have contact with a patient who has active TB, such as relatives, friends, teachers, doctors, nurses and physiotherapists. Pasteurisation of milk prevents transmission of the tubercle to humans from cows.

Treatment

Drug therapy, together with rest, is the treatment for curing TB. Anti-TB drugs used are rifampicin, isoniazid, ethambutol and para-aminosalicylic acid (PAS); these must be taken every day for up to 18 months. The antibiotic, streptomycin, may also be prescribed. Multiple drug regimens are used in the treatment of resistant strains. Uncomplicated pulmonary TB is treated with a relatively short course (i.e. 6–9 months). If other organs are involved, a longer course of treatment may be necessary (e.g. 18 months for bone disease).

Surgery is appropriate only in a very small proportion of patients. If a patient has a resistant tubercle, a lobectomy may be performed, but the patient must still be on a drugs regimen.

The prognosis is good if the patient is not immunosuppressed.

Physiotherapy in pulmonary TB

Physiotherapy is not usually indicated during the rest stage. Once the patient is ambulant, a graded programme of exercises may be required. If it is necessary to give breathing exercises, the physiotherapist should stand behind the patient to avoid droplet infection as the patient coughs. Sputum must be disposed of very carefully so that cross-infection is prevented.

Bronchial and lung tumours

Key point

Tumours may be benign or malignant. The majority are malignant growths that may be primary or secondary.

Tumours arising within the lung (bronchial carcinomas) usually originate within the bronchi, whilst those that spread from other primary sites (e.g. breast, gastrointestinal tract) tend to develop in the lung tissue or the pleura.

In the UK, there are approximately 35 000 deaths from carcinoma of the bronchus each year. Men are more commonly affected than women, although the incidence is increasing in women. The peak incidence is amongst 65-year-olds.

Aetiology

People who smoke tobacco have a much greater risk of developing a malignant tumour than those who do not. The risk depends upon the number of cigarettes smoked, the age of starting to smoke and the timespan of smoking. The concept of pack-years is described at the beginning of this chapter.

The disease is more prevalent in urban dwellers than in rural dwellers. There is also evidence that exposure to carcinogens, either at work or leisure, can result in the development of the disease. Working with radioactive materials, nickel, uranium, chromates or industrial asbestos is associated with an increased risk of bronchial carcinoma.

Pathological changes

The majority of tumours originate in the large bronchi and spread by direct invasion of the lung, chest wall and mediastinal structures. The tumour grows to occlude the lumen of the bronchus and then atelectasis distal to the growth will occur. There are various types (Table 10.4).

Table 10.4 Histology of bronchial tumours

Histology	Proportion of bronchial cancers	Characteristics
Squamous cell	50%	Locally invasive, cavitation sometimes occurs
Oat/small cell	25%	Small lung primary, rapidly dividing, metastasise early
Large cell	12%	Intermediate between squamous and oat/small cell
Adenocarcinoma	12%	Slowly growing, metastasises late, often peripheral lung tumours
Miscellaneous	1%	For example, alveolar oat cell carcinoma

Clinical features

Seventy per cent of patients present with local symptoms. The onset is insidious, and the clinical features may present in a variety of ways:

- *Cough*. This is the most common feature and is often ignored by the patient, who may associate it with smoking. Initially, the cough is dry and irritating but may become productive if infection occurs in accumulated secretions.
- *Haemoptysis*. There are recurrent small spots of blood in the sputum.
- *Dyspnoea*. This is highly variable and may be severe when there is pulmonary collapse or pleural effusion.
- *Pain*. Dull, deep-seated pain is common but it may be pleuritic in nature or intercostal when there is rib disease.
- *Malaise and weight loss*. These are associated with late stages of the disease.
- *Secondary concomitant disease*. Pneumonia or lung abscess may arise as a result of a tumour.
- *Hoarseness of the voice*. This is due to left recurrent laryngeal nerve involvement by tumour of the left hilum.
- *Stridor*. This arises because of narrowing of the trachea or main bronchus.
- *Facial swelling*. This is caused by superior vena caval obstruction following invasion of the mediastinum.
- *Arm and shoulder pain*. These are due to tumour at the apex of the lung (Pancoast tumour) invading the brachial plexus.

Metastases

Metastases are common in patients with bronchial carcinoma and may include the following:

- *Cerebral metastases*. These may cause stroke, headaches and epilepsy.
- *Bone metastases*. The patient may present with spinal cord compression, pathological fracture and bone pain.
- *Liver metastases*. The patient may present with jaundice and hepatomegaly (an enlarged liver).

Non-metastatic presentations include finger clubbing, and neuromuscular and endocrine abnormalities.

Investigations

- *Chest X-ray*. This is essential for any patient presenting with haemoptysis and will demonstrate over 90 per cent of lung tumours. Small tumours or those close to the hilum may be missed.
- *CT scanning*. This may be used to identify smaller lesions. It may also be used to assess suitability for surgery by demonstrating metastatic spread.
- *Histopathology*. Sputum culture may have evidence of tumour cells. Three (early morning) samples should be obtained.
- *Bronchoscopy*. This is used to obtain tissue samples and may also be used to assess operability.

- *Percutaneous needle biopsy*. This may be useful for the histological assessment of a peripheral tumour.
- *Pleural aspiration and biopsy*. These may be used for the patient who presents with a pleural effusion.

Treatment

The appropriate treatment may be surgery, chemotherapy and/or radiotherapy. Drug therapy is essentially to relieve symptoms and includes analgesics, antibiotics and anti-emetics.

- *Surgery*. This involves removing the lobe or lung. It is possible only whilst the tumour remains localised and in the absence of metastases. Stenting is another option for localised disease.
- *Chemotherapy*. Cytotoxic drugs are used with increasing regularity. Results are mixed but anaplastic tumours tend to respond to this type of treatment.
- *Radiotherapy*. This is used symptomatically, particularly to relieve pain and obstruction.
- *Laser phototherapy*. This can be used to treat persistent localised disease.

The prognosis depends upon the type of tumour, but the overall length of survival is around 1 year. Surgery can prolong life in some patients. In the terminal stages attention should be paid to the patient's general well-being and mental state. Some patients benefit from hospice care and adequate opiate analgesia is essential for pain.

Physiotherapy for bronchial and lung tumours

Physiotherapy may be related to three aspects of management of the disease:

- Pre- and postoperative physiotherapy is essential for patients who have a lobectomy or pneumonectomy.
- During and after radiotherapy, when the tumour begins to decrease in size, the patient will begin to expectorate sputum. Positioning and the ACBT should be used for sputum clearance. Percussion and vigorous shaking should not be used, as there is a danger of pathological fractures in ribs or vertebrae in which metastases may be developing. Nor should shaking be used in the presence of haemoptysis.
- During the terminal stage of the disease, where accumulation of secretions is causing distress, modified postural drainage and vibrations with breathing exercises may help to make the patient more comfortable. If coughing is ineffective, suction may have to be used. An active daily programme that fits the patient's requirements may need to be devised, in which case the physiotherapist works in close collaboration with the healthcare team.

Respiratory failure

Definition

Respiratory failure denotes reduction of function of the lungs due to lung disease, or a skeletal or neuromuscular disorder. It is defined in terms of the gas tensions (pressures) in the arterial blood.

Normal arterial oxygen and carbon dioxide pressures (PaO_2 and $PaCO_2$) are 13.0 kPa (97 mm Hg) and 6.1 kPa (46 mm Hg) respectively. There are two types of respiratory failure:

- *Type 1*: A PaO_2 of less than 8.0 kPa (60 mm Hg) is associated with a $PaCO_2$ that is either normal or below 6.7 kPa (50 mm Hg).
- *Type 2*: A PaO_2 of less than 8.0 kPa (60 mm Hg) is associated with a $PaCO_2$ raised above 6.7 kPa (50 mm Hg).

Causes of type 1 respiratory failure

Lung disease results in hypoventilation of the alveoli, leading to a ventilation/perfusion mismatch. The blood supply is normal but there is inadequate oxygen uptake from the affected alveoli. Diseases associated with this type are early chronic bronchitis and emphysema, pneumonia, asthma, acute pulmonary oedema, pulmonary embolism, pulmonary fibrosis and ARDS.

Causes of type 2 respiratory failure

Because of failure of the skeletal or neuromuscular components of the respiratory system there is loss of the pump mechanism essential for ventilation of the lungs as a whole. Therefore, there is a reduced tidal volume or a reduced respiratory rate, leading to a rise in $PaCO_2$ and a fall in PaO_2. Disorders associated with this type are head injuries, polyneuropathies, cervical cord injuries, advanced chronic bronchitis and emphysema, status asthmaticus, crushed chest, muscular dystrophy, myasthenia gravis and kyphoscoliosis.

Clinical features

- *Type 1 due to hypoxaemia*: There may be dyspnoea, restlessness, confusion, central cyanosis, tachycardia, renal failure, pulmonary hypertension.
- *Type 2 due to hypercapnia*: There may be flapping tremor of the hands, confusion, headache, warm peripheries, tachycardia. Dyspnoea occurs initially but the person may become drowsy and comatose if PaO_2 is allowed to rise.

Treatment

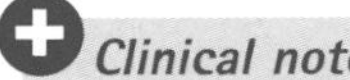

Clinical note

The diagnosis cannot be accurate until arterial blood gases have been measured. Treatment must be directed towards treating the cause.

In type 1 respiratory failure the main problem is the hypoxaemia, so it is important to raise the PaO_2 by giving oxygen therapy, which should be in sufficient amounts to correct the hypoxaemia.

In type 2 respiratory failure there is a danger of reducing the respiratory drive, which is dependent on the anoxic state of the blood stimulating the chemoreceptors in the carotid and aortic arteries. The danger then is that the patient's respiration slows or stops and the $PaCO_2$ rises, resulting in confusion and coma. A Ventimask giving 24 per cent or 28 per cent inspired oxygen may be applied (see the section on oxygen therapy in COPD).

Physiotherapy in respiratory failure

Type 1 failure

It is vital to clear the lung fields of secretions. If the patient is spontaneously breathing, positioning and the ACBT can be used with manual techniques to loosen secretions. If the patient is too weak to cough, suction has to be used. If bronchospasm is evident, a bronchodilator (e.g. salbutamol) may be given in combination with oxygen therapy. If IPPV is applied, a bronchodilator may be administered through the ventilator, and shakings and vibrations should be performed with manual hyperinflation. Suction will be via the endotracheal tube. All treatment is monitored by regular blood gas analysis.

Type 2 failure

It is again necessary to raise the PaO_2 and this is achieved by oxygen therapy using a Ventimask delivering 24 per cent oxygen. If this is not sufficient to raise the PaO_2, the Ventimask may be changed to one delivering 28 per cent oxygen, provided the $PaCO_2$ is not rising from the already high level. If the $PaCO_2$ starts to rise, this is indicative of hypoventilation, usually because the patient is becoming exhausted and NIPPV is indicated. Assisted ventilation may be necessary, although this should be avoided if the patient has a chronic compensated respiratory acidosis. Physiotherapy follows similar principles to that for type 1 failure.

REFERENCES

Abman SH, Ogle JW, Harbeck RJ et al. 1991 Early bacteriologic, immunologic, and clinical courses of young infants with cystic fibrosis identified by neonatal screening. J Paediatr 119: 211–217

Adinoff AD, Hollester JR 1983 Steroid-induced fractures and bone loss in patients with asthma. N Engl J Med 309: 265–268

Amado MC, Portnoy JM 2006 Recent advances in asthma management. Mo Med 103 (1): 60–64

American Thoracic Society 1995 Standards for the diagnosis and care of patients with chronic obstructive pulmonary disease. Am J Respir Care Med 152 (Suppl): S77–S121

Armstrong P, Wilson AG, Dee P, Hansell DM 1995 Imaging of Diseases of the Chest. Year Book Medical: Chicago

Bell SC, Saunders MJ, Elborn JS, Shale DJ 1996 Resting energy expenditure and oxygen cost of breathing in patients with cystic fibrosis. Thorax 51: 126–131

Bellemare F, Grassino A 1982 Effect of pressure and timing of contraction on human diaphragmatic fatigue. J Appl Physiol 53: 1190–1195

Bernard G, Artiglas A, Bringham K et al. 1994 Report on the American–European consensus conference on ARDS: definitions, mechanisms, relevant outcomes and clinical trial coordination. Inten Care Med 20: 225–232

Bollert FG, Paton JY, Marshall TG et al. 1999 Recombinant DNase in cystic fibrosis: a protocol for targeted introduction through *n*-of-1 trials. Scottish Cystic Fibrosis Group. Eur Respir J 13: 107–113

Bone RC 1996 Goals of asthma management: a step-care approach. Chest 4: 1056–1065

Bradley J, Moran F 2006 Pulmonary rehabilitation improves exercise tolerance in patients with bronchiectasis. Aust J Physiotherapy 52 (1): 65

British Thoracic Association 1982 Death from asthma in two regions of England. BMJ 285: 1251–1255

British Thoracic Society 1997 The BTS guidelines on asthma management. Thorax 52 (Suppl 1): S1–S21

Brochard L, Manceebo J, Wysocki M 1995 Non-invasive ventilation for acute exacerbations of chronic obstructive pulmonary disease. N Engl J Med 333: 817–822

Brocklebank D, Ram F, Wright J et al. 2001 Comparison of the effectiveness of inhaler devices in asthma and chronic obstructive airway disease: a systematic review of the literature. Health Techn Assess 5(26): 1–149

Burr ML, Wat D, Evans C et al. 2006 British Thoracic Society Research Committee: Asthma Prevalence in 1973, 1988 and 2003. Thorax 61(4): 296–299

Cecins NM, Jenkins SC, Pengelley J, Ryan G 1999 The active cycle of breathing technique — to tip or not to tip? Respir Med 93: 660–665

Cerny F, Pullano T, Gerd J, Cropp A 1982 Cardiorespiratory adaptations to exercise in cystic fibrosis. Am Rev Respir Dis 126: 217–220

Chang SC, Chang HI, Shiao GM, Perng RP 1993 Effect of body position on gas exchange in patients with unilateral central airways lesions. Down with the good lung? Chest 103: 787–791

Chatham K, Baldwin J, Griffiths H et al. 1999 Inspiratory muscle training improves shuttle run performance in healthy subjects. Physiotherapy 85: 676–683

Chatwin M, Hart N, Nickol AH et al. 2000 Low frequency fatigue induced by a single inspiratory muscle training session. Thorax 55 (Suppl 3): abstract

Christopher F, Chase D, Stein K, Milne R 1999 RhDNase therapy for the treatment of cystic fibrosis patients with mild to moderate lung disease. J Clin Pharm Ther 24: 415–426

Clanton TL, Diaz PT 1995 Focus on ventilatory muscle training: clinical assessment of the respiratory muscles. Phys Ther 75: 983–995

Clarke SW 1991 Chronic bronchitis in the 1990s. Respiration 58 (Suppl): 43–46

Cobos N, Danes I, Gartner S et al. 2000 DNase use in the daily care of cystic fibrosis: who benefits from it and to what extent? Results of a cohort study of 199 patients in 13 centres. DNase National Study Group. Eur J Paediatr 159(3): 176–181

Cochrane GM, Webber BA, Clark SW 1977 Effects of sputum on pulmonary function. BMJ 2: 1181–1183

Cochrane GM, Clark CJ 1990 Benefits and problems of a physical training programme for asthmatic patients. Thorax 1990: 345–351

Cole P 1995 Bronchiectasis. In: Brewis RAL, Corrin B, Geddes DM, Gibson GJ (eds) Respiratory Medicine, 2nd edn. WB Saunders: London

COPD Guidelines Group of the Standards of Care Committee of the BTS 1997. BTS guidelines for the management of chronic obstructive pulmonary disease. Thorax 52 (Suppl 5): S1–S32

Corda L, Bertella E, Pini L et al. 2006 Diagnostic flow chart for targeted detection of alpha$_1$-antitrypsin deficiency. Respir Med 100(3): 463–470

Corless JA, Warburton CJ 2000 Surgery vs non-surgical treatment for bronchiectasis. Cochrane Database Systematic Review CD002180

Corraco WM, Braman SS, Erwin RS 1979 Chronic cough as the sole presenting manifestation of bronchial asthma. N Engl J Med 300: 633–637

Crossley DJ, McGuire GP, Barrow PM, Houston PL 1997 Influence of inspired oxygen concentration on dead space, respiratory drive, and $PaCO_2$ in intubated patients with chronic obstructive pulmonary disease. Crit Care Med 25: 1522–1526

Currie DC 1997 Nebulisers for bronchiectasis. Thorax 521 (Suppl 2): S72–S74

Davies DS 1973 Pharmokinetics of inhaled substances. Postgrad Med J 51 (Supp 7): 69–75

Davis PB, Drumm M, Konstan MW 1996 Cystic fibrosis (state of the art). Am J Respir Crit Care Med 154: 1229–1256

Decramer M 1989 Effects of hyperinflation on the respiratory muscles. Eur Respir J 2: 299–302

Decramer M, De Benedetto F, Del Ponte A, Marinari S 2005 Systemic effects of COPD. Respir Med Suppl B: S3–S10

de Jong W, Kaptein AA, Van der Shands 1997 Quality of life in patients with cystic fibrosis. Paediatr Pulmonol 23: 95–100

Department of Health 1997 Health of the Nation Briefing Pack. leads: DOH

Donahoe M, Rogers RM, Wilson DO, Pennok BE 1989 Oxygen consumption of the respiratory muscles in normal and malnourished patients with chronic obstructive pulmonary disease. Am Rev Respir Dis 140: 385–391

Dransfield MT, Davis JJ, Gerald LB, Bailey WC 2006 Racial and gender differences in susceptibility to tobacco smoke among patients with chronic obstructive pulmonary disease. Respir Med (6): 1110–1116

Driks M, Craven D, Celli C 1987 Nosocomial pneumonia in intubated patients given sucralfale as compared with antacids or histamine type 2 blockers: the role of gastric colonisation. N Engl J Med 317: 1376–1382

Elborn JS, Shale DJ, Britton JR 1991 Cystic fibrosis: current survival and population estimates to the year 2000. Thorax 46: 881–885

Elborn JS, Johnston B, Allen F 1992 Inhaled steroids in patients with bronchiectasis. Respir Med 86: 121–124

Elborn JS, Cordon SM, Shale DJ 1993 Inflammatory responses prior to death in cystic fibrosis. Respir Med 87: 603–607

Elborn JS, Prescott RJ, Stack BH 2000 Elective versus symptomatic antibiotic treatment in cystic fibrosis patients with chronic *Pseudomonas* infection of the lungs. Thorax 55: 355–358

Enright S, Chatham K, Baldwin J, Griffiths H 2000 The effect of fixed load incremental inspiratory muscle training in the elite athlete. Phys Ther Sport 1: 1–5

Enright S, Chatham K, Ionescu AA et al. 2004 Inspiratory muscle training improves lung function and exercise capacity in adults with cystic fibrosis. Chest 126: 406–411

Enright SJ, Unnithan VB, Heward C et al. 2006 Effect of high-intensity inspiratory muscle training on lung volumes, diaphragm thickness, and exercise capacity in subjects who are healthy. Phys Ther 86(3): 345–354

Fleetham JA, Bradley CA, Kryger MH, Anthonisen NR 1980 The effect of low flow oxygen therapy on the chemical control of ventilation in patients with hypoxemic COPD. Am Rev Respir Dis 122: 833–840

Folgering H, von Herwaarden C 1994 Exercise limitations in patients with pulmonary diseases. Int J Sports Med 15 (3): 107–111

Fowler A, Goldman M 1990 Adult respiratory distress syndrome: prognosis after onset. Am Rev Respir Dis 132: 472–478

Freitag L, Bremme J, Schroer M 1989 High frequency oscillation for respiratory physiotherapy. Br J Anaesth 63: 44S–46S

Goldstein RS 1993 Ventilatory muscle training: pulmonary rehabilitation in chronic respiratory insufficiency. Thorax 48: 1025–1033

Green M, Moxham J 1993 Respiratory muscles in health and disease. In: Barnes P (ed.). Respiratory Medicine: Recent Advances. Butterworth–Heinemann Oxford, pp. 252—275

Gross NJ 1995 Airway inflammation in COPD: reality or myth? Chest 107 (Suppl 5): S1–S24

Guell R, Resqueti V, Sangenis M et al. 2006 Impact of pulmonary rehabilitation on psychosocial morbidity in patients with severe COPD. Chest 129(4): 899–904

Hargreave FE, Dolovich J, Newhouse MT (eds) 1990 The assessment and treatm,ent of asthma: a conference report J Allergy Clin Immunol 85: 1098–2011

Hasegawa M, Nasuhara Y, Onodera Y et al. 2006 Airflow limitation and airways dimensions in chronic obstructive pulmonary disease. Am J Respir Crit Care Med 173: 1309–1315

Haworth CS, Selby PL, Webb AK 1999 Low bone mineral density in adults with cystic fibrosis. Thorax 54: 961–967

Hogg JC 2004 Pathophysiology of airflow limitation in chronic obstructive pulmonary disease. Lancet 364: 709–721

Israel E, Rubin P, Kemp JP et al. 1993 The effect of inhibition of 5-lipoxygenase by Ziluteton in mild-to-moderate asthma. Ann Intern Med 119: 1059–1066

Joint Health Surveys Unit 1996 Health Survey for England (1995). HMSO: London

Kaplan TA, ZeBranek JD, McKey RM 1991 Use of exercise in the management of cystic fibrosis. Paediatr Pulmonol 10: 205–207

Kearney CE, Wallace CE 2000 Deoxyribonuclease for cystic fibrosis. Cochrane Database Systematic Review CD001127

Kesten S, Chapman KR 1993 Physician perceptions and management of COPD. Chest 104: 254–258

Kikuchi Y, Okabe S, Tamura G et al. 1994 Chemosensitivity and perceptions of dyspnoea in patients with a history of near-fatal asthma. N Engl J Med 330: 1329–1334

Konstan MW, Berger M 1993 Infection and inflammation of the lung in cystic fibrosis. In: Davis PB (ed.) Lung Biology in Health and Disease. Vol. 64: Cystic Fibrosis. Marcel Dekker: New York, pp. 219–276

Konstan MW, Hillard KA, Norvell TM 1994 Bronchoalveolar lavage findings in cystic fibrosis patients with stable, clinically mild lung disease suggest ongoing infection and inflammation. Am J Respir Crit Care Med 150: 448–454

Lacasse Y, Wong E, Guyatt GH et al. 1996 Meta-analysis of respiratory rehabilitation in chronic obstructive pulmonary disease. Lancet 348: 1115–1119

Levine S, Guillen M 1987 Diaphragmatic pressure waveform can predict EMG signs of diaphragmatic fatigue. J Appl Physiol 62: 1681–1689

Ling SC, Wilkinson JD, Hollman AS et al. 1999 The evolution of liver disease in cystic fibrosis. Arch Dis Child 81: 129–132

Mansoura MK, Smith SS, Choi AD et al. 1998 Cystic fibrosis transmembrane conductance regulator (CFTR) anion binding as a probe of the pore. Biophys J 74(3): 1320–1332

Meecham-Jones DJ, Paul EA, Jones PW, Wedzicha JA 1995 Nasal pressure support ventilation plus oxygen compared with oxygen therapy alone in hypercapnic COPD. Am J Respir Crit Care Med 152: 538–544

Montgomery A, Stager M, Carrico C, Hudson L 1985 Causes of mortality in patients with adult respiratory distress syndrome. Am Rev Respir Dis 132: 485–489

Moxham J 1990 Respiratory muscle fatigue: mechanisms, evaluation and therapy. Br J Anaesth 65: 43–53

Murciano D, Auclair MH, Pariente R, Aubier M 1989 A randomised controlled trial of theophylline in patients with severe chronic obstructive pulmonary disease. N Engl J Med 320: 1521–1525

Nebuliser Project Group of the British Thoracic Society Standards of Care Committee 1997 Current best practice for nebuliser treatment. Thorax 52 (Suppl 2): S1–S3

Newman SP, Pavia D, Clark SW 1981 How should a pressurised beta-adrenergic bronchodilator be inhaled? Eur J Respir Dis 62: 3–21

Newman SP, Pavia D, Garland N, Clarke SW 1982 Effects of various inhalation modes on the deposition of radioactive pressurized aerosols. Eur J Respir Dis 63 (Suppl): 57–65

Nicholson KG, Kent J, Ireland DC 1993 Respiratory viruses and exacerbations of asthma in adults. BMJ 307: 982–986

Nixon PA, Orenstein DM, Kelsey SF, Doershuk CF 1992 The prognostic value of exercise testing in patients with cystic fibrosis. N Engl J Med 327: 1785–1788

O'Callahan C, Barry P 1997 Spacer devices in the treatment of asthma. Br Med J 314: 1061–1062

O'Donnell DE 2006 Hyperinflation, dyspnea, and exercise intolerance in chronic obstructive pulmonary disease. Proc Am Thorac Soc 3(2): 180–184

Office for National Statistics 1997 Mortality Statistics for England and Wales (1996). HMSO: London

O'Neill PA, Dodd M, Phillips B 1987 Regular exercise and reduction of breathlessness in cystic fibrosis. Br J Dis Chest 81: 62–66

Oppenheimer EH, Esterly JR 1975 Pathology of cystic fibrosis: review of the literature and comparison with 146 autopsied cases. Persp Paediatr Pathol 2: 241–248

Patessio A, Iolo F, Donner CF 1993 Exercise prescription. In: Casaburi R, Petty TL (eds) The Principles and Practice of Pulmonary Rehabilitation. WB Saunders: Philadelphia

Pearson MG, Spence DPS, Ryland I, Harrison BD 1993 Value of pulsus paradoxus in assessing acute severe asthma. BMJ 307: 659

Pearson MG, Calverley PMA 1995 Clinical and laboratory assessment. In: Calverley PMA, Pride NB (eds) Chronic Obstructive Pulmonary Disease. Chapman & Hall: London

Peters SP, Ferguson G, Deniz Y, Reisner C 2006 Uncontrolled asthma: A review of the prevalence, disease burden and options for treatment. Respir Med 100(7): 1139–1151

Polkey MI, Green M, Moxham J 1995 Measurement of respiratory muscle strength. Thorax 50: 1131–1135

Porsbjerg C, von Linstow ML, Ulric CS et al. 2006 Risk factors for onset of asthma: a 12-year prospective follow-up study. Chest 129(2): 309–316

Prescott E, Godtfredensen N, Vestbo J, Osler M 2003 Social position and mortality from respiratory diseases in males and females. Eur Respir J 21(5): 821–826

Prior JG, Cochrane GM 1980 Home monitoring of peak expiratory flow rate using a mini-Wright peak flow meter in diagnosis of asthma. J R Soc Med 73: 1329–1334

Prior JG, Webber BA 1979 An evaluation of the forced expiration technique as an adjunct to postural drainage. Physiotherapy 65: 304–307

Quinton PM 1990 Cystic fibrosis: a disease of electrolyte transport. FASEB J 4: 2709–2717

Ramsey BW, Farrell PM, Pencharz P 1992 Nutritional assessment and management in cystic fibrosis: a consensus report. Am J Clin Nutr 55: 108–116

Rees PJ, Clark TJH, Moren F 1982 The importance of particle size in response to inhaled bronchodilators. Eur J Respir Dis 119 (Suppl): 73–78

Rimington LD, Davies DH, Low D, Pearson MG 2001 Relationship between anxiety, depression and morbidity in adult asthma patients. Thorax 56: 266–271

Rosen MJ 2006 Chronic cough due to bronchiectasis: ACCP evidence-based clinical practice guidelines. Chest 129(1): 122S–131S

Roussos C, Zakynthinos S 1996 Fatigue of the respiratory muscles. Inten Care Med 22: 134–155

Rubinfeld AR, Pain MCF 1976 The perceptions of asthma. Lancet i: 882–884

Rudolf M, Riorden JF, Grant BJB et al. 1978 Bromhexine in severe asthma. Br J Dis Chest 72: 307–312

Sahl W, Bilton D, Dodd M, Webb AK 1989 Effect of exercise and physiotherapy in aiding sputum expectoration in adults with cystic fibrosis. Thorax 44: 1006–1008

Senn O, Russi EW, Imboden M, Probst-Hensch NM 2005 Alpha$_1$-antitrypsin deficiency and lung disease risk modification by occupational and environmental inhalants. Eur Resp J Nov 5: 909–917

Silverman EK, Weiss ST, Drazen JM et al. 2000 Gender-related differences in severe, early-onset chronic obstructive pulmonary disease. Am J Crit Care Med 162(6): 2152–2158

Sinuff T, Cook D, Randall J, Allen C 2000 Noninvasive positive-pressure ventilation: a utilisation review of use in a teaching hospital. Can Med Assoc J 163: 969–973

Smith K, Cook D, Guyatt GH et al. 1992 Respiratory muscle training in chronic airflow limitation: a meta-analysis. Am Rev Respir Dis 145: 533–539

Smyth A, Walters S 2000 Prophylactic antibiotics for cystic fibrosis. Cochrane Database Systematic Review CD0011912

Solomon C, Christian D, Welch B, Balmes J 1996 Cellular pulmonary tract and pulmonary function responses to exercise and serial sputum inductions. Am J Respir Crit Care Med 153: A713

Speight AWP 1983 Is childhood asthma being underdiagnosed and undertreated? BMJ 286: 16–20

Stavngaard T, Shaker SB, Dirksen A 2006 Quantitative assessment of emphysema distribution in smokers and patients with alpha$_1$-antitrypsin deficiency. Respir Med 100(1): 94–100

Svanberg L 1957 Influence of posture on lung volumes, ventilation and circulation in normals. Scand J Clin Lab Invest 9: Supp 25

Tashkin DP, Ashutosh K, Bleeker ER 1986 Comparison of the anticholinergic bronchodilator ipratropium bromide with metaproterenol in chronic obstructive pulmonary disease: a 90-day multicenter study. Am J Med 81 (Suppl 5a): 81–90

Thomas SH, O'Doherty MJ, Graham A et al. 1991 Pulmonary deposition of nebulised amiloride in cystic fibrosis: comparison of two nebulisers. Thorax 46: 717–721

Thurlbeck WM 1976 Chronic Airflow Obstruction in Lung Disease. WB Saunders: Philadelphia

Turpin SV, Knowles MR 1993 Treatment of pulmonary disease in patients with cystic fibrosis. In: Davis PB (ed.) Lung Biology in Health and Disease, Vol. 64: Cystic Fibrosis. Marcel Dekker: New York, pp. 236–243

Vender RL 1994 Chronic hypoxic pulmonary hypertension. Chest 106: 236–243

Wark PA, McDonald V 2000 Nebulised hypertonic saline for cystic fibrosis. Cochrane Database Systematic Review CD001506

Webber BA, Hofmeyr JL, Morgan MDL, Hodson ME 1986 Effects of postural drainage, incorporating the forced expiration technique on pulmonary function in cystic fibrosis. Br J Dis Chest 80: 353–359

West JB 1995 Pulmonary Pathophysiology: the Essentials, 5th edn. Williams & Wilkins: Baltimore

Wilson GE, Baldwin AL, Walshaw MJ 1995 A comparison of traditional chest physiotherapy with the active cycle of breathing in patients with chronic suppurative lung disease. Eur Respir J 8: 1715

Yelin E, Katz P, Balmes J et al. 2006 Work life of persons with asthma, rhinitis, and COPD: A study using a national, population-based sample. J Occup Med Toxicol 2 1(1): 2

Zach MS, Oberwaldner B 1989 Chest physiotherapy: the mechanical approach to antiinfective therapy in cystic fibrosis. Infection 15: 381–384

Chapter 11

Adult spontaneous and conventional mechanical ventilation

Sue Pieri-Davies

CHAPTER CONTENTS

INTRODUCTION

This chapter focuses on the ventilatory aspects of the patient in respiratory failure. A basic understanding of all major systems is essential when considering the physiotherapeutic requirements of the ventilated adult, since the initial assessment necessitates identification of the underlying cause. The aim of intervention will then be either correction where possible, and/or alleviation of respiratory symptoms such as breathlessness, reinflation, reduction in the work of breathing and sputum retention.

The detailed undergraduate training in anatomy and physiology places the physiotherapist in an excellent position to manage the respiratory and rehabilitation needs of such complex patients. However, in order to enable an applied approach to the assessment (incorporating problem-solving) findings and necessary intervention, as is the requirement in the emergency on-call duty setting, it is essential to understand the basics of respiratory mechanics in the spontaneously breathing individual.

The section on conventional mechanical ventilation should be read in conjunction with the cardiac and respiratory chapters of this book. It is beyond the scope of a single chapter to detail all appropriate systems, the numerous conditions and causes of ventilatory failure, the concept and uses of non-invasive ventilation, and the specialised area of domiciliary ventilation. A more detailed knowledge of these subjects can be obtained through further private study of the recommended texts and websites provided at the end of this chapter.

SPONTANEOUS VENTILATION

The basics of respiratory mechanics in the spontaneously breathing individual must be understood, since the application of/weaning off mechanical ventilatory support/control will have a direct impact upon respiratory capacity. An ability to recognise and interpret deviations from the normal is of prime importance in maximising and maintaining efficient spontaneous respiratory function, particularly during an episode of critical illness.

The respiratory muscles

The respiratory muscles consist of two main groups:

- the primaries (mostly comprising the diaphragm and intercostals)
- the accessories (mostly comprising the scaleni, abdominals and sternocleidomastoids).

It is also important to remember the effects on oxygenation status and balance of the blood pH with increasing metabolic demands, should the recruitment of additional muscles (for example, the facial muscles with pursed-lip breathing and the shoulder girdle and arm fixators) be required during times of respiratory distress/dysfunction.

The primaries' main role is that of ventilation. The accessories have other functions but are recruited to facilitate ventilation when required. Normally, the respiratory muscles have both ventilatory and non-ventilatory motor functions. For example, the diaphragm acts as the primary respiratory muscle, generating approximately 60–70 per cent of the tidal volume while also being responsible for raising intra-abdominal pressure for postural stabilisation of the torso, parturition and micturition.

Such considerations must be appreciated by the therapist; when the respiratory muscles are required for both motor and ventilatory functions, their ability to assist ventilation is reduced. This is of particular importance when ventilatory support has recently been reduced and motor activity is being encouraged during daytime hours: that is, during the weaning and rehabilitative phases of recovery. Upper limb strengthening exercises may be a primary aim at this stage, so increasing ventilatory support overnight may be appropriate.

The respiratory muscles share the common features of other skeletal muscles, and consist of a mixture of fibre types (Johnson et al. 1973). The proportions of fibre types and their metabolic constituents (e.g. capillaries, glycolytic and oxidative capacities, time of recruitment in contraction) determine a muscle's strength and endurance properties (Moffett et al. 1993) (Table 11.1).

- Type I fibres are important for endurance: slow twitch, high oxidative capacity, recruited first, and most resistant to fatigue.
- Type IIa fibres have a higher oxidative capacity, fast twitch, produce an intermediate level of force, and so are relatively resistant to fatigue.
- Type IIb fibres have a low oxidative capacity, fast twitch, produce greatest force on activation, are the last to be recruited for motor efforts and are easily fatigued when used repeatedly.

Greater knowledge of muscle physiology is required if the aim is to train the respiratory muscles, rather than rest them (via ventilatory support). Muscle training may be an appropriate physiotherapy intervention to facilitate the weaning episode of the prolonged

Table 11.1 Comparison of skeletal muscle fibre types

Characteristics	Type I	Type IIa	Type IIb
Contractile			
Contraction velocity	Slow	Fast	Fast
Myosin adenosine triphosphatase	Slow	Fast	Fast
Twitch duration	Long	Short	Short
Calcium ion sequestration	Slow	Rapid	Rapid
Metabolic			
Capillaries	Abundant	Intermediate	Sparse
Glycolytic capacity	Low	Intermediate	High
Oxidative capacity	High	High	Low
Glycogen content	Low	Intermediate	High
Myoglobin content	High	Intermediate	Low
Fibre diameter	Small	Intermediate	Large
Motor unit size	Small	Intermediate	Large
Recruitment order	Early	Intermediate	Late

(Reproduced from Moffett et al. (1993), with permission.)

ventilatory supported individual where muscle wasting and disuse atrophy are evident, though more research is required in this area.

Respiratory mechanics and airflow

Contraction of the respiratory muscles affects the overall motion of the chest wall. For example, in the upright position, on inspiration, the diaphragm moves downwards on contraction while the abdomen moves out. Synchronicity is achieved when the rib cage and the abdomen move together, increasing in diameter during inspiration and decreasing in diameter during expiration. In supine, most movements are abdominal, with little movement of the rib cage. Body position in both respiratory mechanics and ventilation/perfusion matching is of great importance, as respiratory muscle dysfunction alone — for example, fatigue or weakness — can lead to dyspnoea, hypoventilation, hypercapnoea, reduced oxygenation of body tissues, respiratory failure, metabolic acidosis and, ultimately, death.

Normal resting ventilation is a tricyclical activity consisting of:

- the inward flow of air called inspiration
- the outward flow called exhalation
- the rest phase, which constitutes the zero-flow status.

During the inspiratory and expiratory cycles a volume of air moves in and out of the lungs. These changes occur as a result of pressure gradients between the airway opening (or mouth) and the alveoli. Prior to the beginning of inspiration, the pressures at the airway opening and in the alveoli are equivalent. Since there is no pressure gradient, there is no air movement. (This is known as the resting period of the respiratory cycle, where air neither enters nor leaves the lungs (Figure 11.1).

As inspiration begins, the respiratory muscles contract, causing an upward and outward movement of the chest wall (the bucket and pump handle effects) and the diaphragm descends (Figure 11.2). This is known as the active phase of the breathing cycle and demands effort (termed the work of breathing — see below). The changes in thoracic dimensions create a drop in alveolar pressure; the pressure gradient between the airway opening and the alveoli results in an inward movement of air. The volume change that occurs is called the tidal volume and is on average 500 mL.

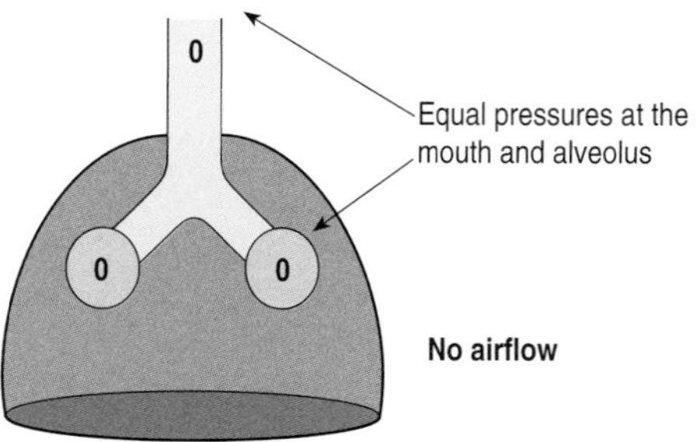

Figure 11.1 Spontaneous breathing: rest phase.

Weblink

Joint guidelines by the British Thoracic Society (www.brit-thoracic.org.uk) and Association for Respiratory Technology and Physiology (http://fp.artpweb2.f9.co.uk) are available for a detailed underpinning of spirometric values and tests. Also downloadable from the web are the American Thoracic Society and European Respiratory Society recommendations for spirometry (www.ersnet.org/ers/lr/browse/viewPDF.aspx? id_attach=7571).

The opposing forces to ventilation

The work of breathing derives from the two resistive forces of the lungs and chest wall: the elastic (Figure 11.3) and frictional forces. Forces within the respiratory system that oppose inflation of the lung and therefore ventilation can be grouped into two categories:

- the elastic opposition to expansion of the lungs
- the frictional opposition or resistance to air movement.

The pressure change that is generated on inspiration must be sufficient to overcome such forces. As we have seen, the effort required and the resulting volume change is termed the 'work of breathing'. Normally, the work of breathing is minimal (healthy lungs). A pressure gradient of 2–5 cm H_2O is typically needed to move the average tidal volume.

Elastic forces

The elastic forces are encountered as a result of both the lungs and chest wall being 'elastic' structures; that is, they resist changes in shape. When they have been inflated or deflated, they tend to return to the same resting/starting position of equilibrium once the driving force has been removed. The lungs naturally want to collapse and the chest wall naturally wants to expand. Thus each exerts a pull on the other. In the absence of other forces (such as muscles), a position is reached in which the opposing forces are balanced.

Due to these opposing forces (of lung and chest wall), the intrathoracic pressure is negative (subatmospheric). To inflate the lungs an extra force must be applied (by the muscles) and intrathoracic pressure falls lower.

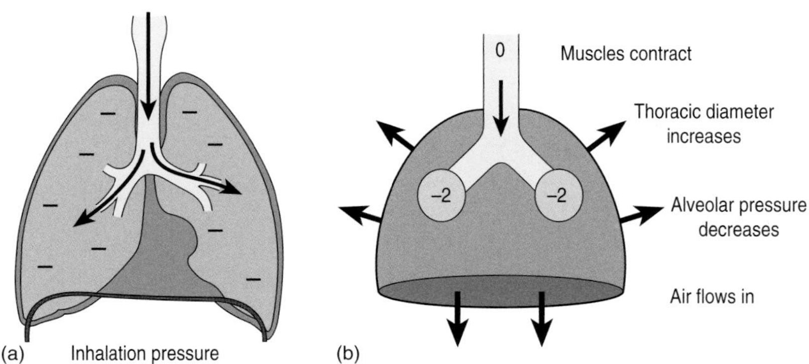

Figure 11.2 Spontaneous breathing: inspiratory phase. (Courtesy of the Johns Hopkins University website.)

Expiration is mostly passive as a result of the elastic forces returning the lungs and chest wall to a balanced position (Figure 11.4). It can, however, be active: for example, in forced breathing and coughing, where the expiratory muscles assist the elastic forces (resulting in a more rapid expiratory rate of flow and faster lung deflation).

The inspiratory muscles perform mechanical work by upsetting the balance of the elastic forces. Hence the harder and faster the respiratory effort is, the more 'elastic' work is required. A certain amount of pressure is required to stretch the lungs to a certain volume. The normal value for elastance is around10 cm H_2O/L. However, in disease states, the lungs become stiffer and the same pressure change may result in a smaller volume change; that is, the elastance of the lung is higher. Pneumonia, ARDS and pulmonary oedema are common lung conditions affecting elastance. Others include fibrotic lung disease, pleural effusion, kyphoscoliosis and obesity.

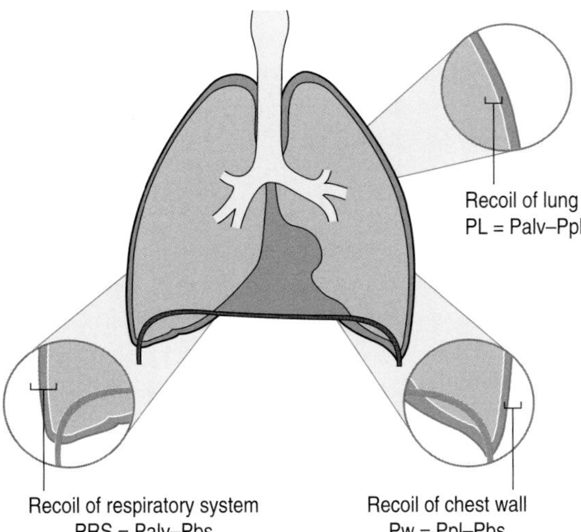

Figure 11.3 The elastic forces of the lung and chest wall. Palv, alveolar pressure (pressure within the alveoli); Pbs, pressure at the body surface; Pl, transpulmonary pressure (pressure difference across the lung); Ppl, pleural pressure; Prs, pressure within the respiratory system; Pw, pleural pressure minus pressure at the body surface (= elastic recoil pressure of chest wall). (Courtesy of the Johns Hopkins University website.)

Compliance

Compliance (demonstrated by the pressure volume curve) is a measure of the distensibility of the lungs or ease with which the lungs inflate (that is, the reciprocal of elastance). It is measured as the change of volume in the lungs in response to a change in pressure. Normal lung and chest wall compliance is ~1 L per kPa (100 mL per cm H_2O). It can be seen from Figure 11.5 that lung compliance is lowered at high and low lung volumes. Hence it is favourable for the patient to sit on the steeply sloped portion of the curve. (It is easier to inflate a partially opened lung than a collapsed lung.)

11

Frictional forces

The second group of opposing forces encountered in ventilation constitute the frictional forces. Impedance to air movement through the airways is called airways

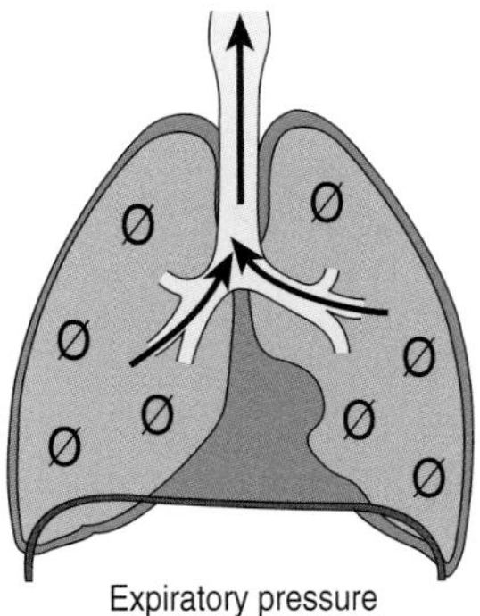

Figure 11.4 Expiratory pressures. (Courtesy of the Johns Hopkins University website.)

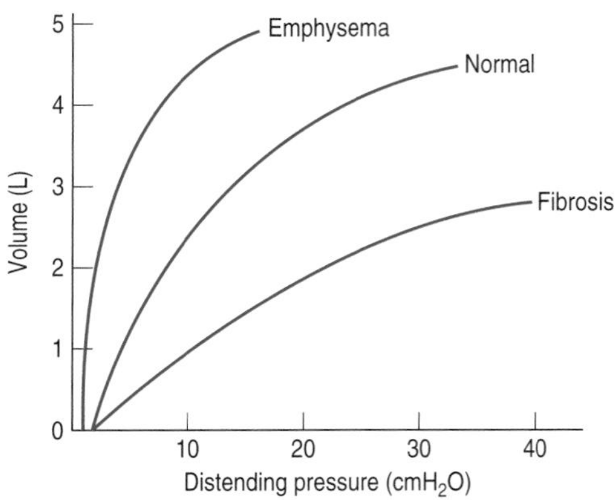

Figure 11.5 Lung compliance curves.

11

resistance. A small but measurable amount of work must be done to maintain the flow. Frictional forces are therefore dependent upon the speed with which air moves through the airway. Resistance is defined as the ratio of the pressure change responsible for air movement and the rate of flow. A normal value for resistance is around 2.5 cm H_2O/L/sec. Factors affecting airways resistance include the size of the airway, its shape and its calibre (Figure 11.5). Different diseases affect such properties, thus altering airway resistance; COPD is the most frequently encountered of these.

With the presence of lung disease, the opposing forces of ventilation are increased. For sufficient lung ventilation, larger patient efforts may be necessary to generate the pressure change needed to overcome the increased elastance or resistance (Figure 11.6). Sustaining large inspiratory efforts may lead to excessive workloads and eventually to respiratory fatigue and failure.

When the work of breathing is excessive because of an increase in the elastic or resistive forces present, respiratory muscle weakness from fatigue may develop.

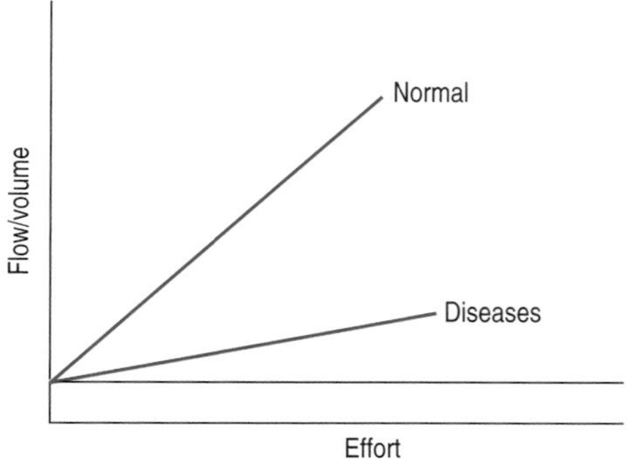

Figure 11.6 The relationship between patient effort and flow/volume.

The strength of the muscles will be inadequate to support normal levels of ventilation and muscle pump effectiveness is diminished, resulting in inadequate ventilation and an increase in $PaCO_2$, which in turn leads to respiratory acidosis. Hypoventilation or respiratory muscle fatigue may also lead to severe hypoxia. Under these conditions, ventilatory support to unload the respiratory muscles and improve ventilation is indicated.

Body positioning, pharmacological management and oxygen therapy are of prime importance to reduce the opposing forces of respiration and maximise ventilation prior to and during the instigation of mechanical support.

RESPIRATORY FAILURE

Respiratory failure occurs when there is an imbalance of ventilatory requirements in relation to neurocardiorespiratory capacity. It is a common medical condition, which occurs when the lungs fail to oxygenate arterial blood adequately (type I respiratory failure) and/or the muscle pump fails to prevent undue CO_2 retention (type II ventilatory failure). While no absolute diagnostic values for arterial PaO_2 and $PaCO_2$ have been defined, values generally quoted are a PaO_2 of less than 8.0 KPa, and a $PaCO_2$ of greater than 6.0 kPa (West 1977).

Arterial blood gas tensions must be measured to make the diagnosis of respiratory failure since many of the accompanying signs and symptoms, such as breathlessness, dyspnoea, cyanosis, agitation and the use of accessory muscles, are not diagnostic of the condition. Oximeters that estimate arterial oxygen saturation (SaO_2), either from the finger or the earlobe, are useful tools for indicating hypoxaemia ($SaO_2 < 90$ per cent), assessing severity and monitoring the patient's condition. Accordingly, all respiratory compromised patients should have oximetry checked. It is important to note, however, that this may be falsely reassuring in the patient receiving supplemental oxygen, since alveolar hypoventilation is not detected. Unconscious patients should therefore have arterial blood gas analysis at initial assessment, to exclude respiratory failure either as a cause or a consequence of neurological depression.

Acute hypoxaemic (type I) respiratory failure (ARF)

This is caused by intrinsic lung disease that interferes with oxygen transfer in the lung. Hypoxaemia results from increased right-to-left shunts (for example, in pneumonia, alveolar collapse, oedema and consolidation) or, more significantly, from ventilation/perfusion ($\dot{V}/\dot{Q}$) mismatch (as in pulmonary parenchymal disease), or from a combination of the two.

Where functional residual capacity (FRC) is reduced, airway closure is present throughout the respiratory cycle since tidal exchange occurs below closing volume. This results in an increased number of underventilated lung units (placing the patient lower down on the compliance curve).

The increased dead space (air in the airways that does not directly contribute to gas exchange) results initially in an increase in total ventilation to maintain a normal $PaCO_2$. This is because in areas of $\dot{V}/\dot{Q}$ inequality, the raised arterial PCO_2 resulting from decreased CO_2 excretion in the underventilated alveoli stimulates the respiratory centre. Relative hyperventilation may ensue in response to severe hypoxaemia with a resultant drop in $PaCO_2$ to below normal range. (The degree of hypoxaemia is restricted by constriction of the blood vessels supplying underventilated alveoli: that is, hypoxic pulmonary vasoconstriction.)

The mechanical disadvantage of a reduced FRC results from the consequential reduction of lung compliance and increased resistance, resulting in a greater work of breathing with a higher metabolic cost. The resultant clinical picture is that of rapid shallow breathing, which in turn further increases both oxygen consumption and carbon dioxide volume for excretion (Table 11.2).

Ventilatory (type II) respiratory failure

This is caused by failure of the respiratory pump (consisting of the respiratory muscles, chest wall, higher centres and nerves), where the amount of CO_2 excreted is less than that produced by metabolism. With respiratory pump failure, even with normal lung pathology, the arterial $PaCO_2$ is raised, with an inevitable fall in alveolar oxygen tension and hypoxaemia (alveolar hypoventilation). Hypoventilation results from a reduced respiratory effort, an inability to overcome resistive ventilatory forces, or an inability to compensate for extra dead space and/or CO_2 production. The respiratory muscle pump is as vital as the heart, failing in the same way and for the same reasons, but a large respiratory reserve is present and function may be markedly impaired without ventilatory failure accompaniment. The resultant clinical picture is summarised in Table 11.3.

Table 11.2 The typical clinical features of type I respiratory failure

- Hypoxia
- Hypocarbia
- Tachypnoea
- Small tidal volumes

Table 11.3 The typical clinical features of absolute type II ventilatory failure

- Hypercarbia
- Hypoxia
- Reduced respiratory rate and/or tidal volumes

Mixed respiratory failure

It is worth noting at this point that a mixed picture of the two types of respiratory failure is frequently seen. While acute hypoxaemic failure may initially present, some cases result in exhaustion. The patient is unable to compensate for the increased dead space, resulting in a raised arterial carbon dioxide tension and mixed respiratory failure. Where individuals are unable to cough effectively or sigh, the risk of alveolar collapse, secretion retention and secondary infection is further increased. Others — for example, unconscious patients or those with bulbar palsy — may be at risk of aspiration, causing further damage to the lungs and further worsening ventilatory function.

11

Pathways to respiratory failure

The causes of respiratory failure are too numerous to detail but can be divided into two major categories:

- a reduction in neuromuscular competence resulting in the inability to generate adequate respiratory muscle force, e.g. reduced central drive, spinal injury, trauma, muscle disease (Figure 11.7)
- an increase in respiratory workload caused by raised ventilatory impedance, e.g. obstructive and restrictive lung defects.

Respiratory muscle dysfunction occurs as a result of various factors (Table 11.4). This can be demonstrated by considering COPD, in which respiratory muscle function is profoundly affected as a result of the increased work of breathing and the increased ventilatory load. The increased work of breathing arises from pathological changes, resulting in raised airway resistance and hyperinflation. At rest, the minute volume of these patients is higher than that of healthy subjects. As a result, the actual cost of breathing in terms of oxygen consumption is markedly increased and the accessory muscles of respiration are recruited.

Hyperinflation also has adverse effects upon the respiratory muscles. The increased lung volumes in COPD are thought to be compensated for by the lowering of the diaphragm or expansion of the rib cage. These changes result in the muscles functioning at a disadvantaged position on the length–tension curve; that is, the diaphragm is at its optimal length for

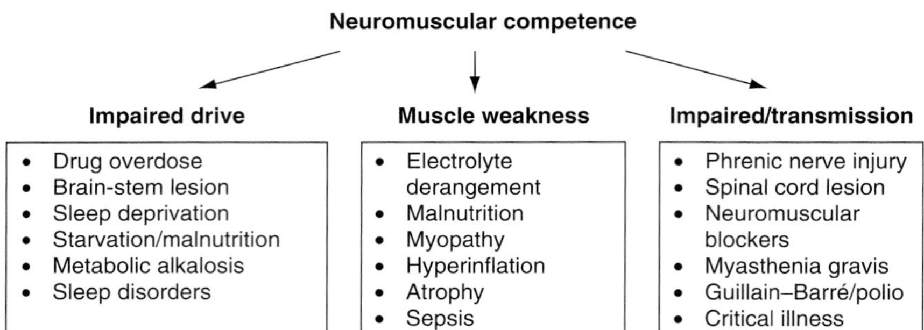

Figure 11.7 Neuromuscular competence.

Table 11.4 Causes of respiratory muscle failure in disease

Obstructive lung diseases
- Upper airflow obstruction (trachea/larynx)
- Generalised disease (asthma/bronchitis/emphysema/cystic fibrosis)

Thoracic restrictive diseases
- Loading (obesity)
- Deformity (pectus/kyphoscoliosis)

Neuromuscular diseases
- Spinal cord (injury/tumour)
- Anterior horn cell (polio)
- Peripheral neuropathy (Guillain–Barré)
- Neuromuscular junction (myasthenia gravis)
- Muscle cell (dystrophies/myopathies)

(Reproduced from Rochester and Arora 1983, with permission.)

providing the maximum contractile force when it is in its resting domed position.

As lung volume increases, the inspiratory muscles shorten and their ability to generate a negative force on inspiration is reduced. Hence the inspiratory effort required to obtain the same tidal volume is greater. A completely flattened diaphragm is incapable of generating any useful pressure and on contraction causes indrawing of the lower rib cage (Hoover's sign), effectively functioning as an expiratory muscle (see PEEPi below).

Respiratory muscle fatigue is an important precursor to respiratory failure. Factors affecting the endurance of the respiratory muscles include energy stores/nutrition, blood substrate concentration, arterial oxygen content, efficiency, mean inspiratory flow, minute ventilation, inspiratory duty cycle, and maximum inspiratory pressure.

When fatigue of the respiratory muscles occurs, rest is indicated rather than exercise. However, a delicate balance between the two must be achieved since there is some evidence that if total rest is applied (through the application of full mechanical ventilation), disuse atrophy may occur, so causing weaning problems.

Increases in both elastic and resistive loads, as present in lung disease, will therefore increase the work of breathing and can lead to respiratory muscle fatigue and weakness, as previously described. When fatigue ensues, hypoventilation will result and weakened muscles will be unable to overcome the opposing forces of respiration to maintain adequate ventilation. Unless ventilatory support is provided to 'unload' the system, respiratory failure results.

The hypoxic drive concept

One of the causes of CO_2 retention in respiratory failure is the use of inappropriate levels of supplemental oxygen. This relates only to a small but important group of patients, in whom the main ventilatory drive is hypoxaemia. Some patients with COPD develop severe hypoxaemia with some CO_2 retention. Due to the degenerative pathological changes within the lungs, this is maintained over long periods of time; while this is not referred to as respiratory failure, an increased work of breathing is usually encountered. Arterial pH is usually at the lower end of the normal range as renal compensation for the raised arterial CO_2 occurs with time and bicarbonate is retained (compensated respiratory acidosis). The cerebrospinal fluid also has a normal pH due to the raised bicarbonate levels, and the main ventilatory drive now arises from the hypoxaemia (despite the raised arterial PCO_2).

The subsequent administration of high inspired oxygen fractions in such cases may pose a potentially lethal clinical scenario, since the hypoxic drive will be abolished while the detrimental effects of the underlying lung condition and increased work of breathing continue. The result is gross respiratory depression with the arterial $PaCO_2$ climbing and arterial blood pH falling to extreme levels if left unnoticed or misinterpreted in the clinical setting.

MECHANICAL VENTILATION

The goals of ventilatory support are clearly defined. They are to:

- improve alveolar ventilation
- decrease the work of breathing
- improve gas exchange.

Mechanical ventilatory support alone will not change the opposing forces of ventilation. The objective of mechanical ventilatory support is to reduce the impact of those forces until the abnormality resolves.

A potted history

Ventilation has a long history of development. There is some descriptive evidence of the artificial ventilation of animals via a reed or cane tube as early as the 1500s (Vesalius 1543). Perhaps the first patient reports date back to the 1700s, when physicians used ironmongers bellows to force air into their patients' lungs. Ventilation truly began in the 1830s, with negative pressure devices being the main ventilatory supports (Woollam 1976; parts 1 and 2). The switch to positive pressure ventilation did not occur until around 1952, when the ability to intubate and tracheostomise patients was established during the polio outbreak of the 1950s. Invasive ventilatory support using positive airway pressure soon became the mainstream treatment, initially using volume-cycled ventilators (Figure 11.8).

Ventilatory support is usually given with the assistance of a mechanical device or ventilator. This can be done in one of two ways:

- invasively, by which the upper airway is bypassed using an endotracheal tube (ETT) or tracheostomy tube
- non-invasively, by which the patient is given ventilatory support via the upper airway (not featured in this chapter) using a mask or similar interface.

In both methods air is mechanically driven through the patient's lungs to assist alveolar ventilation.

Invasive/conventional ventilation

Conventional (invasive) ventilation and the associated methods of cycling have undergone different stages of development. Initially, volume ventilation was the norm, but 'ridged lung' problems were encountered, along with patient and machine asynchrony (hence the expression, 'the patient is fighting the ventilator'). There are two primary methods of cycling used: volume-controlled and pressure-controlled.

Volume-controlled ventilation

This requires a predetermined tidal volume to be delivered to the lungs. A positive pressure is created at the airway, which continues to increase until the specified volume is achieved. Other controls to be set on a volume ventilator include the number of breaths per minute the patient will receive, and the rate of flow at which the volume is delivered to the lungs. A machine delivering a *fixed* rate of flow for a specified time will guarantee a specified tidal volume but is actually *time-cycled*. Where flow-measuring devices are sited at the Y connector, a true volume-cycled machine will compensate for leaks upstream of the connector, where time-cycled will not (Sykes and Young 1996).

Volume ventilation meets the goals of ventilatory support in that it *guarantees* a specified amount of ventilation. This is appropriate today, in the operating theatre setting. The disadvantages of volume-controlled ventilation result from 'setting' (and hence enforcing) the variables of normal breathing: tidal volume (V_t),

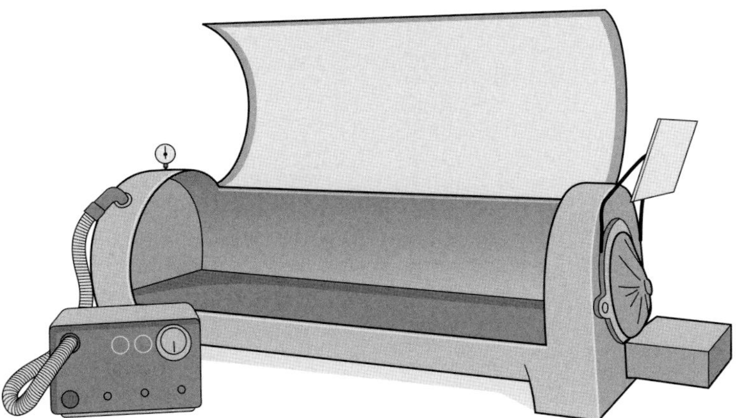

Figure 11.8 Porta lung ventilator. (Courtesy of www.nemc.org/RespCare/portalng.htm.)

respiratory rate (RR) and the I:E ratio (that is, the amount of time spent in inspiration versus expiration). The usual I:E ratio is 1:2, since inspiration is active while expiration is largely passive and thus needs longer time for air to empty from the alveolar units. If expiration is too short, air trapping will occur and intrinsic PEEP (PEEPi) results (thus increasing the risk of lung trauma due to excessive pressure).

With such controlled cycling, the patient must adapt to the ventilator rather than the ventilator adapting to the patient. This may cause dyssynchronisation between machine and patient, sometimes further increasing a patient's work of breathing and indicating the need for sedation with or without drug-induced paralysis until the disease process is resolved. In some instances, the patient may stop interacting with the ventilator. With disuse over time, the respiratory muscles atrophy, and problems may be encountered with weaning through muscle weakness and an inability to endure the requirements of normal resting breathing in an already compromised patient. Ventilating pressures may be high, leading to lung damage, and overventilation may occur if ventilatory requirements are overestimated.

Pressure-controlled ventilation

This is frequently used to guarantee a maximum inflation pressure and reduce the risks of barotrauma (see Complications below). This mode can be used only when a pressure generator delivers increasing pressure throughout inspiration or with a flow generator. Minute ventilation (i.e. respiratory rate (RR) × tidal volume (V_t)) cannot be guaranteed, as with volume-cycled ventilation (Sykes and Young 1996), since a pressure-limited breath is delivered at a set rate. The volume generated is determined by the preset pressure but is also under the influence of the time spent in inspiration, the compliance of the lung and chest wall, and airways resistance. Hence hypoventilation and hypoxaemia may result with inadequate settings. However, the decelerating flow (as airway pressure rises and alveolar volume increases, the rate of flow slows) and maintenance of airway pressure over time are more likely to inflate the more difficult non-compliant lung units.

Ventilation modes

Both volume and pressure control are cycles rather than modes of ventilation. As such, these controlled methods are significantly different to the spontaneous breathing cycle where the inspiratory flow and rate are of the individual's own choosing. In the 1970s and 1980s assisted modes that allowed spontaneous respiratory efforts were introduced, and assist control and synchronised intermittent mandatory ventilation modes were developed for both volume- and pressure-controlled mechanisms. This, in turn, led to the more sophisticated triggering and interactivity microprocessor developments of today's ventilators, resulting in full patient interaction. The ventilator was now becoming an interactive weaning device. However, concern regarding ventilator-induced damage became prevalent throughout the 1990s (Tobin 2001) and protective strategies of alveolar recruitment using PEEP and lower tidal volumes to maintain a higher mean airway pressure and limiting plateau pressure emerged (ARDS Network 2000).

Numerous modes (including dual modes enabling the combination of pressure-limited with volume-guaranteed ventilation) have since been developed with more sophisticated valves and control features: for example, rise time (the speed with which the preset pressure/volume is reached), tube compensation as an automatic feature, and active exhalation valves, to name but a few. The aim of these is to enable improved patient comfort, synchrony and interaction, while allowing greater reductions in the risks of associated ventilatory lung trauma.

Pressure-supported ventilation

In the last 10 years, pressure-supported ventilation (PSV), as opposed to pressure-controlled ventilation (PCV), has become the mode of choice, as it offers better synchrony for the patient and the delivered flow can be more easily changed to suit differing lung and chest wall compliance. In this mode, a preset pressure acts as the limit, while the patient is assisted but remains in control of all respiratory variables. Pressure support serves to reduce the work of breathing in inspiration and results in a larger tidal volume than a spontaneous breath alone, by pushing the patient up the compliance curve. Where FRC is reduced, PEEP/continuous positive airways pressure (CPAP) can also be applied, which serves to restore the resting FRC back to the normal volume.

Advanced pressure modes

- *Airway pressure release ventilation (APRV)* is usually reserved for severe ARDS (where hypoxaemia is a major problem despite a high inspired oxygen fraction), and allows ventilator cycling between two different set CPAP levels (high and low), with the higher level providing the baseline pressure. The pressure is then intermittently 'released' to the lower CPAP level to enable CO_2 elimination.
- *Bilevel ventilation* is the same as APRV but allows spontaneous breathing at either CPAP level, with the spontaneous breaths being supported by either tube compensation or pressure support. The mode is well tolerated and sedation is not usually

necessary. This single mode can be used to provide full support through to the facilitation of weaning.

- *Proportional assisted ventilation (PAV)* is a newer form of ventilation that is fundamentally different from volume and pressure ventilation. In PAV mode, the ventilator generates a pressure change to cause airflow and move volume into the patient's lungs. Unlike conventional ventilation, the pressure is generated in proportion to the patient's own inspiratory efforts. PAV tracks and responds to changes in the patient's breathing pattern/efforts and augments ventilation on a breath-by-breath basis. This means the patient has total control of breathing; the natural effort is simply amplified. The pressure delivered corresponds to changes in elastance, resistance and flow demand.

The complications of mechanical ventilation

Significant pulmonary and non-pulmonary complications may arise at any time as a direct consequence of intubation and mechanical ventilation; some of these are life-threatening. Intubation itself may cause upper airway trauma, loss of teeth, lacerations or trauma (including perforations) to the pharynx, vocal cords or trachea and inadvertent intubation of the oesophagus or right main bronchus. Longer-term intubation may result in sinusitis, necrosis/stenosis of the trachea and glottic oedema. Retained pulmonary secretions are common in the ventilated patient since the cough reflex is impaired, mucociliary transport is reduced and mucus production is increased (Plevak and Ward 1997).

Pulmonary complications

Common pulmonary complications are atelectasis, infection and alveolar overdistension, causing the life-threatening problems of hypotension and barotrauma or volutrauma. The latter is also referred to as atelectrauma.

Atelectasis

This is a common problem in the ventilated individual. Causative factors include aspiration, hypoventilation, mucus plugging and secretion retention. Intubation of the right main bronchus may cause overdistension of the right lung (which may be reflected by high inflation pressures), while the left lung becomes atelectatic. A loss of lung volume, as found with atelectasis and lobar/total lung collapse, will be evident on chest X-ray as a shift towards the affected side with increased opacity and diaphragmatic elevation or tenting.

Aspiration (a particular risk at the time of intubation) is most likely to affect the right lung in the supine position due to the anatomy of the right main bronchus as it branches from the trachea (more vertically than the left). Correct positioning and patency of the endotracheal tube should be checked, along with the auscultation of breath sounds, on a regular basis. The correctly placed tube should be appropriately secured and the weight of the circuit supported to prevent loss of alignment (and subsequent misplacement/accidental extubation, or erosion and trauma) within the trachea.

Ventilator-induced lung injury

This may be divided into barotrauma and volutrauma due to overdistension of the alveolar units.

Barotrauma is the rupture of alveoli, resulting in the tracking of air to the pleura (pneumothorax) or mediastinum (pneumomediastinum). Predisposing risk factors include large tidal volumes and high peak and plateau pressures (in the main/small airways respectively), although predisposing lung pathology may be a better indication of risk. There is usually a gradient between the peak and plateau pressures. However, ventilating pressures below 45 mm Hg and 35 mm Hg respectively are recommended. The I:E ratio is an important consideration in COPD sufferers requiring ventilatory support due to the increased risk of PEEPi development in the presence of increased airways resistance. Manipulation of parameters affecting the I:E ratio may therefore be required, such as increasing the inspiratory flow rate or reducing the ventilatory rate.

Volutrauma (the overdistension of alveoli) has led to the development of lung protection strategies more prevalent today involving the use of lower tidal volumes (6–8 mL/kg). When delivering positive pressure ventilation, air takes the path of least resistance. Thus normal or relatively normal alveoli are ventilated more easily than collapsed or consolidated lung units, and the potential for overdistension (resulting in an increased risk of activating an inflammatory reaction in the normal areas) is established. MacIntyre (2005) emphasises that the forces associated with the repeated opening and closing of alveoli through tidal gas exchanges are linked to worsening inflammatory cascades. In those with acute lung injury or ARDS, protective strategies of PEEP are therefore recommended, with low volumes and a higher plateau airway pressure to avoid such forces, and a speedier wean from ventilation through adherence to respiratory therapy-led weaning protocols (Ely et al. 1998).

In the mechanically ventilated patient, a positive pressure (CPAP/PEEP) may be applied at the end of expiration (Figure 11.9a) in order to recruit the dependent alveoli. In addition to moving the patient on to the more favourable steep portion of the lung compliance

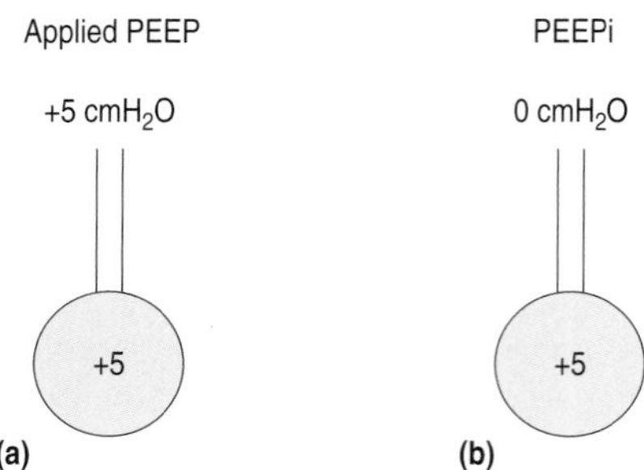

Figure 11.9 Diagram to demonstrate PEEP and PEEPi. (a) Applied PEEP. (b) PEEPi.

(pressure/volume) curve (a mechanically advantageous position for ventilation), this splinting effect on the airway also enables a longer time period for oxygen to diffuse across the alveolar–capillary membrane, thus improving the oxygenation status of the patient.

PEEPi

11

PEEPi (Figure 11.9b) may develop automatically within the airway because of chronic lung diseases, inappropriate settings of applied ventilatory support, or clinical dynamic hyperinflation states such as status asthmaticus, for example. PEEPi occurs when the expiration phase is inadequate in duration for the lung to empty fully prior to the next inspiratory breath (regardless of type). As such, a proportion of each subsequent tidal volume may be retained and, if undetected, result ultimately in barotrauma, volutrauma, hypotension, patient-machine dyssynchrony and even death.

Oxygen toxicity

Oxygen toxicity (due to the production of oxygen free radicals) is associated with higher maintenance levels of inspired oxygen fractions FiO_2 and duration of use. It results in complications such as absorption atelectasis, hypercarbia, tracheobronchitis and diffuse alveolar damage. The lowest level of FiO_2 required is recommended, while maintaining adequate oxygenation, with downward titrations encouraged as soon as possible. The exact level thought to be responsible is as yet unknown, though damage has been reported with maintenance levels of 50 per cent. Again, the application of PEEP may help with the oxygenation status of the individual and the lowering of inspired oxygen fractions, if the pressure is haemodynamically tolerated.

Ventilator-associated pneumonia (VAP)

This life-threatening complication (with reported mortality rates of up to 50 per cent) poses a significant risk and is reported to occur in 13–35 per cent of mechanically ventilated patients. Early-onset pneumonia (within 48–72 hours of intubation) may be due to aspiration at the time of intubation. Most cases are caused by antibiotic-sensitive organisms and flora of the upper airway, such as *Staphylococcus aureus*, *Haemophilus influenzae* and *Streptococcus pneumoniae*. Infections after 72 hours are thought to be caused by antibiotic-resistant pathogens such as *Pseudomonas aeruginosa* (prevalent in percutaneous tracheostomised patients, as shown by Rello et al. 2003) and *Acinetobacter* species. Often precursors to VAP are bacterial colonisation of the aerodigestive tract and aspiration of contaminated secretions into the lower airways (Kollef 2002; Byrd et al. 2006).

VAP should be suspected if there is evidence of pyrexia, radiological changes and purulent pulmonary secretions. Cultures obtained from pulmonary aspirate may not reliably differentiate between pneumonia and tracheal bacterial colonisation. Secretions obtained via fibreoptic bronchoscopy may be useful, but this technique poses the risk of PEEPi development and poor tidal volumes in the ventilated patient (Lawson et al. 2000). (Preparation and ventilatory alterations may be required prior to this procedure; for example, the ETT internal diameter should be at least 2 mm greater than the external diameter of the bronchoscope.) In the longer-term ventilated patient, Baram et al. (2005) found that stable cases with no clinical signs of pneumonia carry a burden of bacteria that is usually greater than the commonly accepted threshold diagnostic of VAP. Georges et al. (2000) also recommend that, in those requiring tracheotomy who show evidence of bronchial colonisation and pyrexia, the procedure should be delayed to prevent the risk of acquiring early VAP.

Predisposing risk factors for acquisition of VAP include surgical procedures (thoracic and upper abdominal), nasogastric tube use, supine position, reintubation, previous antibiotics, chronic lung disease, and use of histamine 2 receptor antagonists and antacids (Celis et al. 1988; Torres et al. 1990). There is recognition that bacterial colonisation of the upper airway may cause contamination of the lower airway, despite the use of a tracheal cuff (Feldman et al. 1999), and that there is usually bacterial colonisation in tracheostomised patients on longer-term ventilatory support (Lusardi et al. 2003).

The literature favours the use of initial broad-spectrum antibiotics until the sensitivities of the causative agents are identified. These will usually be tailored to local organisms and antimicrobial resistance. The aspiration of subglottic secretions is also important in reducing the risk of upper tract colonisation, and vigilant cuff management should be adopted to clear secretions pooling there (Girou et al. 2004). Gastric distension should be avoided and a semi-recumbent position used (Girou et al. 2004) to reduce the risk of aspiration (Orozco-Levi et al. 1995). Avoidance of unnecessary antibiotic administration and rotation of such medication may also be useful in prevention tactics.

Non-pulmonary complications

These include:

- venous thromboembolism (with predisposing risk factors of trauma, immobilisation, obesity, cardiac failure and underlying malignancy) requiring prophylaxis, such as anticoagulation and elastic stockings
- various gastrointestinal problems, as reviewed by Mutlu et al. (2001) (predisposing factors include burns, coagulopathy and head injury) due to stress ulceration, requiring gastric protection strategies
- pressure sores, which may lead to sepsis or osteomyelitis
- neuromuscular weakness and atrophy
- other organ failure.

The cardiovascular system is also inevitably affected in some way by the use of mechanical ventilation. The application of positive pressure ventilation may cause a reduction in preload, stroke volume and cardiac output, which may then reduce renal perfusion and ultimately renal function with fluid accumulation. Maintenance of such positive thoracic pressure can also cause a reduction in the return of blood from the head, resulting in raised intracranial pressure, delirium and agitation, making the already complex multifactorial management even more difficult.

THE ROLE OF THE RESPIRATORY PHYSIOTHERAPIST

The physiotherapist's role in intensive care is considered by many to be an integral part of the overall management of the acutely ill patient, though evidence is scant and varied with further controlled research being required in many areas.

The role is dependent upon many factors, such as country of practice, local requirements, skill mix, knowledge, training, expertise and staffing levels, and varies from unit to unit within the UK. Referral types vary from blanket to consultant only, while treatment interventions range from selected evidence-based methods to prophylaxis intended to minimise the risk of pulmonary complications regardless of the underlying pathophysiology. The more common interventions assumed to be part of the physiotherapist's brief include body positioning, mobilisation, manual hyperinflation and suction, with or without various manual techniques: for example, vibrations, percussion, assisted cough and neuromuscular facilitations to improve lung inflation. Ultimately the aim of physiotherapeutic intervention is to maximise function (motor, ventilatory and psychosocial) and independence for each individual patient. However, it should be remembered that this chapter focuses on respiratory management.

Pulmonary interventions

Interventions should be based upon assessment findings, and must include at least an ability to problem-solve some basic issues with the ventilatory equipment. For example:

- Factors affecting patient machine dyssynchrony (poor coordination of the patient's breathing with the ventilator) (Tobin et al. 2001) and possible corrective measures. An anaesthetist may be required to perform suggested alterations and titrations. Measures aimed at reductions in the work of breathing while on support, if unsuccessful, may also indicate a need for sedation.
- An understanding of ventilator alarms and their significance. For example, low-pressure alarms with reduced tidal volumes are suggestive of a circuit leak.
- Tube displacement and patency, should manual ventilation be difficult.
- With the more advanced clinician, detection or suspicion of PEEPi, through audible wheeze or a prolonged expiration up to delivery of the next breath and a failure of the flow waveform to return to baseline, and so on.

11

In order to do this, a sound knowledge of respiratory mechanics, the background to which has been provided earlier in this chapter, is essential.

If disconnection from the ventilator is required for any reason, the physiotherapist must be able to reinstate ventilatory support safely and to check all mechanical and physiological parameters. This should not be assumed to be the responsibility of the accompanying nurse. Competence with managing the respiratory equipment and monitors (now a legal requirement for all staff involved with their operation) should be gained prior to the first emergency on-call duty.

Suction

Aspiration of pulmonary secretions via the artificial airway is used for secretion clearance only when the patient is unable to do this independently. It should never be used 'routinely' or prophylactically, since research demonstrates undesired effects such as tracheobronchial trauma (Judson and Sahn 1994), hypoxaemia and destabilisation of haemodynamics (Paratz 1992); these may be limited with the use of pre-oxygenation, reassurance and sedation, if required. To avoid unnecessary suction passes, Guglielminotti et al. (2000) explored the bedside detection of retained secretions in the ventilated patient. They recommend that a sawtooth pattern, as seen on the ventilator's flow–volume loop, and/or respiratory sounds over the trachea are good indicators (especially when there is a combined presence) for the need for tracheal suction in the ventilated patient, thus enabling performance of the technique on an 'as-needed' basis.

Positioning

The use of specific body positioning in the intensive care unit is aimed at:

- Optimising oxygen transport via improving ventilation/perfusion ($\dot{V}/\dot{Q}$) matching (e.g. prone positioning in early ARDS).
- Promoting mucociliary clearance (e.g. postural drainage).
- Improving aeration through increased lung volumes (e.g. side-lying with the affected lung uppermost; Stiller et al. 1996).
- Reducing the work of breathing (Dean and Ross 1992; Paratz 1992; Dean 1994). (Upright positioning is required for weaning non-tetraplegic patients since respiratory mechanics are severely altered in the cervical and upper thoracic spinal cord-damaged patient.)

As previously mentioned, the use of a 45° head-up tilt will serve to prevent the risk of gastric reflux and subsequent aspiration, thus contributing significantly to the prevention of VAP.

Manual hyperinflation (MHI)

Definition

Manual hyperinflation is 'a technique that uses a manual bag circuit to deliver a breath of 1.5 times greater than that being delivered by the ventilator, where the ventilator is recording a tidal volume of up to 700 mL' (Clapham et al. 1995; McCarren and Chow 1998).

While evidence is inconsistent concerning the efficacy of this technique (due to variables in studies), it is thought to be particularly useful in reinflating atelectatic areas of lung, thus improving pulmonary compliance (Jones et al. 1992; Clarke et al. 1999) and providing a more efficient breathing pattern. It also facilitates the clearance of troublesome pulmonary secretions when used in combination with other techniques. MHI (which has still not been overtly described due to the many variations in technique used) requires the patient to be disconnected from the ventilator and attached to a manual Mapleson C-type circuit for the purpose of hyperventilating the lungs in order to reinflate atelectatic lung units (via the collateral ventilatory channels). The potential to both hypoventilate and overdistend the lungs exists with this modality, and it is recommended that a simple pressure gauge be used in circuit to minimise the risk of barotrauma (Figure 11.10). A slow deep inspiration should be performed, ensuring that the pressure does not exceed 40–50 cm H_2O (Denehy 1999).

In addition to the advantages of this intervention, rises in intracranial pressure and significant drops in blood pressure have been reported, while the actual tidal volume delivered, airway pressure, amount of PEEP applied, flow rates and *Fi*O2 appear to be very variable (Jones et al. 1992; Denehy 1999; McCarren and Chow (1996, 1998); Glass et al. 1993).

The technique used should ensure that the weight of the tubing and valve is supported to avoid tracheal tube displacement throughout the episode of intervention, and should ideally be performed using a two-handed technique (especially if the hands are small, as the operator may struggle to deliver adequate tidal volume); the hand should be rotated at the reverse of the bag, at a rate that matches the baseline minute ventilation of the patient (Clapham et al. 1995). Observe the chest and listen to feedback from the therapist performing the chest wall vibrations to gauge the lung expansion obtained. The peak inflation volume is held for a couple of seconds to obtain a plateau, and then if utilised, vibrations are begun. Release the bag to allow rapid expiration. Stop the manual vibrations midway through the expiration phase to avoid collapsing the airways down beyond FRC. However, full expiration must occur prior to the next manual hyperinflation, in order to prevent PEEPi development. Repeat manual hyperinflations five to six times and then deliver a submaximal tidal volume for six breaths, before repeating the cycle (as clinically indicated). Baseline parameters should be monitored throughout the process and changes noted. Sudden alterations to the cardiovascular stability of the patient should result in discontinuation of the process and the effects should be documented. Recovery time and any adverse effects should be noted.

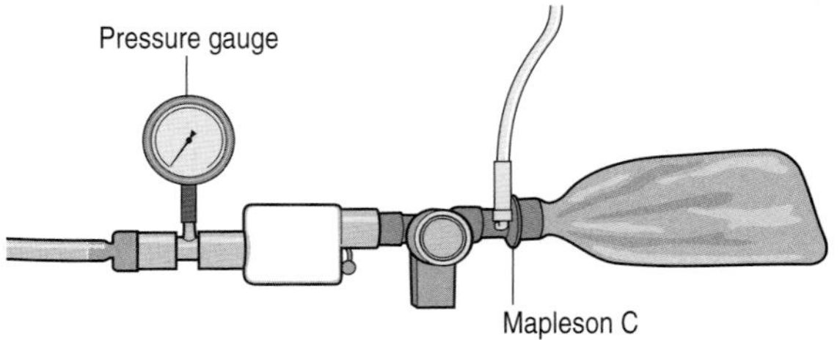

Figure 11.10 Diagram to show integration of a simple pressure gauge in a circuit.

On completion of the intervention (or as indicated, according to physiological status), the patient should be returned to the pre-intervention ventilation regime and observed for cardiorespiratory stability. Outcomes of treatment and the future plan should be clearly recorded.

Key point

Synchronisation (through the use of effective communication skills) between the two operators (i.e. the person bagging and the person performing chest clearance), with the conscious spontaneously breathing patient, is essential to the success of this procedure.

The clearance of oropharyngeal secretions should be undertaken on a daily basis to remove stagnant pooled secretions from the cuff region. It is most effectively done with continuous manual pressurisation of the lower airway to expel secretions as soon as the cuff is deflated to avoid bacterial contamination of the lower respiratory tract. Upon cuff reinflation, the cuff volumes used should be in accordance with findings from occasional cuff pressure checks to avoid tracheal pressure damage, and the volume of air required to seal the cuff adequately should be documented.

Manual techniques

Manual techniques are often used in conjunction with MHI, such as shaking and vibrations to facilitate mucus clearance (Denehy 1999). Few well-designed studies have been performed in this specific area and a more recent animal study (Unoki et al. 2005) is inappropriately misleading in its recommendations regarding the use of external rib cage compression in the ventilated patient. However, care should be taken to ensure that compressions to the chest wall are terminated at mid-expiratory lung volumes to avoid collapsing the airways and reducing FRC.

Percussion appears to have no place in the ventilated patient. It has been shown to have detrimental effects, such as arrhythmias and reduced lung compliance in the critically ill individual (Hammon et al. 1992; Jones et al. 1992 respectively), while the use of vibrations in the intensive care unit to facilitate re-aeration of atelectatic areas is not supported radiographically (Stiller et al. 1996).

Other considerations

While some aspects and combinations of physiotherapy interventions have been considered in light of available evidence (which is somewhat limited in the ventilated patient), other inputs may also form part of the respiratory therapist's role, such as leading on protocols for weaning (the transfer of the work of breathing from the ventilator back to the patient), as recommended by the American task force in 2002. As mentioned previously, faster weaning episodes may be expected with the implementation of respiratory therapy-led protocols (Ely et al. 1998; Marelich et al. 2000; MacIntyre et al. 2001).

The evidence for the role of limb movements, muscle training and mobilisation in the ventilated patient is scarce (if it exists at all). Due to the propensity for adverse effects on both the pulmonary and haemodynamic status of the critically ill patient as a potential complication of various interventions, the therapist's ability to assess and assimilate clinical findings is imperative. Treatment interventions should be tailored to clinical findings at each visit. The need for further research in this area is obvious, particularly in this rapidly changing environment with an increasing blurring of the traditional professional boundaries and development of posts such as consultant therapist, physician and anaesthetic assistant practitioner, enabling an even greater level of autonomy.

FURTHER READING

American Association for Respiratory Care (AARC) Clinical Practice Guidelines (various): www.rcjournal.com/online_resources/cpgs/cpg_index.asp

Heffner JE 2005 Review series. Organization of care for people on long-term artificial ventilation: management of the chronically ventilated patient with a tracheostomy. Chron Respir Dis 2: 151–161: www.CRDjournal.com

Hinds CJ, Watson JD 1995 Intensive Care: A Concise Textbook, 2nd edn. WB Saunders: Philadelphia

MacIntyre NR, Epstein SK, Carson S et al. 2005 Consensus Statement: Management of Patients Requiring Prolonged Mechanical Ventilation. Report of an NAMDRC Consensus Conference. Chest 128(6): 3937–3954

Seaton A, Leitch AG, Seaton D 2000 Crofton and Douglas's Respiratory Diseases, 5th edn. Blackwell: Oxford

Task Force 2002 Evidence-based guidelines for weaning and discontinuing ventilatory support. Respir Care 47(1): 69–90

Tobin MJ 1988 Respiratory muscles in disease. Clin Chest Med 9(2): 263–286

Tobin MJ, Jubran A, Laghi F 2001 Patient–ventilator interaction. Am J Respir Crit Care Med 163(5): 1059–1063

Young D, Adams AP 1999 Respiratory Support in Intensive Care, 2nd edn. BMJ: London

REFERENCES

ARDS Network 2000 Ventilation with lower tidal volumes as compared with traditional tidal volumes for lung injury and the acute respiratory distress syndrome. N Engl J Med 342: 1301–1308

Baram D, Hulse G, Palmer LB 2005 Stable patients receiving prolonged mechanical ventilation have a higher alveolar burden of bacteria. Chest 127(4): 1353–1357

Byrd RP Jnr, Eggleston KL, Takubo T, Roy TM 2006 Mechanical Ventilation: www.emedicine.com/med/topic3370.htm

Celis R, Torres A, Gatell J et al. 1988 Nosocomial pneumonia: A multivariate analysis of risk and prognosis. Chest 93: 318–324

Clapham L, Harrison J, Raybould T 1995 A multi-disciplinary audit of manual hyperinflation technique (sigh breath) in neurosurgical intensive care unit. Intensive and Crit Care Nursing 11(5): 265–271

Clarke RCN, Kelly BE et al. 1999 Ventilatory characteristics in mechanically ventilated patients during manual hyperinflation for chest physiotherapy. Anaesthesia 54: 936–940

Dean E 1994 Oxygen transport: A physiologically based conceptual framework for the practice of cardiopulmonary physiotherapy. Physiotherapy 80: 347–355

Dean E, Ross J 1992 Discordance between cardiopulmonary physiology and physical therapy: toward a rational basis for practice. Chest 101: 1694–1698

Denehy L 1999 The use of manual hyperinflation in airway clearance. Eur Resp J 14: 958–965

Ely EW, Baker AM, Dunagan DP et al. 1998 Effect on the duration of mechanical ventilation of identifying patients capable of breathing spontaneously. N Engl J Med 335 (25): 1864–1869

Feldman A, Kassel M, Cantrell J et al. 1999 The presence and sequence of endotracheal tube colonization in patients undergoing mechanical ventilation. Eur Resp J 13: 546–551

Georges H, Leroy O, Alfandari S, Beaucaire G 2000 Predisposing factors for nosocomial pneumonia in patients receiving mechanical ventilation and requiring tracheotomy. Chest 118(3): 767–774

Girou E, Buu-Hoi A, Stephan F et al. 2004 Airway colonisation in long-term mechanically ventilated patients: Effect of semi-recumbent position and continuous subglottic suctioning. Intensive Care Med 30: 225–233

Glass C, Grap MJ, Corely MC, Wallace Dd 1993 Nurses' ability to achieve hyperinflation with a manual resuscitation bag during endotracheal suctioning. Heart Lung 22: 158–165

Guglielminotti J, Alzieu M, Maury E et al. 2000 Bedside detection of retained tracheobronchial secretions in patients receiving mechanical ventilation. Chest 118(4): 1095–1099

Hammon WE, Connors AF, McCaffree DR 1992 Cardiac arrhythmias during postural drainage and chest percussion of critically ill patients. Chest 102: 1836–1841

Johnson MA, Polgar J, Weightman D 1973 Data on the distribution of fibre types in 31 human muscles: an autopsy study. J Neurol Sci 18: 111–129

Jones AYM, Hutchinson RC, Oh TE 1992 Effects of bagging and percussion on static lung compliance of the respiratory system. Physiotherapy 78: 661–666

Judson MA, Sahn MA 1994 Mobilisation of secretions in ICU patients. Resp Care 39: 213–226

Kollef M 2002 Respiratory Failure: Complications of Mechanical Ventilation. ACP Medicine. Online: www.medscape.com/viewarticle/534431_print

Lawson RW, Peters JI, Shelledy DC 2000 Effects of fibreoptic bronchoscopy during mechanical ventilation in a lung model. Chest 118: 824–831

Lusardi M, Capelli A, De Stephano A et al. 2003 Lower respiratory tract infections in chronic obstructive pulmonary disease outpatients with tracheostomy and persistent colonization by *P. aeruginosa*. Respir Med 97: 1205–1210

MacIntyre NR 2005 Current issues in mechanical ventilation for respiratory failure. Chest 128(5): 561S–567S

MacIntyre NR, Cook DJ, Ely Jr EW et al. 2001 Evidence-based guidelines for weaning and discontinuing ventilatory support: A collective taskforce facilitated by the American College of Chest Physicians, the American Association for Respiratory Care and the American College of Critical Care Medicine. Chest 120 (Suppl): 375S–395S

Marelich GP, Murin S, Battistella F et al. 2000 Protocol weaning off mechanical ventilation in medical and surgical patients by respiratory care practitioners and nurses: Effect on weaning time and incidence of ventilator-associated pneumonia. Chest 118: 459–467

McCarren B, Chow CM 1996 Manual hyperinflation: A description of the technique. Aust J Physiother 42: 203–208

McCarren B, Chow CM 1998 Description of manual hyperinflation in intubated patients with atelectasis. Physiother Theory Pract 14(4): 199–210

Moffett D, Moffett S, Schauf C (eds) 1993 Human Physiology, 2nd edn. Mosby: St Louis, MO

Mutlu G, Mutlu EA, Factor P 2001 GI complications in patients receiving mechanical ventilation. Chest 119(4): 1222–1241

Orozco-Levi M, Torres A, Ferrer M et al. 1995 Semirecumbent position protects from pulmonary aspiration but not completely from gastroesophageal reflux in mechanically ventilated patients. Am J Respir Crit Care med 152: 1387–1390

Paratz J 1992 Haemodynamic stability of the ventilated intensive care patient: a review. Aust J Physiother 38: 167–172

Plevak DJ, Ward JJ 1997 Airway management. In: Burton GG, Hodgkin JE, Ward JJ (eds) Respiratory Care: A Guide to Clinical Practice, 4th edn. Lipponcott: Philadelphia, PA, pp. 555—609

Rello J, Lorente C, Diaz E et al. 2003 Incidence etiology and outcome of nosocomial pneumonia in ICU patients requiring percutaneous tracheostomy for mechanical ventilation. Chest 124(6): 2239–2243

Rochester DR, Arora NS 1983 Respiratory muscle failure. Med Clin North Am 67(3): 573–597

Stiller K, Jenkins S et al. 1996 Acute lobar atelectasis: A comparison of five physiotherapy regimens. Physiother Theory and Pract 12: 197–209

Tobin MJ 2001 Advances in mechanical ventilation. N Engl J Med 344: 1986–1996

Tobin MJ, Jubran A, Laghi F 2001 Patient–ventilator interaction. Am J Respir Crit Care Med 163(5): 1059–1063

Torres A, Aznar R, Gatell JM et al. 1990 Incidence, risk and prognosis factors of nosocomial pneumonia in mechanically ventilated patients. Am Rev Resp Dis 142: 523–538

Unoki T, Kawasaki Y, Mizutami T et al. 2005 Effects of expiratory rib-cage compression on oxygenation, ventilation, and airway secretion removal in patients receiving mechanical ventilation. Resp Care 50(11): 1430–1437

Vesalius A 1543 De Humani Corporis Fabrica Libri Septem.

West JB 1977 Pulmonary Pathophysiology: The Essentials. Williams & Wilkins: Baltimore

Woollam CHM 1976 The development of apparatus for intermittent negative pressure respiration. Anaesthesia 31 (4): 537–547

Chapter **12**

Cardiac and pulmonary rehabilitation

Sushma Sanghvi

CHAPTER CONTENTS

CARDIAC REHABILITATION

Physiotherapists are crucial members of the multidisciplinary cardiac rehabilitation team. This chapter provides key information about research evidence, exercise prescription and planning across the four phases of cardiac rehabilitation. For in-depth information about planning and delivering exercise rehabilitation in special conditions such as in heart failure, with the use of implanted cardioverter-defibrillators (ICDs) and after cardiac transplantation, the reader is advised to refer to the guidelines and texts listed at the end of the chapter.

BACKGROUND

According to the WHO (2007), an estimated 17 million people die of cardiovascular disease (CVD) every year; 7.2 million of these die of coronary heart disease (CHD) and 5.5 million of stroke. CVD is responsible for 10 per cent of the disability-adjusted life-years (DALYs) lost in low- and middle-income countries and 18 per cent in high-income countries. (DALY is defined as the sum of years lost because of premature mortality and years of life lived with disability, adjusted for disability.)

According to British Heart Foundation statistical data (2006), CHD causes over 105 000 deaths in the UK every year. It is also the most common cause of premature death in the UK: 21 per cent in men and 12 per cent in women. Nearly all deaths from CHD are due to myocardial infarction (heart attack). Around 230 000 people in the UK have a myocardial infarction every year. Almost 2 million people in the UK suffer with angina, the most common form of CHD; 675 000 have definite heart failure and these numbers are rising.

There remain huge variations in death rates across the country. Deaths from CHD are highest in Scotland and the North of England. Heart disease is more common in deprived areas and unskilled workers have nearly three times the rate of CHD as skilled workers. South Asians (Indians, Bangladeshis, Pakistanis and Sri Lankans) living in the UK have a higher premature death rate from CHD than average: 50 per cent higher in both men and women. The difference in death rates between South Asians and the rest of the population is increasing.

The government is committed to reducing deaths from CVD by at least 40 per cent by 2010. The overall burden of CVD is now far greater due to more people surviving cardiac illnesses and living much longer than before. Since the introduction of the National Service Framework for CHD, there have been significant improvements in NHS treatment across the UK.

While genetic factors play a part, 80–90 per cent of people dying of CHD have one or more major risk factors influenced by lifestyle. Lack of physical activity, obesity, smoking and diabetes are major risk factors for CHD.

Many people find that making significant lifestyle changes can be difficult; for example, some may be addicted to nicotine. If patients have recently been admitted to hospital with CHD and subsequently need to increase the amount of regular physical activity they undertake, not only do they need to be well motivated; they and their families also need to be confident that exercise is safe.

Like all major illnesses, CHD has a major physical, psychological and behavioural impact on patients and their families. For some, the psychological consequences can be persistent and disabling, and can constitute a barrier to making the lifestyle changes necessary to reduce the subsequent cardiac risk. For example, people with CHD can be afraid to take exercise or participate fully in their daily activities for fear of damaging their heart. After admission to hospital, maybe following a myocardial infarction or for coronary revascularisation, the advice and treatment provision in primary care may not always be sufficient. Many people require more intensive help to understand their illness and its treatment in order to attain the lifestyle changes required and to regain their confidence so that they can enjoy the best possible physical, mental and emotional health and return to as full a normal life as possible.

12

WHAT IS CARDIAC REHABILITATION?

Definition

The rehabilitation of cardiac patients is the sum of activities required to influence favourably the underlying cause of the disease, as well as the best possible physical, mental and social conditions, so that they may, by their own efforts, preserve or resume when lost, as normal a place as possible in the community. Rehabilitation cannot be regarded as an isolated form of therapy, but must be integrated with the whole treatment, of which it forms only one facet. (WHO 1993)

Cardiac rehabilitation is the process by which patients with cardiac disease, in partnership with a multidisciplinary team of health professionals, are encouraged and supported to achieve and maintain optimal physical and psychosocial health (SIGN 2002).

Cardiac rehabilitation is a comprehensive intervention that offers education, exercise and psychosocial support for patients with CHD and their families, and is delivered by many specialist health professionals. It can promote recovery, enable patients to achieve and maintain better health and reduce the risk of death in people who have heart disease.

RESEARCH EVIDENCE FOR CARDIAC REHABILITATION

When provision is good, offering comprehensive and tailored help with lifestyle modification involving exercise training, education and psychological input, cardiac rehabilitation can make a substantial difference by reducing mortality by as much as 20–25 per cent over 3 years.

The Cochrane Review 2004 (Jolliffe et al. 2004) (Table 12.1) established the importance of exercise-based cardiac rehabilitation. Cardiac mortality was reduced by 31 per cent in the exercise-only cardiac rehabilitation and by 26 per cent in comprehensive cardiac rehabilitation groups.

Research has been focused around phase III of rehabilitation and in patients after MI and revascularisation. Many studies still include only low-risk, male, Caucasian, middle-aged MI patients and enroll only a small number of women, the elderly and ethnic minorities. Other cardiac patient groups, such as those who have had cardiac surgery, heart failure or heart transplantation, are excluded, thereby limiting the generalisability of the findings.

Evidence for physical activity and exercise

Physical activity levels are low in the UK. The Health Survey for England data (NHS 1998) show that only 37 per cent of men and 24 per cent of women meet the government guidelines of 30 minutes of moderate physical activity five or more times a week. The WHO estimates that around 3 per cent of all disease burden in developed countries is caused by physical inactivity, and up to 24 per cent of CHD is due to levels of physical activity below 2.5 hours of moderate-intensity activity per week. It is estimated that approximately 36 per cent of deaths from CHD in men and 38 per cent of deaths in women are due to lack of physical activity. Therefore structured exercise as a therapeutic intervention is essential to the cardiac rehabilitation programme.

Table 12.1 Cochrane Review 2004*

Exercise-only rehabilitation	27% reduction in all causes of mortality 31% reduction in cardiac mortality
Comprehensive rehabilitation	13% reduction in all causes of mortality 26% reduction cardiac mortality

*8440 patient meta-analyses (myocardial infarction, revascularisation, ischaemic heart disease).

Evidence for education and psychosocial interventions

Psychological outcomes have been less well studied than the physical and functional effects of exercise training so are less well documented. It is likely that many of the psychological benefits are attributable to group activities, peer support and access to professional advice. It is difficult to measure outcomes for these interventions. Questionnaires have been widely used to measure quality of life and health status. Both generic (for example, Short Form 36, or SF36) and disease-specific (for example, Quality of Life after MI, or QLMI) questionnaires have been used. Short-term benefits have been observed in studies using disease-specific questionnaires.

PATIENT GROUPS IN CARDIAC REHABILITATION

Typically, patients who have had an acute MI or coronary artery bypass graft (CABG) surgery have been referred for cardiac rehabilitation in the past. The National Service Framework recommends that cardiac rehabilitation should be available to people manifesting CHD in various forms. Many more groups are now included in both comprehensive and exercise-based rehabilitation.

Post-revascularisation

The number of patients receiving percutaneous transluminous coronary angioplasty (PTCA) and stenting is increasing. Education for lifestyle modification and exercise training is proven to be beneficial as regards physiological and psychosocial risk factors.

Stable angina

Cardiac rehabilitation improves management of symptoms and exercise training assists in raising the angina threshold so that patients are able to do more before they experience angina.

Chronic heart failure

With advances in the management of CHD, the number of patients presenting with chronic heart failure is increasing. Exercise-based cardiac rehabilitation is beneficial in improving exercise capacity, reducing symptoms and improving quality of life, and patients with mild to moderate heart failure show the biggest improvements.

Special needs groups

An important drawback in most research is the lack of data relating to female and elderly patients; patients' ethnic background is also rarely reported. These under-represented groups need special attention.

Women

The incidence of CHD is rising in women. According to British Heart Foundation statistics (2006), every year in the UK 26 000 women under 74 have an MI. Uptake of cardiac rehabilitation among women is low. When women attend cardiac rehabilitation programmes, the outcomes are as good as or better than for men. Their need may be greater, as they suffer more severe loss of function in relation to return to work, activity and sexuality, and also experience high levels of anxiety and depression. More gender-specific information, individualised and flexible programmes, and suitable environments are required to address the specific needs of this group.

Older adults

Over half of all MIs occur in people over 70 years of age and this figure is set to rise further as the number of older people in the total population increases. Disability rates are very high in these patient populations, particularly in women and those with angina or chronic heart failure. The presence of depression is also a determinant of poor physical functioning. Cardiac rehabilitation has been demonstrated to be safe and to improve aerobic capacity and muscle strength in older adults. Elderly people can derive similar benefits from a comprehensive menu-based cardiac rehabilitation programme. Issues of access, transport, timings and flexible programmes need to be addressed to meet the requirement of this patient population.

Ethnic groups

The incidence of CHD is much higher in some ethnic communities, such as South Asians. It has been suggested that people from ethnic minorities are less likely to be referred to and to join cardiac rehabilitation programmes. Whilst planning rehabilitation strategies for ethnic groups, their heterogeneity, cultural background and linguistic needs must be acknowledged. When a behavioural change is required, it is crucial that the message is clearly understood. Professional knowledge of cultural influences on physical activity and dietary practices would be beneficial to the patient. Similarly, awareness of existing health education material in appropriate languages can enhance the quality of service. It is also helpful to involve health professionals from similar a cultural background, in order to develop and evaluate progress.

A variety of settings appropriate to the targeted communities can be used: for example, community centres, temples, mosques, churches, health centres and so on. Involvement of the family and younger generation is vital.

Other groups

For the following groups individualised assessment and risk stratification are essential.

Cardiac transplant

This group is relatively small. There is some evidence that exercise-based cardiac rehabilitation improves exercise tolerance in this group of patients.

Valve surgery

Supervised exercise training in comprehensive cardiac rehabilitation is beneficial in improving functional capacity, reducing symptoms and improving quality of life.

Congenital heart disease

This group includes young people and children. Supervised exercises improve exercise capacity and psychological function in this patient population.

Implanted cardioverter-defibrillator

The number of patients with an ICD in a cardiac rehabilitation programme may be small, and yet comprehensive cardiac rehabilitation is safe and significantly improves exercise ability and psychological well-being.

PROVISION IN THE UK AND ITS COST-EFFECTIVENESS

The overall level of provision of cardiac rehabilitation programmes in the UK has increased rapidly in the last 20 years. Current data from the British Association of Cardiac Rehabilitation reveal the number of programmes to be 300. The National Service Framework for CHD (2000) has advocated the use of disease registers in primary care to provide long-term follow-up of patients, and has set standards and milestones for secondary prevention.

There are huge variations in programme types, duration, frequency and intensity of exercise training. Many centres are delivering the service in primary care and menu-based programmes are provided by multidisciplinary teams.

One UK estimate suggests a cost of £6900 per quality-adjusted life-years (QALY) and a cost per life-year gained of £15 700 at 3 years from cardiac rehabilitation. This offers good value compared with many other treatments currently provided by the NHS.

COMPONENTS OF CARDIAC REHABILITATION

- Risk factor assessment and modification.
- Education.
- Exercise.
- Psychosocial support.

Operation and delivery

It transpires that cardiac rehabilitation is really a continuum of care from the time the patient is admitted till discharge; it extends to outpatient care, as well as to long-term follow-up in the community. Patient care, of which cardiac rehabilitation forms an essential part, is shared with the cardiology team. Cardiology management includes patient assessment and risk stratification (predicting the likelihood of recurrence of cardiac events and disease prognosis). The patient also undergoes diagnostic tests, is prescribed drug therapy, and may need some form of revascularisation such as angioplasty or a bypass grafting, as appropriate.

Traditionally, cardiac rehabilitation is divided into four phases, progressing from the acute hospital admission stage to long-term maintenance of lifestyle changes:

- Phase I: Inpatient period
- Phase II: Early post-discharge period
- Phase III: Supervised outpatient programme, including structured exercise
- Phase IV: Long-term follow-up/maintenance in primary care.

Phase I: Inpatient period

Cardiac rehabilitation is offered as soon as it is practical as an integral part of care to someone who is admitted (or planned to be admitted) to hospital with CHD. It includes:

- assessment of physical, psychological and social needs
- negotiation of a written informal plan for meeting these identified needs
- initial advice on lifestyle: for example, smoking cessation, physical activity (including sexual activity), diet, alcohol consumption and employment
- mobilisation
- education about prescribed medication, its benefits and possible side-effects
- involvement of the relevant informal carer
- provision of locally written information about cardiac rehabilitation
- discharge planning.

Phase II: Early post-discharge period

This service shows variation from region to region and can range from as little as a telephone helpline to group sessions or individual appointments (Figure 12.1). The National Service Framework recommendation includes:

- comprehensive assessment of cardiac risk, including physical, psychological and social needs for cardiac rehabilitation and a review of the initial plan to meet these needs
- provision of lifestyle advice and psychological interventions according to the agreed plan by the multidisciplinary team
- continuing involvement of the relevant informal carer
- home visits, if appropriate.

Phase III: Supervised outpatient programme, including structured exercise

Traditionally, this phase has been well set up in the form of outpatient hospital-based programmes, although

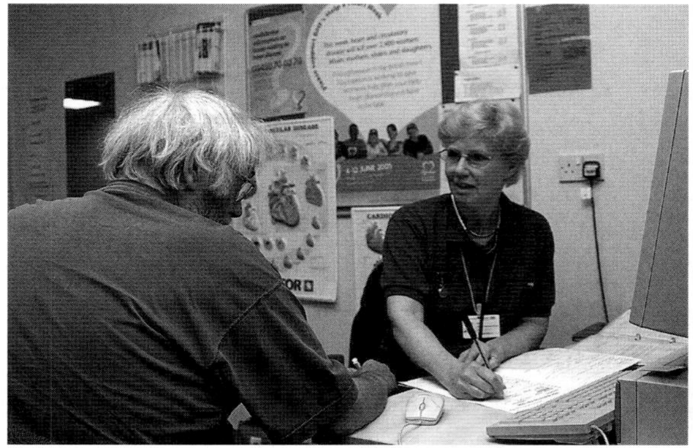

(a)

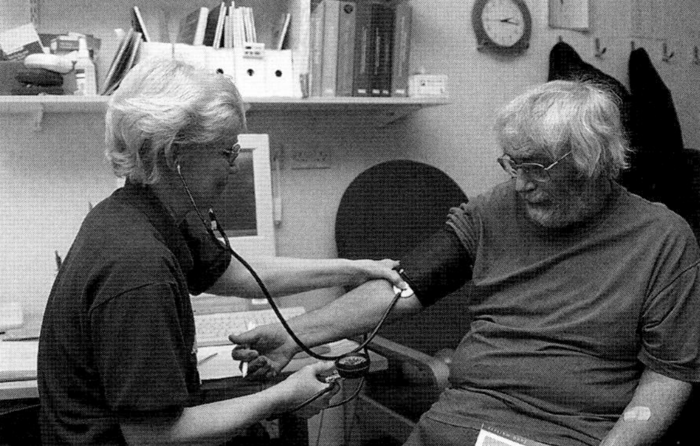

(b)

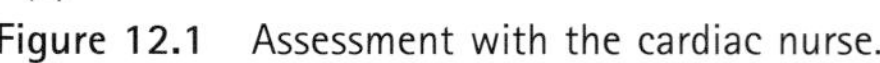

Figure 12.1 Assessment with the cardiac nurse.

more services have now been shifted into primary care. It includes:

- risk stratification and identification of the high-, medium- and low-risk patient for exercise
- individualised progressive exercise prescription and supervised exercise sessions, which vary from 4 to 12 weeks in different regions
- re-evaluation of risk factors for CHD and health promotion advice and education (Figure 12.2)
- psychosocial interventions, such as stress management, counselling and vocational guidance.

Phase IV: Long-term follow-up/maintenance in primary care

This phase is now well established in many districts, with an emphasis on provision of exercise sessions in community or leisure centres. Specialist training to exercise CHD patients in the community is available to exercise instructors from the British Association of Cardiac Rehabilitation (BACR). Phase IV includes:

- long-term maintenance of individual goals
- professional monitoring of clinical status and follow-up of general progress
- ongoing psychosocial support and support groups.

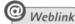

Weblink

British Association of Cardiac Rehabilitation (BACR): www.bcs.com/bacr.

Cardiac rehabilitation team

The cardiac rehabilitation package individualised for each patient requires the expertise and skills of a multidisciplinary collaborative team of professionals (Figure 12.3). This team includes a cardiologist and staff from nursing,

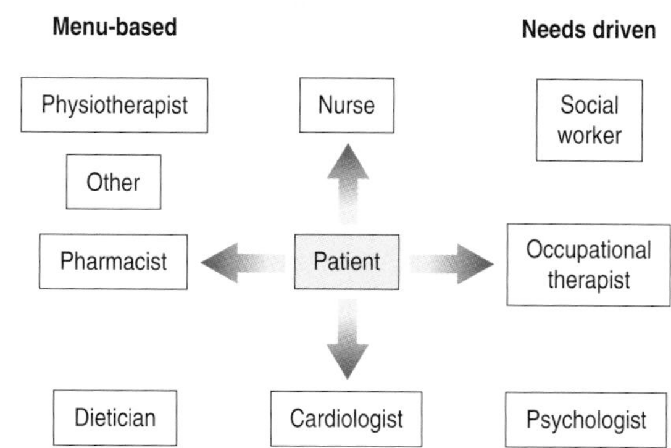

Figure 12.3 The cardiac rehabilitation team.

physiotherapy, dietetics, pharmacy, occupational therapy and psychology who have training in cardiac rehabilitation. Continuation of care in the community involves the primary healthcare team: that is, the GP and cardiac nurse, phase IV exercise specialist and a link person from the local cardiac patient support group.

The role of the physiotherapist

Physiotherapists have the knowledge, assessment skills and clinical reasoning, combined with an evidence-based approach to treatment, to undertake the rehabilitation management of patients with multi-pathology problems. Physiotherapists are also trained to run group sessions and classes. Hence the role of the physiotherapist within the multidisciplinary team should focus on exercise prescription, training and education in phases I–III. Any modification in exercise prescription needs to be discussed with medical and nursing team members. In a group setting where exercise is delivered to CHD patients, teamwork and proper liaison with other team members who are aware of patients' clinical and psychosocial issues are essential.

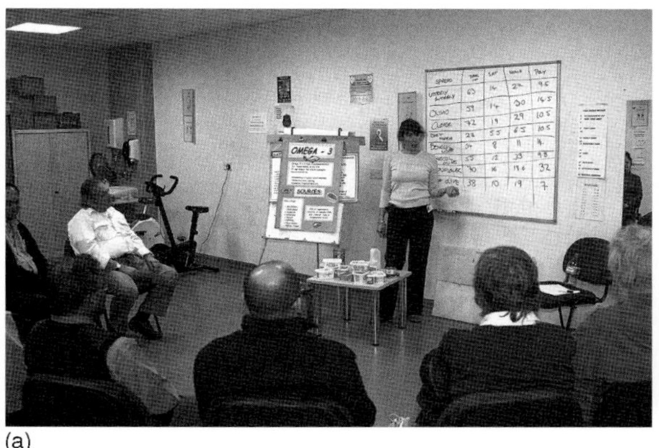

(a)

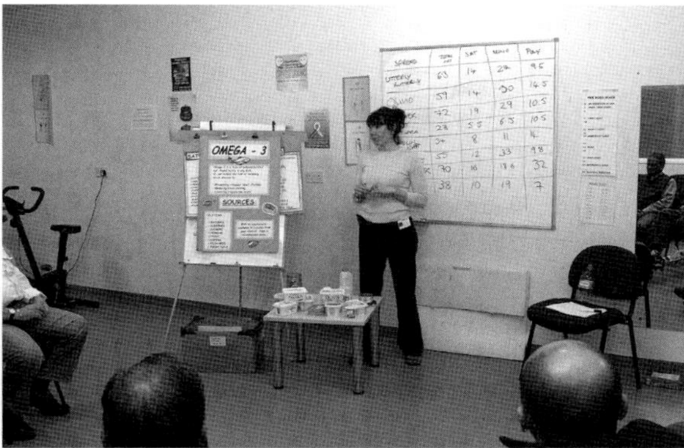

(b)

Figure 12.2 Dietician addressing a group of patients attending a phase III cardiac rehabilitation programme.

Professional development

The Association of Chartered Physiotherapists in Cardiac Rehabilitation (ACPICR) recommends that physiotherapists wishing to specialise in this area should refer to the Skills for Health: Coronary Heart Disease document and consider undertaking professional development in exercise physiology and exercise prescription in cardiovascular disease. Use of clinical and cardiac networks to share experiences – for example, InteractiveCSP (www.csp.org.uk) – is recommended.

BENEFITS OF EXERCISE TRAINING

Definition

The term 'exercise training' applies to a programme of repeated exercises undertaken at a guided or prescribed intensity and frequency over a period of time, usually several weeks. It is based upon aerobic exercise designed to improve physical performance at both maximal and submaximal levels. It may be of low, moderate or high intensity and may also include resistance training.

Research confirms that exercise training improves physical performance (exercise tolerance, muscular strength and symptoms), psychological functioning (anxiety, depression and well-being) and social adaptation and functioning in cardiac patients. It shows reduction in mortality, morbidity, recurrent events and hospital readmissions. It is also found to have a positive impact on patients' physical ability to exercise. Therefore, exercise training as a therapeutic intervention is central to the cardiac rehabilitation programme.

PHYSIOLOGICAL ADAPTATIONS TO EXERCISE TRAINING

In healthy individuals physiological adaptations to aerobic exercise training are central (cardiac) and peripheral (skeletal muscle and vascular).

Adaptations at a submaximal level of aerobic exercise

Adaptations at a submaximal level of aerobic exercise are reduction in heart rate due to decrease in sympathetic activity and increase in parasympathetic activity (vagal tone). The stroke volume increases due to greater left ventricular filling and increase in left ventricular mass. Decrease in resting heart rate and blood pressure implies reduced myocardial oxygen demand. Also, the period of diastole is increased, allowing greater time for blood to flow into the coronary circulation.

Cardiac output (CO = HR (heart rate) × SV (stroke volume)) must always match metabolic demand, but does so with reduced heart rate and increased stroke volume. Systolic blood pressure decreases and there is redistribution of blood flow to trained skeletal muscle and other tissues. Circulating catecholamines decrease and arteriovenous oxygen difference increases.

Key point

As a result of aerobic training, functional and structural changes take place in skeletal muscle, the heart and the circulation. These changes improve the circulatory system's capacity to transport oxygen to the working muscles (central changes) and the capacity of skeletal muscle to extract and use oxygen (peripheral changes).

Central changes as a result of aerobic exercise training

- Increased stroke volume.
- Increased left ventricular mass.
- Increased chamber size.
- Increased total blood volume.
- Decreased total peripheral resistance during maximal exercise.

Peripheral changes as a result of aerobic exercise training

- Increased arteriovenous oxygen difference
- Increased number and size of mitochondria
- Increased oxidative enzyme activity
- Improved capillarisation
- Increased myoglobin.

Increase in $VO_{2\ max}$

Oxygen consumption (VO_2) is expressed either in absolute terms as litres per minute ($L.min^{-1}$) or relative to body weight as millilitres per kilogram per minute ($mL.\ kg^{-1}.\ min^{-1}$). $VO_{2\ max}$ is the highest rate of oxygen consumption attainable during maximal exercise. Aerobic training increases $VO_{2\ max}$. In relative terms, an individual walking at 4 mph uses 17.5 mL of O_2 per kg bodyweight per minute. In absolute terms, a man weighing 70 kg will use 1225 mL or 1.2 L per minute.

Key point

The significance of increased $VO_{2\ max}$ is the reduction in physiological stress evoked by submaximal activity and *not* the ability to perform maximal bouts of exercise.

In CHD patients, the increase in $VO_{2\ max}$ is predominantly due to peripheral adaptations. Central changes are associated with long periods of high-intensity training. Although central changes have been shown with high-intensity training in CHD patients in some studies, this regime is not suitable in conventional rehabilitation programmes. Physical performance improvements are better seen in patients with low exercise tolerance.

Key point

Aerobic exercise training at moderate intensity confers benefit on CHD patients via peripheral adaptations.

Benefits of exercise training in CHD patients (risk factor modification)

The physiological, symptomatic and psychosocial benefits of exercise in CHD patients are summarised in Table 12.2.

Table 12.2 Benefits of exercise training in CHD patients (risk factor modification)

Physiological benefits

- Reduction in systolic and diastolic blood pressure
- Reduction in percentage body fat, increase in lean body mass
- Reduction in fibrinogen levels and platelet aggregation
- Increase in high-density lipoprotein (HDL), reduction in triglycerides
- Increase in insulin sensitivity, improvement in glucose–insulin dynamics

Symptomatic benefits

- Reduced risk of arrhythmias
- Increased ischaemic threshold
- Increased angina threshold
- Improved coronary perfusion
- Reduction in ST wave changes
- Reduced angina episodes/shortness of breath

Psychosocial benefits

- Reduction in anxiety and depression
- Improved sleep patterns
- Improved sense of well-being
- Restoration of self-confidence
- Reduction in illness behaviour
- Improved social communication
- Return to daily activities/hobbies
- Resumption of sex life
- Return to work/vocation
- Compliance with other risk factors

ASSESSMENT FOR EXERCISE PRESCRIPTION

A through assessment is essential in order to plan an individualised and safe exercise prescription for cardiac patients. It should include the following:

- a detailed history of the present condition and clinical presentation
- previous levels of activity and exercise
- physical limitations and disabilities
- signs and symptoms
- risk factor assessment/profile
- screening for relative contraindications
- risk stratification
- functional capacity test
- psychosocial assessment: objectives, beliefs, knowledge, interests, ethnicity
- patient goals and expectations.

Contraindications to exercise

Contraindications to exercise include:

- unstable angina
- resting systolic blood pressure > 200 mm Hg or resting diastolic blood pressure > 110 mm Hg
- orthostatic blood pressure drop > 20 mm Hg with symptoms
- critical aortic stenosis
- acute systemic illness or fever
- uncontrolled atrial or ventricular arrhythmias
- uncontrolled sinus tachycardia
- uncompensated congestive heart failure
- third-degree heart block
- active pericarditis or myocarditis
- recent embolism
- thrombophlebitis
- resting ST segment displacement > 2 mm
- uncontrolled diabetes (resting blood glucose > 400 mg/dL.

EXERCISE PRESCRIPTION: THE FITT PRINCIPLE

To develop an individual exercise training programme, factors known as the FITT principles are considered:

- Frequency **F**
- Intensity **I**
- Time (duration) **T**
- Type of exercise **T**.

Frequency, time and type or mode of exercise are explained later in the chapter, along with activities in different phases of cardiac rehabilitation.

Intensity of exercise

The risk of developing arrhythmias or adverse events such as an acute MI is increased in cardiac patients with vigorous activity. Low- to moderate-intensity exercise training can produce beneficial changes in functional capacity, cardiac function, coronary risk factors and psychosocial well-being, and may possibly improve survival in patients with CHD. For patients with low functional capacity, frequent and short-duration exercise stimulus incorporated throughout the day may be advisable. Intensity is prescribed and monitored by several methods, which can be used independently or in combination with one another.

Heart rate

Each individual patient should have his or her training heart rate calculated, based on thorough assessment and risk stratification. Training intensities for most patients range between 60 and 75 per cent of maximum heart rate for the majority of the population group. The more complex patient will require lower intensities (40–50 per cent), and hence appropriate adjustments to these calculations will be required.

12

In ideal circumstances, the training heart rate is obtained from a maximum or symptom-limited exercise ECG test (exercise tolerance test, or ETT), when this is available. The training heart rate should be set at 60–75 per cent of maximal heart rate or 20 beats below the heart rate at which the symptoms appeared, and should be monitored throughout the exercise session. However, ETT information is not always available to the cardiac rehabilitation team and frequently other methods for determining training intensity are used.

Using heart rate in isolation as a measure of exercise intensity has a number of limitations and hence other methods of monitoring intensity should additionally be followed. This includes the use of a validated rating of perceived exertion scale (RPE) and direct clinical observation for signs of exertion.

Heart rate can remain an appropriate intensity marker, even when patients are influenced by chronotrophic medication such as beta-blockers. In this instance, the resting heart rate and the maximal heart rate are reduced by 20–40 beats per minute and the target heart rate can be recalculated on this basis.

Age-adjusted predicted maximum heart rate formula

This formula uses a predicted maximum heart rate based on age (220 − age) and, as such, can have an error margin of as much as ± 10 beats per minute.

A percentage of this predicted maximum is selected, based on the assessment findings.

Example

- Patient A (low-risk and uncomplicated) is 70 years of age.
- Maximum age-predicted heart rate = 220 − 70 = 150.
  60–75% of predicted maximum heart rate:
  0.60 × 150 = 90
  0.75 × 150 = 112
- Thus, training heart rate = 90–112 beats per minute.

Karvonen formula (heart rate reserve, HRR)

This formula assumes access to a true observed maximum heart rate. This may be obtained, for example, by an ECG tolerance test. This formula is advantageous in that it accounts for the individual's resting heart rate. A percentage of this is selected, based on the assessment findings, noting that 50–70 per cent of HRR is equivalent to 60–75 per cent of maximum heart rate.

HRR is calculated thus:

- HRR = maximum heart rate − resting heart rate.
- Training intensity is selected and calculated, i.e. 50–70 per cent HRR.
- Resting heart rate is added to HRR percentage.

Example

- Patient B (low-risk and uncomplicated) has a resting heart rate of 65 and achieves a maximum heart rate of 160 during an ECG exercise test. Following assessment, the intensity of training has been set at 50–70 per cent of HRR.
- Calculation of HRR = 160−65 = 95
- Selection of percentage of HRR:
  50% of HRR = 0.50 × 95 = 47.5
  70% of HRR = 0.70 × 95 = 66.5
- Add resting heart rate:
  47.5 + 65 = 112.5
  66.5 + 65 = 131.5
- Thus, training heart rate = 112–131 beats per minute.

Rating of perceived exertion (RPE)

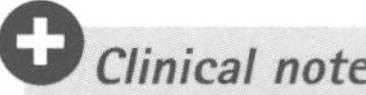

Clinical note

Heart rate monitoring with RPE and observation of the patient during the exercise is an effective way to monitor exercise intensity.

Patients need to develop the ability to perceive their exertion whilst exercising. In other words, they should feel the physical sensation of how hard they are working so that they know the safe limits to which they can exert themselves. In the early stages of rehabilitation, the physiotherapist assists by using the heart rate monitoring method, setting the exercise circuit at a specific work rate and, most importantly, observing the patient's response to exercise. On the 15 point Borg RPE scale (Table 12.3), a rating of 12–13 (or 3–4 on the cardiac rehabilitation-10 (CR-10) scale, Table 12.4) corresponds to 60 per cent $VO_{2\ max}$ or 60 per cent of HRR. A rating of 15 (or 6–7 on the CR-10 scale) corresponds to 75 per cent of $VO_{2\ max}$ or HRR.

In moderate submaximal exercise, muscular sensations and breathlessness relate very closely to exercise stimulus, and so use of the RPE scale is advised in cardiac rehabilitation. The CR-10 scale was developed to focus more on rating individual sensations of strain, exertion or pain. Thus if pain, breathlessness or localised muscle fatigue is the dominant sensation, the CR-10 scale should be used.

Table 12.3 The Borg RPE Scale (Borg 1998)

6	
7	Very, very light
8	
9	Very light
10	
11	Fairly light
12	
13	Somewhat hard
14	
15	Hard
16	
17	Very hard
18	
19	Very, very hard
20	

Table 12.4 The Borg Category Ratio (CR-10) Scale

0	Nothing
0.5	Extremely weak (just noticeable)
1	Very weak
2	Weak
3	Moderate
4	Somewhat strong
5	Strong (heavy)
6	
7	Very strong
8	
9	Extremely strong (almost max)
10	Maximal

Metabolic equivalent (METs)

Metabolic equivalent relates to the rate of the body's oxygen uptake for a given activity expressed as a multiple of resting VO_2. On average, an individual utilises 3.5 mL O_2 per kilo bodyweight per minute ($mL.kg^{-1}.min^{-1}$). One MET therefore equals a VO_2 of 3.5 $mL.kg^{-1}.min^{-1}$. MET value is assigned to an activity by measuring the VO_2 for that activity.

MET values are reported on the ETT. This information is useful to the cardiac rehabilitation physiotherapist as a means of prescribing intensity, as well as identifying the functional capacity of the patient. An individual's exercises can be prescribed and regulated by choice of activities according to the MET values for them (Table 12.5). For example, a patient with a peak capacity of 7 METs cannot be prescribed skipping (8–10 METs). (See also functional capacity, described later in this chapter.)

If an individual walking at 3 mph reports his or her exertion as 12–13 on the RPE scale (12–13 RPE corresponding to 60 per cent of $VO_{2\ max}$), then planning activities of comparable MET value in the exercise prescription will provide the appropriate training stimulus.

Table 12.5 Energy costs of leisure activities

Activity	METs (min)	METs (max)
Cycling		
5 mph	2	3
10 mph	5	6
13 mph	8	9
Dancing		
Ballroom	4	5
Aerobic	6	9
Skipping		
>80/min	8	10
120–140/min	11	11
Swimming		
Breast stroke	8	9
Freestyle	9	10
Tennis	4	9
Walking		
1 mph	1	3
3 mph	3	3.5
3.5 mph	3.5	4
4 mph	5	6

MET values are only estimates and an individual may be working slightly above or below the estimated MET value for a particular task. The variability depends on the complexity of the task. Table 12.5 gives minimal and maximal activity values. Walking is a complex activity that requires balance and the use of arm and trunk movements, and hence there is a variation in the MET value.

Frequency

The ACPICR (2006) recommends exercise training 2–3 times weekly (for example, two supervised classes and one home circuit) for phase III. Exercising 2–3 times per week for a minimum of 8 weeks produces physiological and psychosocial adaptations. However, it should be remembered that to gain the optimum benefits patients will need ongoing exposure to exercise. Phase III should be seen as the beginning of these changes, and after completion of that stage patients should move on to phase IV for continuation and progression. The ultimate aim is to promote life-long adherence to the individual's exercise behaviour.

Time

The conditioning phase (aerobic exercise training) in a phase III cardiac rehabilitation programme should last between 20 and 30 minutes. This should be in addition to the warm-up and cool-down exercises.

Type

Training activity needs to be aerobic and can be delivered in many ways. Initially, endurance training is desirable for CHD patients. Within an individual prescription, incorporating a variety of exercise types will optimise peripheral adaptation, reduce the likelihood of overuse injuries and enhance motivation and compliance.

RISK STRATIFICATION

Exercise-based cardiac rehabilitation is associated with a reduction in coronary mortality and morbidity. As a result of novel treatment approaches now available to CHD patients and of improvement in the management of cardiac patients, the type and number of patients referred for cardiac rehabilitation are increasing.

The risk of adverse cardiac events during exercise is small. In the supervised exercise programmes the risk of exercise-related cardiac events is also small. However, it is essential that the cardiac rehabilitation team responsible for delivering the exercise programme recognise the likelihood of exercise-related incidents and ensure that all reasonable and necessary steps are taken to deliver safe and effective exercise prescription to patients.

Increased myocardial demands of vigorous exercise can precipitate arrhythmias. Risk is increased with extensive cardiac damage, residual ischaemia and ventricular arrhythmias on exercise. All patients should be assessed and have their risk stratified prior to recruitment to the exercise component of cardiac rehabilitation.

> **Clinical note**
>
> For the exercise professional in cardiac rehabilitation the term 'risk stratification' implies thorough evaluation of the patient to assess the degree of risk of further cardiac events associated with exercise. This allows the exercise professional to guide patient management for exercise prescription, monitoring and progression appropriately.

The information required for assessment should include:

- diagnosis and the site and size of infarct/surgery details as appropriate
- current cardiac status
- results of investigations: for example, ETT, echocardiogram report, angiogram
- current medication
- recovery and activity levels since discharge, symptoms
- past medical history, including musculoskeletal, respiratory and neurological problems
- CHD risk factors
- psychosocial status.

Classification

The patients are risk-stratified into low-, medium- and high-risk groups depending on their current cardiac status. This includes the extent of myocardial damage, previous history of MI, complications and associated signs and symptoms. The main risk to patients attending the exercise component of cardiac rehabilitation is ventricular fibrillation. Extensive myocardial damage, residual ischaemia, significant ECG changes, ST segment or arrhythmias on exercise are key factors when predicting risk.

The risk classification given below is based on the guidelines from American Association of Cardiovascular and Pulmonary Rehabilitation (AACVPR 2006).

High risk

The patient is classified at high risk when *any one* of the following risk factors is present:

- decreased left ventricular function (ejection fraction < 40 per cent)

- complex arrhythmias at rest or appearing/increasing during exercise
- abnormal haemodynamics with exercise (especially a decrease in systolic blood pressure during exercise)
- MI complicated by congestive heart failure, cardiogenic shock and complex arrhythmias
- survivor of cardiac arrest
- clinically significant depression.

Moderate risk

Patients are classified as medium-risk when they do not meet the criteria of either high or low risk:

- moderately impaired left ventricular function (ejection fraction 40–49 per cent)
- signs and symptoms, including angina at moderate levels of exercise (5–6.9 METs) or in recovery.

Low risk

The patient is classified as low-risk when *each* of the following risk factors is present:

- no left ventricular dysfunction (ejection fraction > 50 per cent)
- no resting or exercise-induced complex arrhythmias
- uncomplicated MI, CABG, PTCA
- normal haemodynamics with exercise
- functional capacity ≥ 7 METs
- absence of clinical depression.

Functional capacity

Functional capacity (FC) is a strong and independent risk factor of all-cause and cardiovascular mortality, and is the one risk factor that can be improved by training. A low FC of < 6 METs indicates a high mortality group, whereas an FC > 10 METs indicates excellent survival, regardless of occlusive coronary disease or left ventricular function.

Functional exercise testing

The most widely recognised measure of cardiopulmonary fitness is aerobic capacity or maximal oxygen consumption ($VO_{2\ max}$). This variable is defined as the highest rate of oxygen transport and use that can be achieved at maximal physical exertion. Thus it is an expression of the functional health of the combined cardiovascular, pulmonary and skeletal muscle systems. It may be used to prescribe an appropriate training intensity in rehabilitation programmes and to identify improvements in endurance fitness. Determination of $VO_{2\ max}$ during cardiopulmonary exercise testing provides an objective and reproducible assessment of functional capacity in patients with cardiac disease. In clinical practice, $VO_{2\ max}$ is predicted or estimated from treadmill speed and percentage grade, and expressed as METs. Thus ETT can produce an estimated METs value to assess the patient's response to exercise, to guide risk stratification and exercise prescription. It would also serve as an objective outcome measure of the impact of an exercise programme on FC. An ETT is strongly recommended at 3–6 weeks post-event.

ETT can give the following information:

- heart rates and exercise level at peak exercise
- symptoms and/or ECG changes
- RPE
- blood pressure response to exercise
- MET level achieved at training heart rates (e.g. at 60–75 per cent of HR_{max}).

MET values can also be estimated from submaximal protocols recommended for assessing FC. These are externally paced field exercise tests like step test, shuttle walk test and cycle ergometry.

The Chester step test (CST) is a submaximal multistage test lasting for 10 minutes with a choice of four step heights.

The shuttle walking test (SWT) is a low-cost, simple alternative to exercise testing that informs the rehabilitation team on a suitable exercise programme and appropriate training heart rate, and allows assessment of progress during cardiac rehabilitation. The limitation of SWT is that it is not suitable for people with a higher baseline fitness level. It also may not be sensitive to change, demonstrating improvements in functional capacity in the older cardiac population with coexisting pathologies by incremental walking. Thus a variety of outcome measures may be required for the cardiac rehabilitation population. (SWT is described in detail later in this chapter.)

The information obtained from the risk classification is used to determine baseline fitness level; exercise prescription; exercise progression; staff:patient ratio, site of the exercise programme — either supervised or unsupervised, and based in hospital or the community.

EXERCISE PROGRAMMING

Patients should participate in an induction prior to undertaking the phase III exercise component of cardiac rehabilitation. They should not take part if they present with:

- fever and acute systemic illness
- unresolved unstable angina
- resting systolic blood pressure > 200 mm Hg, diastolic blood pressure > 110 mm Hg
- a significant unexpected drop in blood pressure
- tachycardia > 100 beats per minute

- new symptoms of shortness of breath, palpitations, dizziness, lethargy
- a severe respiratory, orthopaedic or metabolic condition that would limit exercise ability.

Warm-up

Strenuous exercise without previous warm-up can produce ischaemic ST segment changes and arrhythmias, even in healthy adults.

Key point

For older adults and cardiac patients, warm-up must be more gradual than for the apparently healthy population.

The warm-up is the preparatory phase of the exercise session. A well-planned and effectively carried out warm-up will improve exercise performance and optimise the safety and effectiveness of the exercise session. For cardiac patients warm-ups should be of at least 15 minutes duration. This time prepares the cardiovascular system for the exercise activity. It allows a gradual increase in myocardial blood supply via vasodilatation of the coronary arteries and achieves a gradual rise in aortic pressure. This reduces the risk of provoking ischaemia and arrhythmias. It also prepares the mind by focusing participants' attention on the activity ahead.

The warm-up consists of pulse-raising exercises, mobilisation of major joints and stretching, and specific warm-up movements.

Pulse-raising exercises

These include rhythmic movements, initially of the lower limbs (for example, walking forwards and back, stepping, sidestepping, step-backs and so on), gradually increasing the heart rate and blood flow to the active muscles.

Mobilising major joints and stretching

The major joints are mobilised by taking each through a normal range of movement (for example, the shoulders are raised and lowered, then circled backwards and forwards; lumbar and thoracic spine are mobilised by bending sideways and turning) (Figure 12.4). This ensures that the joints are well lubricated and blood flow to the structures surrounding the joints increases, allowing a full range of movement. Stretching the large muscles will assist mobilisation.

Muscles that are prone to adaptive shortening due to cardiac surgery or as a result of the ageing process should be stretched for about 10 seconds. Whilst holding a stretch, it is important to keep the rest of the body moving to maintain the pulse rise and to avoid pooling of blood in the lower extremities (venous pooling).

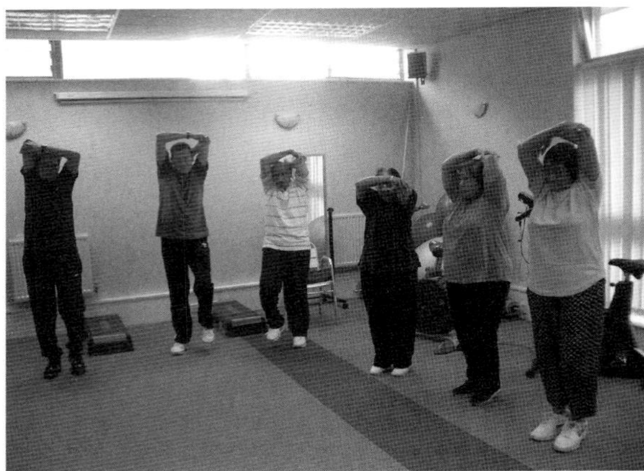

Figure 12.4 A group of phase III patients doing 'warm-up' stretches.

Specific movements

Specific exercises that mimic the movements of prescribed activity at low-intensity levels will assist preparation for the conditioning phase by activating the neuromuscular pathways (for example, alternate legs to side before sidestepping) (Figure 12.5).

Key point

It is recommended that patients should achieve a heart rate within 20 beats per minute of the training heart rate or RPE of 10–11.

Cardiovascular (CV) conditioning

This component includes aerobic exercise training, which produces beneficial physiological effects for both the healthy and the cardiac population. CV training

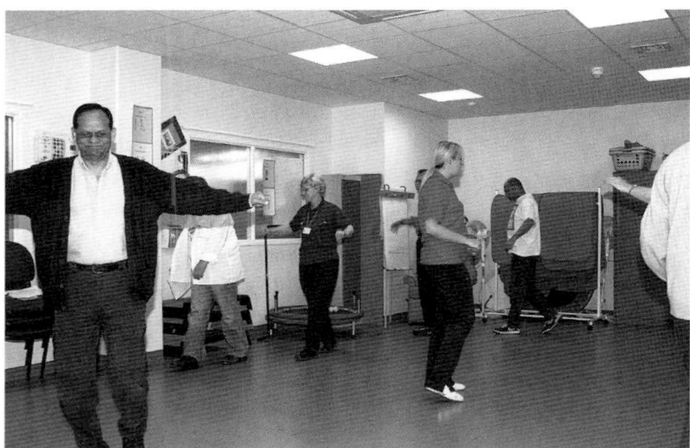

Figure 12.5 Warm-up involving specific movements.

depends on the patient's FC and activity levels, as determined in the assessment. FC may be low for some sedentary patients.

The exercise programme should be designed to produce a training effect that is achieved through varying the frequency, duration, intensity and type/mode of exercise. The principal goal is to improve the duration and efficiency of exercise and then to progress the intensity.

CV conditioning can be executed via a continuous or interval training approach:

- *Continuous training* is an aerobic activity performed at a constant submaximal intensity that is prescribed and monitored: for example, brisk walking, cycling, stepping up and down on a step machine or bench, and walking/running on the treadmill (Figures 12.6 and 12.7).
- *Interval training* consists of bouts of aerobic exercise that are interspersed with periods of lower-intensity work. In cardiac patients, particularly the elderly or those with low FC, a greater amount of work is achieved using an interval training approach than with continuous training. It is also less daunting and encourages compliance. Lower-intensity exercises in interval training are also referred as 'active recovery'.

The CV conditioning period should last for 20–30 minutes. Circuit training is popular as it can be designed with or without equipment. 'Active recovery' stations increase the endurance of specific muscle groups: for example, triceps, pectorals and trapezius.

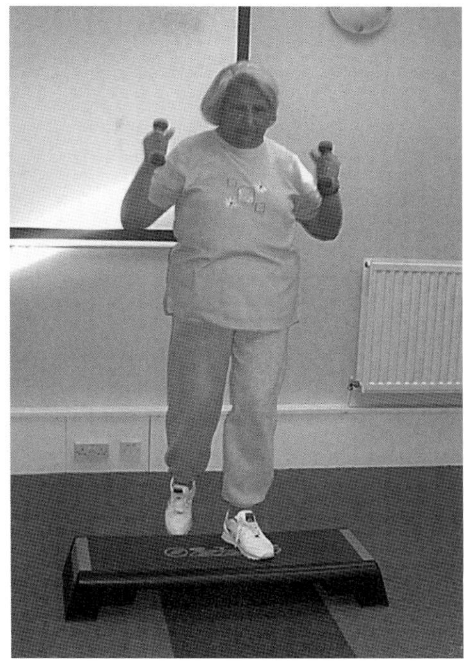

Figure 12.7 A patient performing cardiovascular work.

Individualisation of the CV component is achieved by varying:

- the duration at each CV station
- the intensity
- the period of rest between stations
- the overall duration of conditioning.

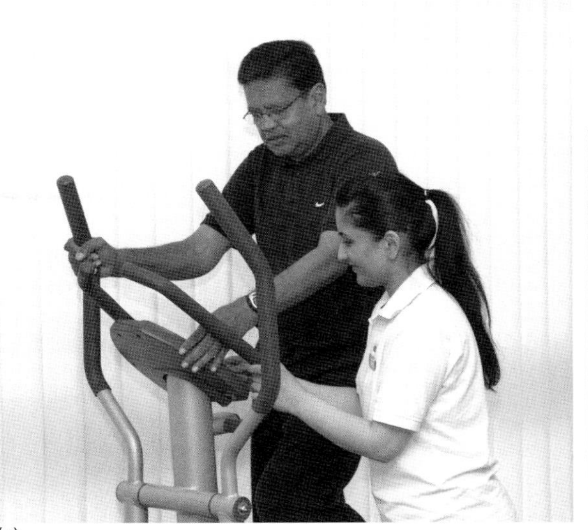

(a)

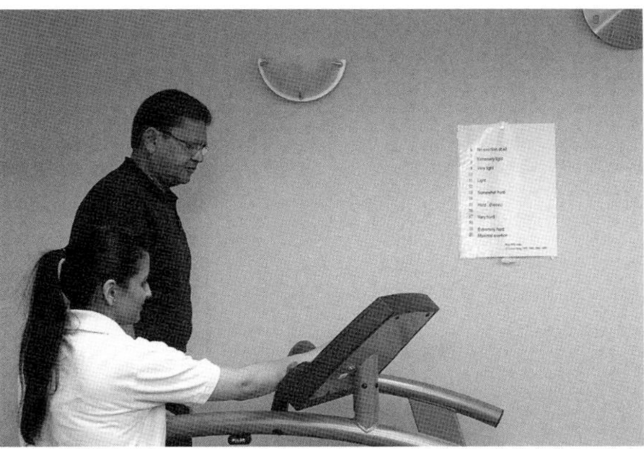

(b)

Figure 12.6 Physiotherapist assisting a patient to set the intensity for exercise training on a treadmill and cross-trainer.

> **Key point**
> In supervised exercise programmes, interval circuit training is better suited to cardiac patients, at least in the initial period. The duration of activity is increased first before raising the intensity.

Exercises performed in a recumbent position should be avoided during the CV conditioning phase. This is because some older adults may experience difficulty in getting up and down. Immediately after vigorous activity, venous return will increase on lying down and will raise myocardial workload. There is also an increased risk of orthostatic hypotension. Floor work when indicated (for example, relaxation exercises and stretching) should be carried out after a cool-down period when the cardiovascular system has recovered.

Class management

Control of the circuits needs to be carefully considered (Figure 12.8). A ratio of 1 member of staff to 5 patients is recommended.

In the type of circuit design shown in Table 12.6, the following elements are included:

- Beginner: 1 minute CV and 1 minute AR
- Intermediate: 1 minute CV, 30 seconds AR and 30 seconds CV alternative
- Advanced: 1 minute CV and 1 minute CV alternative.

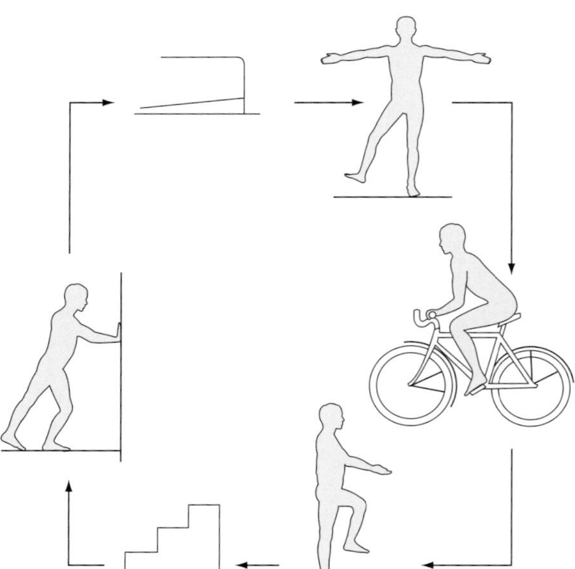

Figure 12.8 An example of a simple circuit set up with cardiovascular and active recovery stations for a beginner in phase III.

Patients complete the circuit twice. The instructor calls out to indicate the 30-second intervals.

Beginners achieve 10 minutes of work, patients at intermediate level achieve 15 minutes of CV work, and advanced level patients achieve 20 minutes of CV work (continuous training).

Cool-down

This consists of pulse-lowering exercises, stretching of large muscle groups, and joint mobilisation at a slower pace with movements of steadily reducing intensity. Its aim is to return the cardiorespiratory system to near pre-exercise levels within 10–15 minutes. It is essentially the reverse of warm-up. A minimum 10-minute period is recommended for cool-down at the end of CV conditioning.

Following sustained aerobic exercise training there is an increased risk of venous pooling. This may also be coupled with effects of medication and can cause hypotension. Cooling down reduces the risk of hypotension, elevated heart rates and arrhythmias.

Post-exercise supervision for 15–30 minutes is recommended. In many programmes the education or relaxation session follows the exercise, giving an opportunity for patient supervision.

Progression

This is achieved by increasing the duration, frequency or intensity of training in order to maintain training stimulus. Ideally, serial exercise testing is used to modify prescription. If this is not available, heart rates and perceived exertion at reference workloads can be compared and the information used to increase any of the three variables or a combination. Progression over a long period towards a more continuous training approach is the aim. Exercise progression will be highly variable between individuals with CHD, depending on the severity of disease, coexisting pathology, patient motivation and compliance.

Resistance training

Health-related physical fitness includes cardiovascular (aerobic) fitness, muscle strength, endurance and flexibility, and body composition (lean to fat ratio). Muscle strength is the ability of a muscle to produce a maximum force at a given velocity of movement. Muscle endurance is the ability of a muscle to perform repeated muscle contractions against a submaximal resistance. Resistance training (RT) increases lean muscle mass and maintains basal metabolic rate when combined with aerobic training, thus aiding in weight management. By improving muscle strength and balance it can reduce the risk of

Table 12.6 An example of circuit design

High-intensity (CV) stations	Active recovery (AR) stations	CV alternative
1. Knee raises	2. Biceps curls	Shuttle walk/jog
3. Treadmill (walking on incline)	4. Lateral arm raises	
5. Step-ups	6. Upright rows	
7. Alternate side taps	8. Forward press with Theraband	
9. Bike	10. Wall press	

falling. Positive effects on bone density are well known with resistance training.

Many activities of daily living, such as carrying shopping and doing housework, require upper body strength. Cardiac rehabilitation professionals often come across patients who are fearful of lifting or of carrying out resistance-based activities. Resistance training is associated with an increase in arterial blood pressure that would increase myocardial workload. Due to these concerns, aerobic exercise training has traditionally been the main focus in cardiac rehabilitation programmes. However, recent research recommends resistance training as part of a supervised exercise programme in cardiac patients. Haemodynamic and cardiovascular responses to resistance training are similar in CHD patients and normal subjects. Because of the increased diastolic pressure, myocardial perfusion may be enhanced. It is now generally agreed that low- and medium-risk cardiac patients can commence resistance exercise after completion of an aerobic exercise programme for 4–6 weeks. This should consist of two sets of 8–10 exercises involving the major muscle groups, performed a minimum of twice per week. Currently in the UK, RT is not included in cardiac rehabilitation programmes for high-risk patients.

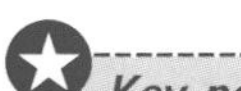

Key point

Resistance training, principally planned to build up muscular endurance, is associated with maintenance of strength and can be performed safely by patients.

Contraindications to resistance training are:

- abnormal haemodynamic responses to exercise
- ischaemic changes during graded exercise testing
- poor left ventricular function
- uncontrolled hypertension or arrhythmias
- exercise capacity of < 6 METs.

Swimming and water-based exercise

Compared to walking, cycling and dancing, the intensity of swimming cannot be reduced so easily. There is only limited research available on water-based activities in CHD subjects. The energy costs required vary hugely, depending on the strokes used. Breast stroke can be modified to achieve the required training intensity, although the intensity of front crawl would be more difficult to control. In water, exertion is not felt to the same extent as on land, and so RPE will not be a reliable indicator.

The horizontal position adopted by swimmers increases the return of blood to the heart, thus increasing central blood volume. This in turn will raise cardiac output and stroke volume and increase myocardial demand. Energy costs for swimming range between 8 and 10 METs. Information on METs obtained from ETT or FC tests should be utilised to assess and prescribe water-based exercises.

12

EXERCISE CONSIDERATIONS FOR SPECIAL POPULATIONS

Heart failure

Heart failure is distinguished by the inability of the heart to pump enough blood (and therefore deliver adequate oxygen) to the metabolising tissues. A patient with heart failure presents with symptoms of breathlessness and fatigue at rest and with swelling of ankles. The New York Heart Association (NYHA) has classified the stages of heart failure based on the severity of symptoms (Table 12.7). The prognosis for heart failure is poor, with 50 per cent of patients dying within 4 years and 50 per cent of those diagnosed with severe heart failure dying within a year.

Key point

Patients with stable heart failure benefit from exercise-based cardiac rehabilitation intervention. Improvement of functional capacity, symptoms (improved NYHA class) and quality of life is reported and is primarily due to peripheral adaptations.

Heart failure patients are classified as a high-risk group, according to the AACVPR stratification criteria. Exercise prescription and training for this group demand rigorous assessment and monitoring. An appropriate

Table 12.7 New York Heart Association functional classification of the stages of heart failure	
Class	**Patient symptoms**
Class I (Mild)	No limitation of physical activity. Ordinary physical activity does not cause undue fatigue, palpitation or dyspnoea (shortness of breath)
Class II (Mild)	Slight limitation of physical activity. Comfortable at rest, but ordinary physical activity results in fatigue, palpitation or dyspnoea
Class III (Moderate)	Marked limitation of physical activity. Comfortable at rest, but less than ordinary activity causes fatigue, palpitation or dyspnoea
Class IV (Severe)	Unable to carry out any physical activity without discomfort. Symptoms of cardiac insufficiency at rest. If any physical activity is undertaken, discomfort is increased

safe environment and system needs to be in place to deliver exercise training. Patients need to be stable, and any change in the clinical status may mean that exercise is contraindicated. Based on risk stratification, an increased staff to patient ratio and close monitoring of symptoms of breathlessness (the Borg CR-10 Scale may be desirable), heart rate and blood pressure pre- and post-exercise should be implemented. Interval training of 1–6 minutes of work/activity (40–60 per cent FC, 11–13 RPE), followed by rest, is recommended.

Contraindications to exercise include:

- uncompensated heart failure
- uncontrolled oedema
- uncontrolled arrhythmias
- symptoms at rest or with minimal exertion (class IV)
- unstable angina
- resting sinus tachycardia (> 120 beats/min)
- hypotension (systolic blood pressure < 90 mm Hg)
- hypokalaemia (serum potassium < 3.0 mEq/L).

Older patients

Many patients referred to cardiac rehabilitation are over 50 years of age. The changes associated with ageing need to be accounted for when prescribing exercise. There is a 1 per cent loss of $VO_{2\ max}$ per year from the age of 25 onwards. Thus the FC can be reduced, depending on activity levels. Maximal heart rate declines with age. Lung elasticity and chest wall expansion decrease with age. Bone density is reduced by about 20 per cent by the age of 65 in women and by 10–15 per cent by the age of 70 in men. Muscle function declines by approximately 25 per cent by the age of 65, as does joint flexibility and range of movement. Lean body mass reduces and body fat increases.

Motor skills

Balance, reaction times and motor coordination decline with age. One-third of people over the age of 65 fall at least once a year. In addition there may be hearing problems. All these can contribute to anxiety and diminished confidence with regard to exercise. The exercise class atmosphere should be social, welcoming, relaxed and non-threatening. Patients need to feel comfortable.

Exercise prescription

- *Frequency*: 2–3 sessions per week.
- *Intensity*: lower end of prescription range (60–75 per cent maximum heart rate); more gradual progression; RPE.
- *Type*: endurance training of longer duration and moderate intensity; resistance training to be introduced later with 40–60 per cent of 1 RM, a maximum of 8–10 repetitions, 1–3 sets, for a minimum of twice per week.
- *Time*: the conditioning period should be 20–30 minutes.

(One repetition maximum (1 RM) is defined as the maximum weight that can be lifted in a smooth continuous movement, using a proper technique and avoiding strain or breath-holding (Daub et al. 1996).)

Extended warm-up and slow and controlled transition between movements should be encouraged. Precautions should be taken regarding extremes of weather.

Hypertension

British Hypertension Society guidelines (Williams et al. 2004) advise antihypertensive therapy at different thresholds as follows:

- Individuals not at high risk of CHD/atherosclerotic disease are classified to be hypertensive and treated at blood pressures of 160/100.
- Individuals with CHD/other atherosclerotic disease are classified to be hypertensive and treated at blood pressures of 140–149/90–99.
- Individuals with diabetes are classified to be hypertensive and treated at blood pressures of $\geq 140/\geq 90$.

Exercise prescription

- *Frequency*: 3–5 sessions per week.
- *Intensity*: reduced to 50–75 per cent of maximum heart rate.
- *Type*: lower resistance/higher repetitions; avoid overgripping equipment; avoid Valsalva manœuvre, isometric work.
- *Time*: increase duration at moderate intensity.

Exercise is contraindicated when systolic blood pressure is > 180 mm Hg or diastolic blood pressure is > 100 mm Hg. Antihypertensive medication may lead to hypotension. Post-exercise extended active recovery with constant feet movement is required to ensure venous return.

Diabetes

Diabetes is a group of diseases marked by high levels of blood glucose resulting from defects in insulin production, insulin action or both.

Diabetes must be stabilised following events such as MI and bypass graft surgery. Diabetic patients may not experience pain and can have silent ischaemia. Close supervision during the session is required.

Exercise prescription

FITT principles apply. Other considerations include the following:

- Monitor blood sugar before and after exercise.
- Insulin may need to be reduced on exercise days.
- Exercise should be avoided when insulin is at its peak effect; insulin uptake is increased if injection is into an exercising limb.
- When the patient is new to exercise, it is advisable to have other people present.
- Autonomic neuropathy may alter heart rate and blood pressure response.
- Monitor for retinopathy.
- Watch for silent ischaemia. Monitor for overexertion.

Peripheral vascular disease

Peripheral vascular disease is also known as atherosclerosis, poor circulation or hardening of the arteries. It presents with intermittent claudication: ischaemic pain on exertion that diminishes with rest. It most commonly affects the legs ('angina' of the legs). In severe cases symptoms include cold, painful feet.

Patients need to be reassured as they suffer from lack of confidence to exercise beyond the point of pain.

Exercise prescription

- *Frequency*: increased frequency; short bouts of exercise are often better tolerated than continuous.
- *Intensity*: increased duration before intensity; peripheral vascular disease (PVD) scales of discomfort are used to monitor patients while exercising (ACSM 2001).
- *Type*: walking/weight bearing.
- *Time*: daily exercise/graduated increase in duration.

Non-weightbearing activities — for example, cycling — can be used to achieve prescribed CV dose and improved compliance.

Obesity

People have traditionally been considered to be obese if they are more than 20 percent over their ideal weight (Figure 12.9). That ideal weight must take into account the person's height, age, sex and build. Obesity has been more precisely defined by the National Institutes of Health (NIH) as a body mass index (BMI) of 30 and above.

BMI is a measure of body fat based on height and weight that applies to both adult men and women: weight (kg) divided by height (m^2). Since the BMI describes bodyweight relative to height, it correlates strongly (in adults) with the total body fat content. BMI categories are as follow:

- underweight = < 18.5
- normal weight = 18.5–24.9

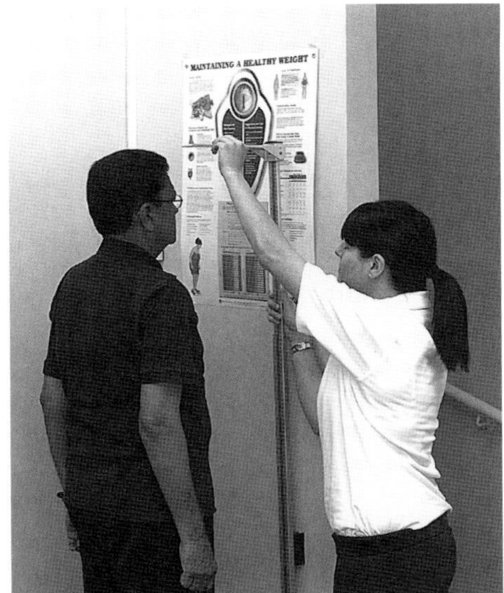

Figure 12.9 Physiotherapist measuring a patient's height to assess body mass index.

- overweight = 25–29.9
- obesity = $\geq$ 30.

Obesity is also measured by measuring the thickness of skin folds. Central obesity is measured by waist:hip ratio ($>$ 0.95 in males, $>$ 0.85 in females).

Exercise prescription

- *Frequency*: 3–5 sessions per week.
- *Intensity*: reduce to 50–75 per cent of maximum heart rate.
- *Type*: combine cardiovascular (CV) work and resistance training (RT) to reduce fat weight and increase lean tissue; avoid high-impact work, which puts stress on joints; provide alternatives and, if necessary, avoid supine positions that can restrict breathing.
- *Time*: increase duration and frequency, as the patient is able.

Osteoarthritis (OA) and rheumatoid arthritis (RA)

OA is a degenerative arthritis caused by wear and tear. It affects discrete joints. RA is a systemic illness characterised by inflammation and can affect multiple joints. Both conditions are marked by inflammation, pain and restricted movement. In RA there may be periods of exacerbation and remission. In advanced arthritis there may be joint deformity.

Exercise prescription

- *Frequency*: 3–5 sessions per week (but rest during RA exacerbations).
- *Intensity*: 60–75/80 per cent maximum heart rate.
- *Type*: mobility/strength work for range of movement and joint stability; low-impact work to avoid stress on joints; non-weightbearing if limited by pain to achieve CV prescription with minimal discomfort; postural alignment.
- *Time*: 20–30 minutes.

Respiratory conditions

These may include asthma, chronic bronchitis and emphysema. Presentation is different in each condition, although the common symptoms are breathlessness and increased work of breathing, with or without excessive sputum production.

Exercise prescription

- *Frequency*: 3–5 sessions per week.
- *Intensity*: based on RPE; assessment on SWT.
- *Type*: endurance work; based on activities of daily living; lower limb activity.
- *Time*: interval training of short duration; increased duration/frequency as able.

EXERCISE PRESCRIPTION AND DELIVERY ACROSS THE FOUR PHASES OF CARDIAC REHABILITATION

Phase I: Inpatient period

Activities for cardiac patients following acute MI or CABG do not typically exceed 2–3 METs in the early stages. These include general mobility exercises and activities of daily living such as standing, walking, dressing and personal hygiene. Before discharge, the patient is advised on progression of physical activity levels. Guidance on convalescence activities over the first 3–4 weeks, including written advice on 'do and don't' activities, should be provided; usually, an incremental walking programme is also given.

Phase II: Immediate post-discharge period

This period is usually between 2 and 6 weeks after discharge. Follow-up varies according to local protocols. Often this is a frightening time for the patient and his or her family, who may feel isolated after the close supervision and support provided in the hospital.

Although progression is individualised for each patient, Table 12.8 may serve as a basis for prescription. The patient should be advised on signs and symptoms of overexertion, chest pain management, timing of exercise (40–50 minutes after meal), and avoidance of temperature extremes.

Structuring exercise sessions

Staff: patient ratio
Room size
Temperature 65–72 degrees F
Humidity – close to 65 per cent
Staff training
Emergency drills.

Phase III: Supervised outpatient programme, including structured exercise

Structured exercise training during this phase is delivered either in hospital or in the community. Access to emergency facilities should be available. Training lasts for 6–12 weeks in most centres. The sessions should be delivered by professional staff with training in cardiology, exercise prescription and emergency procedures. Consideration should be given to the staff:patient ratio. (UK guidelines recommend 1 member of staff to 5 patients.)

Table 12.8 Incremental walking programme

Week	Borg CR-10 scale	Duration (mins)	Distance (yds)	Frequency (per day)
1	2–3	5	200	1–2
2	2–3	10	400–500	2
3	2–3	15	500–750	2
4	3	20	750–1250	1–2
5	3	25–30	1250–1750	1–2
6	3	30–40	1750–3000	1–2

The cardiac rehabilitation team who deliver the exercise sessions should all be trained in basic life support; one member of the team should preferably be trained in advanced life support. There should be access to an automated external defibrillator (AED) and the team should be trained to use it. All staff should have regular practice and updates on emergency drills.

An outcome measures assessment is shown in Table 12.9.

Phase IV: Long-term follow-up/maintenance in primary care

Patients are transferred to phase IV when medically stable and psychologically adjusted. They should have reached their exercise goals and should demonstrate the ability to exercise safely based on an individual exercise prescription and know how to recognise warning signs and symptoms and take appropriate action (that is, stop or reduce the exercise level; take glyceryl trinitrate, GTN).

The exclusion criteria for phase IV are:

- unstable angina
- testing systolic blood pressure > 180, diastolic blood pressure > 100
- significant drop in blood pressure
- uncontrolled tachycardia
- unstable or acute heart failure
- febrile illness.

Table 12.9 Outcome measures: assessment guideline

Functional capacity	Graded exercise test (SWT, CST)
Return to vocation	Work modification
Smoking cessation	Self-reported
Managed blood pressure	Regular average blood pressure recordings
Stress management	HAD scale, self-reported rating
Quality of life	Measure of multiple domains of quality of life
Lipids	Lipid profile
Weight control	Height, weight, BMI, waist:hip ratio

BMI = body mass index; CST = Chester step test; HAD = Hospital Anxiety and Depression Scale; SWT = shuttle walking test.

Discharge planning

Following completion of phase III of cardiac rehabilitation, all patients' individual long-term exercise plans are agreed and arrangements are made for transfer to phase IV. The patient is referred to the primary care service for monitoring of the risk factors. A patient may require further assessment: for example, if experiencing residual ischaemia. In such cases, appropriate cardiology referral and implications for exercise prescription are noted and explained to the patient. All patients should be given information about a long-term helpline and local cardiac support groups.

The cardiac rehabilitation pathway is shown in Figure 12.10.

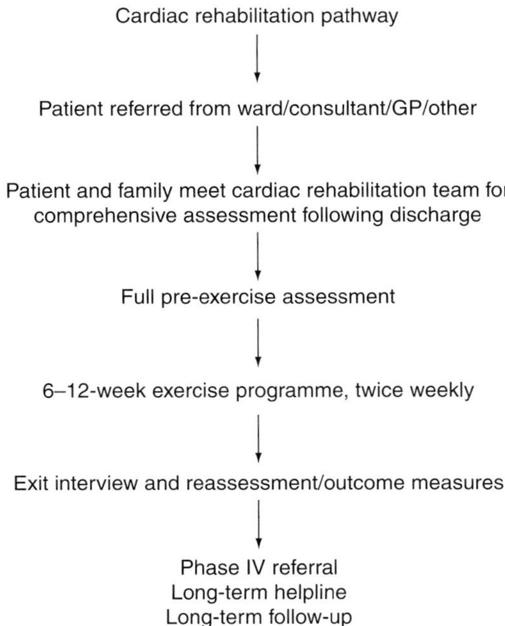

Figure 12.10 The cardiac rehabilitation pathway.

12

CONCLUSION

Comprehensive cardiac rehabilitation is a cost-effective intervention for patients with cardiac disease. The uptake of cardiac rehabilitation still remains low in those who need it most: that is, women, older adults and ethnic groups. Nationwide strategies need to be adopted to offer flexible, menu-driven cardiac rehabilitation packages to these special needs groups. Exercise-based cardiac rehabilitation confers several benefits, including improvement in functional capacity and secondary prevention. Exercise consultation is a vital intervention and should be available and incorporated in all phases of cardiac rehabilitation. Exercise intervention is a behavioural change and the rehabilitation team should utilise counselling skills and deploy strategies in order to promote long-term adherence to exercise and physical activity.

Weblink

www.aacvpr.org
www.ash.org.uk
www.bcs.com/bacr
www.bhf.org.uk
www.bhfactive.org.uk
www.cardiacrehabilitation.org.uk
www.csp.org.uk
www.dh.gov.uk
www.diabetes.org.uk
www.heartstats.org
www.sahf.org.uk
www.sign.ac.uk

PULMONARY REHABILITATION

BACKGROUND

Respiratory disease (meaning all respiratory diseases including lung cancer) is the fourth largest cause of death in the UK (British Heart Foundation 2006). Since 1984, death rates from CHD have steadily declined while death rates from respiratory disease have remained at the same level. For example, between 2002 and 2004, mortality from CHD was reduced by 10 per cent, whereas mortality from lung cancer and respiratory disease was reduced by only 1 per cent. About one-third of the UK population visit their GPs at least once a year with a respiratory condition. Chronic obstructive pulmonary disease (COPD) is the third biggest cause of respiratory death (pneumonia and lung cancer being first and second respectively). According to the Global Burden of Disease study, COPD is projected to be the fifth leading cause of DALY loss worldwide by 2020, behind CHD, major depression, road traffic accidents and cardiovascular disease. The economic and community burden of COPD is shocking. These data call for an urgent need to improve the health status of patients with COPD so that they can achieve optimal functional status and remain productive members of community for as long as possible.

The majority of people with chronic respiratory disability suffer from COPD. Surveys of people with chronic lung disease show that 90 per cent of it is due to chronic airflow limitation. There are approximately 600 000 people with COPD in the UK, most of who present to their doctors with symptoms after the age of 40. Prevalence is beginning to equalise in men and women, and rises with age; in 2000, it was 5 per cent in men aged between 65 and 75, increasing to 10 per cent in men over 75 years. Older patients are likely to suffer multiple disability.

Why rehabilitate patients with chronic respiratory disease?

The predominant symptom of respiratory disease is dyspnoea or breathlessness. Breathlessness is an awareness of the intensity of breathing. Healthy individuals feel breathless on exercise due to increased work of breathing. Dyspnoea is the perception of extreme and unpleasant breathlessness. In other words, dyspnoea is difficult breathing occurring at a level of activity where it would not normally be accepted. It leads to anxiety and fear; fear of becoming breathless leads to inactivity, and this leads to muscle weakness and deconditioning. This in turn will lead to cardiovascular deconditioning, resulting in a further increase in breathlessness. Thus a spiral of inactivity sets in (Figure 12.11). Patients with COPD suffer with a high level of disability and many who experience dyspnoea during normal household chores require help with activities of daily living.

Chronic respiratory disease is characterised by multisystemic effects of illness, such as peripheral muscle weakness, body composition abnormalities and compromised self-management strategies. Patients with COPD report leg fatigue as a symptom that limits their walking. Peripheral muscle weakness in COPD is thought to be due to a combination of inactivity and the systemic effects of chronic hypoxia, hypercapnia, poor nutrition and damage from corticosteroid therapy (see Chapter 10 for more detailed information). COPD is now acknowledged as a disease with systemic effects.

Key point

Activity limitation, secondary breathlessness and peripheral muscle weakness are persistent features of chronic respiratory disease, even when the disease is stable.

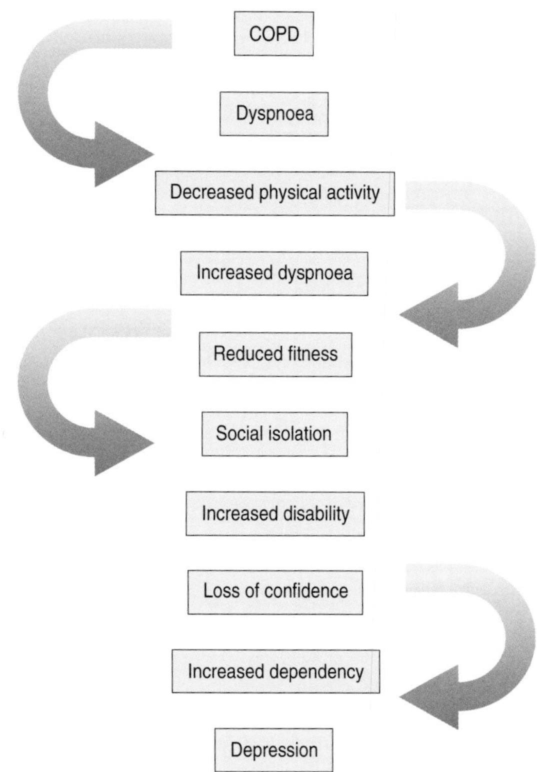

Figure 12.11 Spiral of inactivity in patients with COPD.

WHAT IS PULMONARY REHABILITATION?

In 1999, the American Thoracic Society defined pulmonary rehabilitation as 'a multidisciplinary programme of care for patients with chronic respiratory impairment that is individually tailored and designed to optimise physical and social performance and autonomy'.

A more recent definition proposed by the American Thoracic Society and the European Respiratory Society is as follows: 'It is evidence-based multidisciplinary and comprehensive intervention for patients with respiratory diseases who are symptomatic and often have decreased daily life activities. Integrated into the individualized treatment of the patient, pulmonary rehabilitation is designed to reduce symptoms, optimize functional status, increase participation and reduce healthcare costs through stabilizing or reversing systematic manifestations of the disease.'

The following definition, formulated by the National Institute of Health in 1994 recognises the role of family participation and an interdisciplinary approach to rehabilitation.

Definition

'Pulmonary rehabilitation is a multidisciplinary continuum of services directed to persons with pulmonary disease and their families, usually by an interdisciplinary team of specialists, with the goal of achieving and maintaining the individual's maximum level of independence and functioning in the community' (Cole and Fishman 1994).

General principles of pulmonary rehabilitation

British Thoracic Society (BTS) guidelines (2001) state:

- The goals of rehabilitation are to reduce symptoms and disability and to improve functional independence in people with lung disease.
- Optimum medical management should be achieved or continued alongside the rehabilitation process.
- The rehabilitation process incorporates a programme of physical training, education, and nutritional, psychological, social and 'behavioral intervention.
- Rehabilitation is provided by a multidisciplinary team with involvement of the patient's family and attention to individual needs.
- The outcome of rehabilitation for individuals and programmes should be continually observed with the appropriate measures of impairment, disability and handicap.

12

RESEARCH EVIDENCE FOR PULMONARY REHABILITATION

Evidence for pulmonary rehabilitation is very well established and extensive. Although many studies have focused on patients with COPD, the BTS guidelines (2001) recommend that pulmonary rehabilitation should be available to all patients with chronic respiratory disease who are limited by chronic breathlessness. The benefits of pulmonary rehabilitation include improvement in functional capacity, reduction in sensation of dyspnoea or breathlessness, improvement in health status and quality of life, and a reduction in the usage of health services.

The BTS guidelines and the CSP report on the effectiveness of pulmonary rehabilitation (CSP 2003) give a detailed account of the evidence for the various components of pulmonary rehabilitation. Below is an outline of the levels of evidence for these various aspects. Levels of evidence and grading of recommendations, as described by the National Institute for Clinical Excellence (NICE), are shown in Tables 12.10 and 12.11.

Table 12.10 Levels of evidence and grading of recommendations

Level	Type of evidence
Ia	Meta-analysis of randomised controlled trials
Ib	At least one randomised controlled trial
IIa	At least one well-designed controlled study without randomisation
IIb	At least one other type of well-designed quasi-experimental study
III	From well-designed non-experimental descriptive studies
IV	Expert committee reports of opinions and/or clinical experiences of respected authorities

Table 12.11 Grades of evidence

Grade	Level	Criterion
A	Ia, Ib	Requires at least one randomised controlled trial
B	IIa, IIb, III	Well-conducted clinical studies but no randomised controlled trial
C	IV	Expert committee reports or opinion; indicates absence of directly applicable studies of good quality

Exercise component of pulmonary rehabilitation

- Improvements in functional exercise capacity (level Ia).
- Improvements in functional exercise capacity maintained between 6 and 12 months (level IIb).
- Reduction in the sensation of dyspnoea (level Ia).
- Improvement in peripheral muscle strength and mass (level Ib).
- Reduction in anxiety and depression (level IIb).
- Improvement in health-related quality of life (level Ia).
- Improvement in the ability to perform routine activities of daily living (level IIb).

Psychosocial component of pulmonary rehabilitation

Further research is required to evaluate the impact of physical training and/or psychosocial interventions on mood state. Reduction in anxiety and depression is reported in many studies.

Educational component of pulmonary rehabilitation

Clinical and expert opinion (level IV evidence) suggests that an educational and behavioural component is of value to reinforce and enhance long-term exercise behaviour.

Adjuncts to pulmonary rehabilitation

Non-invasive positive pressure ventilation (NIPPV)

Respiratory muscle support by non-invasive ventilation may have a role in pulmonary rehabilitation. There is some evidence that nocturnal domiciliary administration of NIPPV can augment the effects of rehabilitation in patients with severe COPD. NIPPV administered during exercise training augments exercise tolerance and reduces breathlessness. The evidence for the use of NIPPV as an adjunct to pulmonary rehabilitation is currently at level Ib.

Supplemental oxygen

There is some evidence (level Ib) that patients who desaturate on exercise will benefit from use of supplemental oxygen. A reduction in the sensation of breathlessness is reported.

Respiratory muscle training

Inspiratory muscle strength may be reduced in some patients with COPD. Training the respiratory muscles can improve strength and endurance, but this appears to be task-specific and the effects do not have an impact on overall disability. The level of evidence is currently at level IIb and is inconclusive.

Neuromuscular electrical stimulation (NMES)

The use of NMES as part of a home-based pulmonary rehabilitation programme has recently been developed to improve functional exercise capacity and peripheral muscle strength and reduce the sensation of breathlessness. This may prove to have particular value for severely disabled housebound patients with COPD who respond poorly to aerobic training programmes. Early evidence is at level Ib.

Physiotherapy, relaxation and energy conservation

Physiotherapy advice on sputum clearance, breathing retraining techniques and relaxation is found useful. Energy conservation techniques and practical planning by an occupational therapist also form a part of many pulmonary rehabilitation programmes. Poor nutrition often accompanies advanced lung disease and some patients may be obese. Nutritional advice and intervention may be useful to both groups of patients. However, further research is required in all these areas.

Reduction in the usage of health services

There are reductions in exacerbations (level IIb) and in the number of days spent in hospital (level Ib) with a pulmonary rehabilitation programme. There is strong evidence at level Ia to demonstrate that pulmonary rehabilitation is a cost-effective therapy (level Ia).

PATIENT GROUPS IN PULMONARY REHABILITATION

In the past 10 years it has become increasingly clear, both to clinicians and to patients, what can be expected from pulmonary rehabilitation, although the benefits have been recognised for many years. It is now well known that peripheral muscle weakness and deconditioning contribute a great deal to symptoms and that pulmonary rehabilitation programmes improve the functional capacity and health status of COPD patients.

Pulmonary rehabilitation may therefore benefit all patients whose lifestyle is adversely affected by chronic breathlessness and fatigue, and also those with chronic asthma, bronchiectasis and pulmonary fibrosis. Further research is required to investigate the effect of pulmonary rehabilitation and also to establish how programmes and service delivery will need to be modified in the future.

PROVISION IN THE UK AND ITS COST-EFFECTIVENESS

In 2002 the British Lung Foundation (BLF) and the BTS carried out a survey to produce a comprehensive list of the current provision of services and to establish how widespread these services were. It was found that:

- 160 hospitals/chest clinics provide some form of pulmonary rehabilitation.
- Around 57 per cent of these programmes receive secure funding, while 10 per cent receive no NHS funding.
- Only 15 per cent of programmes provide access to 100 patients or more per year.
- One-third of established programmes are unable to provide an adequate number of physical training sessions.
- About 36 per cent of these programmes provide follow-on care for patients once their pulmonary rehabilitation has been completed.
- Around 44 per cent of programmes have a BLF Breathe Easy group either attached to the hospital or running within the immediate area that patients may attend.

The clinical effectiveness of pulmonary rehabilitation is well established but the cost:benefit ratio depends on the setting. Inpatient programmes tend to increase the overall cost of care. Health benefits produced by pulmonary rehabilitation are cost-effective: that is, they reduce the number of consultations, hospital admissions and length of stay in the hospital. The evidence totally justifies the widespread investment in a pulmonary rehabilitation service. The need for the service is evident and the demand is substantial, yet the capacity to provide the service remains poor (BTS 2002). The proposed development of a National Service Framework for COPD will result in new quality requirements and markers of good practice.

COMPONENTS OF PULMONARY REHABILITATION

Exercise training

This includes in-depth exercise assessment, as well as assessment of dyspnoea, strength training and endurance training.

Education

12

This typically includes:

- anatomy, physiology, pathology and medication (including oxygen therapy)
- dyspnoea/symptom management, chest clearance techniques
- energy conservation/pacing
- nutritional advice
- managing travel
- anxiety management
- goal setting and rewards
- relaxation
- identifying and changing beliefs about exercise and health-related behaviours
- loving relationships/sexuality
- management of exacerbations
- benefits of physical exercise.

Psychosocial and behavioural intervention

Psychological and behavioural intervention is set within the context of rehabilitation programmes through the delivery of education, small group discussions and relaxation therapy. Anxiety and depression, when present, can be improved by rehabilitation. Psychological assessment may prove beneficial in the assessment of motivation since identification of readiness to change may improve compliance with physical training and smoking cessation.

Operation and delivery

Setting or location

Pulmonary rehabilitation is effective in all settings, including hospital inpatient departments, hospital outpatient departments, the community and the home. Hospital outpatient rehabilitation is currently the most efficient form of delivery. The BLF survey (2002) found 80 per cent of programmes in the UK were based in hospital and 9 per cent were community-based. Home programmes promote compliance and longer-term benefits. They also are beneficial for severe COPD patients and relate and focus on the more meaningful daily activities. The disadvantages are the need for supervision specially related to intensity of exercise, lack of peer group support and lower cost-effectiveness for moderate COPD patients. As with cardiac rehabilitation, the location should be determined by patient's needs.

Programme duration and frequency

12

BTS guidelines recommend a minimum of 6 weeks of physical exercise, disease education, and psychological and social intervention for outpatient programmes. The programmes vary between 6 and 12 weeks in duration. The majority of programmes have shown effective change after 6–8 weeks. In the BLF survey it was found that 89 per cent of programmes ran between 6 and 8 weeks. Although improvements in exercise tolerance deteriorate by 12 months, improvements in health-related quality of life appear to persist and are still clinically relevant at 12 months post-rehabilitation.

There is also some evidence that commencing early pulmonary rehabilitation, in the recovery period after hospital discharge after an admission for an acute exacerbation of COPD, leads to significant improvements in functional capacity and quality of life at 3 months, compared with usual care.

Safety issues

For accurate exercise prescription and oxygen needs, a field walking test (monitoring pulse oximetry and heart rate) prior to enrolment in the exercise programme is necessary. Patients need to be assessed against the exclusion criteria, which are:

- unstable angina
- acute left ventricular failure
- uncontrolled hypertension
- uncontrolled cardiac arrhythmias
- medical problems that will severely restrict the ability to exercise, e.g. stroke, arthritis.

In the hospital setting, access to resuscitation equipment and availability of oxygen, along with trained staff who know how to use the equipment, are necessary.

The BTS guidelines recommend that simple first aid medication is available (oxygen, nebulised bronchodilators and GTN), although the back-up of the hospital cardiac arrest team is probably unnecessary. All staff supervising the exercise programme should be trained in basic life support. The minimum staff:patient ratio should be 1:8. The risks must be assessed in all groups when deciding staffing levels, taking into consideration the setting and available help in an emergency, the level of training of the staff, the availability of emergency equipment and the health of the patients.

Supplemental oxygen during exercise training

According to the BTS guidelines, patients who are on long-term oxygen therapy (LTOT) should exercise with supplemental oxygen. Supplementary oxygen should be provided during exercise when clinically important desaturation (SpO_2 < 90 per cent) has been found at the training load in the preliminary test. Clearly, once ambulatory oxygen is recommended for training, then it should be continued for similar activity at home, in line with recent guidelines from the Royal College of Physicians (1999).

Pulmonary rehabilitation team

The holistic nature of pulmonary rehabilitation essentially requires a multidisciplinary, interprofessional approach. Members of the team include physiotherapist and occupational therapist, respiratory nurses and doctors, dietitian and clinical psychologist (Figure 12.12). Strong links with the social worker and other members of the community team are vital for a seamless

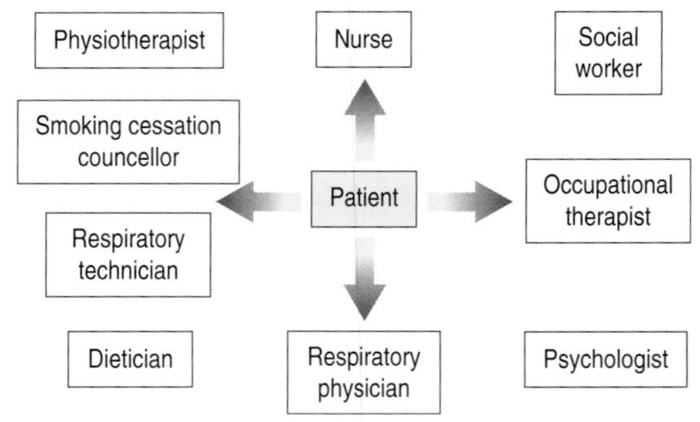

Figure 12.12 The pulmonary rehabilitation team.

delivery of the programme. The BTS suggests that a nominated clinician with an interest in respiratory disease should be responsible for the programme. This clinician should normally be responsible for medical assessment prior to the patient's entry into the programme. The programme should have a responsible officer appointed for the purpose. The coordinator may come from a profession allied to medicine or nursing. Team members should be involved in all aspects of programme delivery. Some blurring of specialist roles is to be expected in the provision of care such as pulmonary and cardiac rehabilitation. Appropriate training in different aspects of rehabilitation, teamwork and excellent communication ensure a seamless service and optimise the benefits for the patient.

The role of the physiotherapist

Exercise training, clearly within the scope of practice for physiotherapists, is identified as an integral component of pulmonary rehabilitation. Thus physiotherapists are ideally placed to play a major part in the provision of pulmonary rehabilitation.

> ***Key point***
>
> Respiratory physiotherapists work with people with breathing disorders, whether they are acute or long-term patients. In managing chronic disorders the focus is often on physical fitness within the limitations of the condition and on coping with breathlessness. In more acute pathologies, then, consideration of the physiology of the whole body is used to maximise the transport of oxygen from the lungs to the tissues (Association of Chartered Physiotherapists in Respiratory Care, ACPRC).

PHYSIOLOGICAL ADAPTATIONS TO EXERCISE TRAINING

Cardiovascular adaptations

As described in earlier in this chapter in relation to cardiac rehabilitation, the physiological adaptations at submaximal levels of exercise that are seen in healthy individuals can also be translated in patients with COPD, provided training intensity is submaximal (60–85 per cent of heart rate maximum). Peripheral and central adaptations are attainable with high-intensity training. However, patients with severe airflow limitation will not be able to exercise at high intensities.

Improvement in functional capacity

Many of the improvements brought about by exercise are likely to be due to enhanced mechanical efficiency, which includes better stride length and gait coordination. To achieve physiological effects with a low-intensity training programme, a longer period of time (a home programme lasting up to a year) may be necessary.

ASSESSMENT FOR EXERCISE PRESCRIPTION

12

As for cardiac rehabilitation, a detailed history of the present condition and clinical presentation, previous levels of activity and exercise, physical limitations and disabilities, and signs and symptoms forms an essential part of the assessment. Baseline measurements such as pulse, oxygen saturation, blood pressure, temperature, spirometry and bodyweight should be noted (Figure 12.13).

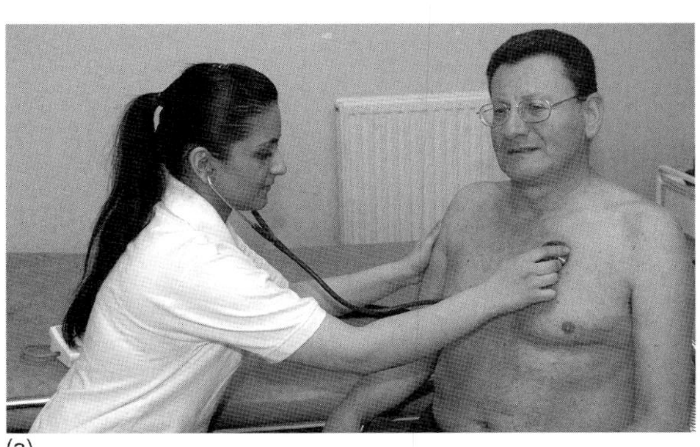
(a)

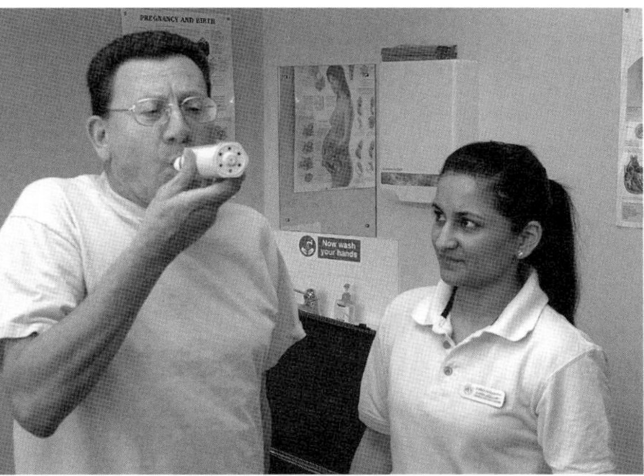

(b)

Figure 12.13 Physiotherapist assessing a respiratory patient for pulmonary rehabilitation.

Assessment of functional capacity

A patient's functional exercise capacity should be assessed to ascertain training intensity, to plan an individually tailored exercise programme and to motivate the patients to continue with their training regimes. It also helps to review the benefits of the exercise programme.

Field exercise tests (FETs)

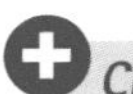

Clinical note

Field exercise tests are submaximal simple tests, which are easy to administer and which use an exercise mode relevant to everyday activities. Submaximal exercise tests can be used to predict $VO_{2\ max}$, to make a diagnosis, to assess functional limitations and to monitor the outcome of interventions such as exercise programmes.

There are two main categories of field test: those that are self-paced and those in which the speed of activity is imposed. These tests have been used increasingly to evaluate different forms of intervention in respiratory medicine and more recently in cardiology. Reproducibility, validity and responsiveness[3] of these tests in some respiratory and cardiac patient groups have been researched. (The term 'reproducibility' refers to the stability of a test when no important change in health has occurred. Responsiveness is the sensitivity of a measure to a clinically relevant change in health. Validity refers to the extent to which a test measures what it is intended to measure. A test is validated when it shows a statistically significant correlation with the gold standard test for a particular physiological variable.)

Self-paced field tests

In the *6-minute and 12-minute walking tests* (6 MWT or 12 MWT), functional exercise capacity is expressed in metres covered by the patient in 6 or 12 minutes. They are usually performed in a corridor with a known track length. Patients are instructed to cover as many metres as possible in the scheduled time. Rest periods are allowed during the test if necessary, and patients are instructed to restart and change the walking speed. The distance covered, heart rate, oxygen saturation and the Borg scale for rating of perceived breathlessness can be obtained throughout the test. The test requires a number of practice walks. It also depends on how motivated the patient is, so lacks standardisation. A change of 54 metres has been suggested as the minimum needed for clinical significance in a properly conducted 6 MWT: that is, for either an improvement or a deterioration in functional exercise capacity.

Externally paced field exercise tests

This type of FET imposes a pace on the patient that reduces the effect of motivation and encouragement.

The *shuttle walk test* (SWT, Figures 12.14 and 12.15) is an incremental externally paced test that stresses the patient to a symptom-limited maximum. The patient walks around a 10-metre course defined by two marker cones (Figure 12.16). The speed of walking is dictated by bleeps played on a cassette recorder and increases every minute until the patient is unable to keep up due to breathlessness and fatigue. The walking distance correlates well with $VO_{2\ max}$. Measurements of heart rate and Borg scores of breathlessness may be obtained throughout the test. A clinical threshold value for the incremental SWT has not yet been identified, although changes in the region of 30–55 per cent have been reported following rehabilitation.

The 12MWT and SWT are compared in Table 12.12.

EXERCISE PRESCRIPTION

Aerobic training

As for the cardiac population, exercise training for pulmonary rehabilitation patients follows the same FITT principle: that is, frequency, intensity, time and type of exercise.

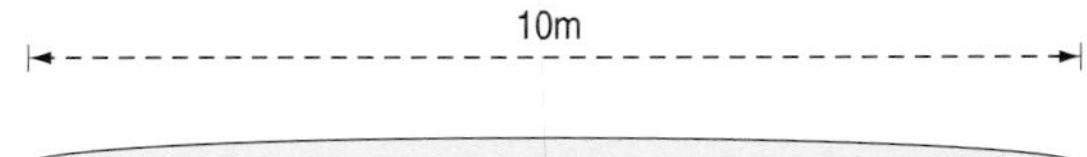

Figure 12.14 The shuttle walk test (SWT).

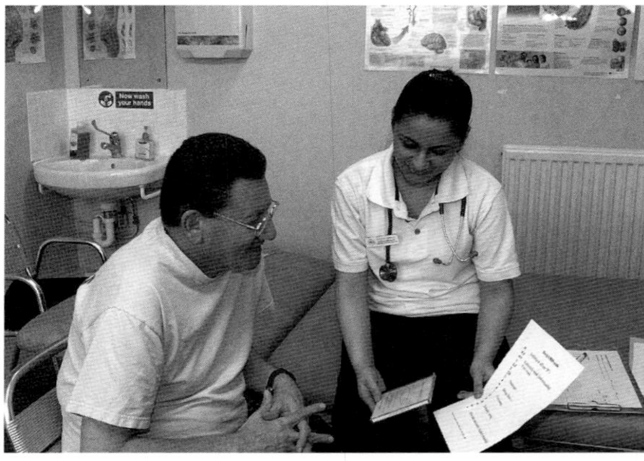

Figure 12.15 Physiotherapist explaining the SWT to a patient.

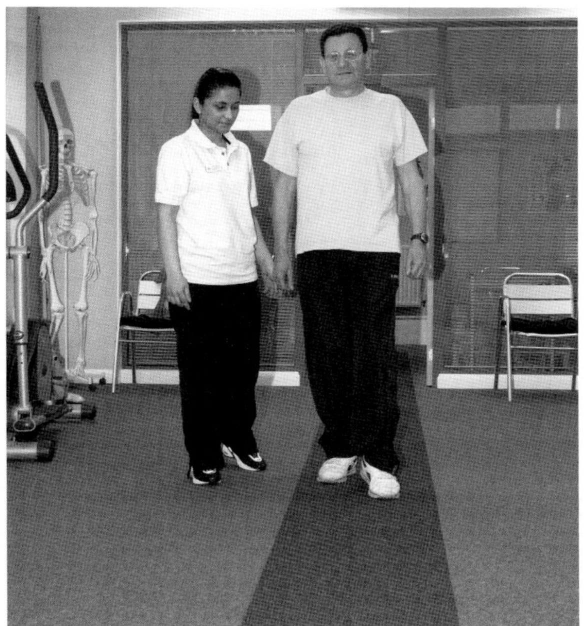

Figure 12.16 The patient walking the 10 metre course.

Training intensity is individualised, based on the results of the SWT or 12MWT. A minimum of 60 per cent and up to 85 per cent of the maximal exercise capacity walk should be used.

High-intensity exercises can be prescribed for patients with moderate obstruction. Breathlessness is affected more by increases in exercise intensity than by duration. Patients with severe COPD will require supervised low-intensity exercises. Intensity is monitored using the BORG scale of breathlessness (see earlier in this chapter), heart rate, and patient signs and symptoms. The period of aerobic exercise should last for 20 minutes. A warm-up must precede the aerobic component.

Progression is best achieved initially by increasing the duration of exercise. Two or three sessions per week are recommended. Home exercise planning and diaries should be given to enhance compliance. The recommended programme duration to achieve an effective change from aerobic training varies between 6 and 12 weeks.

Patients with COPD often report difficulty with tasks involving the upper limbs. Studies have shown that both upper and lower limb training should be performed and that the addition of upper limb training may be helpful in reducing breathlessness. Upper extremity exercise — for example, unsupported arm exercise using weights — may therefore be a useful addition.

As functional exercises form an integral part of pulmonary rehabilitation, the equipment required is simple and dependent upon local resources. For endurance training, hand weights, exercise mats, Therabands and equipment such as an exercise bike and a treadmill may be useful (Figures 12.17 and 12.18).

Table 12.12 Comparison of 12 MWT and SWT

12 MWT	SWT
Self-paced	Externally paced
Requires 3 practice walks	Requires 1 practice walk
Submaximal test	Maximal test limited by symptoms
Weak correlation with $VO_{2\ max}$	Correlates well with $VO_{2\ max}$
Variable depending on patient motivation	Standardised
No equipment required	Requires tape and cassette player
Clinical threshold identified to measure change	No clinical threshold identified

Strength training

Demonstrable skeletal muscle weakness is present even in mild COPD and this can be improved by training. Low-intensity peripheral muscle training is beneficial and training is achievable without injury. Unloaded repetitions may allow severely disabled patients to begin training. The addition of strength training to aerobic exercise improves muscle bulk and strength but does not improve whole-body exercise performance or health status beyond that achieved by aerobic exercise alone.

The principle followed in strength training of specific muscle groups is repetition of isotonic contractions against a fixed weight: usually 60–80 per cent of the maximum weight tolerated by the patient in a single contraction tested by the physiotherapist. A set of ten repetitions can be performed three times with a rest period between sets. Functional strength training — for example, using the individual's own bodyweight as resistance — is implemented in many programmes. The exercises must be preceded by a stretching regime to prevent injuries to muscles, ligaments and tendons.

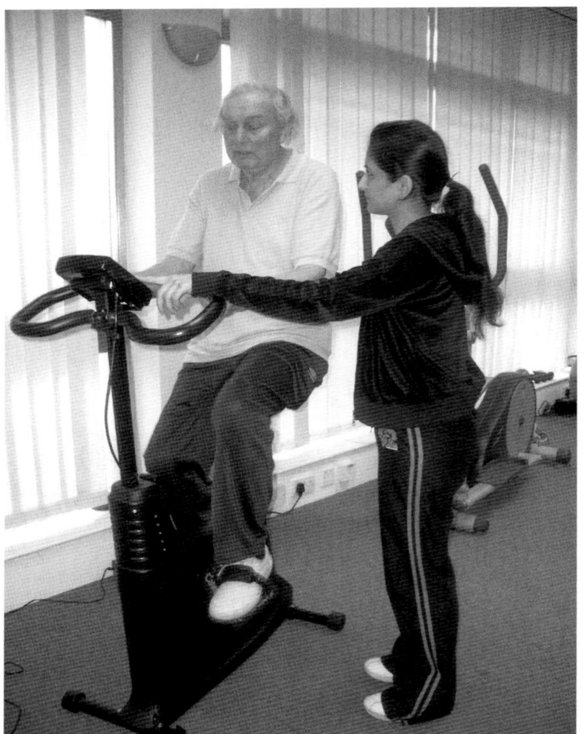

Figure 12.17 Physiotherapist helping a patient to set training intensity on an exercise bike.

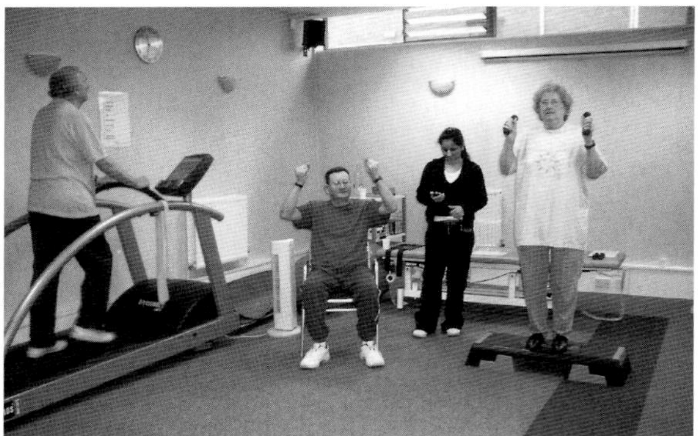

Figure 12.18 Pulmonary rehabilitation group.

Respiratory muscle training

Inspiratory muscle strength may be reduced in some patients with COPD. Training the respiratory muscles can improve strength and endurance, but this appears to be task-specific and the effects do not have an impact on overall disability or handicap. For the present, BTS guidelines do not recommend respiratory muscle training as an essential component of rehabilitation. Respiratory muscle support by non-invasive ventilation may have a role in rehabilitation. Although for most patients exercise alone will be sufficient to achieve functional improvement, for more severely disabled patients or those awaiting lung transplant surgery the addition of NPPV may augment benefit.

ASSESSMENT OF DYSPNOEA

Repeated trials of rehabilitation that incorporates an element of exercise training have shown improvement in dyspnoea using validated measures. There is strong evidence at level Ia to demonstrate that pulmonary rehabilitation programmes that incorporate an exercise component have a beneficial effect on dyspnoea in patients with COPD. Aerobic training with peripheral muscle training confers significant relief of dyspnoea and is associated with improvements in health-related quality of life.

12

Dyspnoea can be measured using graded tools such as the Medical Research Council (MRC) breathlessness score. This is a self-administered scale applied during walking. It grades patients into five levels, grade 5 being for patients considered to be housebound due to breathlessness. The Borg scale of perceived breathlessness and the visual analogue scale (VAS) are the other tools commonly used in pulmonary rehabilitation.

Management of dyspnoea

Pulmonary rehabilitation aims to reduce the perception of dyspnoea through a variety of strategies: increased mechanical efficiency of muscles as a result of training, improved breathing techniques and psychosocial intervention. Physiotherapists deploy techniques such as breathing retraining, which can incorporate diaphragmatic breathing or pursed lip breathing, depending on the severity of COPD.

Dyspnoea is associated with anxiety and fear, which further worsens disability. Relaxation techniques may be beneficial in relieving anxiety, as long as patients are able to apply these techniques to their activities of daily living. An interprofessional approach from the psychologist, respiratory nurse, occupational therapist and physiotherapist would be key to successful implementation of this aspect of pulmonary rehabilitation.

Positioning to relieve breathlessness is taught during the programme and should be translated into meaningful changes in functional activities.

Neuromuscular electrical stimulation is a new area of development for patients with severe COPD.

ASSESSMENT OF ACTIVITIES OF DAILY LIVING (ADL)

Currently one of the following tools is used:

- London Chest Activity of Daily Living Scale
- Manchester Respiratory Activities of Daily Living Questionnaire
- Pulmonary Functional Status and Dyspnoea Questionnaire.

Training in ADL

One of the primary goals of pulmonary rehabilitation is training patients to manage their ADL. Occupational therapists aim to promote economy of movement and effort by teaching pacing, coping skills, work efficiency and time management. By educating patients about their posture, reorganising their work areas and providing simple aids — for example, a perching stool and bath aids — therapists can enable patients to achieve more of their daily routine activities with less effort.

ASSESSMENT OF HEALTH-RELATED QUALITY OF LIFE (HRQOL)

The nature and manifestations of chronic respiratory disease are multifaceted. Research has shown that health status and lung function do not correlate well. In other words, a patient with mild limitation in lung function may still have poor quality of life as a result of limitations imposed by acute dyspnoea. Thus there many tools are employed to deal with the issues associated with COPD.

The HRQoL tools vary from generic questionnaires, such as Short Form 36 (SF36), which measure a number of health-related issues but do not assess any single problem in depth. These forms do allow comparisons between groups of patients. Disease-specific questionnaires are designed to assess one particular problem or a set of related problems. They are used in quantifying health gain following an intervention.

The HRQoL questionnaires used in pulmonary rehabilitation are:

- St George's Hospital Respiratory Questionnaire (SGRQ)
- Chronic Respiratory Disease Questionnaire (CRDQ)
- Breathing Problems Questionnaire (BPQ).

OUTCOME MEASURES

The assessment tools — such as the 6MWT or SWT for functional exercise capacity, MRC breathlessness score for measurement of dyspnoea, the ADL questionnaire and HRQoL questionnaire described above — are also used to measure outcome.

Outcome measures may be simple, depending on the availability of local resources. The BTS recommends that they should reflect the goals of rehabilitation by examination of relevant impairment, disability, handicap and domestic activity.

LONG-TERM EFFECTS OF PULMONARY REHABILITATION

Regardless of the fact that improvements in exercise tolerance deteriorate by 12 months, improvements in HRQoL appear to persist at 12–24 months post-rehabilitation. Maintenance of benefits may depend upon a number of factors, such as patient motivation, disease deterioration, lifestyle change and possible frequency of exacerbations. Audit of the pulmonary rehabilitation programmes, including dropout numbers, is required to give a clearer picture of maintenance of benefits, as it could be true that only motivated and less ill patients participate in follow-up. The Standards in Pulmonary Rehabilitation endorsed by the ACPRC and BTS state that the minimum standard required is an annual audit of a representative sample of patients.

CONCLUSION

Pulmonary rehabilitation is a cost-effective, multidisciplinary intervention. Exercise training is an essential component and confers benefits such as improvement in exercise tolerance, reduction in the sensation of dyspnoea and improvement in HRQoL. Physiotherapists have an integral role in the provision of pulmonary rehabilitation, and this should be in the context either of the outpatient hospital setting or within the community. An education programme aimed at maximising the chance of long-term behavioural change should be included. The evidence justifies urgent investment in pulmonary rehabilitation services for patients with chronic respiratory disease.

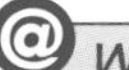

Weblinks

www.aacvpr.org
www.acprc.org
www.lunguk.org
www.brit-thoracic.org.uk
www.csp.org.uk
www.dh.gov.uk

FURTHER READING

Cardiac rehabilitation

American College of Sports Medicine 2006 ACSM's Guidelines for Exercise Testing and Prescription, 7th edn. Lippincott, Williams & Wilkins: Baltimore

Austin J, Williams R, Ross L et al. 2005 Randomized control trial of cardiac rehabilitation in elderly patients with heart failure. Eur J Heart Fail 7(3): 411–417

Bethell HJ, Turner SC, Evans JA, Rose L 2001 Cardiac rehabilitation in the United Kingdom. How complete is the provision? J Cardiopulm Rehabil 21(2): 111–115

Bjarnason-Wehrens B, Mayer-Berger W, Meister ER et al. 2004 Recommendations for resistance exercise in cardiac rehabilitation. Recommendations of the German Federation for Cardiovascular Prevention and Rehabilitation. Eur J Cardiovasc Prev Rehabil 11(4): 352–361

Dalal HM, Evans PH 2003 Achieving national service framework standards for cardiac rehabilitation and secondary prevention. BMJ 326: 481–484

De Bono DP 1998 Models of cardiac rehabilitation: Multidisciplinary rehabilitation is worthwhile, but how is it best delivered? BMJ 316(7141): 1329–1330

DuBach P, Myers J, Dziekan G et al. 1997 Effect of exercise training on myocardial remodelling in patients with reduced left ventricular function after myocardial infarction. Circulation 95: 2060–2067

European Heart Failure Training Group 1998 Experience from controlled trials of physical training in chronic heart failure. Protocol and patient factors in effectiveness in the improvement in exercise tolerance. Eur Heart J 19: 466–475

European Society of Cardiology 2001 Working Group Report: Recommendations for exercise testing in chronic heart failure patients. Eur Heart J 22(1): 37–45

ExTraMATCH Collaborative 2004 Exercise training meta-analysis of trials in patients with chronic heart failure. BMJ 328: 189

Fitchet A, Doherty PJ, Bundy C et al. 2003 Comprehensive cardiac rehabilitation programme for implantable cardioverter-defibrillator patients: a randomised controlled trial. Heart 89(2): 155–160

Franklin BA, Gordon S, Timmins GC 1992 Amount of exercise necessary for the patient with coronary artery disease. Am J Cardiol 69: 1426–1432

Goble AJ, Worcester MUC 1999 Best Practice Guidelines for Cardiac Rehabilitation and Secondary Prevention: A Synopsis. Heart Research Centre: Melbourne on behalf of Department of Human Services, Victoria

Haskell WL 1994 The efficacy and safety of exercise programs in Cardiac Rehabilitation. Med Sci Sports Exerc 26: 815–823

Hunt SA et al. 2005 ACC/AHA guideline update for the diagnosis and management of chronic heart failure in the adult: a report of the American College of Cardiology/American Heart Association Task Force on Practical Guidelines (Writing Committee to Update the 2001 Guidelines for the Evaluation and Management of Heart Failure). J Am Coll Cardiol 46(9): e1–e82

Kobashigawa JA, Leaf DA, Lee N et al. 1999 A controlled trial of exercise rehabilitation after heart transplantation. New Engl J Med 340(4): 272–277

McArdle WD, Katch FI, Katch VL 2001 Exercise Physiology: Energy, Nutrition and Human Performance, 5th edn. Lippincott, Williams & Wilkins: Baltimore, MA

Nieuwland W, Berkhuysen MA, Van Veldhuisen DJ et al. 2000 Differential effects of high-frequency versus low-frequency exercise training in rehabilitation of patients with coronary artery disease. J Am Coll Cardiol 36: 202–207

Oldridge NB 1998 Comprehensive cardiac rehabilitation: is it cost-effective? Eur Heart J 19(suppl O): 42–50

Pollock ML, Gaesser GA, Butcher JD et al. 1998 American College of Sports Medicine Position Stand. The recommended quantity and quality of exercise for developing and maintaining cardiorespiratory and muscular fitness, and flexibility in health adults. Med Sci Sport Exerc 30(6): 975–991

Rees K, Taylor RS, Singh S et al. 2004 Exercise based rehabilitation for heart failure. Cochrane Database Systematic Review (3): CD003331

Singh SJ, Morgan MCDL, Scott S et al. 1992 Development of a shuttle walking test of disability in patients with chronic airways obstruction. Thorax 47: 1019–1024

Smart N, Marwick TH 2004 Exercise training for patients with heart failure: a systematic review of factors that improve mortality and morbidity. Am J Med 116(10): 693–706

Stewart KJ, Badenhop D, Brubaker PH et al. 2003 Cardiac Rehabilitation following percutaneous revascularization, heart transplant, heart valve surgery, and for chronic heart failure. Chest 123: 2104–2111

Sykes K, Roberts A 2004 The Chester step test — a simple yet effective tool for the prediction of aerobic capacity. Physiotherapy 90: 183–188

Thow M 2006 Exercise Leadership in Cardiac Rehabilitation: An Evidence-Based Approach. John Wiley: Glasgow

Weiner DA, Ryan TJ, McCabe CH 1987 Value of exercise testing in determining the risk classification and the response to coronary artery bypass grafting in three-vessel coronary artery disease: a report from the Coronary Artery Surgery Study (CASS) registry. Am J Cardiol 60: 262–266

Williams MA 1994 Exercise Testing and Training in the Elderly Cardiac Patient. Current Issues in Cardiac Rehabilitation Series. Human Kinetics: Champaign, IL

Wood D, Durrington PN, Poulter N et al. 1998 Joint British Guidelines on prevention of coronary heart disease in clinical practice. Heart 80(suppl 2): 1–29

Zigmond AS, Snaith RP 1983 The Hospital Anxiety and Depression Scale. Acta Psychiatr Scand 67: 361–370

Pulmonary rehabilitation

Ambrosino N 1999 Field tests in pulmonary disease. Thorax 54: 191–193

12

American Association of Cardiovascular and Pulmonary Rehabilitation ACCP/AACVPR 1997 Pulmonary Rehabilitation Guidelines panel. Pulmonary rehabilitation. Joint ACCP/AACVPR Evidence-Based Guidelines. Chest 112: 1363–1396

Belman MJ, Botnick WC, Nathan SD et al. 1994 Ventilatory load characteristics during ventilatory muscle training. Am J Respir Crit Care Med 149(4): 925–929

Berry M, Norman A, Sevensky S et al. 1996 Inspiratory muscle training and whole body reconditioning in COPD. Am J Respir Crit Care Med 153: 1812–1816

Bestall JC, Paul EA, Garrod R et al. 1999 Usefulness of the Medical Research Council (MRC) dyspnoea scale as a measure of disability in patients with COPD. Thorax 54: 581–586

Cambach W, Chadwick-Straver RVM, Wagenaar RC et al. 1997 The effects of a community based pulmonary rehabilitation programme on exercise tolerance and quality of life: a randomised controlled trial. Eur Respir J 10: 104–113

Casaburi R, Patessio A, Ioli F et al. 1991 Reductions in exercise lactic acidosis and ventilation as a result of exercise training in patients with obstructive lung disease. Am Rev Respir Dis 143: 9–18

Chartered Society of Physiotherapy 2003 The Effectiveness of Pulmonary Rehabilitation: Evidence and Implications for Physiotherapists. CSP: London

Devito AJ 1990 Dyspnoea during hospitalisations for acute phase of illness as recalled by patients with COPD. Heart and Lung 19: 186–191

Gallefossis F, Bakke PS, Rsgaard PK 1999 Quality of life assessment after patient education in a randomized controlled study on asthma and chronic obstructive pulmonary disease. Am J Respir Crit Care Med 159: 812–817

Garrod R 1998 Pulmonary rehabilitation: the pros and cons of rehabilitation at home. Physiotherapy 84(12): 603–607

Garrod R 2004 Pulmonary Rehabilitation: An Interdisciplinary Approach. Whurr: London

Garrod R, Bestall JC, Paul EA et al. 2000 Development and validation of a standardized measure of activity of living in patients with severe COPD: the London Chest Activity of Daily Living Scale (LCADL). Respir Med 94(6): 589–596

Garrod R, Mikelsons C, Paul EA, Wedzicha JA 2000 Randomised controlled trial of domiciliary non-invasive positive pressure ventilation and physical training in severe chronic obstructive pulmonary disease. Am J Respir Crit Care Med 162(41): 1335–1341

Garrod R, Paul EA, Wedzicha JA 2000 Supplemental oxygen during pulmonary rehabilitation in patients with COPD and exercise hypoxaemia. Thorax 55: 539–543

Griffiths TL, Burr ML, Campbell IA et al. 2000 Results at 1 year of outpatient multidisciplinary pulmonary rehabilitation: a randomised control trial. Lancet 355: 362–368

Guyatt GH, Pugsley S, Sullivan MJ et al. 1984 Effect of encouragement on walking text performance. Thorax 39: 818–822

Guyatt GH, Townsend M, Berman L et al. 1987 A measure of quality of life for clinical trials in chronic lung disease. Thorax 42: 773–778

Kawane H 1997 Smoking cessation in comprehensive pulmonary rehabilitation. Lancet 349: 285

Keilty S, Ponte J, Fleming T et al. 1994 Effect of inspiratory pressure support on exercise tolerance and breathlessness in patients with severe stable COPD. Thorax 49: 990–994

Killian KJ, Leblanc P, Martin DH et al. 1992 Exercise capacity and ventilatory, circulatory and symptom limitation in patients with chronic airflow limitation. Am Rev Respir Dis 146: 935–940

Lacasse YL, Brosseau S, Milne S et al. 2005 Pulmonary rehabilitation for chronic obstructive pulmonary disease (Cochrane review). Cochrane Library Issue 1. John Wiley: Chichester

Lacasse YL, Guyatt GH, Goldstein RS 1997 The components of a respiratory rehabilitation programme. Chest 111: 1077–1088

Larson JL, Covey MK, Wirtz SE et al. 1999 Cycle ergometer and inspiratory muscle training in chronic obstructive pulmonary disease. Am J Respir Crit Care Med 160: 500–507

Man WDC, Polkey MI, Donaldson N et al. 2004 Community pulmonary rehabilitation after hospitalisation for acute exacerbations of chronic obstructive pulmonary disease: randomised controlled study. BMJ 324: 1209–1211

Marcus BH, Owen N 1992 Motivational readiness, self-efficacy and decision-making for exercise. Journal of Community & Applied Social Psychology 22: 3–16

McGavin CR, Artvinili M, Naoe H et al. 1978 Dyspnoea, disability and distance walked — comparison of estimates of exercise performance in respiratory disease. BMJ 2: 241–243

Neder JA, Sword D, Ward SA et al. 2002 Home based neuromuscular electrical stimulation as a new rehabilitative strategy for severely disabled patients with chronic obstructive pulmonary disease (COPD). Thorax 57: 333–337

Nici L 2005 Pulmonary Rehabilitation in the Treatment of Chronic Respiratory Disease. Business briefing: US Respiratory Care. Available from: www.touchbriefings.com/pdf/1132/Nici.pdf. Cited 10 February 07

O'Donnell DE 1994 Breathlessness in patients with chronic airflow limitation. Chest 106: 905–912

Polkey MI, Hawkins P, Kyroussis D et al. 2000 Inspiratory pressure support prolongs exercise induced lactataemia in severe COPD. Thorax 55: 547–549

Redelmeir D, Bayoumi A, Goldstein R et al. 1997 Interpreting small differences in functional status: the six minute walk test in chronic lung disease patients. Am J Respir Crit Care Med 155(4): 1278–1282

Revill SM, Morgan MDL, Singh SJ et al. 1999 The endurance shuttle walk: a new field test for the assessment of endurance capacity in chronic obstructive pulmonary disease. Thorax 54: 213–220

Ries AL, Kaplan RM, Limberg TM et al. 1995 Effects of pulmonary rehabilitation on physiologic and psychosocial outcomes in COPD. Ann Intern Med 122 (11): 823–831

Roomi J, Johnson MM, Waters K et al. 1996 Respiratory rehabilitation, exercise capacity and quality of life in chronic airways disease in old age. Age Ageing 25: 12–16

Salam GF, Mosier MC, Beasley BW et al. 2003 Rehabilitation for patients with chronic obstructive pulmonary disease: meta-analysis of randomised controlled trials. J Gen Intern Med 18: 213–221

Sinclair DJM, Ingram CG 1980 Controlled trial of supervised exercise training in chronic bronchitis. BMJ 280: 519–521

Singh SJ, Morgan MDL, Hardman AE et al. 1994 Comparison of oxygen uptake during a conventional treadmill test and shuttle walk test in chronic airflow limitation. Eur Respir J 7: 2016–2020

Singh SJ, Morgan MDL, Scott S et al. 1992 Development of a shuttle walking test of disability in patients with chronic airways obstruction. Thorax 47: 1019–1024

Van Ede L, Yzermans CJ, Brouwer HJ 1999 Prevalence of depression in patients with chronic obstructive pulmonary disease: a systematic review. Thorax 54: 688–692

Vogiatzis I, Williamson AF, Miles J et al. 1999 Physiologic responses to moderate exercise workloads in a pulmonary rehabilitation program in patients with varying degrees of airflow obstruction. Chest 116(5): 1200–1207

Wedzicha JA, Bestall JC, Garrod R et al. 1998 Randomised controlled trial of pulmonary rehabilitation in severe chronic obstructive pulmonary disease patients, stratified with the MRC scale. Eur Respir J 12: 363–369

Wijkstra PJ, Mark TW, Kraan J et al. 1996 Long term effects of home rehabilitation on quality of life and exercise tolerance in patients with chronic obstructive pulmonary disease. Thorax 50: 824–828

Wijkstra PJ, Mark TW, Kraan J et al. 1996 Long term effects of obstructive pulmonary disease. Am J Respir Crit Care Med 153: 1234–1241

Withers NJ, Rudkin ST, White RJ 1999 Anxiety and depression in severe chronic obstructive pulmonary disease: the effects of pulmonary rehabilitation. J Cardiopulm Rehabil 19: 362–365

REFERENCES

Cardiac rehabilitation

American Association of Cardiovascular and Pulmonary Rehabilitation 2006 Guidelines for Cardiac Rehabilitation and Secondary Prevention Programs, 5th edn. Human Kinetics: Champaign, IL

American College of Sports Medicine (ACSM) 2001 Resource Manual for Guidelines for Exercise Testing and Prescription, 4th edn. Williams & Wilkins: London

Borg GAV 1998 Borg's Perceived Exertion and Pain Scales. Human Kinetics: Champaign, IL

British Heart Foundation 2006 Health Professionals Research and Funding: Coronary Heart Disease Statistics: www.bhf.org.uk/professionals/index. Accessed 5 February 2007

Daub W, Knapik G, Black W 1996 Strength training early after myocardial infarction. J Cardiopulm Rehabil 16(2): 108–110

Jolliffe JA, Rees K, Taylor RS et al. 2004 Exercise-based rehabilitation for coronary heart disease. Cochrane Database for Systematic Reviews 1 (online): www.cochrane.org. Accessed 21 October 2006

National Service Framework 2000 Coronary Heart Disease: Modern Standards and Service models: www.doh.gov.uk/nsf/coronary.htm

NHS Centre for Reviews and Dissemination 1998 Effective Health Care Bulletin: Cardiac Rehabilitation. York: University of York

Scottish Intercollegiate Guidelines Network (SIGN) 2002 Cardiac rehabilitation, no. 57. SIGN: Edinburgh

Standards for the Exercise Component of Phase III Cardiac Rehabilitation 2006 ACPICR (www.csp.org.uk/director/groupandnetworks/ciogs/medicalrehabilitationgroups.cfm)

Williams B, Poulter NR, Brown MJ et al. 2004 British Hypertension Society guidelines for hypertension management (BHS-IV): summary. BMJ 328(7440): 634

World Health Organization 1993 Needs and Action Priorities in Cardiac Rehabilitation and Secondary Prevention in Patients with Coronary Heart Disease. WHO Regional Office for Europe: Geneva

World Health Organization (WHO) 2007 The Atlas of Heart Disease and Stroke. www.who.int/cardiovascular_diseases/resources/atlas/en/. Accessed 10 January 2007

Pulmonary rehabilitation

American Thoracic Society 1999 Pulmonary rehabilitation: an official statement. Am J Respir Crit Care Med 159: 1666–1682

American Thoracic Society and European Respiratory Society 1999 Skeletal muscle dysfunction in chronic obstructive pulmonary disease. Am J Respir Crit Care Med 159(4): S1–S40

Borg GA 1982 Psychophysical basis of perceived exertion. Med Sci Sports Exerc 14: 377–381

British Heart Foundation 2006 Health Professionals Research and Funding: Coronary Heart Disease Statistics: www.bhf.org.uk/professionals/index. Accessed 5 February 2007

British Lung Foundation 2002: www.lunguk.org/downloads/BLF_pul_rehab_survey.pdf

British Thoracic Society (BTS) 2001 British Thoracic Society Standards of Care Subcommittee on Pulmonary Rehabilitation. BTS Statement: Pulmonary Rehabilitation. Thorax 56: 827–834

British Thoracic Society 2002 Pulmonary Rehabilitation Survey (online): www.lunguk.org/downloads/BLF_pul_rehab_survey.pdf. Cited 13 February 2007

Chartered Society of Physiotherapy 2003 The effectiveness of pulmonary rehabilitation: evidence and implications for physiotherapists (online). Chartered Society of Physiotherapy: London: www.csp.org.uk/uploads/documents/evidencebrief_pulmonary_EB05.pdf. Cited 13 February 2007

Cole TM, Fishman AP 1994 Workshop on pulmonary rehabilitation research: a commentary. Am J Phys Med Rehabil 73(2): 132–133

National Institute of Health 1994 Pulmonary rehabilitation research. National Institute of Health workshop summary. Am Rev Respir Dis 48: 825–893

Royal College of Physicians 1999 Domiciliary oxygen therapy services: clinical guidelines and advice for prescribers. Report of a working party. London: Royal College of Physicians

APPENDIX: LONDON CHEST ADL SCORE

THE LONDON CHEST ACTIVITY OF DAILY LIVING SCALE

NAME...

DATE OF BIRTH...

DO YOU LIVE ALONE? YES ☐ NO ☐

Please tell us how breathless you have been during the last few days whilst doing the following activities.

SELF-CARE						
Drying	0	1	2	3	4	5
Dressing upper body	0	1	2	3	4	5
Putting shoes / socks on	0	1	2	3	4	5
Washing hair	0	1	2	3	4	5
DOMESTIC						
Making beds	0	1	2	3	4	5
Changing sheet	0	1	2	3	4	5
Washing windows / curtains	0	1	2	3	4	5
Cleaning / dusting	0	1	2	3	4	5
Washing up	0	1	2	3	4	5
Vacuuming / sweeping	0	1	2	3	4	5
PHYSICAL						
Walking up stairs	0	1	2	3	4	5
Bending	0	1	2	3	4	5
LEISURE						
Walking in home	0	1	2	3	4	5
Going out socially	0	1	2	3	4	5
Talking	0	1	2	3	4	5

How much does your breathing affect you in your normal activities of daily living?

A lot ☐ A little ☐ Not at all ☐

The London Chest Activity of Daily Living Scale (score sheet)

Please read carefully and circle the relevant number next to each activity.

This questionnaire is designed to find out whether there are activities that you can no longer do because of your breathlessness and how breathless the things that you still do make you. All answers are confidential.

If you do not do an activity because it is not relevant, or you have never done it, please answer:
0 – Wouldn't do anyway.

If an activity is easy for you, please answer:
1 – Do not get breathless.

If the activity makes you a bit breathless, please answer:
2 – I get moderately breathless.

If the activity makes you very breathless, please answer:
3 – I get very breathless.

If you have stopped doing this **because of your breathlessness** and ***have no one else to do it for you***, please answer:
4 – I can't do this anymore.

If someone else does this for you, or helps you, BECAUSE you are too breathless, e.g. The home help does your shopping, please answer:
5 – I need someone else to do this.

Chapter 13

Tissue inflammation and repair

Elaine N. Court and Robert W. Lea

CHAPTER CONTENTS

INTRODUCTION

Physiotherapists encounter inflammation or its consequences daily, and it can be considered as both a blessing and a curse. Without it, sprained ankles would never resolve and wounds would never heal, but if the inflammatory response is prolonged or out of proportion to the original injury or disease, that poses problems of its own. For example, it may result in excessive scar tissue, adhesions, prolonged pain and the loss of function so familiar to physiotherapists.

Key point

Inflammation is not just relevant to the sphere of musculoskeletal physiotherapy. A person who has sustained a head injury, has chronic bronchitis or has had a heart transplant will also experience the inflammatory process.

Knowledge of the process and clinical features of inflammation is vital for a physiotherapist to evaluate the degree or stage of a disease effectively. If a reasoned treatment plan is to be constructed, it must take into account the severity, nature and irritability of an injury (see Chapter 2). It is also useful for the physiotherapist to be able to reassure patients confidently that the symptoms they are experiencing are part of the normal healing process (for example, that all surgical scars will show some signs of inflammation).

Our knowledge of inflammation goes back thousands of years. Certainly the condition was well recognised by the Ancient Greeks and Romans. In fact, four components of inflammation described by Cornelius Celsius, a Roman physician in the first century AD, are still regarded as forming the classical clinical signs. These comprise 'calor', indicating heat (relevant primarily to inflammation of the skin); 'rubor', redness; 'dolor',

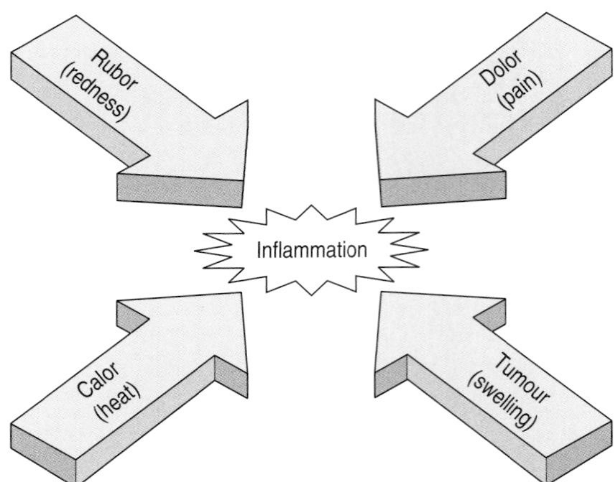

Figure 13.1 Components of inflammation.

pain; and 'tumor', swelling (Figure 13.1). These signs are indicative of the extravasation of plasma and infiltration of leucocytes at the site of inflammation. Later a fifth sign, described by Virchow as '*Functio laesa*' and relating to loss of function, was added.

If we humans are to survive, it is necessary for our bodies to maintain a constant internal environment: a process known as *homeostasis*. The environment, however, contains a multitude of potential dangers — biological, chemical and physical — which are likely to disrupt this delicate balance. As a result, via the process of evolution we have had to develop a complex defence mechanism against these potential insults, which is able to become activated and effective within seconds. A key component of this response is known by the term 'inflammation'.

Inflammation is the immune system's response to tissue damage. The processes involved will occur whether the damage is due to an exogenous source such as a cut or burn or to endogenous failures such as a bone fracture. The principal aim behind inflammation is to repair the tissue and bring it back to its original state.

Inflammation occurs in response to tissue damage, whatever that damage may be, so it is wrong to equate it with 'infection'. This is illustrated by the situations of stress or trauma, where there is no infection yet still inflammation occurs. Similarly, there are numerous situations where an infectious agent does not produce inflammation: for example, in Creutzfeldt–Jakob disease (CJD).

Inflammation has often been described as a complex stereotypical reaction of vascularised living tissue to local trauma. In those regions of the body that do not receive a full blood supply, such as the cornea, a true inflammatory response does not occur, though few would deny that inflammation can be present.

This chapter will describe the process involved in an inflammatory response and how it impacts upon the body. Bear in mind that, when it occurs for only a short period of time, inflammation is a very beneficial sequence of events for the body. Inflammation is an attempt to eliminate antigens and damaged tissue; indeed, in most instances it will probably be occurring without you having any real awareness of the situation. If, however, your body encounters an unusually large amount of antigen or that antigen either is difficult to digest or is sited within an awkward location, or alternatively, if the inflammatory process fails to terminate, then clinical inflammation can be observed.

These symptoms are easy to visualise if, for example, you have just damaged a finger. There are situations, however, where damage is less obvious and so the clinician will need to recognise a number of characteristic symptoms that indicate that a patient has inflammation. The pulse rate is increased, with an associated fever and feeling of general tiredness, and often there is the sensation of pain that is localised to the affected area. For example, in appendicitis the sufferer will experience pain in the right iliac fossa. Upon further investigation, blood tests will reveal a raised neutrophil cell count together with an increase in the concentration of acute-phase proteins (discussed later in this chapter).

TYPES OF INFLAMMATION

Key point

Inflammation is usually subdivided into two types: acute and chronic. The terms relate to the duration of the inflammation and to the nature of the inflammatory response.

Acute inflammation usually lasts for only a few hours to a few days. By the end of this time the accumulated fluid and degraded proteins in the extracellular spaces will have been drained by the lymphatic system, the phagocytic cells will have removed the exudates, debris and fibrin, and the inflammatory cells themselves will undergo cell death or 'apoptosis'. In this way the tissues return to normal. Acute inflammation may be seen, for example, following a surgical incision.

Chronic inflammation is characterised by a persistence of the inflammation, usually beyond 10–14 days, and is accompanied in most instances by fibrosis (the accumulation of synthesised collagen in the tissue). Chronic inflammation can occur, for instance, when the described resolution to the acute inflammatory process is not achieved, possibly through the causative agent not being removed; hence the inflammation becomes prolonged. Chronic inflammation can, however, arise as a low-grade inflammatory process without a preceding acute phase. Rheumatoid arthritis is an example of a chronic inflammatory condition.

ACUTE INFLAMMATION: THE MECHANISMS

Phases of acute inflammation

Three processes are responsible for producing the previously described symptoms involved in acute inflammation.

Firstly, there is a *vascular component* where there is a significant change in blood flow due to dilatation of blood vessels and consequently the amount of blood constituents reaching the affected site. The changes making up this vascular component were described in 1927 by Lewis and are known as the *Lewis triple response*. This flush, flare and wheal effect can be demonstrated by drawing a blunt instrument firmly across the skin (for convenience the forearm is often used) and watching the following sequence of events, which are similar, irrespective of the type of injury:

1. Instantly a white line forms following the 'injury'. This is due to vasoconstriction of the underlying arterioles as a direct response to the injury and is only transient. This vasoconstriction is not considered to be fully part of the inflammatory process.
2. There rapidly follows a flush, seen as a dull red line that occurs as the capillaries dilate. To the naked eye, the vasodilatation can give the impression that the affected tissue actually contains a greater number of blood vessels. This dilatation may last for as long as the inflammatory process persists.
3. An irregular red zone develops, called the flare. This occurs owing to the response of the surrounding arterioles, which have been affected by both nervous and chemical mediators.
4. A 'wheal' (a raised area of skin) develops due to the fluid passing out of the blood vessels and into the extravascular space, so leading to oedema.

Secondly (though it occurs at the same time as the above process), the endothelial cells that form the internal wall of the blood vessels retract such that they no longer form a completely continuous lining of the vessel. Consequently, the vessels become 'leaky' to the extent that fluid — namely, water and some of the salts and smaller proteins (one of these is fibrinogen) contained in plasma — may pass out directly into the extracellular spaces of the damaged area.

Thirdly, the fluid exudate becomes transformed into a cellular exudate. This is achieved through circulating neutrophils leaving the blood vessels and entering the extracellular spaces in the area of tissue damage. In the first 6–24 hours of an inflammatory response it is the neutrophils that predominate. After 24–48 hours they are superseded by monocytes and lymphocytes acting in a similar way.

Detailed consideration of acute inflammation

Initiating events

The tissue becomes physically damaged and may in addition become exposed to micro-organisms as a result of that damage. A complex sequence of events then occurs, in which various mediators are released in order to orchestrate the inflammatory response.

At the site of the tissue damage, three cytokines, interleukin (IL)-1α, tumour necrosis factor (TNF)α and IL-6, are released. These in turn cause the generation of the lipid mediator prostaglandin E_2 (PGE_2), which is believed to act on the hypothalamus, so leading to the rise in body temperature that is often seen with inflammation. This rise in body temperature inhibits the growth of many pathogens and appears to enhance the immune response to the pathogen.

Among the other chemical mediators released in response to tissue damage are various serum proteins known as *acute-phase proteins*. The concentrations of these proteins can increase from between 50 per cent to several-fold over normal levels when there are tissue-damaging infections present. Acute-phase proteins have a wide range of activities; they can neutralise inflammatory cells, help to minimise the extent of local tissue damage, and participate in tissue repair and regeneration. 13

A major acute-phase protein produced by the liver is C-reactive protein. C-reactive protein binds to the C-polysaccharide cell-wall component found on a variety of bacteria and fungi. This binding will activate the complement system (a series of inactive proteins normally present within the blood), which leads to an increased clearance of the pathogen. Other acute-phase proteins include components of the complement cascade and fibrinogen, along with some metal-binding proteins that act to prevent iron loss during infection and injury and additionally minimise the level of haem iron available for uptake by bacteria.

Events at the site of damage

The initial response of the arterioles is vaso*constriction*, but this is transient and the major influence on the circulation is that of vaso*dilatation*. Vasodilatation can be induced by the activation of complement, so leading to the production of the anaphylatoxins C3a and C5a (Figure 13.2).

As mentioned earlier, IL-1α, TNFα and IL-6 are released from the damaged tissue. These, along with released histamine and other mediators, induce vasodilatation and increased capillary permeability.

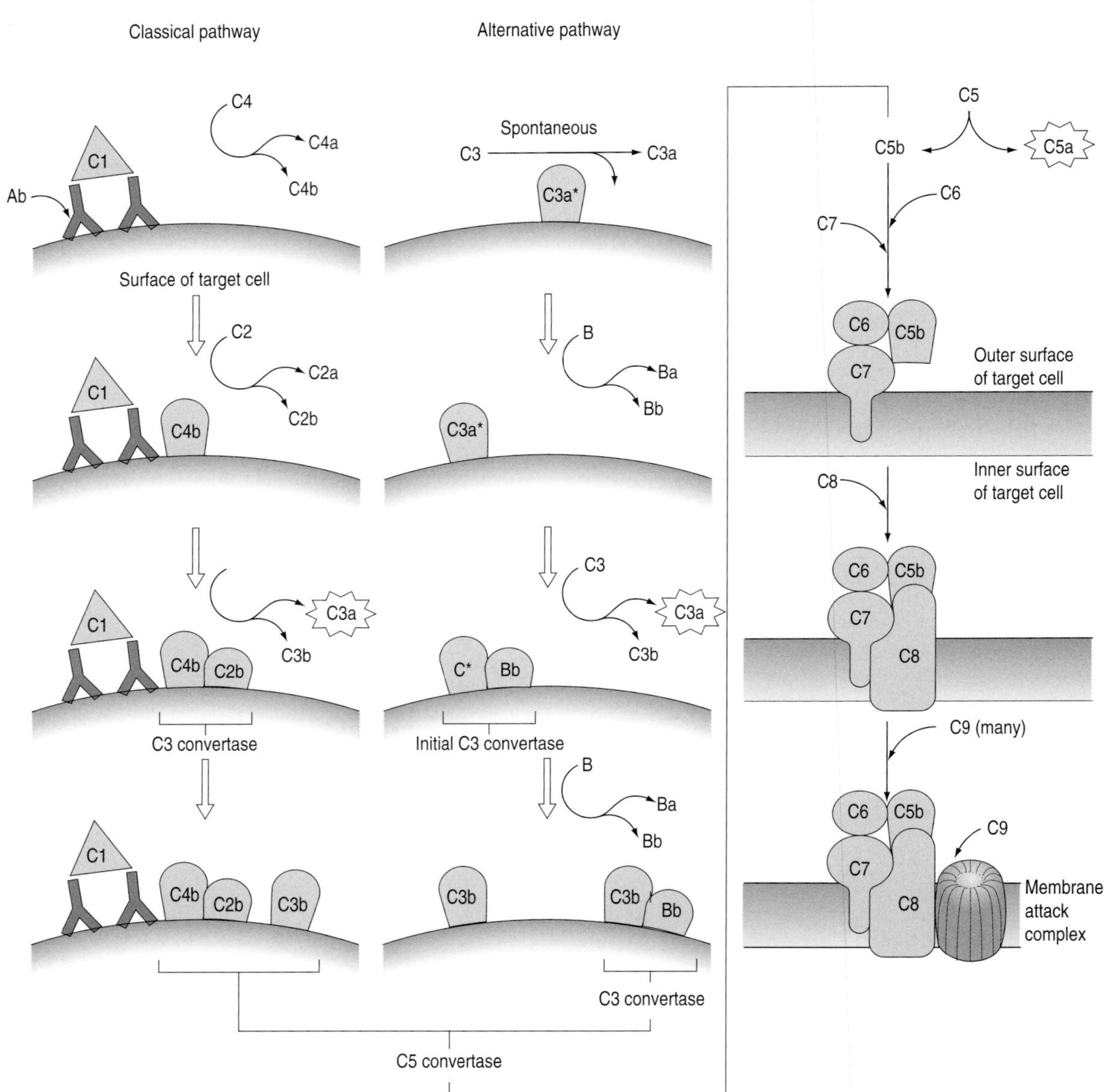

Figure 13.2 Activation of complement. This can be achieved through the activation of the classical pathway (where Ab, either one immunoglobulin (Ig) M is bound, or two IgG molecules are bound in close proximity to one another), as shown on the left-hand side of the figure. This leads to the production of the activated complement factor 1 complex. The alternative pathway (which is initiated by spontaneous decay of C3 but which is unable to continue unless there are specific sites for C* – a C3b-like molecule – to bind with on the target cell) is shown on the right. Whichever pathway is used, a cascade of events occurs such that the activation of one complement protein leads to the activation of the next, and so it continues. Once the C5 convertase complex has been formed, the production of the membrane attack complex (where a hole is inserted through the target cell) occurs through the same process, whichever was the initiating pathway. C3a and C5a are anaphylatoxins, small molecules that can diffuse away from the area. Anaphylatoxins have the ability to cause aggregation of platelets, extravasion and chemotaxis of neutrophils and monocytes, and degranulation of eosinophils, mast cells and basophils – which in turn leads to the release of many mediators, including histamine. The released histamine will induce contraction of smooth muscle and an increased vascular permeability. All these are powerful events in the inflammatory process.

Vasodilatation

The vasodilatation resulting from injury will depend on the level of damage, and it may last from 15 minutes to many hours. This vasodilatation can increase blood flow to the area by up to 10-fold, so providing the appropriate cells and chemicals to the area ready to assist in the inflammatory response.

Increased capillary permeability

Fluid normally passes out of small blood vessels by a process of microfiltration, because of the high hydrostatic pressure at the arteriolar end of the capillaries. Owing to the loss of fluid, but not of large molecules and cells, the colloid osmotic pressure within the capillaries increases. This, coupled with the reduction of hydrostatic pressure at the venous ends of the capillaries, results in the fluid originally removed being returned from the extravascular space into the venous ends of the capillaries (Figure 13.3).

In an inflammatory situation, it is not just fluid that is lost from the vasculature. The retraction of endothelial cells causes intracellular gaps through which larger molecules can pass into the extravascular space. The loss of proteins such as complement factors and immunoglobulins not only assists in the destruction of invading micro-organisms, but also results in the colloid osmotic pressure not being increased as much as normally. Consequently there is no 'driving force' to ensure the re-entry of fluid back into the vasculature, so fluid will remain at the inflammatory site leading to oedema (swelling).

The exudate produced does not just remain at the inflammatory focus. It is drained by the lymphatic channels but is replaced by new exudate. Hence the oedema persists.

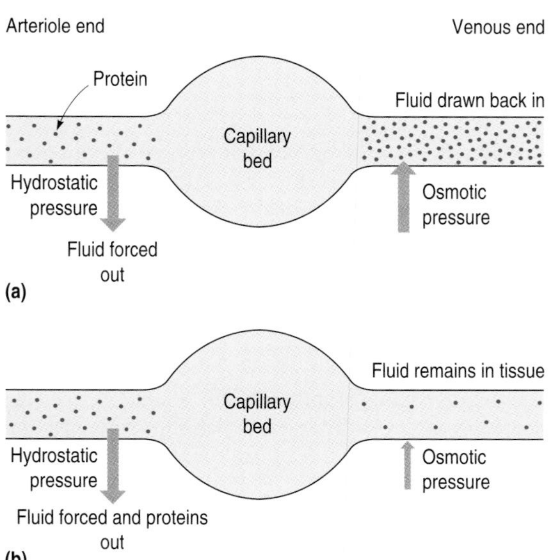

Figure 13.3 Generation of oedema in inflamed tissue. (a) In the normal situation the removal of fluid into the extravascular space at the arteriole end of the capillary bed is balanced by its return to the vasculature at the venule end of the bed. (b) In inflammation, the removal of proteins as well as fluid at the arteriole end of the vascular bed means the driving force for the return of the fluid is not generated, so fluid remains within the tissue.

Cell migration

In the normal situation for any blood vessels larger than capillaries, blood cells (including leucocytes) are kept away from the vessel walls by circulating within the central region of the blood vessel. The area around the vessel wall is in contact mainly with plasma. When there is vasodilatation (and increased capillary permeability) the rate of blood flow decreases, so allowing the blood cells to begin to flow nearer to the endothelium. As a result of this, granulocytes (e.g. neutrophils) come into contact with the endothelium.

The initial events leading to the production of mediators (e.g. activated complement fragments or cytokines that activate the leucocyte and/or endothelial cells) cause specific complementary molecules to be produced on both granulocytes (particularly phagocytes) and endothelium, so allowing them to adhere. As a consequence of activation, one or both cell types become adhesive, leading initially to transient adherence and rolling of the granulocytes along the endothelium (Figure 13.4). This is known as *margination*. With the production of further molecules the granulocytes will become more firmly attached (sticking) to the adhesion molecules produced by the endothelium, and in this 'fixed' position the granulocytes will produce pseudopodia, which enable them to pass through the wall of the endothelium (through the junctions between the cells) — a process known as *emigration*. In this way the cells are able to gain access to the damaged tissue and to any 'invaders' that have occupied the tissue.

Phagocytosis

Definitions

Phagocytosis is the ingestion and destruction by certain cells (phagocytic cells) of other cellular or particulate material.

Chemotaxis is the process through which phagocytic cells are attracted to a substance and then follow the concentration gradient from an area of low concentration moving towards a high concentration.

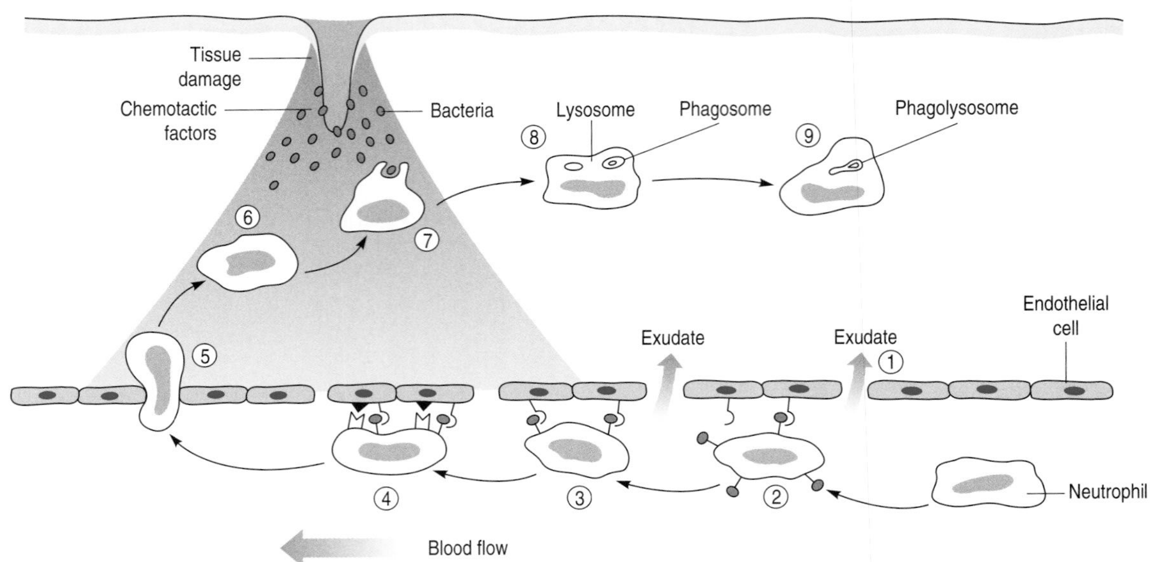

13

Figure 13.4 Schematic illustrating neutrophil margination, emigration, chemotactic attraction and phagocytosis in an inflammatory response. (1) Increased vascular permeability causes fluid to leave the blood vessel. (2) The neutrophils now circulate closer to the endothelium, where the release of TNFα will have caused P- and E-selectins (adhesion molecules) to be synthesised and placed on the surface of endothelial cells. At the same time a complementary adhesion molecule will be generated by the neutrophil. (3) With the aid of the adhesion molecules the neutrophil will start to roll along the endothelium. (4) With the addition of further adhesion molecules, IL-8 receptor on the neutrophil and ICAM-1 on the endothelium, the neutrophil will become firmly fixed. (5) Diapedesis enables the neutrophil to leave the blood vessel. (6) Following the concentration gradient of the chemotactic factors, the neutrophil will approach the site of tissue damage. (7) On encountering material (e.g. bacteria) to be engulfed, the neutrophil produces pseudopodia to encircle the substance. (8) A vacuole is formed within the phagocyte containing the bacteria. (9) A lysosome will fuse with the phagosome, so enabling the engulfed material to be broken down.

Once the phagocytic cells have migrated across the blood vessel wall, chemotactic signals direct the movement of the cells to their required site of action.

A number of chemical factors are known to stimulate leucocyte chemotaxis; examples are the anaphylatoxin C5a (Figure 13.2), platelet-activating factor (PAF) and leukotriene B_4 (LTB_4). All of these agents act through G-protein coupled receptors and cause the movement of the phagocytic cells towards the target area.

On reaching the site of action, the granulocytes (particularly neutrophils) may encounter, for example, damaged tissue or bacteria, either of which will need to be removed. This is achieved by the process of phagocytosis or, for material that is large or difficult to engulf, the release of substances from the phagocytic cell, so leading to extracellular killing. Phagocytosis is achieved by the phagocyte using amoeboid-like movements of its plasma membrane to encircle the foreign material (Figure 13.4). Once this is achieved, the two sides of the membrane combine to form a phagocytic *vacuole* (also known as a *phagosome*). The phagosome then fuses with a lysosome within the cell to form a *phagolysosome*. The lysosome contains powerful enzymes which, coupled with the various reactive oxygen species generated, will now come into contact with the unwanted material, causing it to be broken down. Any usable components produced will be recycled.

In order to assist phagocytosis it is common for opsonisation of the particles to take place.

Definition

Opsonisation is the process whereby a particle becomes coated in another substance, so making it more open to phagocytosis.

One example of an opsonin is generated due to the presence of lipopolysaccharides in the cell wall, which activate the alternative complement pathway. As a result of this activation C3b is generated and binds to the surface of the bacteria (Figure 13.2). The phagocyte contains receptors that will bind to the C3b; this will cause the phagocyte and particle to adhere to one another, so assisting the engulfment process.

A second example of an opsonin is the binding of antibody (immunoglobulin G, IgG) to the particle.

The IgG binds owing to the presence of its variable regions enabling recognition of specific structures present on the bacterium (known as *antigenic determinants*). Once bound by the variable regions (Fab) of the IgG, this effectively labels the bacterium; hence the exposed constant region of the antibody (Fc) is able to bind to complementary receptors on the phagocyte, again allowing adherence between the phagocyte and bacterium that will assist engulfment. These two systems can work in concert, as the binding of two IgG molecules in close proximity with one another will enable the activation of the classical complement pathway, which in turn causes the generation of C3b (Figure 13.2) which binds to the cell, so aiding opsonisation.

For particles unsuitable for ingestion, possibly because they are too large, the phagocyte will use extracellular killing to remove the agent from the system. In this situation the contents of the lysosome are released into the vicinity of the unwanted agent. Whilst this can be an effective means of killing unwanted bacteria, the environment is not as controlled as in the phagolysosome and consequently the agents released can act on surrounding healthy tissue.

To illustrate this, consider two enzymes that are released, elastase and collagenases, which will hydrolyse proteins in bacterial cell envelopes, so leading to death of the bacterium. The elastases can also use collagen cross-linkages and proteoglycans as substrates along with elastin components of blood vessels, ligaments and cartilage. Collagenases are active in cleaving type I and, to a lesser degree, type III collagen from bone, cartilage and tendon. Thus, although the body does have some defence mechanisms in place to help protect it from the damaging effects of the agents released from the phagocytes, these mechanisms can become overwhelmed, leading to damage of otherwise healthy tissue.

Benefits and drawbacks of the inflammatory response

Benefits

The initial passage of fluid exudate into the surrounding damaged tissue immediately delivers further nutrients and oxygen to the damaged site. This extra energy will be vital for any of the body's immune cells that will arrive later. The fluid exudate also has the action of diluting any possible toxins, such as may be produced by certain bacteria, and allows them to be disposed of through the lymphatic system. The exudate may also contain certain specific immunoglobulins that are able to bind with and neutralise potentially harmful pathogens and toxins.

Fibrinogen, which is also contained within this exudate, will initiate fibrin formation. Such an action helps to block the possible movement of micro-organisms and helps to facilitate the chances of these organisms being phagocytosed on the arrival of the body's immune cells.

Drawbacks

The consequent cellular exudate is primarily composed of neutrophils. This cell type is relatively short-lived, perhaps lasting for about only 2 weeks, so must be constantly replaced. Neutrophils are designed chiefly for the phagocytosis of invading micro-organisms and any associated cell debris, and for this reason they contain a number of lysosomal enzymes (as described earlier). In the inflammatory situation, either as a deliberate release process (as described earlier) or perhaps following the death of the neutrophil, these cells may release these lysosomal enzymes. A beneficial consequence of this would be assistance in the digestion of the inflammatory exudate. However, such a release can be harmful in that some of the enzymes may digest normal tissue and result in considerable 'collateral' tissue damage.

In certain situations, swelling of the tissue can cause serious restriction of some of the body's vital actions. One example of this is in *Haemophilus influenzae* infection. Particularly in children, this bacterium can cause epiglottitis (considerable swelling of the epiglottis), which can result in obstruction of the airway.

Inflammatory swelling is very serious whenever it occurs in an otherwise restricted area, such as the skull. For this reason acute meningitis (again perhaps caused by *H. influenzae*) may lead to increased intracranial pressure, impairment of blood flow to the brain, and so ischaemic damage to the brain.

FORMS OF ACUTE INFLAMMATION

Although the term 'inflammation' applies to the processes involved, as outlined in the previous section, the clinical appearance of acute inflammation will vary according to the type of tissue affected. Consequently, a number of terms are employed to describe these different forms of inflammation.

Serous inflammation

Perhaps the most commonly observed instance of serous inflammation is a blister caused by a burn or by the rubbing of an ill-fitting shoe. This form of inflammation is typically characterised by the production of copious exudate, which upon analysis is relatively scarce in cells but which contains comparatively high concentrations of protein.

The source of this fluid may be either plasma (as in the above examples), or the mesothelial cells that line the peritoneal, pleural and pericardial cavities and synovial tissue. Inflammation of this type may be seen, for example, in cases such as acute synovitis, in which the synovial joint is affected, or in peritonitis. In some situations such as conjunctivitis occurring as a response to either a viral or allergic assault (leading to the production of a serous exudate), the typical inflammatory vasodilatation is clearly visible in the form of 'bloodshot' eyes.

Catarrhal inflammation

Acute inflammation of mucous membranes results in the production of a large amount of mucinous (mucus) secretion, the condition being classified as 'catarrhal'. Examples of areas affected are the nasopharynx, lungs, gastrointestinal tract or mucus-secreting glands elsewhere. In tissues it can be seen as large amounts of amorphous stringy material containing some white blood cells, whilst the underlying mucosa shows distension of glands. Probably the best example of such a condition is the common cold.

Fibrinous inflammation

As previously described, the formation of a plasma protein-rich fluid exudate is common in inflammation. When the predominant protein present is fibrinogen, then fibrinous inflammation can occur. Fibrinogen is a large molecule so it requires more severe inflammation if it is to leave the vasculature.

Upon activation of the coagulation process, fibrinogen has the ability to polymerise to form sticky, solid fibrin. This rubbery fibrin may be visible as a variable number of yellow-white strands, or even as thick sheets, which stick out from the surface of the affected site with an irregular (shaggy-like) surface. Fibrinous inflammation is commonly associated with mucosal and serosal membranes and particularly with the pleura and pericardium.

This type of inflammation can be characteristically present in pericarditis, which may, for example, occur as a result of rheumatic fever. In this instance the heart is affected and the parietal and visceral pericardium take on a peculiar appearance often described as 'bread and butter'. Another common situation in which this type of inflammation is usually present is the pneumococcal pneumonias.

Haemorrhagic inflammation

In situations where, for some reason, there is a deficiency in those compounds in the plasma responsible for coagulation, or perhaps where vascular damage is very severe, red blood cells may leave the vessels either through the damaged area or by a process of passive diapedesis, so resulting in haemorrhagic inflammation. Examples of where this might be observed are in meningococcal septicaemia and acute pancreatitis.

This type of inflammation is commonly found mixed with another form, usually either suppurative or fibrinous, or indeed both.

Suppurative inflammation

Suppurative inflammation is also referred to as 'purulent' inflammation, and occurs when there is evidence of copious amounts of pus (or purulent exudate) present. Pus can vary in appearance from yellow-white to grey and from watery to viscous in consistency. Essentially, however, pus consists of some of the damaged tissues, which have become liquefied by the actions of proteolytic enzymes, together with those cells, particularly neutrophils, which had invaded the area and are now dead or dying themselves along with the inflammatory exudate. Such inflammation may occur following infection by a pyogenic organism such as *Staphylococcus*, *Pneumococcus* or *Escherichia coli*.

When a localised collection of pus occurs in a tissue or organ where it has been contained in a membrane of fibrous tissue, then an abscess may be formed. Certain chemicals such as turpentine, and micro-organisms such as *Staphylococcus*, tend to elicit abscesses. Usually, as the abscess progresses, the pressure from the pus will advance in the line of least resistance, so forming a 'point' (fortunately this tracking is usually towards the surface of the body). This 'point' will then burst, allowing the cavity to empty and permitting scar formation in a healing process. On occasion surgical intervention is necessary; the abscess (or boil) is lanced and the pus drained.

If the abscess is deep-seated, pus may also form inside a hollow viscus, such as those found in the appendix or gallbladder. Alternatively a lung infection can spread and lead to the accumulation of pus within the pleural space. Such a condition is described as *empyema* and it can even arise in the subdural cavity in the brain, where it is a significant cause of neurological morbidity and mortality.

Occasionally the pointing of the abscess does not result in tracking towards the surface of the body. When this happens, so-called 'sinus tracts' are sometimes formed which may, for example, spread along the course of veins or in subcutaneous structures. When formed between bone and periosteum, the 'pointing' of the abscess can clearly be hindered and so it tends to result in direct pressure being exerted on the resisting tissue or may lead to the blood supply being cut off to the area. This then allows for sloughing of the parts covering the abscess, and so the pus eventually makes its way through sinus tracts to another cavity. An example of this type of situation is in *Neisseria gonorrhoeae* infection, when it is possible for the abscess to arise in the endometrial cavity and discharge into the peritoneal cavity.

Abscesses will also occasionally form deep in striated muscles, as in the condition *pyomyositis*. In this case the muscle has become infected by pus-producing bacteria, by the bacteria spreading either from a nearby infection in a bone or other tissue or through the blood stream from a distant part of the body. Pyomyositis is more common among people in the tropics but it can also occur in immunocompromised individuals, especially those with AIDS. The muscles most commonly affected are in the thighs, buttocks, upper arms and around the shoulders. Symptoms include cramping pain followed by swelling, mild fever and increasing discomfort, especially when the infected muscle is moved.

Pseudomembranous inflammation

If an inflamed mucosal surface becomes covered by a layer of fibrin, inflammatory cells and necrotic debris, then it can appear as if this has formed a membrane over the affected area — hence the term pseudomembranous inflammation. It occurs on mucosal surfaces such as the pharynx, larynx and other respiratory passages, as well as in the digestive tract. Pseudomembranous inflammation could occur, for instance, following heavy antibiotic therapy which destroys normal flora in the patient's bowels, so allowing colonisation by *Clostridium difficile*; in this case it is known as *pseudomembranous colitis*.

Gangrenous or necrotising inflammation

In this situation the exudate is dominated by the accumulation or induction of tissue necrosis without appreciable fluid or cell exudation. Necrotising inflammation can be observed in many toxic injuries to the gastrointestinal tract or in diseases that induce arterial thrombosis. Oedema produces pressure increases in the surrounding tissues, which in certain situations may lead to closure (occlusion) of the associated blood vessels. This lack of blood supply (and consequently the lack of nutrients which it would normally supply) inevitably leads to widespread necrosis of the tissue. This, together with bacterial invasion, can result in tissue putrefaction, which materialises as gangrene. The above situation arises when the necrotising inflammatory reaction occurs on an epithelial surface; hence it may produce a defect in the epithelium to the level of the basement membrane.

Key point

When epithelial defects occur at levels below the basement membrane, they are referred to as *ulcers*, and the corresponding inflammatory reaction is referred to as *ulcerative*. Ulcers are local defects on the surface of an organ or tissue that have been produced by the sloughing of inflammatory necrotic tissue.

CHRONIC INFLAMMATION

Whereas acute inflammation is characterised by changes in the vasculature and the production of exudate (both fluid and cellular), in chronic inflammation this exudation is less obvious. Chronic inflammation is characterised more by changes in cell and connective tissue proliferation.

Forms of chronic inflammation

Key point

Chronic inflammation is usually subdivided into two forms: *diffuse interstitial* and *granulomatous*.

13

Diffuse interstitial inflammation

Diffuse interstitial inflammation has no particularly characteristic pattern of tissue reaction. The cells involved are monocytes, lymphocytes, plasma cells and fibroblasts (connective tissue cells).

Granulomatous inflammation

In granulomatous inflammation there is an attempt to wall off and so isolate the affected site. The cells involved are the reticulo-endothelial cells and their derivatives (largely macrophages).

Granulomas occur in relatively few diseases: for example, tuberculosis, syphilis, rheumatic fever, rheumatoid arthritis (as subcutaneous nodules) and in foreign-body inflammation. A granuloma is a focal area of granulomatous inflammation that consists of a spherical accumulation of activated macrophages (epithelioid histiocytes) surrounded by lymphocytes, occasional plasma cells and giant cells, and usually connective tissue. Giant cells have been formed in this situation by the fusion of several (10–20) activated monocytes/macrophages; hence the cell contains many nuclei. When the nuclei of the giant cells are sited around the rim of the cell, these giant cells are known as *Langhans cells*.

Causes of chronic inflammation

Chronic inflammation is associated with a large heterogeneous group of diseases, lasting from weeks to months or longer, either as a development of acute inflammation or as a low-grade inflammatory process without a preceding acute phase. This section looks at four causes.

Persistence of infection with micro-organisms

The types of micro-organism that might be causative of chronic inflammation are essentially of low virulence, such as those associated with tuberculosis or syphilis, along with numerous fungi, protozoa and metazoal parasites.

Autoimmunity

Autoimmune-derived chronic inflammation is characterised by macrophages, lymphocytes and plasma cells, such as is observed in rheumatoid arthritis or systemic lupus erythematosus (SLE). In this case there is a 'normal' tissue component, which the immune system now recognises as foreign; thus inflammation occurs in an attempt to remove the self tissue.

Prolonged exposure to either exogenous or endogenous toxins

13

When irritant non-living material becomes implanted into wounds, either accidentally (grit, or splinters of wood, metal or plastic) or deliberately (sutures, surgical prosthesis), then chronic inflammation may begin. The situation may also arise in disease conditions such as osteomyelitis, where a fragment of dead bone (sequestrum) has become detached from sound bone during the process of necrosis.

The morphology of chronic inflammation arising from prolonged exposure to an environmental toxin will depend on the toxin involved. In the case of inhaled silica, for example, there is chronic lung fibrosis. Alternatively, high levels of plasma lipid would lead to atherosclerosis of the arteries.

Persistence of acute inflammation

Chronic inflammation developing from acute inflammation occurs, for example, in alcoholic cirrhosis and gastric peptic ulcers. Commonly, the morphology includes the presence of inflammatory cells more characteristic of chronic inflammation than of acute, such as macrophages, lymphocytes and fibrosis. This type of chronic inflammation can occur where infectious organisms are protected from the host's defence mechanisms and so are able to persist in damaged regions. Such a situation can arise in an undrained abscess cavity where bacteria are continuing to grow in the pus.

SYSTEMIC EFFECTS OF INFLAMMATION

In addition to the localised symptoms of inflammation described in the earlier sections, there are systemic effects that may also have important consequences.

Constitutional symptoms

This term covers a whole range of feelings experienced by the patient. He or she often will feel tired and restless (malaise), often accompanied by nausea. Consequently, during occasions of long-term chronic inflammation, significant weight loss is common. In the 19th century when tuberculosis was relatively common, these symptoms were recognised as being closely associated with such a disorder and given the general term 'consumption'.

Haematological changes

Leucocytosis (an abnormal elevation of the white blood cell count) and lymphocytosis (a high number of normal lymphocytes) occur in chronic infection such as whooping cough. Neutrophilia (increased numbers of neutrophils) occurs in pyogenic infections. Eosinophilia (increased numbers of eosinophils) is found in parasitic infections and allergies. Monocytosis (an abnormal increase in the number of monocytes in the circulating blood) often accompanies bacterial infections.

Anaemia may result from blood lost in the formation of exudates. This is particularly significant in situations such as ulcerative colitis, but anaemia may also be a result of the chronic inflammation actually causing a depression in bone marrow function.

Pyrexia

When activated through the action of phagocytosis, such as occurs during an inflammatory reaction, white blood cells such as macrophages are able to produce so-called 'endogenous pyrogens', which can act upon the hypothalamus to affect the thermoregulatory mechanisms for which this area of the brain is responsible. As a consequence, the general body temperature is increased.

Reactive hyperplasia of the reticulo-endothelial system

This can be seen as lymph node enlargement and is a result of the rapid cell division occurring in these tissues as a consequence of the adaptive immune response's involvement in the inflammatory process. In certain infections such as malaria where blood-borne antigens are involved, a similar effect may be observed in the spleen, a condition known as *splenomegaly*.

Amyloidosis

In situations of long-term chronic inflammation, such as that observed in rheumatoid arthritis, leprosy, tuberculosis and SLE, the elevated levels of the acute-phase protein, serum amyloid A (SAA), often result in the glycoprotein, amyloid, being deposited extracellularly in various tissues around the body. This in turn can lead to secondary (reactive) amyloidosis, which is characterised by the ultimately fatal deposition of insoluble fibrils in a number of tissues, including the spleen, liver and kidney.

FACTORS AFFECTING HEALING

Many factors affect the healing of an individual, from his or her own hormonal status through to deliberate interventions such as the use of a cold compress, ultrasound or drugs.

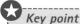

Key point

Whilst it would appear that hormones can have wide-ranging effects on the functioning of the immune system, as yet there is still uncertainty about their actions. Consequently, differing studies can demonstrate apparently opposing actions, some indicating an increased activity of the immune system, others demonstrating decreased responsiveness.

It has been found that, under situations of acute stress, the time taken for recovery of inflammation of bacterial origin is improved. This is possibly achieved through alterations in leucocyte trafficking, such that the leucocytes will be targeted towards the relevant organs. For example, an increase in leucocyte trafficking to the skin is accompanied by a significant enhancement of skin immunity. As a consequence of this, the immune response is more effective and so less damage is potentially done; hence recovery time is reduced.

In contrast to the potential benefits of acute stress, chronic stress will induce the adrenal gland to create additional quantities of cortisol (an endogenous corticosteroid). Cortisol has wide-ranging actions, including controlling blood glucose and lipid levels and influencing blood pressure (too much results in hypertension). In addition to these effects, cortisol will act as a suppressant on the immune system. The mechanism through which this immunosuppression takes place is the same as that initiated by synthetic corticosteroids and is described later under drug therapies.

Sex hormones have also been suggested as influencing inflammation. A study looking at the prevention of systemic inflammation resulting from external perfusion of the blood during corrective cardiac surgery in infants indicated that girls were less likely than boys to develop inflammation. It was suggested that this might be due to the higher levels of progesterone within the girls, which in turn led to raised levels of IL-10 (an anti-inflammatory cytokine).

It has been proposed that the repair process may take longer and be less effective in postmenopausal women owing to the detrimental effects of oestrogen and/or progesterone deficiency in the early stages of healing. The exact relationship between the hormone levels and the phases of inflammation and repair remains unclear, owing to conflicting findings from various studies.

DRUG MANAGEMENT OF INFLAMMATION

Non-steroidal anti-inflammatory drugs (NSAIDs)

NSAIDs are among the most commonly used medicines, being prescribed largely for their anti-inflammatory, antipyretic and analgesic properties. The classic example of this type of agent is aspirin (acetylsalicylic acid), which acts to prevent the production of prostaglandins and thromboxanes, which are powerful pro-inflammatory lipid mediators. There are, however, a multitude of other agents that act in the same way: ibuprofen, naproxen, mefenamic acid, flufenamic acid, piroxicam and others.

NSAIDs work by acetylating cyclo-oxygenase, thereby blocking the conversion of arachidonic acid to prostanoids (Figure 13.5). These mediators are then not available to act to enhance the inflammatory response, so the inflammation decreases.

13

An unfortunate side-effect of NSAIDs arises from their intrinsic toxicity to the gastrointestinal mucosa. They can cause complications ranging from dyspepsia (chronic indigestion) to life-threatening gastrointestinal ulcers. This limits their use, although some (e.g. ibuprofen) carry considerably less risk of these complications than others (e.g. azapropazone).

It has been discovered that there are different isoforms of cyclo-oxygenase, now known as COX-1 and COX-2. COX-1 is the constitutive form of the enzyme. Its concentration remains relatively stable, although small increases can occur when stimulated with hormones or growth factors. COX-2, however, is virtually undetectable in resting cells. Following stimulation by cytokines, endotoxins, growth factors or tumour promoters, COX-2 is induced and can thus be found in, for example, macrophages, fibroblasts, vascular endothelial cells and smooth muscle cells. Consequently, it is believed that in inflammation it is COX-2-dependent prostaglandin production that is the more important of the two isoforms of the enzyme. This has serious implications for the use of selective COX-2 inhibitors in the treatment of inflammation, as, in principle, their use should significantly reduce the incidence of gastrointestinal side-effects (as the prostanoids

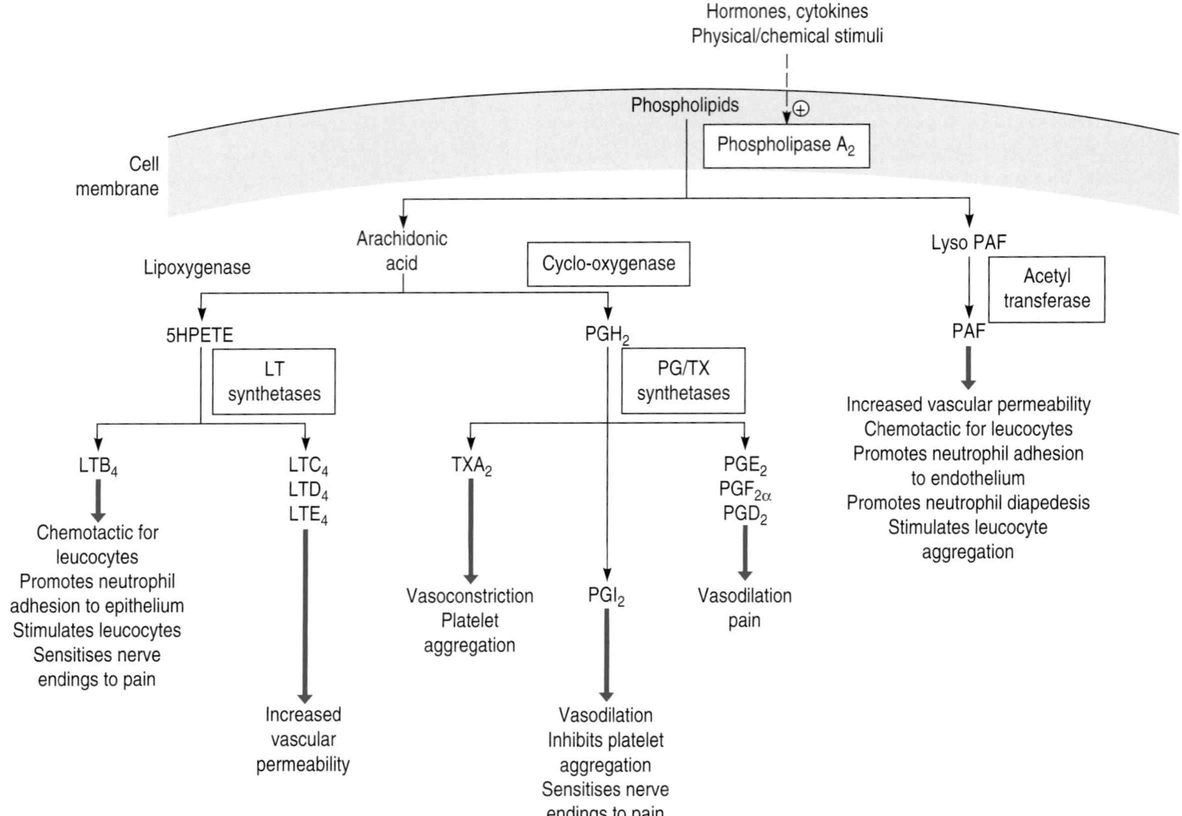

13

Figure 13.5 Production of eicosanoids and platelet-activating factor (PAF). Both eicosanoids and PAF are autocoids (local hormones), which are released from membrane phospholipids. Eicosanoids is the name given to a group of compounds that are formed from polyunsaturated fatty acids (principally arachidonic acid); they include prostaglandins (PG), thromboxane A2 (TXA2) and leukotrienes (LT). PAF is a modified phospholipid that is often coupled with arachidonic acid, such that the release of lyso-PAF from the membrane will also release free arachidonic acid.

in this case are believed to be synthesised via COX-1). Agents within this class are celecoxib and rofecoxib.

Corticosteroids

Physiotherapists encounter the use of steroids in both local and systemic administrations (e.g. injections and inhalers, respectively). Synthetic glucocorticoids are among the most effective anti-inflammatory drugs available; examples include prednisolone, dexamethasone, methylcortisone and methylprednisolone. They are able to affect the immune system in a number of ways that contribute to their powerful anti-inflammatory action.

Corticosteroids induce cells to synthesise the protein lipocortin-1. This lipocortin then acts to inhibit the enzyme phospholipase A_2 (PLA_2). As a result of this inhibition the mediators formed following PLA_2 activation are not produced (Figure 13.5). By preventing the formation of prostanoids, leukotrienes and PAF, these mediators will no longer contribute to the inflammatory response; hence the inflammation is reduced.

In addition to this action, corticosteroids have a number of other actions that contribute to their anti-inflammatory effectiveness. These actions are not fully clear but may include:

- reducing the production of adhesion molecules (so preventing cells from leaving the circulation and entering the target area)
- suppressing activated macrophages
- stabilising membranes (so decreasing the ability of cells to present antigen)
- slowing down cell division (so possibly influencing the overall size of the lymphocyte pool)
- altering the distribution of T lymphocytes (such that the number circulating around the body is considerably decreased).

These actions can prevent the production of antibodies and lymphocyte-mediated destruction of agents recognised as foreign, and consequently prevent an effective mounting of an immune response.

Antihistamines

Key point

There are a number of different subtypes of receptor that histamine can act upon. So, although the term 'antihistamine' is commonly used, it is more accurate to use the term 'histamine H_1 receptor antagonist' when referring to this class of agent.

Examples of agents within this category are diphenhydramine, tripelennamine and promethazine. All these are known as first-generation H_1 antagonists and they have the side-effect of causing decreased alertness, slowed reaction times and sleepiness. Second-generation H_1 antagonists such as terfenadine, astemizole and loratadine have the advantage that they are not sedating as they do not cross the blood–brain barrier.

The principle behind the use of these agents is that, although they do not prevent the release of histamine in an inflammatory response, they will prevent that histamine from being able to act. To achieve this the histamine H_1 receptor antagonist will combine with the H_1 receptors and, although it will not produce a response in its own right, it will prevent histamine from being able to bind to those receptors.

Gold

Gold-based therapies such as auranofin (oral administration), aurothiomalate and aurothioglucose (both given by intramuscular injection) have been used for many years because of their ability to slow the progression of rheumatoid arthritis, along with reducing the symptoms and possibly also decreasing bone/articular cartilage destruction.

The mechanism of action of gold remains unclear. It is known that it is accumulated in lysosomes of macrophages and that it reduces the activity of lysosomal enzymes. Gold compounds will also suppress phagocytosis by polymorphonuclear leucocytes and decrease the release of histamine from mast cells.

FURTHER READING

Belanger A-Y 2002 Evidence-based Guide to Therapeutic Physical Agents. Lippincott, Williams & Wilkins: Philadelphia

Burg ND, Pillinger MH 2001 The neutrophil: function and regulation in innate and humoral immunity. Clin Immunol 99(1): 7–17

Calvin M 2000 Oestrogens and wound healing. Maturitas 34: 195–210

Cook SD, Salkeld SL, Patron LP et al. 2001 Low-intensity ultrasound improves spinal fusion. Spine J 1: 246–254

Da Cunha A, Parizotto NA, Vidal B de C 2001 The effect of therapeutic ultrasound on repair of the Achilles tendon (tendo calcaneus) of the rat. Ultras Med Biol 27: 1691–1696

Dyson M 1995 Role of ultrasound in wound healing. In: McCulloch JM, Kloth LC, Feeder JA (eds) Wound Healing: Alternatives in Management, 2nd edn. FA Davies: Philadelphia, pp. 318–345

Gardner TN, Stoll T, Marks L et al. 2000 The influence of mechanical stimulus on the pattern of tissue differentiation in a long bone fracture: an FEM study. J Biomech 33: 415–425

Ley K 1996 Molecular mechanisms of leukocyte recruitment in the inflammatory process. Cardiovasc Res 32: 733–742

Lundeberg TCM, Eriksson SV, Malm M 1992 Electrical nerve stimulation improves healing of diabetic ulcers. Ann Plast Surg 29: 328–331

Reger SI, Hyodo A, Negami S et al. 1999 Experimental wound healing with electrical stimulation. Artificial Org 23: 460–462

Sluka KA, Christy MR, Peterson WL et al. 1999 Reduction of pain-related behaviors with either cold or heat treatment in an animal model of acute arthritis. Arch Phys Med Rehabil 80(3): 313–317

Speed CA 2001 Therapeutic ultrasound in soft tissue lesions. Rheumatology 40: 1331–1336

Williams AR 1983 Ultrasound: Biological Effects and Potential Hazards. Academic Press: London

Chapter **14**

The physiotherapy management of inflammation, tissue healing and repair

Janette Grey and Gillian Rawlinson

CHAPTER CONTENTS

INTRODUCTION

This chapter will introduce the reader to the processes involved in inflammation and tissue healing and repair, as well as discussing physiotherapeutic interventions that may be used to facilitate this process. The healing and repair process that occurs in response to tissue injury can, in broad terms, be described as a continuum of events that consists of four stages: bleeding, inflammation, proliferation and remodelling.

These stages are not mutually exclusive and will overlap considerably, depending on the nature of the injury and the individual. However, for the purposes of this chapter, these four stages will be considered in sequence as underpinning a return to normal homeostasis and normal function.

Clinical note

The inflammatory and tissue repair processes are fundamental to many pathologies and injuries that are treated by physiotherapists. Treatment of the inflammation itself may be directly affected by physiotherapy modalities or may need to be addressed primarily through drug and medical intervention. For example, the inflammation of the bronchioles in an acute exacerbation of asthma would be managed medically with steroids.

Although inflammation and tissue repair are not exclusive to the musculoskeletal system, it is in this system that the physiotherapist works most closely to influence these processes. This chapter therefore will focus on the sequence of events following soft tissue injury and its physiotherapeutic management. The aims of the chapter are as follows:

- to identify the aims of physiotherapy and to examine how they change throughout the continuum of tissue healing and repair

- to provide the reader with specific physiotherapy examples of managing inflammation and repair
- to develop the reader's ability to use clinical reasoning with regard to the use of core physiotherapy modalities in the management of tissue healing and repair
- to identify where research evidence underpins practice.

In order to clinically reason an appropriate physiotherapeutic approach to treatment for an individual's problem, many factors need to be considered (Fig. 14.1). The physiotherapist needs to understand the anatomical and histological make-up of the different tissues, as well as the normal processes of inflammation, tissue healing and repair. It is also vital that the physiotherapist has excellent assessment and clinical reasoning skills in order to identify the tissues involved and the underlying pathology correctly. The clinical reasoning process also requires the physiotherapist to consider psychological and social factors, which will undoubtedly influence an individual's recovery and rehabilitation. These factors may significantly alter the approach a clinician takes and will maybe even exclude certain treatment modalities that may normally be considered. It is this individualised, holistic and evidence-based approach that makes the physiotherapist an invaluable contributor to the patient's optimal recovery from disease or injury.

At the end of the chapter two case studies will be presented to illustrate the suggested application of physiotherapy interventions discussed in relation to healing and repair processes.

THE CONTINUUM OF TISSUE HEALING AND REPAIR

When any soft tissue is injured, be it through trauma, injury, overuse or surgery, a natural sequence of events follows in order to repair the damaged tissue and restore homeostasis and normal function.

This process starts with a short period of tissue bleeding due to the disruption of small blood vessels and capillaries. Immediately following this period of bleeding a complex cascade of biochemical events proceeds, triggering an inflammatory reaction. The inflammatory process initiates the proliferation of new tissue cells, which eventually remodel with the aim of restoring normal tissue function. This sequence of events is illustrated in Figure 14.2.

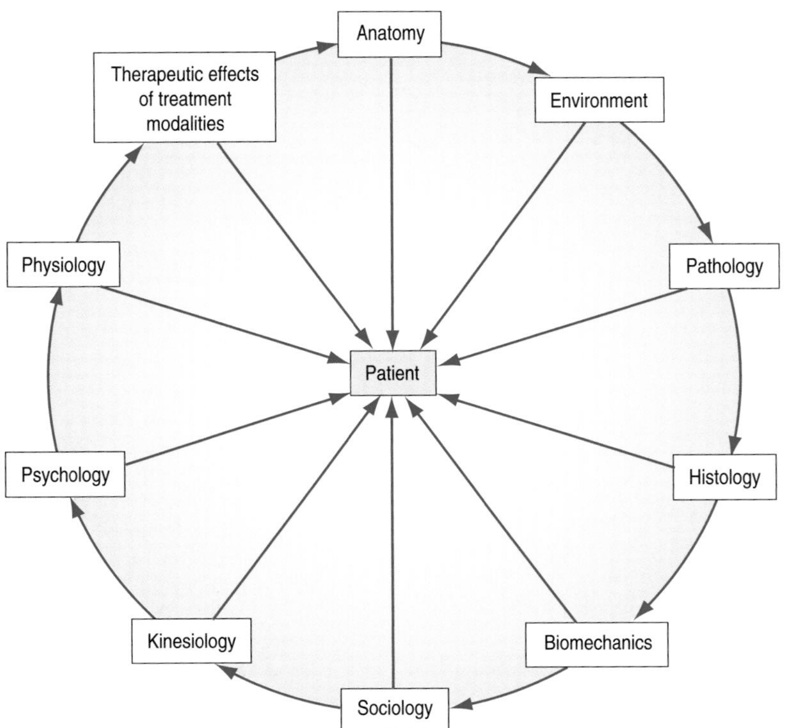

Figure 14.1 Factors influencing the clinical reasoning process in the management of tissue healing and repair.

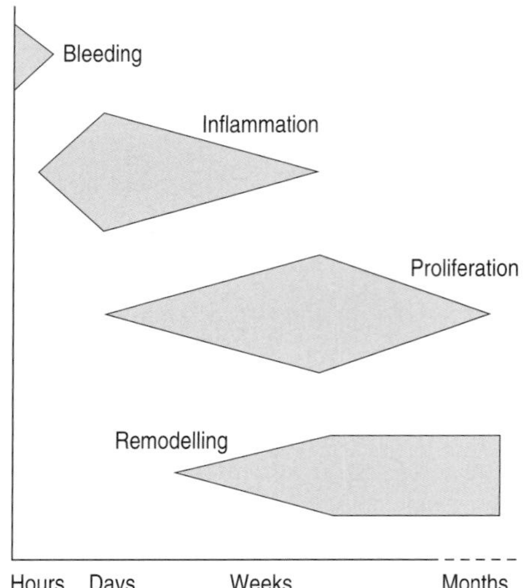

Figure 14.2 Phases and timescale of tissue repair. (Reproduced from Watson 2004, with permission.)

This sequence of events does not follow an exact timescale and it is useful to think of it as a continuum along which each stage of healing will overlap with the next; this depends on many factors, such as severity and nature of the injury, the patient's age and tissue type, and what the individual does or not do in terms of movement, activity and intervention. In many cases these healing processes take place without problems; however, several factors can cause these processes to be delayed or exaggerated, leading to less than optimal tissue structure, pain and ultimately reduced function.

For many years physiotherapists have utilised a wide range of treatment modalities and interventions with the intention of promoting healing and repair. The main aim of using any physiotherapeutic modality or intervention should be to facilitate and progress tissue through this normal healing and repair continuum, thus facilitating early recovery and return to maximum function.

Soft tissue injury

When injury or trauma occurs, producing forces great enough to damage soft tissues, it is important to consider what happens to these tissues at a cellular level. The secondary injury model described by Merrick (2002) considers there to be two stages following tissue injury: namely, the primary and secondary injury response.

- *Primary injury* is considered to be the damage to cells caused by the direct injury mechanism, be it a crush, contusion or strain force. The cells damaged by this mechanical force may have their cell membranes disrupted, causing a loss in homeostasis and subsequent cell death. Many types of tissue may be involved, including ligament, tendon, muscle, nerve and connective tissues.
- *Secondary injury* is thought to occur to cells at the periphery of the damaged tissue as a result of physiological responses to the initial primary injury. It is hypothesised that this damage may occur by two means: hypoxic (which maybe better described as ischaemic) and enzymatic mechanisms.

Ischaemic mechanisms

There are several proposed causes of ischaemia (reduced blood flow) to damaged tissue, including haemorrhage from blood vessels, increased blood viscosity secondary to inflammatory responses, and increased extravascular pressure secondary to oedema. This reduced or absent blood supply will deprive cells that may have survived the primary injury of vital oxygen, causing them to rely on anaerobic energy systems, which have only a short timescale (possibly up to 6 hours). If the ischaemia is prolonged, many of these cells will subsequently die.

Enzymatic mechanisms

The lysosomes of those cells destroyed or damaged in the primary stage of injury will produce enzymes that may damage and destroy neighbouring cells. This often occurs as a result of damage to the cell membrane, which causes the cells to swell and eventually die.

PHASES 1 AND 2 OF TISSUE HEALING AND REPAIR

PHASE 1: BLEEDING (0–10 HOURS)

This is a relatively short phase that will depend upon the initial injury type, the tissues damaged and the severity of injury. If there has been an injury to soft tissues, some degree of bleeding will occur. When capillaries and small blood vessels sustain primary injury, blood will escape into surrounding tissues and, depending on the location, may gradually track distally due to gravity. The type of tissue involved and the type of injury will determine the degree of bleeding, in terms of amount and duration. If very vascular tissue such as muscle is damaged, a larger amount of bleeding will occur in comparison with less vascular tissues like ligament and tendon. The bleeding phase may last for only a few minutes or hours, but in large muscle contusion injuries, for example, bleeding may continue to a small degree for up to 24 hours (Watson 2004).

> **Clinical note**
> When assessing bleeding, it is important to consider the location of the injury, as this will affect where the blood distributes. For example, with a tear of the anterior cruciate ligament, bleeding will be intracapsular in the knee; it is therefore unlikely to present as obvious bleeding and bruising with discoloration, but rather takes the form of a tense swelling which, if aspirated, could be identified as blood causing a haemarthrosis.

PHASE 2: INFLAMMATION (72 HOURS)

Inflammation is a complex biochemical and cellular process, which is still not fully understood. It can be triggered by many factors other than injury, such as infection and pathology.

Following an injury or pathological process there is an immediate inflammatory response. This has been reported to last for several days or even weeks but usually peaks around 2–3 days post-injury. During the inflammatory phase several clinical features may well be evident. These include redness, swelling, pain and loss of function.

During inflammation there is primarily a vascular and cellular response. The vascular response occurs as a result of the action of chemical inflammatory mediators and also via a neural effect on the arterioles. There is an initial vasoconstriction, which lasts only seconds, followed by a more prolonged vasodilatation response. There is also an increase in the permeability of the capillary walls, allowing migration of large plasma proteins into the interstitial space. This alters the osmotic pressure in the tissue and exudate will gather in the interstitial space, causing swelling. As cells migrate across the vessel wall into the interstitial fluid, this will become cellular exudate. This exudate will contain mainly neutrophils initially, and then lymphocytes and monocytes as the inflammatory process progresses (Mutsaers et al. 1997).

The cellular response is mediated and maintained by chemical mediators, resulting in altered cellular activity. These processes will eventually aid the removal of any micro-organisms and damaged tissue debris. Pain is caused both by irritation of damaged nerve endings from these chemical mediators and by pressure on nociceptors due to the increase in exudate.

Clinically, this inflammatory phase is often seen as a hindrance to the repair process, and interventions, which have an anti-inflammatory action, are often employed with the aim of halting and slowing this process. It should be noted, however, that inflammation is in fact a normal response to injury and should be facilitated in order for the patient to progress through the healing and repair continuum.

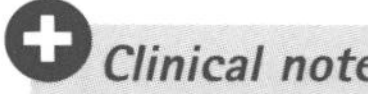

> **Clinical note**
> There is some debate as to whether non-steroidal anti-inflammatory drug (NSAID) therapy should be used in soft tissue injury, as it may slow down this phase of tissue healing, thus slowing overall recovery. Alternatively, there is a suggestion that, if it controls the inflammatory response and prevents it from becoming exaggerated or prolonged, this may in fact facilitate progression through the healing continuum.

Occasionally, individuals will develop a prolonged or exaggerated inflammatory response that fails to resolve within the normal timeframes. The mechanisms behind the development of chronic inflammation are not yet fully understood and are beyond the scope of this chapter.

PHYSIOTHERAPY INTERVENTIONS IN PHASES 1 AND 2 (0–72 HOURS POST-INJURY)

When considering the physiotherapy approaches that we can employ at these early stages of tissue injury, we must consider the physiological processes occurring and the aims and physiological responses to treatment.

When treating any patient with an acute injury — for example, a ligament sprain or a muscle contusion — the aims of treatment must be decided in specific relation to the individual, in order to plan treatment accordingly.

General physiotherapy aims of early-phase management (phases 1 and 2)

The aims are:

- to reduce pain
- to limit and reduce inflammatory exudates
- to reduce metabolic demands of tissue
- to protect newly damaged tissue from further injury
- to protect the newly forming tissue from disruption
- to promote new tissue growth and fibre realignment
- to maintain general levels of cardiovascular and musculoskeletal fitness/activity.

The PRICE principles

PRICE is a mnemonic for the principal interventions commonly used in the early stages immediately following tissue injury. PRICE stands for:

- protection
- rest

- ice
- compression
- elevation.

These interventions together are applied in principle to address the seven aims of early-phase tissue injury and healing management. They are discussed below. The reader is also referred to the guidelines written in conjunction with the Chartered Society of Physiotherapy on the immediate management of soft tissue injury using the PRICE principle (Kerr et al. 1999).

Protection

When soft tissue injury has just occurred, it is important to protect tissues from further damage, both chemical and mechanical (secondary), and also to protect newly forming collagen fibrils in the following days. Measures to prevent tissues from further mechanical damage are generally described as protective modalities and may include treatments such as strapping, use of crutches, slings and braces, and modification of exercises and movements.

The main factors affecting the physiotherapist's decision to use a protective device are the individual's needs, the extent and nature of the tissue injury, and the location of the damage. Devices such as slings may serve the purpose of elevating the limb whilst also having a protective role.

> **Clinical note**
>
> In the case of fasciectomy for release of Dupuytren's contracture, a splint is required immediately after the operation to put the newly cut tissues under stress and to encourage lengthening in order to prevent newly forming tissue from retightening, thus causing continued reduced function of the hand.

Strapping

There are various techniques of strapping that can be applied in the early stages to protect injured areas from further damage whilst allowing the individual to continue with other activities and exercise. When deciding on the use of a strapping technique, it is important to consider the structure(s) damaged and the movement(s) that are likely to stress the damaged area. Strapping can be applied in such a manner as to allow maximal movement whilst giving protection from the movement(s) likely to cause further damage. This again emphasises why it is essential that the physiotherapist has a detailed knowledge of anatomy and human movement when treating injured and healing tissues.

It is important to remember that any strapping applied in these early stages must be able to accommodate any change in size or circumference due to swelling in order to prevent compromise of the circulatory system. Often compression bandaging (as discussed below) will alone restrict movement and may be sufficient to protect from unwanted movement. Alternatively, additional specific strapping may be applied to reinforce and prevent specific movement patterns.

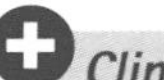

> **Clinical note**
>
> If someone has injured their anterior talofibular ligament in the ankle, it will be necessary in these early stages to protect this structure from stresses caused by inversion and plantar flexion, whilst allowing eversion and dorsiflexion movements. This can be achieved through accurate strapping.

Strapping needs to be re-applied regularly and should also be frequently monitored to ensure its safety and effectiveness. The physiotherapist will need to consider whether the patient is able to re-apply strapping independently or not; if the patient has limited contact with the physiotherapist, this consideration may influence its use.

The patient must also understand the limitations of the strapping. Some individuals may feel able to continue with all activities whilst wearing strapping, when in fact this could be detrimental to the injured and surrounding tissues.

Walking aids

Walking aids will need to be provided if gait is altered. Also, partial weight-bearing may need to be advised in the early phases to protect damaged tissues, which will be stressed excessively during weight-bearing. Remember that the main aim of prescribing a walking aid is to promote a normal gait pattern within the limits of any restricted weight-bearing. This is essential to allow normal movement patterns of adjacent joints and body segments and to minimise any secondary problems.

Rest

Rest, in this context, usually refers to some form of relative rest in terms of general movement and activity to reduce metabolic demands and hence further secondary chemical damage to tissues. Rest from specific activities (relative rest) will also go some way towards protecting damaged and newly forming tissue.

Gauging what exactly is relative rest and what activity would helpful in promoting recovery and preventing other problems requires the physiotherapist to make careful clinical decisions. In the very early stages (0–48 hours), when the tissues are still likely to be bleeding and the inflammatory process will be under way, the patient should be encouraged to rest the injured area fully to prevent increased bleeding and inflammatory response. Therefore the physiotherapist needs to balance these aims of protection and rest carefully with those of promoting movement in order to maintain normal function of adjacent joints and structures.

As this very early phase ends (around 48 hours), very gentle movement is needed to help improve circulation and removal of waste products and to provide the necessary stresses for the correct alignment and orientation of newly forming tissue fibres. This trade-off between rest and activity can often mean conflicting priorities for the patient and the physiotherapist needs to ensure that advice regarding movement and activity is clearly understood by the patient for maximum benefit.

It is worth remembering at this stage that effective physiotherapy practice is underpinned by firm clinical reasoning where individuals' physical, social and psychological needs, their tissue damage and their stage of healing are all considered in light of considered best practice in that treatment area.

Clinical note

It is essential with both elite and recreational athletes that they are advised and managed in terms of maintaining cardiovascular and musculoskeletal fitness. This may require the individual to follow a reduced or non-weight-bearing programme, such as exercise in water, reduced-impact activity or activities not involving the affected area. Remember that athletes may be eager to restart activity prematurely and the physiotherapist must take an active role in ensuring that the patient fully understands the implications of all activities on the likely outcome of their injury/problem.

Cryotherapy (ice therapy)

Cryotherapy is defined as the use of cold and cooling agents for therapeutic benefit. It has long been considered an important part of early tissue injury management. There are various methods of cooling tissues, including application of crushed ice, ice/gel packs, cold compressive devices and ice submersion. The comparative effects of these have not been fully investigated and the method of application is still mainly determined by the nature of the injury, equipment availability and therapist preference. The use of cryotherapy has not been fully explored in terms of scientific research and much of physiotherapy practice in this area is based upon empirical evidence.

The primary reason for applying ice as part of immediate early injury management is to cool the affected tissues and hence reduce the metabolic demands of neighbouring cells. This should enable more cells to survive the ischaemic phase, thus minimising secondary tissue damage. It is suggested that, to maximise the therapeutic effects of cryotherapy, an optimal tissue temperature reduction of 10–15 degrees is required (MacAuley 2001). If application of cryotherapy can reduce the number of cells damaged overall, the healing and repair process will be quicker, hence speeding up return to function.

Traditionally, the application of cryotherapy may have been thought to induce vasoconstriction of the small blood vessels, thus reducing blood supply to the area and hence causing increased ischaemia to the tissues and further secondary damage, as initially described by Knight (1989). Merrick (2002) suggests that the secondary injury model outlined above now better describes the effects of cryotherapy.

The duration, application and frequency of cooling to achieve maximum therapeutic benefits have not yet been determined scientifically, yet these factors will greatly affect the degree of tissue cooling. Clinical guidelines for the application of ice in acute injury management suggest that an application of crushed ice in a damp towel for 20–30 minutes every 2 hours may be the optimal method (Kerr et al. 1999). However, tissues involving more than 2 cm of subcutaneous fat may require cooling in excess of 30 minutes in order to reduce the temperature of the injured tissues sufficiently. Other important points are that the cold application should cover the whole area of injured tissue and a damp towel should be placed between the cooling agent and the skin to avoid skin and tissue damage.

The use of cryotherapy is widespread in practice and it is generally accepted that it is a very safe, easy to use modality, which makes it very popular. However, it is vitally important to remember that direct cold application can cause what are commonly referred to as 'ice burns'. These may be described as superficial frostbite and the symptoms are similar to those of a thermal burn: pain, redness, swelling and blistering. It has been highlighted recently that ice burns are probably under-reported and are much more common than was previously thought.

Key point

Remember to exercise caution when applying cryotherapy and re-assess the patient regularly.

If the patient has reduced sensation or nerve injury is suspected, extreme caution must be used and it is advisable to avoid cryotherapy until this has been fully assessed.

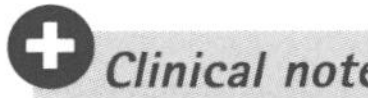

Clinical note

When deciding on the dosage of cryotherapy application always consider:

- the size of the injury
- the depth of the tissues injured and of the subcutaneous fat.

Always check sensation and monitor the skin regularly for evidence of ice burns. Placing a damp towel between the ice pack and skin should avoid damage, as should the use of a cold compression device.

Compression

Compression of the affected tissue and adjacent areas can also be used in the early phases to reduce exudate, protect tissues and possibly reduce pain.

The theory behind the application of compression is that the hydrostatic pressure of the interstitial fluid is raised, thus pushing fluid back into the lymph vessels and capillaries and reducing the amount of fluid that can seep out into surrounding tissues (Rucinski et al. 1991). External compression through the application of an elastic wrap can stop bleeding, inhibit seepage into underlying tissue spaces and help disperse excess fluid (Thorsson et al. 1997).

Compression can be applied using a tubular bandage or some form of elasticated bandage strapping, which may be adhesive or non-adhesive.

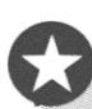

Key point

It is vital that any product used is elasticated in order to accommodate changes in size or circumference of the body part without compromising circulation.

Compression can be used in direct conjunction with cryotherapy in the form of an ice compression device, such as a Cryocuff, which allows simultaneous cooling and compression of tissues. If this method is not used, there is generally some trade-off in terms of using cryotherapy and compression. It is not usually possible to cool tissues sufficiently through a compression bandage; therefore, intermittent use of cooling methods may be applied between compression.

Unfortunately, very few studies look specifically at the effects of applying compression alone in acute soft tissue injury, and again much of contemporary practice is based upon experiential evidence and consensus opinion (Kerr et al. 1999).

Clinical note

When applying compression you will need to consider the following points (Kerr et al 1999):

1. Apply compression as soon as possible after injury.
2. Always apply compression from distally to proximally.
3. Where possible, apply the compression a minimum of 15 cm above and below the affected area.
4. Always follow manufacturer's instructions where available.
5. Do not apply compressive materials with the material at full stretch.
6. Ensure consistent overlap (half to two-thirds of previous turn) of compressive material.
7. Apply turns in a spiral fashion, *never* in a circumferential pattern.
8. Use protective padding such as gauze, underwrap, foam and so on over vulnerable areas such as superficial tendons and bony prominences.
9. Do not apply elasticated leggings in the lying position or in association with elevation.
10. Remove and reapply if the pressure appears not to be uniform or if the patient complains of discomfort; otherwise reapply within 24 hours.
11. Continue compression for first 48 hours when the patient is not lying down.
12. Always check distal areas following compression to check for diminished circulation: that is, colour changes or cold.

Elevation

Another treatment method aimed at reducing bleeding, swelling and thus pain in acutely injured soft tissues is elevation. Some studies have suggested that elevating the injured limb above the level of the heart reduces inter-arterial pressure and enhances draining of extravascular fluid away from the area; however, scientific evidence supporting this is minimal.

It is common practice to combine cryotherapy and compression with elevation in order to minimise swelling and gathering of interstitial fluid (Kerr et al. 1999). However, continuously elevating the limb above the level of the heart is often impractical (especially if it is the lower limb) and may even compromise vascular supply to the body part if combined with compression. It may be more appropriate to advise the patient to elevate the affected limb intermittently during the day when possible and to remove compression at this time.

In the early stages a large amount of swelling is often evident if an individual with lower limb injury (particularly distal injury) stands and walks for a long time with the injured part in a dependent position.

It would seem logical that if patients are advised to minimise the amount of standing and walking they do and to elevate the limb from the earliest point, this may reduce the accumulation of fluid, which can quite quickly become thickened and fibrous due to its high protein content. When an individual does stand and walk around, then the use of compression would seem sensible to continue to minimise the accumulation of exudate in the surrounding tissues.

One practical point to remember when advising elevation is to support the limb adequately during elevation through the use of pillows or a sling (Kerr et al. 1999).

First-line management

Increasingly in modern physiotherapy practice the physiotherapist will constitute the first line of medical assessment, management and advice. This may occur, for example, in the sporting environment, in private practice or via direct access services. These roles require the physiotherapist to have excellent assessment skills and experience, and an understanding of differential diagnoses and indications for onward referral. Several guidelines are in place to aid clinicians in managing and diagnosing injuries and in using investigations such as radiology. Physiotherapists should be aware of these guidelines and implement them appropriately in order to promote best practice. For example, physiotherapists working in these settings should be familiar with the Ottawa guidelines for ankle injury (Bachmann et al. 2003), which guide clinicians as to when to X-ray the ankle to rule out fracture.

Applying the PRICE principles in practice

Having discussed the elements of the PRICE principle, we can see that it is evident that there are sometimes conflicting demands and it is often not possible, or indeed appropriate, to employ all five principles simultaneously. As discussed previously, the research evidence underpinning these interventions is insufficient and much of everyday practice is based upon historical approaches and consensus opinion (Kerr et al. 1999). It is therefore important to take this into account, along with the physiological processes occurring in the tissues, when rationalising a treatment plan for an individual patient. It is also important to make realistic and reasoned treatment decisions considering all biopsychosocial factors. This is illustrated in the case studies at the end of this chapter.

Severity of injury and progression through the healing continuum

The speed of progress and recovery of those who have sustained soft tissue injury will in fact vary, depending on a large number of factors. These will include the type, severity and location of injury, the individual's tissue type and response to injury, and many extrinsic factors such as patient exposure to appropriate treatment and advice in the immediate stages and any other psychosocial factors. For example, a minimal grade I ligament injury, effectively managed in the early stages, may move very quickly through the continuum of tissue injury to repair and remodelling within a few weeks, whereas major tissue injury induced through trauma or surgery may require a much longer process. Those individuals not seeking advice and treatment in the early stages are more likely to develop problems such as chronic swelling and loss of range of movement and function in injured and adjacent structures and may even have compromised the formation of appropriate new tissue.

In view of this, it is desirable that individuals seek early advice from an appropriately trained professional and that they fully understand the advice and treatment approaches taken. Many of the treatment modalities discussed so far can often be implemented by a patient independently at home, and the frequency and accuracy with which they do so will have a large impact on their recovery and progress. It should therefore be ensured that physiotherapy intervention is focused on establishing full patient understanding of the advice and treatment approaches to be implemented at home, especially if the frequency of physiotherapy contact will be limited. If the patient does not fully understand advice and instructions regarding their activities at home, then any benefit gained from a physiotherapy treatment session will be undermined by the patient's behaviour in the intervening period.

When deciding on how long to continue to apply these principles, consideration of the severity and size of the injured area is required. Despite the common descriptions of grades of muscle and ligament injury in use, it is impossible to determine severity accurately without radiological investigation such as ultrasound imaging. This is an area of increasing research; however, its clinical relevance in the management of muscle injuries is still under debate. Without the aid of valid and reliable imaging it would seem sensible to use the patient's level of pain and possibly gentle palpation to assess the size of injury as indicators of when to move rehabilitation forward.

As discussed earlier, it is often suggested that early movement of the injured part should begin at around 72 hours post-injury, as initial pain is reducing, and that the patient should to progress to gradual achievement of a full range of movement of the affected tissues, before moving on to increase normal muscle power, strength, timing and proprioceptive control in light of the patient's individuals needs and abilities.

In the early stages, acute pain is often a sign of further tissue injury and bleeding, and thus activity and movement of the injured area should be discouraged. However, as the continuum progresses, pain is often secondary to problems such as joint stiffness and lack of strength and control, and needs to be respected but not seen as a barrier to progressing rehabilitation. This will be discussed in detail in the following sections.

PHASES 3 AND 4 OF TISSUE HEALING AND REPAIR

This section deals specifically with the management of patients in the later stage of the healing and repair process: that is, beyond the initial bleeding and inflammation stages (the first 1–3 days following injury). Watson (2004) refers to these phases as the stages of proliferation and remodelling. The physiotherapeutic management of patients in these stages of the healing and repair process is still driven by the utilisation of physiotherapeutic measures that complement, support and encourage these normal processes and therefore promote and facilitate repair. The reasoning underpinning physiotherapy in these stages of healing relates to the plastic properties of human tissue.

Plasticity in human tissue

14

> ***Definition***
>
> Plasticity refers to a quality associated with being plastic, malleable, capable of being shaped or formed (Oxford English Dictionary 2007).

Although the term plasticity tends to be most frequently applied in the field of neurology, it is important to recognise that it is a characteristic of all human tissue. Human tissues have the capacity to adapt to the nature and extent of the forces applied to them. For example, if we consider the practice of lifting weights. Over a period of time, within a progressive lifting programme, an individual is able to lift progressively larger weights. The skeletal muscles and tendons loaded by lifting weights adapt over time as the individual progressively lifts more weight. These adaptations affect all components of the musculotendinous apparatus. The contractile component of the muscle grows larger and stronger (Kraemer and Ratamess 2004) and becomes capable of producing increased force. In parallel with this process, the non-contractile components become correspondingly stronger and thicker to accommodate the extra loading (Benjamin 2002). In addition, adaptations occur at the interface between the tendon and the bone so that the bony prominences also develop to withstand the increased force exerted.

Consider an individual who suddenly lifts a weight or engages in an activity where the force generated with the musculotendinous apparatus exceeds that which the muscle, tendon or bone can withstand. In this situation the tissue fails to withstand the force applied and injury occurs. For example, excessive load generated in the quadriceps muscle may lead to muscle damage, patellar tendon damage or avulsion fracture of the tibial tubercle.

Human tissues undergo reversal of these adaptations during the periods of immobilisation/reduced activity that frequently follow trauma. In these situations the effect of immobilisation causes the reverse of the processes identified above. This reduces the ability of the damaged tissues to withstand loading. Physiotherapeutic management of these patients focuses on trying to restore the affected tissues' capacity to withstand normal loading, therefore enabling the individual to return to normal function. It is important to remember that these soft tissue adaptation processes occur in both the injured and the uninjured tissues.

> ***Clinical note***
>
> A patient who sustains a severe second-degree injury to the lateral ligament complex at the ankle and who subsequently has to non-weight-bear will experience soft tissue changes throughout the non-weight-bearing leg and not just in the tissues directly affected by the trauma.

Physiotherapeutic approaches are therefore fundamentally aimed at capitalising on this plastic property of human tissue so that therapy works alongside and enhances the normal healing and repair processes.

Factors influencing the rate of healing in the stages of proliferation and remodelling

One important consideration is that the processes of tissue proliferation and remodelling take place over significant periods of time (Watson 2004). The period of time for the completion of these pathophysiological processes can run into years and is dependent on a number of factors including:

- *Severity of initial trauma*: for example, a severe second-degree ligament sprain of the lateral ligament complex at the ankle will have a more prolonged proliferation and remodelling period than a first-degree ligament sprain affecting the same structure.
- *Early management*, where the approach taken to management has laid the necessary foundations for

proliferation and repair: for example, an appropriate approach has been taken to rest/protection of traumatised tissues (see earlier sections of this chapter). This has the potential to reduce the onset of chronic inflammation where an agent is responsible for the ongoing irritation of an injury and therefore perpetuates the period of the stages of bleeding and inflammation.
- *Tissue vascularity*: for example, skeletal muscle, which is highly vascular, has more potential for repair than a relatively avascular tendon.
- *Age*: for example, a similar grade of injury is likely to take longer in the repair process in an older individual than one who is younger (Myer 2000).
- *Nutrition*: adequate nutrition that is also related to blood flow is required for healing to take place.
- *Medication*: for example, NSAIDs and steroidal drugs slow down proliferation and remodelling processes.
- *Temperature*.
- *Biochemical factors*.
- *Appropriate loading* of healing tissue during rehabilitation.

It is very important for physiotherapists to have a depth of understanding of the pathophysiological processes involved in proliferation and remodelling, as well as the clinical reasoning skills required to make appropriate professional decisions. In addition, in order for treatments to be effective, physiotherapists will also need an ability to apply their knowledge of the clinical effects of a number of physiotherapeutic treatment modalities, as well as a grasp of psychological and sociological theory. In this section short case study examples will be used to illustrate the main points.

Evans (1980) simplified these processes in his 'graphs of hours', 'graphs of days' and 'graph of months'. Although dated, this serves as a useful timeline against which to make judgements about physiotherapy approaches. An understanding of the timeframes involved in this continuum enables the physiotherapist to coordinate an approach to treatment and to capitalise on the normal healing processes whilst ensuring that physiotherapy intervention does not induce further trauma and therefore delay healing and repair.

PHASE 3: TISSUE PROLIFERATION (FIBROUS REPAIR) (1–10+ DAYS POST-INJURY)

Pathophysiology

Cellular processes during this stage include:

- ongoing phagocytosis
- angiogenesis (formation of new blood vessels)
- proliferation of fibroblasts
- production of collagen fibres (initially produced in an unordered and random fashion)
- absorption of inflammatory exudate.

As the initial processes of inflammation begin to lessen, the inflammatory exudate starts to be absorbed. This leads to a decrease in swelling and pain is reduced as a result. An increase in swelling during this stage is usually indicative of a more severe injury. Alternatively, it may be due to inappropriate early management. For example, a patient who has sustained a severe second-degree sprain of the lateral ligament complex at the ankle joint returns to full weight-bearing activity before the injured tissue strength has developed to a point where it is capable of withstanding the forces that walking demands of it.

Tissue proliferation begins to occur as early as 24 hours after trauma. This proliferation initiates the stage of fibrous repair, which usually involves the production of scar (collagen) material. The nature of the tissue that is produced in the proliferation phase is dependent on which elements of the tissues are initially damaged. If the cellular framework (satellite cells) is not damaged, then regeneration of these cells may be possible. If the cellular framework is destroyed, then the tissue is replaced by scar tissue. In addition, if the damaged cells have no capacity to regenerate because they are deemed to be permanent cells (for example, nerve cell bodies or cardiac muscle), then scarring definitely occurs. Scar tissue is a non-differentiated form of fibrous tissue, which may develop some properties of the original tissue but will not function in the same way as the normal tissue would.

By 2–3 weeks after the injury the majority of the scar tissue is in place. After this time the rate of proliferation diminishes but may continue for several months following the injury. There is no hard and fast rule about exactly when this occurs, as the timeframe will vary in accordance with the factors detailed at the beginning of this section; for example, it will occur earlier in vascular tissues.

Around 3–4 days following trauma the process of cell death will be complete and this means that the physiotherapist can assess the injury more objectively. At this stage there is a reduced risk of aggravating/increasing trauma or identifying false positive findings because the patient's pain is masking the real symptoms. It is at this point that the physiotherapist can begin to use therapeutic techniques to promote an increase in circulation and tissue temperature without fear of inducing further tissue damage or further bleeding.

PHYSIOTHERAPY INTERVENTIONS IN PHASE 3 (1–10+ DAYS POST-INJURY)

General physiotherapy aims in the tissue proliferation stage (phase 3)

At this stage in the repair process the aims of physiotherapy might include the following:

1. to decrease pain
2. to decrease swelling
3. to decrease local temperature
4. to prevent further trauma
5. to protect new tissue
6. to increase range of movement
7. to maintain/increase muscle strength/timing and control
8. to prevent soft tissue adaptation in non-injured tissues
9. to improve function.

The above represents an approach to a treatment that is impairment-focused and biomedical. It is essential that this generic approach be modified to reflect the individual nuances of each patient and his or her individual and specific psychosocial needs. For example, aims 6 and 9 could be joined into one function-specific, patient-centred goal — that the patient is able to tie his or her own shoelaces.

In this phase physiotherapeutic treatment approaches are aimed at the achievement of the goals identified above by influencing the pathophysiological processes involved in this stage of healing and repair. Whilst approaches to physiotherapy geared to addressing aims 1–4 have largely been covered when considering the management of the bleeding and inflammation stages of the healing and repair continuum, these are still worthy of mention here. In order to reduce pain, the injury may require a degree of ongoing protection, such as limiting movement to that which is pain-free. However, the degree of protection will slowly be reduced throughout this stage.

Cryotherapy

Cryotherapy can continue to be utilised if the injured area continues to have an elevated temperature. However, in this phase it is likely that it will only be required in more severe injuries. Often the physiotherapist might choose to apply cryotherapy at the conclusion of a treatment session. The clinical reasoning underpinning this is that during this stage the potential to cause minor bleeding and inflammation as a result of treatment is high, due the frail and vulnerable nature of the newly developing tissue. Cryotherapy applied at the end of treatment can potentially minimise this.

Prescribing activity and exercise in the proliferative stage

During this proliferative stage the main input on the part of the physiotherapist is to encourage a graded return to exercise and activity. This is achieved through the prescription of a specific exercise programme tailored to each individual patient's needs. This type of approach, incorporating the active involvement of patients, is valuable as it promotes patient empowerment and prevents them from taking a passive approach to treatment.

The aims of increasing range of movement, maintaining/increasing muscle strength/timing/control, preventing soft-tissue adaptation in non-injured tissues, and improving function are all best achieved through the application of graded exercise and activity. Inevitably function will be improved to some extent by activity to increase range, increase muscle strength and prevent soft tissue adaptation. However, it is important that functional activities pertinent to the individual are targeted specifically within an individual's treatment programme as early as possible. For example, increasing ankle range of movement is unlikely to produce a direct improvement in walking performance without specific rehabilitation activity aimed at improving walking.

Key point

The primary emphasis of activity and exercise in this proliferative phase is to increase range of joint movement.

Grading the level of activity

Ensuring that any activity undertaken by the patient early in the proliferative stage is completed within pain-free limits provides a mechanism to protect newly developing tissues and prevent further secondary damage to those tissues initially traumatised at the time of the injury. It is sensible throughout this proliferative stage of healing and repair to use the patient pain report during activity as an indicator of appropriate levels of activity and exercise. As a rule, any activity or exercise prescribed in the proliferative phase that provokes pain that could be classified with a high SIN (pain **s**everity, **i**rritability and **n**ature) factor should be avoided.

From around the second day post-injury fibroblasts are increasingly prevalent around the site of the trauma. These are the precursors to the formation of new fibrous tissue that will enable the healing process. In the proliferative phase it is inappropriate to perform aggressive activities or exercises involving areas directly affected by trauma, as this will only serve to damage the newly developing tissue further. The use of gentle, active movements, controlled by the patient and within the pain-free range, is appropriate at this point and these will stimulate fibroblast activity and promote the production of collagen tissue. This is an example of the plasticity described earlier in the chapter.

Key point

Caution is needed with some injuries in the proliferative stage so that the movements produced do not promote calcification within the associated soft tissues: for example, so-called dead leg (haematoma of the thigh) following quadriceps contusion. In dead leg the quadriceps muscle is crushed against the femur by a direct blow. This injury commonly damages the periosteum of the femur, which causes osteoblasts to move into the overlying soft tissues (quadriceps). Over-aggressive early movement can promote osteoblastic activity within the muscle, which may develop into myositis ossificans. A large observed difference in uninjured and injured knee range immediately after injury and inability to play on are both key early indicators of myositis ossificans developing as a likely complication (Alonson et al. 2000).

Beyond the fourth day post-injury, as proliferation of newly developed collagen tissue begins to accelerate, healing of the injured tissue is strengthened and, as a result, increasingly greater ranges of pain-free movement can be expected. The physiotherapist needs to encourage patients to practise these movements frequently throughout the day. Taking movements to their pain-free limit will begin progressive loading of the newly developing tissues and will facilitate an inbuilt progression of activity because, as the pain eases, progressively greater ranges of movement will be achievable. This will promote the further formation and alignment of collagen and hence stimulate repair and the development of a functional scar (Watson 2004). However, care must continue to be taken, as during this phase any excessive loading still has the potential to damage the newly formed tissue, thereby provoking further injury and delaying the repair process.

Range of movement exercises will contribute to the maintenance of muscle strength and promote tissue loading, but during this stage it is normal practice to limit the amount of overt strengthening/timing/control exercise recommended to the patient until full non-weight-bearing, pain-free, active and passive ranges of movement are achieved. The use of isometric contractions involving structures not directly affected by the injury can be commenced early in the process.

Clinical note

A patient with a severe second-degree sprain of the lateral complex of the ankle can safely exercise the knee and thigh area during the proliferative stage. The degree to which the muscles of the thigh can be loaded may be influenced by the ability of the patient to weight-bear.

Another available physiotherapeutic technique suitable for this stage is reciprocal inhibition. This can be useful to increase range of movement and tissue length (Waddington 1976). Reciprocal inhibition is the physiological phenomenon that occurs when a skeletal muscle (antagonist) contracts and the opposing muscle (antagonist) relaxes. This technique can be useful when trying to encourage elongation of the musculotendinous apparatus. Its main use is when muscle tension or muscle spasm is identified as the reason for limited range of motion.

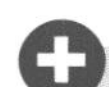

Clinical note

A person with a grade 2 hamstring injury that occurred 6 days ago is likely to be at the stage where some encouragement of increasing length in the hamstrings is desirable to load the newly forming collagen tissue in order to promote further proliferation and repair. In clinical practice this is often difficult due to protective muscle spasm in the affected hamstring group. Reciprocal inhibition, whereby active contraction/shortening of the quadriceps group is used to induce relaxation and lengthening in the hamstrings, can be used. This can be achieved by placing the individual on the unaffected side, fixing the hip of the affected leg in 40 degrees of flexion (thereby ensuring minimal stretch on the hamstrings over the hip joint), moving the knee into extension until slight stretch in the hamstrings is felt and then providing isometric resistance to the quadriceps. As this resistance is applied to the quadriceps, the opposing muscle group (hamstrings) relax reciprocally and allow further elongation. This provides a load to the newly forming fibrous tissue and therefore facilitates repair. The skill involved in this technique lies in ensuring that the lengthening achieved in the hamstrings is slow and controlled. In addition, undue pain in the hamstring group should not be provoked by this technique.

Very gentle passive static stretching of affected tissues can be begun at this stage, as long as precautions are taken not to be over-zealous. Again, the patient's pain report is the main indicator of the amount of stretch that it is safe to apply. Ballistic stretching would not be advocated at this stage, as the potential to overstretch the newly forming tissues and re-injure whilst performing this technique is high.

As the tissues continue to proliferate, more fibrous tissue is laid down and the healing tissues begin to get stronger. During this time corresponding increases in the forces applied to the tissues can be made by augmenting the force of stretch applied, widening the range of movement produced and raising the number of repetitions of any activity.

As a progressively greater load is applied to newly forming fibrous tissue, it begins to remodel in response to the increasing forces applied. In addition, it is proposed that the haphazard arrangement of collagen laid down in the early healing stages begins to take on a more organised pattern as load is applied to it. The collagen fibres begin to align themselves along the lines of stress. It is therefore important that the stresses applied to newly forming tissue are directed along the functional lines of stress normally required by that tissue. This requires physiotherapists to apply their anatomical knowledge in an effective way.

From about the sixth day post-injury onwards, increasing amounts of fibrous tissue are laid down and so increasing levels of activity can be correspondingly promoted. Tissues should be stressed progressively. It is considered to be both safe and advantageous to warm up the affected tissues prior to activity and this has the effect of reducing the amount of load required to stress the tissues (compared with cold tissue); therefore the tissue can be stressed more safely.

14

Electrotherapy in tissue healing and repair

The use of electrotherapy in the healing and repair processes has long been discussed and there is varied evidence to support or discount the use of modalities such as ultrasound, pulsed electromagnetic energy and laser therapy in facilitating these processes. Electrotherapy as a topic is very large and this chapter does not claim to address all the literature and physiology surrounding these modalities fully. The reader is referred to Chapter 18 and to other texts for further information and discussion of these topics.

The most common electrotherapy modalities, which appear to have the potential to have a direct action on the tissue repair process, are ultrasound (US), pulsed shortwave diathermy (PSWD) and laser therapy. There is substantial evidence to support the notion that these modalities all have the capacity to influence the normal physiological processes of tissue repair, particularly the early inflammatory stage; however, clinical trials that

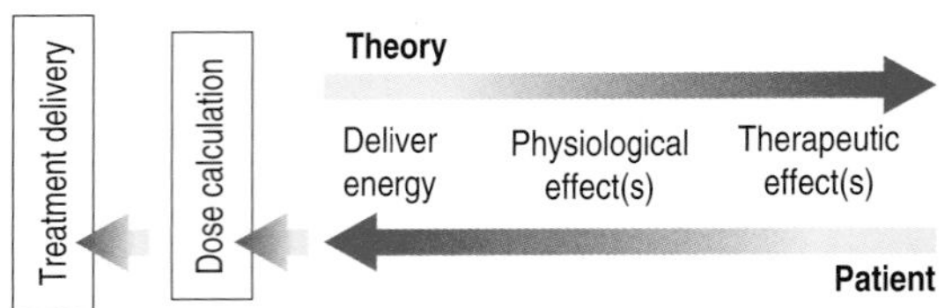

Figure 14.3 A simple model of electrotherapy. (Reproduced from Watson 2006, with permission.)

demonstrate their efficacy in the clinical situation are lacking.

Watson (2006) describes a simple model of electrotherapy (Figure 14.3). This model summarises how machine-generated energy in one form or another is delivered to the tissue. This energy is then absorbed by the tissue (to varying degrees, depending on type), which then results in a change in one or more physiological events. It is the process of the energy being absorbed by the tissues and resulting in a physiological shift that is referred to as the therapeutic effect.

Choosing when and how to use electrotherapy

As with any modality, such as manual therapy, exercise or drug therapy, there is an optimal time to apply it and an appropriate dosage or intensity.

Watson (2006) suggests that the clinical reasoning process behind the use of electrotherapy can be illustrated by working through a reversal of the model shown in Figure 14.3. Starting with the patient and knowing his or her identified physiotherapy problems and stage of healing and repair, the clinician can now work out what physiological effect is required and on what type of tissue. Once this is known, the appropriate modality can be chosen, based on the best available evidence. It must be remembered that if there is no electrotherapy modality suitable for achieving the desired result, then electrotherapy has no place in the management of this condition at this particular time (Watson 2006).

Research suggests that it is the dosage applied and the specific tissue type that appear to influence this physiological shift most greatly. Studies have shown that different modalities applied at different dosages can have very different physiological effects. There does not yet seem to be, at the current time, an optimal dosage identified for any of the modalities for specific tissue types, thus making it difficult for the clinician to justify fully their choice of dosage.

In the proliferation stage it may be appropriate to continue to apply electrotherapeutic modalities, again ensuring that this is only used when an appropriate therapeutic window for the modality selected exists. During this phase the processes of phagocytosis, fibroblast and myofibroblast proliferation, and protein synthesis are prevalent. These processes can be therapeutically enhanced by the use of ultrasound, laser or pulsed shortwave diathermy. All of these modalities have the potential to exert a pro-proliferative effect whereby collagen synthesis is enhanced, if selected appropriately (that is, related to their specific tissue absorption properties), applied at the appropriate time, and given in an appropriate dose. This enables a speeding up of the proliferative phase and therefore can facilitate the rehabilitation process.

PHASE 4: TISSUE REMODELLING (10 DAYS+ POST-INJURY)

Pathophysiology

The key processes involved in the phase of tissue remodelling are:

- ongoing fibroblast activity and collagen production (usually peaking 2–3 weeks following injury)
- absorption of older fibrous tissue
- deposition of new fibrous tissue
- scar tissue contraction
- replacement of type III collagen fibres by type I.

You must remember that the different phases of the healing and repair process do not occur in perfect sequence. The phase of tissue remodelling and soft-tissue contraction overlaps significantly with the earlier proliferation phase (Figure 14.2). The peak of fibrous tissue repair occurs 2–3 weeks after the injury and the whole healing process is a dynamic one, as older fibrous tissue is removed and new scar tissue is laid down. The continued application of physical stress to the developing tissues is one of the most significant factors influencing this phase of the repair process. The newly laid-down fibrous tissues becomes more 'organised', being arranged less randomly and beginning to orientate itself along the lines of stress, thus enabling them to function more normally. This is the beginning of the remodelling phase, which can continue for months and possibly for over a year. It is clear, therefore, that this process continues long after the noticeable healing process and definitely beyond the time for which the patient is in direct contact with the physiotherapist within the active rehabilitation process. This means that therapy, usually in the form of activity and exercise, needs to continue long after an individual has been discharged from the ongoing care of the physiotherapist. Some evidence shows that, even at this stage, remodelling is still ongoing and tissues are not returned to their full functional capacity. Research into anterior cruciate ligament repair in monkeys has indicated that the ligament regained 56 per cent, 76 per cent and 96 per cent of its normal tensile strength 6 weeks, 12 weeks and 24 weeks respectively after repair. Whilst this extent of remodelling may be acceptable in some members of the population, it may not be so in others.

A key feature of the remodelling phase is soft-tissue contraction, the process by which the newly formed tissues begin to shorten physically. There is a potential for the healing tissues to begin to restrict and limit mobility and range of movement in the affected tissue. This process of soft tissue contraction begins to occur around the third week post-injury and continues long into the remodelling phase. Since this continues long after a patient would normally be discharged from the therapist, it is a key influence on the nature of the ongoing prescription of activity and exercise given to patients following discharge.

Key point

The potential for tissue re-injury during the process of soft-tissue contraction is clear. Failure to address this and to plan activity and exercise strategies to avoid it is a key influence on re-injury patterns.

This phase of the remodelling process takes place after the proliferative phase and is referred to as the chronic stage in some texts. Within this chapter this phase is seen as a natural progression following the proliferative stage in an uncomplicated process of proliferation and remodelling.

PHYSIOTHERAPY INTERVENTIONS IN PHASE 4

General physiotherapy aims in the remodelling stage (phase 4)

The aims of physiotherapy in the remodelling stage may include any or all of the following:

- to promote collagen growth and fibre/tissue realignment
- to increase range of movement:
  - active
  - passive
  - accessory
- to increase muscle strength/control/timing
- to prevent soft-tissue adaptation in injured and non-injured tissues
- to maximise function.

These aims can be related to the ongoing pathophysiological processes involved. Fibroblastic activity increases and new collagen fibres continue to be laid down. This process peaks around 2–3 weeks post-injury and continues through to 4–6 weeks following injury, being clearly extended beyond this timeframe in more severe injuries. Ongoing attention is required to progressive activities, as begun in the third to tenth days post-injury. The purpose of the physiotherapeutic treatment is to promote movement and mobility of the injured structures/tissues.

Preventing tissue contraction and adhesion formation

Beginning around the third week post-injury, the healing scar tissue begins to undergo a process known as soft-tissue contraction. This means that the physical length of the tissue actually begins to get shorter. Consider this in the case of a hamstring injury, as described above. At the same time that you are working therapeutically with the patient to lengthen the hamstrings, the remodelling tissue begins to cause the healing scar tissues to shorten. This process can continue for a considerable period of time after the injury. At this stage it is normal for the patient to experience some discomfort during end-range stretching activity.

> ***Clinical note***
> In practice this means that end-of-range stretching should commence at the third week after injury and should continue until the scar tissue contracture process is completed. The reality is that this is a very long-term process, which may need to continue for as long as the remodelling process; as we have seen, this may be in excess of 1 year.

Contractures can sometime become permanent. In this case, it becomes impossible to stretch the scar tissue. This is known as fixed contracture. Fixed contractures develop when the normal connective tissue (which is elastic) is replaced by fibrous tissue (which is inelastic). This means that the tissue will not stretch, thus preventing normal movement. Contractures can occur in any tissue. The key to preventing the development of fixed contractures lies in ongoing therapeutic exercise and activity aimed at ensuring that, as scar tissue forms, it remains a mobile, functionally able structure. At the end of the remodelling stage the injured soft tissue will be repaired by scar tissue. The desired outcome is that this final scar is able to serve as a functional replacement for the tissues initially injured.

Another potential problem during the remodelling phase is the formation of soft-tissue adhesions. This is when newly forming fibrous tissue has been produced between adjacent layers of tissue, such that these layers become bound together. These adhesions, when formed, can severely limit movement and soft-tissue function. Normal movement requires that adjacent layers of tissue are able to move independently; for example, a tendon moves over a bony surface or beneath a fascial band such as retinacula whilst the bone/retinacula stay still. Since the formation of fibrous tissue during the proliferation phase is completely random, the potential for the development of adhesions is a real one. It is movement in the early stages of healing and repair that helps to ensure that the newly forming tissues do not create these adhesions. In some healing processes, where long periods of immobility are part of the patient management, their formation is probably inevitable. Soft-tissue adhesions are normally easily palpable, feeling thickened and immobile to palpation and mobilisation.

> ***Clinical note***
> It is worth considering what happens with soft-tissue repair processes following fracture. A patient sustaining a fracture of the distal radius is normally immobilised within 6–8 hours of the fracture in a plaster cast, which remains in place for a minimum of 4 weeks. During this time the normal soft-tissue repair phases of bleeding, inflammation, proliferation and some remodelling all occur whilst the arm is immobilised. The tissues are not subject, during this time, to any of the beneficial loading described in this chapter. When the plaster is removed, improving mobility and range of movement in the tissues can take significant periods of time.

Passive and accessory mobilisation techniques

Other techniques aimed at restoring full working/functional length in tissues include passive and accessory movement techniques. The application of these demands the application of an in-depth knowledge of human anatomy. This means that the physiotherapist can select the appropriate techniques to attempt to influence a specific structure.

Activity and exercise continue to play a key part in the physiotherapy management. A shift towards an activity and exercise programme placing greater emphasis on improving muscle strength/timing/control is normally seen at this stage. It is important to consider all the ways in which the tissues in question are loaded during normal functional activity. This enables the physiotherapy programme to be tailored appropriately to an individual's need.

Muscle tissue will need to be able to withstand load from active and passive forces, from concentric, eccentric and isometric contractions at varying points within its range. It may need to work in an open-chain or closed-chain environment. It may need to function as an agonist, antagonist, synergist or fixator. It may need to generate strength, power or endurance. All of these factors must be considered when developing patient-specific exercise and activity programmes in the remodelling phase. Only when all of these things are considered and incorporated effectively into an exercise and activity programme is the potential for rehabilitation of individuals back to their full and maximum functional capacity realised.

The context of an individual's normal functional activity is paramount to effective physiotherapy practice, whether it be playing a 90 minute game of football in the Premiership or getting into and out of a car. The key skill that the physiotherapist utilises here is that of movement analysis. By analysing the demands of the activities that an individual aspires to be involved in, the physiotherapist is able to plan rehabilitation to meet individual need with the aim of maximising each individual's capacity. Too often, in the authors' opinion, the lowest common denominator of functional ability is accepted; this becomes the norm and physiotherapeutic intervention fails to enable individuals to achieve their full potential.

> ***Clinical note***
>
> Returning a patient to full road-running function following a second-degree sprain of the hamstring muscles requires full range of motion in the joints of the lumbar spine, hip and knee, appropriate muscle control of the leg musculature (a combination of concentric, eccentric and isometric contractions), and the ability to run at different speeds, on different surfaces (including inclines) and to varying distances. All of these aspects must be covered in the final rehabilitation programme if the individual is to reach maximum potential.

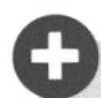

> ***Clinical note***
>
> Returning a patient to playing rugby following a dislocated shoulder requires an analysis not only of the demands of the sport per se but also of the specific position that a player may take on the field. Rugby players need to be able to throw and catch whilst running, run with the ball, tackle and be tackled. In addition, they will need to be able to withstand a direct fall on to the affected arm.

> ***Clinical note***
>
> A window cleaner returning to work after a second-degree sprain of the lateral ligament complex of the ankle requires full range of motion in the joints of the ankle complex and foot, appropriate control of lower leg musculature (a combination of concentric, eccentric and isometric contractions), and the ability to walk at different speeds, on different surfaces and to varying distances. He or she must also be able to balance on a limited base of support, at a variety of heights, for significant time periods whilst cleaning windows. Finally he will probably need to be able to land steadily on his foot when jumping from a height. All of these aspects must be covered in the final rehabilitation programme if the individual is to reach maximum potential.

Tissue remodelling is a prolonged process and this is especially pertinent in young patients who are remodelling and growing at the same time. In this client group remodelling periods are often prolonged beyond the normal periods for adult members of the population.

> ***Clinical note***
>
> It should be acknowledged that, whilst this chapter identifies the key influences that physiotherapy could have on the process of tissue healing and repair, in cases of severe and extensive soft-tissue trauma a degree of permanent loss of function of the affected tissues is inevitable. This loss of function within the tissues may lead to a degree of long-term disability for the individual affected.

CASE STUDIES

The following case studies apply the principles covered in this chapter to two common soft-tissue lesions in the lower limb. The case studies have been chosen in an attempt to demonstrate the similarities and differences in managing patients with soft-tissue trauma affecting different tissues. Read through them, along with Tables 14.1–14.2, and try to relate them to the phases of tissue healing and repair.

CASE STUDY: AN INJURED HAMSTRING

Joe is a 25-year-old university student who plays football on a weekly basis. He injured his right hamstring whilst playing football yesterday. He describes a sudden onset of pain in the posterior thigh whilst he was running. He was unable to play on and hobbled off the pitch. There was no first aid advice available. He spoke to a friend, who recommended that he go to see a local physiotherapist. Joe has self-prescribed ibuprofen and paracetamol. He is otherwise well and has had no previous injuries.

Joe attends the physiotherapy clinic the next day and limps into the clinic, weight-bearing only through his toes on the affected leg.

CASE STUDY: AN INJURED ANKLE

Margaret is a 55-year-old hotel receptionist who slipped whilst coming down the stairs this morning, sustaining an inversion injury to her left ankle. She is unable to weight-bear and has severe pain in her foot and ankle; she is therefore attending the accident and emergency department at her local hospital. X-ray has revealed no bony injury. She is provided with crutches and taught to non-weight-bear. She is given an appointment to see the physiotherapist in A&E that afternoon.

Table 14.1 Case study: An injured hamstring

Treatment aim	Treatment intervention
To protect newly damaged tissue from further damage	Cryotherapy: apply ice pack or ice compression device to injury site (20 mins minimum duration regularly through day)
To reduce metabolic demands of tissue	Compression application of elasticated strapping (as described above)
To prevent and reduce swelling	Elevate affected limb for intermittent periods. Beware of combination with prolonged extensive compression
To reduce pain	Use of crutches initially to protect injured area and to encourage weight-bearing as pain allows
To protect newly forming tissue from disruption	
To prevent soft-tissue adaptation in non-injured tissues	Pain at the early stage should be seen as a protective mechanism to protect and prevent further damage. Encourage movements of hip and knee within pain limits. Anything that provokes pain at anything other than a minimal level should be discouraged initially
To promote collagen growth and fibre realignment	
To increase and restore normal joint range of movement (passive, active and accessory)	Increase passive and active movements of the hip and knee and then combine movement of both joints to increase stretch and load on tissues
To maintain and increase muscle strength, timing and control	Progress active and dynamic activity, looking at lower limb and pelvis as whole
To increase proprioception of affected lower limb	Increase activity/football-specific tasks to increase proprioception, timing and neuromuscular control
To increase tensile strength of new collagen tissue	
To restore and encourage optimal function in relation to patient's needs	

Table 14.2 Case study: An injured ankle

Treatment aim	Treatment intervention
To protect newly damaged tissue from further damage	Cryotherapy: apply ice pack or ice compression device to ankle/foot (? 15 mins minimum duration regularly through day). Monitor for reactions, remembering tissues are superficial and there is minimal subcutaneous fat
To reduce metabolic demands of tissue	
To prevent and reduce swelling	Compression: apply elasticated strapping, particularly when patient is mobilising and not elevating distal limb (as described above)

(Continued)

Table 14.2 Case study: An injured ankle—cont'd

Treatment aim	Treatment intervention
	Elevate affected limb for intermittent periods. Beware of combination with prolonged extensive compression Advise on minimising walking and standing in first 5 days to reduce accumulation of swelling
To reduce pain To protect newly forming tissue from disruption To prevent soft-tissue adaptation in non-injured tissues To promote collagen growth and fibre realignment To increase and restore normal joint range of movement (passive, active and accessory)	Teach safe use of crutches initially to protect injured ankle, with weight-bearing as pain allows Pain at the early stage should be seen as a protective mechanism to protect and prevent further damage. Encourage movements of knee, ankle and foot within pain limits. Anything that provokes pain at anything other than a minimal level should be discouraged initially Encourage normal gait pattern without use of crutches as pain and acute stage ends Increase passive and active movements of the knee, ankle and foot and then increase stretch and load on tissues Consider using accessory joint mobilisations to maintain/increase range of movement at the distal tibiofibular, talocrural, subtalar and mid-tarsal joints
To maintain and increase muscle strength, timing and control To increase proprioception To increase tensile strength of new collagen tissue To restore and encourage optimal function in relation to patient's needs	Progress active and dynamic activity, looking at lower limb and pelvis as whole. Increase activity/specific tasks to improve proprioception, timing and neuromuscular control of lower limb, particularly around the foot and ankle Consider occupation and return to work. Can job be adapted initially to allow early return to work or is time off appropriate? Consider all patient's needs in terms of sport and activities

REFERENCES

Alonson A, Hekeik P, Adams R 2000 Predicting recovery time from the initial assessment of a quadriceps contusion injury. Aust J Physiother 46(3): 167–177

Bachmann LM, Kolb E, Koller MT et al. 2003 Accuracy of Ottawa ankle rules to exclude fractures of the ankle and mid-foot: systematic review. BMJ 326: 417–425

Benjamin M 2002 Tendons are dynamic structures that respond to changes in exercise levels. Scand J Med Sci Sports 12(2): 63–64

Evans P 1980 The healing process at cellular level. Physiotherapy 66(8): 256–259

Kerr KM, Daily L, Booth L 1999 Guidelines for the Management of Soft Tissue (Musculoskeletal) Injury with Protection, Rest, Ice, Compression and Elevation (PRICE) the first 64 hours. Chartered Society of Physiotherapy: London

Knight KL 1989 Cryotherapy in sports injury management. Int Perspect Physiother 4: 163–185

Kraemer WJ, Ratamess NA 2004 Fundamentals of resistance training: progression and exercise prescription. Med Sci Sport Exerc 36(4): 674–688

MacAuley D 2001 Ice therapy: how good is the evidence? Int J Sports Med 22: 379–384

Merrick M 2002 Secondary injury after musculoskeletal trauma: a review and update. J Athl Train 37(2): 209–217

Mutsaers SE, Bishop J, McGrouther G et al. 1997 Mechanisms of tissue repair: from wound healing to fibrosis. Int J Biochem 29(1): 5–17

Myer AH 2000 The effects of aging on wound healing (wound care and seating). Topics Geriatric Rehabil 16(2): 1–10

Oxford English Dictionary 2007: http://dictionary.oed.com

Rucinski TJ, Hooker DN, Prentice WE et al. 1991 The effects of intermittent compression on oedema in post-acute ankle sprains. J Orthop Sports Phys Ther 14(2): 65–69

Thorsson O, Lilja B, Nilsson O et al. 1997 Immediate external compression in the management of an acute muscle injury. Scand J Med Sci Sports 7: 182–190

Waddington PJ 1976 PNF Techniques. In: Hollis M, Fletcher-Cook P (eds) 1999 Practical Exercise Therapy. Blackwell Science: Oxford

Watson T 2004 Soft Tissue Wound Healing Review. www.electrotherapy.org

Watson T 2006 Electrotherapy and tissue repair. Sportex Med 29: 7–13

Chapter **15**

Neurological physiotherapy

Julie Rigby, Christine Smith and Anita Watson

CHAPTER CONTENTS

INTRODUCTION

The challenges facing physiotherapists working in the clinical field of neurology are many and varied. The complex nature of the human nervous system and the vast array of neurological conditions found in clinical practice place heavy demands on physiotherapists. The onset of a neurological condition, as a result of disease or trauma, has a devastating effect not only on the patient but also on families. It is essential that any approach to management encompasses the needs of the patient and significant others. Many neurological conditions are progressive and longstanding and result in some element of residual impairment. There are many challenges in the rehabilitation process from diagnosis to discharge. The longstanding nature of many neurological conditions means that professionals are involved in management and rehabilitation over many years.

Historically, there has been a lack of research in the field of rehabilitation, and regarding the role of the physiotherapist in particular. There is now a growing evidence base that supports a variety of approaches to the rehabilitation of the neurologically impaired patient. The role and function of the physiotherapist is contextualised within a team approach to the treatment and rehabilitation of neurologically impaired adults. The importance of a collaborative approach to rehabilitation is widely supported within the literature (Edwards 2002; Plum and Morissey 2002; Fawcus 2000; Stokes 1998). Neurological dysfunction can result in the disruption of normal physical, psychological, cognitive and social functions. Consequently, this demands the collaboration and co-ordination of a number of rehabilitation professionals. No one professional group can offer all the expertise required to enable patients to reach their maximum level of recovery. It is vital that a truly holistic approach to the management and treatment of patients and their families be adopted, with clinical reasoning and problem-solving at its centre.

This chapter begins by outlining the principal causes of neurological dysfunction and then describes some of the commonly occurring clinical features. The clinical features have been grouped together into categories to aid cross-reference within the assessment process. Some of the general principles of physiotherapy assessment and treatment are discussed in relation to present-day clinical practice. The variations in approaches to rehabilitation add to the complexity and challenges facing the physiotherapist working in neurology. The section on the general principles of physiotherapy offers the reader an eclectic approach to rehabilitation and is not intended to promote any one approach over another.

Measurement of outcome is an important aspect of neurological rehabilitation. The chapter provides a section on outcome measurement and goal-setting in relation to the International Classification of Function framework set out by the WHO in 2001. The most commonly used outcome measures have been critically appraised in relation to their psychometric properties.

The chapter concludes with an overview of the more commonly known neurological conditions, namely stroke, Parkinson's disease, multiple sclerosis, motor neurone disease and traumatic brain injury. These sections are not intended to be exhaustive, and readers can consult the list of further recommended reading at the end of the chapter.

Background knowledge

Readers are also advised to refer to appropriate literature for details of the anatomy of the central nervous system (CNS) in relation to its function (Figure 15.1). A thorough understanding of the structure and function of the CNS and the neural control of movement will be needed to manage patients with complex neurological dysfunction effectively.

Glossary

Towards the end of this chapter is a glossary of some of the terms used within neurology.

NEUROLOGICAL DYSFUNCTION: BASIC ISSUES

Principal causes of neurological dysfunction

The most commonly occurring neurological dysfunction is that which occurs as a result of dysfunction

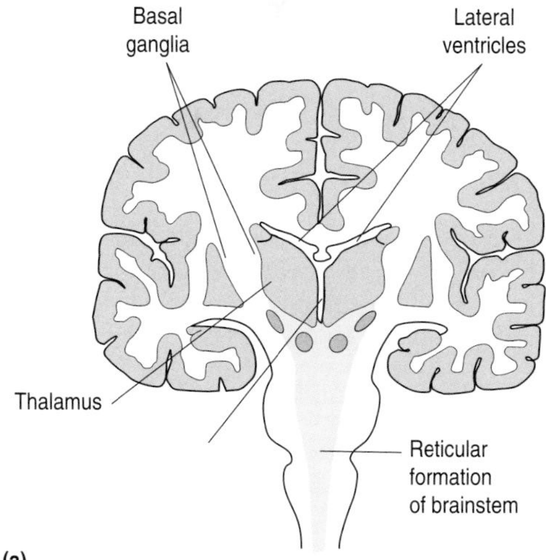

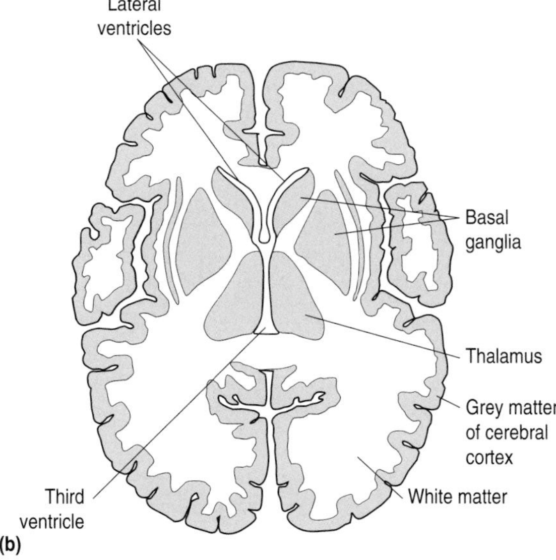

Figure 15.1 Internal appearance of the brain and brainstem. (Reproduced from Palastanga et al. 2002, with permission.)

within the circulatory system: namely, stroke (detailed more fully later). Other causes of neurological dysfunction include trauma, as in head injury or spinal injury, where direct or indirect trauma results in temporary or (if there has been destruction of nerve tissue) permanent damage. Diseases can affect the nervous system and some seem to have an affinity for a particular part of the system. Examples of diseases that can affect the nervous system are meningitis, syphilis and (less commonly) tuberculosis and poliomyelitis. Diseases of unknown origin that affect the CNS include multiple sclerosis, motor neurone disease and Guillain–Barré. Multiple sclerosis and motor neurone disease are discussed later in the chapter.

Congenital defects such as spina bifida, inherited conditions such as Huntington's chorea, vitamin B deficiency, neoplasms and toxic substances such as lead, arsenic and mercury can all have a detrimental effect on the nervous system too. However, these are less common occurrences and therefore will not be covered within this chapter. Peripheral neuropathies and fibromyalgia are also not covered.

Clinical features of damage to the CNS

The clinical features of disruption to the CNS are determined partly by the site(s) and the severity of the damage. However, the CNS is integrative in nature and so damage to one part will result in a disruption in function of other parts. The site of damage alone is not necessarily a predictor of the clinical features with which patients will present. No two patients' nervous systems are the same and how each patient responds to any given damage will also be different. Despite the fact that patients do not present in exactly the same way, there are common clinical features that arise. Some of the main features are covered below.

Physical dysfunction

Smooth and efficient movement is reliant upon intact sensory and motor pathways. Any disruption to these pathways will lead to movement disorders.

Incoordination of movement

Weakness or paralysis of muscle groups will result in an imbalance of activity and therefore incoordination of movement.

Ataxia

Movements are jerky and patients have difficulty grading or controlling movements. Sometimes this can be due to a loss of postural control and an inability to produce co-contraction within muscle groups. The type of ataxia is determined by the system affected. The various forms of ataxia are listed in Table 15.1.

Involuntary movements (dyskinesia)

Dystonia (previously known as athetosis)

Movements are writhing and slow and are often brought on by attempts to move. Generalised dystonia may produce gross movements of the arms and legs. Focal dystonias usually involve the eyes, neck or upper limbs. They are thought to occur as a consequence of damage to the basal ganglia. There may also be disruption in facial and tongue movements. It is thought that these movements may be due to a disturbance in reciprocal inhibition.

Table 15.1 Types of ataxia and associated motor disorder

Sensory ataxia	A 'high-stepping' gait pattern More reliance on visual or auditory information about leg or foot position
Vestibular ataxia	Disturbed equilibrium in standing and walking Loss of equilibrium reactions A wide-based, staggering gait pattern
Cerebellar ataxia	Disturbance in the rate, regularity and force of movement Loss of movement coordination Overshooting of target (dysmetria) Decomposition of movement (dyssynergia) Loss of speed and rhythm of alternating movement (dysdiadochokinesia) Incoordination of agonist–antagonist muscles and loss of the continuity of muscle contraction (tremor, e.g. intention tremor)

(Reproduced from Stokes 1998, with permission.)

Chorea

Although patients with chorea also present with jerky movements, these movements tend to occur more randomly throughout the body. The absence of sustained abnormal posturing distinguishes this condition from dystonia.

Ballismus

The movements are large and sudden and can affect one side of the body (hemiballismus).

Tremor

These are fine, rapidly oscillating, unwanted movements. Tremors are often classified in relation to the circumstances in which they occur. For example, an intention tremor is made worse by voluntary movement of the limb, particularly at the end of a movement. The precise mechanisms related to tremors are continuing to be explored. A condition in which tremor often features is Parkinson's disease.

Disturbances in muscle tone

Tone can be defined as 'a state of readiness'. Each person has his or her own particular state of readiness that changes according to the circumstances. Muscle tone consists of both neural and non-neural components. Both tonic reflex activity and the visco-elastic components of the muscle are important to consider. In clinical practice muscle tone may be abnormally increased (hypertonia) or decreased (hypotonia), or more commonly a combination of the two.

Sensory disturbances

Disturbances in cutaneous sensation result from a disruption in afferent information. This can be classified as *paraesthesia*, or *anaesthesia* when there is diminished or absent afferent information. An increase in cutaneous sensitivity is termed *hyperaesthesia* and can be an equally troublesome feature. The presentation depends on the site of the lesion and the severity of the damage.

Pain is a feature of some neurological conditions. The source of the pain can vary, ranging from disturbances in nerve endings and/or pathways, to pain caused by secondary complications such as malalignment of joints. It is important to carry out a comprehensive assessment to identify the cause of pain. Effective management of the pain is essential, as patients who present with pain will report that this is the symptom that most concerns them.

Cognitive/emotional changes

Occasionally patients may present with altered cognitive function. For many patients this type of impairment can be more disabling than physical impairments. Even some mild cognitive difficulties can result in individuals being unable to live independent lives. Rehabilitation for these types of difficulty is also usually less established. Damage to the frontal lobes, such as following some types of head injury, tends to predispose patients to these types of change. Examples include altered levels of arousal, reduced attention span and memory impairment. Changes in behaviour can include agitated states, disinhibition and reduced motivation. Emotional changes can present in the form of emotional lability, depression or euphoria.

Key point

Care must be taken to distinguish emotional changes that occur as a direct result of the pathology and those that are the person's reaction to the newly acquired or diagnosed condition.

Perceptual disturbances

This is a non-specific term that describes the way in which the individual perceives sensory information. Perception requires the interaction of visual and spatial components. Types of perceptual disturbance include disruption in figure–ground differentiation, spatial awareness, inattention or neglect, disturbances in constructional abilities, and many other forms. The reader is advised to consult texts specifically focused on this type of difficulty, as these areas can be particularly complex to assess and treat.

Visual disturbances

Many neurological conditions affect visual pathways. Examples include hemianopia, in which the patient loses vision in half the visual field of each eye, diplopia (double vision), nystagmus (incoordination of eye movements) and optic neuritis (lesions of the optic nerve).

Auditory disturbances

Deafness directly related to neurological conditions is relatively uncommon in neurological patients. When it does occur, it is usually due to trauma to the structures of the auditory system.

Communication disturbances

These can be particularly frustrating and disturbing for patients, particularly those who have a good insight into their difficulties. Communication involves both receptive and expressive components. Examples of communication disorders are dysarthria (motor disturbance), dysphasia (receptive and expressive language disorder) and dyspraxia. Collaboration with a speech and language therapist is required in order to be fully informed of the patient's level of difficulty.

Autonomic disturbances

Dysfunctions may be due to damage affecting autonomic areas or pathways. Following spinal cord injury, some patients can present with autonomic dysreflexia. This is a sympathetic nervous system discharge producing hypertension, bradycardia, sweating, skin vasoconstriction, headache, pilo-erection and capillary dilatation. This response is often triggered by impaired bladder or bowel function or other noxious stimulus.

APPROACH TO PHYSIOTHERAPY

Rehabilitation and team working

The patient's main goal is usually to achieve as high a degree of independence and quality of life as possible. This will depend on many factors:

- the environment in which the person will be functioning
- the extent of damage to the central nervous system
- the rehabilitation programme available
- the patient's motivation to achieve his or her goals.

Physiotherapists need to employ a problem-solving approach to the rehabilitation of patients with neurological damage, wherever possible engaging the patient in this process. Many different approaches to the rehabilitation of patients are emerging and an eclectic approach to neurological rehabilitation is becoming increasingly accepted. Emerging approaches to neurological rehabilitation include:

- constraint-induced movement therapy
- robot-assisted therapy
- virtual reality-based therapy
- locomotion training, using devices for automating bodyweight support
- functional electrical stimulation (FES).

Key point

The increasing amount of research in the field of neurological rehabilitation and the growing acceptance and knowledge of the mechanisms of neuroplasticity are informing modern therapies. Physiotherapists need to stay abreast of new developments and the emerging evidence base on which to base their practice.

Physiotherapists need to be able to make a comprehensive assessment of the patient's neurological deficit and remaining abilities in order to formulate an appropriate programme of rehabilitation. This can only come from a sound understanding of the control of human movement, the likely implications of damage to areas of the nervous system, and knowledge of the types of treatment approach available and when best to apply them. Advantages and disadvantages of the various types of intervention need to be considered.

15

There is increasing acceptance that the nervous system and the musculoskeletal system cannot be separated, as they work harmoniously together to meet the demands placed upon them. Hence many concepts previously utilised exclusively within each of these fields are becoming commonly used in both areas.

Physiotherapists have a key role in all aspects of patients' management. This might be selecting the most appropriate treatment programmes for patients, implementing review programmes to maintain patients at their optimum level of functioning, or delaying deterioration in the case of progressive neurological conditions. Realistic goals that are measured and time-framed, and that consider the whole person and the family/carers need to be negotiated.

Therapy programmes should be carried out in the environment that is most appropriate for the patient, taking into account the nature of the patient's goals, the stage of the rehabilitation process and the facilities available. This might mean that treatment is implemented in the hospital setting or in the community. The shift of programmes towards community settings allows therapists to choose the most appropriate location for treatment, be it the patient's home, the place of employment, the gymnasium or the supermarket!

Key point

Using a team approach within rehabilitation is considered standard practice these days. However, the composition of the team and the model of team working adopted can vary.

ASSESSMENT OF NEUROLOGICAL PATIENTS

Irrespective of changes in approaches to rehabilitation, the one factor that remains consistent is the need to carry out a comprehensive assessment of the patient and the environment in which he or she is likely to be functioning. Many members of the healthcare team will carry out assessments. Wherever possible, joint assessments with exchange of information, sometimes in the form of shared case notes, will be carried out.

Assessment is an ongoing process that, in reality, is an integral part of treatment. Assessment of neurological patients is complex and multifaceted, and contains many interrelated elements. Often assessment occurs over a number of sessions with the patient, because carrying out a full assessment in one attempt can frequently be too tiring for the patient. Gathering the necessary information over a longer period of time invariably gives a much more accurate picture of the patient's strengths and difficulties.

Clinical interview (subjective history)

As in all assessments, obtaining a thorough subjective history is vital. This can come from a variety of sources: the medical notes, nursing notes, the patient, relatives and carers. Initial interviews can be very important, not just for gathering information, but also because this is where establishing a rapport with the patient and carers begins.

Physiotherapists need to draw on all aspects of their communication skills to allow the patient and family to be at ease. Increasingly, in appropriate cases, initial interviews take place in the patient's home. This not only ensures that the person is more relaxed, but also allows assessment of the patient's functional environment. Later, when home programmes are being devised, knowledge of the patient's home can be invaluable.

When assessing patients with communication disorders, it is important to find alternative or supplementary methods of communicating with them. Collaboration with the speech and language therapist is invaluable at such times.

Whilst interviewing the patient, important clues can be observed with regard to physical abilities, communication, cognition, emotion, hearing, vision and attention span.

It should also be noted how much the patient changes position, attends to posture and so on. Assessment thus begins the minute contact is made with the patient.

The assessment should include both background history and also components specific to physiotherapy. Background history should include demographic details, past medical history, diagnosis, the present condition and its history, medication, social factors (housing, family, lifestyle, care circumstances) and details of the involvement of other healthcare professionals.

Clinical examination (objective history)

The main purpose of the clinical examination is to gather information about the patient's movement disorder and level of functional ability (Freeman 2002). Initially, observe the patient and try to draw conclusions about what he or she is able to do unaided. It is important to bear in mind the fact that at no point must the patient be put at risk. It is part of the physiotherapist's role to 'risk-assess' what it is reasonable to allow patients to attempt independently and what they need help with in order to be safe. Once patients have been given the opportunity to demonstrate what they can do unaided, assistance can then be given to ascertain what they can achieve with help. This is where assessment and treatment begin to merge into one and the same thing. By conducting an assessment in this manner, it is possible to see how the patient responds to handling, albeit in the short term. It is not uncommon for physiotherapists' eyes to tell them one story and their hands to tell them something quite different!

It is prudent to begin the assessment wherever the person happens to be when initial contact is made. For instance, observing patients' gait when they walk into the room often gives a more accurate picture of functional gait pattern than when they are asked to walk whilst being watched.

Wherever possible, observations should be backed up by clinical or other forms of measurement. In this way, baseline information on which to build interventions and evaluation of effectiveness is made more reliable.

Outline of an assessment format

For simplicity, the assessment outlined here is based on an initial contact with a patient sitting in a wheelchair. The assessment is by no means exhaustive and is intended to be used as a guide for students. Many other assessment formats exist. It is prudent to use the one that most closely applies to your situation.

Database

- Personal details:
  Name, address, date of birth, consultant, GP.
- Medical diagnosis
- Investigations carried out:
  CT, MRI, blood tests and so on.
- Medication:
  Can impact on treatment effects, e.g. antispasmodic medication.
- Previous medical history:
  Operations, illnesses, conditions.

Clinical interview (subjective history with patient and carer where appropriate)

- Patient's and carer's perception of their difficulties:
  What are they finding difficult, including reason(s) why — personal activities of daily living, premorbid fitness, levels of fatigue and so on?
- History of present condition (HPC):
  Onset of condition and how it has progressed to date; might include previous physiotherapy treatment and how the patient responded to it.
- Social history/home circumstances:
  Occupation/lifestyle, family/partner support, general health of partner, input from support agencies, type of accommodation, toilet — upstairs/downstairs, bedroom — upstairs/downstairs, hand rail — which side, transport and so on.
- Equipment/adaptations:
  Stair lift, small equipment, wheelchair, walking aids and so on.
- Vision:
  Glasses, hemianopia, diplopia, nystagmus and so on.
- Communication:
  Dysarthria, dysphasia, dysphonia, dyspraxia.
- Swallowing and nutritional status.
- Hearing aid.
- Cognition, perception, behaviour, emotional status:
  Attention or memory deficits, speed of processing information, neglect, spatial awareness, emotionally lability and so on.
- Continence:
  Bladder, bowel function.
- Pain:
  When, where, aggravating factors, methods of relief, irritability and so on.
- Expectations of intervention:
  What do the patient/carer expect to gain from this episode of treatment?

Clinical examination (objective history in supported sitting)

- Posture:
  Alignment of body parts (e.g. head, shoulder girdles, pelvis, spinal curves, trunk creases, weight-bearing aspects), symmetry vs asymmetry, acceptance of supporting surface, ability to move within base

of support, dominated by flexion/extension/mixture of the two and so on.

- Muscle tone (observe then handle) of upper limb, trunk and lower limb:
  Hypertonicity, hypotonicity, combination of tone, associated reactions (e.g. on preparation for movement, during movement — note movement precipitating them or whether present continuously).
- Active movement:
  Observe all areas, e.g. trunk, arms, head and legs, what can be done without/with assistance and so on.
- Passive range of movement:
  What is the available joint range?
  If limited, what is it limited by, e.g. adaptive muscle shortening, joint stiffness, pain and so on?
  Use joint 'end-feel' to assist decision.

At this point in the assessment, the person can be asked to move out of the chair and on to a plinth, if deemed appropriate. By now the information needed to assess how much assistance the person requires to complete the transfer safely should have been collected. If assistance is required, the opportunity arises to evaluate the degree to which assistance is required and how effective that assistance might be. During the transfer, assessment of how effectively the patient moves from sitting to standing, along with his or her ability to transfer bodyweight and take steps, can be carried out. Finally, analysis of how the person sits down can also be completed.

15

Transferring from chair to bed

- Sit to stand sequence:
  What components of movement did patients manage by themselves and what did they need assistance with?
  If assistance was required, what was needed and why?
  Level/type of associated reactions?
- Once in standing (assess here or later):
  Balance reactions, posture, awareness of midline, alignment of body parts, muscle tone and so on.
- During moving from chair to bed:
  Do patients effectively transfer bodyweight, awareness of midline, control of placement of non-weight-bearing leg, control of stability on weight-bearing leg?
  Were they independent or did they need assistance?
  Were they safe?
- Standing to sitting:
  Is the person able to control all aspects of the movement sequence?
  Does he/she sequence the movement correctly?
  Does he/she compensate, and if so, how and why?
- Unsupported sitting:
  Re-examine the patient's posture. Has it changed? If so, why?
  Has the patient readily accepted the new base of support and is he/she able to sit independently?
  Assess all aspects of sitting balance, use of arm support, level of muscle tone and so on.
- Function whilst in unsupported sitting (if appropriate):
  For example, getting undressed. Observe changes in muscle tone, balance reactions, weight transference, compensations, strategies employed to achieve the task, sequencing of task, ability to attend to multiple tasks and so on.

Sitting to lying and supine lying

- Sitting to lying:
  Can the patient lie down independently or is assistance needed?
  How was the task achieved?
  Did the patient compensate, and if so, why?
  Did the patient influence the level of tone?
- In lying:
  Posture, acceptance of new base of support, testing of passive and active range of movement, sensory testing and so on.
- Moving within lying:
  Is the patient able to roll to either side?
  Compare analysis of movement with normal movement sequences. Does the patient compensate? Effort involved? Changes in level of tone? Functional?
- Lying to sitting:
  Can the patient sit up independently on to the side of the bed or is assistance needed? Identify any assistance required and reasons why.
  Analysis of movement sequence and comparison with normal. Functional? Can the patient move into sitting to either side?

Sitting to standing and standing to sitting

- Sitting to standing:
  Which components of the movement could the person do independently and which needed assistance? What type and why?
  Did the person move using both sides equally?
  Comparison of movement sequences with normal. Did you observe any associated reaction? If so, where and why? Functional and safe?
- Standing to sitting:
  Which components of the movement could the person do independently and which needed assistance? What type and why?

Did the person move using both sides equally?
Comparison of movement sequences with normal. Did you observe any associated reaction? If so, where and why? Functional and safe?

Standing and moving in standing

- In standing:
  What can the person do independently?
  Is the patient symmetrical? Overall posture, alignment of limbs, level of muscle tone once in standing.
  Is the patient accepting the new base of support? Compensating in any way? If so, how?
- Standing balance:
  What balance mechanisms are used?
  How do these compare with normal balance strategies?
  Why does the patient choose those particular strategies?
  Compensations, and if so, how and why?
  Functional tasks in standing?
- Moving in standing:
  Can the patient transfer weight laterally from one leg to another?
  Move weight in an anterior–posterior direction?
  Maintain own trunk, hip and knee extension?
  Compensation in any way?
- Moving in standing:
  Able to step forwards, backwards, across midline with either leg?
  Able to use saving reactions? If not, why not?
  Level of muscle tone during tasks?
  Able to maintain stability on weight-bearing leg?

Walking

- Is walking functional?
- Analyse the quality of the gait pattern.
- Use of a walking aid? If so, is it being used correctly?
- Able to walk in different directions, on different surfaces, in different environments (with distractions)?
- Is walking an effort (energy expenditure)?
- Any associated reaction? If so, when, where and why?
- Walking pattern (stance phase on each leg):
  Stability over stance leg, maintenance of hip extension and abduction, stability of hip and knee
  Are all stages of stance phase (heel strike to toe off) equally as good?
  Muscle tone?
  Compensatory strategies?
- Walking pattern (swing phase of each leg — from toe off to heel strike):
  Able to alter tone from stance phase?
  Analyse movement sequences in comparison to normal.
  Able to clear the floor? If not, why not?
  Recruitment of appropriate muscle groups? Timing of recruitment?
  Able to place either leg appropriately?

It is important during any assessment not to lose sight of the fact that many patients, following neurological damage, will have to compensate in some way. As long as the level of compensation is an appropriate one and does not rob the patient of any further recovery, this is an acceptable and often necessary compromise. Understandably, most patients' main goal is to gain as much functional independence as possible.

List of problems and goals

Now the assessment is complete, a problem and goals list needs to be formulated. It is important to bring the problems identified as a physiotherapist together with the patient's/carer's perceived problems. Problems and goals need to be agreed with the patient and family. At the end of the day it is important to remember that the goals should be the patient's, not the physiotherapist's.

- Problem list (with date set in order of priority)
- Reason for problems
- Agreed goals (in order of priority)
- Review date
- Treatment plan
- Date goal achieved, signature and job title. If not achieved, state reason why.

PHYSIOTHERAPY INTERVENTIONS

Many physiotherapists adopt an eclectic approach to rehabilitation, rather than adhering to one specific model of therapy. Historically, research into the numerous treatment approaches has been sparse and there is little evidence in the literature to support the superiority of one treatment approach over another in terms of outcome. Treatment of adults who suffer neurological injury or disease after they have reached full physical maturity is aimed at recovering function or training the patient to compensate for loss of activity. Physiotherapy management follows a problem-solving approach and involves rehabilitation/re-education of movement, maximising function and prevention of secondary complications; it should take account of social/psychological factors. Readers are directed to Edwards (2002), Carr and Shepherd (1998), Partridge (2002) and Bobath (1990) for details of specific treatment approaches.

In addition to the physiotherapist addressing problems arising from disturbance of motor and sensory function, many patients with neurological conditions may require intensive care in the acute stages of rehabilitation. With such patients, the main goals of treatment are:

- To prevent the build-up of respiratory secretions and enhance oxygenation of the brain. For intubated patients this may include the use of bagging, suction and positioning.
- To preserve the integrity of the neuromuscular system in order to prevent or minimise adaptive muscle shortening and contractures. This may include the use of passive movements, correct positioning, postural management, appropriate handling and prophylactic splinting in conjunction with appropriate drug management for spasticity.
- To provide an appropriate level of stimulation by handling and the use of sensory stimulation regimes as required.
- To provide early family education and support via involvement in aspects of the patient's care, providing time to discuss progress and potential outcomes of intervention, advice on support groups and sources of information.

For patients who are managed in a less intensive environment and those in the later stages of rehabilitation, the goals of physiotherapy are:

- To facilitate the recovery of active movement and to integrate movement into functional activities
- To maximise cardiovascular and respiratory function, muscle strength and range of movement
- To prevent secondary complications, including soft tissue adaptations
- To prevent unnecessary compensatory movement strategies
- To encourage social and vocational reintegration
- To provide advice to the patient, family, carers and other members of the team on aspects of ongoing management.

A typical time history for rehabilitation is shown in Table 15.2.

15

OUTCOME MEASURES AND GOAL-SETTING

Once the assessment is complete, key problems need to be identified by using clinical reasoning processes. Goals of treatment, with appropriate timescales, can be formulated with the patient and the family. Goals need to be negotiated and discussed with all parties, including the rehabilitation team, so that there is a clear understanding of what is involved in achieving them. Failure to go through this process can lead to frustration and misunderstanding for all parties, particularly the patient and the family.

Note on terminology

The WHO model of illness provides a useful framework and common terminology for describing and measuring the consequences of disease and the impact that rehabilitation may have on them (Edwards 2002).

The original WHO International Classification of Impairments, Disabilities and Handicap from 1980 has been replaced by the International Classification of Functioning (ICF). This change has shifted the emphasis away from impairment, handicap and disability to a more positive focus on body function, activity and participation. Table 15.3 compares the old and new terminologies.

- *'Body function'* considers the loss or abnormality of body structure, or of a physiological or psychological function.
- *'Activity'* refers to the nature and extent of functioning at the level of the person. It may be limited in nature, duration or quality .It considers whether a person can perform a task and how well they do it.
- *'Participation'* refers to the nature and extent of a person's involvement in life situations in relation to impairment, activities, health conditions and contextual factors.

This classification provides the underlying framework for which healthcare interventions can be determined and outcome measures developed.

The principle of outcome measurement

One of the responsibilities of healthcare professionals is to provide evidence of the effectiveness of their treatment and management. The introduction of the clinical governance framework within the NHS and the implications this has with regard to accountability and clinical effectiveness have meant that knowledge, understanding and use of outcome measurements is of growing importance.

Measurement implies the quantification of data in either absolute or relative terms. Determining the effectiveness of an intervention by measuring its effect on an outcome provides the basis for evidence-based healthcare (Edwards 2002). Outcome measures take the guesswork and subjectivity out of evaluation and can assist the physiotherapist in proving clinical effectiveness.

Outcome measures also provide a method of communication. The importance of a language of universal use among clinicians must be promoted. The focus on multidisciplinary care and the blurring of traditional professional boundaries require at the very least a system of measurement that can be understood by and utilised by the whole interdisciplinary team.

Table 15.2 Typical time history for rehabilitation

Stage	Definition	Typical management
Acute	Immediate period following the event	Initial assessment of basic systems Physiotherapy intervention for respiratory system Initial dialogue with patient and carers about the nature of the condition Assessment of patient's environment and social milieu
Intermediate	Period that commences once the patient is medically stable, conscious and actively engaged in the rehabilitation process	Regular identification and assessment of agreed rehabilitation objectives Active engagement in physiotherapy intervention programme Formulation and adherence to self-treatment strategies
Discharge and transfer	Period immediately prior to and following discharge from formal rehabilitation	Assessment of residual disability Physiotherapy intervention for agreed discharge objectives Modifications to the patient's environment Management of transfer of skills between environments Review and monitoring of self-treatment strategies Determination of the pattern of rehabilitation once the patient has returned home or when community physiotherapy stops
Long-term		May include: Regular review of patient status Task-specific treatment sessions Review and modification of self-treatment strategies

(Reproduced from Stokes 1998, with permission.)

15

Table 15.3 Comparison of the old and new WHO terminologies

Terminology prior to 2002	Terminology after 2002
Impairment	Body function
Disability	Activity
Handicap	Participation

A wide range of outcome measures is available and care is required when deciding which outcome measure to use, and when. The general principles to follow when developing and/or considering the use of outcome measures are:

- Identification of what needs to be measured
- Selection of the appropriate outcome measure
- Establishing whether it measures what you want it to measure (reliability, validity and sensitivity)
- Establishing whether it is easy to use on a day-to-day basis (clinical utility).

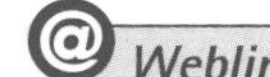

Weblink

The Chartered Society of Physiotherapy (CSP) has provided a summary of the outcome measures currently available that have relevance to physiotherapy care interventions. It can be found on the CSP website at www.csp.org.uk.

Outcome measures should be sensitive enough to allow for measurement of changes over time. The use of a suitable outcome measure for all physiotherapy interventions is an essential part of the treatment and management process, and the clinical area of neurology is no exception.

Outcome measures in context

Physiotherapy outcome measures should be considered in the wider context of rehabilitation. Rehabilitation can be considered a problem-solving and educational process aimed at reducing disability and enhancing function in people who are affected by disease (Wade 1992).

Rehabilitation principles are based upon the enhancement of activity by restoring skills and capabilities through functional retraining and environmental adaptation. Rehabilitation promotes independence and aims to facilitate the fullest potential physically, psychologically, socially and vocationally for a patient. Rehabilitation involves the recovery or improvement of function as well as prevention of disability and the maintenance of social role.

Irrespective of the approach taken towards rehabilitation, the ability to quantify the function is the key to successful treatment. This process involves assessment, treatment planning, goal-setting and evaluation of outcome. The WHO ICF classification and the process of rehabilitation together provide the context in which outcome measurement is used in physiotherapy.

Table 15.4 provides a summary of the outcome measures commonly used within neurology. It is not meant to be comprehensive and the reader is directed to the recommended reading list at the end of the chapter.

The types of measure available include functional, technical and quality-of-life measures:

- *Functional measures* are concerned with the level of ability or dependency. It is the change in the functional status of the patient and in the amount of caring and assistance required by the patient that tends to be the aim of neurological rehabilitation (Stokes 1998). At this time there is no standard outcome measurement available. Examples of the outcome measures currently used are the Barthel Index, Functional Independence Measure (FIM), Gross Motor

15

Table 15.4 Outcome measures frequently used within the clinical setting

Dimension	Outcome measure	References
Impairments		
Muscle strength	Hand-held dynamometer	Bohannon et al. (1995)
	MRC grades	Medical Research Council (1976)
Range of motion	Goniometry	Norkin and White (1975)
Tone	Modified Ashworth Scale	Bohannon and Smith (1987)
Sensation	Stereognosis	Lincoln and Edmans (1989)
Fatigue	Fatigue Severity Scale	Petajan et al. (1996)
Disability		
Global disability		
Generic	Barthel Index	Mahoney and Barthel (1965)
	Functional Independence Measure	Granger et al. (1993)
Disease-specific	Motor Assessment Scale for Stroke	Carr et al. (1985)
Focal disability		
Gait	10-metre timed walking test	Wade (1992)
	Hauser Ambulatory Index	Hauser et al. (1983)
Mobility	Rivermead Motor Assessment Scale	Lincoln and Leadbitter (1979)
Balance	Functional reach test	Duncan et al. (1990)
	Timed get-up-and-go test	Podsialo and Richardson (1991)
Upper limb function	Nine-hole peg test	Mathiowetz et al. (1985)
	Action Research Arm Test	Crow et al. (1989)
	Frenchay Arm Test	Sunderland et al. (1989)
Handicap	London Handicap Scale	Harwood and Ebrahim (1995)
	Environmental status scale	Mellerup et al. (1981)
Quality of life		
Generic	36-item Short Form Health Survey	Ware et al. (1993)
	Nottingham Health Profile	Hunt et al. (1981)
Disease-specific	39-item Parkinson's Disease Questionnaire	Peto et al. (1995)
	Functional assessment of multiple sclerosis	Cella et al. (1996)

(Reproduced from Edwards 2002, with permission.)

Function Measurement (GMFM) and the Motor Assessment Scale (MAS).
- *Technical measures* are concerned with the level of body function. Examples of these are muscle tone measurement, range of movement and muscle performance measurement.
- *Quality-of-life measures* are concerned with the level of participation and the patient's ability to function in the community and interact with society. Examples of these are the Nottingham Health Profile and Short Form 36 (Stokes 1998).

Goal-setting

Definition

Goal-setting refers to the identification and agreement of targets that the patient, therapist and team will work towards over a specified period of time (Wade 1999a,b).

The planning of goals is necessary to ensure that the rehabilitation effort is as effective and efficient as possible (Elsworth et al. 1999). Outcome is better if the goals involve the patient, are challenging and are set at different levels.

The evidence relating to goal-setting is limited, but there is a general trend towards its inclusion in the rehabilitation process (Wade 1999c). With the emphasis on patient-centred care and inclusion of the patient in the decision-making processes, a formal process of goal-planning will help to improve the coordination and cooperation of all those people involved. Cooperative goal-setting makes the process of rehabilitation more patient-focused and helps to motivate the patient through the long period of rehabilitation and beyond. In other words, the effects of treatment will be long-lasting and will continue to be evident when treatment has ceased.

Good rehabilitation practice should involve SMART goals (**s**pecific, **m**easurable, **a**chievable, **r**ealistic, **t**ime-framed):

1. Set meaningful and challenging but achievable goals.
2. Involve the patient and carers.
3. Include short-term and long-term goals.
4. Set goals both at a team and an individual professional level.

Key point

Patients may or may not be present at the goal-planning meeting but it is obviously important that their wishes be represented. Being present at the actual meeting may be too stressful for the patient.

It is common practice to set goals for the long, medium and short term. In summary the terms commonly used to document goals are:

- long-term goals = aims
- medium-term goals = objectives
- short-term goals = targets.

Wade (1999a) defines these terms as in Table 15.5.

In summary, goal-setting allows for the alignment of patient and professional goals. It is a method of ensuring that the rehabilitation team focuses on the needs of an individual patient and can help to motivate patients. It should lead to an overall improvement in treatment effectiveness and provide a method of measuring the effectiveness of treatment interventions (Edwards 2002; McGrath and Adams 1999).

STROKE (CEREBROVASCULAR ACCIDENT)

Introduction

Each year in England and Wales 110 000 people have their first stroke and 30 000 go on to have further strokes (Department of Health (DoH) 2001). Stroke is the single biggest cause of severe disability and the third most common cause of death in the UK. A substantial proportion of health and social care resources is devoted to the immediate and continuing care of people who have had a stroke (DoH 2001) and approximately 5 per cent of all hospital costs can be attributed to stroke care (Fawcus 2000). Stroke accounts for 10–12 per cent of all deaths in industrialised countries, and 88 per cent of stroke deaths occur in patients over the age of 65 years (Bonita 1992).

A stroke (cerebrovascular accident) has a major impact on a person's life. It can lead to long-term

Table 15.5 Aims, objectives and targets

Aim	Describes a state Is for the patient and family Is in terms of a social role or functioning or well-being
Objective	Is set within the medium term Involves direction of change as much as achieving a specific state Is framed in terms of patient behaviour and environment
Target	Is set within the short term Is specific and often involves only one named person/profession May be set at any level or in terms of the rehabilitation process

(Reproduced from Wade 1999b, with permission.)

15

disability and necessitate long-term care. Patients who have suffered a stroke present healthcare professionals with a variety of complex physical, psychological and social problems. The sudden loss of any capacity causes severe stress not only to the patient but also to the family. The resultant neurological deficit can have a devastating outcome.

The signs and symptoms associated with a stroke (see below) are dependent upon the size and location of the lesion.

A stroke usually results in hemiplegia (paralysis of one side of the body). This hemiplegia is contralateral to the side of the brain in which the lesion occurs. An interruption of blood flow to the brain leaves the patient with a focal loss of function of varying severity. The most common deficit is a motor deficit. Other neurological deficits can include:

- visual
- perceptual
- sensory
- communication
- swallowing.

Definition

Stroke can be defined as an interruption of blood flow (of vascular origin) to the brain, resulting in a range of focal neurological deficits that last longer than 24 hours (Lundy-Ekman 1998). WHO defines stroke as 'a condition with rapidly developing clinical signs of focal loss of cerebral function, with symptoms lasting longer than 24 hours or leading to death, with no apparent cause other than that of vascular origin' (Fawcus 2000).

These can be seen in isolation or in any combination and vary widely between patients. Disorders of balance and posture are a commonly occurring feature (Fawcus 2000).

The neurological deficit ranges from a temporary loss of function followed by complete recovery, to permanent life-altering impairment and disability, to death. It is generally referred to as a *non-progressive lesion*; that is, the severity of signs and symptoms is worse initially and declines with time and treatment intervention.

Key point

Eighty-four per cent of strokes are ischaemic in origin and 16 per cent result from a haemorrhage. The prevalence is 2 per 1000 of the population. Forty per cent of sufferers have a residual neurological deficit, 30 per cent die and 30 per cent make a full recovery.

Early diagnosis of a stroke is vital to ensure that the most appropriate treatment is provided. The development of the Face Arm Speech Test (FAST) by the Stroke Association allows a simple and quick diagnosis to be made. FAST requires an assessment of three specific symptoms of stroke, all of which should be tested:

- *Facial weakness* — can the person smile? Has the mouth or eye drooped?
- *Arm weakness* — can the person raise both arms?
- *Speech problems* — can the person speak clearly and understand what you say?

Transient ischaemic attack (TIA)

A number of people suffer from a brief focal loss of function with full recovery occurring in 24 hours. This is known as a *transient ischaemic attack*. This may lead to a major stroke and is sometimes seen as a warning event. Approximately 5–10 per cent of people who have a TIA will go on to have a major stroke. Some people have a mild residual deficit, which persists for days or weeks. This is referred to as a *minor stroke* or a *reversible ischaemic neurological deficit* (RIND; Hume-Adams and Graham 1998). The Primary Care Concise Guidelines for Stroke (RCP 2004) state that it is important for people who suffer a TIA to commence a daily dose of 300 mg aspirin once their symptoms have resolved. This helps to reduce the risk of a further TIA or stroke.

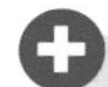

Clinical note

Strokes can occur at any age but are more common in the elderly. There are several risk factors associated with cerebrovascular disease, listed in Table 15.6.

Pathology

Strokes are non-progressive in nature and are caused by ischaemia or haemorrhage. A small number are caused by congenital abnormalities of the blood vessels and can result in spontaneous intercranial haemorrhage. These defects of the blood vessels are known as

Table 15.6 Risk factors for stroke

Major risk factors	Minor risk factors
■ Hypertension	■ Contraceptive pill
■ Raised cholesterol	■ Excessive alcohol consumption
■ Atherosclerosis	■ Physical inactivity
■ Diabetes mellitus	■ Obesity
■ Cardiac disease	
■ Smoking	

(Reproduced from Weiner and Goetz 1994, with permission.)

arteriovenous malformations (AVMs). They are liable to subsequent bleeding and surgical intervention is the treatment of choice (Stokes 1998; Fawcus 2000).

Ischaemic stroke

Ischaemic stroke occurs when an embolus (a migrating clot) or thrombus (a fixed clot) lodges itself in a blood vessel, obstructing the blood flow to the area distal to the blockage. This causes an abrupt interruption to blood flow and leads rapidly to cell death and focal neurological deficit. The thrombus is usually due to atherosclerosis and is often associated with hypertension, diabetes mellitus, and coronary or peripheral vascular disease. The symptoms of ischaemia develop over a few minutes.

The area affected by the stroke will depend upon the distribution of the artery and the degree of anastomosis by other cerebral arteries. The addition of oedema at the site of the lesion will add to the focal deficit. Once the oedema has reduced, the residual deficit will become apparent. Patients will complain of headache with hemiplegia, and there may be a disruption of speech. The hemiplegia is initially hypotonic but may develop into hypertonicity within a few days of the stroke.

Haemorrhagic stroke

A haemorrhagic stroke occurs when there is a rupture of a blood vessel into the brain tissue. This can occur as a result of hypertension that leads to lipohyalinosis in the small arteries of the brain, causing micro-aneurysms to form. These then rupture. The onset is dramatic, with severe headache, vomiting and loss of consciousness.

Subarachnoid haemorrhage

This occurs when there is bleeding into the subarachnoid space following the rupture of a berry aneurysm near the circle of Willis. There is a sudden intense headache associated with vomiting and neck stiffness. Loss of consciousness may occur. Ten per cent of people will die within a few hours, and 40 per cent within 2 weeks (Stokes 1998). Surgical intervention is the best hope of recovery, followed by intensive rehabilitation.

Brain imaging (RCP 2004) should be undertaken within 24 hours of onset of symptoms to allow early detection of the type of stroke. This will allow the most appropriate medical intervention to be delivered.

Clinical features

The clinical manifestations of occlusion of the cerebral arteries are shown in Table 15.7.

The clinical features depend on the size and severity of the lesion and are extremely varied. Many of the clinical features of damage to the CNS can be manifested (see earlier in this chapter). Generally there will be a mixture of these features. The list is not exhaustive and it is beyond the scope of this text to cover every possibility; however, it is important to note that no two patients are alike. The recommended reading at the end of the chapter lists texts that deal with these signs more comprehensively.

Management

There are three stages of management: medical management, rehabilitation and prevention of further strokes (Fawcus 2000). The increase in chronic disease

15

Table 15.7 Arteries involved in cerebral vascular occlusion

Artery	Features
Middle cerebral artery (supplies most of the convexity of the cerebral hemispheres)	Dense contralateral hemiplegia Contralateral homonymous hemianopia Cortical type of sensory loss Speech problems in left hemisphere lesions, with neglect of contralateral side Lesions in the right hemisphere result in parietal damage, visuospatial disturbances and left-sided neglect
Posterior cerebral artery	Visual disturbance Contralateral homonymous field defect Memory disturbance and contralateral sensory loss
Anterior cerebral artery	Contralateral monoplegia Cortical sensory loss Sometimes behavioural abnormalities associated with frontal lobe damage

*The initial presentation is one of hypotonus. Hypertonus may develop over time. (Reproduced from Stokes 1998, with permission.)

generally has led to extra emphasis on health promotion strategies.

Medical management

It is important to establish the type of stroke that has occurred because medical management will depend on whether it is ischaemic, haemorrhagic or subarachnoid. The national clinical guidelines for stroke (RCP 2004) outline the recommended treatments and management.

The diagnosis of stroke is primarily dependent upon the clinical presentation. Medical management usually consists of the treatment of any underlying pathology (e.g. hypertension) and the prevention of secondary complications.

In the UK there are recommendations for the type of service provision stroke sufferers can expect. Research suggests that stroke patients do better when treated in a specialised stroke unit that has a coordinated multidisciplinary stroke team (Fawcus 2000; Edwards 2002). This type of service should be expected within the first 6 months; after that time patients can be cared for equally well in a community or general hospital setting.

Physiotherapy management

The physiotherapy-specific national guidelines for stroke (RCP/CSP 2004) should be viewed as a framework to guide clinical decisions rather than as rigid rules. The guidelines are continually updated in the light of new evidence. The national clinical guidelines should be referred to for guidance on the involvement of carers and families, discharge planning, long-term management and service evaluation. The following key factors have been identified by Ashburn (1997) as the important features of physical recovery following stroke:

1. Recovery is most rapid in the first few months and movement patterns recur in similar hierarchal patterns in most patients.
2. The timing and achievement of independent sitting balance are key indicators of functional independence.
3. The initial level of motor dysfunction and the time interval between paralysis and return of movement are important indicators of movement recovery.
4. Studies have shown a link between unilateral neglect and poor function.
5. There is a paucity of evidence with regard to the extremes of motor function. Why do some patients do very well and others do not?
6. The description of active selected movement recovery has so far been neglected.
7. Knowledge of long-term movement patterns is limited.

Key point

Physiotherapy management is based upon a holistic problem-solving multidisciplinary approach aimed at the promotion of independence, improved function, maximisation of activity, amelioration of symptoms and prevention of abnormality.

PARKINSON'S DISEASE AND PARKINSONISM

Introduction

Parkinson's disease (PD) is a progressive, primary neurodegenerative disorder first described as 'the shaking palsy' by James Parkinson in 1817. *Parkinsonism* is the collective term for a group of conditions called *motor system disorders* that includes PD as the most common manifestation, along with: other degenerative brain disorders, such as progressive supranuclear palsy (PSP) and multiple systems atrophy (MSA); secondary effects of a primary neurological condition, such as multiple cerebral infarction; trauma, from boxing, for example; and drugs (Stokes 1998).

The four primary symptoms of PD and Parkinsonism are:

- tremor at rest
- rigidity
- bradykinesia (slowness of movement)
- hypokinesia (poverty of movement).

The aetiology of these diseases is unknown, but different theories *that have not been proven and remain speculative* continue to emerge. The following are examples of some of these theories:

- free radicals, which contribute to cell death via a process of oxidation
- external or internal toxins, e.g. pesticides, which selectively destroy dopaminergic neurones
- genetic predisposition
- acceleration (accelerated ageing) of the degeneration of the dopamine-producing cells
- a combination of oxidative damage, environmental toxins, genetic predisposition and accelerated ageing.

Regardless of its cause, PD affects men and women in equal numbers and there are no known social, economic or geographic variations. It is a disease of late middle age, usually affecting people over the age of 50. The average age of onset is 60 years, but 1 in 7 patients with PD is diagnosed under the age of 50 (Caird 1991).

There is no specific diagnosis for PD, which differentiates it from other forms of Parkinsonism. Early signs of the disease are subtle and develop gradually, with family and friends often noticing problems before the patient. Classically, tremor is the first sign that leads patients to seek medical advice, as it begins to interfere with activities of daily living. Early minor symptoms may be:

- fatigue, tiredness and general malaise
- shaking
- soft voice
- spidery handwriting
- forgetfulness
- irritability/depressed mood.

Pathology

PD is a slowly degenerating condition affecting the CNS and is the most common basal ganglia disorder. It is caused by death of cells that produce dopamine in the substantia nigra and the corpus striatum (caudate nucleus and putamen). Approximately 80 per cent of dopamine-producing cells are estimated to have been lost before the presentation of clinical features of the disease.

Key point

Dopamine is an inhibitory chemical neurotransmitter responsible for the transmission of impulses between the substantia nigra and the corpus striatum. The action of dopamine acts as a counterbalance to the excitatory neurotransmitter, acetylcholine.

Neurotransmitters transmit electrical impulses across a synapse from one neurone to another. In the normal state, a balance between excitation and inhibition of the motor cortex via the basal ganglia exists, resulting in the production of smooth, purposeful muscle activity. The depletion of dopamine in PD leads to a lack of inhibition on the cholinergic neurones, with unopposed excitation and loss of the normal balance of excitatory and inhibitory neurotransmitters acting on the neurones. In addition, the loss of dopamine results in a reactive increase in the production of acetylcholine in the basal ganglia. The combined effect of the deficiency in dopamine, reactive increase in acetylcholine and subsequent degeneration of the pigmented neurones in the substantia nigra results in the lack of normal movement control, with patients unable to direct or control their movements.

The lack of inhibition of the reticulospinal and vestibulospinal pathways results in excessive contraction of postural muscles. The disturbance of inhibition and excitation results in the classical clinical features outlined below.

Clinical features

Onset of the disease is usually slow, often with unilateral presentation of signs and symptoms, later becoming bilateral. The rate of progression varies between patients, with some people becoming severely affected whilst others develop only minor symptoms. Diagnosis is usually made on the presentation of the characteristic signs of the disease: tremor, rigidity, bradykinesia and hypokinesia.

Tremor

The tremor associated with Parkinson's disease is a resting tremor, which disappears on movement and is often seen when the individual is under stress. It is usually unilateral and can affect the arm and the leg, but is more commonly observed in the hand. Hand tremor is often described as a *pill-rolling tremor* (because it resembles the action of a pill being rolled between the thumb and the tips of the fingers) and is highly characteristic of the condition.

Developments in imaging and computing have led the way for a revival in functional sterotactic surgery for PD. Stimulation of key areas within the brain (subthalamic nucleus, thalamus and globus pallidus) can lead to significant improvements for patients with severe tremor.

Rigidity

Rigidity is defined as an increased resistance to stretch and the inability to achieve complete muscle relaxation (Wichmann and DeLong 1993). The rigidity is the result of an increase in muscle tone with disruption of normal reciprocal inhibition. Reciprocal inhibition refers to the lower levels of activity that occur in muscles opposing the prime movers, which allow movement to take place in a controlled manner. When this is disturbed, all muscle groups can be equally active, leading to stiffness within a limb. It is difficult for the patient to perform active movements or for the limbs to be moved passively. Rigidity contributes to the pain associated with PD and to the impoverished movement found in this disease.

Two types of rigidity are seen in people with PD:

- *Lead pipe rigidity* manifests as a uniform resistance to movement throughout the range of movement.
- *Cogwheel rigidity* presents as an intermittent on/off resistance throughout the range of movement, making movements jerky.

Bradykinesia

Bradykinesia is the term used to describe slowness in the execution of movement and loss of spontaneity of movement. This contributes to problems with posture and balance and affects the patient's ability to carry out activities of daily living. The unpredictability of the bradykinesia can be very frustrating to patients.

Bradykinesia occurs as a result of loss of normal basal ganglia function. All movements become slow and are reduced in speed, velocity and range. Automatic movements are affected and repetitive movements are difficult (Stokes 1998; Hume-Adams and Graham 1998; Wiener and Goetz 1994). This leads to the patient to walk with short, hesitant steps and to speak with a slow, quiet voice; handwriting can become small and untidy. Blinking and facial expressions are reduced, resulting in the typical mask-like expression. Swallowing can also be affected, leading to difficulty with eating and drinking, and patients may be unable to control their saliva.

Hypokinesia

These clinical features have a detrimental effect on the movement, postural stability, balance and gait of people with PD. The patient is unable to make quick compensatory movements and so has a tendency to fall. Patients tend to develop a typical gait with small shuffling steps because they are unable to shift the centre of gravity during walking. They may tend to lean too far forwards or sometimes backwards. Posture is usually flexed, with flexion at the hips and knees, rounded shoulders and neck flexion, and is described as 'simian'. The patient often tries to correct head posture by hyperextending the upper cervical spine, leading to a 'poking chin'. Individuals' upper bodies may lean too far forwards, in standing or when walking, such that they have to take steps forwards, appearing to chase their centre of gravity. This phenomenon is called 'festination' and so the typical Parkinson's gait is called a 'festinating gait'.

There can also be characteristic difficulties with 'freezing' during the gait cycle, particularly when coming across obstacles, doorways or a change in walking surface. In addition, the effectiveness of the drugs used to manage PD can fluctuate, leading to 'on/off' states.

Non-motor problems

PD also leads to symptoms not related to motor disturbance, which tend to be more problematic in the later stages of the condition. These can include depression, dementia, emotional changes, incontinence and disturbance of sleep. Pain and autonomic disturbances can also lead to significant problems.

Management

Improvements in the treatment of PD means that life expectancy is usually not shortened. A coordinated, multidisciplinary approach to the management of the condition means that care should be provided at the right time and by the most appropriate healthcare professional.

The general principles of management are to:

- improve function
- improve safety
- delay the loss of independence.

Assessment involves identifying the underlying impairments, functional limitations and abilities of the individual. Multidisciplinary goal-setting is integral to the success of intervention strategies, which can be both *compensatory* and *preventative*. Treatment must include management of the musculoskeletal, cardiopulmonary and neurological systems.

Medical management

The medical management of PD consists primarily of prescribing drugs that aim to replace the lost dopamine or reduce the signs and symptoms associated with a loss of dopamine. Because the disease manifests itself differently in different patients, it can take time before the most appropriate drug regimen is established. The main drug used in PD is the dopamine precursor, *levodopa*.

Levodopa is the standard symptomatic medication for PD. It is usually given with carbidopa or benserazide, which increases the amount of levodopa that can cross the blood–brain barrier. Levodopa is especially effective against the bradykinesia and the impoverished voluntary movement (Cutson et al. 1995), but can lead to the development of involuntary movements or dyskinesias.

Other drugs used to treat PD are:

- bromocriptine — mimics the role of dopamine
- selegiline — delays the breakdown of dopamine and enhances the effects of levodopa
- anticholinergics — to control tremor and rigidity by blocking the action of acetylcholine
- amantadine — used in the later stages to decrease dyskinesia.

In the later stages of PD, medication management can become increasingly difficult, with patients experiencing more episodes of dyskinesia or 'off' time, dependent on the timing of the drugs. At this stage apomorphine injections can be used to decrease the 'off' time when severe motor complications occur.

The importance of accurate timing for administration of medication cannot be underestimated, both in terms of lifestyle management and for maximising therapy sessions.

Physiotherapy management

The normal model of delivery of treatment for patients with PD is a combination of individual treatment sessions and group work. Treatment may be specifically targeted towards the different stages of the disease, with advice and fitness training in the early stages and education of compensatory strategies to help overcome the difficulties in the later stages. If the patient is severely affected by PD, treatment may need to address respiratory status, functional aids and adaptations, and palliation of the signs and symptoms (Turnbull 1992; Banks and Caird 1982; Kamsma 1995).

The main aims of physiotherapy (National Collaborating Centre for Chronic Conditions 2006) are related to:

- gait re-education and improving balance and flexibility
- improving aerobic capacity
- facilitating initiation of movement
- increasing functional independence
- ensuring safety within the home.

Assessment

Physiotherapy assessment focuses on movement and function, and is ideally carried out in the patient's usual surroundings. Motor impairments such as tremor, bradykinesia, hypokinesia, akinesia, rigidity and postural instability should be assessed in relation to the functional abilities of the patient. The physiotherapist should assess the patient performing a variety of activities, including walking, turning, sitting, standing, going up and down stairs, and performing upper limb activities. Assessment of pain, muscle strength, range of movement, respiratory function and posture should be included as appropriate (Table 15.8).

Treatment approaches

Physiotherapists draw upon a wide range of approaches when managing patients with PD. For example, theories of learning, and neurophysiological and biomechanical approaches are utilised. The dominant treatment concept has been termed METERS (**m**ovement **e**nablement **t**hrough **e**xercise **r**egimes and **s**trategies; Plant et al. 2000).

Table 15.8 Assessment guidelines for Parkinson's disease

Background history	Demographic details, past medical history, years since onset of symptoms, years since diagnosis, presenting problems
Motor impairment	Tremor, bradykinesia, akinesia, dyskinesia, rigidity
Functional status	Walking, sit to stand, turning, change in direction, bed mobility, stairs, car transfers, upper limb function (e.g. reaching, grasping, writing, manipulation of objects), postural instability, use of mobility aids
Specific tests	Muscle strength, range of movement, posture, pain, respiratory status

Treatment techniques include the use of general exercise regimens and specific exercise programmes (Table 15.9). General exercises help to preserve overall fitness to maintain functional ability and support an active lifestyle. Specific exercise regimens help to improve individual problems and can promote increased flexibility, which will help to prevent secondary problems associated with a loss of flexibility (Partridge 2002). Specific exercises have also been shown to promote psychological well-being (Palmer et al. 1986).

Degeneration of the basal ganglia results in the inability to perform complex motor sequences and therefore produce skilled movement. Treatment approaches include the use of compensatory strategies. These strategies involve breaking down complex movement sequences into smaller component parts. These components are then arranged sequentially and are performed at a conscious level.

Key point

It is important to avoid simultaneous motor and cognitive tasks.

Physiotherapists also use mental rehearsal techniques and cueing strategies to help the client function more effectively within the limits of the disease. The cues used may be visual, auditory, proprioceptive and cognitive (Table 15.10). External and internal cues utilise cortical mechanisms to activate and sustain movement (Morris 2000).

A range of other techniques can be used as appropriate if the patient is presenting with pain or pulmonary problems. General physiotherapy techniques can be used to alleviate these symptoms. Examples are massage, electrotherapy modalities and mobilisation techniques.

To provide a comprehensive service that supports patients with PD, a multidisciplinary approach is essential. The service needs to span primary, secondary and intermediate health and social care settings. A wide range of healthcare professionals will be involved in the management in a variety of settings. Multidisciplinary goal-setting is recommended and the use of appropriate outcome measures is essential. Table 15.11 provides examples of the outcome measures that may be used when managing clients with PD.

Table 15.9 Exercise guidelines for Parkinson's disease

General exercises	Specific exercises
▪ For the trunk, upper and lower limbs, and face ▪ Speech and breathing exercises ▪ Gait re-education ▪ Balance training and re-education ▪ Transfer practice and training ▪ Relaxation techniques	▪ Individual home exercise programmes aimed at specific functional problems ▪ Strengthening exercises for the trunk with aerobic exercise to improve stability ▪ Individual programmes to improve flexibility and to improve overall function ▪ Balance and lower limb strengthening to prevent falls ▪ Slow stretching regimes

Table 15.10 Cueing strategies for Parkinson's disease

Cues	Examples
Visual	Strips of card on the floor can assist step length and initiation problems Strategically placed cue cards containing a key word help to activate movement
Auditory	A musical beat or voice can help with gait
Proprioceptive	Rocking from side to side or taking a step backwards before walking can help to overcome freezing
Cognitive	Memorising the separate parts of a movement and rehearsing them mentally can be helpful

Table 15.11 Outcome measures in Parkinson's disease

Measurement of	Outcome measure
Function	Parkinson's Activity Scale Rivermead Mobility Index Timed get-up-and-go test
Balance	Berg balance test Functional reach test
Gait	Clinical gait assessment 10-metre walk test

MULTIPLE SCLEROSIS

Introduction

Multiple (disseminated) sclerosis (MS) is a progressively degenerative disease of the CNS, of unknown cause, whose pathological trademarks are inflammation and demyelination. The presenting clinical features can be very varied, resulting in a complex combination of physical, psychological and cognitive problems. This highly variable presentation (and often unpredictable condition) poses a major challenge to therapists if they are to assist individuals in managing the condition as effectively as possible.

The prevalence of MS varies worldwide, with the lowest amongst populations living nearest to the equator. The condition appears to be most common in temperate climates. People who emigrate before the age of 15 years exhibit the rate of incidence of their adopted country (Dean and Kurtzke 1971). These facts seem to suggest that there may be an environmental trigger that allows the disease to develop through a genetic or immunological susceptibility in children below the age of about 15 that is no longer present in adults.

Approximately 15 per cent of individuals with MS have an affected relative. This risk rises to 1:50 for offspring and 1:20 for siblings of affected persons (Sadovnick et al. 1988).

Another possible contributing factor to the onset of MS could be gender. MS is more common in women than men in a ratio of approximately 2:1. Race appears to have an influence, with black and Asian populations having a lower incidence. Other suggested factors are diet and socioeconomic status; the higher the standard of living, the higher the risk of developing MS.

Key point

In the UK, an estimated 80 000 people have been diagnosed with MS. This makes it the second highest cause of neurological disability in young adults. Approximately 1 per 800–1000 of the population is affected, with the average onset of the condition being at 30 years of age (Sadovnick and Ebers 1993). The range of onset is extremely broad, from 10 years to 59 years.

Pathology

Acute stage

Breach of the blood–brain barrier is one of the first significant events to occur at this stage. T-lymphocytes, in particular, are targeted against the vascular wall.

They are responsible for the secretion of cytokines, which then recruit other cells, including macrophages. The lymphocyte makes a hole in the endothelium and enters the CNS. This results in a perivascular inflammatory lesion that leads to tissue damage, particularly of myelin.

This inflammatory stage can vary in its duration from days to a month. The intensity and duration of the attack will determine the overall extent of the damage. This phase is associated with vasogenic oedema that ultimately resolves over a matter of weeks, with repair of the blood–brain barrier. A residual fibrous scar is then left on the myelin sheath, termed a *plaque* or *sclerosis*.

Later stages

In the early stages of the condition, it is not demyelination that is the main cause of symptoms, but rather the inflammation itself. However, as the condition progresses, repeated onset of the attacks results in more permanent damage. Over a period of time the CNS combats this damage via a number of compensatory mechanisms, but eventually the extent to which it can compensate for the deficits is superseded by the structural damage. Permanent deficits are the final outcome of this run of events.

Forms and diagnosis of MS

- About 45 per cent of sufferers initially present with a *relapsing–remitting* form of the condition (RRMS). An acute flare-up, lasting from a few days to a few weeks, is followed by a period of remission where no symptoms are displayed. The periods of relapse and remission can vary in themselves, with an acute relapse being followed by a period of remission lasting weeks to months.
- About 40 per cent of the people who initially presented with RRMS will go on to develop a secondary stage of progression with or without superimposed relapses — known as *secondary progressive MS* (SPMS). The person appears to exhibit a steady deterioration, without any noticeable acute periods to account for this.
- The third main form of the condition, known as *primary progressive MS* (PPMS), presents as a steadily deteriorating condition from the onset, with no identifiable relapses or remissions. The rate of deterioration can be fairly rapid in some cases. About 10–15 per cent of cases are in this category.
- Two further categories need to be included for completeness: *benign* (10–12 per cent of cases), with no significant disability due to MS 10 years after onset; and *malignant* (Marburg's disease).

In spite of the increasing reliance on MRI as a diagnostic tool, clinical evaluation continues to be the main method of diagnosing MS. Other investigations used are evoked potentials and, less commonly, analysis of cerebrospinal fluid by way of a lumbar puncture. The most widely used diagnostic criteria are those of Poser et al. 1983; (Table 15.12).

Clinical features

Any part of the CNS may be affected, so unsurprisingly symptoms vary tremendously. Some of the most common clinical features will be described here, but readers may need to refer to other texts for more detailed information.

Weblink

Multiple Sclerosis International Federation: www.msif.org.

Table 15.12 Diagnostic criteria in multiple sclerosis

	Minimum number of			
Category	Relapses	Deficits	Paraclinical evidence	Oligoclonal bands
Clinically definite	2	2		
	2 and	1		
Clinically probable	2	1		
	1	2		
	1	1 and	1*	+
Lab-supported definite	2	1 or		+
Lab-supported probable	1	1 and	1	+
	2		+	

*Progression of MRI abnormalities over time also constitutes paraclinical evidence for diagnosis of laboratory-supported definite MS.
(Reproduced from Poser et al. 1993, with permission.)

Vision

The optic nerve, cervical cord, brainstem and cerebellar peduncles are most commonly affected. Frequently at onset the first feature is optic neuritis of varying severity. Pain is felt behind the affected eye, with some element of visual disturbance occurring. In 58 per cent of cases acuity is affected without pain. However, overall more than 9 per cent of cases recover the majority of their visual acuity. Later on, other symptoms affecting eye movement are dysmetria, nystagmus, internuclear ophthalmoplegia (slowing of adduction) and ocular flutter. Diplopia might be experienced.

Sensation

Sensory symptoms are common early on in the course of the condition. Numbness, pins and needles, tightness around a limb and other more unusual sensations, such as of water running down a limb, are the most frequently experienced. Later on joint proprioception is also commonly affected.

Motor function

Motor symptoms are more common than sensory symptoms and are usually more disabling in the long run. Changes in muscle tone, weakness, tremor, poor coordination and ataxia are all impairments that often result in difficulties with movement. Neurological conditions where the white matter is affected often result in considerable spasticity. Spasticity, most commonly in the legs, may be present with or without accompanying weakness. Other than cerebellar ataxia, spasticity is frequently the most disabling feature in people with MS. Individuals may report spasms, sometimes at night, which can be painful. Cerebellar ataxia can result in arm movements being uncoordinated (intention tremor), a wide-based gait pattern and speech disturbances. The reader is asked to refer to the clinical features section at the start of this chapter for more specific details on each of the above symptoms.

15

Swallowing

Individuals entering the later stages of MS may experience swallowing difficulties (dysphagia). An underestimation of the degree of swallowing difficulties may result in bronchopneumonia and ultimately can therefore be potentially life-threatening. Swallowing is a highly complex motor skill that requires careful assessment by a speech and language therapist, dietitian and radiographer. Videofluoroscopy using a modified barium swallow is an essential investigation if comprehensive assessment of dysphagia is to be made. Assessment of the individual's posture during swallowing should not be overlooked. Ultimately, if severe difficulties persist with oral feeding, then alternatives such as a gastrostomy may need to be considered.

Bladder and bowel

Bladder disturbances in MS are very common and often take the form of either detrusor hyperreflexia or detruso-sphincter dyssynergia. Urgency, frequency, nocturnal disturbances and urge incontinence are the various types of bladder presentation. People often report that social trips have to be strategically planned around where the nearest toilet might be. Detrusor hyperreflexia rarely occurs without the presence of spasticity in the legs. Detruso-sphincter dyssynergia presents as delay or inability to void, frequency, urgency and an inability to empty the bladder fully. This may result in urinary retention and the susceptibility to urinary tract infections.

Treatment is often successful in the form of muscle relaxants, anticholinergic drugs and self-catheterisation.

Constipation is the main bowel problem and is relatively straightforward to treat.

Pain and fatigue

People with MS tend to be more susceptible to pain syndromes such as trigeminal neuralgia, myelopathies and musculoskeletal-type pain. The latter is usually a result of poor posture and poor alignment of joints — sometimes through soft tissue adaptations and overstressed joints.

Key point

One of the most common and usually most disabling symptoms is that of fatigue. Fatigue in its truest sense, for people with MS, is usually described as 'a deterioration in performance with continuing effort' (Barnes 2000).

As the day progresses, any activities involving physical effort are often increasingly difficult to carry out. Fatigue is a significant feature of most people with MS. This is an important consideration when it comes to planning physiotherapy treatment interventions.

Cognition

Cognitive difficulties, such as disturbances in functional memory, reduced information processing speeds and impaired intellectual function, are more common in people with MS than is widely recognised. Cognitive impairments may contribute significantly to any reduction in functional capability. Although these types of impairment are more common in people with long-standing MS, they have also been shown to exist at a time when there are relatively few physical symptoms (Van den Burg et al. 1987).

Management

Medical management

> **Clinical note**
> Medical management can be divided into interventions that may influence the condition directly and those that help to manage the symptoms.

In acute relapses, rest and steroid therapy are the mainstays of medical management. In spite of the widespread use of steroids in MS there remains little consensus in the UK over the most appropriate dose and mode of administration. Steroid therapy is most commonly administered in the form of 1 g of intravenous methylprednisolone for 3–5 days, with or without a reducing dose of steroids. The most common oral regimen is prednisolone 60 mg daily, reducing to zero over 1–3 weeks. Low-dose oral steroids are generally better tolerated, but evidence of efficacy is less robust.

Steroids have been shown to shorten the recovery time during relapses, although they do not seem to have an overall effect on the long-term progress of the condition. Longer-term use of steroids is less well supported in the literature and any potential benefits must be weighed against the potentially harmful side-effects of steroid therapy.

Interferon-α has now unequivocally been proven to be of benefit to some people with MS, by reducing the number of relapses that occur in relapsing–remitting MS and thereby delaying progression of the condition.

Many other types of medical intervention are utilised to manage the consequences of the disease process, such as antispasmodic medication to reduce the effects of spasticity and referral for further investigations depending upon the presenting symptoms. For example, an ultrasound scan of the bladder may be needed to establish incomplete voiding of the bladder.

Physiotherapy management

The key to any successful intervention is a comprehensive and ongoing assessment of the person's difficulties and needs. A coordinated interdisciplinary approach is also crucial if the condition is to be managed effectively (Ko Ko 1999). Rehabilitation programmes must be tailored to meet the needs of the individual and carers, who should be at the centre of the goal-setting approach.

Individuals with MS often feel their needs are best served by services that allow direct access to them at the time of need. They also often feel they benefit most from a consistent approach on an ongoing basis that allows continuity of management rather than episodes of care (Robinson et al. 1996).

The main aims of any physiotherapy intervention must be to keep the individual as functionally independent as possible. In order to do this, often in the face of increasing disability, it is vitally important that the physiotherapist works with the person on a psychological as well as physical level. Timing of interventions is crucial and is one of the main reasons for the need for ongoing monitoring of this group of patients. The importance of early contact with patients cannot be overstated. This allows time for an effective rapport to be established, which will become invaluable as the disease progresses. Even in the early stages, the more aware the patient is of the condition, the more effective the management is likely to be. Physiotherapists need to be proactive in the area of patient education by consulting with the evidence base in conjunction with an informed knowledge of the condition, to ensure this component of the management programme is as effective as possible. Establishing and encouraging early self-management with the patient will pay dividends in the long run.

Additional goals of a physiotherapy programme are to minimise abnormalities of muscle tone, preserve the integrity of the musculoskeletal system by preventing secondary problems (Thompson 1998), improve posture along with advice on postural management, and facilitate the use of efficient functional movement patterns, including re-education of gait.

Measurement

The most frequently used measurement tools to monitor outcomes of treatment for people with MS are:

- Functional Independence Measure (FIM)
- Barthel Index
- Rivermead Motor Assessment Scale
- SF-36
- Health-Related Quality of Life (HRQoL) scale
- Multiple Sclerosis Quality of Life (MSQoL) scale
- Kurtzke Expanded Status Scale (Kurtzke 1981, 1983).

MOTOR NEURONE DISEASE

Introduction

Motor neurone disease (MND) is characterised by progressive degeneration of motor neurones:

- anterior horn cells in the spinal cord, resulting in lower motor neurone (LMN) lesions
- corticospinal tract cells, resulting in upper motor neurone (UMN) lesions
- motor nuclei in the brainstem, resulting in both upper and lower motor lesions.

Key point

'Motor neurone disease' is in fact a global term mainly used in the UK and Australia. In other parts of the world the condition is often referred to as 'amyotrophic lateral sclerosis'.

Although MND is primarily a disease of the motor neurones, there may be occasional involvement of other areas of the CNS. The autonomic nervous system, sensory nerves, lower sacral segments of the spinal cord and the three cranial nerves that control movement of the eyes are usually unaffected.

The aetiology of the condition is unknown, although 5 per cent of people have a familial form (Figlewicz and Rouleau 1994). It is a condition that usually affects people in later life, starting at between 50 and 70 years, with a marginally higher occurrence in males.

Key point

Precise figures for incidence and prevalence are not known. The incidence is thought to be 2 per 100 000 per year, whilst the prevalence is estimated to be 7 per 100 000. The approximate number of people with MND in the UK is 5000 (MND Association 2000).

Clinical features and diagnosis

The onset of MND is usually insidious and the exact presentation depends upon the areas of the CNS affected. Where there is LMN degeneration, the main features are weakness, muscle wasting and fasciculation of the nerves undergoing degeneration. Degeneration of UMNs usually results in spasticity with accompanying weakness and muscle wasting.

Forms of MND

The following is a broad categorisation of the forms of MND, but in reality there is often considerable overlap.

Amyotrophic lateral sclerosis (ALS)

This is the most common form of the condition (65 per cent). It is more common in males and involves both upper and lower motor neurones. It is characterised by spasticity, muscle weakness and hyperactive reflexes, with possible bulbar signs of dysarthria, dysphagia and emotional lability. The hands tend to be affected initially, with the person reporting clumsiness; there is evidence of thenar eminence wasting, with the shoulder also often being involved early on. With bulbar involvement, speech, swallowing and the tongue are affected. The average survival rate is 2–5 years.

Progressive bulbar palsy

This affects 25 per cent of people with MND, with slightly older people and women being more commonly affected. Both upper and lower neurones may be involved. Dysphagia and dysarthria are characteristic of this form of the condition, owing to LMN damage causing nasal speech, regurgitation of fluids via the nose, tongue atrophy, pharyngeal weakness and fasciculation. Life expectancy is usually between 6 months and 3 years.

Progressive muscular atrophy

This affects approximately 7.5 per cent of people with MND and there is predominantly LMN involvement. Males are more affected than females in a ratio of 5:1. Muscle wasting and weakness with weight loss and fasciculation are the main presenting features. Mental deterioration and dementia are found in fewer than 5 per cent of people (Tandan 1994). Life expectancy is usually more than 5 years.

Primary lateral sclerosis

This is a rare form of the condition that affects mainly the UMNs. It is characterised by spastic quadriparesis, pseudobulbar symptoms, spastic dysarthria and hyperreflexia. A survival rate of 20 years or more can be expected.

Diagnosis

As with many other progressive diseases, no one specific test exists for the diagnosis of MND. Investigations often include imaging (MRI), myelogram (EMG), blood tests, and clinical investigations to exclude the possibility of other conditions such as syringomyelia or cervical spondylosis (Swash and Schwartz 1995).

Management

Medical management

Medical and healthcare professionals have a significant role to play in the management of this condition, owing to its complex and potentially rapidly deteriorating course. Owing to the high number of professionals involved in the person's care, it is vitally important that interventions be coordinated in some way. As in many cases where a high number of professionals from various agencies are involved, individuals with MND and their families often report that one of the most frustrating aspects of their management is the lack of coordination of service provision.

The family and their long-term needs must be considered. It is vitally important that the person with MND maintains as much control over his or her life as possible. Timely interventions, speedy responses, advice and support, ongoing assessment, and access to equipment and services are the main needs for this group of people.

> **Rilutek**
>
> In 1996 a drug called Rilutek, whose active ingredient is riluzole, became the first licensed drug treatment available for people with MND. It is not a cure for the condition but has been reported to extend life by several months (National Institute for Clinical Excellence 2001).

Physiotherapy management

Assessment of the person's needs on an ongoing basis is a prerequisite of any treatment interventions. Again, a multidisciplinary team assessment and approach is necessary for this group of people.

Early and medium stages

In the early stages, information on MND and support agencies, advice on appropriate exercise programmes, support for the person with MND and the family, and providing a point of contact will be the main physiotherapy interventions.

As the condition progresses — and this will vary from person to person — physiotherapy interventions will take the form of advice on exercise programmes and how best to incorporate these into everyday activities. This will ensure that the movement is as functional as possible. Active assisted exercises may be required if the person needs assistance to move. The main aim at this stage is to keep the person as independent as possible for as long as possible. To this end, assistive devices may be needed and again the physiotherapist may need to liaise with the occupational therapist, orthotist and rehabilitation engineers in the case of environmental control systems.

As movement becomes more difficult through weakness or spasticity, passive movements are indicated to prevent secondary impairments of the musculoskeletal system. It is vital that carers be involved in this process, if they so wish, in order to assist in the process of maintenance. A large part of the physiotherapist's role will be teaching and advising carers and other members of the team. One aspect of advice from the physiotherapist might be how to move and position the client in the most appropriate manner. The client is likely to be increasingly reliant on other forms of mobility during this stage of the condition and, as such, will need advice on the type of wheelchair (often powered) required.

In the case of individuals with dysphagia it is important that the physiotherapist works closely with the speech and language therapist and nursing staff to ensure optimum positioning for a safe swallow. Monitoring of respiratory function will also be necessary for this group of clients.

Terminal stage

In the terminal stage of the disease the person may be cared for at home or admitted to a hospice. Management of any prevailing symptoms and ensuring the person is as comfortable as possible are the main aims. It is of vital importance that both practical and emotional support is forthcoming for the family and carers. Deterioration is often rapid, with the most common cause of death being respiratory tract infection leading to respiratory failure.

TRAUMATIC BRAIN INJURY

Introduction

Acquired brain injury (ABI) refers to any acute brain injury caused by:

- trauma
- vascular accident
- cerebral anoxia, e.g. as a result of cardiac arrest
- toxic or metabolic conditions, e.g. hypoglycaemia
- infection, e.g. meningitis.

The brain injury may be direct as a result of physical injury to the brain, or indirect if a situation arises where cerebral perfusion pressure reaches a critical low and regulatory mechanisms are lost leading to ischaemic damage (Mendlow et al. 1983). Alternatively, intracranial causes can be the result of damage, such as acute traumatic haematomas, raised intracranial pressure (ICP) and infection.

Traumatic brain injury (TBI) describes a wide range of conditions and has in the past been used interchangeably with the term 'head injury'. The prefix of traumatic differentiates this group of people from those who have an ABI as a result of the other causes identified above. In addition to the damage that leads to the TBI, there are often associated injuries, such as limb fractures and internal organ damage. Skull fractures may be simple or compound, undisplaced or depressed.

Brain injury can be classified according to the Glasgow Coma Scale duration of coma, by the length of post-traumatic amnesia (PTA), or by results from a CT scan (Table 15.13; Jennett and Teasdale 1981). PTA is defined as 'the length of time between injury and the restoration of continuous day-to-day memory' (Russell and Smith 1981).

Table 15.13 Classification of brain injury

Classification	Score on Glasgow Coma Scale (GCS)	Duration of coma	Length of PTA
Mild	13–15	< 20 mins	< 1 hour
Moderate	9–12	< 6 hours	1–24 hours
Severe	3–8	> 6 hours	> 24 hours

Key point

The annual attendance of patients with TBI at Accident & Emergency departments is approximately 1778 per 100 000 a year in England and Wales. Studies in England, Wales and Scotland indicate an admission rate in the order of 270–310 cases per 100 000 per year (Jennett and MacMillan 1981). The most frequently admitted groups are children and small babies. Men aged 15–24 have the most serious head injuries and account for more than 30 per cent of all deaths in this age group; road traffic accidents and sporting injuries are the other most common cause of TBI, but alcohol consumption and recreational drug use may be contributing factors.

Pathology

15

The most common causes of TBI are direct blows to the head, deceleration and rotational forces. *Contrecoup lesions* can occur as a result of falls or direct blows to the head where there may be contusions at the site of impact along with contusions at the opposite side to the impact. Often the frontal lobes are most prone to damage owing to their proximity to the orbital ridges. Vascular damage usually occurs from subarachnoid bleeding with intracerebral and subdural haematomas appearing at the time of injury.

Potential problems following TBI

Post-traumatic epilepsy

This can be present in up to 40 per cent of cases, depending on the severity of brain injury. 'Anticonvulsants may be prescribed during the first 7 days following TBI for the prevention of early seizures' (RCP and BSRM 2003, p. 33). More commonly prescribed medication includes carbamazepine and valproic acid owing to their reduced side-effects in comparison to phenobarbital and phenytoin. Many anticonvulsants can produce significant side-effects.

Post-traumatic hydrocephalus

This refers to enlargement of the ventricular system and generally is non-obstructive. If hydrocephalus is diagnosed, ventricular shunting is the usual treatment.

Neuroendocrine and autonomic disorders

These types of problem include hypertension, hypothalamic–pituitary disorders and hyperthermia. Hypertension can occur as a new condition in 10–15 per cent of patients but is usually transient and can be managed effectively with beta-blockers.

Cranial neuropathies

These are a common occurrence following TBI, with cranial nerves I and III, and less commonly IV, VI and VIII, being affected.

Gastrointestinal and nutritional needs

Nutritional needs in the acute stages of TBI are reported to increase by an estimated 25 per cent. Long-term outcomes have been more favourable owing to the nutritional needs of patients being met (Young et al. 1987). Alternative methods of feeding may need to be considered in the early stages to achieve this aim. Problems with dysphagia occur in approximately 25 per cent of patients and this might also be another reason why alternative methods of feeding may need to be adopted.

Orthopaedic and musculoskeletal complications

Fractures are a common feature of TBI, with occult fractures (where there is no evidence of fracture on initial X-ray) being amongst the most serious problems. Peripheral nerve injuries are frequently underdiagnosed, and heterotopic ossification occurs in 76 per cent of cases.

Continence

Urinary incontinence following TBI is very common for a number of reasons but is primarily due to disinhibition.

Sexual dysfunction

The most common occurrence is oligomenorrhoea: that is, infrequent or light menstruation. Other complications include impotence and altered libido, along with difficulties created by any behavioural changes.

Motor function

Disturbances in the CNS can lead to hypertonicity, contractures and disordered movement. Hypertonicity can predispose patients to adaptive muscle shortening (contractures). Timely and effective management of hypertonicity can ultimately avoid the need for surgical intervention. Movement disorders encountered might be rigidity, tremors, ataxia, akathisia (feeling of inner restlessness and inability to sit still) and dystonias including chorea.

Sensation

Disturbances in sensory function can present in the form of diminished or absent cutaneous sensation (paraesthesia/anaesthesia), or various agnosias such as sensory neglect. Certain sensory disturbances can be addressed to some extent within the rehabilitation programme. However, longstanding sensory disturbances tend to persist.

Cognition

As mentioned earlier, altered behaviour can be the most troublesome aspect of a patient's rehabilitation and long-term social reintegration. Commonly occurring features include disturbances in level of arousal, speed of processing of information, memory, abstract reasoning and flexibility, self-awareness, distractibility and limited attention span. Behavioural deficits and psychosocial adjustment after TBI include depression, poor social awareness, agitation, aggressive behaviour and difficulties initiating activities (Prigatano 1992; Wood 1990).

Management

Early medical management

The management immediately after trauma involves primarily life-support measures. It is important that levels of consciousness be recorded and measured using a scale such as the Glasgow Coma Scale. In conjunction with this, on transfer to an acute hospital setting, further investigations such as a skull X-ray, CT scan or MRI may be necessary. In some cases, intracranial monitoring will be necessary to ensure that further damage or deterioration in the patient's condition does not occur. Certain patients will require neurosurgical intervention, which cannot be covered in any detail within this text. Readers are referred to NICE Clinical Guideline 4 (2003), Black and Rossitch (1995) and Teasdale et al. (1990) for further information.

In summary, the overall goals in the acute setting are:

- gaining medical stability
- clearing post-traumatic amnesia
- reducing behavioural and physical dependence.

If the patient does not require a high level of medical input, a less medically acute setting with intensive therapy services may be more appropriate.

Later-stage medical management

As with many complex neurological conditions, patients are best managed by an experienced interdisciplinary rehabilitation team, using a patient-centred, goal-orientated approach. By this stage, patients should have been transferred to an environment that is conducive to intensive rehabilitation. It is increasingly common for patients with complex disabilities to be managed using a key worker or case manager approach in order to provide more effective continuity of the services delivered.

Patients can present with a wide variety of impairments, depending on the site of the damage. Those with severe physical impairments early on in their rehabilitation improve significantly. However, by far the overriding residual problem is that of cognitive impairment, including disruption of executive functions. These types of impairment, and the resultant psychosocial implications, can lead to significant limitations in social interactions and can be the main barriers to individuals returning to independent living (Lezak 1986; Brooks and McKinlay 1983; Oddy and Humphrey 1980; Oddy et al. 1978).

The effectiveness of rehabilitation is still under review. However, some evidence exists that suggests that rehabilitation is effective in improving patients' levels of independence (Malec and Basford 1996; Cope 1995; Hall and Cope 1995).

Physiotherapy management

Acute stage

The main priority at this stage is to ensure the patient is medically stable. However, it is also important not to lose sight of the fact that proactive management of potential secondary complications can ultimately enhance patient outcomes. It is necessary to optimise the patient's respiratory function if secondary cerebral damage is to be avoided. All interventions during this stage need to be carefully balanced against the risk of raising the intracranial pressure (Ada et al. 1990).

Later stage – after months or years

The cognitive abilities and behavioural presentation of individuals with TBI will have an impact upon their level of function. It is therefore vital that these elements be assessed and taken into account when agreeing goals for interventions. Historically, physiotherapists have failed to take sufficient account of these factors, and subsequent physiotherapy interventions have perhaps been less effective than they might have been. Access to a neuropsychologist, who can assess and advise on the most effective way to deal with these factors when planning treatment, is invaluable.

Measurement

The most frequently used measurement tools to monitor outcomes of treatment for people with TBI are:

- Glasgow Outcome Scale (Jennett and Bond 1975)
- Disability Rating Scale (Rappaport et al. 1982)

- Functional Independence Measure (FIM) and Functional Assessment Measure (FAM)
- Glasgow Coma Scale (Teasdale and Jennett 1974).

Glossary of terms

The following glossary is intended to provide a brief description of some of the terminology found in this chapter:

Agnosia Loss of knowledge or inability to perceive objects
Anaesthesia Absence of sensation
Ataxia Loss of coordination affecting functional movement
Babinski sign Abnormal response of the plantar reflex (great toe turns upwards on testing)
Bradykinesia Slowness of movement
Clonus Succession of intermittent muscular relaxation and contraction usually resulting from a sustained stretch
Diplopia Double vision
Dysarthria Incoordination of speech
Dysphagia Difficulty in swallowing
Dysphasia Disruption of expressive (produce) and or receptive (understand) speech
Dyspraxia Inability to execute volitional purposeful movements
Dystonia Involuntary movement characterised by twisting and repetitive movement
Flaccidity Absence of muscle tone
Hemianopia Loss of visual field in one half of each eye
Hemiplegia Paralysis of one side of the body
Hypertonicity Increased muscle tone
Hypotonicity Decreased muscle tone
Nystagmus Involuntary rhythmic oscillation of one or both eyes
Paraesthesia Disruption of sensation causing abnormal sensation
Ptosis Drooped eyelid
Rigidity Stiffness of neurological origin, increased resistance to stretch throughout the range
Tone The active resistance of muscle to stretch
Tremor Fine type of involuntary movement (several types seen in neurological dysfunction)

15

FURTHER READING

It is outside the scope of this chapter to provide the reader with details of each different general approach to neurological rehabilitation, or to advocate the use of or extol the strengths of any specific approach. Readers are directed to Edwards (2002), Partridge (2002) and Stokes (1998) for more comprehensive information on the different approaches.

Readers are referred to Edwards (2002) for a detailed account of abnormal muscle tone.

General

Brincat CA 1999 Managed care and rehabilitation: adopting a true team approach. Top Stroke Rehabil 6(2): 62–65
Carr JH, Shepherd RB 1998 Neurological Rehabilitation: Optimizing Motor Performance. Butterworth–Heinemann: London
Edwards S 2002 Neurological Physiotherapy: A Problem-Solving Approach, 2nd edn. Churchill Livingstone: London
Greenwood R, Barnes MP, Mcmillan TM, Ward CD (eds) 1993 Neurological Rehabilitation. Churchill Livingstone: Edinburgh
Partridge C (ed.) 2002 Neurological Physiotherapy: Bases of Evidence for Practice. Whurr: London
Reinkensmeyer D, Lum PS, Winters J et al. 2002 Emerging technologies for improving access to movement therapy following neurological injury. Emerging and Accessible Telecommunications, Information and Healthcare Technologies. IEEE: New York
Stokes M 1998 Neurological Physiotherapy. New York: Mosby International

Stroke

Alexander H, Bugge C, Hagen S 2001 What is the association between the different components of stroke rehabilitation and health outcomes? Clin Rehabil 15: 207–215
Ashburn A 1997 Physical recovery following stroke. Physiotherapy 83: 480–490
Bosworth H, Horner R, Edwards L, Matchar D 2000 Depression and other determinants of values placed on current health state by stroke patients: evidence from VAS Acute Stroke (VAS+) study. Stroke 31: 2603–2609
Royal College of Physicians/Clinical Effectiveness and Evaluation Unit 2004 National Clinical Guidelines for Stroke, 2nd edn. RCP: London

Parkinson's disease

Deane KHO, Jones D, Ellis C et al. 2001 Physiotherapy for patients with Parkinson's disease (Cochrane review). Cochrane Library: Oxford
Morris M 2000 Movement disorders in people with Parkinson's disease: a model for physical therapy. Phys Ther 80: 578–597
Plant R et al. 2000 Physiotherapy for People with Parkinson's Disease: UK Best Practice. Institute of Rehabilitation: Newcastle upon Tyne
Schenkman M, Cutson TM, Kuchibhatla M et al. 1997 Reliability of impairment and physical performance measures for persons with Parkinson's disease. Phys Ther 77: 19–27
Suteeraiva Hananon M, Protas EJ 2000 Reliability of outcome measures in individuals with Parkinson's disease. Physiother Theory Pract 16: 211–218

Multiple sclerosis

Barnes D 2000 Multiple Sclerosis: Questions and Answers. Merit: Hampshire

Motor neurone disease

Motor Neurone Disease Association 2000 A Patient and Carer Centred Approach for Health and Social Professionals: Motor Neurone Disease Resource File. MND Association: Northampton

Traumatic brain injury

Campbell M 2000 Rehabilitation for Traumatic Brain Injury: Physical Therapy Practice in Context. Churchill Livingstone: London

REFERENCES

Ada L, Canning C, Paratz J 1990 Care of the unconscious head-injured patient. In: Ada L, Canning C (eds) Key Issues in Neurological Physiotherapy. Butterworth–Heinemann: Oxford, p. 249

Ashburn A 1997 Physical recovery following stroke. Physiotherapy 83: 480–490

Banks MA, Caird FI 1982 Physiotherapy benefits patients with Parkinson's disease. Clin Rehabil 3: 11–16

Barnes D 2000 Multiple Sclerosis: Questions and Answers. Merit: Hampshire

Black P, Rossitch E 1995 Neurosurgery: an Introductory Text. Oxford University Press: Oxford

Bobath B 1990 Adult hemiplegia: evaluation and treatment. 3rd edn. Butterworth–Heinemann: Oxford

Bohannon RW, Smith MB 1987 Interrater reliability of a modified Ashworth scale of muscle spasticity. Phys Ther 67: 206–207

Bohannon RW, Cassidy D, Walsh S 1995 Trunk muscle strength is impaired multidirectionally after stroke. Clin Rehabil 9: 47–51

Bonita R 1992 Epidemiology of stroke. Lancet 339: 342–343

Brooks DN, McKinlay WW 1983 Personality and behavioural change after severe blunt head injury: a relative's view. J Neurol Neurosurg Psychiat 46: 336–344

Caird FI (ed.) 1991 Rehabilitation in Parkinson's Disease. Chapman & Hall: London

Carr JH, Shepherd RB 1998 Neurological Rehabilitation: Optimizing Motor Performance. Butterworth–Heinemann: London

Carr JH, Shepherd RB, Nordholm L, Lynne D 1985 Investigation of a new motor assessment scale for stroke patients. Phys Ther 65: 175–180

Cella DF, Dineen K, Arnason B et al. 1996 Validation of the functioning assessment of multiple sclerosis quality of life instrument. Neurology 47: 129–139

Cope DN 1995 The effectiveness of traumatic brain injury rehabilitation: a review. Brain Inj 9: 649–670

Crow JL, Lincoln NB, Nouri FM, De Weerdt W 1989 The effectiveness of EMG feedback in the treatment of arm function after stroke. Int Disabil Studies 11: 155–160

Cutson TM, Laub KC, Schenkman M 1995 Pharmacological and non-pharmacological interventions in the treatment of Parkinson's disease. Phys Ther 75: 363–373

Dean G, Kurtzke JF 1971 On the risk of multiple sclerosis according to the age at immigration to South Africa. BMJ 3: 725–729

Department of Health (DoH) 2001 National Service Framework for Older People. DoH: London

Duncan PW, Weiner DK, Chandler J, Studenski S 1990 Functional reach: a new clinical measure of balance. J Gerontol 45: 192–197

Edwards S (ed.) 2002 Neurological Physiotherapy: a Problem-Solving Approach, 2nd edn. Churchill Livingstone: London

Elsworth JD, Marks JA, McGrath JR, Wade DT 1999 An audit of goal planning in rehabilitation. Top Stroke Rehabil 6(2): 51–61

Fawcus R (ed.) 2000 Stroke Rehabilitation: a Collaborative Approach. Blackwell Scientific: Oxford

Figlewicz DA, Rouleau GA 1994 Familial disease. In: Williams AC (ed.) Motor Neurone Disease. Chapman & Hall: London, pp. 427–450

Freeman JA 2002 Assessment, outcome measurement and goal setting in physiotherapy practice. In: Edwards S (ed.) Neurological Physiotherapy, 2nd edn. Churchill Livingstone: London, pp. 21–34

Granger CV, Cotter AC, Hamilton BB, Fiedler RC 1993 Functional assessment scales: a study of persons after stroke. Arch Phys Med Rehabil 74: 133–138

Hall KM, Cope DN 1995 The benefit of rehabilitation in traumatic brain injury: a literature review. J Head Trauma Rehabil 10(5): 1–13

Harwood R, Ebrahim S 1995 Manual of the London Handicap Scale. Department of Health Care of the Elderly: University of Nottingham

Hauser SL, Dawson DM, Lehrich JR et al. 1983 Intensive immunosuppression in progressive multiple sclerosis: a randomised three-arm study of high-dose intravenous cyclophosphamide, plasma exchange and ACTH. N Engl J Med 308: 173–180

Hume-Adams J, Graham DI 1998 An Introduction to Neuropathology, 2nd edn. Churchill Livingstone: Edinburgh

Hunt SM, McKenna SP, Williams J 1981 Reliability of a population survey tool for measuring perceived health problems: a study of patients with osteoarthritis. J Epidemiol Commun Health 35: 297–300

Jennett B, Bond M 1975 Assessment of outcome after severe brain injury: a practical scale. Lancet 2: 81

Jennett B, MacMillan R 1981 Epidemiology of head injury. BMJ 282: 101–104

Jennett B, Teasdale G 1981 Management of Head Injuries. FA Davis: Philadelphia

Kamsma YPT, Brouwer WH, Lakke JPW 1995 Training of compensational strategies for impaired gross motor skills in Parkinson's disease. Physiother Theory Pract 11: 209–229

Ko Ko C 1999 Effectiveness of rehabilitation for multiple sclerosis. Clin Rehabil 13 (suppl 1): 33–41

Kurtzke JF 1981 A proposal for a uniform minimal record of disability in multiple sclerosis. Acta Neurol Scand 64 (suppl 87): 110–129

Kurtzke JF 1983 Rating neurologic impairment in multiple sclerosis: an expanded disability status scale (EDSS). Neurology 33: 1444–1452

Lezak MD 1986 Psychological implications of traumatic brain damage for the patient's family. Rehabil Psychol 31: 241–250

Lincoln NB, Edmans JA 1989 A shortened version of the Rivermead Perceptual Assessment Battery. Clin Rehabil 3: 199–204

Lincoln NB, Leadbitter D 1979 Assessment of motor function in stroke patients. Physiotherapy 65: 48–51

Lundy-Ekman L 1998 Neuroscience: Fundamentals for Rehabilitation. WB Saunders: London

Mahoney FI, Barthel DW 1965 Functional evaluation: the Barthel Index. Maryland State Med J 14: 61–65

Malec JF, Basford JS 1996 Postacute brain injury rehabilitation. Arch Phys Med Rehabil 77: 198–207

Mathiowetz V, Weber K, Kashman N et al. 1985 Adult norms for the 9-hole peg test of finger dexterity. Occup Ther J Res 5: 24–37

McGrath JR, Adams L 1999 Patient-centered goal planning: a systematic psychological therapy? Top Stroke Rehabil 6(2): 43–50

Medical Research Council 1976 Aids to the Examination of the Peripheral Nervous System. HMSO: London

Mellerup E, Fog T, Raun N et al. 1981 The socio-economic scale. Acta Neurolog Scand 64: 130–138

Mendlow AD, Teasdale GM, Teasdale E et al. 1983 Cerebral blood flow and intracranial pressure in head injured patients. In: Ishii S, Nagai H, Brock M (eds) Intracranial Pressure. Springer: Berlin, pp. 495–500

Morris M 2000 Movement disorders in people with Parkinson's disease: a model for physical therapy. Phys Ther 80: 578–597

Motor Neurone Disease Association 2000 A Patient and Carer Centred Approach for Health and Social Professionals: Motor Neurone Disease Resource File. MND Association: Northampton

National Collaborating Centre for Chronic Conditions 2006 Parkinson's Disease: National Clinical Guidelines for Diagnosis and Management in Primary and Secondary care. Royal College of Physicians: London

National Institute for Clinical Excellence 2001 Technology Appraisal: Guidance on the Use of Riluzole for the Treatment of Motor Neurone Disease. Appraisal no. 20. National Institute for Clinical Excellence: London

National Institute for Clinical Excellence 2003 Head Injury: Triage, Assessment, Investigation and Early Management of Head Injury in Infants, Children and Adults. National Institute for Clinical Excellence: London

Norkin CC, White DJ 1975 Measurement of Joint Motion: a Guide to Goniometry. FA Davies: Philadelphia

Oddy M, Humphrey M 1980 Social recovery during the year following severe head injury. J Neurol Neurosurg Psychiat 43: 798–802

Oddy M, Humphrey M, Uttley D 1978 Subjective impairment and social recovery after closed head injury. J Neurol Neurosurg Psychiat 41: 611–616

Palastanga N, Field D, Soames R 2002 Anatomy and Human Movement, 4th edn. Butterworth–Heinemann: Oxford

Palmer SS, Mortimer JA, Webster DD et al. 1986 Exercise therapy for Parkinson's disease. Arch Phys Med Rehabil 67: 741–745

Partridge C (ed.) 2002 Neurological Physiotherapy: Bases of Evidence for Practice. Whurr: London

Petajan JH, Gappmaier E, White AT et al. 1996 Impact of aerobic training on fitness and quality of life in multiple sclerosis. Ann Neurol 39: 432–441

Peto V, Jenkinson C, Fitzpatrick R, Greenhall R 1995 The development and validation of a short measure of functioning and wellbeing for individuals with Parkinson's disease. Qual Life Res 4: 241–248

Plant R, Joneo D, Ashburn A et al. 2000 Physiotherapy for People with Parkinson's Disease: UK Best Practice. Institute of Rehabilitation: Newcastle upon Tyne

Plum H, Morissey D 2002 Cross-speciality collaboration. Physiotherapy 88: 530–533

Podsialo D, Richardson S 1991 The timed 'up and go': a test of basic functional mobility for frail elderly persons. J Am Geriatr Soc 39: 142–148

Poser CM, Paty DW, Scheinberg LC et al. 1983 New diagnostic criteria for multiple sclerosis: guidelines for research protocols. Ann Neurol 13: 227–231

Prigatano GP 1992 Personality disturbances associated with traumatic brain injury. J Consult Clin Psychol 60: 360–368

Rappaport M, Hall KM, Hopkins K et al. 1982 Disability rating scale for severe head trauma: coma to community. Arch Phys Med Rehabil 63: 118–123

Robinson I, Hunter M, Neilson S et al. 1996 A Dispatch from the Front Line. The Views of People with Multiple Sclerosis about their Needs: a Qualitative Approach. Brunel MS Research Unit: London

Royal College of Physicians/British Society of Rehabilitation Medicine (Turner-Stokes L, ed.) 2003 Rehabilitation following acquired brain injury: national clinical guidelines RCP/BSRM: London

Royal College of Physicians/Clinical Effectiveness and Evaluation Unit 2004 National Clinical Guidelines for Stroke, 2nd edn. RCP: London

Russell WR, Smith A 1981 Post-traumatic amnesia in closed head injury. Arch Neurol 5: 16–29

Sadovnick AD, Baird PA, Ward RH 1988 Multiple sclerosis: updated risks for relatives. Am J Med Genet 29: 533–41

Sadovnick AD, Ebers GC 1993 Epidemiology of multiple sclerosis: a critical review. Can J Neurol Sci 20: 17–29

Stokes M 1998 Neurological Physiotherapy. Mosby: New York

Sunderland A, Tinson D, Bradley L, Langton Hewer R 1989 Arm function after stroke: an evaluation of grip strength as a measure of recovery and a prognostic indicator. J Neurol Neurosurg Psychiatr 52: 1267–1272

Swash M, Schwartz MS 1995 Motor neurone disease: the clinical syndrome. In: Leigh PN, Swash M (eds) Motor

Neurone Disease: Biology and Management. Springer: London, pp. 1–17

Tandan R 1994 Clinical features and differential diagnosis of classical motor neurone disease. In: Williams AC (ed.) Motor Neurone Disease. Chapman & Hall: London, pp. 3–27

Teasdale G, Jennett B 1974 Assessment of coma and impaired consciousness: a practical scale. Lancet ii: 81–83

Teasdale GM et al. 1990 Risks of acute traumatic intracranial haematoma in children and adults: implications for managing head injuries. BMJ 300: 363–367

Temkin NR, Kikmen SS, Wilensky AJ et al. 1990 A randomized double-blind study of phenytoin for the prevention of post-traumatic seizures. N Engl J Med 323: 497–502

Thompson A 1998 Symptomatic treatment in multiple sclerosis. Curr Opin Neurol 11: 305–309

Turnbull GI (ed.) 1992 Physical Management of Parkinson's Disease. Churchill Livingstone: New York

Van den Burg W, Van Zomeren AH, Minderhoud JM et al. 1987 Cognitive impairment in patients with multiple sclerosis and mild physical disability. Arch Neurol 44: 494–501

Wade DT 1992 Measurement in Neurological Rehabilitation. Oxford University Press: Oxford

Wade DT 1999a Goal planning in stroke rehabilitation: how? Top Stroke Rehabil 6(2): 16–36

Wade DT 1999b Goal planning in stroke rehabilitation: what? Top Stroke Rehabil 6(2): 8–15

Wade DT 1999c Goal planning in stroke rehabilitation: evidence. Top Stroke Rehabil 6(2): 37–42

Ware JE, Snow KK, Kosinski M et al. 1993 SF-36 Health Survey: Manual and Interpretation Guide. Health Institute, New England Medical Center: Boston, MA

Weiner WJ, Goetz CG 1994 Neurology for the Non-neurologist. 3rd edn. Lippincott: Philadelphia

Wichmann T, DeLong MR 1993 Pathophysiology of parkinsonian motor abnormalities. Adv Neurol 60: 53–61

Wood RLI 1990 Neurobehavioural paradigm for brain injury rehabilitation. In: Wood RL (ed.) Neurobehavioural Sequelae of Traumatic Brain Injury. Taylor & Francis: New York, pp. 3–17

Young B, Ott L, Twyman D et al. 1987 The effect of nutritional support on outcome from severe head injury. J Neurosurg 67: 668–676

Chapter **16**

Massage

Joan M. Watt

CHAPTER CONTENTS

INTRODUCTION

Massage is the starting point of the physiotherapy profession. Swedish massage was the basis for the strokes and principles used by the first members of the Chartered Society of Physiotherapists. There is evidence of massage being used in many ancient civilisations. The word massage may derive from the Arabic word *mass*, meaning 'to press', or the Greek word *massien*, meaning 'to knead'.

Definition

Massage is an age-old process that involves stimulation of the tissues by rhythmically applying both stretching and pressure (Watt 1999). Holey and Cook (2003) defined therapeutic massage as 'the manipulation of the soft tissues of the body by a trained therapist as a component of a holistic therapeutic intervention'.

PREPARATION 

Preparation encompasses the treatment room, couch, self, patient and contact medium.

Treatment room

The room needs to be kept at a comfortable temperature to ensure the patient is not subjected to chills or draughts. It must also afford the necessary privacy without contravening the patient's rights. There must be a treatment couch, small arm table and chair.

Couch DVD

In the clinical setting most treatment couches/plinths can have their height adjusted to suit the individual therapist. To achieve a good height for performing massage, stand side-on to the couch, resting your hand on it with the fingers loosely flexed at the metacarpophalangeal

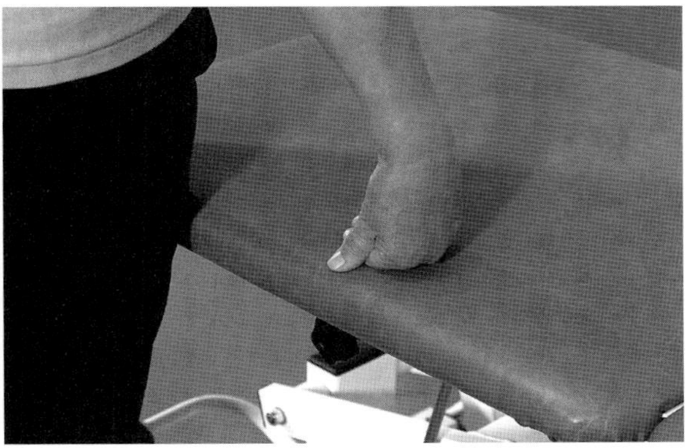

Figure 16.1 Setting the plinth to the correct height.

joints and elbow not quite fully extended. Adjust the height of the couch until you can comfortably rest your hand as above. It takes time, trial and error to find the optimum position (Figure 16.1).

The couch should have a fresh clean cover, as well as a paper couch roll. There should be pillows, a face hole or face pillow, and a blanket or towels to cover the patient.

Self-preparation

Stance

It is very important to ensure that your stance allows you to reach all the parts to be massaged in a specific stroke without having to keep altering position. Stand in the lunge position to perform long strokes such as effleurage and stroking (Figure 16.2). To reach across the patient assume a similar position facing the couch (Figure 16.3). Do not stand still; let your whole body go with the stroke and always keep your pelvis tucked and knees slightly bent to protect your back. Ensure your shoulders are relaxed, comfortable and not hunched.

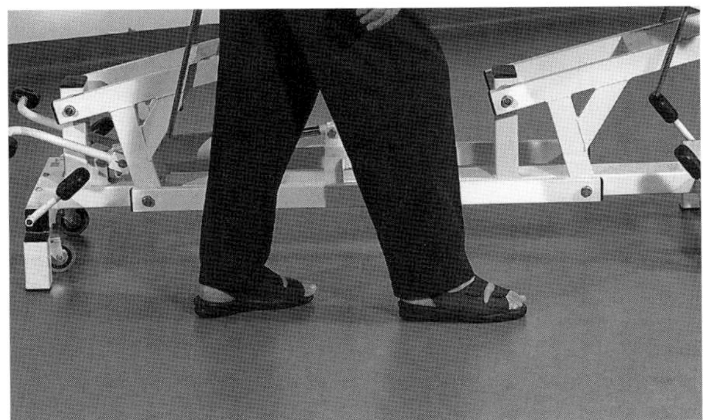

Figure 16.2 Lunge stance.

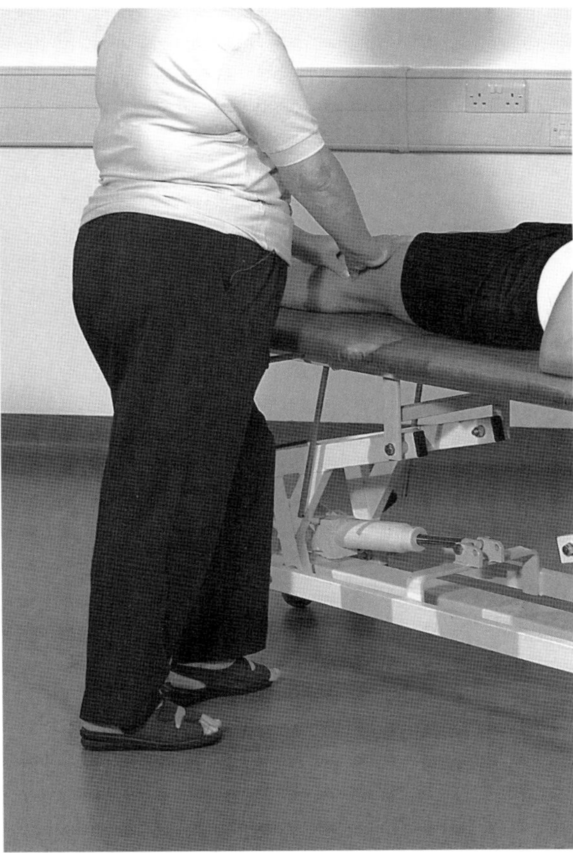

Figure 16.3 Reaching the patient.

Clothing

Clothing should be loose enough to allow unrestricted movement whilst looking neat and professional. Hair should not be allowed to come into contact with the patient. If your hair is long enough to touch your collar, it should be tied back.

Hands

Hands are your most important tool for massage. They must be clean and smooth, with skin that is well nourished by the regular use of hand creams. Nails should be free from polish and cut short, so they do not show above the fleshy finger pad. A very thin wedding ring may be worn, provided the patient does not experience any irritation from it. All other rings, bracelets, bangles and watches must be removed.

It is also important to practise exercises to improve the ranges of movement of your hands. Hollis (1998) advocates full abduction/extension of the thumb to give a wide grasp of an octave span; full flexion and extension of the wrists or at least 80 degrees of each movement; and full pronation and supination of the radioulnar joints.

Exercises DVD

1. Make a fist and then spread the fingers and thumbs as wide as possible; hold for 5–10 seconds.
2. Bring the fingertips of one hand in contact with the fingertips of the other and press, so that thumbs and little fingers are as widely spaced as possible.
3. Push two, three and then four fingers between two adjacent fingers of the other hand. Repeat in each space of both hands.
4. Put the palms together, with fingers and thumbs in contact and the elbows bent at chest level. Slowly turn your hands to point the fingers to ground. Return to start position.
5. Put the backs of your hands together, arms out straight, and bend the elbows up towards your chin to flex the wrists.
6. Clasp your hands with the wrists crossed, keeping your elbows straight (Figure 16.4a). Bend your elbows to bring your hands up to your chin (Figure 16.4b), then straighten your elbows again (Figure 16.4c). Keep the hands firmly clasped at all times. Do not force; go only as far as is comfortable.

Practising your rhythm

Sit with a pillow on your knee, with your hands open and relaxed. Try to clap as rhythmically as possible. Repeat with the ulnar borders of your hands, with clenched fists and ulnar borders of your fists (Figure 16.5).

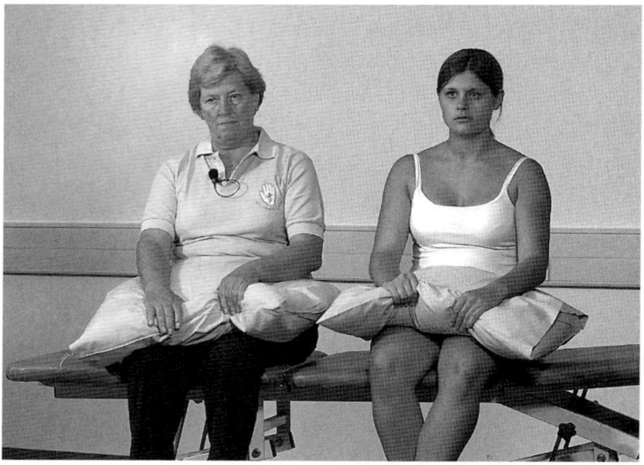

Figure 16.5 Practising your rhythm.

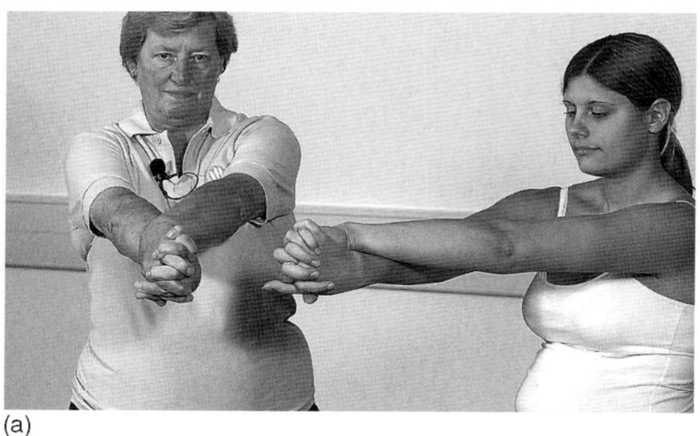

(a)

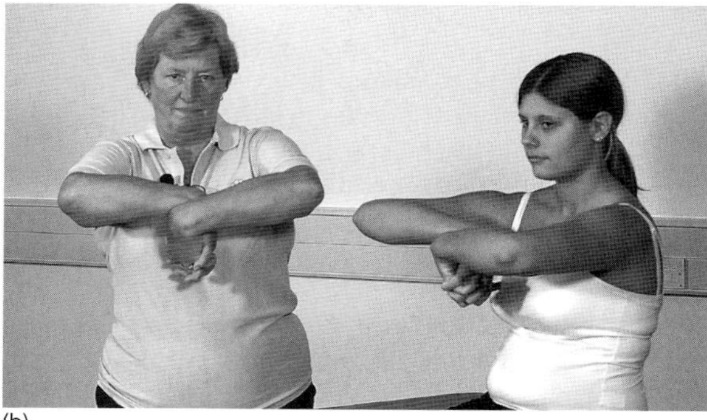

(b)

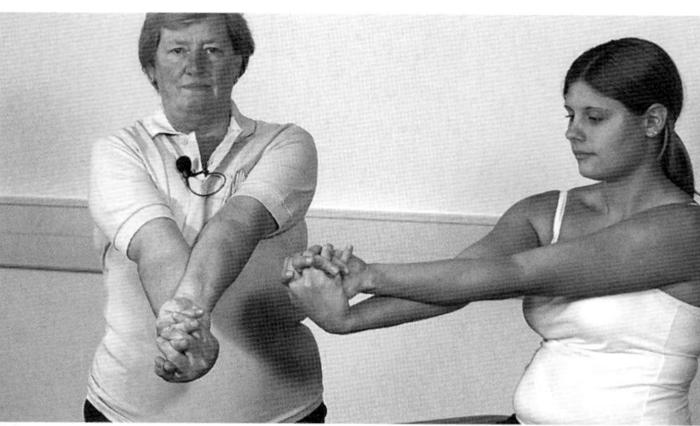

(c)

Figure 16.4 Pre-massage exercises.

16

Practising your strokes

Sit with a pillow on your knees. Grasp the outer edge of the pillow with lightly clenched hands and alternately push and pull it with your hands (Figure 16.6).

Palpation

The sense of touch and palpation skills must be highly developed in the person performing massage. It requires practice to attune and improve our sense of touch and thus our palpation skill. Start by feeling the differing textures of various types of material. Sit with a pillow on your knees and feel the pillow slip between your fingers and thumb; then do the same with a towel (Figure 16.7). Once you are confident that you can easily tell one type of fabric from another, repeat the exercise with your eyes closed.

Use your own body to identify anatomical landmarks and accustom your hand to the feel of differing tissues. Start by feeling the point of your elbow first with your thumb tip, then with each finger, both separately and together, and then with the palm of the hand. Repeat with each hand in turn. Close your eyes and focus on the message you receive from your hands. Try the same routine on the calf, shin, anterior aspect of the thigh, forearm, neck, shoulders and abdomen.

The sense of touch can be improved by many different methods. Put a selection of different round objects of various sizes and textures into a bag and then try to identify each by touch only. As this becomes easier, choose smaller articles with more closely related textures and time how long it takes to identify each one correctly.

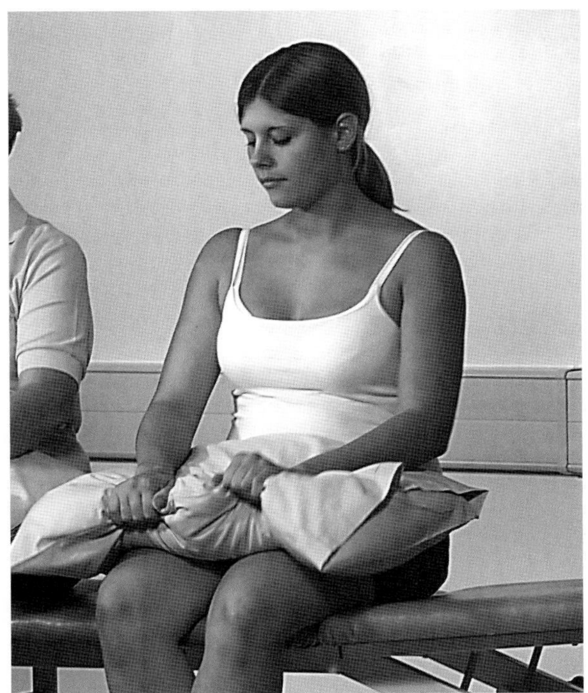

Figure 16.6 Practising strokes.

It is also important to learn depth of contact. Too light a pressure can be uncomfortable and ticklish and is frequently referred to as 'skin polishing'. Too heavy or firm a pressure may well produce trauma and damage tissue. Again, you can practise depth on your own skin. Try to move your hand across your leg as lightly as possible and then increase depth until you feel it is producing pain. Try this out on a friend or colleague and agree a score rate, with 1, say, being very light and 5 being heavy. Make your mind up what depth/number you are using for contact, then ask your model for his or her own answer. Always listen to what the model tells you and alter the pressure to achieve the score he/she has given.

Patient preparation

It is important that the patient is fully informed of exactly what the massage session will involve. Consent is dealt with in the section on legal aspects below and must always be in place before any massage starts.

> ***Key point***
>
> It is vital to request the patient to remove specific pieces of clothing as required to permit treatment. Always explain the reasons behind these requests. The patient's sense of decency and modesty has to be respected at all times. Never remove any article of the patient's clothing without asking their specific permission to do so. Remember it is possible to apply some forms of massage through one layer of clothing or over a thin cloth or towel.

Neither the physiotherapist nor the patient should ever feel uncomfortable, threatened or embarrassed by the manipulations being used. Always tell the patient exactly what you are doing and why. Explain why strokes have to be taken right up into the lymph drainage areas and make sure the person is happy for you to do so.

Draping or covering of the patient has to be properly carried out. Use shorts, towels of various sizes, towelling robes and togas (Figure 16.8). The patient's own clothing can also be very useful. Again, explain why you want the towel tucked in and, wherever possible, encourage patients to do this for themselves.

Coupling media DVD

Many and varied products are used as coupling media in massage. Massage oils, creams, gels, powders and aromatherapy products are readily available.

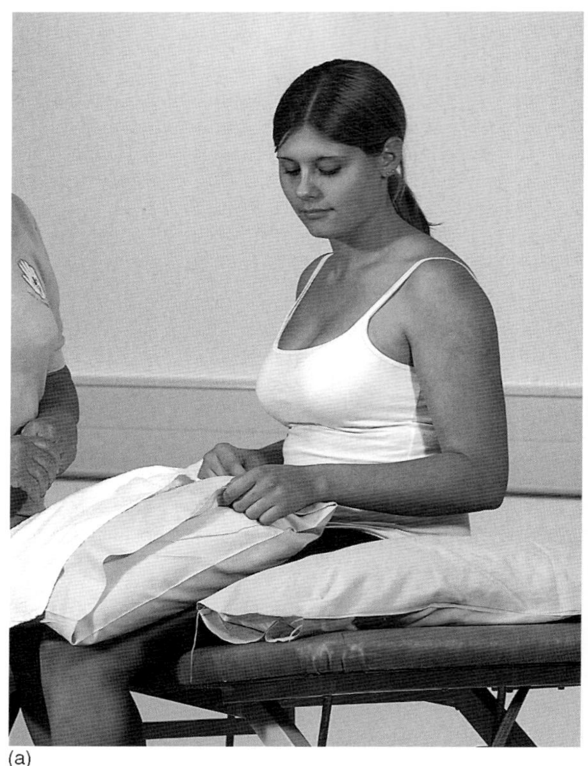

(a)

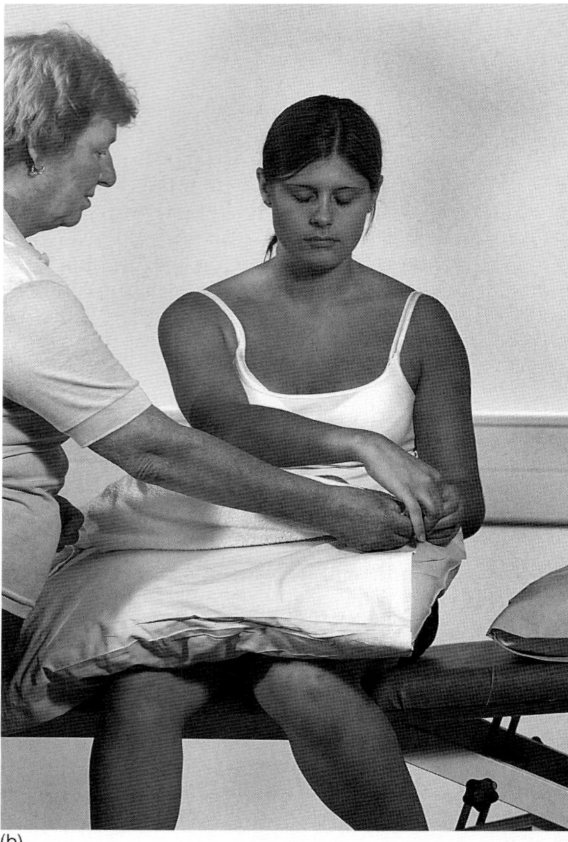

(b)

Figure 16.7 Assessing textures

16

The first and most important step is to ensure that the lubricant selected is acceptable to both patient and masseur and that there are no contraindications to its use. Full information on the contents of the chosen product is essential, especially if the recipient or masseur has any allergies. Many massage oils/creams use nut oils as a base and obviously these must never be applied in cases of nut allergy. Very hairy skin can be irritated and damaged by the use of powder or too little lubricant during massage. Powder should never be applied to hot sweaty skin as it clogs pores and tends to form hard lumps on the surface.

Ice massage can be extremely useful but great care must be taken to ensure the skin is not damaged by the effect of the ice. Always ensure the ice is kept moving and that you regularly check skin colour and reaction. Stop if the patient reports feeling uncomfortable or is cooling too fast.

Apply oils directly to your hands and do not use too much. Always make sure the whole area to be treated is clean before starting and also clean thoroughly at the end of the massage.

Water alone or with soap can be used to good effect as a lubricant. The addition of a small amount of oil can be beneficial when dealing with dry, scaly skin.

Never apply any heating agent/cream when you are treating any area where there has been tissue damage and healing. A hot cream may produce too much superficial increase in skin temperature and create further damage.

LEGAL ASPECTS DVD

It is mandatory to acknowledge and implement all pertinent legal requirements before, during and after using massage.

The practitioner must explain the reasons for applying massage and outline exactly what is involved. Written informed consent must be obtained.

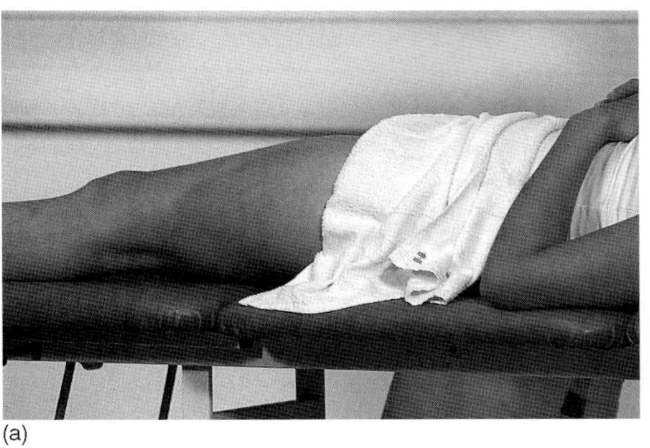
(a)

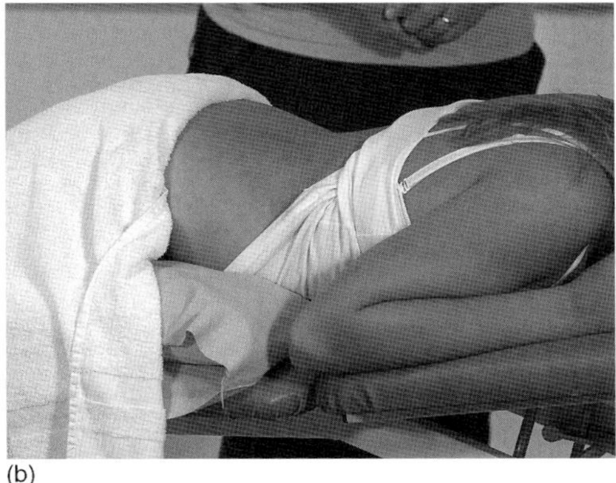
(b)

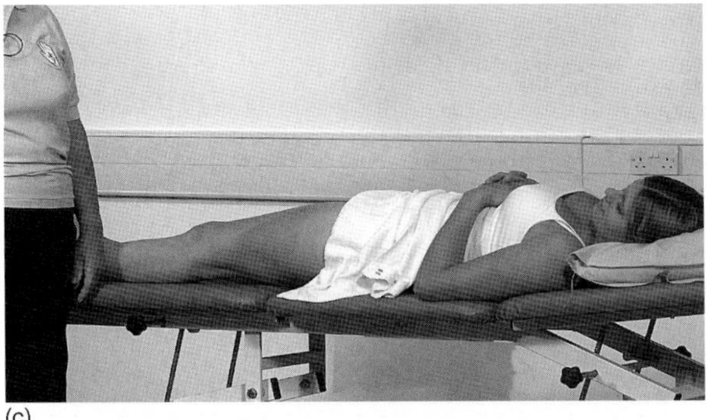
(c)

Figure 16.8 Covering the patient.

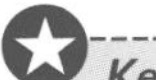

Key point

To apply massage without written informed consent can be construed as assault. All child protection, chaperone and local laws must be obeyed.

Throughout the whole treatment both patient and physiotherapist must be totally comfortable and at ease with the methodology. Keep enquiring if the patient is happy with the proceedings.

Remember to keep accurate, legible, dated and signed treatment notes. Do not just write 'massage'; give a short description of the techniques you have used and list the outcomes.

CONTRAINDICATIONS (DVD)

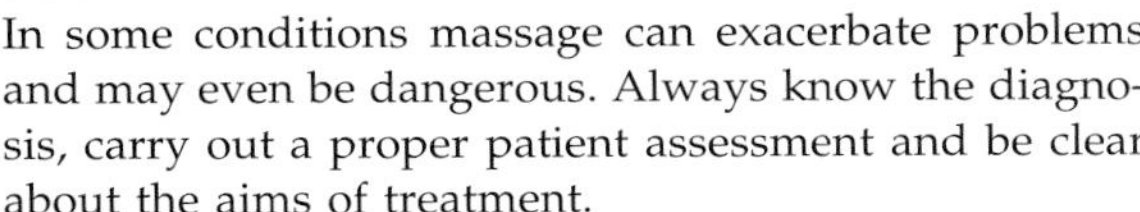

In some conditions massage can exacerbate problems and may even be dangerous. Always know the diagnosis, carry out a proper patient assessment and be clear about the aims of treatment.

1. Skin infections of viral, fungal or bacterial origin are contraindications to massage. Any type of skin infection in the area to be massaged or involving the hands of the physiotherapist would preclude the application of massage.
2. Open wounds should not be massaged. Apart from being painful, massage can damage the healing tissue and restart bleeding, and may cause infection.
3. Circulatory problems can be adversely affected by massage, which increases blood flow and manipulates the blood vessels. Bleeding disorders such as haemophilia, arteriosclerosis, haemorrhage, thrombosis and artificial blood vessels are all contraindications to massage. Remember that deep venous thrombosis (DVT) is a total contraindication to massage.
4. If massage is applied too early in the healing process in the context of a recent injury, it will cause further damage. At this stage it will cause trauma to the fragile healing tissue, leading to delay in repair, further bleeding and resultant excess scar tissue. It is recommended that massage should not be started until 48 hours after injury. Always ensure bleeding has stopped. Proceed with great care and use very gentle strokes initially.
5. Tumours can be mechanically stimulated by massage, which speeds up metabolism and so causes

the tumour to spread. Do not massage directly over or close to a tumour. Remember, though, that massage can be very effective and has proved to be an invaluable aid to cancer victims and in palliative care.

6. Massage is contraindicated in acute inflammation, as the inflammatory process can be worsened by its effects.
7. Myositis ossificans should not be massaged directly. This can cause increased formation of bony cells and further damage the soft tissues surrounding the site. Vigorous deep massage has been known to separate small bony particles from the site of ossification.
8. Although diabetes is not a total contraindication to massage, great care must be taken. It is usual for the peripheral circulation to be affected in diabetes, and as a result, blood vessels and skin can be easily damaged.
9. Alteration of skin sensation can be a contraindication to the use of massage. Massage may be used in certain circumstances, provided the experienced practitioner has an accurate diagnosis and knows the extent and reason for the changes. Loss of sensation, heightened sensation, presence of tingling, or neurological skin alteration all contraindicate massage.

ESTABLISHED TECHNIQUES (DVD)

Massage manipulations may be grouped under various headings. The three listed below are the main components of basic massage:

1. stroking manipulations
2. pressure manipulations or petrissage
3. percussive manipulations or tapotement

Stroking manipulations

There are two subcategories in this group: stroking and effleurage.

Stroking

As the name suggests, a stroking movement is performed, traditionally from distal to proximal in the direction of the lymph drainage (Figure 16.9a). This manipulation can also be performed in the opposite direction or in a crossover method. It can be applied using the pads of the fingers, the thumbs or one, two or alternate hands (Figure 16.9b).

One specific type of stroking is termed 'thousand hands', and was first described by Hollis. In this case one hand is used to perform a short stroke and then the second hand performs the same movement, overlapping the first. This is a fairly light touch but must not be so light as to irritate or tickle. It can be applied in fast or slow strokes.

Effects of stroking

- Accustoms the patient to your touch.
- Allows assessment of the state of the skin and tissues of the area to be treated.
- Improves sensory analgesia.
- Slow stroking will relax and sedate, and decreases muscle tone.
- Faster strokes will stimulate superficial blood flow, accelerating lymph drainage.

Stroking is therefore used at the start and the end of a session.

Effleurage

The meaning of this word is stroking; in massage it is used specifically to indicate a deeper form of stroking

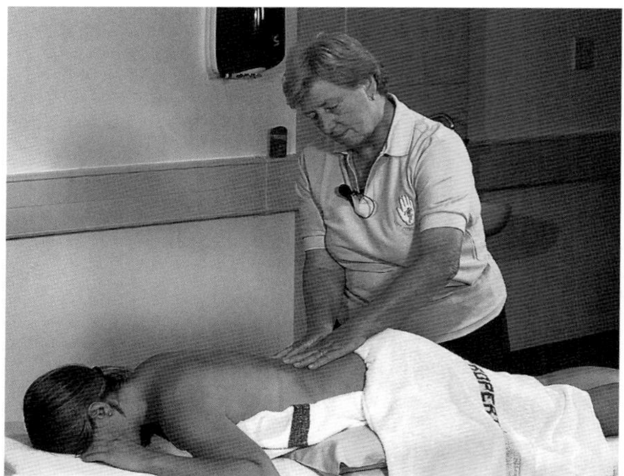

(a)

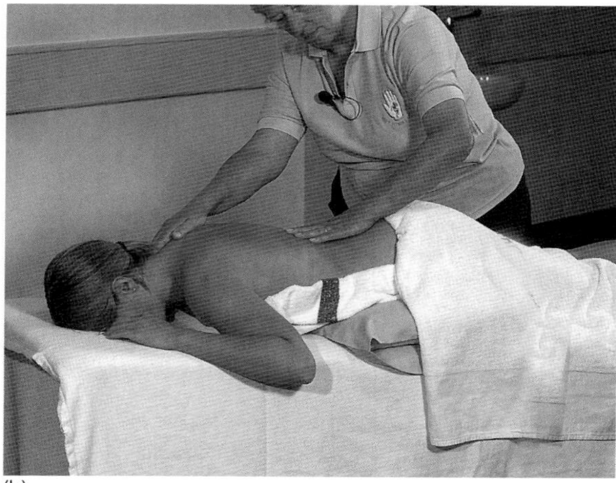

(b)

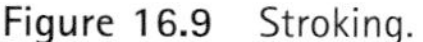

Figure 16.9 Stroking.

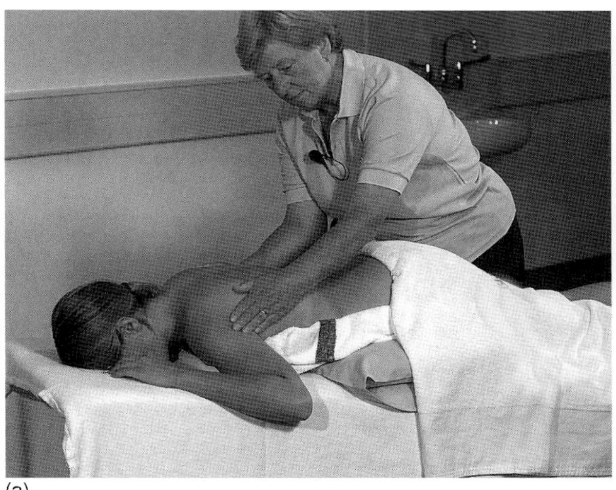
(a)

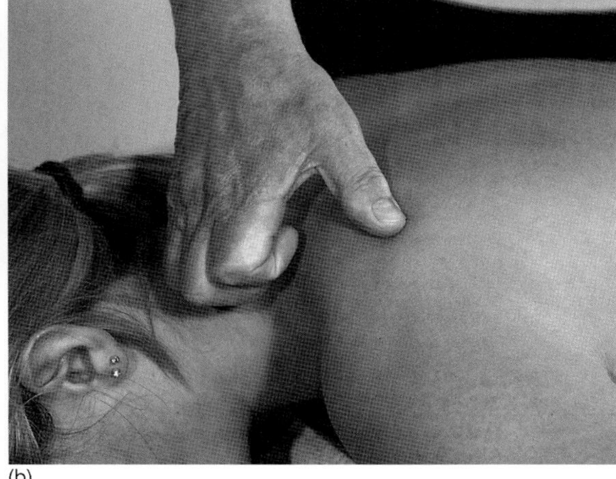
(b)

Figure 16.10 Effleurage.

(Figure 16.10a). As such, it can be applied as described for stroking or reinforced using one hand over the other or a lightly clenched fist (Figure 16.10b) or forearm. Because this manipulation goes deeper it can be graded.

- Grade 1 is sufficient to influence flow in superficial vessels.
- Grade 2 affects deeper vessels.
- Grade 3 applies to reinforced effleurage, with one hand on top of the other.

Effleurage can be applied in the direction of the lymph glands or in the opposite direction; all sorts of patterns can be employed, from a figure 7 or 8, to a circular or T shape.

Effects of effleurage

- Assists lymphatic and venous return.
- Assists interchange of tissue fluid.
- Assists removal of waste product and chemical irritants.
- Passively stretches muscle fibres.
- Restores mobility at tissue interfaces.
- Light strokes decrease muscle tone.
- Deep strokes increase muscle tone.

It is used at the start and end of a session, and in between other manipulations.

Clinical note

Precautions should be observed for both stroking and effleurage. The general contraindications listed above apply. In addition, ensure enough pressure and contact to prevent tickly sensations and apply sufficient lubricant to allow smooth movement over the skin at all depths.

Pressure manipulations or petrissage 

The petrissage group is made up of five categories: kneading, picking up, wringing, rolling and shaking.

Kneading

The tissues are compressed against the underlying structures during this manipulation. The kneading action is performed in a circular movement, either from proximal to distal or distal to proximal (Figure 16.11). The whole hand (one, both or alternate), finger and thumb tips, or finger and thumb pads may be used to perform kneading. The stroke can also be superimposed or reinforced by placing one hand or other fingers on top of the contact.

The action is to perform a circular movement with pressure on the upward part for about 25 per cent of the circumference. Contact must be maintained for the rest of the circle and only be lifted to move on to the next circle.

Kneading is classed in three grades:

- Grade 1 is sufficient to influence superficial vessels and compress superficial tissues on underlying structures.
- Grade 2 effects deeper tissue drainage and will compress deep tissue on underlying structures.
- Grade 3 is applied to superimposed or reinforced strokes. It may be applied as strongly as can be tolerated by the patient without producing tissue damage.

Effects of kneading

- Stimulates venous and lymphatic flow.
- Increases mobility of fibrous tissues.
- Helps interchange of tissue fluids.

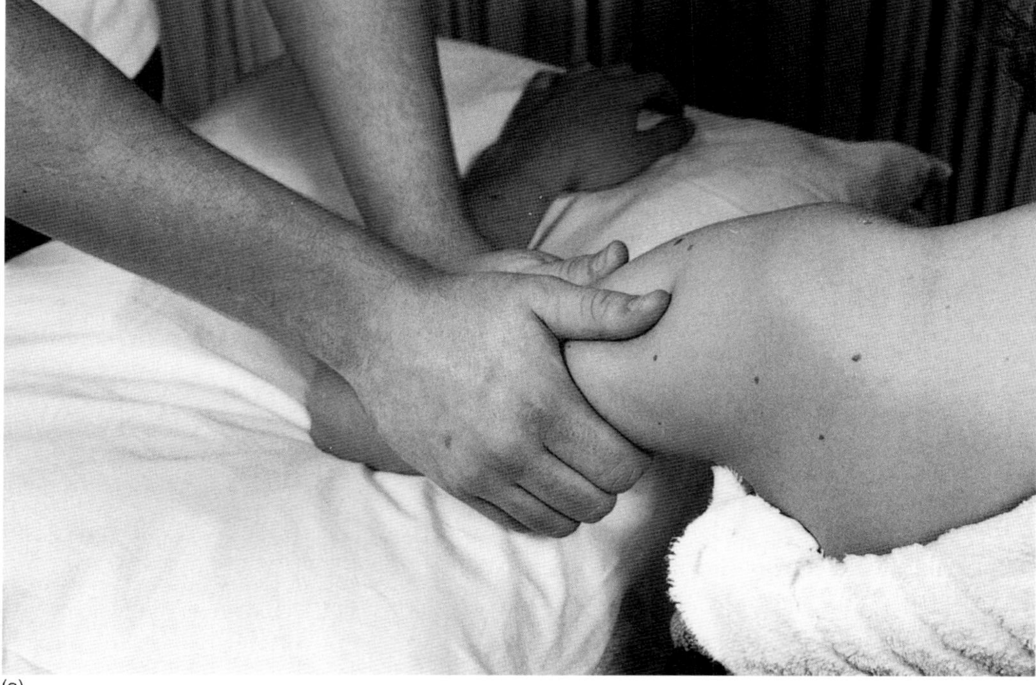
(a)

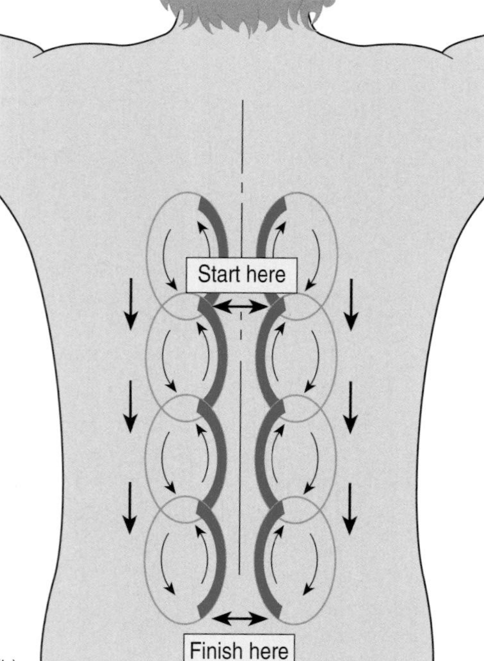

(b)

Figure 16.11 Kneading.

- Helps prepare soft tissue for exercise.
- Helps removal of waste products.
- Increases length and strength of connective tissues.
- Provokes somatovisceral reflex effects.
- Restores mobility between tissue interfaces.

Clinical note

The general contraindications listed above apply to kneading. Be careful not to compress too heavily or to nip tissue by squeezing too hard.

Picking up

The tissues are compressed against underlying structures, then 'picked up', lifted, squeezed and released. The manipulation can be single-handed in a C-shape (Figure 16.12), double-handed in alternate C-shapes and V-shapes (Figure 16.13) or double-handed in a V-shape. For a C-shape the thumb is held away from the palm so that the web between it and the first finger form a C-shape. In a V-shape the web forms a letter V.

Grading for picking up is the same as for kneading. Grade 3 is only used in the double-handed manipulation and will only be tolerated over very muscular areas.

Effects of picking up

These are exactly the same as for kneading. Picking up is particularly good for mobilising soft tissues, and is used after effleurage and kneading.

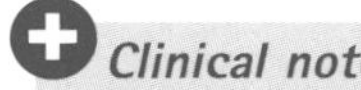

Clinical note

The general contraindications as listed apply to picking up. Be sure there is no recent soft tissue trauma. Be aware that if skin contact is lost during this manipulation a pinching action will result.

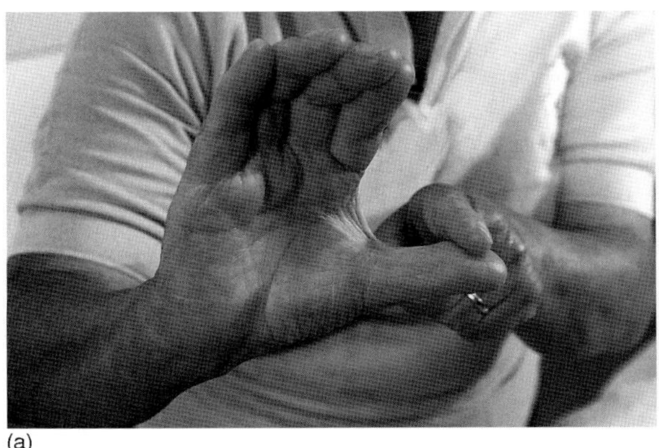

(a)

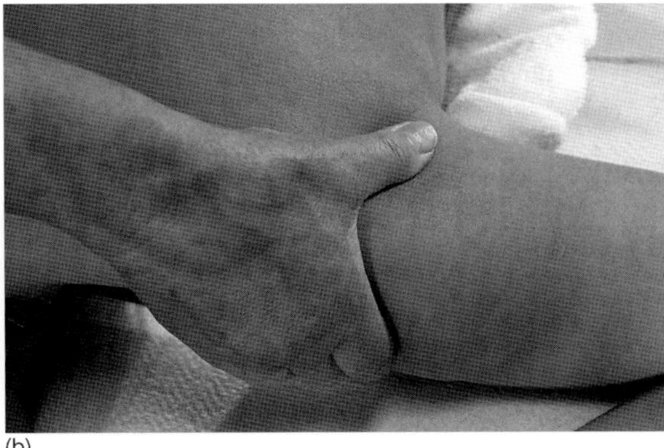

(b)

Figure 16.12 Picking up: single-handed C. (a) Hand position. (b) On the patient.

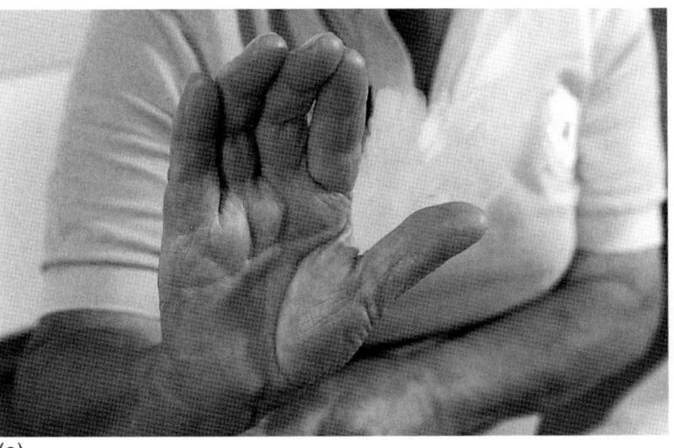

(a)

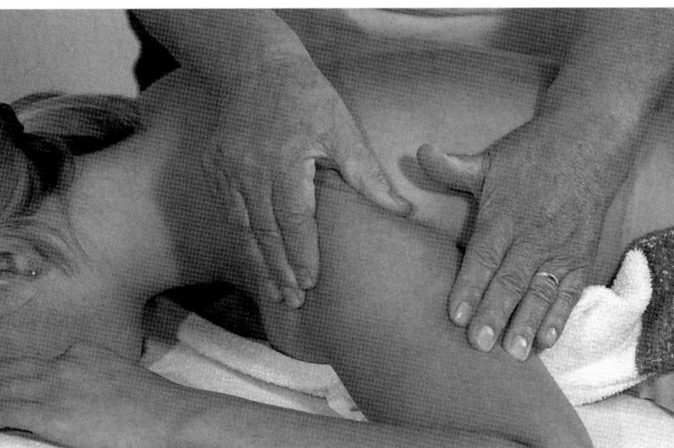

(b)

Figure 16.13 Picking up: single-handed V. (a) Hand position. (b) On the patient.

Wringing

In wringing the tissues are compressed against underlying structures, then one hand pulls towards the physiotherapist while the other hand pushes away.

Fingers and thumb can be used in wringing, with the tissues being compressed between them. The tissue is then lifted and pulled towards you with one hand and pushed away from you with the other. Full hands are also used in this stroke (Figure 16.14).

There are only two grades for wringing:

- Grade 1 is usually applied to finger strokes only
- Grade 2 uses the whole hand.

There is no grade 3 as it would be too painful to tolerate.

Effects of wringing

These are as stated for kneading. Wring is particularly good for separating superficial and deep adherent tissues.

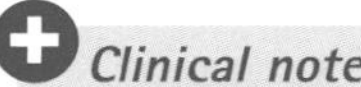

> ***Clinical note***
>
> The usual general contraindications apply. Be aware of tissue damage if wringing is used on recently injured tissue. Grasping tissue too tightly will produce a nipping effect.

Rolling

In this manipulation both hands are used. Contact is made with both palms. The thumbs are held away from the fingers, while the tips of the thumbs are close to or touching each other (Figure 16.15). The fingers pull the tissue towards the thumbs and then the thumbs squeeze and lift to push the tissue away.

There are two types of rolling: skin rolling and muscle rolling. In muscle rolling the roll action is not so marked and the action is more of a push with the fingers and a pull back with the thumbs.

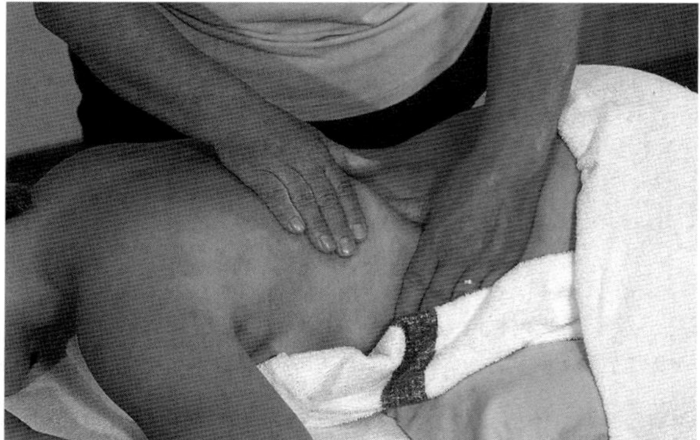

Figure 16.14 Wringing.

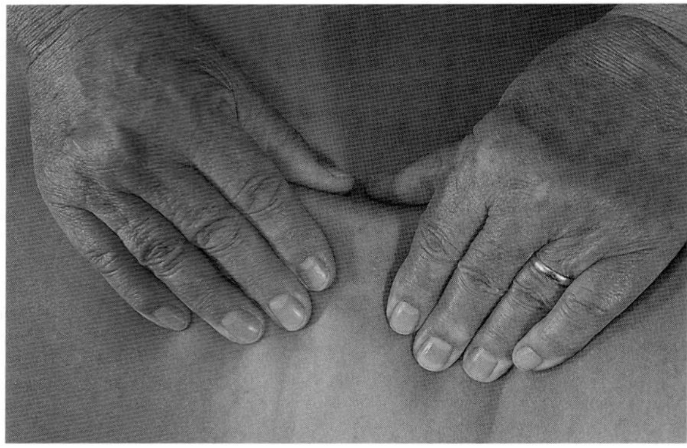

Figure 16.15 Rolling.

- Skin rolling constitutes grade 1.
- Muscle rolling constitutes grade 2.

Again, there is no grade 3 because it would be too painful.

Effects of rolling

These are as stated for kneading. Rolling also mobilises scar tissue. When performed slowly, it has a stretch effect on the tissues being manipulated.

> ***Clinical note***
>
> The usual contraindications apply. Take care not to nip tissues on applying a rolling action. Do not be too vigorous when working with recent scar tissue.

Shaking

In this manipulation muscle or more superficial tissue can be shaken from side to side. The tip of the thumb and tips of one or more fingers are used when treating small areas. The full length of the thumb and all fingers is used in larger areas (Figure 16.16). In a very large area such as the buttocks or thighs, the whole flat hand can be placed on the area and shaken, after applying gentle compression. In the final type of shaking — whole limb shaking — the leg or arm is lifted, gently supported and then shaken.

- Grade 1 shaking is used to describe thumb and fingertip shaking.
- Grade 2 applies to use of the full thumb and fingers and also to the flat hand.
- Grade 3 is whole limb shaking.

Effects of shaking

- Produces a feeling of invigoration and stimulation.
- Increases tissue mobility.
- Assists in breaking down tissue adhesions.

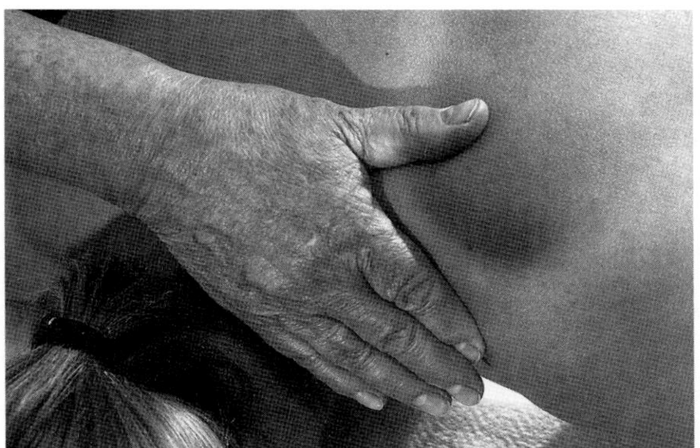

Figure 16.16 Shaking.

- Stimulates lymphatic and venous flow.
- Helps prepare soft tissues for stretch and exercise.

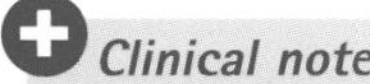

Clinical note

The usual contraindications apply, with specific care being taken to ensure the tissues are not nipped when using fingers and thumb. In whole limb shaking it is important for the patient to be relaxed. There should be no 'kick back' produced in any joint nor any feeling of strain experienced by the patient.

Percussive manipulations or tapotement 

In this category of massage strokes there are five main headings: hacking, clapping, beating, pounding and vibration. In some cases the last-mentioned stroke could be applied to the petrissage group but that tends to relate to more specific massage for sport and not the general concept.

Hacking

To perform this manipulation the arms are held abducted with the elbows bent. The area to be massaged is then hit by the medial border of the hands and/or fingers (Figure 16.17). The action is produced by pronation and supination of the radioulnar joints. It is important that the practitioner's shoulders and hands are relaxed and not held in any tension. The rhythm of all percussion strokes should be practised to ensure it is consistent.

- Grade 1 uses only the medial borders of the fingers.
- Grade 2 uses the medial borders of hands and fingers.
- Grade 3 uses the medial borders of hands and fingers more deeply and slowly.

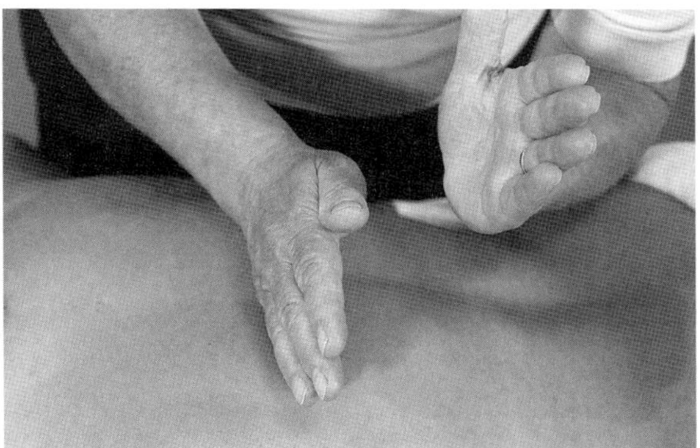

Figure 16.17 Hacking.

Effects of hacking

- Stimulates local circulation.
- Stimulates muscle tone.
- Gives a generalised feeling of stimulation.
- Provokes muscle and tendon reflexes.
- Light strokes affect superficial tissue.
- Deeper strokes aid the evacuation of the lungs.

Clinical note

All the usual contraindications apply. When using the deep technique it is good practice to cover the area with a thin cloth to prevent any skin irritation.

Clapping

To perform this stroke the hands are held loosely cupped and the area is struck by the palmar aspect of the hands and fingers (Figure 16.18). The action is produced by alternately flexing and extending the wrist joints.

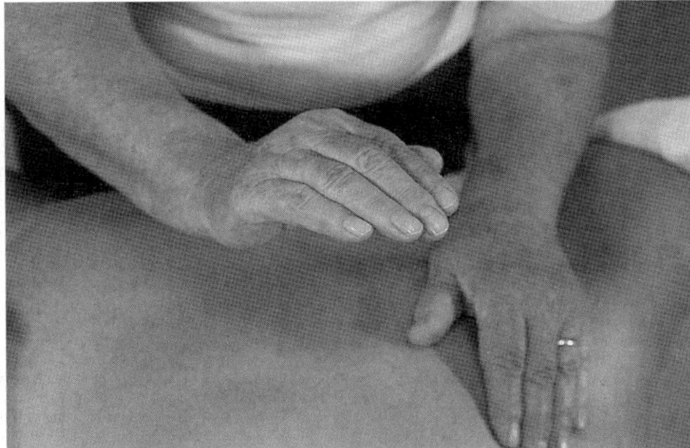

Figure 16.18 Clapping.

- Grade 1 clapping is very superficial and is often called skin clapping. This is performed at a fairly fast pace with minimal contact.
- Grade 2 clapping is deeper, slower and firmer.
- Grade 3 clapping is very firm and may involve elbow as well wrist action.

Effects of clapping

These are the same as for hacking, with the exception of provoking a tendon or muscle reflex.

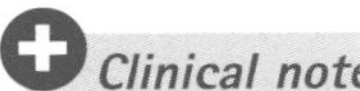

Clinical note

All the usual contraindications apply. Always ensure the hands are relaxed or the patient will find that contact produces pain. In grade 3 clapping, cover the area with a light cloth.

Beating

This form of tapotement involves the use of lightly clenched fists to hit the area. The action involved is wrist flexion and extension, with the finger/palmar area making contact with the treatment area (Figure 16.19).

- Grade 1 beating is performed at a fast rate, with fairly light contact.
- Grade 2 is slower, with firmer contact.
- Grade 3 is very deep and the rate can be varied as required.

Effects of beating

These are identical to clapping.

Clinical note

The usual contraindications apply. Ensure that hands are relaxed during the stroke. In grade 3 beating always make sure you cover tissue with a light cloth.

Pounding

In this stroke the hands are held in lightly clasped fists with the thumbs resting against the first fingers. The action is to pronate and supinate the radioulnar joints and make contact with the patient using the ulnar border of the hand (Figure 16.20).

- Grade 1 of this stroke applies to a fast rate with light contact.
- Grade 2 is used at a slower rate with firmer contact
- Grade 3 is deeper, with varying rates.

Effects of pounding

These are exactly the same as for clapping.

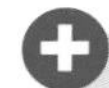

Clinical note

The same precautions should be applied as for clapping.

Vibrations

In this manipulation the tissues are pressed and moved up and down, or away from and towards the manipulator, and then released. At the same time small oscillations of the whole arm produce a trembling effect. A single hand or both hands (Figure 16.21) may be used and the hands should be held slightly in flexion.

- Grade 1 applies to light rapid movements.
- Grade 2 is firmer and slower, with more tissue movement.
- Grade 3 is as firm a pressure as can be tolerated and uses a very slow action.

Effects of vibrations

- Stimulates muscle tone.
- Stimulates the local circulation.
- Provides a feeling of well-being.
- Aids peristalsis.

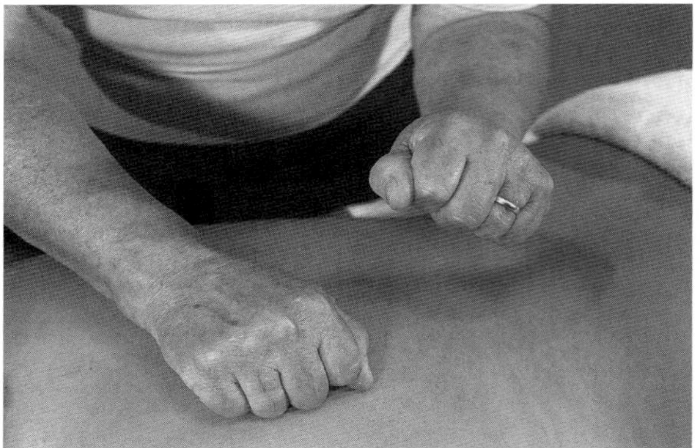

Figure 16.19 Beating.

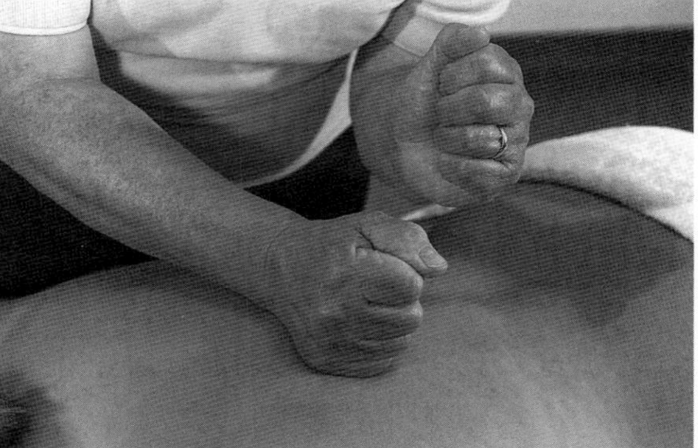

Figure 16.20 Pounding.

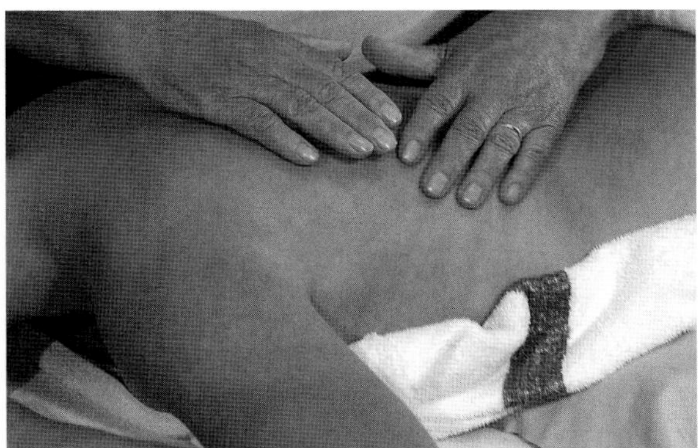

Figure 16.21 Vibrations.

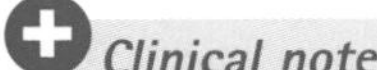

Clinical note

The usual contraindications apply. The hands must make firm enough contact to avoid producing a ticklish sensation.

NEWER TECHNIQUES

Massage is still evolving and as a result newer types of manipulation are being practised. With the increase in good scientific research we are now able to understand what these can do. We shall consider myofascial release, frictions, trigger pointing and acupressure here, but this is in no way a comprehensive list. As long as massage is a well-used, practised and evaluated skill, it will continue to develop and new skills will evolve.

Myofascial release (DVD)

As the name suggests, this type of manipulation is used to produce change in the myofascia, both superficial and deep. Myofascia is continuous throughout the body and is made up of collagen fibres. Superficial fascia underlies the skin and deep fascia covers, separates and protects skeletal muscle. The functions of the fascia are to form, support, provide boundaries, guide, mould, compartmentalise and control.

Problems associated with the fascia that respond to myofascial massage manipulations are:

- adhesion formation
- restricted or prevented movement
- alterations to the internal muscle structure
- fibrositis
- tissue contraction and scarring.

Strokes used in myofascial release include myofascial spread, fascial lift and roll, and myofascial mobilisation.

Myofascial spread

This manipulation is basically a stretch technique. Fingertips or hands, either in a line or crossed, can be used. The hands/fingers are laid on the tissue and pressed in until a slight resistance is felt; the hands are then drawn apart evenly until the tissue will go no further. This position is held until the resistance gives and the hands slide further apart (Figure 16.22). The movement is slow, steady and sustained.

- Grade 1 applies to release of superficial fascia.
- Grade 2 deals with deep fascia.

Effects of myofascial spread

- Makes fascia more fluid.
- Releases collagen bonds.
- Lengthens fascial layers.
- Restores mobility.
- Decreases effects of adhesions and scars.

Clinical note

All the general contraindications apply to the use of myofascial techniques. Caution should be used when dealing with flaccid paralysis, and with lax or unstable joints. Be aware that some advanced arthritic joints are held by fascial splinting.

Fascial lift and roll

This technique is very similar to skin and muscle rolling but is aimed at the fascia. Both hands are placed over the area, and the tissue is lifted until a very slight resistance is felt below the skin level. The tissue is then lifted slowly and pressed by the thumbs towards the fingers (Figure 16.23).

- Grade 1 only applies, as this technique is limited to superficial fascia.

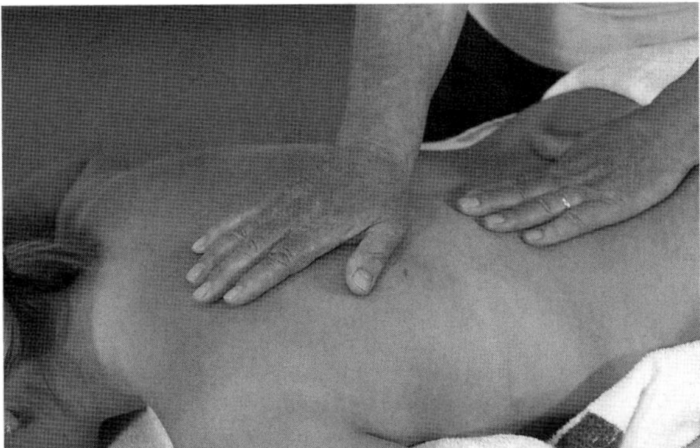

Figure 16.22 Myofascial spread.

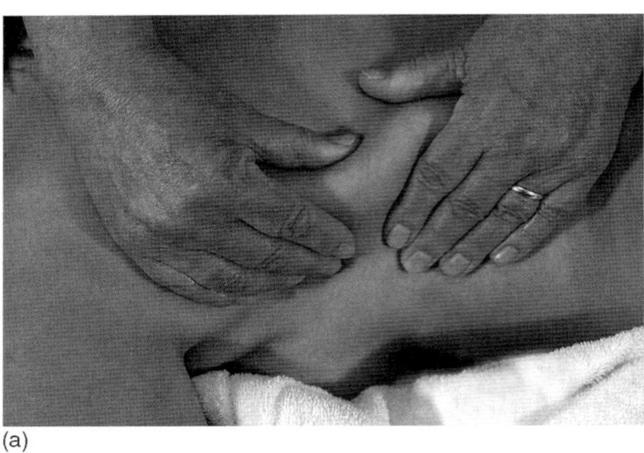

(a)

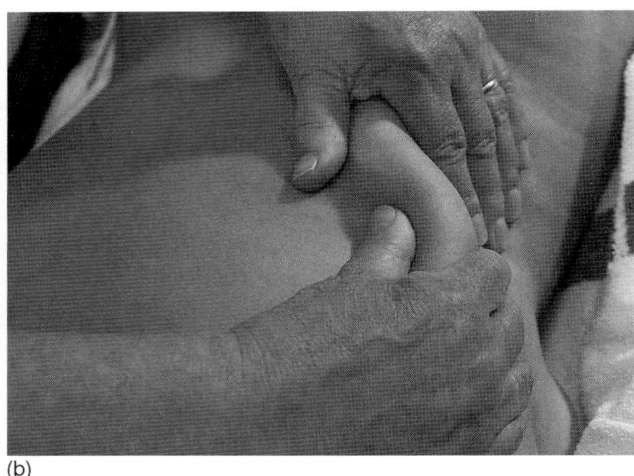

(b)

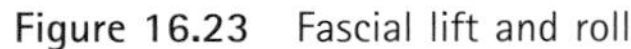

Figure 16.23 Fascial lift and roll.

Effects of fascial lift and roll

- Releases adherent areas in the superficial fascia.

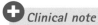

Clinical note

Precautions should be exactly as for myofascial spread. Never force the tissue.

Myofascial mobilisation

To perform this stroke, the fingers, knuckles, palms or forearm are placed on the surface. Pressure is applied and the myofascia is moved against the underlying structures. The action can be forwards/backwards or circular in pattern (Figure 16.24).

- Grade 1 is light and is used for the superficial fascia.
- Grade 2 is deeper and mobilises the deeper fascia.

Effects of myofascial mobilisation

- Frees myofascia that is adhering to itself or to underlying tissues.
- Re-establishes the ability of tissues to slide freely over each other.

Clinical note

Precautions are as for myofascial spread. The technique should not produce pain.

Frictions DVD

This massage technique was developed by Dr James Cyriax to treat soft tissue lesions (Cyriax 1993). It is a localised manipulation applied at the injury point and aims to give a stretching across the fibres to separate them and restore mobility.

To perform this stroke the fingertips or thumbs are applied, either alone or reinforced by the adjacent finger. The action is then to move across the tissue — transverse friction (Figure 16.25) — or to follow a circular pattern — circular friction.

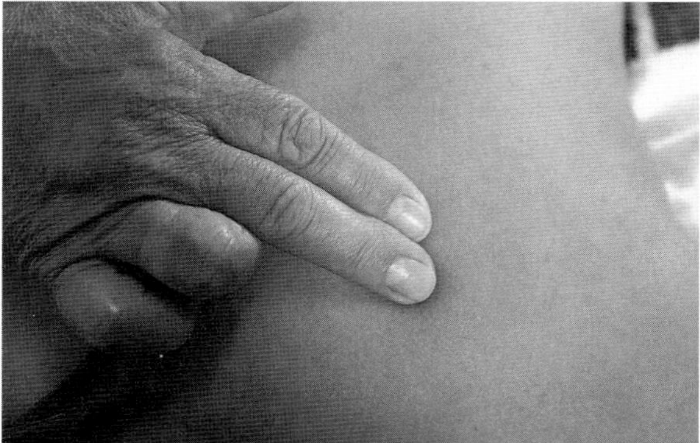

Figure 16.24 Myofascial mobilisation.

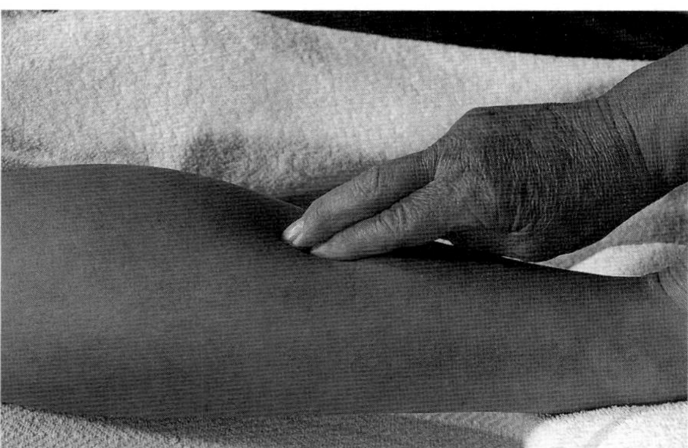

Figure 16.25 Deep transverse friction to the gastrocnemius musculotendinous junction.

- Grade 1 does not apply to this technique as it is aimed at deeper structures.
- Grade 2 is sufficient to affect deep tissue and cause compression.
- Grade 3 applies to reinforced and most transverse frictions and may produce pain before causing numbing.

Effects of frictions
- Restore tissue mobility.
- Stimulate local circulation.
- Aid the resolution of inflammation.
- Reduce pain as a counter-irritant effect.
- Stretch fibrous tissue.

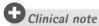

Clinical note
All the usual contraindications apply. Friction must be applied to the exact site of damage. The skin must move with the finger/thumb tips. Use little or no lubricant. Warn the patient that the treatment can cause pain until numbing takes place – about 2 minutes. Always apply within the patient's tolerance.

Trigger pointing (DVD)

Trigger points in the myofascia were first identified by Travell and Simons (1992). These points are bands within a muscle that have become ischaemic and fibrous because they have been held in excess spasm or tone for some time. The cause can be postural or mechanical and may be affected by metabolic, nutritional or other factors.

Trigger points are easily identified by palpation; pressure produces pain and this can follow a particular pattern of referral, as described by Travell and Simons.

To apply the trigger pointing technique, deep stroking is performed with the tips of the fingers or thumbs. Direct pressure may be applied to the specific point via the thumb, fingertip or elbow (Figure 16.26). Hold for 8–12 seconds, treat the area of referred pain and always stretch afterwards. When the full range has been restored, the trigger point will no longer be active.

- There is no Grade 1.
- Grade 2 applies to the stroking technique.
- Grade 3 is as much pressure as the patient can tolerate.

Types of trigger point
There are various types of trigger point and it is important to address all of them during treatment:

- active — produces pain at rest
- latent — only pain on palpation
- primary — response to trauma, acute or chronic overload

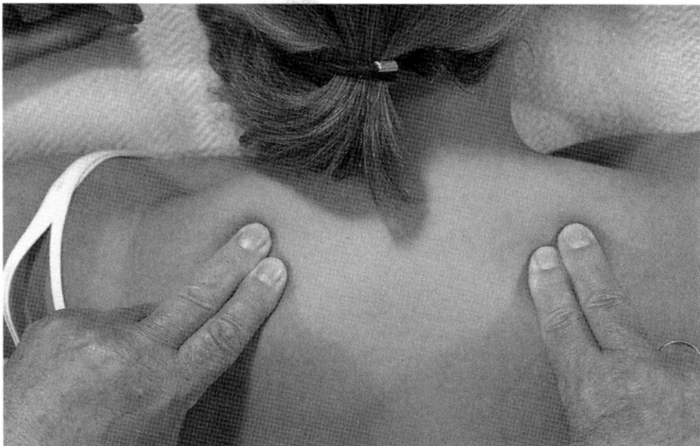

Figure 16.26 Trigger pointing.

- key — activates or neutralises satellites
- satellite — activated by key, situated in area of referral or antagonist or synergist
- general — near centre of muscle fibre
- attachment — in tendon or aponeurosis.

Effects of trigger pointing
- Gives pain relief.
- Reduces muscle spasm.
- Helps restore normal muscle tone.
- Allows full stretch of tissue.

Clinical note
The usual contraindications apply. Trigger pointing must always be applied within the patient's tolerance.

16

Acupressure

This technique is very similar to trigger pointing in which direct pressure is applied. In acupressure the pressure is applied to points on the acupuncture meridian lines, with the aim of producing effects on the tissue without using needles.

Effects of acupressure
- Relieves pain via release of endorphins.
- Stimulates local circulation.
- Stimulates lymphatic flow.

Clinical note
Contraindications apply as before. Acupressure should not be used on any patient with heart disease or visceral conditions. The practitioner must have full knowledge of acupressure points, an understanding of energy points, and a grasp of the philosophy behind this oriental belief.

SPECIFIC USAGE OF MASSAGE

Tension headaches (DVD)

Tension headaches respond well to treatment with massage techniques.

Start off with effleurage to identify particular tension spots and accustom the patient to your touch. Address the mid-scapular, trapezius and levator scapulae areas with trigger pointing (Figure 16.27a). Then treat the base of the skull with pointing and gentle circular thumb/finger kneading (Figure 16.27b). The length of time it takes for relaxation to be experienced will vary, and may be anything from 4 or 5 minutes up to 10.

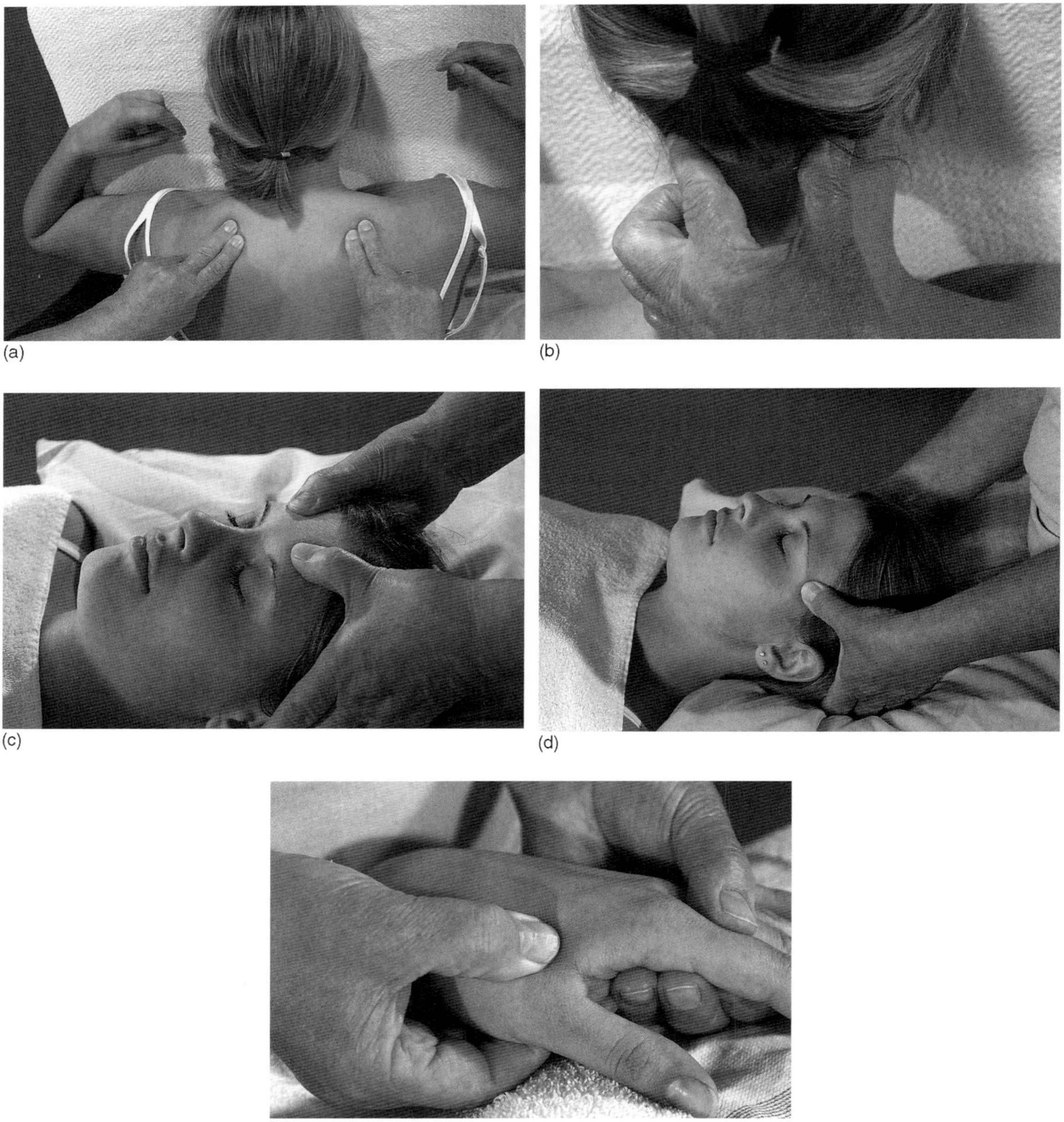

(a)

(b)

(c)

(d)

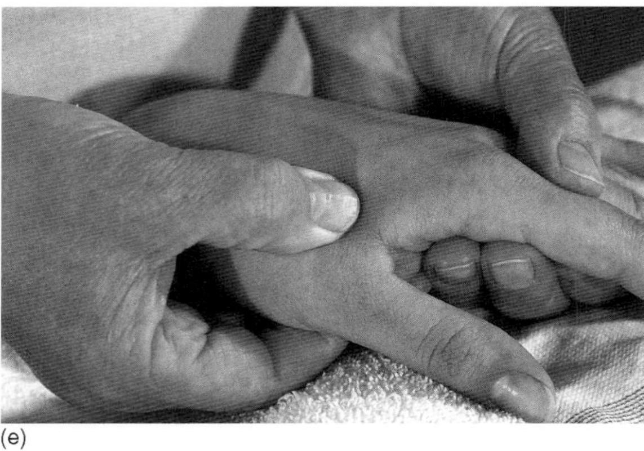

(e)

Figure 16.27 Management of tension headaches with massage techniques.

When the tension releases, return to the use of effleurage for the whole upper posterior shoulder area and then turn the patient into supine. In this position start with the two acupressure areas immediately above the inner eyebrows (Figure 16.27c); trigger for 20 seconds on, then 20 seconds off. Four times is usually sufficient. Then move to the two points at the side of the temple (Figure 16.27d) and repeat the same routine. Finally go to the point in the posterior web of each thumb (Figure 16.27e) and use the 20 seconds on/off method for four repetitions.

It is also good to teach patients to administer these trigger point routines themselves.

Specific frictions for tennis elbow

Identify the centre of the pain by asking the patient to extend the wrist against resistance. Once this is located, start with circular friction to accustom the patient to the touch and gradually deepen (Figure 16.28a). Then change to transverse friction (Figure 16.28b), warning the patient that he or she will experience pain and ensuring that you are working within the patient's tolerance. After a maximum of 2 minutes, the spot should become numb and the patient may well say the pain has gone. Teach stretching exercises to do at home. Explain that ice massage may also be of some help. The treatment can be repeated as often as the patient can tolerate but deep transverse friction may preclude further intervention for 3–4 days.

Friction of tendo Achilles

Frictions are used very successfully in the treatment of Achilles tendonitis. Start with the patient's foot resting over a rolled-up towel (Figure 16.29a). Isolate the tendon and, ensuring you are clear of the bursa, use a circular pattern, alternating between finger and thumb. Increase depth as the patient can tolerate but always work within his or her tolerance (Figure 16.29b). Follow with full-range passive stretch, then assisted stretch and finally active stretch and eccentric exercises.

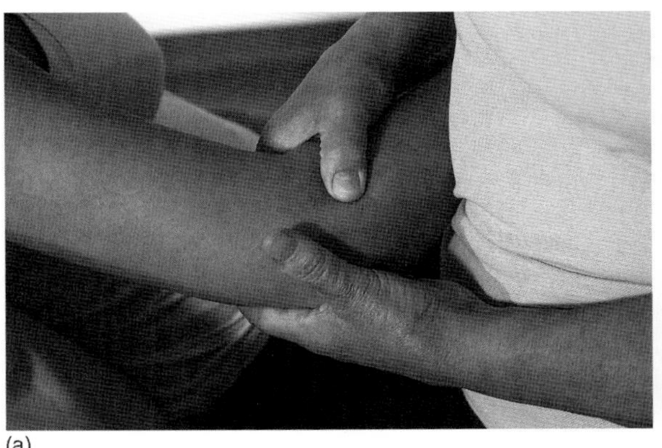
(a)

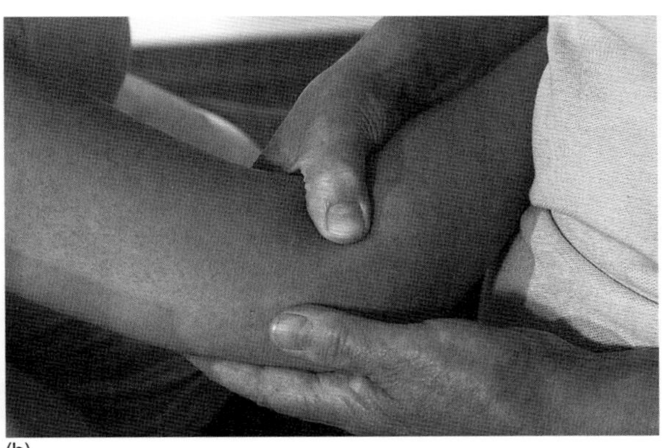
(b)

Figure 16.28 Frictions for lateral epicondylitis (tennis elbow).

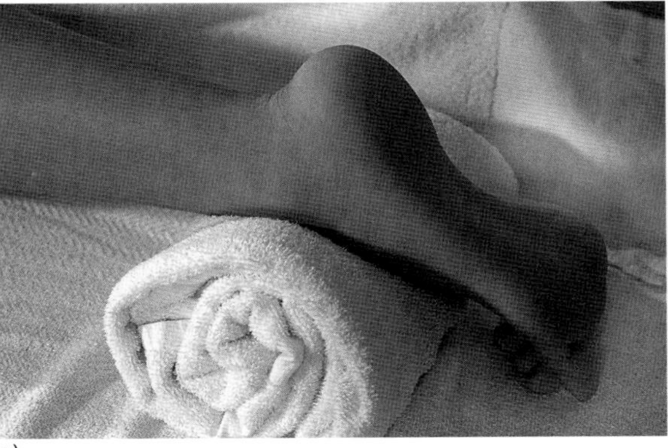
(a)

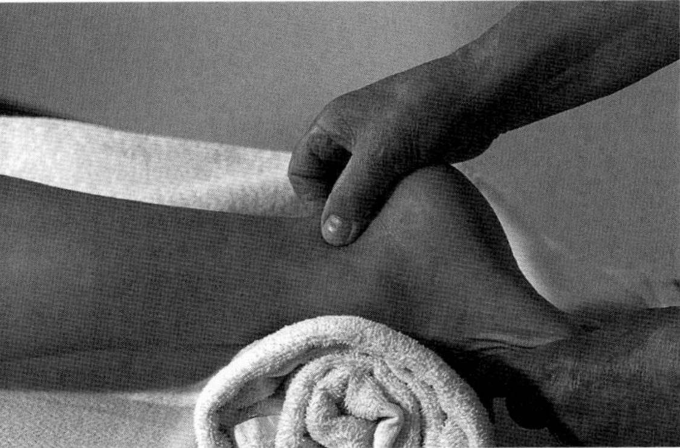
(b)

Figure 16.29 Frictions for Achilles tendonitis.

16

Massage for lymphoedema (DVD)

Post-mastectomy lymphoedema can be reduced by the careful administration of massage. The patient should be seated with the arm in elevation (Figure 16.30a). Start by clearing the distal areas with short, light effleurage strokes (Figure 16.30b). As you begin to approach the axilla the patient may well tense up, as this area can be extremely tender and sensitive. Explain what you are doing and start at the posterior aspect of the upper arm, again using short effleurage no greater than grade 1 (Figure 16.30c). Slowly work to the lateral, anterior and finally medial aspects. Finish with full-arm effleurage, deeper distally, and easing as you near the drainage areas (Figure 16.30d).

CONCLUSION (DVD)

- We still do not fully or scientifically understand the total effects of touch. Be aware that by releasing, relaxing and easing soft tissue the practitioner may also cause emotional release. It is not unusual for patients to cry or feel very drowsy after treatment.
- Always have permission to touch and make sure the informed consent form is signed. Remember that failure to do so can be construed as assault or even battery.
- Explain exactly which areas you will touch and why.
- Never proceed if you feel uncomfortable or embarrassed about the procedure, or if the patient feels that way.

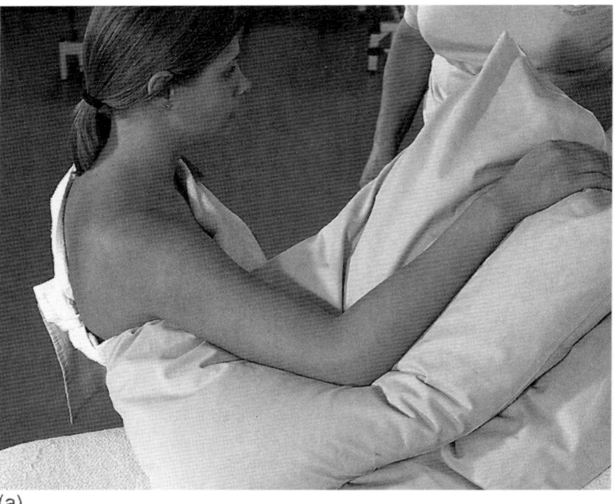
(a)

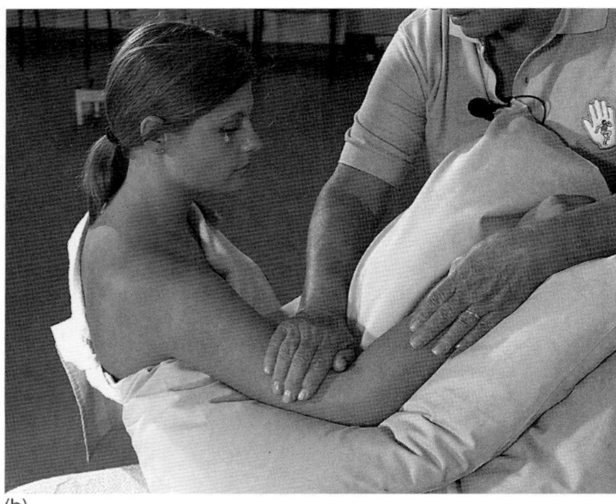
(b)

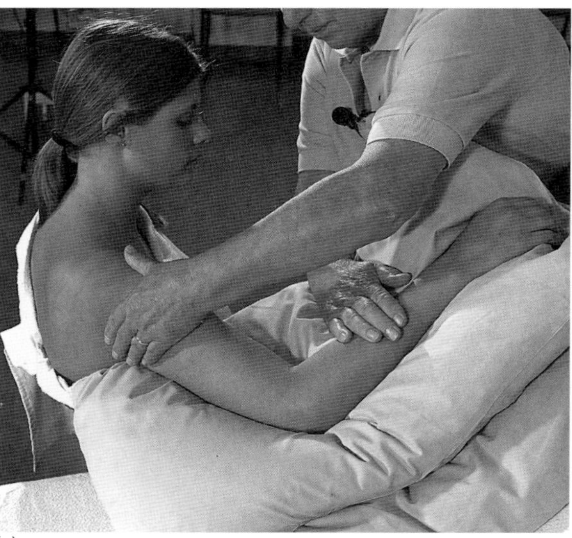
(c)

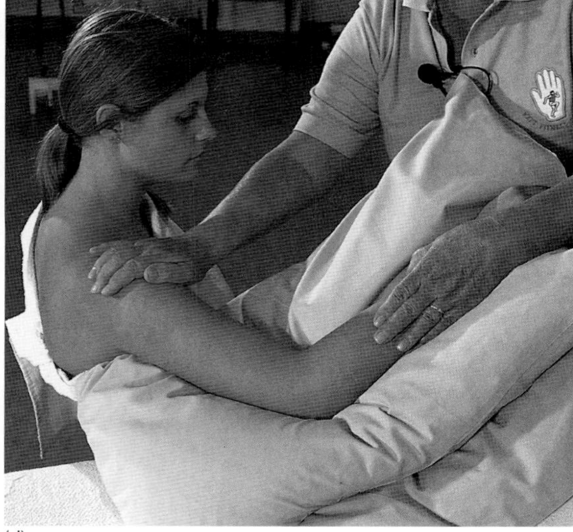
(d)

Figure 16.30 Massage for lymphoedema.

- Respect the patient's privacy and expose only the areas required. Use draping in such a way that your hands cannot disappear under it during the performance of any techniques.
- Request the patient's permission to remove or undo any clothing.
- Get the patient to tuck in towels or other drapes themselves.
- Remember to respect all legalities, including child protection and chaperonage.
- Ask regularly if the patient is comfortable and happy with the massage.
- Protect your own back and hands.

FURTHER READING

Andrade C-K, Clifford P 2000 Outcome-Based Massage. Lippincott Williams & Wilkins: Philadelphia

Benjamin B, Sohnen-Moe C 2004 The Ethics of Touch. Sohnen-Moe Associates: Tucson AZ

Jarmey C, Tindall J 2006 Acupressure for Common Ailments. Gaia: London

Neil-Asher S 2005 The Concise Book of Trigger Points. Lotus: Chichester

REFERENCES

Cyriax J 1993 Textbook of Orthopaedic Medicine, vol. 2. Baillière Tindall: London

Holey E, Cook E 2003 Evidence-Based Therapeutic Massage. Churchill Livingstone: Edinburgh

Hollis M 1998 Massage for Therapists, 2nd edn. Blackwell Science: Oxford

Travell J, Simons D 1992 Myofascial Pain and Dysfunction, 2 vols. Lippincott, Williams & Wilkins: Philadelphia

Watt J 1999 Massage for Sport. Crowood: Ramsbury

Chapter **17**

Exercise in rehabilitation

Duncan Mason

CHAPTER CONTENTS

INTRODUCTION

Exercise is one of the cornerstones of rehabilitation, widely used by many types of health professional, to manage an even wider range of medical conditions. It could be defined as 'using voluntary muscle activity produced by the integration of higher centres, cardiovascular, pulmonary and neuro-musculoskeletal components to rehabilitate these systems'. The aims and reported effects of exercise are also numerous. During this chapter we will see an evidence-based overview and rationale behind some of the more commonly encountered types of exercise.

Exercise is frequently used to enhance recovery rate of all components of the movement control system: namely musculoskeletal and central nervous system, to increase range of motion, increase muscle strength, develop a higher level of proprioceptive feedback and overall to develop an improvement in sensorimotor control. However, the list of benefits does not end here. Exercise is used in rehabilitation of the cardiovascular and pulmonary systems (Rees et al. 2004), which are required to provide the raw fuels for the physiological processes involved in muscle contraction. Exercise has also been shown to have beneficial effects on the higher centres, reducing the effects of some mental illnesses (Galper et al. 2006). This explains its invaluable use in the field of mental illness.

Exercise can be delivered in a variety of ways: in the clinic setting or by teaching home exercises; to individuals or in a group setting; on land or in water. All approaches need to be considered in order to select the most appropriate for the individual requirements of each patient. The way in which the exercise is taught or delivered to an individual is also important in the ultimate success of this modality; this too will be discussed in the course of this chapter.

To summarise, exercise is a widely used treatment modality that has been shown to be effective in the management of many medical conditions, when appropriately selected and applied.

Glossary of Terms

The following glossary is intended to provide a brief description of some of the terminology found in this chapter:

Delayed-onset muscle soreness (DOMS) A dull or often more severe aching sensation that follows unaccustomed muscular exertion. It is often associated with athletic activity. Eccentric exercise activity is said to provoke symptoms more readily due to microtrauma. Soreness usually peaks 24–48 hours after exercise (Cheung et al. 2003)

Kinetic chain exercise (a) Closed kinetic chain: an exercise performed where the distal segment of the limb is fixed (e.g. knee squats with feet on the floor). (b) Open kinetic chain: an exercise where the distal segment of the limb is able to move freely in space (e.g. a biceps curl with a free weight)

Muscle contracture The adaptive shortening of muscle or other soft tissues that cross a joint, which results in limitation of range of motion (Kisner and Colby 1996)

Muscle spasm A persistent muscle contraction that cannot be voluntarily released

Muscle spasticity A condition associated with hyperactivity of the stretch reflexes and tendon stretch receptors, due to loss of inhibitory influences on the alpha-motor neurones on the motor unit (Mense et al. 2001)

Muscle tension (also sometimes referred to as **muscle stiffness**) An increase in resistance to passive movement of a joint

Muscle tone The resting activity level or tension of a muscle, clinically determined as resistance to passive movement or to deformation

Myalgia Pain felt within a muscle

Proprioception The specialised variation of the sensory modality of touch that encompasses the sensation of joint movement (kinaesthesia) and joint position (joint position sense) (Lephart et al. 1997)

Stretching Any therapeutic manœuvre designed to lengthen pathologically shortened soft-tissue structures and thereby increase range of motion (Kisner and Colby 1996)

STRENGTHENING EXERCISES

Introduction

Strengthening exercises are aimed at increasing the torque-producing capacity or endurance of a specific muscle or muscle group.

Adequate muscle strength is necessary to perform many activities of daily living, whether it is to achieve self-care, or to accomplish occupational or recreational tasks. As a result of many pathologies, muscle strength can be lost, whether directly caused by trauma resulting in a disruption in the motor control mechanism, or indirectly — for example, as a result of pain inhibition or disuse atrophy.

An evaluation of muscle strength is usually performed as part of a patient's objective examination. This should lead the therapist to a diagnosis and enable rationalisation of an appropriate point from which to start strengthening rehabilitation.

As a strengthening exercise programme is undertaken, physiological changes occur within the muscle to increase its capacity to produce torque and sustain muscle contractions. This allows exercises to be progressed in turn to further overload and strengthen the muscle.

Therapists commonly employ several types of strengthening exercise:

- free active
- isometric, concentric, eccentric
- open/closed kinetic chain
- resisted.

These will be discussed in further detail in the remainder of this section and will be used according to the strength requirements of the individual.

Other factors, such as the number of repetitions, how often they are performed (that is, number of sets), frequency per day and the load applied, are also important factors in determining intended outcomes.

Measurement of muscle strength

Key point

It is important for a physiotherapist to measure muscle strength objectively when assessing an individual, in order to obtain a baseline level from which future improvements (or lack of them) can be gauged. This allows the therapist to devise an individual exercise plan and to evaluate the effectiveness of a prescribed exercise regimen.

Muscle strength can be evaluated in a number of ways: manually, functionally or mechanically.

The Oxford scale

The Oxford Scale has been devised to assess muscle strength manually and is widely used by physiotherapists. According to the Oxford Scale, muscle strength is graded from 0 to 5. Table 17.1 summarises the grades.

There are limitations to the usefulness of the Oxford Scale. These include:

- a lack of functional relevance
- non-linearity (the difference between grades 3 and 4 is not necessarily the same as the difference between grades 4 and 5)
- a patient's variability with time (alternating between grades)
- a degree of subjectivity between assessors
- assessment of muscles acting only concentrically
- the difficulty of applying the scale to all cases in clinical practice (so that strength is rarely evaluated throughout the full range since many individuals seen by physiotherapists do not possess full range in the first place).

Due to these shortcomings, modified versions of the Oxford Scale are commonly seen in clinical practice.

Functional tools

Functional tools or scales can be used to evaluate strength and can be related to a specific activity or to one of its components. These tools are commonly employed when rehabilitating sportsmen and women back to competition. Sport-specific activities can be monitored by a physiotherapist with a working knowledge of the demands of a particular sport, its training and competitive requirements.

17

Isokinetic assessment

Isokinetic assessment has been used with increasing frequency since its inception in the 1970s. It involves computerised evaluation of movement when exercising at a preset angular velocity on the isokinetic equipment (Figure 17.1). This means that the subject can push as hard or as little as desired and the machine will move only at the preset velocity. It is therefore the resistance provided by the machine that varies.

Use of isokinetics has functional relevance since it can evaluate both eccentric and concentric activity through range.

Table 17.1 The Oxford Scale

Grade	Muscle contraction
0	No contraction
1	Flicker of a contraction
2	Full-range active movement with gravity eliminated (counterbalanced)
3	Full-range active movement against gravity
4	Full-range active movement against light resistance
5	Normal function/full-range against strong resistance

> **Key point**
> Isokinetic machines are used for treatment as well as assessment. They produce objective, reproducible and quantifiable data and therefore have obvious advantages over other methods of evaluating strength.

Drawbacks

The drawbacks of isokinetics relate to its function, as natural human movements rarely occur at fixed velocities. Also, the machine operates on a fixed axis of movement, which does not replicate the instantaneous axis of movement found in most normal joints. The equipment can also be time-consuming to set up and not all physiotherapists will have access to it.

Additional limitations have been acknowledged by Lieber (1992). These include the time required to recruit muscle fibres (50–200 milliseconds), making the data obtained during this period unusable. Another drawback is the limb striking the testing bar at the end of

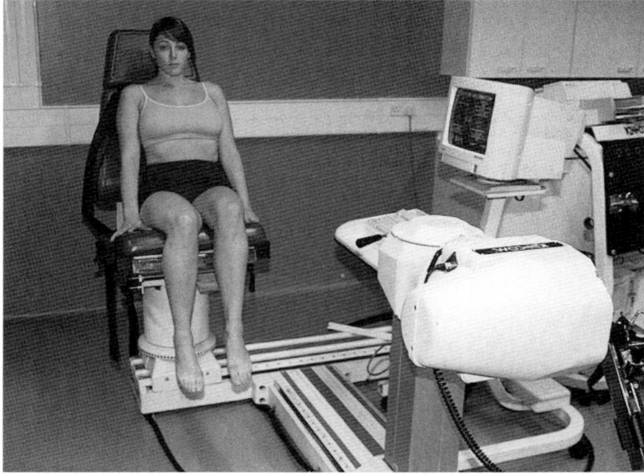

Figure 17.1 A typical isokinetic machine.

the movement, although some isokinetic units employ a damping mechanism to prevent this.

Key point

While isokinetics can give the physiotherapist an idea of any underlying deficiencies in the musculoskeletal system, there is no single tool to evaluate strength that is both totally functional and quantifiable.

Strength training

Benefits

Strength training can include free active exercise or resistance training, when the body must overcome this resistance to produce movement. This may be simply via use of bodyweight or free weights or via use of other equipment such as exercise machines in a multigym. Resistance training can also refer to submaximal and endurance work. All aspects of resistance training can be incorporated into various rehabilitation programmes. Some of the reported physiological benefits of resistance training are:

- increased cross-sectional area of muscle
- increased muscle fibre size
- increased or maintained bone density
- increased tensile strength of tendons and ligaments
- decreased heart rate.

In order for a muscle or muscle group to develop sufficient strength gains, it must be loaded progressively; otherwise strength improvements will be limited. This factor can often be overlooked when rehabilitating an individual, and failure to progress exercise may result in a lack of improvement on the part of the patient.

Initial improvement in strength, when measured objectively, may be rapid without noticeable changes in physical characteristics. This is due to enhanced neuromuscular coordination and utilisation of previously redundant motor units. More motor units are recruited within a given muscle and a stronger contraction of the muscle is therefore produced. This neural adaptation occurs before other physical and physiological changes that result from resistance training. It can be therefore said that there are two mechanisms that we try to employ when applying strengthening exercises: firstly, the physiological adaptations occurring in the muscles, which take 6–8 weeks, and secondly, the neural adaptations to facilitate increase of motor units within a muscle, which happens a lot sooner.

Free active exercise

These strengthening exercises are performed when the only external resistance to be overcome is that resistance provided by the weight of the body part. These exercises are used when the individual is at grade 2 or 3 or below on the Oxford Scale for the targeted muscle group. Certain strategies are employed when dealing with an individual with this level of disability. The muscle's mid-range is the most effective part of the range for facilitating muscle activity, followed by inner range and then outer range. Muscles are also more effective at generating torque when the angle of pull is at 90 degrees so the joint may be placed in this position to facilitate activity. The use of overflow can also facilitate muscle activity: for instance, when applying a force at another muscle in the region that normally works functionally with the targeted muscle, or by working the corresponding muscle on the other side of the body. Muscle contractions can also be enhanced by use of afferent input to the CNS, touching the corresponding dermatome (an area of skin sharing the same nerve root innervation), vocal encouragement, visual feedback and use of biofeedback units such as EMG; all these are useful in facilitating activity in redundant motor units. The type of muscle contraction used can also have a bearing on the effectiveness of the exercise.

Muscle contractions

Muscles can contract in three different ways: concentrically, eccentrically and isometrically. The characteristics of these different types of contraction are summarised in Table 17.2.

17

Table 17.2 Types of muscle contraction

Type of contraction	Characteristics
Isometric	Muscle maintains the same length throughout the contraction
Concentric	Muscle contracts from a relatively lengthened position to a shorter position Performed either against gravity or against load/resistance Outer range to inner range
Eccentric	Muscle contracts from a relatively shortened position to a longer position Performed either with gravity or with a controlled release of a load/resistance Inner range to outer range

Key point

Sometimes the terms *isotonic shortening* and *isotonic lengthening* may be seen instead of concentric and eccentric contraction. These are best avoided, as they imply that one contraction is an opposite of the other, whereas physiologically their characteristics vary greatly.

Individual muscles often exhibit more than one type of contraction at a time. Consider the muscle work occurring in the hamstring muscles in Figure 17.2. The proximal part of the muscle is lengthening (controlling hip flexion), and the distal part is shortening, controlling tibial movement.

When compared to concentric exercise, eccentric exercise is mechanically and metabolically more efficient; more negatively, however, it is less resistant to fatigue and may result in delayed onset muscle soreness (DOMS), microtrauma inflammation between sarcomeres. See Table 17.3 for further examples of eccentric activity.

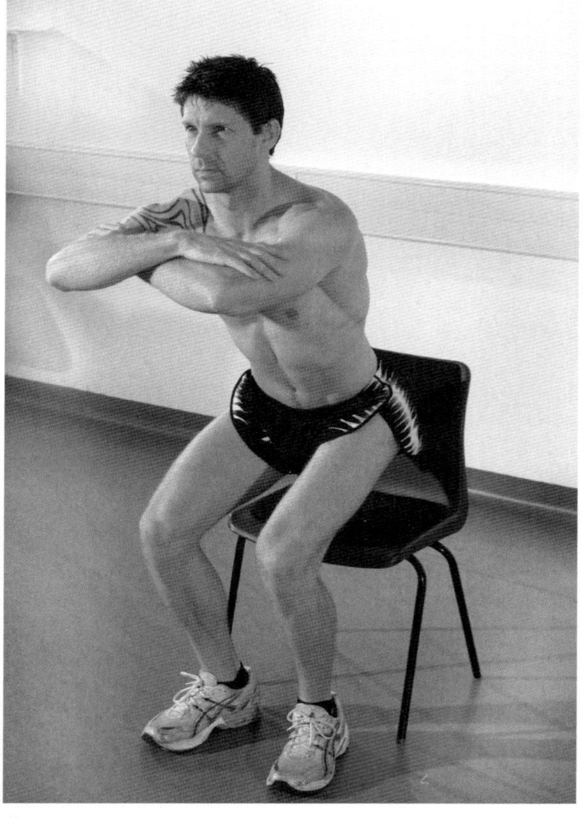

Figure 17.2 Concurrent dual contraction during a squat.

17

Table 17.3 The functions of eccentric muscle work

Function	Example
Deceleration of a limb part	Kicking a football; the hamstrings act to decelerate hip flexion and knee extension
Force absorption	Landing from a jump; the quadriceps contract, absorbing some of the ground reaction force and thus reducing the joint reaction forces
Controlling a movement against gravity	Sitting down in a chair; gluteus maximus and the upper part of the hamstrings are controlling hip flexion

DOMS is a dull aching sensation that follows unaccustomed muscular exertion. It is a key characteristic occurring after eccentric muscle activity, and should be differentiated from other types of muscle soreness that arise during or soon after exercise owing to metabolic factors such as lactate build-up.

DOMS is typically felt most acutely 48 hours after eccentric exercise has been completed (Leger and Milner 2001; Howell et al. 1993; Rodenberg et al. 1993). This commonly occurs in certain muscles of individuals infrequently undertaking a particular activity that has quite a high eccentric component. Examples include fell-running (quadriceps in the downhill component) or playing squash (gluteus maximus when reaching for a low shot).

DOMS is effectively the occurrence of local microtrauma within the muscle. A key site for this inflammation is between adjacent sarcomeres or within the Z bands. Evidence for this inflammatory reaction can be found in increased levels of creatine kinase (CK) in the blood following exercise. This enzyme is released into the blood stream following a muscular injury. Occasionally, the high CK levels found after eccentric exercise can confuse the clinical picture of a patient in whom CK levels may be used as a means of informing clinical diagnosis (Gralton et al. 1998). Saxton et al. (1995) have also reported a decrease in proprioceptive function with high-level eccentric exercise.

Despite many suggestions of dietary, medicinal and exercise remedies, there is conflicting evidence as to how best to enhance recovery from DOMS (Racette et al. 2005; Rahnama et al. 2005; Close et al. 2005; Bennett et al. 2005).

Treatment with eccentric exercise

Eccentric exercise has been identified as a key treatment technique when rehabilitating tendon injuries such as in the tendo Achilles. Stanish et al. (1985) proposed treatment protocols with eccentric exercise, involving alteration in both load and speed.

The benefits of using eccentric exercise programmes for tendon injuries are thought to include:

- increasing the tensile strength of the tendon
- stressing healing tissue in a functional manner to influence collagen deposition
- influencing the organisation of collagen in a structure.

Knowledge of the types of contraction, whether eccentric, concentric or isometric, is required when planning strengthening exercises. Eccentric contractions are capable of producing more torque than isometric, which in turn are stronger than concentric contractions. Isometric exercises are particularly useful when an area is immobilised — for instance, when a joint is immobilised in plaster of Paris — provided the contraction does not further damage soft tissues or destabilise fracture sites, as active movement certainly would. It is useful to apply eccentric and concentric exercises in a functional context during rehabilitation. The functions of eccentric exercise are the deceleration of limb part — for example, hamstrings braking knee extension when kicking a football; the absorption of force — for example, when landing from a jump; and controlling a movement with the recoil of resistance or with gravity — for example, during sit to stand (Figure 17.3).

Open-chain and closed-chain kinetic strengthening

A kinematic chain is an engineering term used to describe a system of links connected by joints. They may be opened or closed (Figure 17.4). Open-chain exercise is defined as an exercise where the distal end of the segment is not against a constraint or a resistance. In closed-chain exercise, the terminal segment is restrained. A squat is an example of a closed-chain exercise (Figure 17.5). A leg curl from sitting in a chair is an example of an open-chain exercise (Figure 17.6).

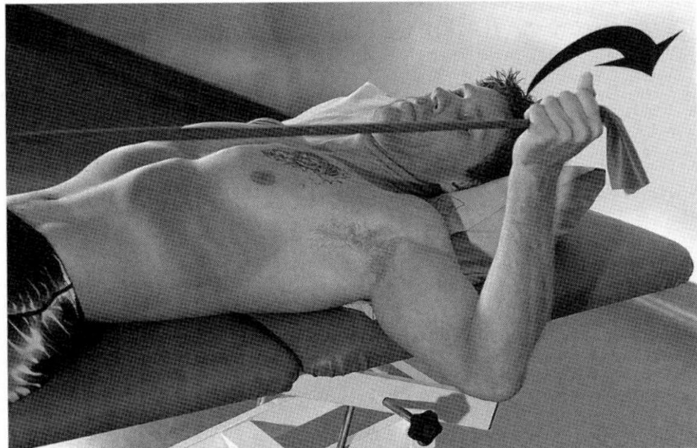

Figure 17.3 Eccentric training of the lateral rotators for throwing activities.

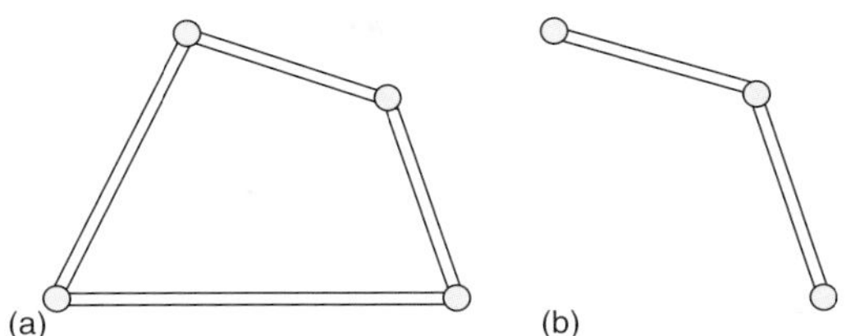

Figure 17.4 (a) Closed kinetic chain; (b) open kinetic chain.

The emphasis on closed kinetic chain exercises has grown stronger since the onset of accelerated protocols for anterior cruciate ligament (ACL) rehabilitation. A closed kinetic chain exercise occurs when the distal part of the limb (upper or lower) is fixed on a firm surface. Squatting is a commonly quoted example of a closed-chain kinetic exercise, but performing a leg press exercise with the feet in contact with a metal footplate is also a valid example. Contemporary postoperative management of ACL reconstruction currently involves a combination of open and closed kinetic chain exercise; this reflects the mixture of open and closed kinetic functions in the knee and the lower limb as a whole.

The following are some of the proposed benefits of closed-chain exercises in the lower limb:

- The shear force acting at the knee joint is reduced compared with the last 30 degrees of open-chain extension (Wilk et al. 1996).
- They encourage more functional movement patterns.
- They stimulate co-contraction of the hamstrings, helping to reduce anterior tibial translation (important in ACL rehabilitation).
- They increase shoulder stability in the upper limb by stimulating co-contraction of surrounding muscles.

Closed kinetic chain exercises are not just a valuable part of lower limb rehabilitation; they are also widely used to good effect in the upper limb, particularly when addressing scapular or glenohumeral stability problems.

Resisted exercise

Resisted exercise is a more progressive form of strengthening exercise, used in the more advanced stages of rehabilitation to achieve grade 5 on the Oxford Scale. It is also an essential component of

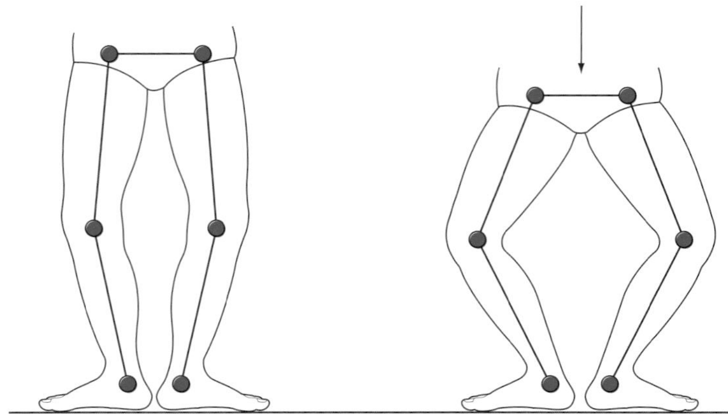

Figure 17.5 A squat.

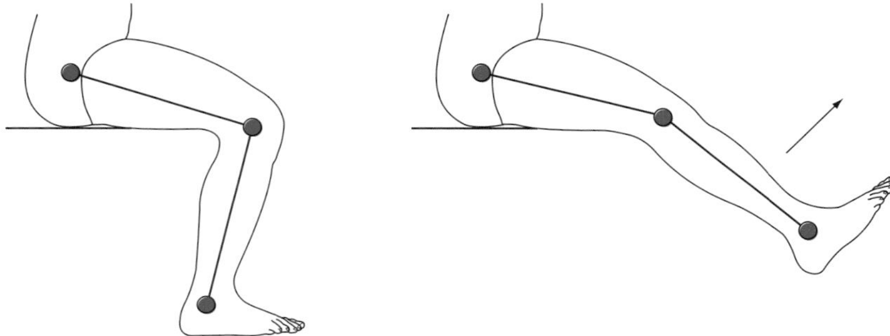

Figure 17.6 A leg curl.

the training regimes of athletes, aimed at enhancing performance and preventing onset of injuries. As the name suggests, it is an activity during which an external resistance must be overcome to complete the exercise. This external resistance could be provided by the therapist during treatment, but more commonly is provided by equipment. The conventional means for this is by application of weight training with use of free weights or weight-training equipment as found in gymnasia. However, other equipment, such as medicine balls, elastic tubing, or wrist and ankle weights, can be equally effective if used selectively. As larger weights are applied in this type of training, it essential to ensure that patients have been progressively advanced to this stage of rehabilitation and must be closely supervised during the exercise, particularly when the loads are progressed. This type of training can be used to promote power or endurance in muscles; this will be discussed in more detail in the following sections.

Types of muscle fibre

There are three main types of muscle fibre, usually called I, IIa and IIb. Newer subdivisions are now being described, such as Ic, IIc and IIab (Scott et al. 2001). Individual muscles are composed of all fibre types but have different proportions of each. Some of the differences in the physiological make-up of these muscle fibres are listed in Table 17.4.

The exact proportion of different fibre types is not consistent between muscles or between individuals. These characteristics are generally thought to be partly genetically determined and are part of the reason for the natural selection that sees individuals excel in different sports or play in different positions within a team. They are also influenced by training applied to the muscle (Scott et al. 2001). Some general points can be made, however

- Postural muscles such as soleus are involved in maintaining position rather than in dynamic activity and therefore have a higher number of type I fibres.

Table 17.4 Some characteristics of the muscle fibre types			
	Type I	Type IIa	Type IIb
Fitness component	Cardiorespiratory fitness	Muscular endurance	Strength/power
Energy system utilised	Aerobic	Anaerobic	Anaerobic
Contraction speed	Slow	Fast	Fast
Numbers of mitochondria	Many	Moderate	Low
Resistance to fatigue	High	Moderate	Low

- Muscles that may be involved in more dynamic activity, such as the gastrocnemius, will have proportionately greater numbers of fast-twitch fibres — types IIa and IIb.
- With age the number and size of type II fibres decrease (Rogers and Evans 1993), making tasks that require a quick burst of strength more difficult. This should be an important consideration when rehabilitating elderly patients.
- There is evidence that muscle fibres can convert from one fibre type to another. This occurs particularly between types IIa and IIb (Scott et al. 2001). This is known as *plasticity*.

Number of repetitions

How many repetitions of a particular exercise are performed, along with load applied, determines the type of muscle training effect. Resistance training includes pure strength work as well as endurance work, and as a consequence the number of repetitions will be based on the required outcome.

There is little clear evidence on the number of repetitions that should be used, but there are many protocols that can be used or adapted. A group of repetitions is known as a *set*, with three or four sets of an exercise usually being performed. This allows physiological recovery of the muscle to occur and delays the effects of fatigue.

Instructing a patient to perform 10 repetitions may be the most appropriate number to prescribe for the particular weight and exercise, but there needs to be a method of determining the weight required for these repetitions. It is important not to lose sight of the purpose of resistance training, particularly strength training — one of progressive overload to increase muscle strength and improve function. Progressive overload will not occur with repetitions using a weight that is too light and as a consequence recovery will be slower.

The majority of protocols that are in existence for strength training are based upon what are known as the 'one repetition maximum' (1RM) and the '10 repetition maximum' (10RM). The 1RM is the weight that can be lifted once and only once in an exercise, further completed effort being prevented by fatigue (Cahill et al. 1997). Determining the 1RM therefore prevents a challenge in the clinical environment and perhaps explains the sometimes arbitrary nature of repetitions given. The 10RM is similarly calculated: that is, the weight that can be lifted 10 times. Once the 1RM or 10RM is established, weight-training protocols can be calculated using percentages of this figure.

Clinical note

Sets consisting of 10 repetitions are commonplace within exercise prescription. However, this is often just an arbitrary number. Avoid giving 'sets of 10' without any underlying rationale. It is often better when prescribing and teaching an exercise to observe the patient for signs of fatigue and substitution before deciding on the number of repetitions in a set; if this happens to be 10, then that is fine, but more often than not this will not be the case.

The number of repetitions prescribed is determined by the objective of the exercise. If the aim is to increase power, then relatively few repetitions will be required, with long rests between sets, to achieve gains, provided a high load is applied. Muscles with a higher proportion of type IIa and IIb muscle fibres with a mobiliser function will respond to this type of regime. If the aim is to increase endurance, then lower loads will be required, but longer holds and higher frequencies of repetitions will be necessary for suitable gains. These exercises will be suitable for muscles with stability or postural function and a relatively higher proportion of type I fibres.

Further study

For more detail on exact protocols consult a weight-training text.

Resistance training in different populations

The elderly. Physical strength decreases with age. Some of the reported reasons for this decline are:

- a decrease in the number of actual muscle fibres
- muscle fibre atrophy
- impaired excitation–contraction coupling
- an inability or decreased ability to recruit type II motor units (Rogers and Evans 1993).

It is important to appreciate these long-term declines when addressing rehabilitation programmes with this section of the population. The issues outlined above related to progressive overload are just as significant but can be forgotten. An increase in basic strength may mean improved performance in functional tasks.

Children and adolescents. There is currently no evidence to suggest that resistance training in children is harmful, provided it is well supervised. The vast majority of adverse incidents have been related to poor technique and/or unsupervised activity. There have been no reports of growth plate fractures in studies related to youth strength training programmes.

The American Academy of Pediatrics has produced a series of recommendations in this area that stress supervision and numbers of repetitions of between 8 and 15. Practising technique with no load is also highlighted.

From a clinical viewpoint it is important to consider appropriate resistance training programmes when rehabilitating children and adolescents, adhering to the same principles of progressive overload.

17

MOBILISING EXERCISES

Introduction

These are exercises aimed at moving a targeted anatomical structure a precise amount in order to gain a treatment effect.

Soft-tissue extensibility is a prerequisite for normal functioning. Unfortunately, following injury, inflammation, prolonged abnormal postures and other factors such as exercise history, age and gender, this extensibility can be lost.

Physiotherapists regularly encounter people who have well-established limitation of movement, and need to be able to recognise this presentation and act accordingly to restore the length of the soft tissues involved. It is also important that the physiotherapist is able to identify the muscles and soft tissues that are most prone to shorten and lose mobility. The following sections of this chapter discuss the key concepts in the use of mobilising exercises in physiotherapy.

Mobilising exercises are a fundamental component of the rehabilitation process since they enhance normal tissue healing and are necessary to load the soft tissues progressively; ultimately the resultant scar tissue is stronger (Melis et al. 2002) and this enables it to withstand the stresses and strains it encounters during normal functional use more effectively (Hunter 1998).

Mobilising exercises can be used to maintain or increase range of movement, when this is restricted, for which the causes are numerous. These causes include:

- contractures of the joint capsule
- adhesions within the soft tissues
- muscle spasm or tightness
- neural sensitivity and inhibition due to pain.

Physiotherapists often use mobilising exercises in conjunction with other treatment modalities such as passive movements, heat, electrotherapy and soft-tissue techniques, depending on the presenting symptoms of the client.

For the purposes of this chapter, exercises are divided into the following classes:

1. passive
2. active assisted
3. auto-assisted
4. active
5. stretching (including hold/relax).

Classes of mobilising exercise

Passive exercises

Passive exercises can be defined as exercises in which movement is produced entirely by an external force, with the absence of voluntary muscle activity on behalf of the patient. This external force may be supplied by the therapist (as is the case with passive movements), or by a machine. For example, continuous passive motion (CPM) units might be used following total knee arthroplasty or other knee surgical procedures or in stroke rehabilitation (Lynch et al. 2005) to enhance recovery of the shoulder.

Passive exercises are typically employed in the early stages of rehabilitation after the onset of trauma, provided that affected structures are stable enough to sustain movement without vulnerability to further injury and provided that the exercise is not unduly painful. They may also be used to maintain range of movement in soft tissues during periods of joint inactivity. They are commonly utilised in conjunction with stretching exercises to increase further the ranges achieved.

Active assisted exercises

These are exercises in which the movement is produced *in part* by an external force, but is completed by use of voluntary muscle contraction. These exercises are of obvious value when strengthening a weakened muscle, but with the assistance given by the external force they can also be used to increase range of movement whilst allowing the individual to maintain control of the exercise.

Clinical note

All manner of equipment is used to facilitate active assisted exercises. Common examples are pulleys, slings and poles for shoulders, and re-education boards for knees and elbows, as well as many other external adjuncts. The physiotherapist should be as innovative as required.

Another important factor to be considered is *gravity*. If the exercise is performed with assistance from gravity, this may increase its effect on mobilising the targeted structure (Figure 17.7).

Auto-assisted exercises

These exercises can be either passive or active assisted, as described above, and occur when the external force is applied by the individual rather than by the physiotherapist. This may be through use of exercise equipment: for example, shoulder mobilisation using auto-assisted pulleys.

Active exercises

Also known as *free active exercises*, these are activities in which the movement is produced solely by use of the individual's voluntary muscle action. They can be used either as strengthening for grade 2 and above on the Oxford Scale (discussed later), or to mobilise structures — as is the case with dynamic stretching exercises.

Key point

With any exercise the correct choice of starting position is important. For example, for a mobilising exercise aiming to increase range of movement, gravity may well need to be counterbalanced or the body part positioned so that gravity assists the movement. If an exercise is performed against gravity, it will have more emphasis on strengthening.

A clinically useful feature of active exercises is that they can be performed without the use of equipment, so they can be practised anywhere and can easily form the basis of a home exercise programme.

Stretching exercises

Stretching exercises, if performed appropriately, may be a simple yet very effective form of treatment. For example, in the elderly a loss of hip extension during walking implies the presence of functionally significant hip flexor tightness (Kerrigan et al. 2001) and predisposes individuals to falls and subsequent femoral neck fractures. Overcoming hip tightness with specific stretching exercises as a simple intervention shows some improvement in walking performance and possibly fall prevention in the elderly (Kerrigan et al. 2003).

Stretching is commonly employed within the athletic population. Increasing the range of motion available at a joint has obvious advantages in increasing function and performance. It is suggested that regular stretching improves force, jump height and speed, although there is no evidence that it improves running

17

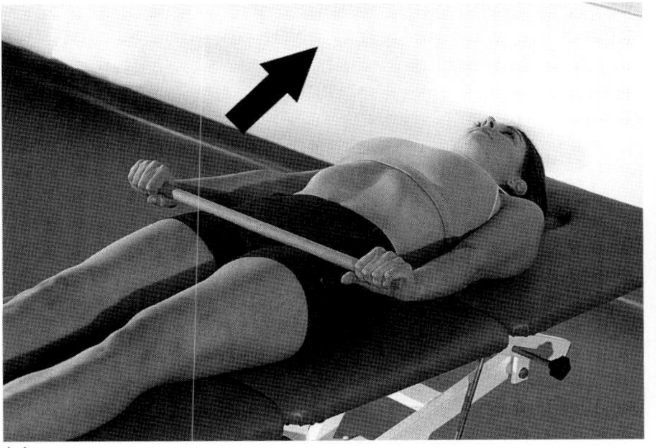

(a)

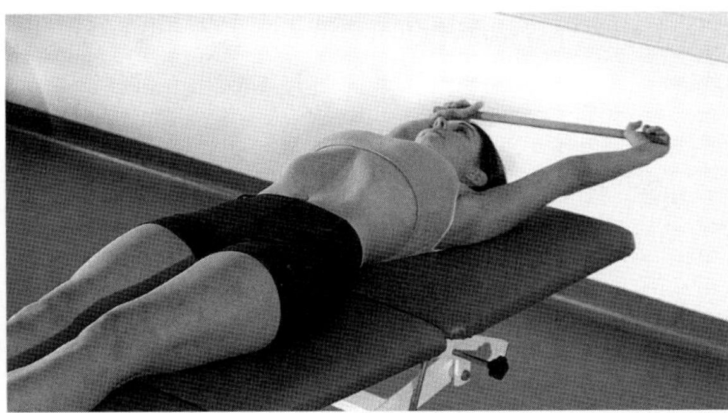

(b)

Figure 17.7 Active assisted shoulder elevation, demonstrating the use of gravity and the other arm (via a pole) to gain range of movement.

economy (Shrier 2004). It has also been suggested that it contributes to injury prevention, although at present research does not suggest that stretching reduces risk of injury or reduces the effects of DOMS (Herbert and Gabriel 2002).

Key point

Stretching exercises are normally used to mobilise neural and muscle tissue to the limits of the available range. There are many forms of stretching exercise and techniques commonly used in combination; therefore consensus as to their effects is difficult to ascertain within the published evidence.

Stretching exercises are performed with the target structure moving towards a lengthened position. The stretching exercise will involve further movement in this direction, so as to lengthen the structure further. Collagen fibres realign rapidly as a result of stretching forces and become aligned (and therefore stronger) in the direction of the stretching force (Melis et al. 2002). The limiting factors to further movement, such as the degree of pain experienced, will govern the extent to which any further movement is possible. Stretches are commonly used to increase range of movement by mobilising restrictions within soft tissue (such as scar tissue), and are specifically used in the lengthening of tight muscles.

The time at which stretching is commenced after an injury needs careful consideration. After any soft-tissue injury the length of the immobilisation depends on the grade of injury and must be optimised so that the scar can bear the pulling forces operating on it without re-rupture. Mobilisation of soft tissues by stretching will aid resorption of the connective tissue scar and recapillarisation of the damaged area (Kujala et al. 1997).

17

Stretching may also be used as a preventative measure: to stop joint contractures, for example. However, whilst the primary intervention for the treatment and prevention of contracture is to stretch the soft tissues regularly, and the rationale behind this intervention appears sound, the effectiveness of stretching has not been verified with well-designed clinical trials on subjects who have sustained soft-tissue injury (Shrier and Gossal 2000). One such trial (Malliaropolous et al. 2004) looked at frequency of stretching protocols in athletes with hamstring injuries and found a significant difference in rate of recovery when the protocol was applied three times daily, as compared to once a day. However, lack of a control group limits our insight into the effectiveness of this modality and lack of longer-term surveillance obscures its effect on re-injury rates.

Stretches may be applied in one of two ways: either dynamically or statically (Table 17.5).

Dynamic stretching

This involves gaining range by an active movement and should not be confused with ballistic stretching (see below), which involves the use of repetitive, bouncing, dynamic, rhythmic movements performed at higher velocities. Dynamic stretching involves progressively increasing the range through successive movements until the end of range is reached.

Dynamic stretching is especially useful when dealing with more advanced sports-related rehabilitation problems. The exercises enhance dynamic function and neuromuscular control through repetition and practice, thereby training motor patterning and enhancing the movement memory. If the patient is suitable, this form of stretching can be highly effective to mobilise soft tissues and enhance motor control.

Note on ballistic stretching. Ballistic stretching uses repeated, successive movements and *momentum* to gain range. The drawbacks to using this type of exercise with most individuals encountered in the hospital setting are that patients are typically not conditioned to use ballistic stretching effectively or *without sustaining further injury*.

During ballistic stretching, the stretch reflex is normally initiated to resist the change in muscle length and to protect the muscle from injury. This occurs due to stimulation of the non-contractile elements of muscle spindles, which send afferent information about the length of muscles to spinal cord level. This in turn causes stimulation of the extrafusal fibres via the alpha-motor neurone, resulting in a muscle contraction (see Figure 17.17 later in the chapter).

Table 17.5 Stretching exercises: a summary

	Dynamic stretch	Static stretch
Feature of stretch technique	Faster, rhythmic, higher velocity, motor control, functional	Slow, controlled, emphasis on postural awareness, bodily alignment
Duration of stretch	Repetitive, progressive	Sustained 30-second hold
Stage employed	End-stage rehabilitation Training motor patterning	Early, middle and end-stage rehabilitation
Client types	Sportspersons, active persons	All

Should this muscle contraction coincide with the next ballistic movement, it is suggested that a muscle unconditioned to cope with that stress may become injured. As a result, patients are normally instructed not to 'bounce' whilst performing their stretching routines.

Static stretching

As the name suggests, this involves maintaining a position for a sustained period to gain the desired effect (Figure 17.8). It is widely agreed that an effective time to hold a static stretch is at least 30 seconds (Bandy et al. 1997). This gives time for the muscle spindle to adapt to the new length and will also result in an increase in functional length of viscoelastic structures such as muscles, albeit temporary (Magnusson 1998).

Static stretching is a controlled, slow movement with emphasis on correct bodily alignment. Static stretching protocols are commonly used and, for example, have been shown to be effective in terms of improving flexibility of muscle (Chan et al. 2001). An element of fine motor control and postural awareness is important during static stretching exercises and this can be enhanced by the use of feedback and correction from the physiotherapist, as well as mirrors. Exercise forms such as Pilates, tai chi and yoga employ many of these principles and can be used effectively within a patient's exercise programme.

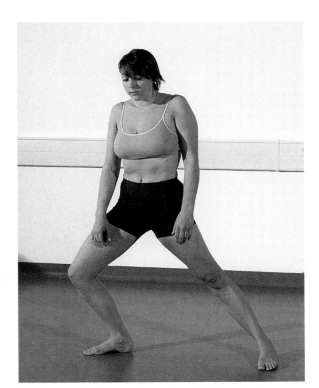

Figure 17.8 Static stretching of the right hip adductors.

> **Key point**
>
> Correction of this type of exercise is frequently required to ensure an effective stretch is produced in the targeted tissue.

Therapeutic stretching or strengthening exercises are successful only if the target muscle is properly isolated (Gluck and Liebenson 1997), particularly when the tissue concerned crosses more than one body segment. Problems are often encountered when stretching two joint muscles. For example, when stretching the hamstrings, pelvic alignment needs to be controlled as well as considering hip flexion and knee extension components in order to stretch effectively.

The *order* in which the components are added can also influence the effect, depending on which area of the muscle's structure is to be targeted. For example, if the aim is to target the distal portion of rectus femoris, one may wish to employ a stretch that extends the hip then flexes the knee, whilst proximally the components may be added alternatively (Figure 17.9).

It is also important to consider the functional anatomy of the area being targeted, particularly when contemplating the addition of rotational components to stretching exercises. Using the hamstrings as an example, the medial hamstrings (semimembranosus and semitendinosus) would require a component of lateral rotation to stretch them effectively. To stretch biceps femoris effectively, an element of medial rotation would be required due to its ability to act as a lateral rotator of the knee.

Spinal position

Many upper- and lower-limb muscles at the scapula and pelvis take their origins from the axial skeleton, so spinal position can influence limb position. Consequently, throughout many stretching exercises it is important to consider any lumbopelvic, scapulothoracic or spinal movement to ensure that it is controlled throughout the exercise. Where possible there should be no spinal movement, ensuring a 'neutral' posture is maintained throughout, the 'neutral' position being the position of optimal alignment and stability (Richardson et al. 2004). For example, in the lumbar spine this would equate to a gentle curve in the lumbar lordosis. In the cervical spine, again there would be a gentle cervical lordosis with a right angle between the mandible and anterior neck. The spine would then be maintained in this position for the duration of the stretch to prevent unwanted spinal movement and potential limitation of treatment effectiveness.

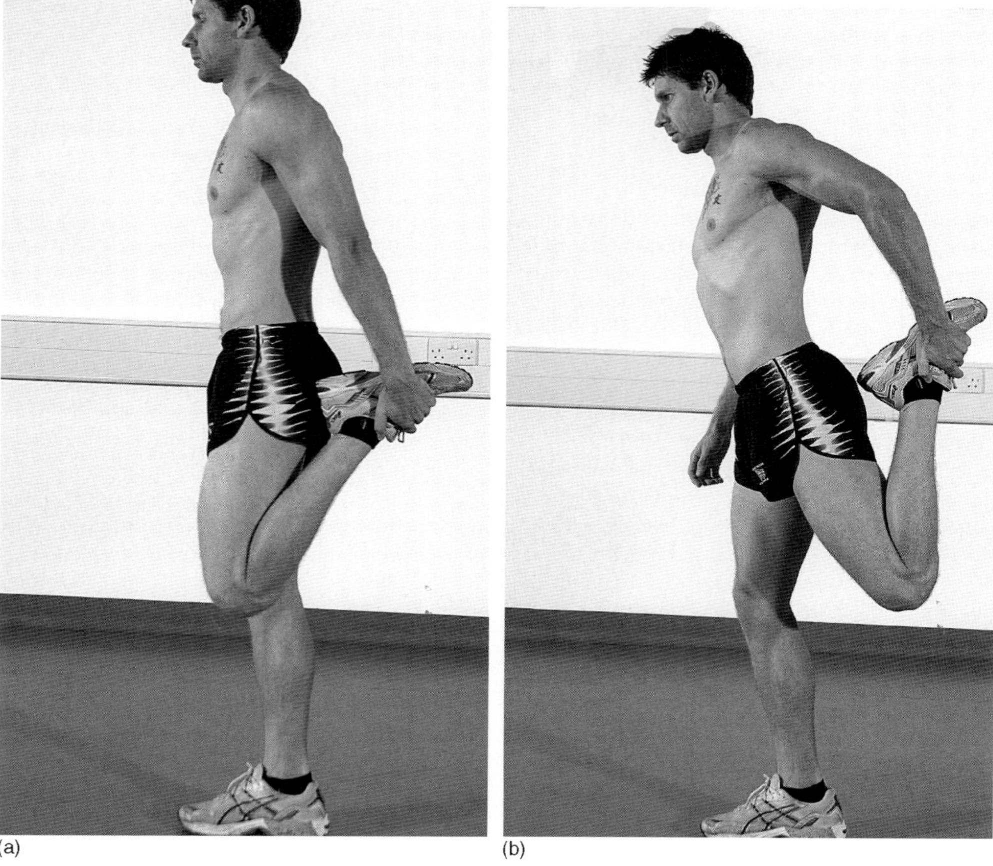

(a) (b)

Figure 17.9 Demonstrating the order effect of adding components to a stretch of rectus femoris. (a) Knee flexion then hip extension; (b) hip extension then knee flexion. Note that the lumbar spine should remain in neutral throughout.

Teaching stretching exercises: a practical guide

Before performing the stretch:

- Ensure that your assessment has not identified any contraindications to stretching.
- Ensure that there is a logical, reasoned basis for your stretching programme. For example, if there is a bony block to movement caused by osteophytes, stretching is not appropriate (see Chapter 2 on end-feel).
- Explain to patients how and why they are performing the stretch to ensure maximum compliance and benefit.
- Explain to patients what they should experience during the treatment: i.e. how far to stretch,
- degree of discomfort to expect.
- Consider how the stretch might be made more comfortable prior to stretching (e.g. use of a hot pack or hydrotherapy).

During the stretch:

- Maintain spinal position in neutral throughout.
- The patient should perform the stretch across all joints at the same time for two or more joint muscles.
- Make the stretch slow and sustained; do not bounce.
- The patient should experience a pulling sensation, not pain.
- Hold the position for 30 seconds.
- If tension releases, take the movement a little further.
- Release slowly.

After the stretch:

- Warn the patient what feelings to expect.
- Remember that, once movement has been regained, active muscle control throughout that range will be needed as well as some form of maintaining the stretch in the long term.

Contraindications to stretching

These are some of the contraindications:

- bony block or end-feel to movement on passive assessment of the joint in question
- recent or unstable fractures
- the presence of infection or haematoma in the tissues
- some recent surgical repairs and other procedures, such as skin grafting and tendon repair
- patient refusal.

Key point

Although static stretching is widely believed to cause an increase in a muscle's functional length, recent investigations suggest otherwise. It has been suggested by Magnusson et al. (1998) that the viscoelastic properties of muscles remain unaltered in the long term following stretching, and rather that it is the muscle's *tolerance* to stretch that is increased. Such details, along with further developments in the area, need to be considered when prescribing stretching exercises.

Hold/relax techniques

Proprioceptive neuromuscular facilitation (PNF), also commonly referred to as hold/relax and contract/relax, can have effective results when trying to mobilise muscles. PNF stretching techniques may produce greater increases in range of motion than passive, ballistic or static stretching methods (Spernoga et al. 2001). PNF is a form of treatment devised to rehabilitate movement manually in specific patterns using a number of physiological principles to enhance its effectiveness.

A core principle of PNF is that, after a muscle has contracted maximally, it will then relax maximally. This principle can be used when prescribing exercises to mobilise muscles that are in a shortened position. The patient is asked to contract the tight muscle strongly and hold the contraction isometrically for around 10 seconds, then relax. Following a short period of 2–3 seconds the physiotherapist then applies a stretch to the muscle, which is maintained for 30 seconds. Following a period of recovery this sequence is repeated.

Another useful principle used in PNF is that of *reciprocal inhibition*, which states that when a muscle (the agonist) contracts maximally, its opposite counterpart (antagonist) will relax maximally. This can be used by asking the patient to perform maximal contraction of the agonist to the muscle to be mobilised, followed by application of a stretch.

This principle of reciprocal inhibition can also prove useful and is worth considering during static stretching exercises where a contraction of the muscle's antagonist can act to relax and lengthen it.

PROGRESSION OF EXERCISE

An exercise programme without planned progression will quickly become ineffective. It is essential to review the exercise programme regularly and revise it to match the patient's status. There are various ways to progress exercises, including:

1. changing the starting position
2. changing the length of the lever
3. changing the speed at which the exercise is performed
4. altering the range through which the movement is performed
5. applying resistance.

Starting position

Changing the starting position may change the base of support and may affect the difficulty of an exercise. Reducing the base of support will normally have the effect of advancing the difficulty of the exercise, from a neuromuscular control perspective, and vice versa. For example, performing an exercise whilst standing on one leg will require more hip abductor control than when standing on two legs.

A change in starting position can also change a body segment's relationship to gravity, which will change the nature of an exercise. An exercise performed against gravity will require concentric muscle work and eccentric work to return to the starting position; it will therefore be a strengthening exercise.

With more grossly weakened muscles (Oxford Scale 2 and below), exercises performed in a gravity-counterbalanced position will be more effective. Exercises performed in this position will also be more effective in mobilising structures.

If an exercise is performed with the assistance of gravity, it may have a strong mobilising effect upon reaching the end of the available range of movement due to the weight of the body part. An example of this is performing squats from a standing starting position to increase the range of knee flexion, using the effects of gravity and bodyweight to increase knee flexion (Figure 17.10). Another example is shoulder flexion in lying and standing (Figures 17.11 and 17.12).

17

Length of the lever

Changing the length of the lever will affect the forces applied to the body during exercise (Figure 17.13).

A lengthened lever will result in a higher force being exerted at the fulcrum of the movement, so more muscle work will be needed to produce or control the movement. This will also result in a higher force being applied to structures during mobilising exercises.

Levers may be shortened or lengthened by flexing or extending joints, most commonly the elbow or knee

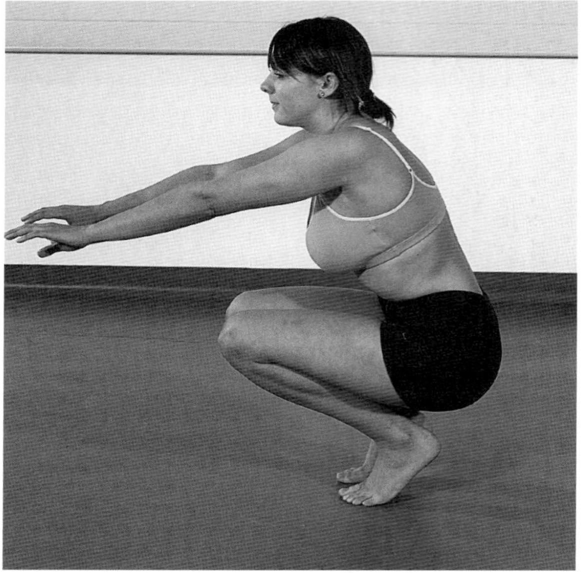

Figure 17.10 Squats in standing using gravity to mobilise knee flexion.

joints. They may also be lengthened by holding or attaching an object to the end of a limb — such as holding a weight at arm's length.

The positioning of the application of resistance along the lever will also affect the muscle work required. Resistance applied distally will require more effort and will reduce when the same resistance is applied more proximally. In mobilising exercises a resistance applied distally on the lever will have a greater mobilising effect than resistance applied proximally.

Speed of movement

A change in the speed at which a movement is performed will change the nature of an exercise. When altering the speed, the physiotherapist must be clear as to the desired effect. An exercise performed slowly requires a great deal of precision and postural control. An exercise performed at higher velocities will produce a greater mobilising effect at the end of range, but the client will require adequate neuromuscular control to perform this without risking further injury.

Range of movement

A change in the range through which an exercise is performed will alter its difficulty. Muscles are at their strongest in middle range and weakest in outer range (a more lengthened position). This is discussed in more detail in the context of muscle-strengthening exercises.

Resistance to movement

The final way to progress an exercise is to apply resistance to strengthen a muscle (Figure 17.14). Resistance can be applied in a number of ways. These are related to the desired effect — whether the aim is to produce a change in power or in endurance, as discussed.

DEALING WITH MOVEMENT DYSFUNCTION DVD

When dealing with movement dysfunction we are interested in the kinetic chain, a series of successive joints or segments, and the way each segment's movement and orientation influence the rest. Movement dysfunction can give rise to acute muscle strain (Emery 1999) and overuse injuries due to abnormal stresses caused by abnormal movement patterning. When patients present with symptoms resulting from movement dysfunction, exercise is used to rehabilitate them. Sahrman (2002) states that either maintenance or restoration of precise control of each segment is necessary to manage pain of a musculoskeletal origin.

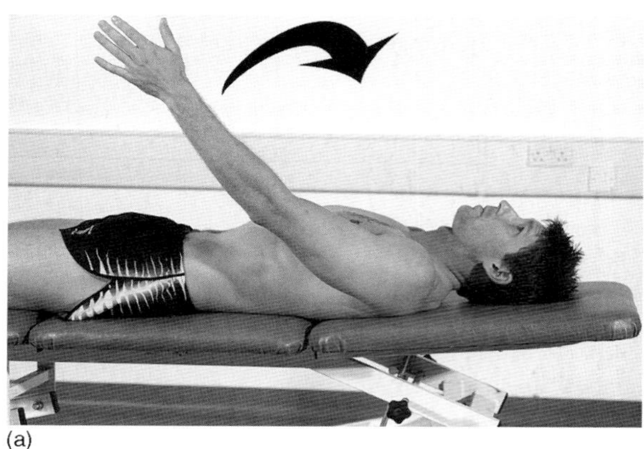

(a)

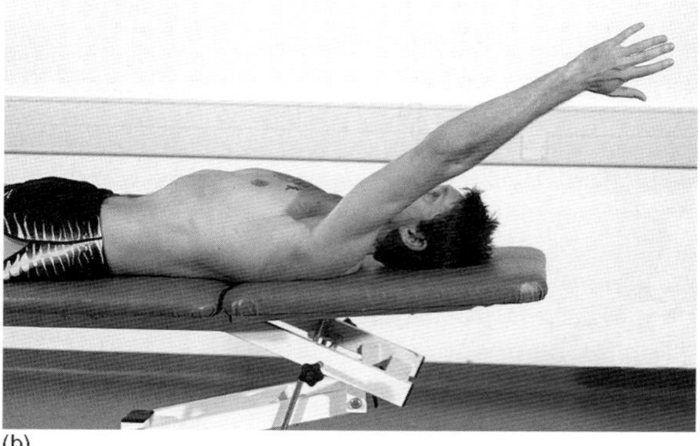

(b)

Figure 17.11 Shoulder flexion in lying.

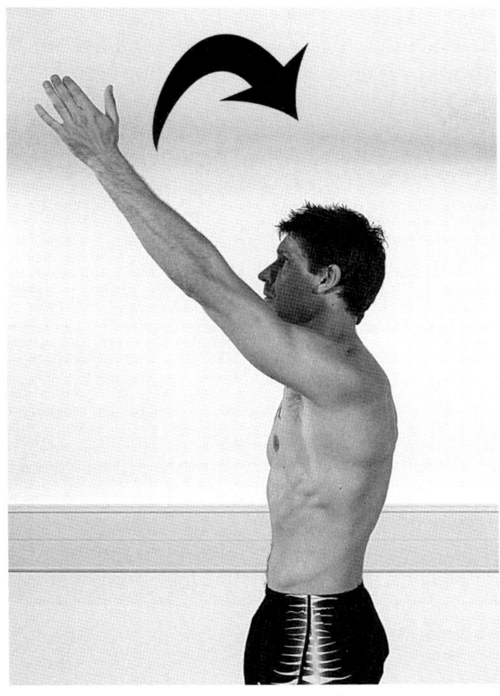

Figure 17.12 Shoulder flexion in standing. Gravity resists the movement throughout the range in standing, even though the movement is the same as in Figure 17.11.

Several muscle imbalance classifications have been suggested relating to muscles' structure, function and response to injury. Movement dysfunction is said to at occur both a segmental or *local* or single-joint level and at a *global* level, affecting many segments of a region (Bergmark 1989).

Muscles can be classified as either stabilisers or mobilisers, depending on their structure and function (Table 17.6). It is not always clear, though, which group all muscles belong to, and difficulties in classification may result from some muscles having dual characteristics and quite possibly dual roles.

Key point

Stabiliser muscles characteristically are deep, have broad, aponeurotic attachments, and their primary function is one of postural and dynamic control. They have a higher proportion of type I muscle fibres.

Mobiliser muscles have features that enable them to fulfil their role as the main producers of force to generate a particular movement. They tend to be more superficially situated and have long, cylindrical muscle bellies. They have a higher proportion of type IIa and IIb muscle fibres.

In the presence of pain, pathology, disability or dysfunction these two classes of muscle can change their relative recruitment patterns, and typically this results in an alteration in function. This can happen at a local level, resulting in delayed or deficient recruitment and leading to loss of control of a segment (Hodges and Richardson 1996). It can also occur at a global level; the stabilisers become inhibited and weakened, and have increased functional length, whereas the mobilisers become increasingly facilitated and overactive, and have shortened functional length. This is sometimes termed 'muscle imbalance'.

These changes in muscle function may eventually cause muscle imbalance problems such as altered function and damage to the muscles involved as well as to the soft tissues implicated by changes in movement

17

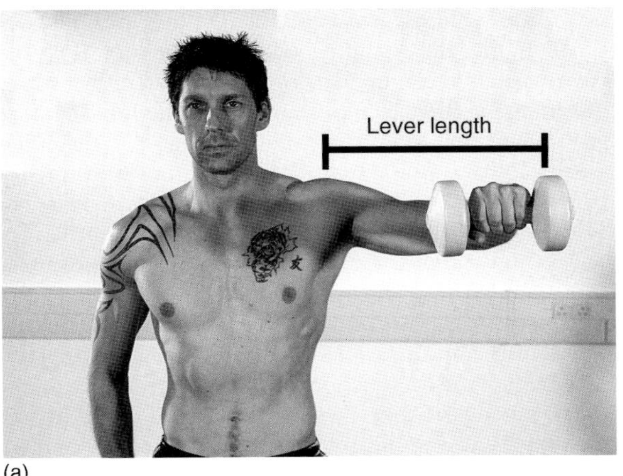

(a)

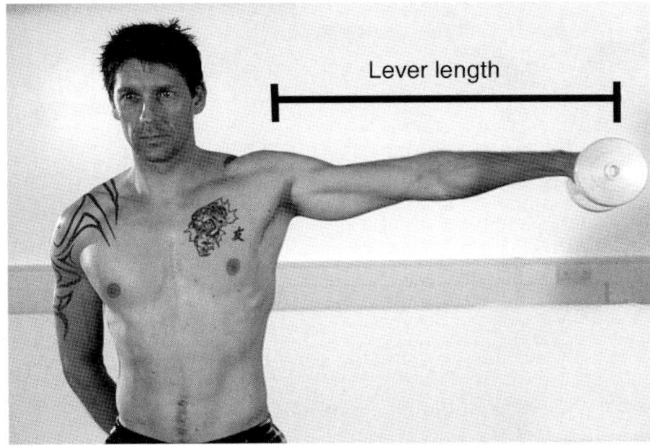

(b)

Figure 17.13 (a) Shoulder abduction with a shortened lever. (b) Shoulder abduction with a long lever. The muscle work of shoulder abduction is greatly increased by increasing the lever length.

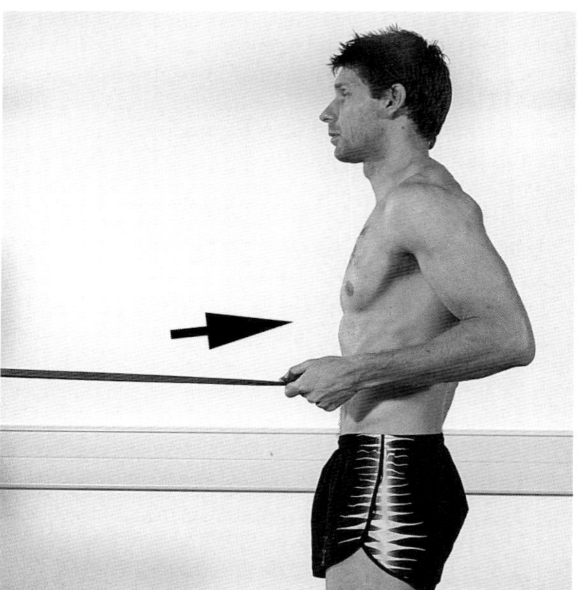

Figure 17.14 A resistance exercise to strengthen shoulder extensors.

Table 17.6 The muscle groups commonly affected by muscle imbalance
Muscles prone to tightness (mobilisers)
▪ Sternocleidomastoid
▪ Scalene muscles
▪ Levator scapulae
▪ Pectoralis minor
▪ Rhomboids
▪ Erector spinae
▪ Rectus abdominis
▪ Hamstrings
▪ Vastus lateralis
▪ Tensor fasciae latae
▪ Rectus femoris
▪ Piriformis
▪ Gastrocnemius
Muscles prone to weakness (stabilisers)
▪ Deep cervical flexors
▪ Serratus anterior
▪ Lower fibres of trapezius
▪ Subscapularis
▪ Transversus abdominis and internal obliques
▪ Gluteus medius and minimus
▪ Vastus medialis
▪ Psoas major
▪ Multifidus

patterns. A shortened muscle in a region shows a lowered irritability threshold and is recruited first in a movement, causing changes in motor programming (Norris 1995).

When movement dysfunction is identified, changes in movement patterns are influenced by structures that produce either a 'give' or a 'restriction' (Comerford and Mottram 2001). A give is excessive or uncontrolled movement while restriction is reduced movement. This can happen at a local level — that is, in a single segment — or at a global level — that is, in a region (several segments). These structures may not just be muscular; they may be also bony, such as joint surfaces or osteophytes, or they could be articular, giving rise to changes in ligaments or capsular laxity and tightness. The factors influencing movement could also be neurological, as is the case with neural irritability. Consideration of myofascial, articular and neural components needs to be included in the assessment and continued management of these problems. Pain is often clinically associated with movement dysfunction, as it is usually pain that causes the patient to seek treatment initially.

Treatment

Treatment of this type of problem involves re-education of sensorimotor control and stability function to allow the patient to control the position of the affected joint, thus controlling the segmental 'give'. For example, in the case of scapulothoracic instability, this would involve positioning of the scapula in its correct alignment and progressing through a variety of starting positions. There are no hard and fast rules as to which position to start in; this will depend on an individual's movement profile and functional deficit.

The next stage in treatment involves progressively challenging the stability with movement. This may involve moving into a restriction and, here again, sensorimotor control is important. Using the same example as above, this would involve 'setting' the scapula in neutral, then (whilst maintaining this position) moving the glenohumeral joint into a previously restricted range.

As the stability is recruited more readily, exercises are then progressed to gain through-range control of the stabilisers, first into inner then into outer range, involving concentric then eccentric work respectively. As the stabiliser function improves through exercise, it is perceived that these muscles are more readily recruited during normal functional activity and the normal recruitment patterns return.

The final treatment priority is to lengthen the mobilisers. This will often occur as a result of increased stability and more 'normal' movement patterns.

Rehabilitation using this approach can be lengthy, as the problems of movement dysfunction are likely to have built up over a considerable time.

Further study

The topic of movement dysfunction has been outlined briefly here. Further reading should be undertaken prior to practicing the techniques suggested.

REHABILITATION OF SENSORIMOTOR CONTROL

Exercises are aimed at accessing the sensorimotor control loop (Figure 17.15) to develop and enhance movement control.

Introduction

Normal proprioception is essential to everyday functioning, whether it involves simply placing a cup on a table or running around a football field. Definitions of proprioception have been the cause of some debate within the literature as proprioception is only a part of the process of sensorimotor control. Therefore some authors include the motor response as well as the initial sensory input within their definition.

Definition

Proprioception is 'specialised variation of the sensory modality of touch and encompasses the sensations of joint movement (kinaesthesia) and joint position (joint position sense)' (Lephart and Henry 1995).

The above definition implies that proprioception is very much an *afferent* (sensory) response. However, motor response has also been incorporated into other definitions of proprioception (Jerosch and Prymka 1996), and proprioception is an example of afferent input entering the CNS.

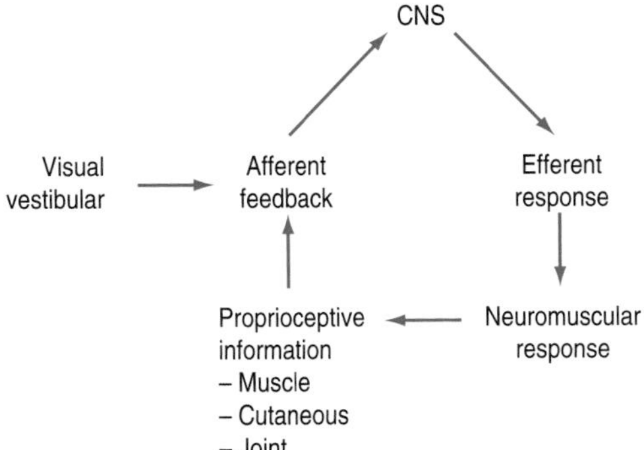

Figure 17.15 Diagrammatic representation of the mechanism of sensorimotor control.

Physiotherapists are concerned with the normal functioning of this afferent response, but more importantly it is the efferent (motor) response to this sensory input that physiotherapists are most involved with from a rehabilitation point of view.

Loss of proprioception is a commonly encountered clinical problem and disturbs the continual feedback of accurate afferent information; it therefore has a knock-on effect on motor control. The key areas where proprioceptive deficits have been identified through research are presented in Table 17.7. The first column in the table illustrates the importance of being aware of the potential scope of proprioceptive loss, and how important appropriate sensorimotor rehabilitation is to a large percentage of patients.

It is primarily the muscle spindles that play a significant role in providing afferent proprioceptive feedback during movement (Proske 2005). It is the articular receptors that provide more information in outer range when the structures in which they are embedded are put on stretch (Jerosch and Thorwesten 1998). It has also been hypothesised that proprioceptive deficiency could in fact precipitate degenerative joint changes (Barrett et al. 1991).

Key point

Proprioception could also play a vital role in prevention of injury as well as in reducing symptoms of pathology. Caraffa et al. (1996) found a seven-fold reduction in ACL injuries in a group of 300 semi-professional and amateur footballers who undertook a proprioceptive training programme, when compared to a matched control group.

17

Table 17.7 Conditions commonly exhibiting reduced proprioception

Proprioceptive deficits identified in	Clinical example
Osteoarthritis	Particularly joint degeneration in the lower limb, the knee encountered most commonly
Ageing	Any elderly patient
Immobility	Patients on bed rest or immobilised due to illness or trauma
Trauma	Anterior cruciate ligament (ACL) injuries, glenohumeral dislocation and instabilities, lateral ligament injuries of the ankle

The mechanism of proprioception

There are many *receptors* within joints, muscles and skin that continually convey information to the CNS. Using this information, we continually make subconscious and conscious modifications to how we move, allowing us to carry out normal functional activities. Each receptor supplies a different type of information: for example, joint pressure, joint acceleration/deceleration and joint velocity. When the receptors are stimulated through movement or other forces, they act as transducers and convert this mechanical deformation into an electrical sensory impulse (Barrack et al. 1994). This sensory impulse then passes on to the CNS, triggering the appropriate motor response.

A practical illustration of this can be seen in Figure 17.16. When walking on uneven ground the muscles of the foot and ankle continually have to adjust in order to keep the body upright and prevent a fall. The peronei and anterior tibials, for example, will be continually controlling the movement of the foot and ankle, responding to constant positional changes. This example illustrates the nature of proprioception, as a continuous process occurring at different levels of the CNS at the same time.

Consider all the potential tasks that you might undertake whilst walking, such as carrying a rucksack, using a walking pole or exercising a dog. All of these tasks will be bombarding the CNS with many sources of afferent information. If the responses to this information were all at the conscious level it would be a slow walk. This is a key point to understand when rehabilitating a patient with a proprioceptive deficit — many actions need to function at a subconscious level.

17

Receptors, as well as having different functions, also have different properties. For example they may react at different speeds, and can be rapidly or slowly adapting (Barrack et al. 1994; Borsa et al. 1994). The impulse from a rapidly adapting receptor drops off quickly, whereas that from a slowly adapting receptor fires for longer periods. Some examples are presented in Table 17.8.

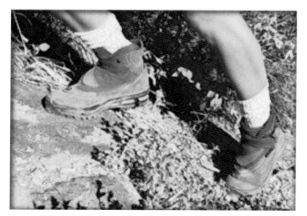

Figure 17.16 Subconscious muscular action to control the ankle when walking on uneven ground.

Importantly, many joint receptors are also only active at the beginning and the end of range. Therefore, as a joint moves through a range of movement, it is reliant on other receptors to keep the CNS informed of its activity. Particularly important in maintaining this function are the muscle spindles (Figure 17.17).

The large volume of proprioceptive information entering the CNS is utilised at three different levels:

- *Spinal level*. Reflex contractions occurring at this level contribute to reflex stability within a joint, helping to reduce the risk of injury from sudden forces acting on the joint.
- *Brain stem*. This is the part of the brain that receives input from the vestibular centres in the eyes and ears and helps to control balance.
- *Motor cortex, cerebellum and basal ganglia*. These are responsible for control of complex movement patterns.

Instability

The word 'instability' is frequently encountered when dealing with patients who display reduced proprioception. Instability can effectively be divided into two types:

- *Mechanical (true) instability*. Disruption of the passive control system (articular and ligamentous) of a joint results in instability. This is the type of instability detected by manual testing — for example, valgus stress testing at the knee to test the medial collateral ligament, or an anterior drawer to test for shoulder instability.
- *Functional instability*. Passive control systems are intact, with no laxity detected through manual testing. The patient will, however, complain of symptoms such as 'giving way' (lower limb) or 'pain' and 'heaviness' (upper limb). The problem is one of poor neuromuscular control and was initially described by Freeman et al. (1965) with reference to ankle inversion injuries.

The above definitions illustrate the fact that joint stability is multifactorial and relies significantly on dynamic as well as passive control (Waddington and Shepherd 1996). This is a key point and has major implications for the rehabilitation process. Functional instability is, however, the type of instability most commonly encountered by physiotherapists. Recent work on ankle injuries has shown that the majority of patients suffer from functional instability only (Richie 2001). The potential courses of functional instability are presented in Table 17.9.

Table 17.8 Examples of receptors and their functions

Receptor	Type	Function
Ruffini end organs	Slowly adapting	Monitoring position of the limb in space
Pacinian corpuscles	Slowly adapting	Detection of acceleration and deceleration or sudden mechanoreceptor deformation
Muscle spindles	Rapidly adapting	Changes in muscle length
Golgi tendon organs	Slowly adapting	Changes in muscle tension

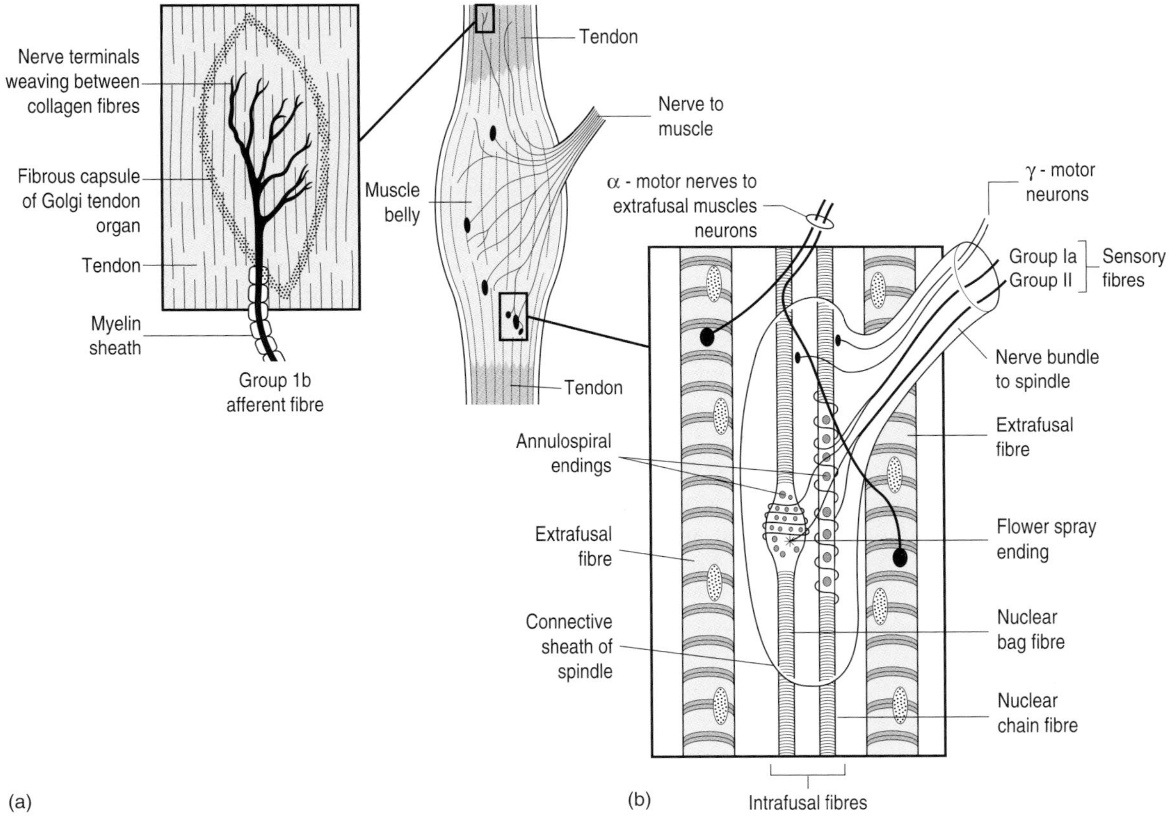

Figure 17.17 (a) The Golgi tendon organ. (b) The muscle spindle.

Correcting functional instability is the primary aim during functional rehabilitation (Lephart et al. 1997) and is particularly important before undertaking rapid dynamic activities, such as sudden deceleration, which are seen in many sports but, just as importantly, may also be seen in many occupations.

It is possible in some situations to reduce or even alleviate the symptoms of mechanical instability through appropriate neuromuscular training. In others a referral for surgery may be necessary to correct the defect. If functional instability is not addressed, chronic injury syndromes can develop.

Key point

Individuals suffering from mechanical instability are also likely to develop functional instability – a breakdown in the sensorimotor control loop results in lack of muscular control around the joint.

Table 17.9 Potential causes of functional instability within a joint

Cause	Rationale	Reference
Articular deafferentation	Articular mechanoreceptors are damaged, reducing the afferent impulse to the CNS, resulting in a decreased motor response	Freeman et al. (1965)
Differentiation	Trauma can result in direct damage to the motor supply, resulting in a decreased muscular response to perturbation	Wilkerson and Nitz (1994)
Neurogenic inflammation	Thought to be related to joint inflammation and inflammatory mediators directly affecting the motor endplate and therefore the motor response	Wilkerson and Nitz (1994)
Capsular distension	Joint effusion following trauma can cause muscle inhibition, leading to instability	Wilkerson and Nitz (1994)

Assessing proprioception

Assessment of proprioception takes several forms, many of which rely on complex equipment. There is currently a lack of validated tests that can be used easily within the clinical setting. The key measurements of proprioception often quoted in a research context are discussed below.

Threshold to detection of passive movement (TTDPM)

Isokinetic dynamometers are usually used to assess this component of proprioception. To take the ankle as an example: the blindfolded subject sits on the machine and the dynamometer starts to move the ankle passively. The subject then indicates the point at which movement has been sensed (normally by pressing a button). This result is compared to the unaffected side.

Reproduction of positioning

17

Reproduction of passive positioning (RPP)

In this instance the joint is moved passively to a position and back (usually by an isokinetic dynamometer or similar device). The patient then presses a button, which takes the joint back towards the position and stops the machine when the subject feels the identical position has been reached.

Reproduction of active positioning (RAP)

This is less frequently used, and involves the subject actively moving a joint to a given position.

Measurement of reflex latency

This involves the use of electromyography (EMG) to record the electrical activity of muscles through electrodes positioned over motor points. The time of onset of contraction in response to a perturbation or planned movement is recorded, as are the recruitment patterns of the muscles around that segment. Beard et al. (1994) tested anterior cruciate-deficient knees, and suggested that a latent or slow muscle contraction of hamstrings in response to sudden movement could be used as an assessment method. In terms of functional significance this is a very useful test but it requires equipment to produce quantifiable data.

An appreciation of the presence of latency of contraction can be observed when comparing functional movements of affected and non-affected limbs. The affected limb will often exhibit a tremor or lack a smooth pattern to movement when compared to the more normal unaffected side.

REHABILITATION OF SENSORIMOTOR CONTROL OF THE LIMBS

Issues

The key aims of rehabilitation to sensorimotor control are:

- to provide early afferent input to a joint. This will limit further damage and reduce further losses through inactivity.
- to restore reflex stability. This is the coordinated, co-contraction of all stabilising muscles around a segment when called upon to move.
- to restore normal neuromuscular coordination. This is the correct sequencing of muscle activity necessary to perform normal movement.
- to enhance the neuromuscular response. This is to facilitate control through the sensorimotor control loop.

Early commencement of proprioception can sometimes be neglected in rehabilitation. In the case of the lower limb, partial weight-bearing at least is sometimes incorrectly seen as a prerequisite of proprioceptive training. Wobble board work in sitting is an exercise that can be started early and progressed (Figure 17.18). Sensorimotor control exercises need to be functional and are usually a combination of open and closed kinetic chain exercises. Closed kinetic chain exercises

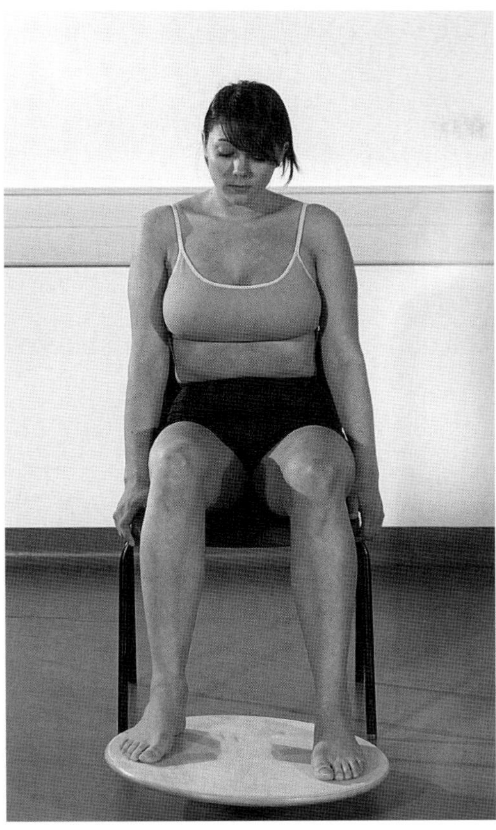

Figure 17.18 Wobble board work in sitting.

are useful in that they gain co-contraction of stabiliser muscles and hence segmental control and in that they give high-quality proprioceptive feedback as the fixed distal segment gives a reference point from which the CNS can work.

A wide variety of equipment is available to facilitate rehabilitation of the sensorimotor system. There are numerous types of balance board, from simple unidirectional rocker boards to air cushions. Wobble boards are a good way of bombarding the CNS with afferent input in the early stages of rehabilitation, but they are not a functional piece of equipment and it is important to progress from these types of apparatus as required. Other equipment, such as low-friction surfaces, can be a useful adjunct for enhancing dynamic functional stability. It should also be borne in mind that this equipment could be used just as effectively in the upper limb as in the lower. The only limit to devising proprioceptive exercises should be your imagination.

There are several means available to the physiotherapist to progress proprioceptive exercises. These include:

- removing visual stimulus
- altering the base of support
- increasing weight-bearing
- increasing speed of an activity
- making an exercise more complex, e.g. adding perturbation

Visual input provides additional afferent input to the CNS. Without it, any given exercise becomes more difficult to perform, as the subject will have to rely more heavily on proprioceptive information, even with wobble board activities in sitting.

Examples of altering the base of support are illustrated in Figures 17.19–17.21. This activity progressively requires greater neuromuscular control and strength to maintain a given position.

Key point

It is important during rehabilitation to place the joint(s) in situations that encourage the reflex stability required to meet the functional demands of the individual. Stability work should therefore be progressed to place joints in more challenging and functional positions.

The lower limb

Proprioceptive exercises in the lower limb in the early stages of rehabilitation are progressions towards full weight-bearing. In the latter stages more dynamic stop–start activities can be added that require aspects of eccentric control with acceleration, deceleration and strong reflex stability around the ankle and knee. As detailed above, they can be progressed in several ways (see section on progression of exercise).

Figure 17.2 earlier in this chapter llustrates a typical exercise for the lower limb. It is important to remember that this is not a particularly functional exercise as the limb remains static, so will require progression by the end-point of rehabilitation. The more dynamic activities outlined above can be described as proprioceptive as they stress the joints in challenging positions and encourage the reflex actions that are required.

The upper limb

Key point

The objective of proprioceptive rehabilitation is to 'enhance cognitive appreciation of the respective joint relative to position and motion, and to enhance muscular stabilisation of the joint in the absence of structural restraints' (Borsa et al. 1994).

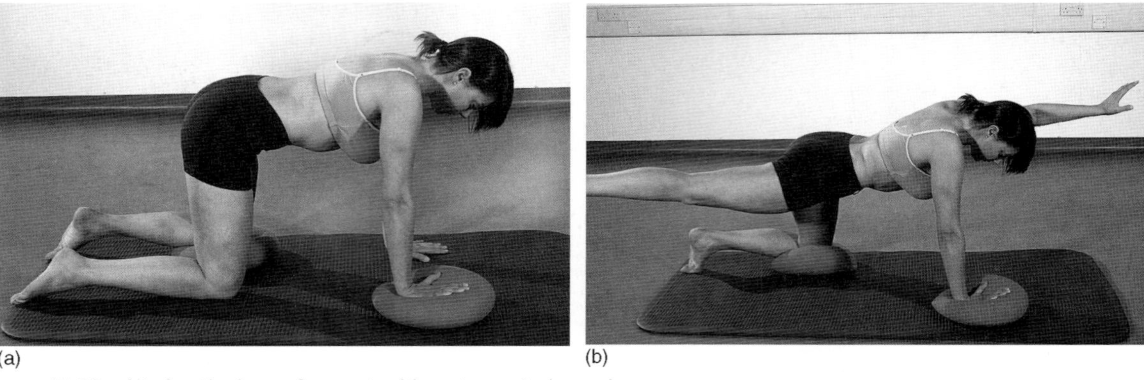

(a) (b)

Figure 17.19 Altering the base of support with motor control exercises.

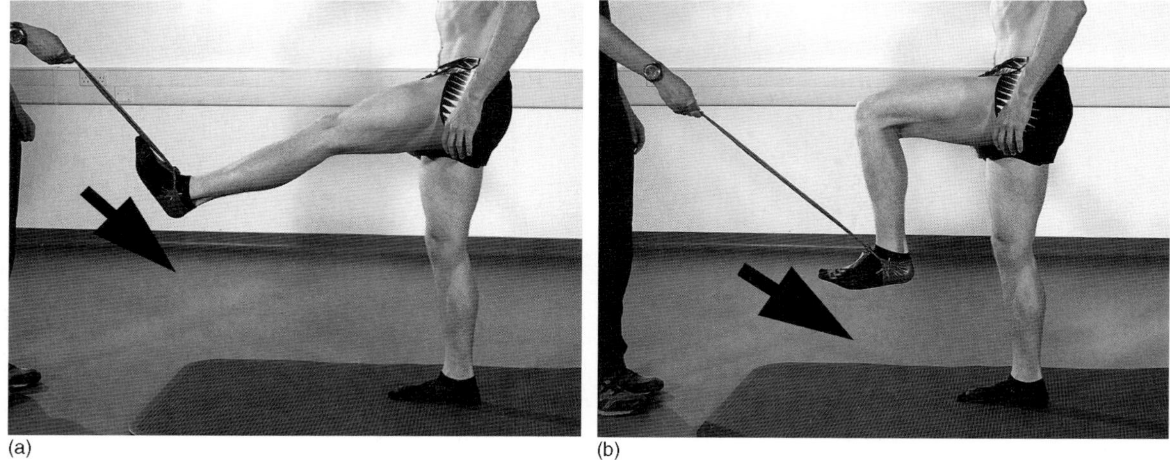

(a) (b)

17

Figure 17.20 Eccentric control of hip extension using rubber tubing. The speed at which the exercise and resistance of the tubing can be changed to suit the aims of the exercise and increase specificity.

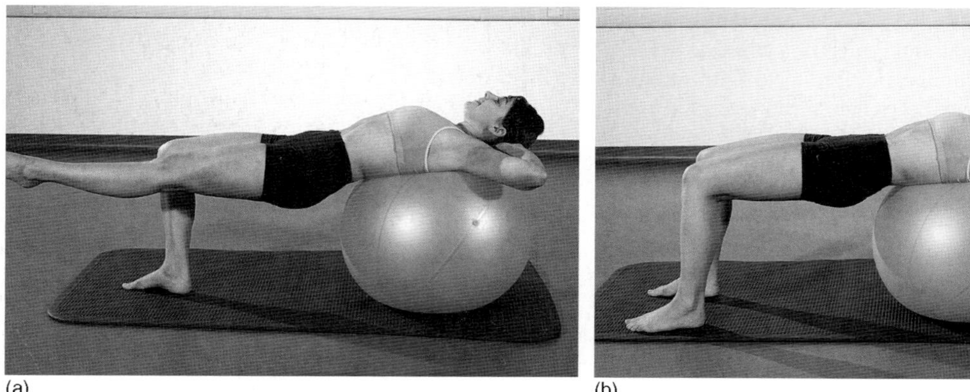

(a) (b)

Figure 17.21 Example of lower limb motor control exercises.

The above quotation refers to rehabilitation of unstable shoulders and perhaps highlights the potential differences in the nature of pathologies between the upper and lower limb. The shoulder is inherently more unstable than the joints of the lower limb, and is therefore much more vulnerable to mechanical as well as functional instability. Consequently, a comprehensive assessment needs to be undertaken when rehabilitating the shoulder to ascertain the exact cause of the problem.

Owing to this potential level of instability, closed-chain exercises are often a useful starting point, as they help to encourage joint stability through co-contraction of the surrounding muscles induced by the axial compression (Davies and Dickoff-Hoffman 1993). Variations of the four-point kneeling position are commonly used to achieve this (Figure 17.19). These positions are also useful in rehabilitating scapula stability, which will also be affected with (or be a cause of) many shoulder problems.

When rehabilitating older patients or those in poorer physical condition, four-point kneeling may not be an appropriate position and variations of closed-chain exercises can be used. These can include resting the hand on a wobble board in sitting, or resting the hand against a wall or table, to allow a degree of weight-bearing and then moving the shoulder.

Reflex stabilisations can also be used and are aimed at eliciting the correct motor response at the appropriate speed and in the most functional position. These consist of a sustained isometric contraction in a specific range in the joint's motion. These particular exercises and variations of them could be used with an athlete who would require shoulder stability in a vulnerable position, such as a rugby player when making a tackle.

The weighted-pan exercise is another example of an exercise based upon function. The patient is asked initially to observe weights being dropped into the pan that he or she is holding. The arm is placed progressively in more challenging positions, and the patient is instructed not to let the arm drop. The patient then closes his or her eyes and the exercise is repeated. This helps restore reflex stability in the upper limb.

Once a degree of control has been restored, more functional exercises can be taught. These may be occupation- or sports-specific to ensure that patients can withstand the stresses they encounter during their lives.

Rehabilitating the sensorimotor system requires adequate strength and endurance within the muscle. Many of the exercises illustrated can also be viewed as strengthening exercises; and although much of the preceding discussion has emphasised sensorimotor rehabilitation in isolation, the need for an accompanying strength and endurance programme is paramount. Indeed, muscular fatigue has been shown to induce proprioceptive deficits (Voight et al. 1996).

There is no definitive way to rehabilitate the sensorimotor system, and issues of progression depend on functional need, pain, swelling and an appropriate strength base.

REHABILITATION OF SENSORIMOTOR CONTROL OF THE SPINE (DVD)

The spine needs an effective neuromuscular control system and also benefits from sensorimotor control rehabilitation. The term 'core stability' is used with reference to back rehabilitation — 'core' referring to the trunk as the central control point of all movement. Research has shown that the muscles that stabilise the spine can become defacilitated and wasted (Hides et al. 1996) and have delayed recruitment during functional movements (Hodges and Richardson 1996). Loss of control of the core, it is hypothesised, leads to loss of segmental stability due to loss of core stability mechanisms. These mechanisms include increase of intra-abdominal pressure (Cresswell et al. 1992) and a stabilising effect through tensioning the thoracolumbar fascia (Hodges and Richardson 1997).

If core stability is impaired, it could have a detrimental effect on many other anatomical structures along the kinetic chain. This may be proximally in the pelvic and shoulder girdles or more distally in the limbs. Dynamic postural control requires reflex stabilisation of the trunk musculature that controls core stability. Specific transversus abdominis and multifidus re-education is required, progressed into dynamic movements and then function. The emphasis is on maintaining a neutral spinal position during exercise (Panjabi 1992), thus reducing shear forces around the spinal segments and facilitating stabiliser activity. Swiss ball exercises are commonly used to help restore this dynamic control (Figure 17.22).

Key point

Panjabi (1992) uses the phrase 'clinical instability' when referring to a decrease in the effectiveness of the passive and dynamic stabilisers within the spine.

Conscious appreciation of spinal position and associated muscle activity has been aided by the use of equipment such as the stabiliser pressure biofeedback device (Chattanooga, Australia). This is a simple device consisting of an air-filled chamber and an attached dial that monitors pressure changes. Patients are instructed to perform exercises while maintaining a constant pressure reading or altering the pressure through exercise (Figure 17.23).

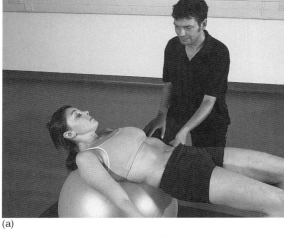

(a)

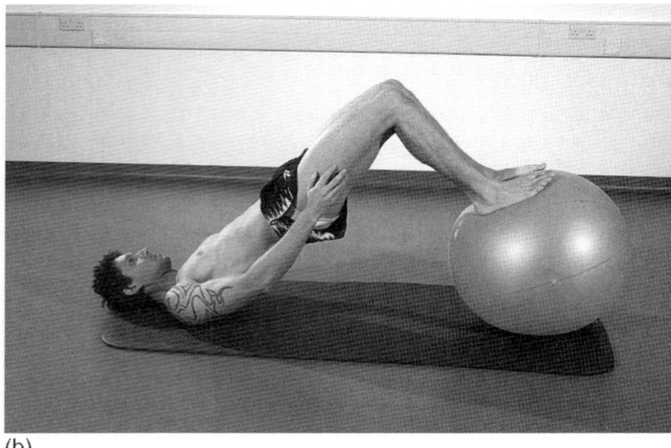

(b)

Figure 17.22 Swiss ball exercises. (a) Designed to develop neuromuscular control around the trunk; (b) aiming to integrate trunk and hip control.

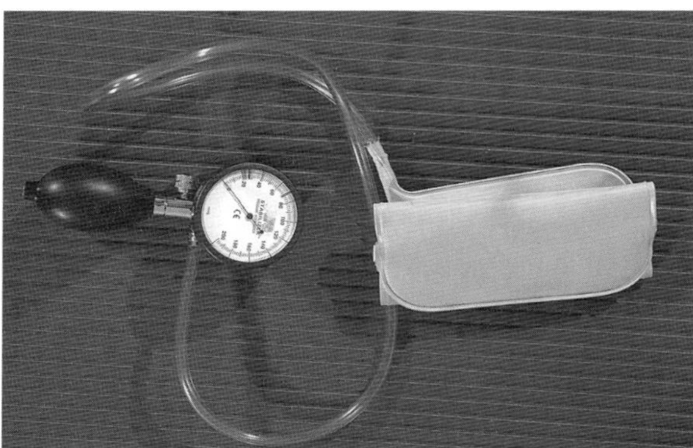

Figure 17.23 Pressure biofeedback maintains the correct degree of deep abdominal contraction.

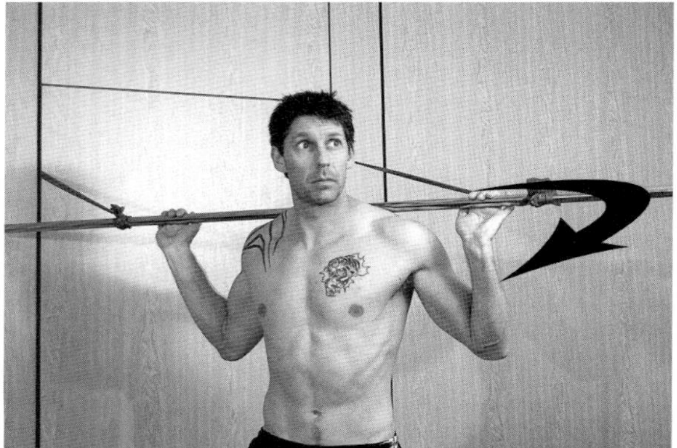

Figure 17.24 Pole rotation resisted by rubber tubing to enhance trunk control.

Pain is often the major concern in these patients and a neuromuscular training programme will aim to decrease or alleviate this. The mechanisms of spinal pain are, however, varied and often poorly understood.

Core stability should not be confused with core strength, as is commonly the case. Core stability refers to a level of low-threshold activity in the trunk stabiliser muscles, which results in functionally stable sensorimotor control of the trunk. Core strength refers to the effective production of torque in the trunk muscles and does not relate to finer levels of sensorimotor control. An example of a more advanced core stability exercise can be see in Figure 17.24, where the patient controls trunk rotation whilst overcoming the resistance applied from rubber tubing.

PLYOMETRIC EXERCISES DVD

Plyometric exercises are normally incorporated into the later stages of a rehabilitation programme and are aimed predominantly at those individuals who require more dynamic neuromuscular control as part of their normal functional activities: for example, athletes. Plyometrics are also used as part of athletes' training programmes, as they have been found to enhance performance (Sinnett et al. 2001; Swanik et al. 2002).

Plyometric exercises utilise the stretch shortening cycle to produce an enhanced concentric contraction. A plyometric activity consists of a rapid eccentric contraction followed by an immediate concentric contraction. Typically, these exercises are performed in the lower limb and involve various jumping-type activities. They can also be performed in the upper limb. Successful performance involves a rapid change from eccentric to concentric contraction. The time between the eccentric and concentric contractions is known as the *amortisation phase*; the quicker this phase, the more powerful the muscular concentric contraction.

Consider the jumping activity in Figure 17.25. As the feet hit the floor, the knees flex and result in a stretch in what is known as the series elastic component. The series elastic component consists of three structures: DVD

- Z lines
- myosin hinges
- Sharpey's fibres (located at the site of tendon insertion into bone).

With these three structures acting together, the series elastic component behaves like an elastic band that is stretched quickly; it stores up energy that can be suddenly released. This energy is added to the stretch reflex that occurs in the quadriceps on landing and, together with the following concentric contraction, combines to provide a more powerful contraction.

Plyometrics are used in the upper limb and certainly have functional applications. Medicine ball drills are often incorporated into upper limb exercises, as are activities with rubber tubing. Medicine ball work can involve paired throwing activities or use of a trampoline (Figure 17.26). DVD

The stated benefits of plyometric exercise are:

- increased power of muscular contraction
- enhanced neuromuscular coordination.

Before deciding to use plyometric exercises in the clinical situation, this checklist should be considered:

1. Is the person free of pain?
2. Is there an absence of recurrent swelling?
3. Does the person demonstrate a sufficient level of stability?

Despite the emphasis of plyometrics being on advanced rehabilitation, it can also play a role in improving the neuromuscular response following injury.

Latency of contraction is commonly seen in the peronei following an inversion injury to the ankle. The principles of plyometrics can be used, with the aid of

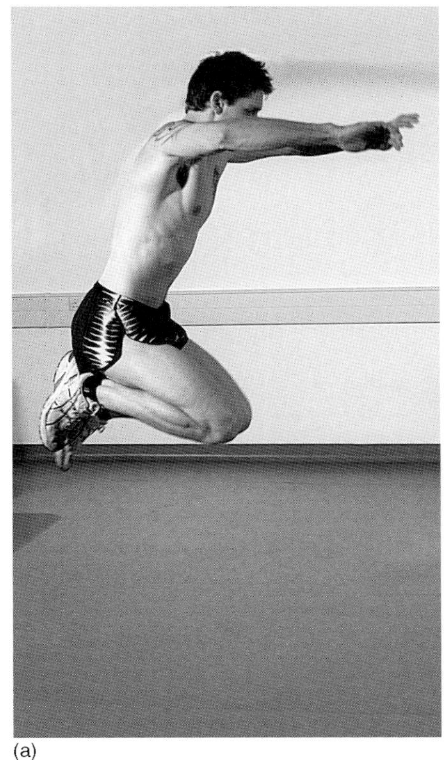

(a)

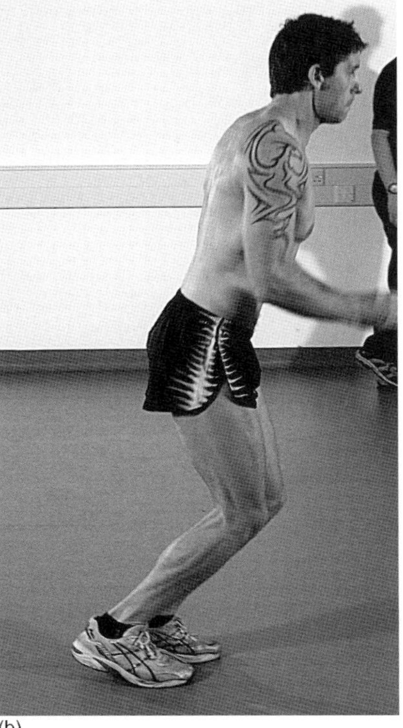

(b)

Figure 17.25 A plyometric drill for the lower limb.

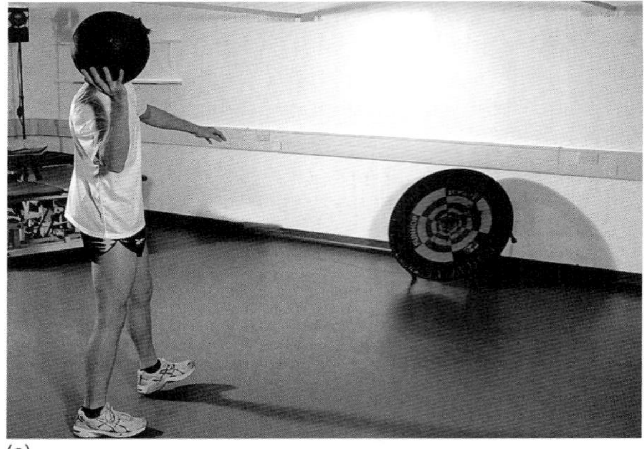

(a)

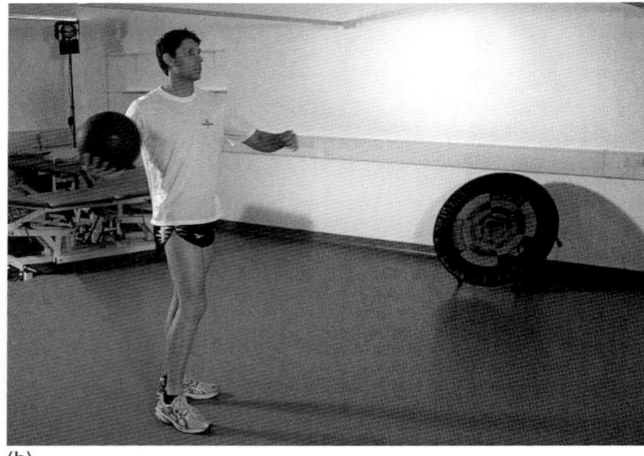

(b)

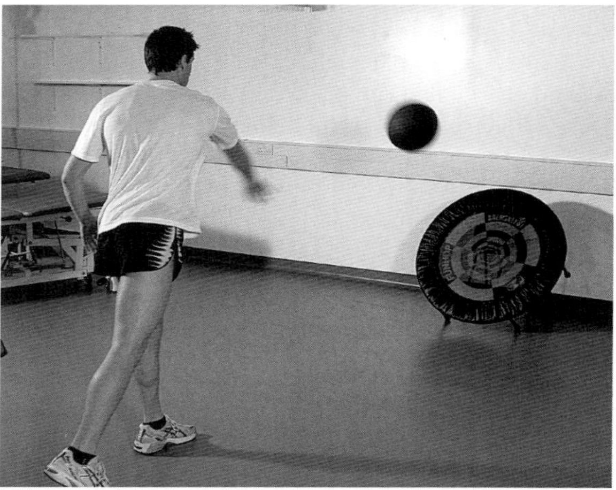

(c)

Figure 17.26 Plyometric drill using a trampette.

rubber tubing, to work on improving the neuromuscular response and strengthening the peronei at the same time. The patient takes the strain on the rubber tubing, holding the foot in an everted position. He or she is then instructed to release the tension on the rubber and then immediately evert the foot again. The condition of the ankle needs to be carefully assessed before commencing this type of exercise, in the same way as the inclusion criteria are checked for weight-bearing exercises. Similar activities could be used in the upper limb for shoulder medial rotators (Swanik et al. 2002).

There is little information on the number of repetitions that should be completed with plyometric exercises. Foot contacts have been suggested as an effective way of measuring the intensity of activity (Tippet and Voight 1995) in lower limb exercise, with a beginner counting 75–100 foot contacts and progressing up to 200–250 of low to moderate intensity. No values have been stated for the upper limb. Common sense should also prevail in monitoring performance, looking out for loss of quality of performance, obvious fatigue, increase in time of the amortisation phase, and so on.

Plyometric exercises should be performed no more than two or three times per week. The eccentric component is likely to cause a degree of DOMS and the muscle will need adequate time to recover.

FUNCTIONAL TESTING AND REHABILITATION

All rehabilitation should be geared towards a return to normal functional activity. In the latter stages of rehabilitation the functional aspects are perhaps of greatest importance.

Rehabilitation should not be measured as complete solely by outcomes such as bilateral symmetry of strength and range of movement, or an individual's ability to balance on a wobble board on the injured leg for a predetermined time. The physiotherapist needs to have a clear insight into the specific occupational, sporting and functional requirements of an individual to make sure the person is rehabilitated to the correct level. Such demands may involve working with large loads, working in challenging environments or playing professional sport.

Functional testing is an extension of functional rehabilitation and plays a major role in determining an individual's ability to return to pre-injury levels. This can take the form of one particular drill that encompasses several of the most difficult aspects of the individual's occupation or sport. For example, a soccer player needs to be able to run quickly, accelerate and decelerate, change direction and jump. A circuit could be set up similar to the one illustrated in Figure 17.27 to test any number of skills. This circuit could be timed over a number of sessions to determine improvement, or may simply be used as a one-off test to determine a return to full training.

Functional tests can be used as a measure of progress and are commonly employed as a requirement for return to work in physically challenging occupations or for return to play in sport. A functional test will establish a baseline to measure future improvement, identify risk factors predisposing to injury or re-injury and provide motivation to the individual, as it is a measurable outcome. Such a test consists of the performance, usually involving maximal effort, of a series of tasks.

In an assessment of functional tests the individual's ability to be able to respond to and tolerate functional demands is observed. The way the body part contributes to the body's overall movement and sensorimotor performance is also assessed.

There are several validated and widely used functional performance tools in existence but it may be necessary to design a functional test. If this is the case, careful planning is required. The first consideration is to identify the appropriate task, whether it is specific to strength, motor control or sports. It will then need to be decided what environment the task needs to be performed in; replicating functional environments enhances specificity. Once the tasks are established, it is necessary to plan how they will be measured and what equipment will be required for this: for example, video, surface EMG or a stopwatch.

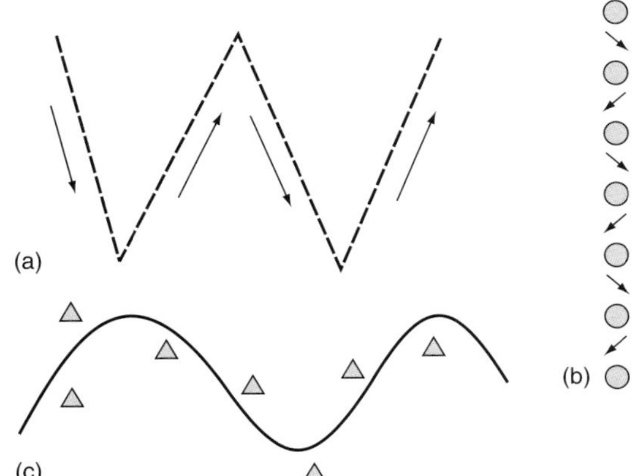

Figure 17.27 Example of a timed circuit.

Once the planning has been completed, all that remains is to perform the test, then collect, analyse and interpret the data. Analysis should consider performance of all phases of the whole task. For example, video analysis should include observation of starting position, preparatory position, approach, execution of task and termination of activity (such as landing). Once the task has been analysed, you can proceed to interpretation and analysis of how the individual has shown improvement and whether this sufficient to withstand the rigors of a return to competition or work.

> **Key point**
>
> When devising functional tests it is useful to apply the SMART principle: specific, measurable, achievable, realistic and timed. In this way the test can be developed as a valuable objective measure. There is a large scope for development of such tests, but it is also important that, once such tests are devised, they are seen to be reliable and valid.

Figure 17.28 illustrates a fireman undergoing specific functional rehabilitation whilst wearing full kit, thus replicating the working environment.

Functional rehabilitation allows a more objective measure of fitness to return to work. However, unless you are working in a specialist centre, it may not always be possible to duplicate a particular working environment as described above completely. In this situation the physiotherapist needs to be inventive and reproduce the tasks to be undertaken in the working environment as closely as possible, using any equipment or apparatus that may be available. This can include benches, wall bars, air cushions, rubber tubing, rucksacks, and sports-specific equipment such as tennis racquets. Further occupational tests are presented in Figures 17.29. In these situations the fireman has to perform timed functional tests, based upon set criteria.

Functional testing does not always need to be used as a measure for determining return to full function; it may instead be used as a baseline measure of functional ability. Examples of this include the various timed and distance hop tests that are used to test

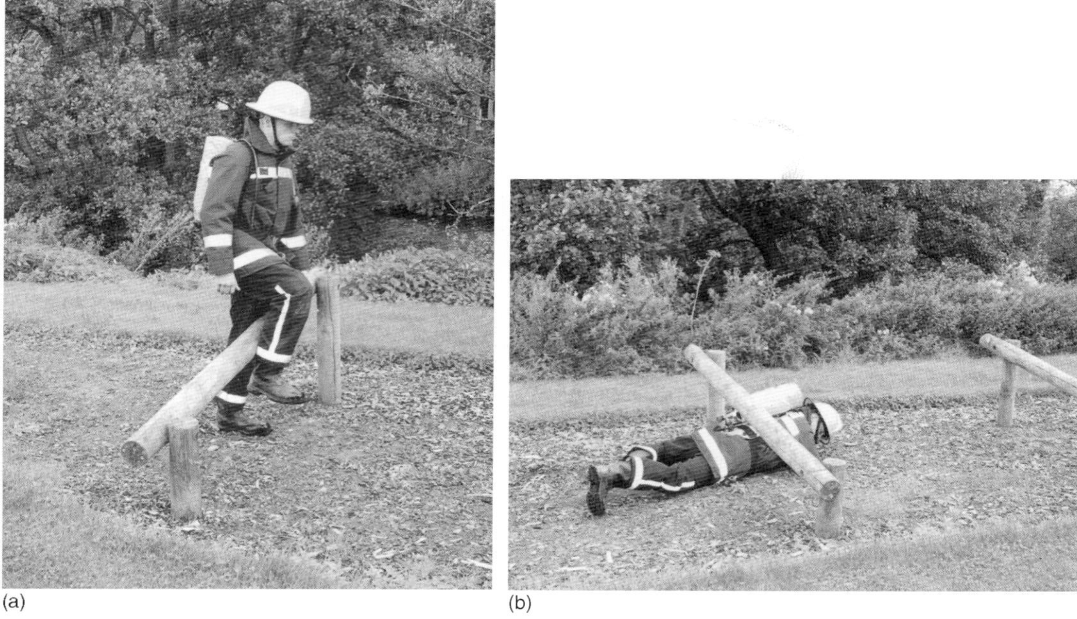

(a) (b)

Figure 17.28 A firefighter undergoing specific functional rehabilitation. (Courtesy of Fire Brigade Rehabilitation Centre, Penrith, UK.)

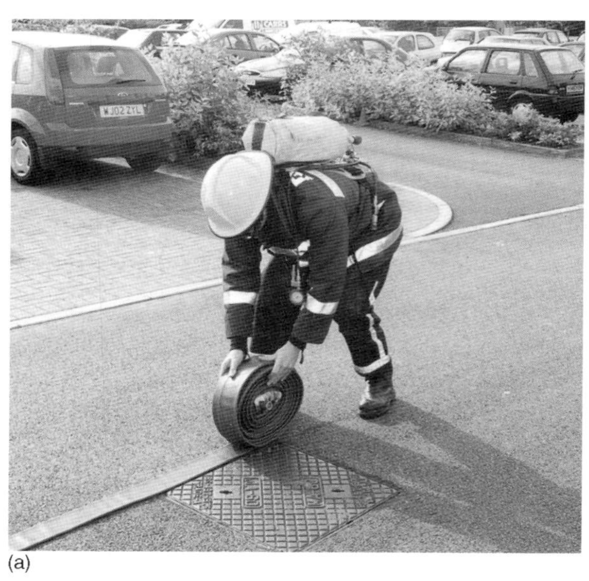

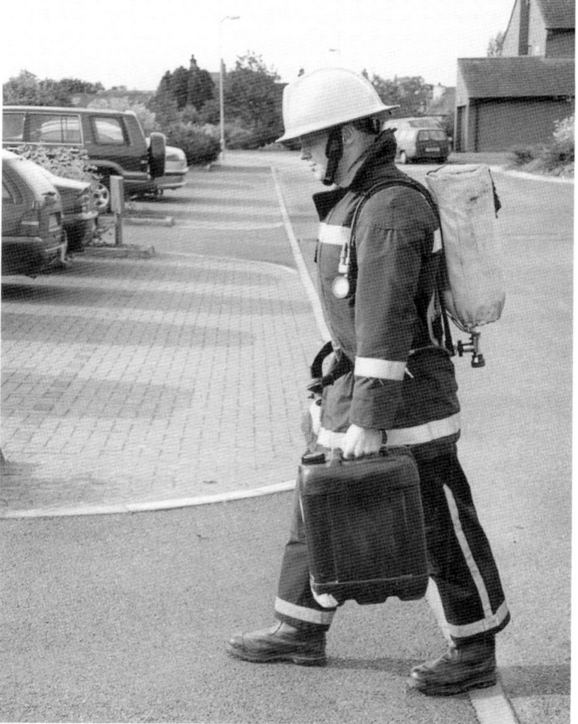

(a) (b)

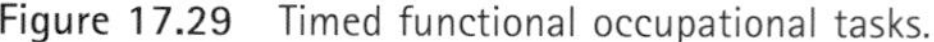

Figure 17.29 Timed functional occupational tasks.

ACL-deficient knees. Tippet and Voight (1995) suggest the following times when functional testing is undertaken within a sports environment:

- pre-season training
- during rehabilitation
- immediately after injury.

Although the examples highlighted above involve quite dynamic activities, functional testing and rehabilitation can be applied to all populations. An example of functional testing in the elderly population is the sit-to-stand test (Figure 17.30) or a walk of fixed distance. This can be either timed or judged on the number of repetitions.

Functional testing also provides psychological as well as physical benefits, not only in confirming progress but in improving confidence levels. It must be remembered that there is no substitute for 'live' conditions and functional testing can only go so far in preparing individuals for full function.

GROUP EXERCISE

Group exercise sessions are used widely, especially with more recent moves towards physiotherapists working in primary care as part of their educational or advisory role (Crook et al. 1998). Group work can take the form of exercise classes in a gym, in a hydrotherapy pool or as part of an educational programme, during which patients not only exercise but are also informed about the nature of their condition (Figure 17.31).

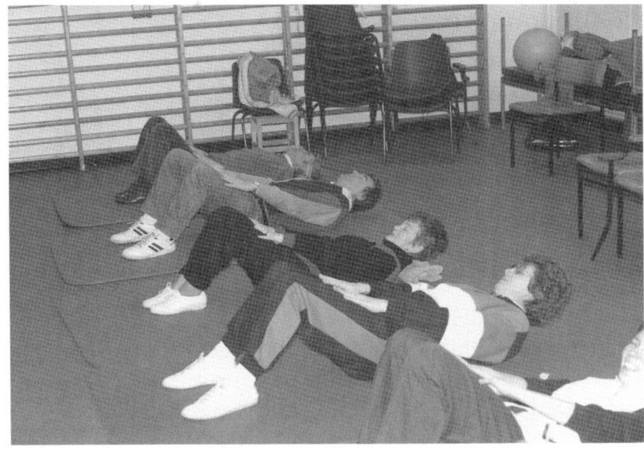

Figure 17.31 Group exercises in a chronic back pain management programme.

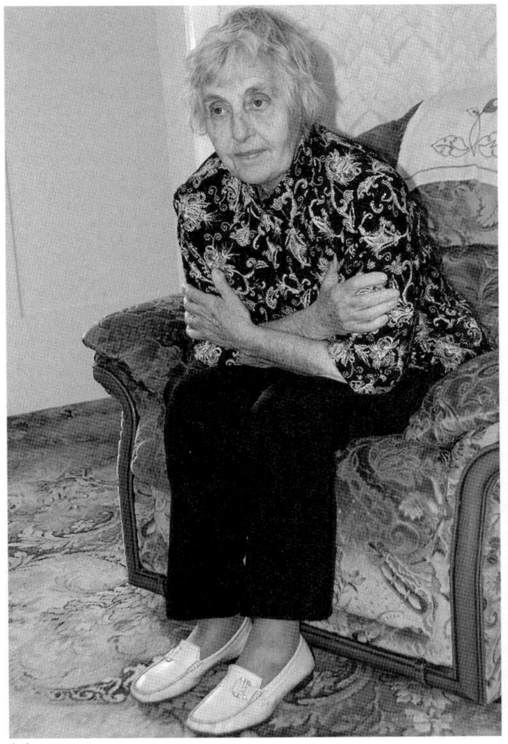

(a)

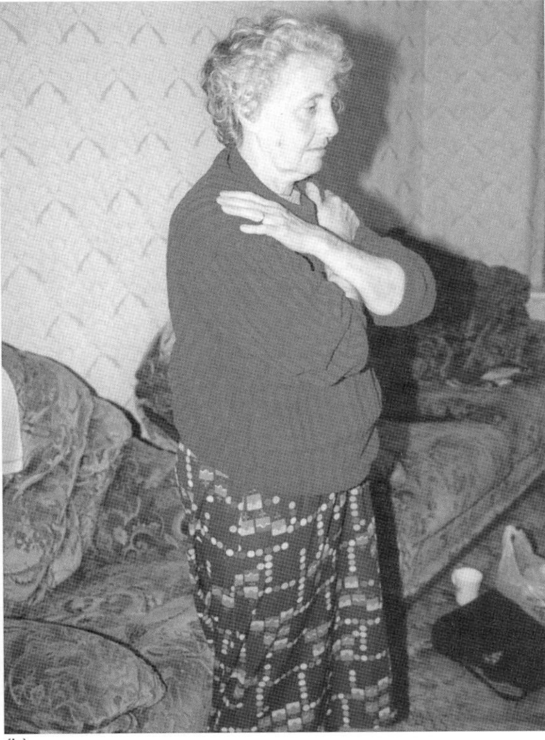

(b)

Figure 17.30 The sit to stand functional test. An example of a simple functional test requiring no equipment.

Educational programmes are commonly employed with the more longstanding pathologies and they encourage patients to take responsibility for the continued management of their condition (for example, back education programmes or osteoarthritis knee schools).

There are advantages and disadvantages to group work (Table 17.10).

Benefits and drawbacks

Provided that members are carefully selected, there are several advantages to treating patients in groups. Exercising with patients who have experienced similar problems can provide peer support, encouragement, reassurance and camaraderie. It is also more economically effective if the therapist is able to supervise several people at once.

The disadvantages of group work are that certain individuals may not respond to the group environment. In particular, they may be embarrassed or dislike the interaction. Many clients will respond better to individual attention from their therapist, particularly in the early stages of rehabilitation; this is not possible in group work.

If groups are used solely as a way of treating large numbers of patients with diverse pathologies, they will prove ineffective. This factor, along with a poorly organised treatment session, could lead to demotivation. There need to be clear objectives and goals for each class, with defined inclusion criteria.

Finally, it is important that participants in the group do not become too competitive, thereby reducing the effectiveness of the exercise and also risking further injury.

17

Planning group work

Careful planning is necessary if group work is to be effective. The aims of the group session must be clearly planned and stated so that selection criteria for participants can be agreed. This will ensure that the session is both safe and effective. Factors such as age, gender, psychological status, stage in rehabilitation, past medical history and general fitness need to be considered. The facilities and equipment that are available must be appropriate for the activities planned. Important considerations are the space available and the layout and temperature of the room or gym — the aim being to provide not only a suitable environment, but also a safe place to exercise.

Format of a group session

This should include:

1. patient assessment for suitability for group exercise (at an individual appointment)
2. warm-up session
3. main exercise session
4. cool-down period.

A warm-up is commonly used at the start of a session in order to improve circulation and increase body tissue temperature, thereby preparing the participants for exercise physically as well as mentally. Warm-up exercise may also limit the build-up of metabolites and subsequent acidosis during intense exercise (Kato et al. 2000). It is also interesting to note that proprioception has been found to be significantly more sensitive after warm-up (Bartlett and Warren 2002).

Following the warm-up come the main exercises, and then it is important to also allow time for cooling down, particularly following vigorous exercise, to assist with removal of lactic acid and waste products of metabolism.

Circuit training

Circuit training is often used in group work. It involves an exercise programme in which exercises are performed

Table 17.10 Advantages and disadvantages of group exercises

Advantages	Disadvantages
▪ Competitive element can be useful in increasing a person's performance ▪ A variety of exercises is possible ▪ Group exercise can be fun if properly organised ▪ Helps the individual to feel less isolated if meeting people with similar problems ▪ Provides a good opportunity for the physiotherapist to educate and inform the group about the condition ▪ Specialist groups such as ankylosing spondylitis or cardiac rehabilitation groups provide social support	▪ Difficult to pitch the exercises at a level suitable for all group members ▪ Temptation to put inappropriate individuals in the group to save time and relieve overburdened staff ▪ Difficult to monitor all of the people all of the time ▪ Difficult to progress all the members of the group appropriately ▪ Competitive element may be counterproductive or dangerous ▪ Some people do not respond well in a group situation

at successive stations either with a predetermined number of repetitions or for a set duration. Timed rest follows each exercise period prior to moving to the next station.

The exercises forming the circuit could be chosen from any of the aforementioned exercise types. The exercises included as part of the circuit must each form part of the client's overall rehabilitation goals. There will also usually be a cardiovascular element to circuit training, which is commonly used for cardiac or pulmonary rehabilitation programmes.

Key point

During group work the physiotherapist facilitates the session by giving feedback and motivation to all participants to ensure that they benefit fully from the session. Also, it is important that the participants have a home exercise programme to ensure their progress is continued at home.

The order of exercises in a circuit needs to be planned from a safety aspect so that group members do not endanger each other. Exercises also need to be ordered to achieve optimum effectiveness. For example, two exercises targeted to achieve similar effects should not be adjacent on a circuit, as that might cause excessive fatigue of the muscle groups involved.

HYDROTHERAPY

Hydrotherapy involves exercising in water. The same principles that apply to exercising on dry land, as discussed in this chapter, generally hold true for exercising in water. It is normal to have clients performing individually devised exercises, concurrently and under supervision, in order to gain the advantages of group activity and to make maximal use of this resource without the drawbacks of a class setting. This still, however, requires careful planning.

Hydrotherapy is used in the treatment of a wide range of conditions to enhance cardiovascular fitness, to mobilise, to strengthen, to coordinate movement, and to regain function of the neuro-musculoskeletal system. Many hospital departments have purpose-built heated hydrotherapy pools. The warm environment may allow the muscles to work more effectively owing to a rise in temperature and to relaxation of any muscle spasm. It will also have a pain-relieving effect. Conditions commonly managed by hydrotherapy are wide-ranging, from rheumatological conditions such as rheumatoid arthritis and ankylosing spondylitis, to trauma cases and neurological conditions.

Contraindications and precautions are important when considering patients for any exercise programme, and more so with hydrotherapy. This is mainly due to the warm environment in which they are exercising and the dangers of slipping or drowning. Contraindications include the presence of certain medical disorders, such as recent or severe neurological conditions (including uncontrolled epilepsy), certain cardiovascular problems and kidney failure. Hydrotherapy is also contraindicated with debilitating disease, and in the presence of infections that may be exacerbated or transmitted to other patients.

The starting positions used to exercise in the pool will be different from those commonly used on dry land. Patients commonly exercise in standing or sitting in the pool or perform more dynamic exercises such as walking or swimming, but they can also be treated whilst being floated in lying. Floats are placed around the neck and waist to support the patient, allowing him or her to exercise freely. Floats may also be placed around the limbs.

Other than starting position, the factors that need to be considered which change the nature of the exercise are buoyancy, turbulence and streamlining.

Buoyancy

This results from the relative density of the body or body part and the higher density of water. Buoyancy produces an apparent loss of weight of an object when it is placed in the water and it may be used to either assist or resist movement. It will be of particular advantage in reducing the effect of gravity on the body, particularly on load-bearing joints. Buoyancy may increase the function or the range of movement that is possible: for example, hip and knee flexion in standing. It may also be utilised to increase range of movement as a mobilising exercise, an effect that can be further enhanced by the use of a float or inflatable wrist or ankle bands: for example, to mobilise shoulder flexion with a wrist float in sitting.

Buoyancy can also be used in strengthening exercises. *Buoyancy-resisted* exercise involves pushing against buoyancy. Again, the effect can be increased by adding floats: for example, hip extension whilst being floated in supine against an ankle float.

Key point

The greater the buoyancy of the float, the greater the mobilising effect of the exercise. These types of exercise are classed as *buoyancy-assisted.*

As the exercises are progressed, the inflatable bands can be further blown up. Alternatively, the position of the float on the lever can be adapted, thereby changing the buoyancy effect on the limb; that is, the effect will be increased with a distal float placement. If buoyancy is to be counterbalanced, the patient will need to exercise along the pool surface.

Turbulence

As limbs move through water they meet resistance; turbulence is created, resulting in the production of currents. Turbulence results in an area of low pressure behind the moving body or body part. Faster movements will produce more turbulence. These currents may act to make movement more difficult and so this principle is of value when progressing an exercise, if exercises are performed rapidly. Also, therapist-created turbulence can be used in re-education of movement, particularly in the weight-bearing muscles of the lower limb. Clients are subjected to turbulence during standing and must maintain their position.

Streamlining

This refers to the surface area of the body part that is exposed to the water when moving through it. The simplest example is the orientation of the upper limb during exercise. If the hand moves with the palm facing the resistance of the water, more effort is required than when the limb is rotated so that the ulnar border leads. Moving from streamlined to non-streamlined positions can be used to strengthen progressively. This principle can be further progressed by use of hand-held bats or by placing flippers on the feet.

> **Further Study**
>
> For information on specific treatment techniques such as Bad Ragaz and Halliwick, further reading or study is required.

17

EXERCISE PRESCRIPTION AND COMPLIANCE

In this chapter we have considered many types of exercise, for varying populations and conditions. For prescription of exercise to be effective as a treatment modality, selection of the programme needs to be appropriate, as does how the exercises are delivered. The way in which exercises are taught will enhance their effectiveness by promoting compliance and accurate performance.

It is good practice when teaching exercise, as with any treatment intervention, to obtain informed consent. Not only does this conform to legal requirements but also it serves to educate patients about their condition by presenting the rationale behind the treatment approach. Education can only enhance compliance with the exercises (Lee and Yoo 2004), as can active encouragement (Prasad and Cerny 2002). When teaching the exercises, it may help to demonstrate the intended exercise to the patient, before giving detailed instruction and feedback on performance. There is no point in allowing an exercise to be performed incorrectly, as it will not effectively achieve its intended goal. It may benefit patients to be given a clear written copy of their exercises, using lay terms. This should, however, be a personalised exercise programme; all to often patients are given printed sheets with little thought to individual requirements. Written instructions should include information on how to perform the exercise: for example, speed, number of repetitions, sets and duration of recovery.

It is important for the therapist to observe the performance of exercise closely in order to detect signs of substitution or fatigue. Substitution strategies may present with movement dysfunction and it is necessary to inhibit overactive muscles in order to correct abnormal recruitment patterns. Fatigue will also affect performance, so once early signs of fatigue are noted, it is best to allow the muscles to rest and recover prior to performing further sets. Feedback is necessary, but should be given in a way that does not reduce the effectiveness of the treatment and so cause demotivation. It should also be given positively to reinforce good performance.

A positive outlook, high-quality education and constructive feedback will all serve to improve motivation; in turn, a patient that is highly motivated will be more likely to comply with the exercise programme.

As a final point, it is also good practice to give a patient a home exercise programme, to review it at each consultation and to progress it as the patient's improvement allows. This will give good returns in rehabilitation rates, as the patient can participate actively and regularly in the recovery and maintenance of their condition.

> **Key point**
>
> For exercise to be successful:
>
> - Provide clear instructions.
> - Give regular constructive feedback and encouragement on performance.
> - Educate patients on the reasons behind their exercise.

ACKNOWLEDGEMENTS

With thanks to Sean Kilmurray, Lecturer at the University of Central Lancashire, for his contribution to the original chapter in the 13th edition of this book.

FURTHER READING

Crook P, Stott R, Rose M et al. 1998 Adherence to group exercise: physiotherapist-led experimental programmes. Physiotherapy 84: 366–372

Jerosch J, Prymka M 1996 Proprioception and joint stability. Knee Surg Sports Traum Arthrosc 4: 171–179

Kato Y, Ikata T et al. 2000 Effects of specific warm-up at various intensities on energy metabolism during subsequent exercise. J Sports Med Phys Fitness 40(2): 126–130

Kisner C, Colby LA 1996 Therapeutic Exercise: Foundations and Techniques, 3rd edn. FA Davies: Philadelphia

Lieber 1992 Skeletal Muscle Structure and Function: Implications for Rehabilitation and Sports Medicine. Williams & Wilkins: Baltimore

Mense S, Simons DG, Russell J (eds) 2001 Muscle Pain: Understanding its Nature, Diagnosis and Treatment. Lippincott, Williams & Wilkins: Philadelphia

Richardson C, Hodges PW, Hides J 2004 Therapeutic Exercise for Lumbopelvic Stabilization: A Motor Control Approach for the Treatment and Prevention of Low Back Pain, 2nd edn. Churchill Livingstone: London

Richie DH 2001 Functional instability of the ankle and the role of neuromuscular control: a comprehensive review. J Foot Ankle Surg 40: 240–251

Tippet SR, Voight ML 1995 Functional Testing in Functional Progressions for Sport Rehabilitation. Human Kinetics: Champaign, IL

REFERENCES

Bandy WD, Irion JM, Briggler M 1997 The effect of time and frequency of static stretching on flexibility of the hamstring muscles. Phys Ther 77: 1090–1096

Barrack RL, Lund PJ, Skinner HB 1994 Knee joint proprioception revisited. J Sport Rehabil 3: 18–42

Barrett DS, Cobb AG, Bentley G 1991 Joint proprioception in normal, osteoarthritic and replaced knees. J Bone Joint Surg 73B(1): 53

Bartlett MJ, Warren PJ 2002 Effect of warming up on knee proprioception before sporting activity. Br J Sports Med 36(2): 132–134

Beard DJ, Kyberd PJ, O'Connor JJ et al. 1994 Reflex hamstring contraction latency in anterior cruciate ligament deficiency. J Orthopaed Res 12: 219–228

Bennett M, Best TM, Babul S et al. 2005 Hyperbaric oxygen therapy for delayed onset muscle soreness and closed soft tissue injury. Cochrane Database of Systematic Reviews 4

Bergmark A 1989 Stability of the lumbar spine: a study in mechanical engineering. Acta Orthopaed Scand Suppl 230: 1–54

Borsa PA, Lephart SM, Kocher MS, Lephart SP 1994 Functional assessment and rehabilitation of shoulder proprioception for glenohumeral instability. J Sport Rehabil 3: 84–104

Cahill BR, Misner JE, Boileau RA 1997 The clinical importance of the anaerobic energy system and its importance in human performance. Am J Sports Med 25: 863–872

Caraffa A, Cerulli G, Projetti M et al. 1996 Prevention of anterior cruciate ligament injuries in soccer: a prospective controlled study of proprioceptive training. Knee Surg Sports Traum Arthrosc 4: 19–21

Chan SP, Hong Y, Robinson PD 2001 Flexibility and passive resistance of the hamstrings of young adults using two different static stretching protocols. Scand J Med Sci Sports 11(2): 81–86

Cheung K, Hume P, Maxwell L 2003 Delayed onset muscle soreness: treatment strategies and performance factors. Sports Med 33(2): 145–164

Close GL, Ashton T, Cable T et al. 2005 Effects of dietary carbohydrate on delayed onset muscle soreness and reactive oxygen species after contraction induced muscle damage. Br J Sports Med 39(12): 948–953

Comerford MJ, Mottram SL 2001 Masterclass. Functional stability re-training: principles and strategies for managing mechanical dysfunction. Manual Ther 6(1): 3–14

Cresswell AG, Grundstrom H, Thorstensson A 1992 Observations on intra-abdominal pressure and patterns of abdominal intra-muscular activity in man. Acta Physiol Scand 144(4): 409–418

Crook P, Stott R, Rose M et al. 1998 Adherence to group exercise: physiotherapist-led experimental programmes. Physiotherapy 84: 366–372

Davies GJ, Dickoff-Hoffman S 1993 Neuromuscular testing and rehabilitation of the shoulder complex. J Orthopaed Sports Phys Ther 18: 449–558

Emery CA 1999 Does decreased muscle strength cause acute muscle strain injury in sport? A systematic review of the evidence. Phys Ther Rev 4(3): 141–151

Freeman MAR, Dean MRE, Hanhan IWF 1965 The aetiology and prevention of functional instability of the foot. J Bone Joint Surg 47B: 678–685

Galper DI, Trivedi MH, Barlow CE et al. 2006 Inverse association between physical inactivity and mental health in men and women. Med Sci Sports Exerc 38(1): 173–178

Gluck NI, Liebenson CS 1997 Clinical implications of paradoxical muscle function in muscle stretching or strengthening. J Bodywork Mov Ther 1: 219–222

Gralton E, Wildgoose J, Donovan WM, Wilkie J 1998 Eccentric exercise and neuroleptic malignment syndrome. Lancet 352: 1114

Herbert RD, Gabriel M 2002 Effects of pre- and post-exercise stretching on muscle soreness, risk of injury and athletic performance: a systematic review. BMJ 325(7362): 468–472

Hides JA, Richardson CA, Jull GA 1996 Multifidus recovery is not automatic following resolution of acute first episode low back pain. Spine 21: 2763–2769

Hodges PW, Richardson CA 1996 Inefficient muscular stabilization of the lumbar spine associated with low back pain: a motor control evaluation of transversus abdominis. Spine 21: 2640–2650

Hodges PW, Richardson CA 1997 Feedforward contraction of transversus abdominis is not influenced by the direction of arm movement. Exp Brain Res 114(2): 362–370

Howell JN, Chlebourn G, Conaster R 1993 Muscle stiffness, strength loss, swelling and soreness following eccentric induced exercise in humans. J Physiol 464: 183–196

Hunter G 1998 Specific soft tissue mobilization in the management of soft tissue dysfunction. Manual Ther 3(1): 2–11

Jerosch J, Prymka M 1996 Proprioception and joint stability. Knee Surg Sports Traum Arthrosc 4: 171–179

Jerosch J, Thorwesten L 1998 Proprioceptive abilities of patients with post-traumatic instability of the glenohumeral joint. Zeitschrift für Orthopädie und Ihre Grenzgebiete 136(3): 230–237

Jull GA, Janda V 1987 Muscles and motor control in low back pain. In: Twomey LT, Taylor JR (eds) Physical Therapy of the Low Back. Churchill Livingstone: Edinburgh, pp. 253–278

Kato Y, Ikata T et al. 2000 Effects of specific warm-up at various intensities on energy metabolism during subsequent exercise. J Sports Med Phys Fitness 40(2): 126–130

Kerrigan DC, Lee LW, Collins JJ et al. 2001 Reduced hip extension during walking: healthy elderly and fallers versus young adults. Arch Phys Med Rehabil 82: 26–30

Kerrigan DC, Xenopoulos-Oddsson A, Sullivan MJ et al. 2003 Effect of a hip flexor-stretching program on gait in the elderly. Arch Phys Med Rehabil 84(1): 1–6

Kisner C, Colby LA 1996 Therapeutic Exercise: Foundations and Techniques, 3rd edn. FA Davies: Philadelphia

Kujala UM, Orava S et al. 1997 Hamstring injuries: current trends in treatment and prevention. Sports Med 23: 397–404

Lee SJ, Yoo JS 2004 The effects of a physical activity reinforcement program on exercise compliance, depression, and anxiety in continuous ambulatory peritoneal dialysis patients. Daehan Ganho Haghoeji 34 (3): 440–448

Leger AB, Milner TE 2001 Muscle function at the wrist after eccentric exercise. Med Sci Sports Exerc 33: 612–620

Lephart SM, Henry TJ 1995 Functional rehabilitation for the upper and lower extremity. Orthoped Clin N Am 26: 579–592

Lephart SM, Pincivero DM et al. 1997 The role of proprioception in the management and rehabilitation of athletic injuries. Am J Sports Med 25: 130–137

Lieber 1992 Skeletal Muscle Structure and Function: Implications for Rehabilitation and Sports Medicine. Williams & Wilkins: Baltimore

Lynch D, Ferraro M, Krol J et al. 2005 Continuous passive motion improves shoulder joint integrity following stroke. Clin Rehabil 19(6): 594–599

Magnusson SP 1998 Passive properties of human skeletal muscle during stretch manoeuvres. Scand J Med Sci Sports 8(2): 65–77

Malliaropoulos N, Papalexandris S, Papalada A, Papacostas E 2004 The role of stretching in rehabilitation of hamstring injuries: 80 athletes follow-up. Med Sci Sports Exerc 36(5): 756–759

Melis P, Noorlander ML, van der Horst CM et al. 2002 Rapid alignment of collagen fibres in the dermis of undermined and not undermined skin stretched with a skin-stretching device. Plast Reconstr Surg 109: 674–680

Mense S, Simons DG, Russell J (eds) 2001 Muscle Pain: Understanding its Nature, Diagnosis and Treatment. Lippincott, Williams & Wilkins: Philadelphia

Norris CM 1995 Spinal stabilisation. 4: Muscle imbalance and the low back. Physiotherapy 81(3): 127–138

Panjabi MM 1992 The stabilising system of the spine. Part II: Neutral zone and stability hypothesis. J Spinal Dis 5: 390–397

Prasad SA, Cerny FJ 2002 Factors that influence adherence to exercise and their effectiveness: application to cystic fibrosis. Pediatr Pulmonol 34(1): 66–72

Proske U 2005 What is the role of muscle receptors in proprioception? Muscle & Nerve 31(6): 780–787

Racette R, Peronnet F, Massicotte D, Lavoie C 2005 Metabolic response to prolonged cycling with (13)C-glucose ingestion following downhill running. Eur J Appl Physiol 93(5–6): 598–605

Rahnama N, Rahmani-Nia F, Ebrahim K 2005 The isolated and combined effects of selected physical activity and ibuprofen on delayed-onset muscle soreness. Randomized Controlled Trial. J Sports Sci 23(8): 843–850

Rees K, Taylor RS, Singh S et al. 2004 Exercise based rehabilitation for heart failure. Cochrane Database of Systematic Reviews 3

Richardson C, Hodges PW, Hides J 2004 Therapeutic Exercise for Lumbopelvic Stabilization: A Motor Control Approach for the Treatment and Prevention of Low Back Pain, 2nd edn. Churchill Livingstone: London

Richie DH 2001 Functional instability of the ankle and the role of neuromuscular control: a comprehensive review. J Foot Ankle Surg 40: 240–251

Rodenberg JB, Bär PR, De Boer RW 1993 Relations between muscle soreness and biochemical and functional outcomes of eccentric exercise. J Appl Physiol 74: 2976–2983

Rogers MA, Evans WJ 1993 Changes in skeletal muscle with aging: effects of exercise training. Exer Sports Sci Rev 21: 65–102

Sahrman S 2002 Diagnosis and Treatment of Movement Impairment Syndromes. Mosby: St Louis, MO

Saxton JM, Clarkson PM, James R et al. 1995 Neuromuscular dysfunction following eccentric exercise. Med Sci Sports Exerc 27: 1185–1193

Scott W, Stevens J, Binder-Macleod SA 2001 Human skeletal muscle fibre type classifications. Phys Ther 81(11): 1810–1816

Shrier I 2004 Does stretching improve performance? A systematic and critical review of the literature. Clin J Sport Med 14(5): 267–273

Shrier I, Gossal K 2000 Myths and truths of stretching. Physician Sports Med 28(8):

Sinnett AM, Berg K, Latin RW, Noble JM 2001 The relationship between field tests of anaerobic power and 10-km run performance. J Strength Cond Res 15(4): 405–412

Spernoga SG, Uhl TL, Arnold BL, Gansneder BM 2001 Duration of maintained hamstring flexibility after a one-time, modified hold–relax stretching protocol. J Athlet Train 36(1): 44–48

Stanish WD, Curwin S, Rubinovich M 1985 Tendinitis: the analysis and treatment for running. Clin Sports Med 4(44): 593–609

Swanik KA, Lephart SM, Swanik CB et al. 2002 The effects of shoulder plyometric training on proprioception and selected muscle performance characteristics. J Shoulder Elbow Surg 11(6): 579–586

Tippet SR, Voight ML 1995 Functional Testing in Functional Progressions for Sport Rehabilitation. Human Kinetics: Champaign, IL

Voight ML, Hardin JA, Blackburn TA et al. 1996 The effects of muscle fatigue on and the relationship of arm dominance to shoulder proprioception. J Orthop Sports Phys Ther 23: 348–352

Waddington GS, Shepherd RB 1996 Ankle injury in sports: role of motor control systems and implications for prevention and rehabilitation. Phys Ther Rev 1: 79–87

Wilk KE, Escamilla RF, Fleisig GS et al. 1996 A comparison of tibiofemoral joint forces and electromyographic activity during open and closed kinetic chain exercises. Am J Sports Med 24(4): 518–527

Wilkerson GB, Nitz AJ 1994 Dynamic ankle instability: mechanical and neuromuscular interrelationships. J Sport Rehabil 3: 43–57

Chapter **18**

Electrotherapy

Tim Watson

CHAPTER CONTENTS

INTRODUCTION

Electrotherapy has been a component of physiotherapy practice since the early days of our profession. Modern electrotherapy use needs to be evidence-based and the modalities must be chosen judiciously. When employed appropriately, electrotherapy modalities have a demonstrable capacity to achieve significant benefit. Used unwisely, they either will do no good at all or, worse still, will aggravate the clinical condition. In addition to the delivery skills of each modality, there is a critical skill in making the appropriate clinical decision as to which modality to use and when.

With regard to the mechanisms by which each modality achieves its effects, it is important to realise that it is not the modality per se that brings about the therapeutic benefit. The applied energy stimulates or induces a physiological response. It is the physiological response in turn that brings about the therapeutic effects. The key to the application of electrotherapy is the relationship between these concepts. The therapist working with an electrotherapy modality is using, or manipulating, the physiological changes in order to achieve the desired effect. This may seem to be a pedantic argument, but it is a critical point. The outcome of the therapy is achieved through physiological manipulation and this is true for the application of all electrotherapy modalities.

A further very important concept is that the electrotherapy intervention is only one component of the overall treatment package. It is rarely appropriate for a patient to receive electrotherapy in isolation. It is most usually combined with a range of manual therapies, exercise, advice and education. The elements of the treatment package need to be complementary. Careful construction of treatment programmes will permit the most effective outcome. It may be that the electrotherapy components are only utilised for the first few sessions, or indeed, only for the sessions later in a series. Electrotherapy is not an essential component for all patients and should only be used when and where it is appropriate.

The evidence to support the use of electrotherapy is an important part of the clinical decision-making process. It may not be possible at the present time to give a full explanation of how every effect of each modality is achieved (as is the case with almost all aspects of therapy). Clearly, where valid published research exists, it should be taken into account.

Scope

The aim of this chapter is to enable the reader to identify the key issues in electrotherapy, using commonly employed modalities as examples. It does not purport to examine or explain the evidence fully for every modality, and there are many 'modalities' that will hardly be mentioned. This does not mean that they are unimportant or worthless; it is a realistic reflection of the complexity of modern electrotherapy practice and the limits of what can be achieved in a single chapter. In terms of clinical practice, the most widely used modalities in the UK are ultrasound, interferential therapy, transcutaneous electrical nerve stimulation (TENS) and pulsed shortwave, with laser following close behind. The interested reader will be referred throughout to appropriate review material.

MODEL OF ELECTROTHERAPY

Electrotherapy modalities follow a very straightforward model that is presented in Figure 18.1. The model identifies the delivery of energy from a machine or device as the starting point of the intervention. Energy delivery to the tissues results in a change in one or more physiological events. Some are very specific whilst others are multifaceted. The capacity of the energy to influence physiological events is key to the processes. The physiological shift that results from the energy delivery is used in practice to generate what are commonly referred to as therapeutic effects.

The clinical application of the model is best achieved by what appears to be a reversal of this process. Starting with the patient and his or her problems, identified

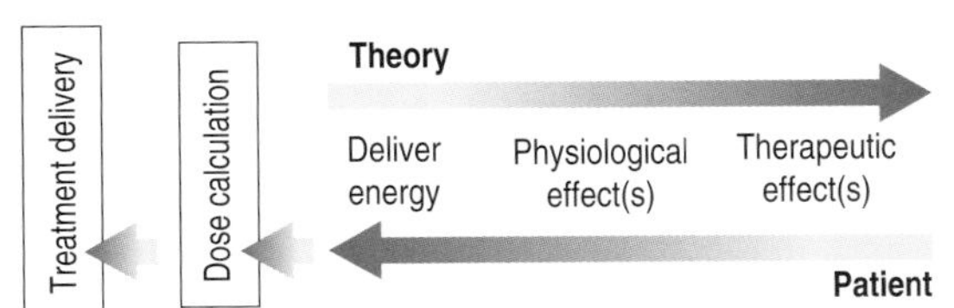

Figure 18.1 A simple generic model of electrotherapy.

from the clinical assessment, the treatment priorities can be established and the rationale for the treatment determined. Having established the therapeutic target (or aim), move one step back through the model and identify which physiological events/processes need to be activated or stimulated in order to achieve the outcome. Once the required physiological changes have been identified, moving one step further back will enable a modality decision to be made. This is based on the existing evidence as to which modalities stimulate which physiological effects. If there is no electrotherapy modality that is capable of achieving the intended effects, then electrotherapy would have no founded use in the management of this particular patient. The effects of electrotherapy appear to be modality-dependent. This is a critical decision, in that each modality has a limited subset of effects that are fundamentally different from another modality. It is certainly not the case that some modalities are universally 'better' than others; what is true is that some modalities are more effective at achieving particular therapeutic effects.

Once you have identified the modality that is best able to achieve the effects required, the next clinical stage is to make a 'dose' selection. Not only is it critical to apply the right modality; it must also be applied at the appropriate 'dose' in order for maximal benefit to be achieved. There is a substantial and growing body of evidence that if the same modality is applied at different doses, the results will be different. An example might be the use of ultrasound energy. Applied at a low 'therapeutic' dose, it can stimulate tissue repair and healing. Applied at a much higher dose (high-intensity focused ultrasound, or HIFU), it is used to ablate tumour tissue. The energy form is the same, but if the therapist varies the applied 'dose', the outcome clearly differs.

One might argue that this is an extreme example, and in some ways it is; the point, though, is that the effects of the therapy are both modality- and dose-dependent. There are 'therapeutic windows' in electrotherapy (as there are in almost all therapeutic interventions)- and in order to achieve the 'best' outcome, it is essential to come as close to this window as one possibly can.

The fundamental model we are using to explain electrotherapy could be applied to many interventions: drug therapy, manual therapy or exercise therapy, for example. All involve the use of an intervention in order to achieve a physiological shift or change. It is this change that is the therapeutic tool. The treatment is just a tool to stimulate the physiological change and electrotherapy is therefore little different from manual therapy or any other intervention. It is a tool that, when applied at the right time at the right dose and for the right reason, has the capacity to be beneficial. Applied inappropriately, it is not at all surprising that it has the capacity to achieve nothing or in fact to make things worse. The skilful practitioner uses the available evidence combined with experience to make the best possible decision, taking into account the psychosocial and holistic components of the problem. It is not a simple reductionist solution.

THERAPEUTIC WINDOWS

Windows of opportunity are topical in many areas of medical practice and are not a new phenomenon at all. It has long been recognised that the 'amount' of a treatment is a critical parameter. This is no less true for electrotherapy than for other interventions. There are literally hundreds of research papers that illustrate that the same modality applied at a different 'dose' will produce a different outcome.

Given the research evidence, there appear to be several aspects to this issue. Using a very straightforward model, there is substantial evidence, for example, that there is an *'amplitude' or 'strength' window*. An energy delivered at a particular amplitude has a beneficial effect, whilst the same energy at a lower amplitude may have no demonstrable effect. Laser therapy offers an obvious example; one level will produce a distinct cellular response whilst a higher dose can be considered to be destructive. Karu (1987) demonstrated and reported these principles in relation to laser energy and the research produced since has served to reinforce the concept (Vinck et al. 2003). Further examples of amplitude windows can easily be found in the work of Hill et al. (2002), Reher et al. (2002) and Cleary (1987).

Along similar lines, *'frequency windows'* are also apparent. A modality applied in a specific frequency or pulsing regime might have a measurable benefit, whilst the same modality applied using a different pulsing profile may not appear to achieve equivalent results. Examples can be found in many papers, including Young and Dyson (1990a,b) and Sontag (2000).

Electrical stimulation frequency windows have been proposed and there is clinical and laboratory evidence to suggest that there are frequency-dependent responses in clinical practice. TENS applied at frequency X appears to have a different outcome to TENS applied at frequency Y in an equivalent patient population. Studies by Sluka et al. (2006), Han et al. (1991) and Palmer et al. (1999) illustrate the point.

Assuming that there are likely to be more than two variables to the real-world model, some complex further work needs to be invoked. There is almost certainly an *energy- or time-based window* (e.g. Hill et al. 2002) and then another factor based on treatment frequency (number of sessions a week or treatment intervals). Work ontinues to identify the more and less critical parameters for each modality across a range of clinical presentations.

ELECTROTHERAPY MODALITY GROUPING

No matter which classification of the numerous electrotherapy modalities is adopted, it can easily be criticised. The groupings used in Figure 18.2 constitute one way of looking at the scope of electrotherapy, though it is not presented as the 'right' model. The division into three main subgroups — electrical stimulation, thermal modalities and non-thermal modalities — is the theme that will be followed in this chapter.

The *electrical stimulation modalities* have a common mode of action in that their primary effect will be on nerve (and in some circumstances, muscle) tissue. Commonly employed forms of electrical stimulation include transcutaneous electrical nerve stimulation (TENS), interferential therapy (IFT), various forms of muscle stimulation (e.g. neuromuscular electrical stimulation — NMES, functional electrical stimulation — FES), and many others that will not be considered in any detail in this chapter. Microcurrent therapy is 'different' in that its primary mode of action is to influence tissue repair rather than stimulate nerve, and thereby it falls into an overlap zone between categories.

The *thermal modalities* group includes various forms of heating that have been used for many years in therapy: infrared therapy, conductive heating, wax therapy, hot packs and the 'deeper' heating modalities — shortwave diathermy (SWD) and microwave diathermy (MWD). Use of the heating modalities has diminished in clinical practice over recent years. Much as some of the interventions employed in the past may lack evidence, there are nevertheless compelling reasons to keep heat therapies in the clinical repertoire, and there are areas where the use of heat-based therapies is likely to re-emerge as a strongly evidence-based intervention. Examples of modern heat therapy applications are given in Michlovitz et al. (2004) and Usuba et al. (2006).

The *non-thermal modalities* are grouped together on the basis that, if delivered at sufficiently high levels, any of them *could* produce a significant or even destructive heating effect in the tissues. If they are delivered at sufficiently low dose, they are considered to be 'non-thermal' in their primary effect. This is somewhat misleading, in that any energy delivered to the tissues that is subsequently absorbed will achieve a heating effect. The non-thermal label is derived from the fact that there is no gross thermal change, and the patient is not able to perceive a thermal effect. More properly, these should possibly be referred to as *microthermal* or *subthermal* modalities. Ultrasound (US), pulsed shortwave therapy (PSWT) and laser therapy fall most obviously into this

Electrical stimulation modalities	Thermal modalities	Non-thermal modalities
Transcutaneous electrical nerve stimulation (TENS)	Infra red radiation (IRR)	Therapeutic ultrasound (US)
Interferential therapy (IFT)	(Continuous) shortwave diathermy (SWD)	Laser therapy
Neuro muscular electrical stimulation (NMES)	Pulsed shortwave therapy (PSWT)	Pulsed shortwave therapy (PSWT)
Functional electrical stimulation (FES)	Microwave diathermy (MWD)	Magnetic therapy
'Russian' stimulation	Hydrocollator (hot) packs	Microcurrent therapy
Diadynamic therapy	Wax therapy	
Others including: H wave therapy, Rebox therapy, Microcurrent therapy	[Therapeutic ultrasound]	

Figure 18.2 Electrotherapy modalities classification.

group, and various forms of magnetic therapy that are gaining ground in the literature would also be best suited to this area. The current clinical use of these modalities is primarily directed at enhancing the process of healing and tissue repair. Ultrasound presents a dilemma in that some practitioners use it as a modality that is employed with the deliberate intention of heating the tissues, though the evidence would support its 'non-thermal' use over and above its thermal application.

ELECTRICAL STIMULATION MODALITIES

General principles of electrical stimulation

The general principles of electrical stimulation (ES) in the context of commonly employed electrotherapy modalities focus on the use of electrical currents (usually in the form of discrete pulses) to initiate action potentials in nerves. This would be true for modalities like TENS, NMES in its various forms, and interferential therapy (though this modality does not employ discrete pulses). There are other forms of intervention that employ alternative mechanisms; these include iontophoresis (which uses a direct or pulsed direct current to enhance the delivery of a chemical substance or drug through the skin) and microcurrent-type therapies, which are delivered at a level that is insufficient to stimulate a nerve action potential but which do appear to have an effect on the repair responses in wounds and damaged tissues.

Nerve action potentials

Assuming that the majority of ES modalities work by means of nerve activation, a brief examination of how this is achieved would be beneficial. A nerve, in its resting state, is said to be *'polarised'*. When an action potential is transmitted along a nerve, the membrane at the point of the action potential is momentarily *depolarised* before returning to its normal state (*repolarisation*). Essentially, the employment of an electrical current or pulse is a means to initiate an action potential along the course of the nerve. Once the action potential has been initiated by this exogenous signal, then it will continue along the nerve (whether sensory or motor) in the normal fashion; electrical stimulation is simply an initiator of the activity. If the nerve is stimulated 10 times a second, then 10 action potentials a second will be initiated. If stimulated 100 times a second, predictably, it will fire 100 times a second. There are some constraints to this relationship, based on refractory periods and threshold potentials that are beyond the scope of this chapter, but these are usefully reviewed in most standard electrotherapy texts (Robertson et al. 2006; Kitchen 2002a).

The nerve being stimulated is effectively unable to differentiate between different types of electrical stimulation. It is simply responding to an external (exogenous) stimulus and will fire accordingly. There is no evidence to suggest (all else being equal) that the effect of TENS at 80 Hz, interferential therapy at 80 Hz and neuromuscular stimulation at 80 Hz will have a different outcome. If they are all applied at the same frequency and at the same amplitude (strength), then the outcome will be the same. The use of different forms of electrical stimulation relates to the evidence that different nerve types appear to respond preferentially to variations in stimulation parameters, and this is what the different types of machine are best able to achieve.

Bearing these principles in mind, we will consider the commonly employed ES modalities in brief and their primary clinical applications will be described. There are many alternative and additional widespread uses of these modalities that are evidenced, but are beyond the scope of this overview chapter. References are provided for those with further interest in this area.

Transcutaneous electrical nerve stimulation (TENS)

18 TENS is a method of electrical stimulation that primarily aims to provide a degree of pain relief (symptomatic) by specifically exciting sensory nerves and thereby stimulating the pain gate mechanism and/or the opioid system (Sluka and Walsh 2003; Walsh 1997). Strictly speaking, any form of electrical stimulation applied with surface electrodes that stimulates nerves can be referred to as TENS, but in clinical practice, the term is most commonly employed in the context identified above.

The different methods of applying TENS relate to these different physiological mechanisms. Success is not guaranteed with TENS, and the percentage of patients who obtain pain relief will vary, but it would typically be in the region of 65 per cent or more for acute type pains and 50 per cent or more for more chronic pains. Both of these are better than the placebo effect.

The technique is non-invasive and has few side-effects when compared with drug therapy. A few patients experience an allergic-type skin reaction and this is almost always due to the material of the electrodes, the conductive gel or the tape employed to hold the electrodes in place. Most TENS applications are now made using self-adhesive, pre-gelled electrodes (Figure 18.3), which have several advantages, including lower allergy incidence, reduced cross-infection risk, ease of application and lower overall cost.

Machine parameters

The main parameters (or settings) on a TENS machine are those that are influential in terms of sensory nerve stimulation, the primary aim of the modality. The location of these controls on a typical TENS machine is illustrated in Figure 18.4.

The current intensity (A on the figure) (strength) will typically be in the range of 0–80 mA, though some machines may provide higher outputs. Although this is a small current, it is sufficient because the primary targets for the therapy are the sensory nerves; as long as sufficient current is passed through the tissues to depolarise these nerves, the modality can be effective.

The machine will deliver electrical 'pulses', and the rate of delivery of these pulses can be varied. The pulse rate (B) will normally range from about 1 or 2 pulses per second (pps) up to 200 pps or more. To be clinically effective, it is suggested that the TENS machine should cover a range from 2–150 Hz.

In addition to the stimulation rate, the duration (or pulse width) of each pulse (C) may be varied from about 40 to 250 microseconds (μs). Recent evidence would suggest that this is possibly a less important control than the intensity and frequency. Short-duration pulses are effective because sensory nerves have a relatively low threshold and will respond well to short-duration, rapidly changing pulses. There is generally no need to apply a prolonged pulse in order to force the nerve to depolarise, and stimulation for less than a millisecond is sufficient.

Most modern machines will offer a 'burst' mode (D) in which the pulses will be delivered in bursts or 'trains', usually at a rate of 2–3 bursts per second. Finally, a modulation mode (E) may be available, which employs a method of making the pulse output less regular and therefore minimising the accommodation effects that are often encountered with this type of stimulation.

Machines commonly offer a dual channel output; that is, two pairs of electrodes can be stimulated simultaneously. In some circumstances this can be a distinct advantage, though it is interesting that most patients and therapists tend to use just a single channel application.

The pulses delivered by TENS stimulators vary between manufacturers, but tend to be asymmetrical biphasic modified square wave pulses. The biphasic nature of the pulse means that there is usually no net direct current (DC) component, thus minimising any skin reactions due to build-up of electrolytes under the electrodes.

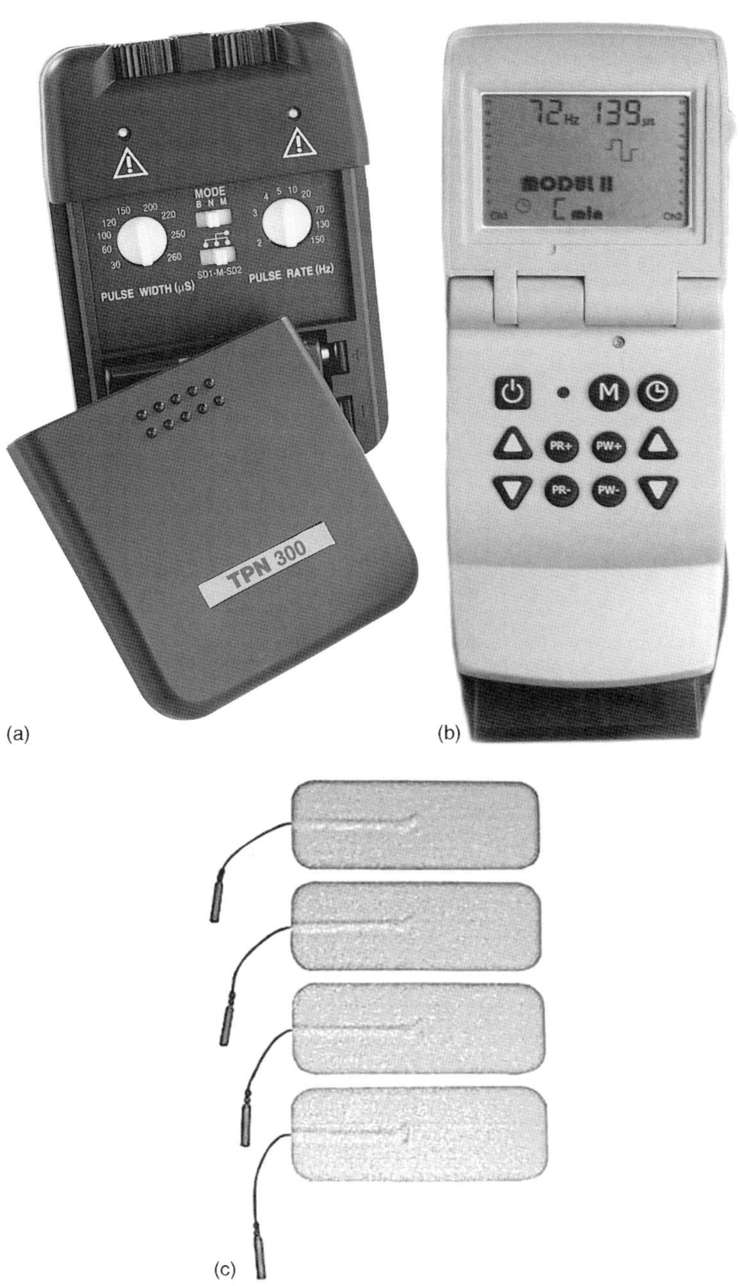

Figure 18.3 TENS machines and electrodes. (a) Analogue TENS (PhysioMed); (b) digital TENS (Nature's Gate); (c) self-adhesive electrodes (SKF).

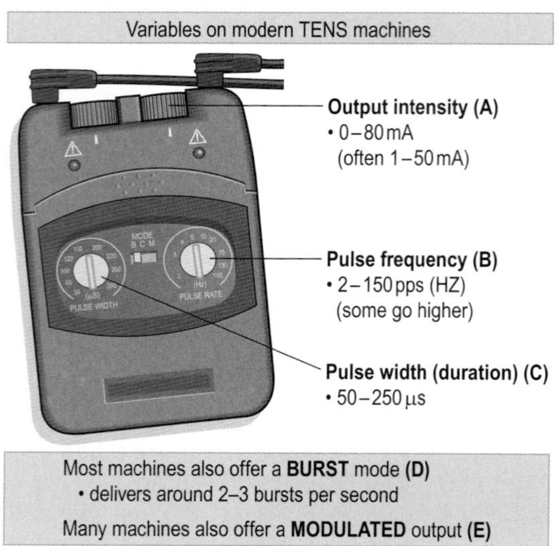

Figure 18.4 Typical analogue TENS machine and treatment settings.

Mechanism of action

The type of stimulation delivered by the TENS unit aims to excite (stimulate) the sensory nerves and, by so doing, activate specific natural pain relief mechanisms. For convenience, we may consider there to be two primary pain relief mechanisms that can be activated: the pain gate mechanism and the endogenous opioid system. The variation in stimulation parameters used to activate these two systems will be briefly considered (see also Chapter 19).

Pain relief by means of the pain gate mechanism primarily involves activation (excitation) of the A-beta (Aβ) sensory fibres, thus reducing the transmission of the noxious stimulus from the 'C' fibres through the spinal cord and on to the higher centres. The A-beta fibres appear to respond preferentially when stimulated at a relatively high rate (in the order of 80 or 90–130 Hz). It is difficult to find support for the concept that there is a single frequency that works best for every patient, but this range appears to cover the majority of individuals (Walsh 1997). This TENS mode is delivered with high-frequency (traditional or normal) TENS.

An alternative approach is to stimulate the A-delta (Aδ) fibres, which respond preferentially to a much lower rate of stimulation (in the order of 2–5 Hz); this will activate the opioid mechanisms and provide pain relief by causing the release of an endogenous opiate (encephalin) in the spinal cord, reducing the activation of the noxious sensory pathways (Walsh 1997; Han et al. 1991; Sluka et al. 2006). This TENS mode is delivered with low-frequency (acupuncture or AcuTENS) TENS.

A third possibility is to stimulate both nerve types at the same time by employing a burst mode stimulation. In this instance, the higher-frequency stimulation output (typically at about 100 Hz) is interrupted (or burst) at the rate of about 2–3 bursts per second. When the machine is 'on', it will deliver pulses at the 100 Hz rate, thereby activating the A-beta fibres and the pain gate mechanism, but by virtue of the rate of the burst, each burst will produce excitation in the A-delta fibres, therefore stimulating the opioid mechanisms. For some patients this is by far the most effective approach to pain relief, though as a sensation, numerous patients find it less acceptable than the other forms of TENS.

Traditional TENS (high TENS, normal TENS)

Usually this uses stimulation at a relatively high frequency (90–130 Hz) and employs a relatively narrow pulse width (often about 100 µs, though, as identified above, there is less support for manipulation of the pulse width in the current research literature and the use of a fixed-pulse duration of around 200 µs may be the most efficient). The stimulation is delivered at 'normal' intensity (see below). A period of 30 minutes is probably the minimally effective time, but it can be delivered for as long as needed. The main pain relief is achieved during the stimulation, with a limited 'carry-over' effect: that is, limited pain relief after the machine has been switched off (Chesterton et al. 2002).

Acupuncture TENS (low TENS, AcuTENS)

TENS is used at a lower stimulation frequency (2–5 Hz) with long-duration pulses (200–250 µs). The intensity employed will usually need to be greater than with traditional TENS — a definite, strong sensation but still one that is not painful (see below). A minimally useful stimulation of 30 minutes should be delivered. It takes some time for opioid levels to build up with this type of TENS and hence the onset of pain relief may be slower than with the traditional mode. Once sufficient opioid has been released, however, it will keep on working after cessation of the stimulation. Many patients find that stimulation at this low frequency at intervals throughout the day is an effective strategy. The 'carry-over' effect may last for several hours in the clinical setting, though time frames of rather more limited duration have been demonstrated by Chesterton et al. (2002).

Brief intense TENS

This is a TENS mode that can be employed to achieve rapid pain relief, but some patients may find the strength of the stimulation too intense and will not tolerate it for sufficient duration to make the treatment worthwhile. The pulse frequency applied is high (in the 90–130 Hz band) and the pulse width is also high (200 μs plus). The current is delivered at or close to the tolerance level for the patient, such that they would not want the machine turned up any higher. In this way, the energy delivery to patients is relatively high when compared with the other approaches. It is suggested that 15–30 minutes at this stimulation level is the most that would normally be used. Pain relief onset is rapid and marked if the patient can cope with the stimulation intensity (Walsh 1997; Sluka and Walsh 2003).

Burst mode TENS

As described above, the machine is set to deliver traditional TENS but the burst mode is switched on, interrupting the stimulation outflow at a rate of 2–3 bursts/second. The stimulation intensity will need to be relatively high, though not as high as in brief intense TENS — more like acupuncture TENS.

Frequency selection

With all of the above mode guides, it is probably inappropriate to identify very specific frequencies that need to be applied to achieve a particular effect. If there was a single frequency that worked for everybody, it would be much easier, but the research does not support this concept. Patients (or therapists) need to identify the most effective frequency for their pain, and manipulation of the stimulation frequency dial or button is the best way to achieve this. Patients who are told to leave the dials alone are less likely to achieve optimal effects. Frequency ranges within which the 'ideal' is likely to be found are identified above.

Stimulation intensity

It is not possible to describe the treatment current strength in terms of how many (milli)amps should be applied. The most effective intensity management appears to be related to what the patient feels during the stimulation, and this may vary from session to session, though it will tend to be fairly consistent for any individual patient. As a general guide, it appears to be effective to go for a 'definitely there but not painful' level for the normal (high) TENS, and a 'strong but not painful' level for the acupuncture (low) mode (Sluka and Walsh 2003). The location of these effective settings is illustrated in Figure 18.5.

Electrode placement

In order to achieve maximal benefit with the modality, target the stimulus at the appropriate spinal cord level (appropriate to the pain). Placing the electrodes on either side of the lesion or pain areas is the most common mechanism employed to achieve this. There are many alternatives that have been researched and found to be effective, most of which are based on the appropriate nerve root level/spinal cord segment:

- stimulation of appropriate nerve root(s)
- stimulation of the peripheral nerve (proximal to the pain)
- stimulation of the motor point (innervated by an appropriate nerve root level)
- stimulation of trigger point(s) or acupuncture point(s)
- stimulation of the appropriate dermatome, myotome or sclerotome.

It is beyond the scope of this chapter to detail specific electrode combinations for specific clinical problems, and it would probably be inappropriate to do so anyway. The TENS literature covers electrode placement in some detail and the interested reader is referred to useful specific texts in this context (Walsh 1997; Johnson 2002).

If the pain source is vague, diffuse or particularly extensive, both channels can be employed simultaneously. A two-channel application can also be effective

18

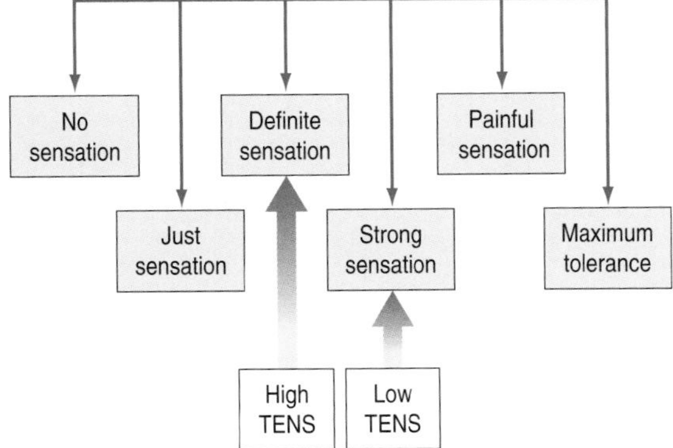

Figure 18.5 Stimulus strength for TENS clinical application.

for the management of a local plus a referred pain combination, with one channel being used for each component. Most standard machines do not allow different stimulation parameters to be set for each channel, though there are some devices that will allow this possibility: for example, channel A on low-frequency opioid setting and channel B on higher-frequency pain gate setting.

Interferential therapy (IFT)

The basic principle of IFT is to utilise the strong physiological effects of low-frequency ($\cong < 250$ pps) electrical stimulation of muscle and nerve tissues without the associated pain encountered with low-frequency stimulation (Palmer and Martin 2002; Watson 2000).

IFT is delivered using either dedicated main-powered interferential devices (Figure 18.6), portable battery-powered devices (Figure 18.7), or multi-mode units that include IFT stimulation amongst several other treatment modes (Figure 18.8).

For the production of low-frequency effects of sufficient intensity at depth, patients may experience considerable discomfort in the superficial tissues (that is, the skin). This is due to the compound impedance of the skin being inversely proportional to the frequency of the stimulation. The lower the stimulation frequency, the greater the resistance to the passage of the current, and so more discomfort is experi-enced. The skin impedance at 50 Hz is approximately 3200 Ω whilst at 4000 Hz it is reduced to approximately 40 Ω. The result of applying this higher frequency is that it will pass more easily through the skin, requiring less electrical energy input to reach the deeper tissues and giving rise to less discomfort.

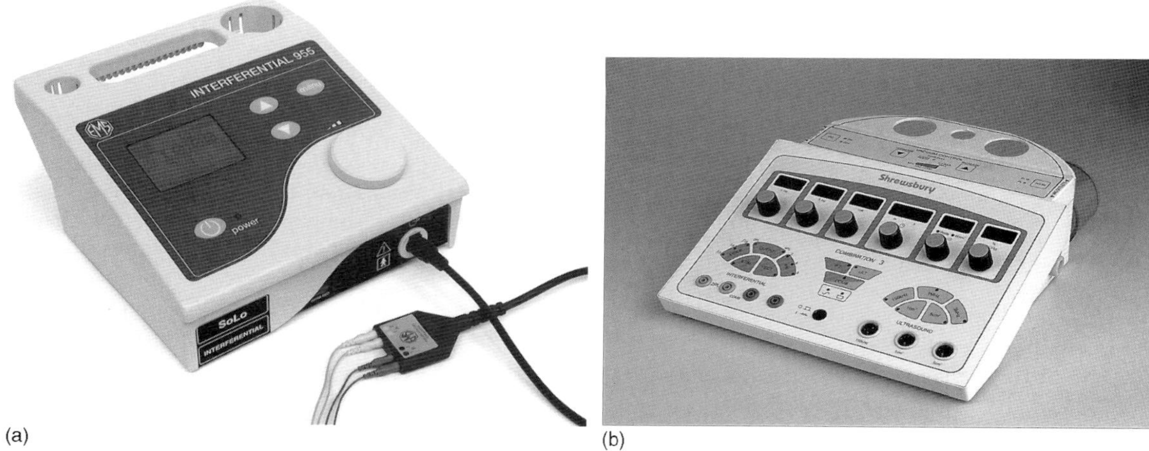

(a) (b)

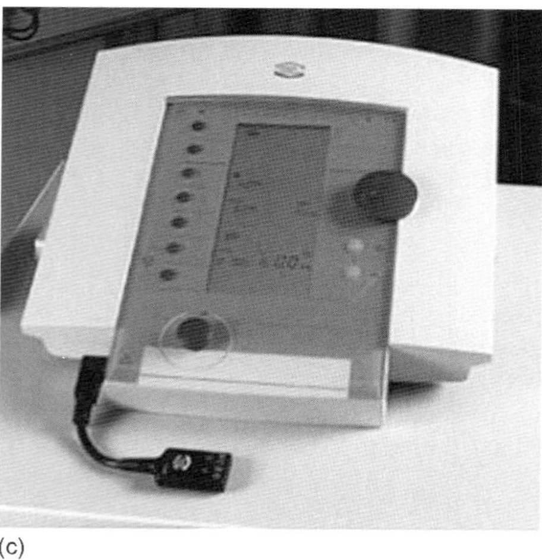

(c)

Figure 18.6 Mains-powered dedicated interferential devices. (a) EMS IFT device; (b) Shrewsbury IFT device (CME); (c) Enraf IFT device (Mobilis).

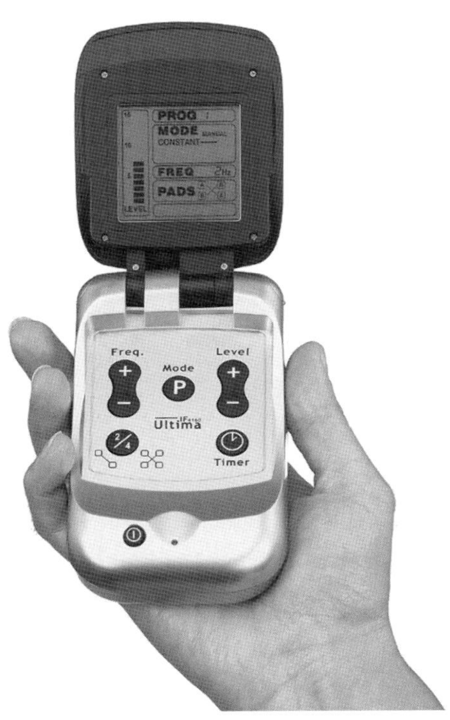

Figure 18.7 Portable (battery-powered) IFT device: Portable IFT (Tenscare).

The effects of tissue stimulation with these 'medium-frequency' currents (medium frequency in electromedical terms usually being considered as 1 KHz–100 KHz) are not fully understood; and while there is likely to be an effect, little detail is currently known, though medium-frequency currents are assumed not to stimulate nerve directly.

IFT utilises two of these medium-frequency currents, passed through the tissues simultaneously; they are set up so that their paths cross and they literally interfere with each other. This interference gives rise to an interference (beat frequency) that has the characteristics of low-frequency stimulation; in effect, the interference mimics a low-frequency stimulation.

The exact frequency of the resultant interference (or beat frequency) can be controlled by the input frequencies. If, for example, one current were at 4000 Hz and its companion current at 3900 Hz, the resultant beat frequency would be at 100 Hz, carried on a medium-frequency 3950 Hz amplitude modulated current (Figure 18.9).

By careful manipulation of the input currents it is possible to achieve any beat frequency that is needed clinically. Modern machines usually offer beat frequencies of 1–150 Hz, though some offer a choice of up to 250 Hz or more. Some machines offer a range of 'carrier' frequencies: that is, other than 4000 Hz. The evidence would suggest that the higher the carrier frequency, the less discomfort will be experienced by the patient; therefore, where there is a choice, the higher carrier frequency should be employed.

The use of two-pole IFT stimulation is made possible by electronic manipulation of the currents. The interference occurs within the machine instead of in the tissues. There is no known physiological difference between the effects of IFT produced with two- or four-electrode systems. The key difference is that, with a four-pole application, the interference is generated in the tissues, and with a two-pole treatment, the current is 'pre-modulated': that is, the interference is generated within the machine unit.

Whichever way it is generated, the treatment effect is generated from low-frequency stimulation, primarily involving the peripheral nerves. Low-frequency nerve stimulation is physiologically effective (as with TENS and NMES) and this is the key to IFT intervention.

Frequency sweep

Nerves will accommodate to a constant signal and a sweep (or gradually changing frequency) is often used to overcome this problem. The principle of using the sweep is that the machine is set to vary the effective stimulation frequency automatically using either pre-set or user-set sweep ranges. The sweep range employed should be appropriate to the desired physiological effects (see below). It has been repeatedly demonstrated that 'wide' sweep ranges are ineffective in the clinical environment. The clinical advantage of the sweep treatment application, beyond that of minimising the accommodation effects, is that a range of treatment frequencies can be automatically applied (Watson 2000).

> ***Key point***
> Care needs to be taken when setting the sweep on a machine in that, with some devices, the user sets the actual base and top frequencies (e.g. 90 and 130 Hz) and, with other machines, the user sets the base frequency and then how much needs to be added for the sweep (e.g. 90 and 40 Hz).

The pattern of the sweep makes a significant difference to the stimulation received by the patient. Most machines offer several sweep patterns, though there is very limited 'evidence' to justify some of these options. In the classic 'triangular' sweep pattern, the machine gradually changes from the base to the top frequency, usually over a time period of 6 seconds — though some machines also offer 1- or 3-second options. In the example illustrated (Figure 18.10), the machine is set to sweep

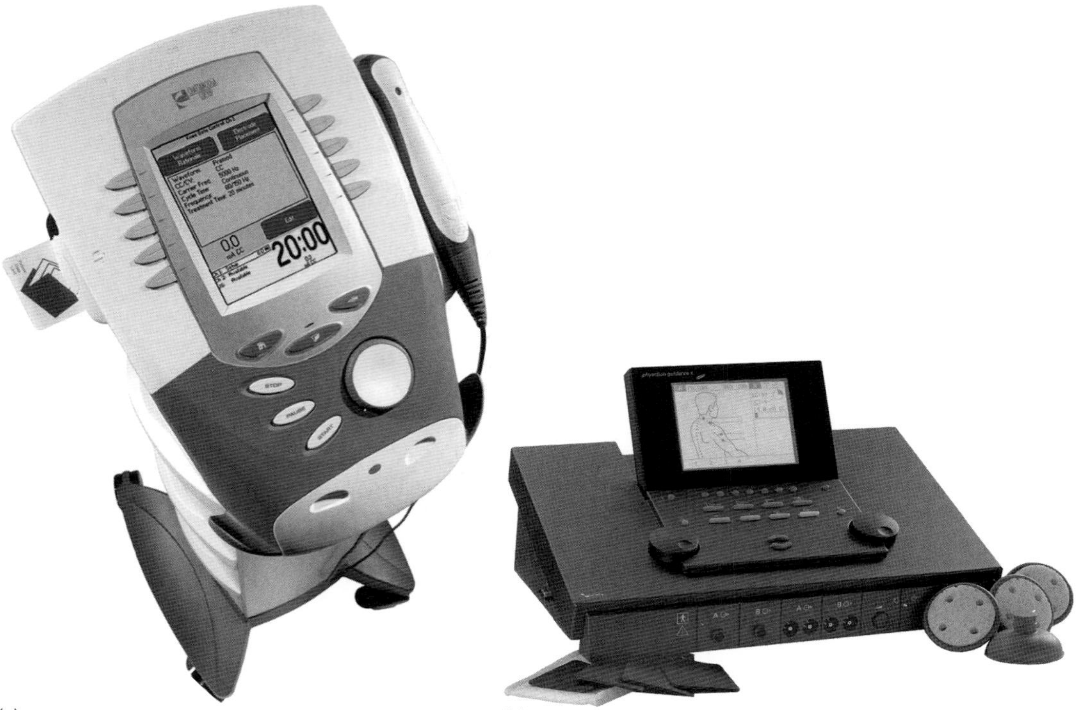

(a) (b)

Figure 18.8 Multi-mode units that include IFT. (a) Chatanooga Intelect System (SKF); (b) Uniphy Guidance (CME).

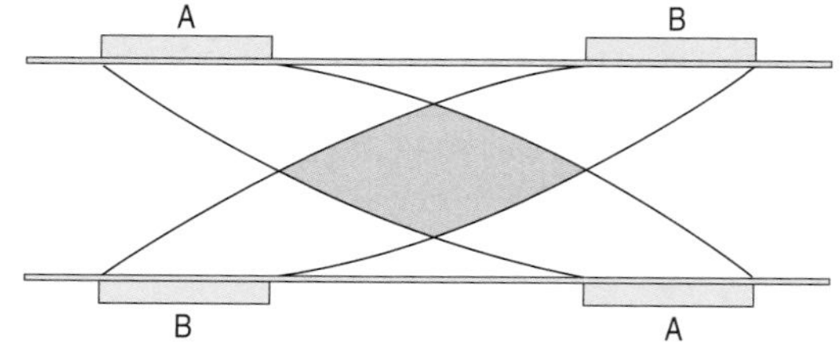

Figure 18.9 Basic principles of interferential current production. Current 'A' is at 4000 Hz and current 'B' is at 3900 Hz. Interference current (beat frequency) is generated in the central zone at the difference between input currents, which would be 100 Hz.

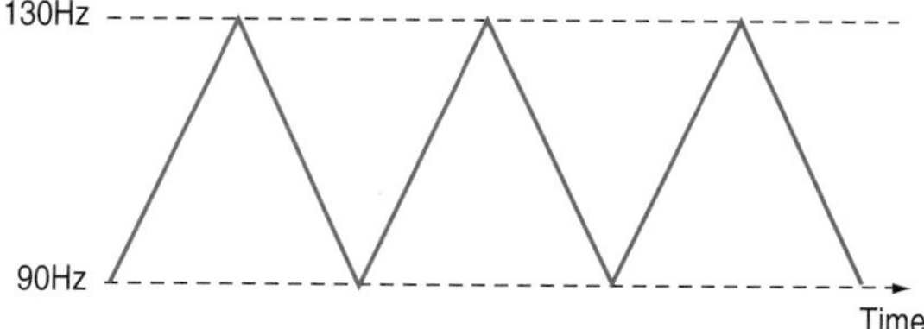

Figure 18.10 90–130 Hz triangular frequency sweep pattern with IFT.

from 90 to 130 Hz, employing a triangular sweep pattern. All frequencies between the base and top frequencies are delivered in equal proportion.

Other patterns of sweep can be produced on many machines: for example, a rectangular (or step) sweep. This produces a very different stimulation pattern in that the base and top frequencies are set, but the machine then 'switches' between these two specific frequencies rather than gradually changing from one to the other. Figure 18.11 illustrates the effect of setting a 90–130 Hz rectangular sweep.

There is a clear difference between these examples, even though the same 'numbers' are set. One will deliver a full range of stimulation frequencies between the set frequency levels and the other will switch from one frequency to the other. There are numerous other variations on this theme, and the 'trapezoidal' sweep (Figure 18.12) is effectively a combination of these two.

The only sweep pattern for which 'evidence' appears to exist is the triangular sweep. The others

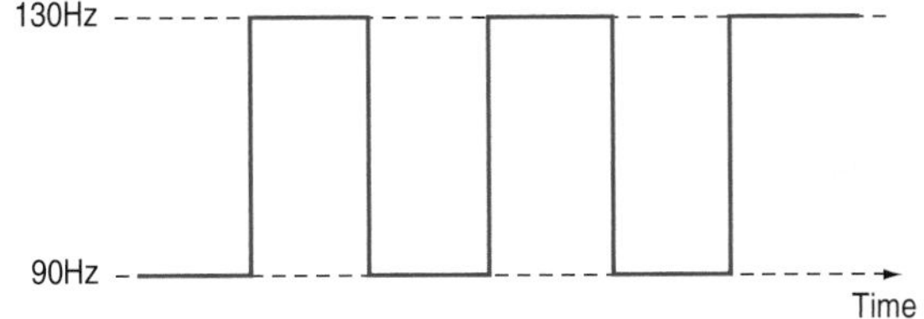

Figure 18.11 90–130 Hz rectangular frequency sweep pattern with IFT.

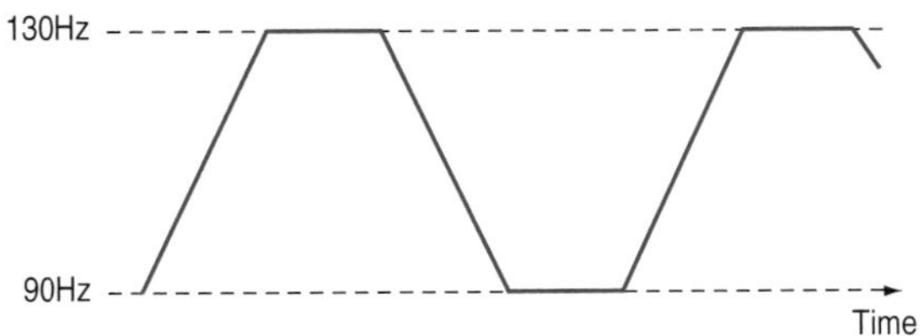

Figure 18.12 90–130 Hz trapezoidal frequency sweep pattern with IFT.

are perfectly safe to use, but whether they are clinically effective or not remains to be shown.

Physiological effects and clinical applications

It has been suggested that IFT works in a 'special way' because it is 'interferential', as opposed to 'normal' stimulation. The evidence for this special effect is lacking and it is most likely that IFT is just another means by which peripheral nerves can be stimulated. Many patients regard it as more acceptable than other forms of electrical stimulation because it generates less (skin) discomfort.

The clinical application of IFT is based on peripheral nerve stimulation (frequency) data, though it is important to note that much of this information has been generated from research with other modalities, and its transfer to IFT is assumed rather than proven. There is a lack of IFT-specific research compared with other modalities such as TENS and NMES.

The are four main clinical applications for which IFT appears to be used:

- pain relief
- muscle stimulation
- increased local blood flow
- reduction of oedema.

In addition, claims are made for its role in stimulating healing and repair, though these are not specifically covered in this section. As IFT acts primarily on nerve, the strongest effects are likely to be those that are a direct result of such stimulation (that is, pain relief and muscle stimulation). The other effects are more likely to be secondary consequences of these.

Pain relief

Electrical stimulation for pain relief has widespread clinical use, though the direct research evidence for the use of IFT in this role is limited. Logically, one could use the higher frequencies (90–130 Hz) to stimulate the pain gate mechanisms and thereby mask pain symptoms. Alternatively, stimulation with lower frequencies (2–5 Hz) can be used to activate the opioid mechanisms, again providing a degree of relief. These two different modes of action can be explained physiologically and will have different latent periods and varying duration of effect (as for TENS). It remains possible that relief of pain may be achieved by stimulation of the reticular formation at frequencies of 10–25 Hz or by blocking 'c' fibre transmission at $>$ 50 Hz. Although both of these latter mechanisms have been proposed with IFT, neither has been categorically demonstrated (Palmer and Martin 2002).

A good number of recent studies (e.g. Hurley et al. 2004; Johnson and Tabasam 2003; Walker et al. 2006; McManus et al. 2006; Jorge et al. 2006) provide substantive evidence for a pain relief effect of IFT.

Muscle stimulation

Stimulation of the motor nerves can be achieved with a wide range of frequencies. Clearly, stimulation at low frequency (e.g. 1 Hz) will result in a series of twitches, whist stimulation at 50 Hz will result in a tetanic contraction. There is limited evidence at present for the 'strengthening' effect of IFT, though this evidence exists for some other forms of electrical stimulation and the paper by Bircan et al. (2002) suggests that it might be a possibility for IFT. On the basis of the current evidence, the contraction brought about by IFT is no 'better' than would be achieved by active exercise, though there are clinical circumstances where assisted contraction is beneficial: for example, to assist the patient to appreciate the muscle work required (similar to surged Faradism, as used in the past — but much less uncomfortable). For patients who cannot generate useful voluntary contraction, IFT may be beneficial, as it would be for those who, for whatever reason, find active exercise difficult. There is no evidence that has demonstrated a significant benefit of IFT over active exercise. The choice of treatment parameters will depend on the desired effect. The most effective motor nerve stimulation range with IFT appears to lie between approximately 10 and 20 or maybe 25 Hz.

Caution should be exercised when employing IFT as a means of generating clinical levels of muscle contraction in that the muscle will continue to work for the duration of the stimulation period (assuming sufficient current strength is applied). It is possible to continue to stimulate the muscle beyond its point of fatigue and short stimulation periods with adequate rest are probably a preferable option. Some IFT devices are capable of generating a 'surged' stimulation mode, which might be advantageous in that fatigue would be minimised. This surged intervention would be similar to but more comfortable than Faradism.

Blood flow

There is very little, if any, quality evidence demonstrating a direct effect of IFT on local blood flow changes. Most of the work that has been done involves laboratory experimentation on animals or asymptomatic subjects, and most blood flow measurements are superficial: that is, skin blood flow. Whether IFT is actually capable of generating a change (increase) in blood flow at depth remains questionable. The elegant experimentation by Noble et al. (2000) demonstrated vascular changes at 10–20 Hz, though it was unable to identify the mechanism for this change clearly. The stimulation was applied via suction electrodes, and the outcome could therefore be a result of the suction rather than the electrical stimulation, though this is largely negated by virtue of the fact that other stimulation frequencies were also delivered via the suction electrodes without significant flow changes. The most likely mechanism is via muscle stimulation effects (IFT causing muscle contraction, which brings about a local metabolic and thus vascular change). The theory that the IFT is acting as an inhibitor of sympathetic activity remains a theoretical possibility rather than an established mechanism.

Based on current available evidence, the most likely option for IFT use as a means to increase local blood flow remains via the muscle stimulation mode, and thus the 10–20 Hz or 10–25 Hz frequency sweep option appears to be preferable.

Oedema

IFT has been claimed to be effective as a treatment to promote the reabsorption of oedema in the tissues. Again, the evidence is very limited in this respect and the physiological mechanism by which it could be achieved as a direct effect of the IFT remains to be established. The preferable clinical option, in light of the available evidence, is to use IFT to bring about local muscle contraction(s); combined with local vascular changes, thiscould be effective in encouraging the reabsorption of tissue fluid. The use of suction electrodes may be beneficial, but also remains unproven in this respect.

A study by Jarit et al. (2003) demonstrated a change in oedema following knee surgery in an IFT group, though the Christie and Willoughby study (1990) failed to demonstrate a significant benefit on ankle oedema following fracture and surgery. The treatment parameters employed are unlikely to be effective, given the information now available. If IFT has a capacity to influence oedema, current evidence and physiological knowledge would suggest that a combination of pain relief (allowing more movement), muscle stimulation (above) and enhanced local blood flow (above) is most likely to be effective.

Treatment parameters

Stimulation can be applied using several different electrode systems (Figures 18.13–18.15). Pad electrodes and sponge covers are commonly employed, though

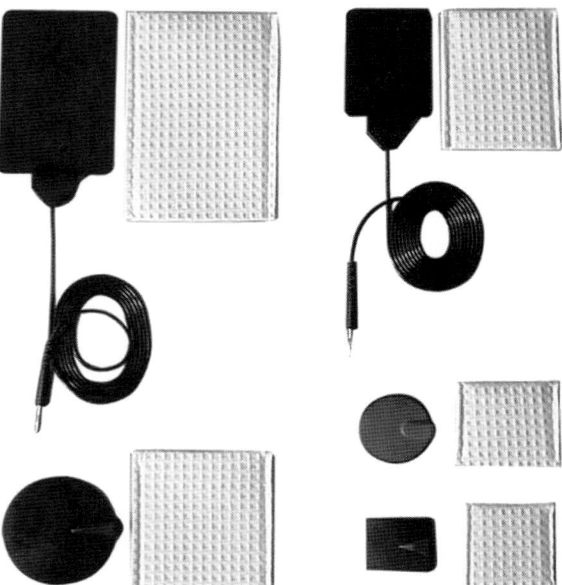

Figure 18.13 IFT rubber and sponge pad electrode system (SKF).

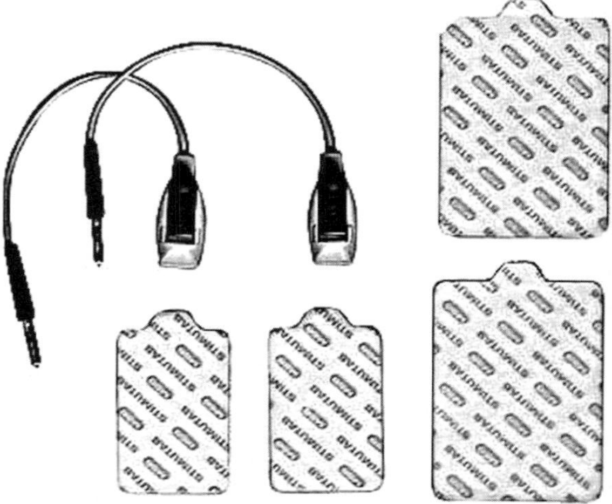

Figure 18.14 Self-adhesive, pre-gelled IFT electrodes (SKF).

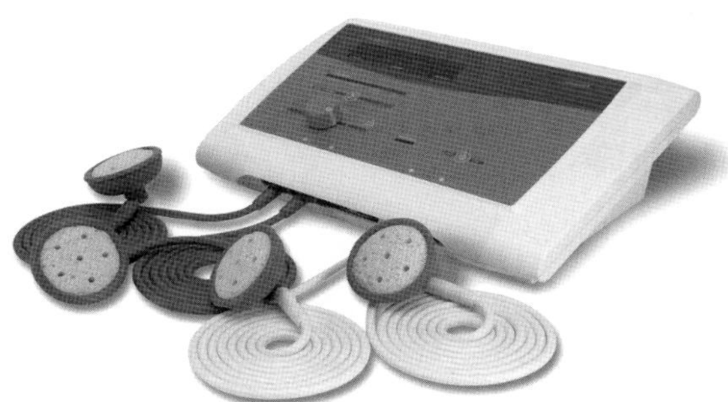

Figure 18.15 IFT vacuum electrode system (PhysioMed).

electroconductive gel is an effective alternative. The sponges should be thoroughly wet to ensure even current distribution. Self-adhesive pad electrodes are also available (similar to the newer TENS electrodes) and make IFT application easier in the view of many practitioners. The suction electrode application method has been in use for several years, and whilst it is useful, especially for larger body areas like the shoulder girdle, trunk, hip and knee, it does not appear to provide any therapeutic advantage over pad electrodes. Care should be taken with regard to maintenance of electrodes, electrode covers and associated infection risks (Lambert et al. 2000).

Electrode positioning should ensure adequate coverage of the area for stimulation. In some circumstances, a bipolar method is preferable if a longitudinal zone requires stimulation rather than an isolated tissue area. Placement of the electrodes should be such that a cross-over effect is achieved in the desired area (when using the four-pole application).

Treatment times vary widely, according to the usual clinical parameters of acute/chronic conditions and the type of physiological effect desired. In acute conditions, shorter treatment times of 10 minutes may be sufficient to achieve an effect. In other circumstances, it may be necessary to stimulate the tissues for 20–30 minutes. It is suggested that short treatment times are initially adopted, especially with the acute case, because of the possibility of symptom exacerbation. The times can be progressed if the aim has not been achieved and no untoward side-effects have been produced. There is no research evidence to support the continuous progression of a treatment dose in order to increase or maintain its effect.

Muscle stimulation modalities

Historically, motor nerve stimulation in order to generate muscle contraction was a commonly employed modality, most usually in the form of Faradism. More recently, this intervention has become somewhat 'out of favour'. There are, in fact, still circumstances where it could be of significant benefit, but in clinical practice, using IFT (preferably in a surged mode) is probably a more effective means to the same end.

There has been a significant increase in the use of portable or mains-powered muscle stimulators, which are effectively the modern replacement for Faradism. Figure 18.16 illustrates some examples of dedicated battery-powered and multimodal mains-powered devices.

There is a growing range of chronic (meaning 'not short-term') electrical stimulation devices that are aimed at stimulating the motor nerve and hence bringing about muscle activity/contraction. This form of therapy goes by several names, but those most commonly applied are neuromuscular electrical stimulation (NMES), chronic NMES and neuromuscular stimulation (NMS). NMES is probably the preferred generic term.

A growing body of evidence suggests that gains in strength, endurance capacity and function can be achieved with these types of stimulation. Much of the early work has been conducted in laboratory studies and also with athletes rather than typical patient groups. There are recent papers, however, that have demonstrated significant clinical benefit with patient groups, including strengthening of peripheral musculature (Callaghan and Oldham 2004; Lyons et al. 2005; Stevens et al. 2004; Talbot et al. 2003), work with shoulder problems in stroke patients (Ada and Foongchomcheay 2002; Chantraine et al. 1999), COPD/cardiac patients (Neder et al. 2002; Vivodtzev et al. 2006; Zanotti et al. 2003) and various forms of incontinence (Amaro et al. 2003; Barroso et al. 2004; Indrekvam et al. 2001). Useful reviews of this field of intervention are included in McDonough (2002), Robertson et al. (2006) and Lake (1992).

So-called functional electrical stimulation (or FES) constitutes a further branch of neuromuscular-based stimulation. In this branch of electrotherapy, the explicit intent of the stimulation is to achieve controlled muscle activation in order to facilitate some aspect of functional activity. The range of applications is growing swiftly, especially with recent advances in computer-controlled stimulators. One of the early and most successful areas is the dropped foot stimulator (Taylor et al. 1999; Sheffler et al. 2006), which assists patients — most often following a stroke — to achieve ankle dorsiflexion during the swing phase of gait utilising stimulation of the anterior tibial nerve (Figure 18.17). Modern devices incorporate a range of foot switches or pressure detectors, which enable stimulation to be active at exactly the right part of the gait cycle. Other forms of FES include standing and gross walking activity with paraplegic patients, which is also making significant gains with computerised control systems.

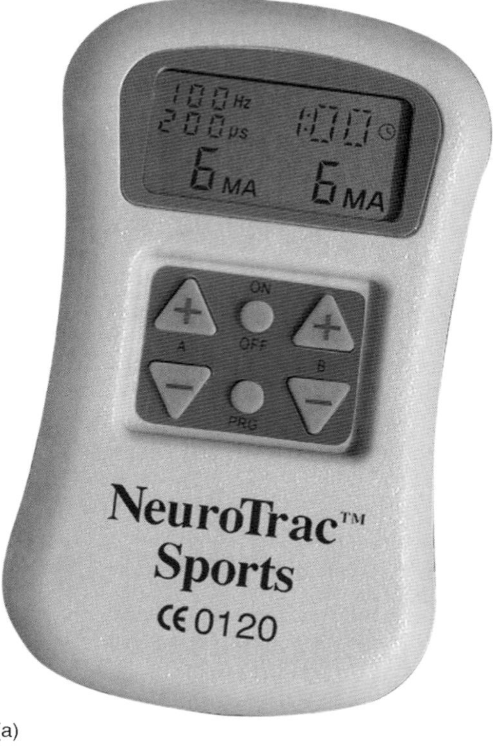

(a)

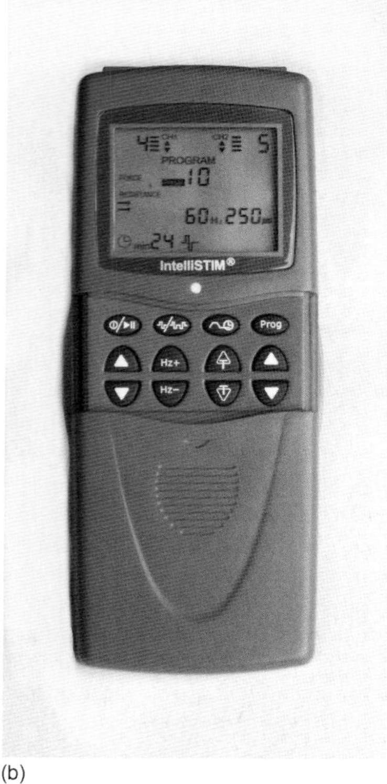

(b)

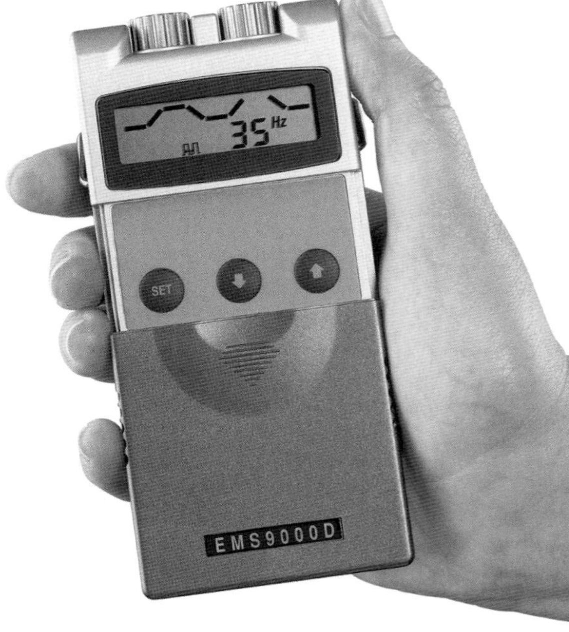

(c)

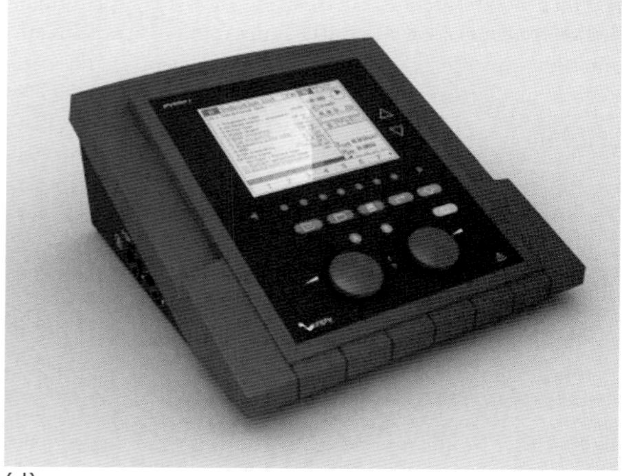

(d)

Figure 18.16 Battery-powered (portable) muscle stimulators are shown in (a)–(c), and a multimodal mains-powered device that will deliver muscle-stimulating currents in (d). (a) NeuroTrac Sports (SKF); (b) IntelliSTIM (Natures Gate); (c) DigiStim (PhysioMed); (d) Phyaction Multimodal system (CME).

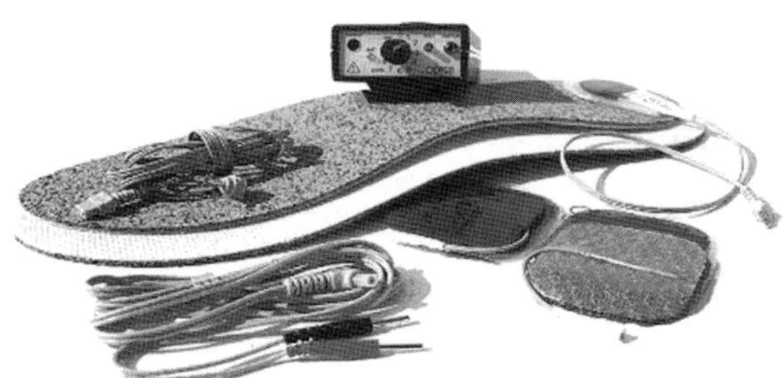

Figure 18.17 Odstock dropped foot stimulator. The Salisbury ODFS111 stimulator, inner soles, foot switch, electrode pads and leads. The stimulator is a single-channel device designed primarily for gait assist. (Courtesy of the Department of Clinical Science and Engineering, Salisbury District Hospital, UK.)

Other forms of electrical stimulation

There are probably more 'new' electrical stimulation-type devices that come out in a year than new equipment in any other area of electrotherapy. Many of them are actually based on one of the three main areas identified in the previous sections (TENS, IFT or NMES), though there are, of course, machines that do indeed deliver a 'different' form of stimulation; others are simply a variation on a theme — or a combination of themes. Examples of other electrical stimulation modalities in clinical use would be:

- *Russian stimulation*: burst-modulated medium-frequency current used primarily for muscle stimulation
- *H wave therapy*: twin-pulse low-frequency stimulation used for pain relief and oedema reduction
- *Diadynamic currents*: rectified and or modulated low-frequency stimulation used for pain relief and muscle stimulation
- *Iontophoresis*: DC or pulsed DC employed to promote the movement of chemical agents across the skin.

In addition, combination therapy involves the simultaneous delivery of ultrasound and IFT, and thereby achieving the effects of both modalities, although there is no evidence that any additional effects will occur by using this combination approach. Ultrasound is sometimes combined with other electrical stimulation modes (e.g. Diadynamic currents, TENS).

Microcurrent therapy is probably worth a mention, if for no other reason than it appears to break all the 'rules' that were identified earlier in this chapter. It is not delivered with the intention of stimulating nerve, but rather plays to the bioelectric environment of the tissues, and therefore has a primary effect in terms of tissue repair (Watson 2006b). The general characteristics of this type of therapy are that it utilises a direct current, pulsed or continuous, delivered at a very low amplitude (literally in the microamperage range), which is subsensory from the patient perspective. This type of therapy has already been shown to be effective in several clinical areas, most notably fracture repair (Ciombor and Aaron 2005; Simonis et al. 2003) and healing of open wounds (Evans et al. 2001; Watson 1996, 2002b); soft tissue repair research is now evolving and has shown strong future potential.

It is not possible in a general chapter such as this to identify all possible combinations and variations. The interested reader might try investigating the major texts in the area (Robertson et al. 2006; Kitchen 2002a), reading the current literature (though many of these 'new' devices are yet to have specific research published as regards their efficacy), or utilising a Web-based resource (though, as with any Web-based material, one needs to be both critical and selective with regard to the information accepted).

THERMAL MODALITIES

Introduction

Thermal-based treatments have been popular in the past but have somewhat lost favour in more recent times, being considered old-fashioned and ineffective. There is little doubt that the application of heat to the body tissues generates significant physiological effects (Lehmann 1982; Michlovitz 1996; Kitchen 2002a). Applied with good reason and utilising the appropriate forms of thermal energy (contact or induction methods), it is capable of being useful in therapy.

General principles of thermal treatments

The general principles of heat transfer to the body are well covered in the standard texts and only a brief summary will be included here. Essentially, thermal energy can be applied by using contact methods (hydrocollator or hot packs, wax therapy), by using radiant heat sources (infrared) or by applying electromagnetic energy that is absorbed in the tissues, resulting in heat generation (e.g. shortwave and microwave therapies).

Some modalities (e.g. laser and ultrasound) can generate heating effects if applied at sufficient energy levels, but these modalities appear to be more effective in the clinical environment when applied at 'non-thermal' levels.

Therapeutic effects of heating therapies

The effects of tissue heating can be effectively described in general terms rather than repeating the same information in subsequent sections. These effects are described and evidenced in much more detail in specialist texts

(Lehmann 1982; Kitchen 2002a; Michlovitz 1996), but are summarised below for quick reference. Those effects listed are considered to be local rather than systemic. Systemic effects are usually minor in relation to the therapeutic application of heat, and are detailed in the same sources as identified above.

The effects of tissue heating are, then:

- increased metabolic activity of cells/tissues
- increased local blood flow (volume)
- increased collagen extensibility
- reduction in local muscle tone
- reduced pain perception
- (possible) increased rate of tissue healing (almost certainly a secondary effect).

Infrared radiation

Infrared is one of the least used heat modalities in modern practice. Radiation is delivered using luminous (combined infrared and visible red radiation) or non-luminous (infrared only) sources. Whichever is employed, the effective penetration depth of the electromagnetic energy is a matter of 1 or 1.5 mm at best, and hence this is a very superficial form of heating. It is argued that, even though the heat is generated in superficial tissues only, the effect in terms of pain relief is significant, as many sensory nerve endings are found in these tissues; when these are stimulated, they can be used to achieve pain relief by means of the pain gate mechanism. Furthermore, the heating of superficial tissues gives rise to local increases in blood flow, which can in turn induce a reduction in pain by increasing the absorption of inflammatory metabolites, decreasing local muscle spasm, encouraging the reabsorption of oedema and possibly increasing tissue repair by means of metabolic stimulation. Whether these effects are of sufficient magnitude to be of clinical value remains controversial, though there is little doubt that the local application of such superficial heat does give rise to pain relief and the patient will often report valuable pain relief as a result (Kitchen and Partridge 1991; Kitchen 2002a).

Wax therapy

In a similar way to infrared therapy, wax therapy has become far less widely used than in the past. It does, however, still have some specialist applications, most notably in hand therapy and peripheral nerve lesion rehabilitation (Brosseau et al. 2002).

In principle, melted wax is applied to the part to be treated using a 'dunk' technique, in which the hand or foot (for example) is repeatedly dipped into a bath of molten wax at around 45–50 degrees C, each layer of wax being allowed to cool slightly before the next is applied. Alternatively, the wax can be applied using a bandage application or ladled on to the part to be treated.

As the wax solidifies from its melted state, thermal energy is released (latent heat), which is subsequently transferred to the superficial tissues. Tissue temperatures can be raised by a useful 3–4 degrees C to a possible depth of up to 2 cm, thereby providing a 'deeper' treatment effect than infrared therapy, for example.

In addition to the direct heating effect, it is argued that the deeper tissues will also heat up as a result of the conduction of thermal energy from the superficial tissues. The applied wax also contains a variety of oils, and these have beneficial effects in terms of improving skin condition and facilitating exercise and massage therapies that usually follow the wax treatment.

It is suggested that a similar heating level can be achieved in the tissues using a hot pack (see below) or hot water immersion, but many patients find that the application of therapeutic wax has perceived benefits over and above the heat part of the treatment, and will certainly prefer it as a form of therapy to other forms of heating. This appears to be especially true for patients with long-term or chronic conditions, low-grade, chronic inflammatory conditions and non-acute degenerative joint problems.

Further details are available in most standard electrotherapy or thermal therapy texts (Robertson et al. 2006; Kitchen 2002a; Lehmann 1982; Michlovitz 1996).

Hot packs

Hot packs used in therapy go by several names, but are most commonly called hydrocollator packs or simply hot packs. This type of heat application is sometimes referred to as 'moist' heat, in that the pack is heated by immersion in hot (70 degrees C) water to bring the pack up to therapeutic temperature. The pack (Figure 18.18) is wrapped, typically in towelling, prior to being placed against the skin of the patient. The skin surface temperature of the pack will be significantly lower than

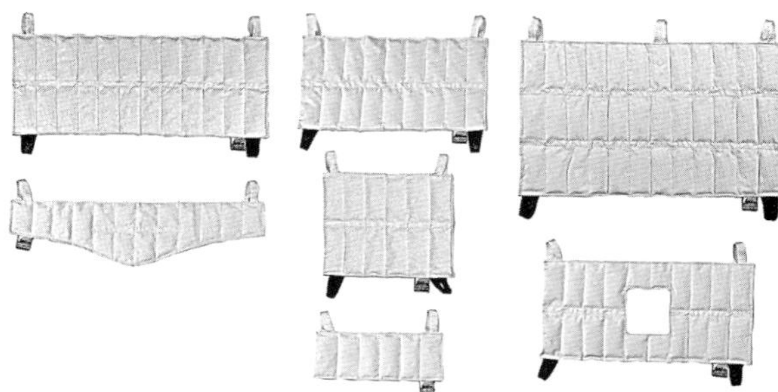

Figure 18.18 Hydrocollator treatment packs in various forms (PhysioMed).

70 degrees C due to the insulating nature of the towels, which are essential.

Key point

Hot packs should never be applied directly to the skin surface.

The tissue temperature rises associated with hot pack therapy are of sufficient magnitude to achieve changes in the 'therapeutic range' (Lehmann 1982), and will produce sufficient heating to be of clinical value down to a depth or 2–3 cm at least.

Treatment durations of 15–20 minutes appear to be clinically effective and the rise in tissue temperature will achieve effects in common with other thermal modalities.

Shortwave and microwave diathermy

Both continuous shortwave diathermy (SWD) and certainly microwave diathermy (MWD) have shown a significant reduction in clinical popularity in recent years (Pope et al. 1995). Recent surveys have shown that almost no departments in the UK routinely use microwave diathermy, and most departments and practices do not even have the machines available. Continuous shortwave, once a highly utilised modality, has also undergone a reduction in clinical use, though many departments do still have the equipment available (Al Mandeel and Watson 2006).

Both modalities bring about tissue heating by means of the introduction of electromagnetic energy into the tissues, and tissue temperature rises occur as a result of increased molecular activity. It is an indirect form of heating (as opposed to conductive-type heating previously described).

SWD utilises high-frequency (around 27 MHz) electromagnetic energy, which is applied using either capacitor plate-type electrodes or a monode/drum applicator. Although attached to the same treatment unit, each of these electrode types brings about heating in a slightly different way, and importantly, there is a fundamental difference in the types of tissue in which the heat is produced.

The interested reader is referred to the detail in electrotherapy texts, but in summary, the capacitor plate-type application results in high-frequency energy being delivered to the tissues (electrostatic), the dissipation of this energy being primarily in the tissues of high impedance; thus a very high proportion of the heating effect is generated in the skin, fat and other 'insulating' superficial tissues. The previous claim that this was a deep form of heating is questionable, and in terms of current clinical application, its demise is probably appropriate.

The alternative mode of application employs the monode or drum applicator (as per pulsed shortwave). The energy delivered from this type of applicator is effectively an electromagnetic (as opposed to electrostatic) field, oscillating at high frequency. The delivered energy is primarily absorbed in tissues of low impedance (such as muscle, nerve or tissue where there is significant water content), and it is here that the most significant heating effects are achieved.

It is suggested that, when applying continuous shortwave in the clinical environment with the deliberate intention of heating the tissues, the monode or drum applicator should routinely be used unless the primary tissue in which the heating is desired is the skin or superficial fat layers.

NON-THERMAL MODALITIES

Introduction

There has been significant debate in more recent years as to the potential for various electrotherapy modalities to have their primary mode of action by 'non-thermal' means. There is a growing body of evidence that supports the contention that it is not necessary to provide sufficient energy actually to 'heat' the tissues in order to generate therapeutic benefit. Modalities such as ultrasound, shortwave, laser and microwave therapies, when applied at sufficiently low intensity, appear to bring about significant clinical effects without generating perceptible thermal change. This is a difficult area, as when any energy is delivered to the body and absorbed in sufficient quantity, there will be a thermal effect. What is generally meant by the clinical term 'non-thermal' is that neither the patient nor the therapist is able to detect any significant temperature change.

Various authors have argued that the therapeutic benefits of generating tissue 'stimulation' without overt heating are advantageous in many circumstances (Watson 2000, 2006a; Kitchen and Dyson 2002). This is not to denigrate the therapeutic benefits of heating as a therapeutic tool, but rather to add a non-thermal aspect. Clearly, all the modalities identified in this section *could* generate significant heating if applied at sufficient levels. Their application, as described here, is in the clinically non-thermal mode.

Therapeutic ultrasound (US)

US therapy is one of the most commonly employed electrophysical treatment in many countries. Both mains-powered and battery treatment units are available; additionally, it is reasonably common to find US as one modality offered on multimodal electrotherapy machines (Figure 18.19).

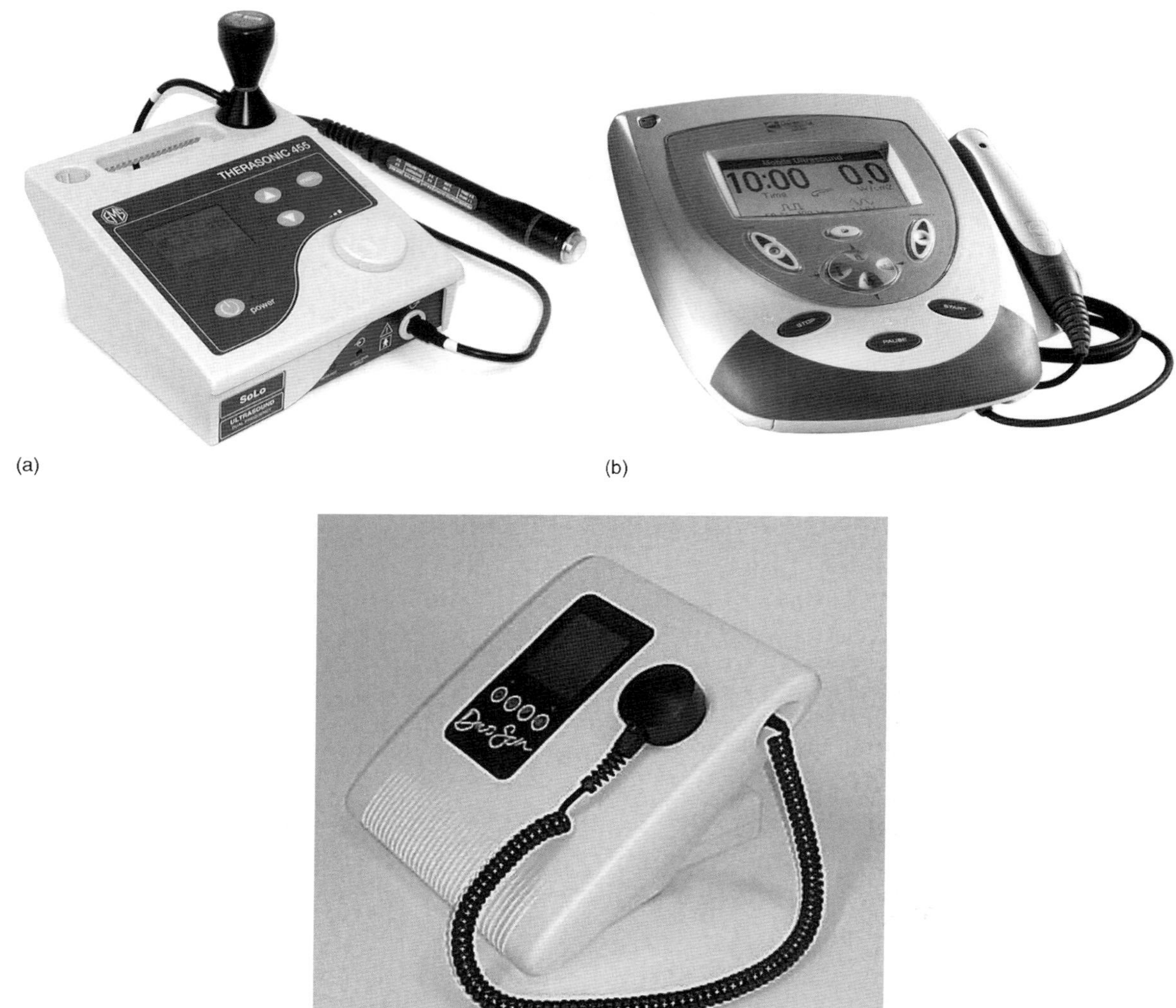

Figure 18.19 Examples of clinical ultrasound therapy machines. (a) EMS US machines; (b) Chatanooga Portable US device (SKF); (c) long-wave US machine (Orthosonics).

US is a form of mechanical (vibration) energy and vibration at increasing frequencies is known as sound energy. The normal human sound range is from 16 Hz to something approaching 15–20 000 Hz. Beyond this upper limit, the mechanical vibration is known as ultrasound. The frequencies used in therapy are typically between 1.0 and 3.0 MHz (1 MHz = 1 million cycles per second) and is clearly beyond the human sound detection range. Some therapy devices offer application frequencies at other rates: for example, 1.5 MHz, 0.75 MHz and long-wave ultrasound devices that operate in the kilohertz range (for example, 48 kHz and 150 kHz). The effect of long-wave ultrasound is beyond the scope of this section, which will concentrate on 'traditional' US.

Sound waves are longitudinal waves consisting of zones of compression and rarefaction. Particles of a material, when exposed to a sound wave, will oscillate about a fixed point. Clearly, any increase in the molecular vibration in the tissue can result in heat generation, and US can be used to produce thermal changes in the tissues, though current usage in therapy does not focus on this phenomenon (Baker et al. 2001; ter Haar 1999;

Nussbaum 1997; Watson 2000). In addition to thermal changes, the vibration of the tissues has effects that are considered to be 'non-thermal' in nature, though, as with other modalities, there must be a thermal component, however small. As the US wave passes through a material (the tissues), the energy levels within the wave will diminish as energy is transferred to the material.

Ultrasound transmission through the tissues

All materials (tissues) will present impedance to the passage of sound waves. The specific impedance of a tissue will be determined by its density and elasticity. In order for the maximal transmission of energy from one medium to another to occur, the impedance of the two media needs to be as similar as possible. The greater the difference in impedance at a boundary, the greater the reflection that will occur, and therefore, the smaller the amount of energy that will be transferred.

The difference in impedance is greatest for the steel/air interface, which is the first one that US has to overcome in order to reach the tissues. To minimise this difference, a suitable coupling medium has to be utilised. If even a small air gap exists between the transducer and the skin, the proportion of US which will be reflected approaches 99.998 per cent, which in effect means that there will be no transmission.

The coupling media used in this context include water, various oils, creams and gels. Ideally, the coupling medium should be fluid so as to fill all available spaces, be relatively viscous so that it stays in place, have an impedance appropriate to the media it connects, and should allow transmission of US with minimal absorption, attenuation or disturbance. At the present time gel-based media appear to be preferable to oils and creams. Water is a good medium and can be used as an alternative but clearly it fails to meet the above criteria in terms of its viscosity. There is no realistic (clinical) difference between the gels in common clinical use (Poltawski and Watson 2007).

Absorption and attenuation

The absorption of US energy follows an exponential pattern; that is, i.e. more energy is absorbed in the superficial tissues than in the deep tissues. In order for energy to have an effect, it must be absorbed, and at some point this must be considered in relation to the US dosages applied to achieve certain effects. Because the absorption (penetration) is exponential, there is (in theory) no point at which all the energy has been absorbed, but there is certainly a point at which the US energy levels are not sufficient to produce a therapeutic effect. As the US beam penetrates further into the tissues, a greater proportion of the energy will have been absorbed and therefore there is less energy available to achieve therapeutic effects. The half-value depth is often quoted in relation to US and represents the depth in the tissues at which half the surface energy remains available.

As it is difficult, if not impossible, to know the thickness of each specific tissue layer in an individual patient, average half-value depths are employed for each frequency. The 'average' half-value depths of commonly employed US frequencies are:

- 3 MHz = 2.0 cm
- 1 MHz = 4.0 cm.

Table 18.1 provides an estimate of the ultrasound energy remaining at various tissue depths. To achieve a particular US intensity at depth, account must be taken of the proportion of energy that has been absorbed by the tissues in the more superficial layers. The table gives an approximate reduction in energy levels with typical tissues at two commonly used frequencies.

@ Weblink

More detailed information and absorption tables are available at www.electrotherapy.org and in Watson (2002c).

As the penetration (or transmission) of US is not the same in each tissue type, it is clear that some tissues are capable of greater US absorption than others. Generally, tissues with a higher protein content will absorb US to a greater extent; thus tissues with high water content and low protein content (e.g. blood and fat) absorb little of the US energy, whilst those with a lower water content and a higher protein content will absorb US far more efficiently. It has been suggested that tissues can therefore be ranked according to their tissue absorption (Figure 18.20).

Although cartilage and bone are at the upper end of this scale, the problems associated with wave reflection mean that the majority of US energy striking the surface of either of these tissues is likely to be reflected. The best-absorbing tissues in terms of clinical practice are those with high collagen content: ligament, tendon,

Table 18.1 Ultrasound intensity at various tissue depths based on average half-value data

Depth (cm)	3 MHz	1 MHz
2	50%	
4	25%	50%
6		
8		25%

18

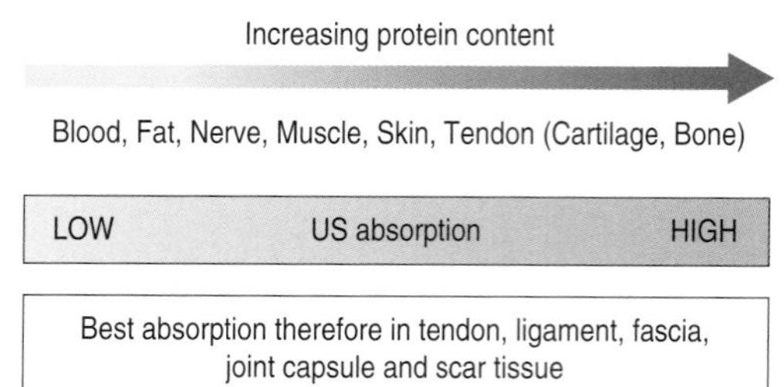

Figure 18.20 US absorption in different tissues.

fascia, joint capsule and scar tissue (Watson 2000; ter Haar 1999; Nussbaum 1998; Frizzell and Dunn 1982).

The application of therapeutic US to tissues with a low energy absorption capacity is less likely to be effective than the application of the energy to a more highly absorbing material. Recent evidence of the ineffectiveness of such an intervention can be found in Wilkin et al. (2004), whilst application in tissue that is a better absorber will result in a more effective intervention (e.g. Sparrow et al. 2005; Leung et al. 2004).

Pulsed ultrasound

Most machines offer the facility for pulsed US output. Typical pulse formats are 1:1 and 1:4, though others are available. In 1:1 mode, the machine offers an output for 2 ms followed by 2 ms rest. In 1:4 mode, the 2 ms output is followed by an 8 ms rest period. The effects of pulsed US are well documented and this type of output is preferable, especially in the treatment of the more acute lesions. The duty cycle (percentage of time during which the machine gives an output) will be 50 per cent for the 1:1 mode and 20 per cent for the 1:4 mode. Table 18.2 illustrates the equivalent pulse ratios and duty cycles (as a percentage).

Clinical uses of ultrasound therapy

One of the therapeutic effects of US relates to tissue healing. It is suggested that the application of US to injured tissues will, amongst other things, speed the rate of healing and enhance the quality of the repair; this will be focus of the following section.

Table 18.2 Pulse ratios and equivalent duty cycle percentage for clinical US machines

Mode	Pulse ratio	Duty cycle
Continuous		100%
Pulsed	1:1	50%
	1:2	33%
	1:3	25%
	1:4	20%
	1:9	10%

The therapeutic effects of US are generally divided into thermal and non-thermal.

Thermal effects and uses

In thermal mode, US will be most effective in heating dense collagenous tissues and will require a relatively high intensity, preferably in continuous mode, to achieve this effect.

Many papers have concentrated on the thermal effectiveness of US and, much as it can be used effectively in this way when an appropriate dose is selected (continuous mode $> 0.5\ \mathrm{W\ cm^{-2}}$), the focus of this chapter will be on the non-thermal effects. Both Nussbaum (1998) and ter Haar (1999) have provided some useful review material with regard to the thermal effects of US. Comparative studies on the thermal effects of US have been reported by several authors (Draper et al. 1993, 1995a,b) with some interesting and potentially useful results.

It is too simplistic to assume that, with a particular treatment application, there will be either thermal or non-thermal effects. It is almost inevitable that both will occur, but it is furthermore reasonable to argue that the dominant effect will be influenced by treatment parameters, especially the mode of application (pulsed or continuous). Baker et al. (2001) have argued the scientific basis for this issue coherently.

Non-thermal effects and uses

The non-thermal effects of US are now attributed primarily to a combination of *cavitation* and *acoustic streaming* (ter Haar 1999; Baker et al. 2001; Williams et al. 1987). There appears to be little by way of convincing evidence to support the notion of *micromassage*, though it does sound rather appealing. Details of these primary physical effects of US are detailed in appropriate texts and papers (Young 2002; Robertson et al. 2006).

The result of the combined effects of stable cavitation and acoustic streaming is that the cell membrane becomes 'excited' (up-regulates), thus increasing the activity levels of the whole cell. The US energy acts as a trigger for this process, but it is the increased cellular activity that is, in effect, responsible for the therapeutic benefits of the modality (Figure 18.21) (Watson 2000; Dinno 1989; Leung et al. 2004).

Ultrasound application in relation to tissue repair

The process of tissue repair is a complex series of cascaded, chemically mediated events that lead to the production of scar tissue, which constitutes an effective material to restore the continuity of the damaged tissue. The process is more complex than may be described here and there are numerous recent review papers, including Watson (2003; 2006b).

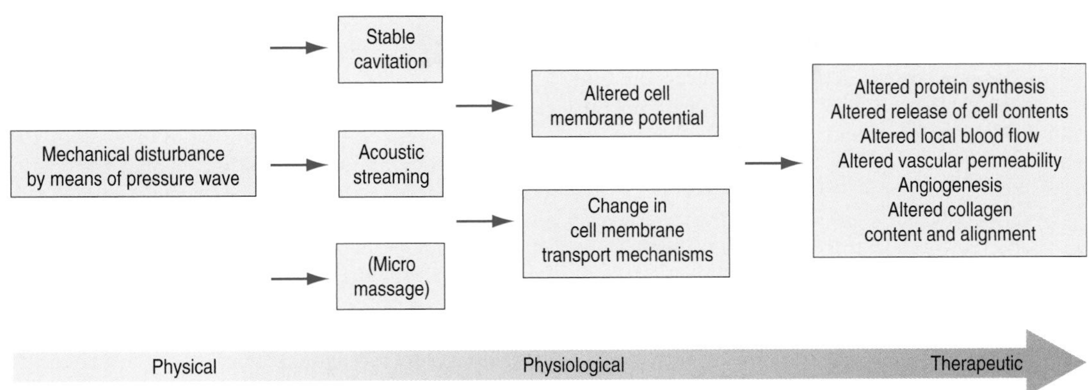

Figure 18.21 Mechanisms of US action.

Inflammation

During the inflammatory phase, US has a stimulating effect on mast cells, platelets, white cells with phagocytic roles and macrophages (Nussbaum 1997; ter Haar 1999; Maxwell 1992). For example, the application of US induces the degranulation of mast cells, causing the release of arachidonic acid, which itself is a precursor for the synthesis of prostaglandins and leukotrienes, which act as inflammatory mediators (Mortimer and Dyson 1988; Nussbaum 1997; Leung et al. 2004). By increasing the activity of these cells, the overall influence of therapeutic US is certainly pro-inflammatory rather than anti-inflammatory. The benefit of this mode of action is not to 'increase' the inflammatory response as such (though if applied with too great an intensity at this stage, it is a possible outcome — Ciccone et al. 1991), but rather to act as an 'inflammatory optimiser'. The inflammatory response is essential to the effective repair of tissue, and the more efficiently the process can complete, the more effectively the tissue can progress to the next phase (proliferation). US is effective at promoting the normality of the inflammatory events, and as such has a therapeutic value in promoting the overall repair events (ter Haar 1999). A further benefit is that the chemically mediated inflammatory events are associated with stimulation of the proliferative phase, and hence the promotion of the inflammatory phase also acts as a promoter of repair.

Employed at an appropriate treatment dose, with optimal treatment parameters (intensity, pulsing and time), the benefit of US is to make the earliest repair phase as efficient as possible, and thus have a promotional effect on the whole healing cascade. For tissues in which there is an inflammatory reaction, but in which there is no 'repair' to be achieved, the benefit of US is to promote the normal resolution of the inflammatory events, and hence resolve the 'problem'. This will be most effectively achieved in the tissues that preferentially absorb US: that is, the dense collagenous tissues (Watson 2006a).

Proliferation

During the proliferative phase, US also has a stimulative effect (cellular up-regulation), though the primary active targets are now the fibroblasts, endothelial cells and myofibroblasts (Ramirez et al. 1997; Mortimer and Dyson 1988; Young and Dyson 1990a,b; Nussbaum 1997, 1998; Dyson and Smalley 1983; Maxwell 1992). These are all cells that are normally active during scar production and US is therefore pro-proliferative in the same way that it is pro-inflammatory; it does not change the normal proliferative phase, but maximises its efficiency, producing the required scar tissue in an optimal fashion. Harvey et al. (1975) demonstrated that low-dose pulsed US increases protein synthesis, and several research groups have demonstrated enhanced fibroplasia and collagen synthesis (Enwemeka 1989; Enwemeka et al. 1990; Turner et al. 1989; Huys et al. 1993; Ramirez et al. 1997). Recent work has identified the critical role of numerous growth factors in relation to tissue repair, and some accumulating evidence has identified that therapeutic US has a positive role to play in this context (Reher et al. 1999).

Remodelling

During the remodelling phase of repair, the somewhat generic scar that is produced in the initial stages is refined such that it adopts functional characteristics of the tissue that it is repairing. This is achieved by a number of processes, mainly related to the orientation of the collagen fibres in the developing scar and also to the change in collagen type, from predominantly type III collagen to a more dominant type I collagen (Watson 2006a).

The application of therapeutic US can influence the remodelling of the scar tissue in that it appears to be capable of enhancing the appropriate orientation of the newly formed collagen fibres and also the collagen profile change from mainly type III to a type I construction, thus increasing tensile strength and enhancing scar mobility (Nussbaum 1998). US applied to tissues enhances the functional capacity of the scar tissues (Nussbaum 1998; Huys et al. 1993; Yeung et al. 2006). The role of US in this phase may also have the capacity to influence collagen fibre orientation, as demonstrated in an elegant study by Byl et al. (1996).

The application of US during the inflammatory, proliferative and repair phases is not of value because it changes the normal sequence of events, but because it has the capacity to stimulate or enhance these normal events and thus increase the efficiency of the repair phases (ter Haar 1999; Watson 2006a). It would appear that, if a tissue is repairing in a compromised or inhibited fashion, the application of therapeutic US at an appropriate dose will enhance this activity. If the tissue is healing 'normally', the application will speed the process and thus enable the tissue to reach its endpoint faster than would otherwise be the case. The effective application of US to achieve these aims is dose-dependent.

There has recently been a strong range of research papers that have identified the potential for low-intensity ultrasound to promote the process of fracture repair. Detailed analysis and review is beyond the scope of this chapter, but those with an interest in this field are referred to key summary review papers (Busse et al. 2002; Warden et al. 2000, 2006).

Treatment doses

It appears to be important to make an accurate dose selection when applying therapeutic US. There are numerous research papers that have demonstrated no value when using the modality, and part of the reason for this would appear to be that there is a dose dependency in terms of therapeutic outcome.

The detail of making dose selections is beyond the remit of this chapter. Essentially, it involves the variation of frequency, pulsing ratio (duty cycle), intensity and time.

Weblink

Details of calculation methods have been published (such as Watson 2002a) and are also available at various web resources and manufacturers' sites (e.g. www.electrotherapy.org).

Pulsed shortwave therapy

Pulsed shortwave therapy (PSWT) is a widely used modality in the UK (Al Mandeel and Watson 2006), though it is often called pulsed electromagnetic energy (PEME). The latter is less than fully appropriate, in that many modalities come under the heading of PEME, PSWT being only one of them; use of this term should be avoided. The older term, pulsed shortwave diathermy, is not really appropriate either, in that the modality is not primarily employed as a diathermy (literally, 'through heating').

PSWT employs the same operating frequency as traditional SWD: that is, 27.12 MHz. The output from the machine is pulsed such that the 'on' time is considerably shorter than the 'off' time. Thus the mean power delivered to the patient is relatively low, even though the peak power (during the 'on' pulses) can be quite high (typically around 150–200 watts peak power with modern machines).

The control offered by the machine will enable the user to vary (a) the mean power delivered to the patient and (b) the pulsing parameters governing the mode of delivery of the energy. It would seem from current research that the mean power is probably the most important parameter (Hill et al. 2002).

When using PSWT in the clinical environment, there are two 'modes' of application. The information in this section relates to application using the 'monode' or 'drum' electrode (Figure 18.22) rather than the capacitor plate delivery system, which lacks supportive evidence.

Main machine parameters

Pulse repetition rate (Hz or pps)

The pulse repetition rate controls the number of pulses of shortwave energy that are delivered to the patient in a second. The units are often denoted in Hertz (Hz), though pulses per second (pps) is probably a more appropriate term. Most, if not all machines offer a preset range of widely varying pulse repetition options. For example, the Megapulse machine (EMS) offers a range of 100/200/400/600/800 pps, whilst the Curapulse machine (Enraf) offers 26/35/46/62/82/110/150/200/300/400 pps. There is no evidence that the actual value of the pulse rate is critical, but the ability to deliver more or fewer pulses per second does enable the user to influence the mean power (see below).

Pulse duration (width)

The pulse duration (often called the pulse width) refers to the duration, in microseconds, of each individual pulse of shortwave energy. Most, but not all machines allow the therapist to adjust the pulse duration using a range of pre-set options. For example, the Megapulse machine (EMS) offers pulse durations of 20/40/65/100/200/400 μs, whilst the Curapulse machine (Enraf) offers durations of 65/82/110/150/200/300/400 μs. There is no evidence that the actual duration is a critical

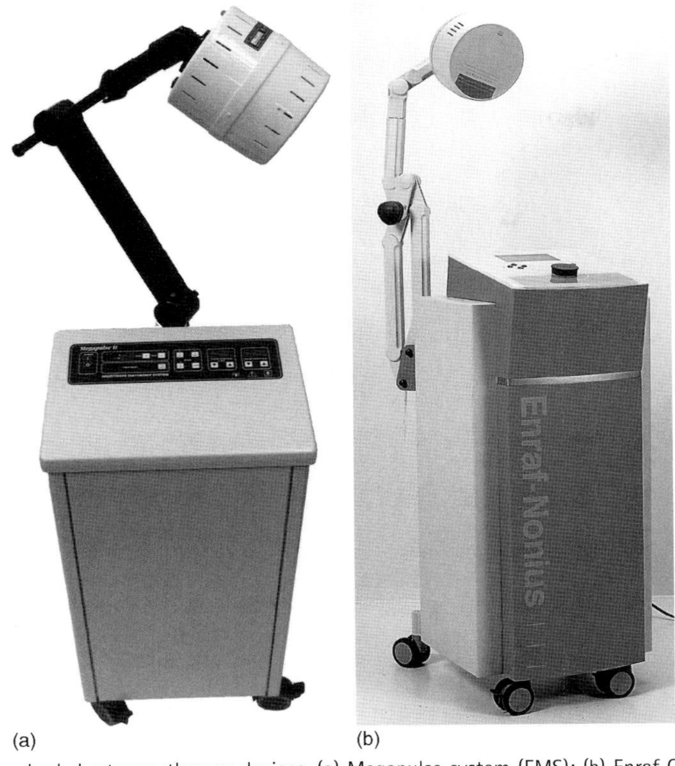

(a) (b)

Figure 18.22 Examples of pulsed shortwave therapy devices. (a) Megapulse system (EMS); (b) Enraf Curapulse system (Mobilis).

measure; it is simply a means of influencing mean power delivery.

Power output of the machine

The combination of having the facility to determine both the repetition rate of the pulses and the duration of each pulse enables the user to influence the mean power delivered to the patient.

The peak power (which can sometimes, but not always, be controlled by the operator) is typically around 150–200 watts in modern machines. This is the 'strength' of the shortwave whilst the pulse is on — that is, energy is delivered to the patient. The 'mean power' takes account of the fact that there are on and off phases — the energy delivery is intermittent — and thereby describes the average power output rather than the power output at any one moment in time (which might be maximum or zero).

The relationship between pulse parameters and power levels is illustrated in Figure 18.23.

The applied mean power appears to be the critical dose parameter. Each different type of pulsed shortwave machine will have a 'mean power' table associated with it, and it is from this table that the therapist is able to establish the settings required to deliver a mean power of XXX watts. If, for example, it is intended to deliver a mean power of 5 watts with the machine in use, the therapist should consult the appropriate table for the machine to determine exactly which combination of pulse repetition rate and pulse duration will provide

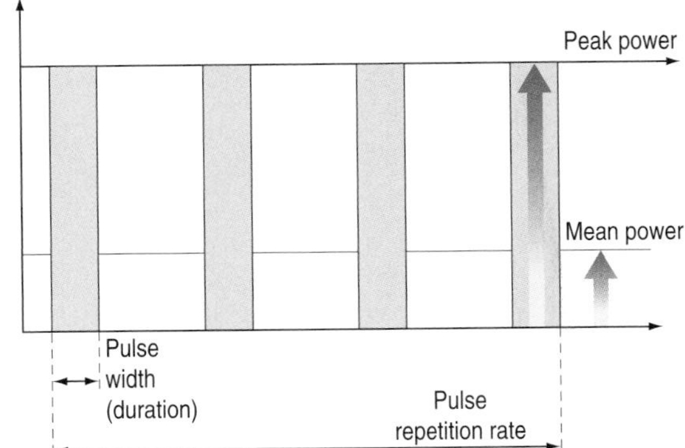

Figure 18.23 The relationship between pulse parameters and power levels with pulsed shortwave therapy.

the required mean power. It is important to note that these tables are not transferable between machines.

Tissue heating

With respect to the effects of pulsed shortwave, there is an element of tissue heating which occurs during the 'on' pulse, but this is dissipated during the prolonged 'off' phase and therefore it is possible to give treatment with no *net* increase in tissue temperature. Figure 18.24a demonstrates no accumulation of either thermal or non-thermal effects. In Figure 18.24b, the pulses are sufficiently close to generate an accumulative non-thermal effect, while in Figure 18.24c there is an accumulation of both thermal and non-thermal effects. The settings applied on the machine will determine which of these is achieved in a particular treatment, with the mean power appearing to be the most critical parameter. The 'non-thermal' effects of the modality are generally thought to be of greater significance. They appear to accumulate during the treatment time and have a significant effect after a latent period, possibly in the order of 6–8 hours. It is suggested (Hayne 1984) that the energy level required to produce such an effect in humans is low.

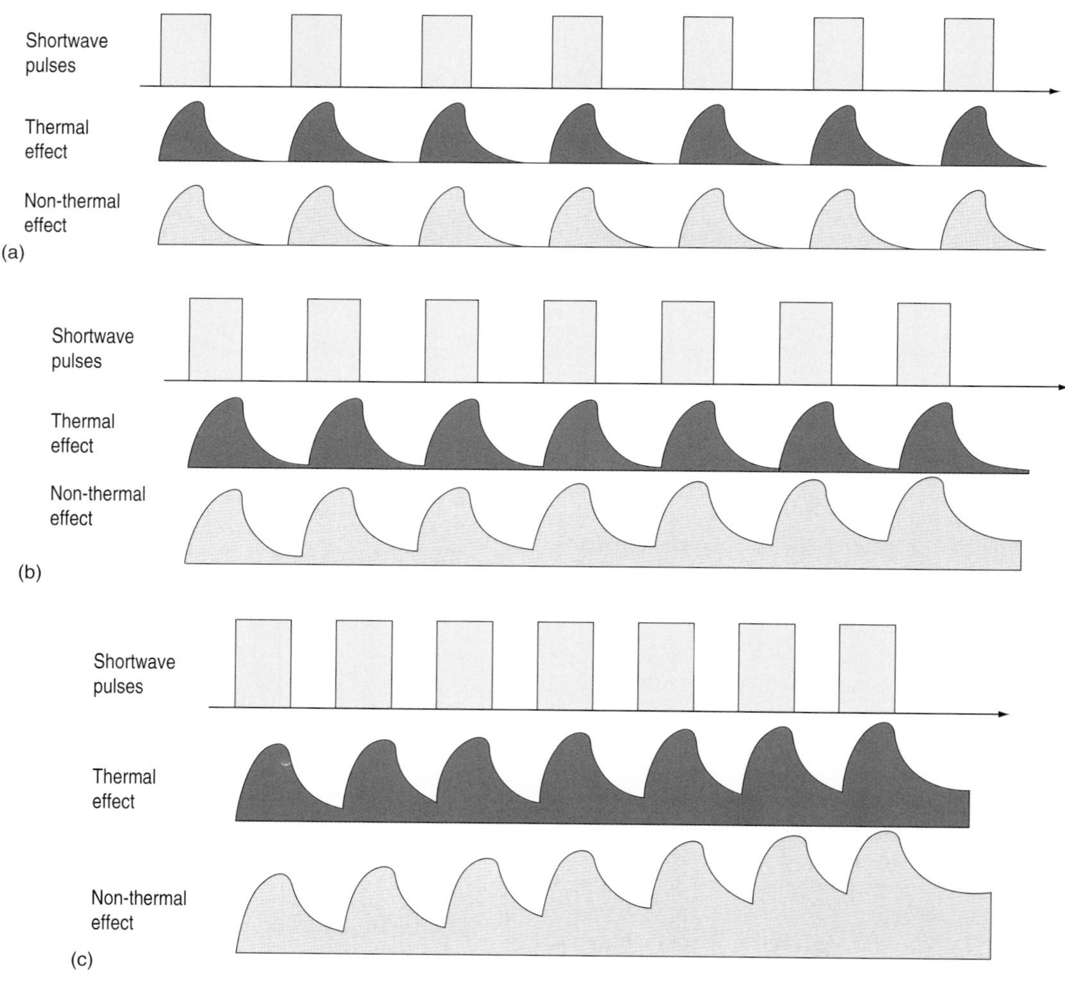

18

Figure 18.24 Effect of varying the pulse parameters on the accumulated heat generated in the tissues. (a) Pulses at sufficient distance – no accumulative effect; (b) pulses closer together – accumulating non-thermal effect, no thermal accumulation; (c) pulses closer still—accumulation of thermal and non-thermal effects.

Research has been conducted over several years relating to the thermal nature of PSWD. It was unclear just what power levels were required to bring about real tissue heating, and in fact, the opinion has been that PSWD was a non-thermal modality per se. Research has demonstrated (Bricknell and Watson 1995) that PSWD does have a thermal component, and real tissue heating can occur at different treatment settings. This is important in that, if the modality is to be applied in circumstances where the heating would be inappropriate or contraindicated, it is essential to know the power/energy levels at which the thermal effects begin. This research shows that a measurable heating effect can be demonstrated at power levels over 5 watts, though on average, it will become apparent at some 11 watts mean power. More recent work by Seiger and Draper (2006) suggests that it may still be safe to apply higher mean power levels than previously thought, even with metal in the tissues.

If a 'non-thermal' treatment is the intended outcome of the treatment, it is essential that the mean power applied remains below a level that is likely to induce significant heating effects, and at present, this is taken as being at 5 watts mean power. If a thermal effect is an intentional outcome of the intervention, then it may be perfectly appropriate to deliver power levels in excess of 5 watts, but if doing so, the therapist must ensure that precautions are taken, as for any other thermal intervention.

Effects of PSWT

These can be basically divided into two types: those of the electric field and those of the magnetic field. There appears to be almost no literature/research concerning the effects of pulsing the electric field (using condenser plate electrodes), and all the research identified here is concerned with the therapeutic effects of the magnetic field (monode type) electrode.

The primary effect of the pulsed magnetic field appears to be at the cell membrane level and is concerned with the transport of ions across the membrane. Some interesting publications have strongly supported the 'non-thermal' effects at cell membrane level (Luben 1996; Cleary 1996).

Normal cell membranes exhibit a potential difference due to the relative concentration differences of various ions on either side of the membrane (reviewed in Charman 1990). It is argued that the application of energy that is absorbed at cell membrane level results in cellular 'up-regulation' and thereby increased levels of cellular activity. This is not a change in role, but effectively an increase in work rate.

Cells involved in the inflammatory process demonstrate a reduced cell membrane potential and consequently, the cell function is disturbed. The altered potential affects ion transport across the membrane, and the resulting ionic imbalance alters cellular osmotic pressures. The application of PSWT to cells affected in this way is claimed to restore the cell membrane potential to 'normal' values and also to restore normal membrane transport and ionic balance. The mechanism by which this effect is brought about is not yet established, but two theories suggest that this is either a direct ionic transport mechanism or an activation of various pumps (sodium/potassium) by the pulsed energy. Evidence (Luben 1996; Cleary 1996) supports the contention that the energy is absorbed in the membrane and that, via a mechanism of signal transduction, it stimulates or enhances intracellular effects.

There appears to be a strong similarity in the mechanism of effect of US, laser and PSWT. All three modalities appear to have their primary effect at cell membrane level, with the resulting 'up-regulation' of cellular behaviour being the key to the therapeutic effects.

Clinical effects

The clinical effects of PSWT are primarily related to the inflammatory and repair phases in musculoskeletal/soft tissues. Goldin et al. (1981) list the effects of the modality (following research in soft tissue repair after skin graft application). Other papers have similarly identified the list of effects, which are most easily reviewed in the standard electrotherapy texts (Kitchen 2002a; Robertson et al. 2006; Watson 2006a).

Suggested treatment doses

In the light of current research, it is suggested that the minimum energy required to achieve a therapeutic effect should be utilised. Specific detailed research (clinical and laboratory) is essential for further validation of the treatment, which is currently criticised for being unfounded. There is also a strong argument that the concentration of electromagnetic energy is likely to be critical, and it may be that, in the near future, PSWT doses are described in terms of mean power concentration (W cm^{-2}) rather than just in watts. This would be in keeping with US and laser therapies.

The general guide below is based on both clinical and research evidence wherever possible.

Acute conditions

Apply a *mean power* of less than 3 watts. The more acute the lesion presentation, the lower the delivered mean power (that is, 3 watts is maximal for this group). Using shorter-duration (narrower) pulses and a higher repetition rate may be beneficial and the typical treatment time is between 10 and 15 minutes.

Subacute conditions

Apply a *mean power* of between 2 and 5 watts; as the condition becomes less acute, use of longer-duration (wider) pulses appears to be preferable. Treatment time would typically be in the region of 15 minutes.

Chronic conditions

Application of a mean power greater than 5 watts is usually required in order to achieve a reasonable tissue response. As noted previously, when such mean powers are employed, it is important to remember that the 'thermal' effect of pulsed shortwave becomes apparent at power levels greater than 5 watts, and therefore appropriate thermal precautions need to be taken. Pulses of longer duration are probably of benefit if there is a choice, and treatment times are typically between 15 and 20 minutes.

Laser therapy

The term LASER is an acronym for **l**ight **a**mplification by **s**timulated **e**mission of **r**adiation. In simple yet realistic terms, the laser can be considered to be a form of light amplifier, it providing enhancement of particular properties of light energy (Figure 18.25).

Laser light behaves according to the basic laws of light, in that it travels in straight lines at a constant velocity in space. It can be transmitted, reflected, refracted and absorbed. It can be placed within the electromagnetic spectrum according to its wavelength/frequency, which will vary according to the particular generator under consideration (Figure 18.26).

There are several aspects of laser light that are deemed to be special and are often referred to in the literature. These include *monochromacity*, *coherence* and *polarisation*. There remains some doubt as to exactly how essential these particular aspects of laser light are in relation to the therapeutic application of this energy form. Monochromacity is probably the most important factor, as many of the therapeutic effects have been noted in various trials with light that is non-coherent. Additionally, it is thought that polarisation is soon lost within the tissues and it may therefore be less important than was thought at first.

Therapy lasers have several common characteristics, which are summarised below.

Terms

Therapy lasers tend to fall into a particular category of laser light known as 3A or 3B. More recently, the terms low-level laser therapy (LLLT) and low-intensity laser therapy (LILT) have been adopted. Ohshiro and Calderhead suggest that LLLT involves treatment with a dose that causes no detectable temperature rise in the treated tissues and no macroscopically visible change in tissue structure. Essentially, the energy can cause in increase in temperature and a change in tissue structure, but that is not the intention with therapy laser, which is applied at levels below that needed to achieve these more overt effects (compared with surgical laser).

Parameters

Most LLLT apparatus generates light in the red visible and near-infrared bands of the electromagnetic spectrum (Figure 18.27), with typical wavelengths of 600–1000 nm. The mean power of such devices is generally low (1–100 mW), though the peak power may be much higher than this.

The treatment device may be a single emitter or a cluster of several emitters (Figure 18.28), though it is common for most emitters in a cluster to be the non-laser type of device. The beam from single probes is usually narrow (Ø1 mm to 6 or 7 mm) at the source. A cluster probe will usually incorporate both higher- and lower-power emitters of different wavelengths.

The output may be continuous or pulsed, with narrow pulse widths (in the nano- or microsecond ranges) and a wide variety of pulse repetition rates from 2 Hz up to several thousand Hz. It is difficult to identify the evidence for the use of pulsing from the research literature, though it would appear to be a general trend that lower pulsing rates are more effective in acute conditions whilst higher pulse rates work better in more chronic conditions.

Many texts make reference to the types of generator, according to the gas contained within the tube, but in therapy applications most modern apparatus utilises laser diodes. These are most commonly made of gallium aluminium arsenide (GaAlAs), in which the ratio of the constituents determines the wavelength of the output; alternatively, laser LEDs of various kinds are employed.

Light absorption in the tissues

As with any form of energy used in electrotherapy, the energy must be absorbed by the tissues in order to have some effect. The absorption of light energy within the tissues is a complex issue, but generally, the shorter wavelengths (ultraviolet and shorter visible) are primarily absorbed in the epidermis by the pigments, amino acids and nucleic acids. The longer infrared radiation wavelengths (> 1300 nm) appear to be rapidly absorbed by water and therefore have a limited penetration into the tissues. The band between (i.e. 600–1000 nm) is capable of penetration beyond the superficial epidermis and is, in part at least, available for absorption by other biological tissues.

When applied to the body tissues, LLLT delivers energy at a level sufficient to disturb local electron orbits and result in the generation of heat, initiate chemical change, disrupt molecular bonds and produce free radicals. These are considered to be the primary mechanisms by which LLLT achieves its physiological and therefore therapeutic effects and the primary target is effectively the cell membrane (see below).

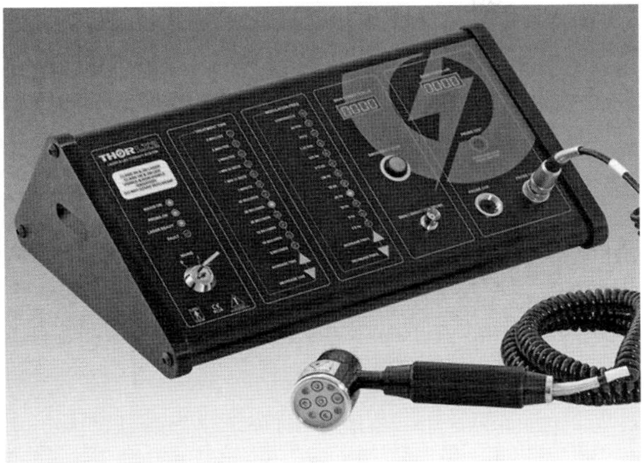

(a) 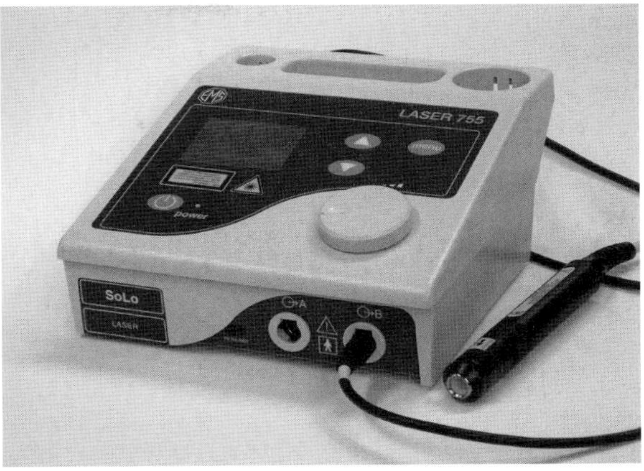 (b)

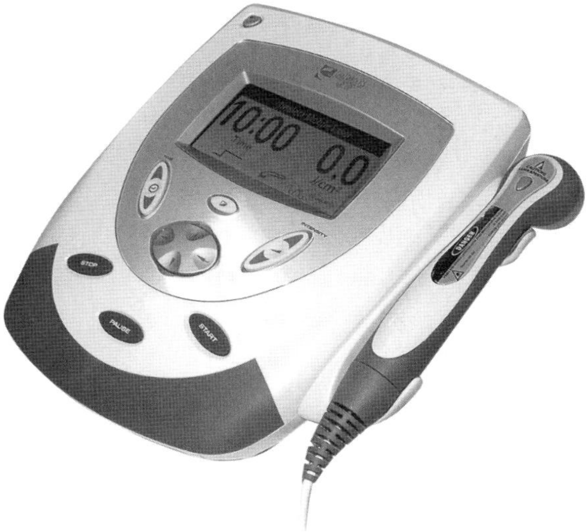

(c)

Figure 18.25 Typical laser therapy devices. (a) THOR – LX2 laser; (b) EMS laser; (c) Chatanooga laser module (SKF).

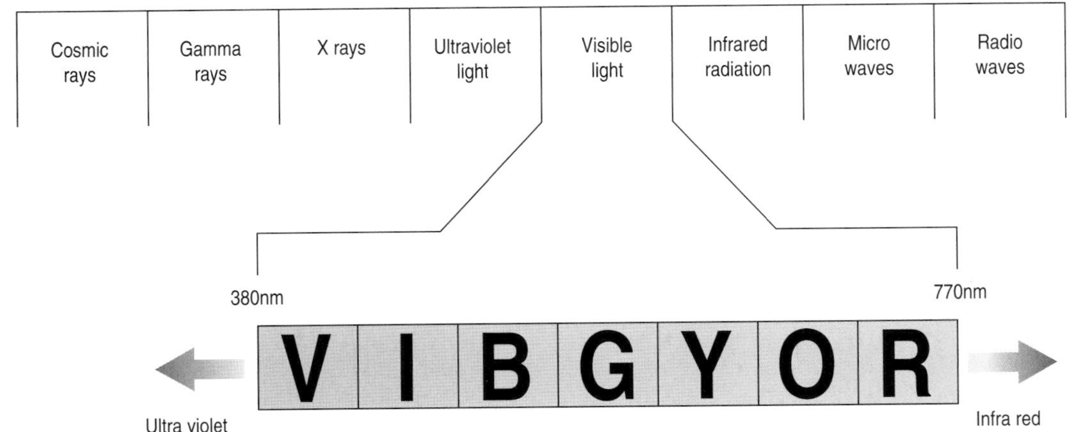

Figure 18.26 Light energy as a part of the electromagnetic spectrum.

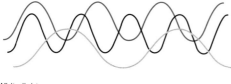

White light
Multiple wavelengths
Non coherent
(a)

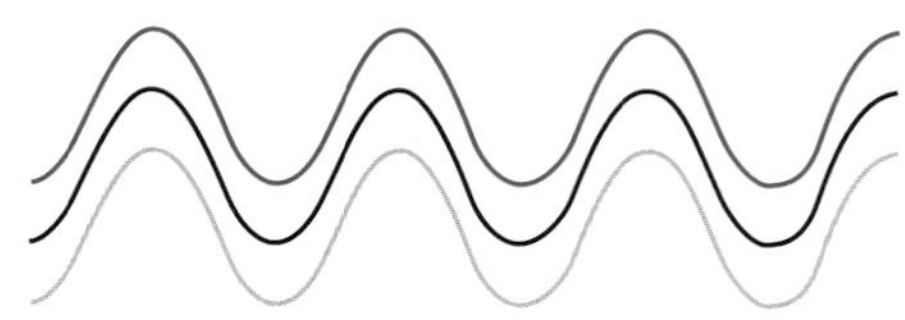

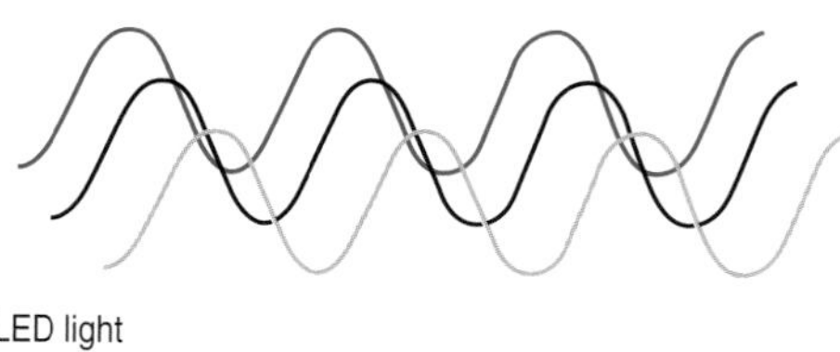

Figure 18.27 Characteristics of various light forms. (a) 'Normal' white light; (b) true laser light; (c) light-emitting diode (LED)-type laser light.

Although much of the applied laser light is absorbed in the superficial tissues, it is proposed that deeper or more distant effects can be achieved, probably as a secondary consequence via some chemical mediator or second messenger systems, though there is limited evidence to support this contention fully.

The actual penetration of LLLT at common wavelengths is a widely debated point and it is common to find widely varying values cited in the literature. It is often claimed that, because laser light is monochromatic, polarised and coherent, it is capable of greater penetration than 'normal' (or non-coherent) light. This should give penetration depths of 3–7 mm for visible red light and some 30–40 mm (at best) for IRR laser light. The fact that the polarisation appears to be lost in the tissues — as is much, if not all, of the coherence — will result in a shallower penetration. King (1990) cites the penetration depth for 630 nm light as 1–2 mm, whilst at 800–900 nm penetration depths of 2–4 mm are expected. (Penetration depth in this context refers to the depth of the tissues to which 37 per cent of the light at the surface is able to penetrate.) A very small percentage of the light energy available at the surface will be available at 10–15 mm into the tissues.

Laser–tissue interaction

Definition

Photobioactivation is a commonly used phrase in connection with LILT. It means the stimulation of various biological events using light energy but without significant temperature changes.

Much, if not all, of the cited work on therapeutic laser considers its photobioactivation effects. Some authors have proposed that other terms are preferable, including *photobiostimulation* and *photobiomodulation*. It provides for a great semantic argument, but let us assume at this point that these terms are generally interchangeable.

Many of the early ideas about photobioactivation were proposed by Karu, who reported and demonstrated several key factors. She notes in her 1987 paper that some biomolecules change their activity in response to irradiation with low-intensity visible light, but that these molecules do not appear to absorb the light directly. The cell membrane appears to be the primary absorber of the energy, which then generates intracellular effects by means of a second messenger/cascade-type response. The magnitude of the photoresponse was deemed to be determined at least in part by the state of the cells/tissues prior to irradiation, summarised in a simple statement that 'starving cells are more photosensitive than well-fed ones.' The laser light irradiation of the tissues is seen, then, as a trigger for the alteration of cell metabolic processes, via a process of photosignal transduction. The often-cited Arndt-Schults Law supports this proposal (Karu 1987, 1998).

The following list of physiological and cellular level effects is compiled from several reviews and research papers (such as Baxter 2002; Tuner and Hode 2004) and does not claim to be complete or guaranteed for the in vivo situation. It does, however, illustrate the range and scope of photobioactivation effects:

- altered cell proliferation
- altered cell motility
- activation of phagocytes
- stimulation of immune responses

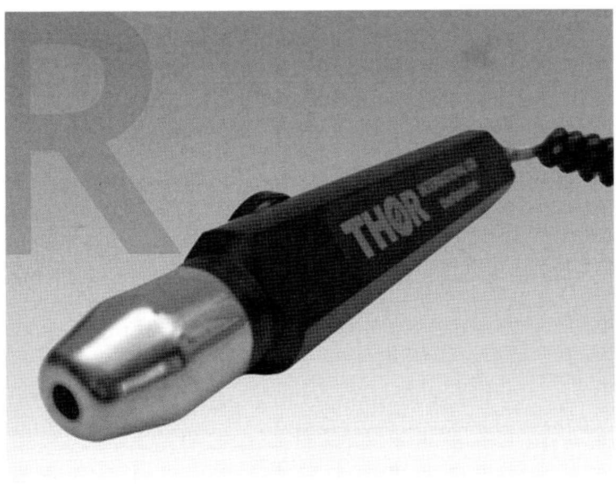

(a)

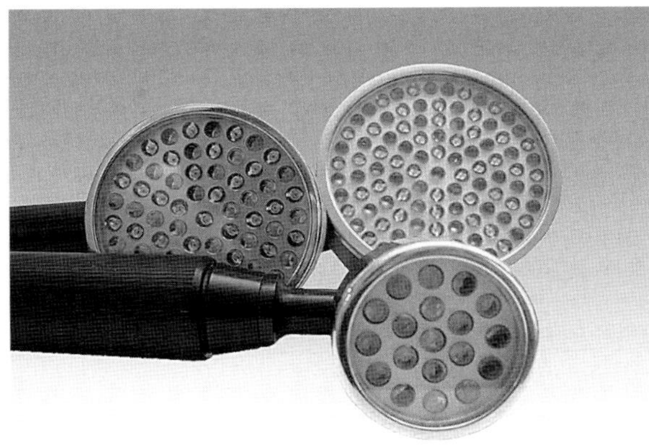

(b)

Figure 18.28 Laser therapy applicators. (a) Single probe (Thor); (b) cluster probes (Thor).

- increased cellular metabolism
- stimulation of macrophages
- stimulation of mast cell degranulation
- activation and proliferation of fibroblasts
- alteration of cell membrane potentials
- stimulation of angiogenesis
- alteration of action potentials
- altered prostaglandin production
- altered endogenous opioid production.

Treatment doses

Most research groups and many manufacturers recommend that the dose delivered to a patient during a treatment session should be based on the *energy density* rather than the power or other measure of dose. Energy density is measured in units of joules per square centimetre (J/cm^2). One of the most significant inhibitors to the more widespread adoption of laser therapy in the clinical environment relates to the difficulty in getting these 'effective' laser doses to work on a particular machine. Few devices enable the practitioner to set the dose in J/cm^2. Some will provide joules, some watts, and some $watts/cm^{-2}$. It is currently argued that joules (i.e. energy) may in fact be the most critical parameter rather than energy density. The debate is not yet resolved and so energy density will be used here, mainly because the published research almost exclusively cites it; therefore, it may be of more use when it comes to trying to replicate an evidence-based treatment dose.

Some machines offer 'on board' calculations of this dose, whilst other machines require the operator to make some calculations based on known machine parameters:

- output power (watts)
- irradiation area (cm^2)
- time (seconds)
- if pulsed — pulse width, frequency and power settings.

$$\text{Energy density } (J/cm^2) = \frac{\text{Total amount of energy}(J)}{\text{Irradiation area}(cm^2)}$$

$$\text{Total energy}(J) = \text{Average power(watts)} \times \text{time(sec)}$$

$$\text{Average power (watts)(pulsed output only)} = \text{Peak power (W)} \times \text{frequency (Hz)} \times \text{pulse duration (sec)}$$

There are various alternative methods for calculating these doses, but those cited above offer a reasonably simple method, should one be needed.

Most authorities suggest that the energy density per treatment session should generally fall in the range of 0.1–12.0 J/cm^2, though there are some recommendations which go up to 30 J/cm^2. Again, as a generality, lower doses should be applied to the more acute lesions, which would appear to be more energy-sensitive.

Clinical applications

The recent research, both laboratory-based and clinical trials, is found to concentrate on a few key areas. Most dominant amongst these are wound healing, inflammatory arthropathies, soft tissue injury and the relief of pain. There is supportive research for the clinical use of LLLT in these and other circumstances but, as with many treatment modalities, the evidence remains somewhat controversial at the present time.

Open wounds

There is a growing body of evidence in this context, with some mixed results, but on the whole, they are positive outcome trials. There are useful sections in Baxter (1994) and more recently in Tuner and Hode (2004). A general summary might conclude that a treatment programme could be thus: treat to the floor of the ulcer/pressure sore/wound, preferably using a cluster probe to cover the area, typically up to 2 J/cm^2. Also treat the margin/periphery normally using a single probe with a dose typically up to 4 J/cm^2.

Inflammatory arthropathies

There have been several trials involving the use of LILT and various inflammatory problems in joints. As with the wound work, there are mixed results, but the general trend appears to be supportive. The recent Ottawa Panel (2004) review was supportive of laser therapy in rheumatoid arthritis.

Soft tissue injury

There is a fairly widespread use of LILT in a variety of soft tissue treatments. Some results are excellent and others poor. It is possible that the weak results relate to incorrect doses or possibly to the use of laser therapy for injuries that are simply beyond the reach of the energy delivered (see penetration section above). Tuner and Hode (2004) describe multiple examples of effective (and less effective) soft tissue treatments with LILT and identify some of the key research in this area.

Pain

It has been broadly assumed (until recently) that the effect of laser therapy with regard to pain relief was primarily a secondary effect of dealing with the inflammatory state. Whilst this may well be true (to some extent at least), there is growing evidence that laser therapy can have a more direct effect on nerve conduction characteristics and hence may result in reduced pain as a more direct effect of the therapy. A recent example of a paper along these lines would be Vinck et al. (2005).

The therapeutic use of laser has increased slowly in the general practice of therapy, though there are specialist areas where it is strongly advocated — for example, wound healing. One of the key issues limiting the more widespread uptake of the modality is the apparent difficulty in deciding on an effective clinical dose, and then setting the machine to deliver such a dose. It is hoped that with improvements in technology, this will become an easier task, and thus, the clinical application of laser therapy is likely to increase in the short- to medium-term future.

CONCLUSION

In summary, electrotherapy has an evidence-based role in physiotherapy practice. It has been the subject of considerable debate over recent years, but the evidence base identifying what it is (and what it is not) capable of achieving is substantial. This chapter has attempted to summarise the key modalities in use in the current clinical environment, and has alluded to others.

Each modality will have a range of specific physiological effects, and these can be employed in turn to bring about therapeutic effects. Modalities have some commonality in terms of their modes of action, and the modalities have been grouped together in this chapter on that basis: electrical stimulation modalities, thermal modalities and 'non-thermal' modalities.

By employing an evidence-based clinical decision-making model, it is possible to make rational and evidenced therapeutic decisions as regards which modality (if any) to use and when. The details of dose-based decisions have been largely omitted from this text, but making the appropriate decision as to which modality to employ in particular circumstances is the first and probably the critical choice. Once the most appropriate modality has been identified, the specific treatment 'dose' needs to be pinned down. Research papers and standard electrotherapy texts are available in addition to online resources to facilitate these detailed decisions.

The overuse of electrotherapy in the past has resulted in the demise of this area of practice. This chapter has attempted to identify the key issues for commonly available modalities, to illustrate their potential clinical applications based on the available evidence, and to identify detailed sources for further information.

FURTHER READING

Weblink

- Electrotherapy on the Web (author: T Watson): www.electrotherapy.org

REFERENCES

Ada L, Foongchomcheay A 2002 Efficacy of electrical stimulation in preventing or reducing subluxation of the shoulder after stroke: a meta-analysis. Aust J Physiother 48(4): 257–267

Al Mandeel M, Watson T 2006 An evaluative audit of patient records in electrotherapy with specific reference to pulsed short wave therapy (PSWT). Int J Ther Rehabil 13(9): 414–419

Amaro JL, Oliveira Gameiro MO et al. 2003 Treatment of urinary stress incontinence by intravaginal electrical stimulation and pelvic floor physiotherapy. Int Urogynecol J Pelvic Floor Dysfunct 14(3): 204–208; discussion 208

Baker KG, Robertson VJ et al. 2001 A review of therapeutic ultrasound: biophysical effects. Phys Ther 81(7): 1351–1358

Barroso JC, Ramos JG et al. 2004 Transvaginal electrical stimulation in the treatment of urinary incontinence. BJU Int 93(3): 319–323

Baxter D 1994 Therapeutic Lasers: Theory and Practice. Churchill Livingstone: Edinburgh

Baster D 2002 Low Intensity Laser Therapy. In Kitchen S (ed.) Electrotherapy: Evidence Based Practice. Elsevier: Oxford

Bircan CO, Senocak O, Peker O et al. 2002 Efficacy of two forms of electrical stimulation in increasing quadriceps strength: a randomized controlled trial. Clin Rehabil 16(2): 194–199

Bricknell R, Watson T 1995 The thermal effects of pulsed shortwave therapy. Br J Ther Rehabil 2(8): 430–434

Brosseau L, Robinson V et al. 2002 Efficacy of thermotherapy for rheumatoid arthritis: a meta analysis. Physical Therapy Reviews 7: 5–15

Busse JW, Bhandari M et al. 2002 The effect of low-intensity pulsed ultrasound therapy on time to fracture healing: a meta-analysis. CMAJ 166(4): 437–441

Byl NN, Hill Toulouse L et al. 1996 Effects of ultrasound on the orientation of fibroblasts: an in-vitro study. Eur J Phys Med Rehabil 6(6): 180–184

Callaghan MJ, Oldham JA 2004 Electric muscle stimulation of the quadriceps in the treatment of patellofemoral pain. Arch Phys Med Rehabil 85(6): 956–962

Chantraine A, Baribeault A et al. 1999 Shoulder pain and dysfunction in hemiplegia: effects of functional electrical stimulation. Arch Phys Med Rehabil 80(3): 328–331

Charman RA 1990 Bioelectricity and electrotherapy — towards a new paradigm? Part 2: Cellular reception and emission of electromagnetic signals. Physiotherapy 76(9): 509–516

Chesterton LS, Barlas P et al. 2002 Sensory stimulation (TENS): effects of parameter manipulation on mechanical pain thresholds in healthy human subjects. Pain 99: 253–262

Christie AD, Willoughby GL 1990 The effect of interferential therapy on swelling following open reduction and internal fixation of ankle fractures. Physiotherapy Theory and Practice 6: 3–7

Ciccone C, Leggin B et al. 1991 Effects of ultrasound and trolamine salicylate phonophoresis on delayed-onset muscle soreness. Phys Ther 71: 666–675

Ciombor DM, Aaron RK 2005 The role of electrical stimulation in bone repair. Foot Ankle Clin 10(4): 579–593

Cleary SF 1987 Cellular effects of electromagnetic radiation. IEEE Eng Med Biol 6(1): 26–30

Cleary SF 1996 In vitro studies of the effects of nonthermal radiofrequency and microwave radiation. Non-thermal effects of RF electromagnetic fields. ICNIRP: Munich

Dinno M 1989 The significance of membrane changes in the safe and effective use of therapeutic and diagnostic ultrasound. Phys Med Biol 34: 1543ff

Draper D, Sunderland S et al. 1993 A comparison of temperature rise in human calf muscle following applications of underwater and topical gel ultrasound. JOSPT 17: 247–251

Draper DO, Ricard MD 1995a Rate of temperature decay in human muscle following 3 MHz ultrasound: the stretching window revealed. J Athl Train 30(4): 304–307

Draper DO, Schulties S et al. 1995b Temperature changes in deep muscles of humans during ice and ultrasound therapies: an in vivo study. J Orthop Sports Physical Ther 21(3): 153–157

Dyson M, Smalley D 1983 Effects of ultrasound on wound contraction. In: Millner R, Rosenfeld E, Cobet U (eds) Ultrasound Interactions in Biology and Medicine. Plenum: New York, pp. 151–158

Enwemeka CS 1989 The effects of therapeutic ultrasound on tendon healing. A biomechanical study. Am J Phys Med Rehabil 68(6): 283–287

Enwemeka CS, Rodriguez O et al. 1990 The biomechanical effects of low-intensity ultrasound on healing tendons. Ultrasound Med Biol 16(8): 801–807

Evans RD, Foltz D et al. 2001 Electrical stimulation with bone and wound healing. Clin Podiatr Med Surg 18(1): 79–95, vi

Frizzell LA, Dunn F 1982 Biophysics of ultrasound. In: Lehmann J (ed.) Therapeutic Heat and Cold. Williams & Wilkins: Baltimore

Goldin JH, Broadbent N et al. 1981 The effects of Diapulse on the healing of wounds: A double blind randomised controlled trial in man. Br J Plast Surg 34: 267–270

Han JS, Chen XH et al. 1991 Effect of low- and high-frequency TENS on Met-enkephalin-Arg-Phe and dynorphin A immunoreactivity in human lumbar CSF. Pain 47(3): 295–298

Harvey W, Dyson M et al. 1975 The stimulation of protein synthesis in human fibroblasts by therapeutic ultrasound. Rheumatol Rehabil 14: 237

Hayne CR 1984 Pulsed high frequency energy: its place in physiotherapy. Physiotherapy 70: 459–464

Hill J, Lewis M et al. 2002 Pulsed short-wave diathermy effects on human fibroblast proliferation. Arch Phys Med Rehabil 83(6): 832–836

Hurley DA, McDonough SM et al. 2004 A randomized clinical trial of manipulative therapy and interferential therapy for acute low back pain. Spine 29(20): 2207–2216

Huys S, Gan BS et al. 1993 Comparison of effects of early and late ultrasound treatment on tendon healing in the chicken limb. J Hand Ther 6: 58–59

Indrekvam S, Fosse OA et al. 2001 A Norwegian national cohort of 3198 women treated with home-managed electrical stimulation for urinary incontinence — demography and medical history. Scand J Urol Nephrol 35(1): 26–31

Jarit GJ, Mohr KJ et al. 2003 The effects of home interferential therapy on post-operative pain, edema, and range of motion of the knee. Clin J Sport Med 13(1): 16–20

Johnson M 2002 Transcutaneous Electrical Nerve Stimulation (TENS). In: Kitchen S (ed.) Electrotherapy: Evidence-Based Practice. Elsevier: Oxford

Johnson MI, Tabasam G 2003 An investigation into the analgesic effects of different frequencies of the amplitude-modulated wave of interferential current therapy on cold-induced pain in normal subjects. Arch Phys Med Rehabil 84(9): 1387–1394

Jorge S, Parada CA et al. 2006 Interferential therapy produces antinociception during application in various models of inflammatory pain. Phys Ther 86(6): 800–808

Karu TI 1987 Photobiological fundamentals of low power laser therapy. J Quantum Electronics QE 23(10): 1703–1717

Karu T 1998 The Science of Low-Power Laser Therapy. Gordon and Breach: Amsterdam

King PR 1990 Low level laser therapy: a review. Physiother Theory Pract 6: 127–138

Kitchen S 2002a Electrotherapy: Evidence-based Practice. Churchill Livingstone: Edinburgh

Kitchen SS 2002b Infrared Irradiation. In: Kitchen S (ed.) Electrotherapy: Evidence-based Practice. Churchill Livingstone: Edinburgh

Kitchen S, Dyson M 2002 Low Energy Treatments: Non-thermal or Microthermal. In: Kitchen S (ed.) Electrotherapy: Evidence-based Practice. Churchill Livingstone: Edinburgh

Kitchen SS, Partridge CJ 1991 Infra-red therapy. Physiotherapy 77(4): 249–254

Lake DA 1992 Neuromuscular electrical stimulation: An overview and its application in the treatment of sports injuries. Sports Med 13(5): 320–336

Lambert I, Tebbs SE et al. 2000 Interferential therapy machines as possible vehicles for cross-infection. J Hosp Infect 44(1): 59–64

Lehmann J 1982 Therapeutic Heat and Cold. Williams &Wilkins: Baltimore

18

Leung KS, Cheung WH et al. 2004 Low intensity pulsed ultrasound stimulates osteogenic activity of human periosteal cells. Clin Orthop Rel Res 418: 253–259

Luben RA 1996 Effects of microwave radiation on signal transduction processes of cells in vitro. Non-thermal effects of RF electromagnetic fields. ICNIRP: Munich

Lyons CL, Robb JB et al. 2005 Differences in quadriceps femoris muscle torque when using a clinical electrical stimulator versus a portable electrical stimulator. Phys Ther 85(1): 44–51

Maxwell L 1992 Therapeutic ultrasound: its effects on the cellular and mollecular mechanisms of inflammation and repair. Physiotherapy 78(6): 421–426

McDonough S, Kitchen S 2002 Neuromuscular and Muscular Electrical Stimulation. In: Kitchen S (ed.) Electrotherapy: Evidence-based Practice. Churchill Livingstone: Edinburgh

McManus FJ, Ward AR et al. 2006 The analgesic effects of interferential therapy on two experimental pain models: cold and mechanically induced pain. Physiotherapy 92(2): 95–102

Michlovitz S 1996 Thermal Agents in Rehabilitation. FA Davis: Philadelphia

Michlovitz S, Hun L, Erasala GN 2004 Continuous low-level heat-wrap therapy is effective for treating wrist pain. Arch Phys Med Rehabil 85: 1409–1416

Mortimer AJ, Dyson M 1988 The effect of therapeutic ultrasound on calcium uptake in fibroblasts. Ultrasound Med Biol 14(6): 499–506

Neder JA, Sword D et al. 2002 Home based neuromuscular electrical stimulation as a new rehabilitative strategy for severely disabled patients with chronic obstructive pulmonary disease (COPD). Thorax 57(4): 333–337

Noble JG, Henderson G et al. 2000 The effect of interferential therapy upon cutaneous blood flow in humans. Clin Physiol 20(1): 2–7

Nussbaum E 1998 The influence of ultrasound on healing tissues. J Hand Ther 11(2): 140–147

Nussbaum EL 1997 Ultrasound: to heat or not to heat — that is the question. Physical Therapy Reviews 2: 59–72

Ottawa Panel 2004 Ottawa panel evidence-based clinical practice guidelines for electrotherapy and thermotherapy interventions in the management of rheumatoid arthritis in adults. Physical Therapy 84(11): 1016–1043

Palmer S, Martin D 2002 Interferential Current for Pain Control. In: Kitchen S (ed.) Electrotherapy: Evidence-based Practice. Churchill Livingstone: Edinburgh

Palmer ST, Martin DJ et al. 1999 Alteration of interferential current and transcutaneous electrical nerve stimulation frequency: effects on nerve excitation. Arch Phys Med Rehabil 80(9): 1065–1071

Poltawski L, Watson T 2007 Relative transmissivity of ultrasound coupling agents commonly used by therapists in the UK. Ultrasound Med Biol 33(1): 120–128

Pope GD, Mockett SP et al. 1995 A survey of electrotherapeutic modalities: ownership and use in the NHS in England. Physiotherapy 81(2): 82–91

Ramirez AJ, Schwane A et al. 1997 The effect of ultrasound on collagen synthesis and fibroblast proliferation in vitro. Med Sci Sports Exerc 29: 326–332

Reher P, Doan N et al. 1999 Effect of ultrasound on the production of IL-8, basic FGF and VEGF. Cytokine 11(6): 416–423

Reher P, Harris M et al. 2002 Ultrasound stimulates nitric oxide and prostaglandin E2 production by human osteoblasts. Bone 31(1): 236–241

Robertson VJ, Ward A et al. 2006 Electrotherapy Explained: Principles and Practice. Butterworth–Heinemann: Oxford

Seiger C, Draper DO 2006 Use of pulsed shortwave diathermy and joint mobilization to increase ankle range of motion in the presence of surgical implanted metal: A case series. J Orthop Sports Phys Ther 36(9): 669–677

Sheffler LR, Hennessey MT et al. 2006 Peroneal nerve stimulation versus an ankle foot orthosis for correction of footdrop in stroke: impact on functional ambulation. Neurorehabil Neural Repair 20(3): 355–360

Simonis RB, Parnell EJ et al. 2003 Electrical treatment of tibial non-union: a prospective, randomised, double-blind trial. Injury 34(5): 357–362
Sluka KA, Walsh D 2003 Transcutaneous electrical nerve stimulation: basic science mechanisms and clinical effectiveness. J Pain 4(3): 109–121
Sluka KA, Lisi TL et al. 2006 Increased release of serotonin in the spinal cord during low, but not high, frequency transcutaneous electric nerve stimulation in rats with joint inflammation. Arch Phys Med Rehabil 87(8): 1137–1140
Sontag W 2000 Modulation of cytokine production by interferential current in differentiated HL-60 cells. Bioelectromagnetics 21(3): 238–244
Sparrow KJ, Finucane SD et al. 2005 The effects of low-intensity ultrasound on medial collateral ligament healing in the rabbit model. Am J Sports Med 33(7): 1048–1056
Stevens JE, Mizner RL et al. 2004 Neuromuscular electrical stimulation for quadriceps muscle strengthening after bilateral total knee arthroplasty: a case series. J Orthop Sports Phys Ther 34(1): 21–29
Talbot LA, Gaines JM et al. 2003 A home-based protocol of electrical muscle stimulation for quadriceps muscle strength in older adults with osteoarthritis of the knee. J Rheumatol 30(7): 1571–1578
Taylor P, Burridge J et al. 1999 Clinical audit of 5 years provision of the Odstock dropped foot stimulator. Artif Organs 23(5): 440–442
ter Haar G 1999 Therapeutic Ultrasound. Eur J Ultrasound 9: 3–9
Tuner J, Hode L 2004 The Laser Therapy Handbook. Prima: Grangesberg, Sweden
Turner S, Powell E et al. 1989 The effect of ultrasound on the healing of repaired cockerel tendon: is collagen cross-linkage a factor? J Hand Surg 14B: 428–433
Usuba M, Miyanaga Y et al. 2006 Effect of heat in increasing the range of knee motion after the development of a joint contracture: an experiment with an animal model. Arch Phys Med Rehabil 87(2): 247–253
Vinck EM, Cagnie BJ et al. 2003 Increased fibroblast proliferation induced by light emitting diode and low power laser irradiation. Lasers Med Sci 18(2): 95–99
Vinck E, Coorevits P et al. 2005 Evidence of changes in sural nerve conduction mediated by light emitting diode irradiation. Lasers Med Sci 20(1): 35–40
Vivodtzev I, Pepin JL et al. 2006 Improvement in quadriceps strength and dyspnea in daily tasks after 1 month of electrical stimulation in severely deconditioned and malnourished COPD. Chest 129(6): 1540–1548
Walker UA, Uhl M et al. 2006 Analgesic and disease modifying effects of interferential current in psoriatic arthritis. Rheumatol Int 26(10): 904–907
Walsh D 1997 TENS: Clinical Applications and Related Theory. Churchill Livingstone: Edinburgh
Warden SJ, Bennell KL et al. 2000 Acceleration of fresh fracture repair using the sonic accelerated fracture healing system (SAFHS): a review. Calcif Tissue Int 66(2): 157–163
Warden SJ, Avin KG et al. 2006 Low-intensity pulsed ultrasound accelerates and a nonsteroidal anti-inflammatory drug delays knee ligament healing. Am J Sports Med 34(7): 1094–1102
Watson T 1996 Electrical stimulation for wound healing. Physical Therapy Reviews 1(2): 89–103
Watson T 2000 The role of electrotherapy in contemporary physiotherapy practice. Manual Ther 5(3): 132–141
Watson T 2002a Current concepts in electrotherapy. Haemophilia 8: 413–418
Watson T 2002b Electrical stimulation for wound healing: a review of current knowledge. In: Kitchen S (ed.) Electrotherapy: Evidence-based Practice. Churchill Livingstone: Edinburgh
Watson T 2002c Ultrasound dose calculations. In Touch 101: 14–17
Watson T 2003 Soft tissue healing. In Touch 104: 2–9
Watson T 2006a Electrotherapy and tissue repair. Sportex Medicine 29: 7–13
Watson T 2006b Tissue repair: The current state of the art. Sportex Medicine 28: 8–12
Wilkin LD, Merrick MA et al. 2004 Influence of therapeutic ultrasound on skeletal muscle regeneration following blunt contusion. Int J Sports Med 25(1): 73–77
Williams A, McHale J et al. 1987 Effects of MHz ultrasound on electrical pain threshold perception in humans. Ultrasound Med Biol 13: 249–258
Yeung CK, Guo X et al. 2006 Pulsed ultrasound treatment accelerates the repair of Achilles tendon rupture in rats. J Orthop Res 24(2): 193–201
Young S 2002 Ultrasound Therapy. In: Kitchen S (ed.) Electrotherapy: Evidence-based Practice. Churchill Livingstone: Edinburgh, pp. 211–230
Young SR, Dyson M 1990a The effect of therapeutic ultrasound on angiogenesis. Ultrasound Med Biol 16(3): 261–269
Young SR, Dyson M 1990b Effect of therapeutic ultrasound on the healing of full-thickness excised skin lesions. Ultrasonics 28(3): 175–180
Zanotti E, Felicetti G et al. 2003 Peripheral muscle strength training in bed-bound patients with COPD receiving mechanical ventilation: effect of electrical stimulation. Chest 124(1): 292–296

MANUFACTURERS' LINKS

Central Medical Equipment Ltd (CME)
Unit 32A, Atcham Business Park, Atcham, Shropshire SY4 4UG
Web: www.physiobuyer.com

EMS Physio Ltd
Wantage, Oxfordshire OX12 9FE
Tel: 01235 772272
Web: www.emsphysio.co.uk

Mobilis Healthcare Group
100 Shaw Road, Oldham, Lancashire OL1 4AY
Tel: 0161 678 0233
Web: www.mobilisphysiotherapy.com/

Nature's Gate
P.O. Box 371, Basingstoke, Hampshire RG24 8GD
Tel: 01256 346060
Web: www.naturesgate-uk.com/

Orthosonics Ltd Europe
Bremridge House, Bremridge, Ashburton Devon TQ13 7JX
Tel: 01364 652426
Web: www.orthosonics.com

Physio-Med Services Ltd
7–23 Glossop Brook Business Park, Surrey Street, Glossop, Derbyshire SK13 7AJ
Tel: 01457 860 444
Web: www.physio-med.com

SKF Services Ltd
Unit 18 Huffwood Trading Estate, Billingshurst, West Sussex RH14 9UR
Tel: 01403 785111
Web: www.skfservices.com

Tenscare Ltd
PainAway House, Epsom, Surrey KT17 1DT
Tel: 013 7272 3434
Web: www.tenscare.co.uk

THOR International Head Office UK
Old British Schoolhouse, East Street, Chesham HP5 1HQ
Tel: 01494 797 100
Web: www.thorlaser.com/

Chapter **19**

Pain

Lester Jones and G. Lorimer Moseley

CHAPTER CONTENTS

INTRODUCTION

Pain is a common and normal human experience. It helps us to learn safe behaviour when our body has been injured and adopt protective behaviour when it is threatened. Pain usually seems like a reasonably predictable experience. In a normal state, receptors in the tissues of the body respond at reasonably predictable thresholds of stimulation. When they do respond, they initiate action potentials, which travel along peripheral neurones into the spinal cord. Neurotransmitters released from these neurones often activate secondary neurones, which send action potentials up the spinal cord to the brain. The brain then evaluates this information. Often, pain is perceived in the tissues that were stimulated. This might seem simple, but it is not.

Definition

The International Association for the Study of Pain (IASP) defines pain as 'an unpleasant, sensory and emotional experience associated with actual or potential tissue damage, or described in terms of such damage' (Merskey and Bogduk 1994).

There are several key parts of this definition:

- Firstly, although the nociceptive system is critical for detecting dangerous stimuli and alerting the brain, pain is not simply the transmission of noxious sensory information (nociception). (Nociceptive neurones are so important that people born with a particular genetic mutation, in which nociceptive neurones do not function normally, do not experience pain when they receive a noxious stimulus (Cox et al. 2006).) Rather, pain has potentially profound cognitive and emotional influences, just like other perceptual states (even vision — think of your favourite visual illusion and notice that what you see is not necessarily an accurate reflection of the light that is hitting the light receptors on your retina).

- Secondly, pain is not a measure of tissue damage, which means that tissue can be injured but not painful, and painful but not injured.
- Thirdly, pain is about threat to body tissue, not about a particular mode of sensory input. This sets pain apart from other information that is sent from our tissues to our brain, the so-called somatic senses. It is this threat-specific quality that makes pain critical for protection and preservation of the body; pain seems to be the conscious component of a complex defence system.
- Finally, there are many unconscious components of this defence system, all of which can influence each other, and influence pain. Thus, pain is a fundamentally conscious process, which is preceded and accompanied by a range of responses, most of which are not conscious. According to this model of pain, when people are in pain, we can be sure that their brain is concluding that tissue is in danger and that they should take some sort of action to get the tissues out of danger (Butler and Moseley 2003; Wall 1999).

THE PHYSIOLOGY OF PAIN

This section will discuss the physiology of pain in three categories:

1. activation of the nociceptive system
2. modulation of the nociception/pain system
3. sensitisation of the nociception/pain system.

Within each category, we will separate peripheral from spinal and brain mechanisms, when it is appropriate to do so.

Activation of the nociceptive system

Peripheral mechanisms

19

The peripheral nervous system is well studied but not completely understood. Many types of neurone in the periphery are thought to contribute to nociception (Meyer et al. 2006). The most important of these neurones are probably A-delta and C fibres — conventionally called nociceptors — although many Aδ and C fibres also respond to non-noxious inputs (Craig 2002).

For the sake of clarity, we will classify Aδ and C fibres (Table 19.1) as *primary nociceptors*.

Nociceptors are found in most tissues of the body and can be considered to have the principle role of detecting dangerous thermal, mechanical or chemical stimuli. Studies have attempted to identify activation thresholds for different noxious stimuli (the activation threshold being the lowest intensity of a stimulus that produces an action potential in the nociceptor). While there is variability between individuals, there seems to be a predictable range of activation thresholds for primary nociceptors in healthy pain-free individuals.

Thresholds of unsensitised nociceptors

- *Mechanical* — two classes:
  Mechanically sensitive afferents — early response (e.g. to pinch)
  Mechanically insensitive afferents — > 600 kPa (Raja et al. 1999)
- *Thermal*:
  Heat: 41–49°C (Tillman et al. 1995, cited in Raja et al. 1999; Kelly et al. 2005)
  Cold: 6.7°C (hand)–11.8°C (forearm); 0°C (Kelly et al. 2005)
- *Chemical* (concentrations that have elicited pain):
  Acetylcholine 1% solution (Schmelz et al. 2003)
  Capsaicin 0.1% solution (Schmelz et al. 2003).

Spinal mechanisms

Primary nociceptors terminate in the dorsal horn of the spinal cord. The dorsal horn consists of numerous layers, which are defined according to the projections and the structural and functional properties of their neurones. The majority of nociceptors terminate in laminae I (Aδ fibres usually terminate here), II (C fibres

Table 19.1 Comparison of the characteristics of Aδ and C fibres

Characteristic*	Aδ	C
1a. Conduction speed	Fast (4–36 m/s)	Slow (0.4–2 m/s)
1b. Pain onset	First/fast pain	Second/slow pain
2a. Accommodation (adaptation)	Fast	Slow
2b. Pain duration	Brief	Long
3a. Receptive field	Small	Large
3b. Localisation	Precise	Diffuse
4. Sensory quality	Sharp, pricking	Aching, dull, burning
5. CNS response	Reflex, analysis	Emotional, suffering

*Characteristics referred to by the letter 'a' are physiological, while 'b' describes the consequences for the nature of the pain. (Reproduced from Van Griensven 2005; see also Craig 2002; Meyer 2006.)

usually terminate here) and V (Aδ, C and Aβ fibres all terminate here). Lamina II neurones project to other laminae and can be excitatory or inhibitory. Because peripheral input on to lamina I fibres is almost exclusively nociceptive (Aδ), the neurones that project from here are called *nociceptive-specific* second-order neurones. Because peripheral input on to lamina V second-order neurones includes Aδ, C and Aβ fibres, lamina V second-order neurones tend to respond over a wide range of stimulus inputs, which is why they are called *wide-dynamic-range neurones*.

Transmission from the dorsal horn to the brain

There are five ascending pathways for nociceptive information. The largest is the *spinothalamic tract*, which includes neurones that originate in laminae I and V. Other pathways include the spinoreticular, spinomesencephalic, cervicothalamic and spinohypothalamic tracts. Importantly, there is not a single nociceptive pathway; nor is there a single target location (a 'pain centre') in the brain. Rather, there are many sites within the CNS at which nociceptive input is processed and modulated.

Brain mechanisms

The brain is defined here as that part of the CNS that lies above the spinal cord. There are several important characteristics of how nociception is handled by the brain.

Parallel processing

Many brain areas are involved in pain. Most often, the thalamus, insula, and primary (S1) and secondary (S2) somatosensory and pre-frontal cortices are involved. These areas are called the pain matrix (Apkarian et al. 2005) (Figure 19.1). However, these areas are never the only areas involved and they are not always all involved. The pattern of brain activation varies greatly between and within individuals.

Different aspects of pain seem to involve different brain areas

In an attempt to clarify the potential roles of different brain areas in pain, some authors conceptualise two systems.

The *medial nociceptive system* includes the medial thalamic nuclei, anterior cingulate and dorsolateral prefrontal cortices. It is described as slow and only broadly somatotopic, which means it does not have the capacity to code in detail the location in the body at which the stimulus occurred. Activity in this system has been proposed to subserve the affective-emotional dimensions of pain: that is, the unpleasantness of pain rather than the intensity and quality.

The *lateral nociceptive system* includes the lateral thalamic nuclei and the primary (S1) and secondary (S2) somatosensory cortices. It is described as fast and is highly somatotopic, which means it is able to code, in great detail, the tissue location at which the stimulus occurred. Activity in this system is proposed to subserve the sensory-discriminative aspects of pain: that is, the intensity of the pain and the sensory characteristics of the stimulus (e.g. warm, sharp, deep, superficial). The intensity and unpleasantness of pain can be independently manipulated (e.g. Moseley and Arntz 2007).

Multiple inputs — the neuromatrix theory

Melzack (1990) proposed the neuromatrix theory as a way of conceptualising how myriad inputs and factors affect pain and nociception. Inputs and factors in that theory include previous learning and past experiences, immune and endocrine states and responses, activity in the autonomic nervous system, and information coming from nociceptors and other sensory receptors. The theory suggests that pain will occur when all these elements are evaluated and a specific network of neurones in the brain is activated. Melzack calls each particular network of neurones a neurosignature (or neurotag — Butler and Moseley 2003), which is analogous to the representation concept used in cognitive neuroscience literature (see Damasio (2000) for review of representation theory). Remember that this is a theory and that the brain physiology underpinning pain and consciousness is not well understood.

Pain is in the brain

Both Melzack's 'neuromatrix model' and the IASP definition of pain highlight the need to use a biopsychosocial approach in evaluating and treating a person's pain. They also reinforce the concept of pain being created by the brain as a result of multiple influences, in particular the detection or perception of danger to the body's tissues. Tissue damage, along with the resultant nociception, is just one of these influences. As is suggested by the IASP definition, tissue damage is neither sufficient nor necessary for pain.

Modulation of nociception/pain

Anecdotal evidence that somatic, psychological and social factors modulate pain is substantial — sport-related and war-related stories are common (see Butler and Moseley 2003 for several examples). However, numerous experimental findings corroborate the

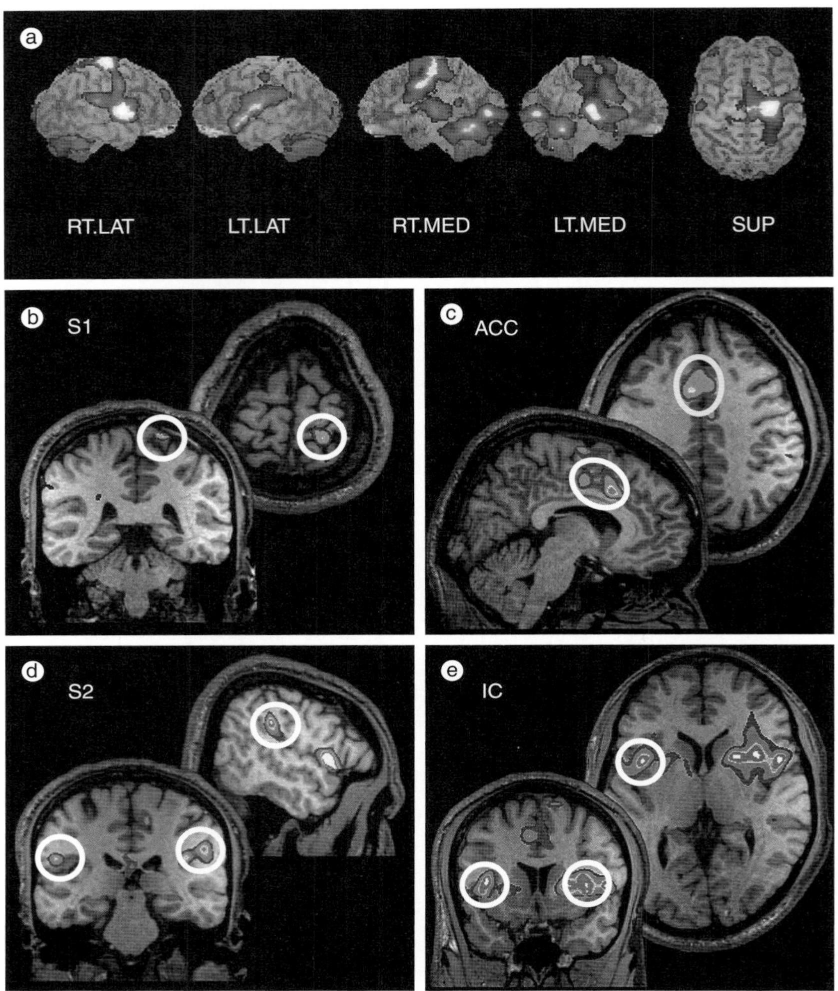

Figure 19.1 Pain evoked activation in the human brain. (a) Surface-rendered image obtained using positron emission tomograms (PET). They show areas of the brain that are more active during painful thermal stimulation than they are during non-painful thermal stimulation. (b)–(e) Images obtained using functional MRI of a similar stimulus. This time, cross sectional views are shown so that we can see activation of primary and secondary somatosensory cortices (S1 and S2), anterior cingulate and insular cortices (ACC and IC). Because the areas shown in each image are more active during pain than during non-painful heat, we take them to be important in producing pain. (Figure (a) reproduced from Casey et al. 2001; (b)–(e) adapted from Bushnell et al. 1999, with permission.)

anecdotal evidence (see Fields et al. 2006 for a review of CNS mechanisms of modulation).

Experiments that manipulate the psychological context of a noxious stimulus often demonstrate clear effects on pain, although the direction of these effects is not always consistent. For example, a large amount of literature concerns the effect of attention on pain, and of pain on attention (Asmundson et al. 1997; Crombez et al. (1996, 1997, 1998, 1999); Duckworth et al. 1997; Eccleston 1994; Eccleston and Crombez 1999; Eccleston et al. 1997; Matthews et al. 1980; McCracken 1997; Moseley and Arntz 2007; Naveteur et al. 2005; Peters et al. 2000). Despite the wealth of data, consensus is lacking; some data suggest that attending to pain amplifies it and attending away from pain nullifies it, but others suggest the opposite. Most likely, the effect depends on the coping style of the individual and the wider context of the experiment or situation.

Anxiety also seems to have variable effects on pain. Some reports link increased anxiety to increased pain during clinical procedures (Gore et al. 2005; Klages et al. 2006; Pud and Amit 2005; Schupp et al. 2005) and during experimentally induced pain (Tang and Gibson 2005), but other reports suggest no effect (Arntz et al. (1990, 1994)). Relevant reviews conclude that the influence of anxiety on pain is probably largely dependent on attention (Arntz et al. 1994; Ploghaus et al. 2003).

Expectation also seems to have variable effects on pain. As a general rule, expectation of a noxious stimulus increases pain if the cue signals a more intense or more damaging stimulus (Chua et al. 1999; Fields 2000; Keltner et al. 2006; Moseley and Arntz 2007; Ploghaus et al. 1999; Sawamoto et al. 2000) and decreases pain if the cue signals a less intense or less damaging stimulus (Benedetti et al. 2003; Pollo et al. 2001). There are several informative reviews on the influence of expectation on pain (e.g. Fields 2000; Wager 2005).

The common denominator of the effect of attention, anxiety and expectation on pain seems to be the underlying evaluative context, or *meaning* of the pain. That is demonstrated by the consistent effect that some cognitive states seem to have on pain. For example, catastrophic interpretations of pain are associated with higher pain ratings in both clinical and experimental studies (see Sullivan et al. 2001 for review). Believing pain to be an accurate indicator of the state of the tissues is associated with higher pain ratings (Moseley et al. 2004), whereas believing that the nervous system amplifies noxious input in chronic pain states increases pain threshold during straight leg raise (Moseley 2004).

The social context of a noxious stimulus also affects the pain it evokes. For example, when men have blood taken by a woman, it hurts less than when it is taken by another man (Levine and De Simone 1991). The effects are variable but again seem to be underpinned by the underlying evaluative context or meaning (see Butler and Moseley 2003 for a review of pain-related data and Moerman 2002 for exhaustive coverage of the role of meaning in medicine and health-related interactions).

To review the very large amount of literature on somatic, psychological and social influences on pain is beyond the scope of this chapter. However, it is appropriate, and clinically meaningful, to reiterate the theme that emerges from that literature: the influences on pain perception, tolerance and report are variable, and seem to depend on the evaluative context of the noxious input.

Sensitisation of the nociception/pain system

The nociceptive system is dynamic. If the system becomes more sensitive than usual, it often results in hyperalgesia (things that hurt now hurt more) and allodynia (things that did not hurt now do).

Definitions

Hyperalgesia An increased response to a stimulus that is normally painful.

Allodynia Pain due to a stimulus that does not normally provoke pain (Merskey and Bogduk, 1994).

Hyperalgesia and allodynia might be expected and seem intuitively sensible after recent damage to tissue, but they are also a predominant feature of persistent pain. It is unlikely that the same processes are involved in hyperalgesia and allodynia in acute post-injury pain and hyperalgesia and allodynia in chronic pain.

Peripheral mechanisms

Peripheral mechanisms that increase the pain evoked by a standardised stimulus include the presence of inflammatory mediators, decreased circulation (which increases the local concentration of H^+ ions), the presence of immune mediators and activation of certain genes (see Figure 19.2 and Meyer et al. 2006 for an exhaustive review of peripheral mechanisms of modulation). Inflammatory mediators are released by tissue damage and by activation of nociceptors (neurogenic inflammation). This sensitisation, driven by peripheral mechanisms, is called peripheral sensitisation, and the hyperalgesia that follows is called primary hyperalgesia.

Spinal cord mechanisms

Second-order nociceptors can also become sensitised. The N-methyl-D-aspartate (NMDA) receptors in the dorsal horn respond to persistent or intense stimulation by opening channels to allow greater post-synaptic activity. This means that the same input from the periphery will result in greater activation of the second-order nociceptor, which means that more messages of danger to body tissue will be sent to the brain.

Dorsal horn mechanism

NMDA receptors are important in central sensitisation. They are normally blocked by magnesium, but prolonged nociceptive activity and release of peptides can remove the block and allow glutamate to bind to the receptor. The resultant activation of voltage-sensitive channels allows an influx of calcium into the second-order neurone. This process can lead to a change in the NMDA receptor so that the magnesium block then becomes less effective, which means that, next time, the sensitisation will happen more quickly.

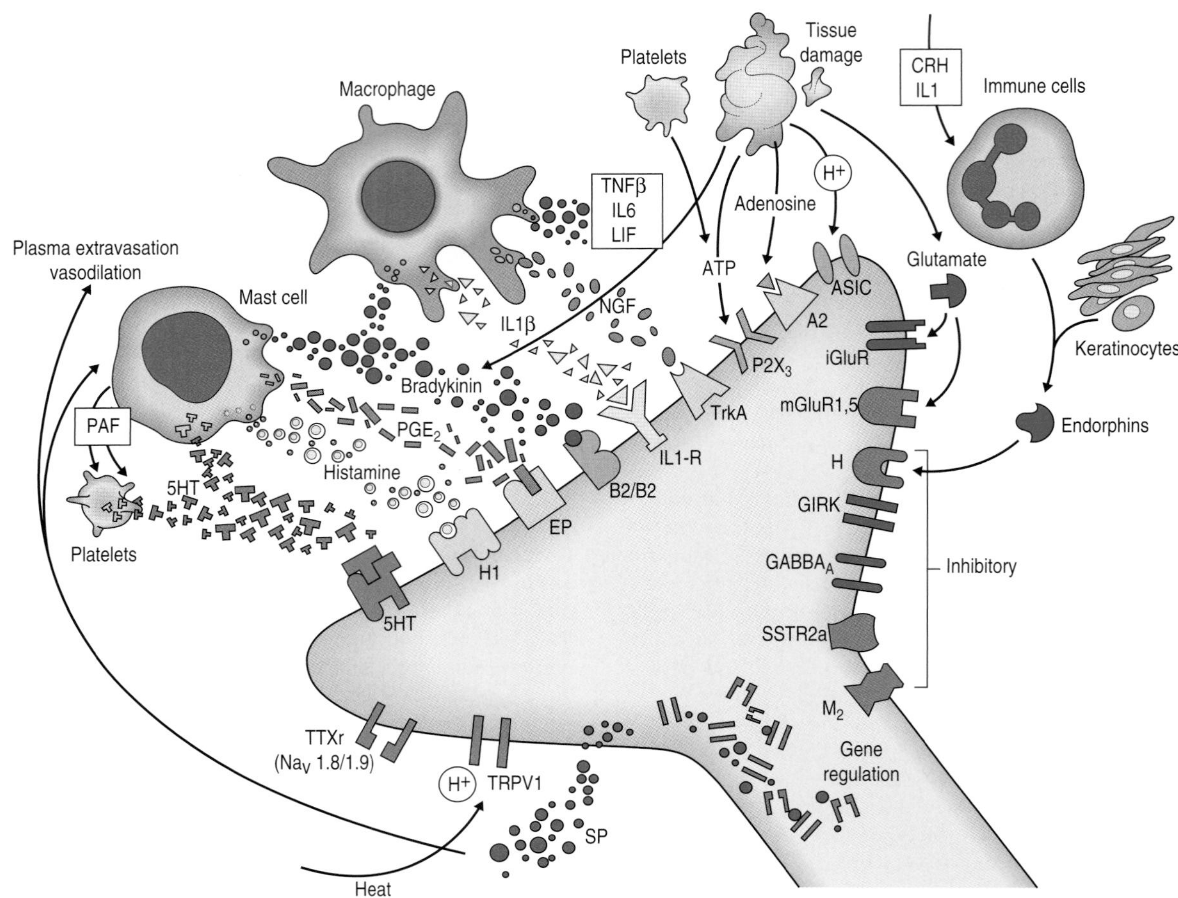

Figure 19.2 Potential peripheral mediators of peripheral sensitisation after inflammation. The point of this figure is not so that the reader can remember everything that happens, but to illustrate that even peripheral sensitisation, which occurs almost every time we injure tissue, is extremely complex. The interested reader should refer to the cited text because to discuss all of these processes here is beyond the scope of the chapter. (Artwork by Ian Suk, Johns Hopkins University, adapted from Woolf and Costigan 1999.)

19

There are other mechanisms in the dorsal horn that can sensitise the nociceptive system. Wide-dynamic-range neurones in the laminae of the dorsal horn provide an interaction of the processing for nociception and other sensory information. This may be important in how people describe their pain, sometimes referred to as the 'quality' of pain. It also provides a potential mechanism for further sensitivity of the nociceptive system, whereby the responses to normally non-painful stimuli, such as touch, are now painful. This may be because the wide-dynamic-range neurones synapse with sensitised neurones. Another mechanism of sensitisation involves the sprouting of neurones across laminae. Such sprouting may link a non-nociceptive peripheral nerve fibre (e.g. Aβ fibre) with an interneurone that would normally respond to noxious stimulation. This is probably more likely to occur after peripheral nerve injury or death. Butler and Moseley's *Explain Pain* (2003) discusses these mechanisms in an accessible but reasonably detailed way.

Neuropathic pain

The pain associated with nerve damage is known as neuropathic pain and may include descriptions such as 'burning' or 'electric shock'. CNS damage, such as stroke, can result in centrally mediated neuropathic pain that reduces the inhibition of the nociceptive system. Peripherally, damage to an axon or the myelin covering of a nerve can lead to spontaneous transmission of impulses from the damaged area of the dorsal root ganglion (DRG). Such damage will usually result in hypersensitivity to mechanical input. This sensitivity forms the basis for tests such as Tinel's sign, sometimes considered as an indicator of neuropathic pain.

Damaged neurones alter their genetic expression (Butler 2000). This means that the affected neurone may increase production of certain chemoreceptors. If this occurs, the neurone will become more sensitive to that chemical. For example, increased production of adrenoreceptors will cause increased neuronal firing when the blood concentration of adrenaline (epinephrine) is increased, or when the sympathetic nervous system is activated. There is mounting evidence that interactions between the immune system, endocrine system and autonomic nervous system are important in all types of pain, including neuropathic pain (Watkins and Maier 2000).

ASSESSMENT AND MEASUREMENT OF PAIN

Pain is an essentially personal experience, which means that measurement of pain relies on the person in pain communicating their experience. Therefore, any measure of pain, including report of pain, is really a measure of pain behaviour. Clinicians and researchers make a judgement according to how well they think the measure of pain behaviour might reflect pain, but ultimately this relies on assumptions that as yet cannot be verified. This limitation also applies to physiological measures such as brain imaging.

Earlier in this chapter, we argued that pain depends on many modulating factors and can be expressed in many ways. Moreover, we argued that pain is one output of the brain that serves to protect the tissues. Those arguments mean that assessment and measurement of people in pain encompasses more than measurement of their pain. One framework that is useful in assessment of people in pain is the World Health Organization International Classification of Functioning, Disability and Health (WHO ICF).

World Health Organization International Classification of Functioning, Disability and Health (WHO ICF)

This section uses the WHO ICF as a framework for assessment and treatment planning of patients in pain. This framework is advocated by the IASP (Merskey and Bogduk 1994). The WHO ICF focuses on how a person is functioning and evaluates outcomes using the person's actual performance in the real-life environment. This makes it especially useful for those patients for whom pain relief is not the only, and possibly not the most important, objective.

The WHO ICF has three components: the body (function and structure), activities and participation, and contextual factors (for example, environmental factors that might influence function). Each component is classified at a level of severity (none, mild, moderate, severe, complete) and interactions between components are evaluated (WHO 2002). As it relates to pain patients, the three components of the ICF broadly mirror the components of the biopsychosocial model, which considers tissue-based, psychological and social influences on pain.

The interview

Most therapeutic processes will start with an interview (Table 19.2). The interview aims to capture information about the patient in terms of the ICF. Physiotherapy interviews have conventionally focused on symptoms:

Table 19.2 Content summary of structured interview for biopsychosocial assessment

Area of examination	Information gained
Orientation	Nature and location of symptoms; patient's story from onset to present, expectations of physiotherapy, questions and concerns about problem
Previous intervention	Investigations and understanding, treatment effects, advice received, causal beliefs
Medical history	Comorbidity and effect on function, special questions (red flag screening), medication
Effects on function and participation	Current social and employment situation, typical day, effects on work, restrictions on activity, assistance required, aids and adaptations, downtime, sleep
Coping strategies	Current coping strategies: active and passive, perceived consequences of change (e.g. increasing activity, exercise, pacing)
Socioeconomic	Effect on finances, benefits, medico-legal
Effect on family	Beliefs, responses, nature of support provided
Emotion	Nature and extent, effect on motivation
Pre-examination	Body chart, behaviour of symptoms

(Reproduced from Goldingay (2006b), with kind permission of S Goldingay and the CNS Press.)

location, intensity, quality, temporal patterns, and signs. This information is very important, but it is not sufficient. According to the ICF, this information relates to the *body*, the biopsychosocial model's equivalent of the tissues. However, we advocate, as do other reviews in this area (e.g. Gifford et al. 2006), that the interview must also provide information about activities, participation and contextual factors (that is, the 'psychosocial'), and how these issues may interact with pain and the state of the tissues (Goldingay (2006a, 2006b)). The aim of the interview, then, is to identify factors, from across biopsychosocial domains, which activate or sensitise the nociceptive or pain system.

Measures and scales

Self-report measures

Assessing pain is a key aspect of the assessment process. Self-report measures are considered the gold standard in assessing pain intensity, location, quality and temporal variation.

Definitions

Quality of pain This refers to characteristics such as aching, burning, stabbing and cramping, which a patient attributes to his/her pain.

Temporal aspects of pain Commonly, this refers to 24-hour behaviour of pain but might also relate to other influences such as menstrual cycle or seasonal changes.

Visual analogue scales (VAS) and numerical rating scales (NRS) are most common and useful. A VAS consists of a horizontal line, usually 100 mm long. At each end is a term of reference for the patient, called an *anchor*. The left anchor is usually 'No pain' and the right 'worst pain' or 'worst pain imaginable'. Patients mark a point on the line in answer to a question about their pain, and the distance from the mark to the left anchor is used as a measure of their pain. An NRS uses numbers instead of a line, such that 0 = 'no pain' and 10 = 'worst pain'. The VAS is probably more sensitive to change, less vulnerable to perseveration (remembering what you said last time and responding the same way), and more difficult to measure. The NRS is easier to use clinically and is probably sufficiently sensitive to detect clinically meaningful changes (a clinically meaningful change is usually considered to be about 2 points on a 10-point scale (McQuay et al. 1997).

Several tools assess the quality of pain. The most widely used is the short form of the McGill Pain Questionnaire (MPQ) (Melzack 1975b). The MPQ lists a variety of words that are grouped as being about the sensory-discriminative aspect of pain (e.g. sharp, burning, intense), the affective aspect of pain (e.g. punishing) or its evaluative context (e.g. annoying). There are many other measures that emphasise different aspects of pain.

Notes on pain scales

McGill Pain Questionnaire (Melzack 1975b)

Attempts to measure pain as a multi-dimensional experience.

- 20 categories of adjectives.
- 4 subclasses – sensory/affective/evaluative/miscellaneous.
- Patients select adjectives that best describe pain experience.
- Adjectives are weighted and a score – the pain rating index – is calculated for each subclass.
- Valid and reliable in range of contexts.
- Takes a long time to fill out (a short version is also available).
- Patients may prefer to use other words to describe the quality of pain.

Brief Pain Inventory (Cherny and Portenoy 1999; Keller et al. 2004)

- Patients self-categorise social status and current work situation.
- Boxes are checked to indicate pain history.
- Pain location is marked on a body chart.
- Pain intensity and quality are determined by ratings on 0–10 scales or yes/no responses.
- Seven questions are specific to the impact of pain: function, mood, life enjoyment.
- Easily administered.

Chronic Pain Index (Von Korff et al. 1994)

- Patients respond to 8 questions about pain intensity and interference with life activities.
- Pain intensity and interference of activity are seen as a single dimension reflecting severity.
- Scoring method and grading system completed by assessor.

Behavioural measures

Although self-report measures are behavioural measures, they are generally considered as a separate category. Non-self-report behavioural measures are useful as a corroborator of self-report measures, or when the patient is unable to use the measure (as with children), or when the clinician considers the patient's report is dubious. Behavioural measures include observation (by a covert or overt observer) and performance (for example, functional, endurance, speed or load tests). Full review of behavioural measures is beyond the scope of this paper, but the interested reader is referred to the *Handbook of Pain Assessment* (Turk and Melzack 2001) and *Manage your Pain* (Nicholas et al. 2002) for examples.

Measures of the impact of pain

Critical to the ICF framework and to the biopsychosocial model is evaluation of other factors that might be modulating pain or the behavioural response to pain, or both. Numerous measures have been devised and tested. The following is a brief account of the most widely used and documented.

Measuring potential impact of beliefs and thoughts

The importance of evaluation of the threat to body tissue has been mentioned earlier. Inherent to this evaluation is fear of movement and (re)injury. A large amount of research has investigated the role of pain-related fear avoidance behaviour. There are many specific findings that relate fear and catastrophic thought processes to pain intensity, disability and self-efficacy, but the *principle* can be summarised thus: people who have heightened concerns about pain, its cause and its consequences often have a sense of helplessness and adopt a passive coping style. As a result, they have a lower criterion for a movement or activity to be considered potentially painful or potentially injurious. They therefore avoid those movements and activities — 'fear-avoidance'. Avoidance of activity leads to disuse and hampers healing and recovery, which leaves the patient in a vicious circle of progressive depression, disuse and disability (Figure 19.3). According to the fear-avoidance model, most people do not follow this path because they have a more accurate and appropriate level of concern and thus do not tend to avoid movement and activity (Vlaeyen and Linton 2000). See Vlaeyen and Linton (2000) for a review of fear-avoidance beliefs and pain and Sullivan et al. (2001) for a review of catastrophic thought processes and pain.

Fear-avoidance beliefs can be gauged via the interview, but can be quantified via the fear-avoidance beliefs questionnaire (Waddell et al. 1993) or the Tampa scale of kinesiphobia (kinesiphobia meaning 'fear of movement') (Miller et al. 1991). Data for both tools are available from a range of patient and non-patient populations. Catastrophic thought processes can also be gauged via the interview, but can be quantified via the pain catastrophising scale (Sullivan et al. 1995), which also has a large amount of data available. Other measures that are psychometrically robust and widely used in research, but are less popular clinically, include the survey of pain attitudes (Jensen et al. 1987), the pain beliefs and perceptions inventory (Williams et al. 1994) and the pain anxiety symptoms scale (McCracken et al. 1992).

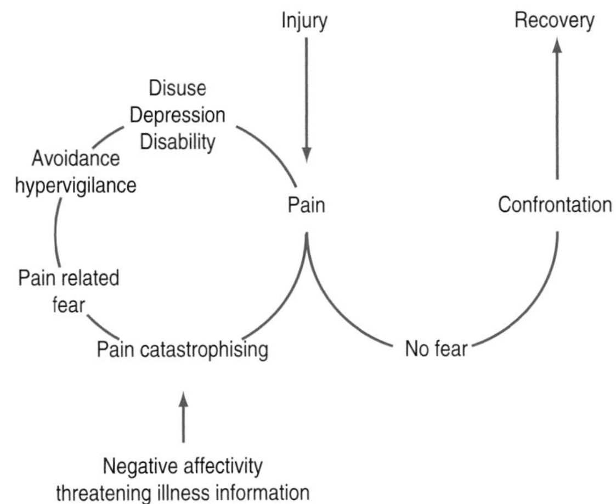

Figure 19.3 The fear-avoidance model.

> **What about the clinician's thoughts and beliefs?**
>
> There is some evidence that the clinician's thoughts and beliefs about pain modulate the effect of the treatment. For example, researchers undertook a placebo-controlled double blind study of fentanyl (a powerful analgesic) during wisdom teeth removal (Gracely et al. 1985). Although all patients had the same likelihood of receiving fentanyl, the researchers told some of the dentists that the patient would not receive fentanyl. This was a lie. When the clinician thought that the patient might get fentanyl (which was true), pain dropped by 2 points after the placebo injection. When the clinician thought that the patient could not get fentanyl (which was a lie), pain increased by 5 points after the placebo injection. This difference (~7 points!) was due to the belief of the dentist!

Other studies have shown that the fear-avoidance beliefs of patients with back pain are similar to those of their rheumatologists (Poiraudeau et al. 2006) and that rheumatologists' fear-avoidance beliefs affect the decisions they make about their patients' management (Coudeyre et al. 2006).

Self-efficacy

Self-efficacy is the belief individuals have about their ability to perform a task using their current resources. Because self-efficacy depends on appraisal of the demands of a particular task and of the individual's own capacity to meet them, self-efficacy depends on evaluative factors relating to pain and injury. Self-efficacy is therefore affected by inappropriate or inaccurate appraisals. However, self-efficacy can be assessed as a separate construct that is sensitive to treatment and is closely related to function (Nicholas et al. 1991). For more information on self-efficacy as it relates to pain assessment and management, see Nicholas et al. (2002).

Red, yellow, blue and black flags

Red flags are those signs and symptoms that should alert the physiotherapist to seek other specialist opinion. A useful resource for patients with back pain is Greenhalgh and Selfe's *Red Flags* (2006).

'Yellow' flags are thought to be signs and symptoms, beliefs and attitudes that increase the risk of acute pain developing into a disabling chronic pain condition. This approach was devised to assess for risk of pain-related disability in patients with acute (recently occurred) back pain. Increasingly it is being used in patients who report pain in other anatomical locations. The purpose of assessing in this manner is to identify patients who have unrealistic and unhelpful beliefs about their pain and prognosis (Kendall et al. 1998). While there are standardised questionnaires available, carefully selected questions can also be used effectively during interview (Watson and Kendall 2000).

As an adjunct to yellow flags, a more comprehensive consideration of occupational factors can be achieved by considering assessment of 'blue' and 'black' flags. 'Blue' flags would be indicated if a person has work-related concerns about how he/she as an individual might be impeded in returning to work. For example, there may be a perception that the managers do not want this person to return to work. 'Black' flags are indicated if work processes and policy, which influence all workers, may impede the person returning to work. An example of this would be where an employer does not have any occupational health processes in place, such as workplace assessment or return to work plans.

Measures of functional limitation and disability

There are a large number of self-report tools that aim to measure the functional impact of a person's pain. A large proportion of those tools concern back pain (e.g. the Roland Morris disability questionnaire (Roland and Morris 1983) and the Oswestry questionnaire (Fisher and Johnston 1997)) or neck pain (e.g. neck disability index (Vernon and Mior 1991)). These tools are widely used and a large amount of data exists from patient and non-patient populations. There are also disability questionnaires that are not anatomically focused: for example, the task-specific tools, whereby patients select a task or activity that they are unable to perform because of pain, and rates their ability to perform that task over the course of treatment. An advantage of such a tool is that it can be used with different populations. A disadvantage is that it makes direct comparison between treatments or between patients difficult.

MANAGEMENT OF PAIN

European guidelines for the management of low back pain, based on the best available research evidence, have been published. Included are guidelines for people with pain of recent onset, for people with pain that is persistent and for people with pain that is threatening to lead to ongoing disability (Airaksinen et al. 2004; van Tulder et al. 2002). Elements of these guidelines will be presented below (see Airaksinen et al. 2006 for application in physiotherapy). It is important to recognise that these are specific to low back pain, but in the absence of guidelines they may also provide a basis for the management of other painful conditions.

Promoting optimal function with reference to WHO ICF

Within the ICF framework, the range of factors influencing a person's function will be considered as treatment targets. For example, the physiotherapist may recognise that a person with back pain has restricted movement. If, when considering restriction in *activities and participation*, it is also identified that the person is afraid of walking up the front stairs at home because there is no rail, the focus of treatment might change to incorporate this context. Thus, the clinician must reason as to the most achievable goal; addressing the restriction in movement may resolve the fear about the stairs. Alternatively, the patient may need a handrail. Optimally, the physiotherapist assists the patient in becoming confident to climb stairs without a rail. This will lead to generalisation to confidence in other environments. The important issue is that focusing on body structure and function alone will not guarantee that function is restored, and using the ICF prompts clinicians to explore and resolve other barriers to rehabilitation.

Clinical note

Warning: you can make things worse! These behaviours on the part of the clinician have been linked to worse outcomes (Kouyanou et al. 1998):

- over-investigation
- over-treatment
- unhelpful treatment
- disconfirmation of pain
- unhelpful advice.

Awareness of analgesics

In some places the physiotherapist has a prescribing role. However, it is more common for physiotherapists to liaise with other healthcare professionals to ensure effective pain relief is available and is administered to the patient. Different analgesic drugs act differently, stay in the blood stream for different durations and have different side-effects. It is important that physiotherapists know about the analgesics that are prescribed to the patients with whom they work.

Deactivating/desensitising the nociceptive system

One of the main purposes of treatment of pain is to deactivate and desensitise the nociception and pain systems.

Deactivating peripheral mechanisms of nociception

Peripheral sensitisation is a normal and necessary sequel to injury. Because inflammation is the main cause of peripheral sensitisation, limiting inflammation should help desensitise the nociceptive system. Normally, the body's response to injury, which includes motor, immune and vascular responses as outlined earlier, limits the period of inflammation.

There are also techniques available to the clinician that aid in reducing inflammation and its effects. The convention has been initially to cool the area, elevate and immobilise it (**r**est, **i**ce, **c**ompression and **e**levation) and subsequently to promote a gradual increase in movement and activity. There are also pharmacological means to reduce or limit inflammation. The broad class of drugs that are most often used to reduce inflammation are aptly called 'anti-inflammatories', although there are three important considerations with regard to their use:

- Firstly, the clinician must evaluate the relative importance of inflammation in initiating the healing process. This depends on sound knowledge of biological mechanisms associated with healing, nociception and pain.
- Secondly, the site of analgesic effect of anti-inflammatories has not been established; it is unlikely that their only effect is at the tissues.
- Thirdly, even if their main effect is at the tissues, they cannot be confined to the target area because they are administered systemically (for example, orally, by injection) or transported remotely in the circulation (for example, topical agents). This is why most drugs have unwanted side-effects. Thus, advice about any drug should not be given without appropriate expertise and medico-legal jurisdiction.

An important method by which inflammation and its effects are normally limited is movement. Movement promotes blood flow, oxygen supply, waste product removal and appropriate forces to guide healing. One common barrier to movement is the conscious decision of the patient not to move. Such decisions depend on the patient's evaluation of the importance and risks of doing so, and this is where the clinician can be key to normal recovery — effectively removing the barriers to normal recovery. Of course, strategies that enhance a person's motivation to move should be considered in light of a sound understanding of tissue healing and within a clinical reasoning framework.

Strategies that are used to enhance motivation include reassurance and education (Butler and Moseley 2003; Moseley et al. 2004), training diaries and overt monitoring of self-initiated rehabilitation (Moseley 2006a), challenging unhelpful cognitions and offering new ones (effectively, cognitive therapy principles), careful and graded exposure to movements or activities of which the patient is fearful (Vlaeyen and Linton 2000), and reinforcement of helpful behavioural responses (effectively, behavioural therapy principles (Nicholas and Sharp 1997)). A number of these strategies are discussed later.

Clinical note

Motivation is sometimes used to describe the opposite to laziness. However it should be considered as a term that describes the outcome of a person's evaluation of influences on the decision to act or not. A challenge for the clinician is to help resolve barriers to action and enhance resources. Together, these might swing the balance and enhance a person's motivation.

Deactivating spinal mechanisms of nociception

The dorsal horn laminae have, for many years, been thought able to inhibit the nociceptive system.

According to the 'gate control theory', this occurs in lamina II (Melzack and Wall 1965). While the theory is more than 40 years old and our understanding of neurophysiology has developed further in that time, the basic premise that sensory information is received and modified in the dorsal horn by competing stimulation and descending information holds true. Thus, there are two broad mechanisms that can desensitise spinal nociceptive neurones: shifting the balance of descending modulation towards inhibition and providing novel peripheral input that activates Aβ neurones. The former can be promoted by all the same strategies for removing the barriers to normal recovery of movement and activity, which are outlined above. The latter can be utilised in varying degrees of sophistication, from 'rubbing it better' to trancutaneous electrical nerve stimulation (TENS), which was developed as a direct application of the gate control theory (Melzack 1975a). There is good evidence that TENS reduces acute pain, but not chronic pain (McQuay et al. 1997).

Deactivating brain mechanisms of nociception and pain

The mechanisms by which nociception and pain can be decreased by the brain are not well understood. However, the *principle,* which depends on the conceptualisation of pain as the conscious correlate of the implicit perception of threat to body tissues (see Moseley 2007 for review), is well understood. We argued earlier that pain depends on evaluative factors, which means that any input that alters the brain's evaluation of threat to body tissue should modulate pain. In the same way that evaluative factors should change pain, they should also change descending modulation of nociceptive circuits. Comprehensive coverage of the strategies that are advocated within the literature is beyond the scope of this chapter, but it is appropriate to mention some of them.

Cognitive-behavioural therapy

Cognitive-behavioural therapy probably began as a combination of cognitive therapy and behavioural therapy. Cognitive therapy focuses on identifying, challenging and replacing cognitions (thoughts, beliefs and emotional processes) that might be contributing to the patient's pain or functional limitations, perhaps via fear or avoidance of movement and re-injury, or simply by elevating the perception of threat to body tissue. Once identified, thoughts and beliefs can be challenged by pointing the patient to material, experiences or situations that contradict that belief. Ultimately, unhelpful thoughts and beliefs need to be replaced by more accurate or helpful ones.

Clinical note

The psychological construct of self-efficacy is likely to be important. As we have seen, self-efficacy is the belief someone has about his or her ability to perform a task using current resources. Education might help the person realise an underestimation of resources (for example, thinking his/her back is fragile) and an overestimation of challenges or demands (for example, thinking he/she has to wait until the pain is gone before he starts moving). A more realistic view of these, a reconceptualisation, will allow the person to feel more confident about doing things that use his/her back more normally. The person's self-efficacy for this will have improved.

Apart from reconceptualisation, there are a number of other ways that self-efficacy can be enhanced. Physiotherapists tend to be good at them all, although they may not always recognise it. Verbal persuasion, encouraging someone to attempt something, gives a person a sense that he/she can do it. Mastery of a task is often an outcome of physiotherapy. Physiotherapists often help guide patients through increasingly difficult but safe activities in order to master a functional task. These could be seen as behavioural experiments, where the new view a person has of pain is tested out. Each time a person achieves a step along the way, self-efficacy will be enhanced, but especially if that person believes it has been achieved independently. The raised self-efficacy is often evident, as the person persists at increasingly difficult tasks.

Lastly, physiotherapists often group together people with similar health or function problems. In these groups, individuals often see people in very similar circumstances to themselves. Modelling from others is another strategy for enhancing self-efficacy, and to be effective, the 'model' has to share characteristics with the person. So, physiotherapists are creating the perfect environment for a person to see someone, who he/she can identify as similar, perform tasks successfully. Having seen this success the person is likely to increase his/her own self-belief about performing the task.

Behavioural therapy was first applied to the management of people in pain several decades ago (Fordyce 1970, 1973). In that work, operant conditioning principles guided treatment such that behaviours consistent with decreased pain or disability were reinforced and those consistent with increased pain or disability were not.

Modern cognitive-behavioural pain management is far wider in its application than cognitive and behavioural therapy combined. There are many strategies that are incorporated into a cognitive-behavioural pain management approach. Cognitive-behavioural principles within the context of physiotherapy practice is comprehensively presented in Nicholas and Tonkin (2004).

Explaining pain biology

Intensive education about the biology of pain is one way in which unhelpful cognitions about pain, injury and activity can be challenged and replaced. Explaining pain biology in detail has been shown to change beliefs and attitudes about pain, movement and activity (Moseley et al. 2004), increase pain threshold during relevant tasks (Moseley 2004) and, combined with movement-based physiotherapy, decrease pain and disability in the long term (Moseley 2002, 2003). By educating someone effectively, the person is given a new perspective on which to base thoughtful action. This involves the acceptance, by the person, that the information he or she had before has been superseded by the newly presented information. Patients are given new concepts that include neural sensitivity and central processing, to replace old ones about tissue vulnerability. The material that is used to explain pain is presented in the aptly named book, *Explain Pain* (Butler and Moseley 2003).

Relaxation

Relaxation is best performed at times when people are still in control of their pain but feel that it is worsening. Often it is targeting the emotional response to pain or the expectation of pain. As such, it is important to ensure patients have a strategy that can be used at such times, preferably without interruption to any task that they might be doing. Physiotherapists often prefer muscular hold-relax techniques but teaching more meditative techniques is perhaps more valuable, as they can be applied in many different contexts and environments.

Clinical note

Relaxation should be seen as a skill that needs to be practised. A useful technique is described by Nicholas et al. (2003). Firstly, there is a focus on breathing and 'loosening up' with exhalation. Secondly, the person is encouraged to imagine the tension leaving the muscles with each exhalation. The third step involves linking the relaxation to a word the person says to himself or herself (such as 'relax') and an image of a peaceful scene. The word and the image may facilitate further relaxation, but through repetition they will also become triggers to relaxation (via classical conditioning).
A person is then able to use the word or the image to bring on a relaxed state quickly.

Pacing

Pacing is essential for people who have persistent pain and find it difficult to plan ahead because they are unsure of how their pain might affect activity. An example is where a person is highly active on days when the pain is mild, but inactive on days when the pain increases. Sometimes called the 'boom or bust cycle', it prevents a person from attending regular employment as well as interfering with planning of social activities.

Resolution of the 'boom or bust cycle' can be achieved by pacing activity to a level that the person knows can be achieved, despite pain. When pain is increased, the person should attempt to use strategies, such as thought challenging and relaxation, to push the activity up to the planned level. When the pain is mild, the person must resist increasing activity above the planned level.

Clinical note

It is useful, when giving exercise advice to a person with persistent pain or a sensitised nervous system, to consider the use of exercise quotas: that is, to use a pre-determined duration or number of repetitions as a limit to activity, rather than using pain or discomfort as the guide. This will reinforce the message that activity is beneficial and that pain is not a sign of ongoing damage.

Setting quotas entails establishing a baseline of tolerance for the exercise or activity. The first quota should be below this (80 per cent of baseline) to ensure the person is confident of achieving it. Then the person should work at gradually increasing activity past the baseline towards a more desirable level. It is essential that people plan the next quota in advance. Initially this might be just the day before; then as patients become more confident in their activity levels, they can plan the upcoming week in advance.

Setbacks may occur and sometimes quotas may not be achieved. In such cases, the person should be encouraged to use active coping strategies to try to improve performance. If this fails, the quota may need to be slightly decreased. It is important to assist people with their self-motivation by providing successful experiences and it should also be clear to them that the activity is the focus, not the pain (Nicholas and Tonkin 2004).

On first coming to physiotherapy, individuals will have a sense of the level of activity they can achieve. That sense may be exaggerated or, more likely, underestimated. A more realistic level may only be achieved after education, successful behavioural experiments and reconceptualisation. Optimum levels of activity will be achieved when the skills of thought-challenging, relaxation and pacing are well developed and consistently applied.

Graded activity versus graded exposure

Physiotherapists will often employ a graded activity programme to help someone return to full function. The assumed benefits of this are generally considered to be physical: that is, the person is getting gradually stronger or more flexible and therefore is able to do more. Another benefit is confidence, or self-efficacy, and graded activity can enhance self-efficacy by allowing the person to achieve successful performance at increasingly more difficult levels. Assessment of performance should always include these influences, and changes in performance should not just be considered in terms of strength and range of movement.

Further to this is the influence of fear or phobias on confidence and on performance. As previously mentioned, fear-avoidance behaviour can lead to severe disability. An effective psychological strategy that has been employed to reduce fear is graded exposure. This involves first finding a baseline that does not elicit fear and then introducing gradual exposure to increasingly more fearful experiences that have been identified and ranked by the patient. If someone is fearful of pain on movement, then the experiences often will involve physical activities. For example, someone with a complex regional pain syndrome in his/her right upper limb may start by imagining the hand being touched by someone else. The person may then progress to stroking a rough texture, to shaking hands with someone, to lifting a bag full of shopping.

By integrating graded exposure and graded activity, the physiotherapist is likely to help the person to reach physical goals that relate to strength, range of movement and function, as well as psychological goals that relate to decreasing fear and increasing self-efficacy, participation and function.

Targeting cortical representations of the body

Emerging data suggest that there may be another strategy by which supraspinal mechanisms of nociception/pain can be desensitised. That strategy relates to the one way in which the brain changes when pain persists — alterations in the representation of the affected part in primary sensory cortex (S1) (see Flor et al. (2006) and Moseley (2006b) for review). The mechanisms by which this occurs may be activity-dependent, but may also relate to inhibition of non-noxious sensory input at the thalamus (Rommel et al. 1999). That S1 representation changes cause pain is argued (Harris 1999) but not empirically demonstrated (Moseley and Gandevia 2005). Notwithstanding, it is clear that normalisation of S1 representation is associated with reduced pain (Flor 2003; Maihofner et al. 2004; Pleger et al. 2005), that tactile acuity relates to pain and to S1 representation changes (Flor 2003), and that training tactile discrimination increases tactile acuity and reduces pain, at least in some patient groups (such as those with phantom limb pain — Flor et al. 2001) and complex regional pain syndrome (Zalucki et al. 2006). The role of normalising S1 representation is yet to be established. However, it seems reasonable to suggest that a role may emerge.

Clinical note

There is a large amount of data that shows that (a) you can improve tactile acuity via training; (b) when you improve tactile acuity, you do so by altering the firing properties of neurones in the brain; and (c) improving tactile acuity is therefore associated with altered representation of the trained body part in the brain.

There seem to several important aspects to training tactile acuity:

1. *Sensory stimulation.* The body part in question must be stimulated.
2. *Attention.* Training is more effective if the subject attends to the input. A useful way to ensure that this occurs is to provide a task that requires that a person attend. This is what Flor and colleagues (2001) and Moseley and colleagues did (Zalucki et al. 2006). In those studies, patients were required to discriminate between stimuli of different types and at different locations.
3. *Gaze direction.* Training is better if the subject directs the head toward the body part being stimulated.
4. *Visual input.* Training is better if the subject can see the body part being stimulated.

LIMITATIONS AND OPPORTUNITIES

This chapter attempts a monumental task — to synthesise volumes of pain research from basic and clinical sciences, into a digestible package appropriate for clinical physiotherapy practice. The complexity of the human experience, which is exemplified in the human experience of pain, means that this chapter can only provide an introduction. We considered it most important that the reader conceptualises pain in a manner that is consistent with what is known about human biology. Entire books have been written about the peripheral nociceptor and entire libraries could be filled with books on the spinal cord and brain, so we have attempted to convey what we think is sufficient evidence for adopting a certain way of thinking about pain. We think the following points are justified on the basis of the available research, and can be considered the key 'take-home messages'.

Key points

1. The science shows clearly that pain depends on the brain's appraisal of threat to body tissue. Nociception is a very important informant in this regard, but it is neither sufficient nor necessary for pain.
2. Many factors from sensory, psychological and social domains modulate pain.
3. The effect of these factors can be understood via the principle that pain is the conscious correlate of the implicitly perceived threat to body tissues.
4. It is possible to identify and estimate the impact of various factors on pain by questioning the patient carefully in the interview and by using self-report questionnaires.
5. Once issues have been identified, they should be addressed in management.
6. Physiotherapists have a wide range of skills and resources with which to deactivate and desensitise the nociception and pain systems at various levels: tissue, spinal and brain.
7. This chapter is a starting place. We have referred the reader to better and more comprehensive sources of information.

When we evaluate the large amount of research in pain sciences and management, two things seem clear. Firstly, the field is progressing rapidly. With a better understanding of the complexity of pain we are encountering new opportunities for pain management. Secondly, physiotherapists are ideally trained and resourced to be intimately involved with these new developments; physiotherapists, perhaps more than any other professional group, can access every domain that contributes to pain, from the tissues to society as a whole.

ACKNOWLEDGEMENTS

Lester Jones is an honorary senior lecturer in pain sciences at the University of Sydney. G. Lorimer Moseley is supported by the Nuffield Dominions Trust and is on leave from University of Sydney.

FURTHER READING

Butler D, Moseley GL 2003 Explain Pain. NOI: Adelaide

Gifford L (ed.) Topical Issues in Pain, vols 1–5. CNS: Falmouth

Jones L, Wang A 2007 Pain management. In: Partridge C (ed.) Recent Advances of Physiotherapy. Wiley: London, pp. 133–179

Moseley GL 2007 Painful Yarns: Metaphors and Stories to Help Understand the Biology of Pain. Dancing Giraffe: Canberra

REFERENCES

Airaksinen O, Brox J, Cedraschi C 2004 European guidelines for the management of chronic non-specific low back pain. European Commission, Research Directorate General: Brussels

Airaksinen O, Brox JI, Cedraschi C et al. 2006 Chapter 4 European guidelines for the management of chronic nonspecific low back pain. Eur Spine J 15: S192–S300

Apkarian AV, Bushnell MC, Treede R-D, Zubieta J-K 2005 Human brain mechanisms of pain perception and regulation in health and disease. Eur J Pain 9: 463–484

Arntz A, Vaneck M, Heijmans M 1990 Predictions of dental pain - the fear of any expected evil, is worse than the evil itself. Behav Res Ther 28: 29–41

Arntz A, Dreessen L, De Jong P 1994 The influence of anxiety on pain: Attentional and attributional mediators. Pain 56: 307–314

Asmundson GJ, Kuperos JL, Norton GR 1997 Do patients with chronic pain selectively attend to pain-related information? Preliminary evidence for the mediating role of fear. Pain 72: 27–32

Benedetti F, Pollo A, Lopiano L et al. 2003 Conscious expectation and unconscious conditioning in analgesic, motor, and hormonal placebo/nocebo responses. J Neurosci 23: 4315–4323

Butler D 2000 The Sensitive Nervous System. NOI: Adelaide, p. 431

Butler D, Moseley GL 2003 Explain Pain. NOI: Adelaide, p. 114

Cherny NI, Portenoy RK 1999 Cancer pain: principles of assessment and syndromes. In: Wall PD, Melzack R (eds) Textbook of Pain, 4th edn. Churchill Livingstone: Edinburgh

Chua P, Krams M, Toni I et al. 1999 A functional anatomy of anticipatory anxiety. Neuroimage 9: 563–571

Coudeyre E, Rannou F, Tubach F et al. 2006 General practitioners' fear-avoidance beliefs influence their management of patients with low back pain. Pain 124: 330–337

Cox JJ, Reimann F, Nicholas AK et al. 2006 An scn9a channelopathy causes congenital inability to experience pain. Nature 444: 894–898

Craig A 2002 How do you feel? Interoception: the sense of the physiological condition of the body. Nature Rev Neurosci 3: 655–666

Crombez G, Eccleston C, Baeyens F, Eelen P 1996 The disruptive nature of pain: an experimental investigation. Behav Res Ther 34: 911–918

Crombez G, Eccleston C, Baeyens F, Eelen P 1997 Habituation and the interference of pain with task performance. Pain 70: 149–154

Crombez G, Eccleston C, Baeyens F, Eelen P 1998 Attentional disruption is enhanced by the threat of pain. Behav Res Ther 36: 195–204

Crombez G, Eccleston C, Baeyens F, van Houdenhove B, van den Broeck A 1999 Attention to chronic pain is

19

dependent upon pain-related fear. J Psychosom Res 47: 403–410
Damasio A 2000 The Feeling of what Happens: Body and Emotion in the Making of Consciousness. London: Vintage, pp. 386ff
Duckworth MP, Iezzi A, Adams HE, Hale D 1997 Information processing in chronic pain disorder: A preliminary analysis. J Psychopathol Behav Assess 19: 239–255
Eccleston C 1994 Chronic pain and attention: a cognitive approach. Br J Clin Psychol 33: 535–547
Eccleston C, Crombez G 1999 Pain demands attention: a cognitive-affective model of the interruptive function of pain. Psychol Bull 125: 356–366
Eccleston C, Crombez G, Aldrich S, Stannard C 1997 Attention and somatic awareness in chronic pain. Pain 72: 209–215
Fields H, Basbaum A, Heinricher M 2006 CNS mechanisms of pain modulation. In: McMahon SB, Koltzenburg M (eds) Textbook of Pain. Churchill Livingstone: Edinburgh, pp. 125–143
Fields HL 2000 Pain modulation: expectation, opioid analgesia and virtual pain In: Mayer EA, Saper CB (eds) Biological Basis for Mind Body Interactions. Elsevier: Amsterdam, pp. 245–253
Fisher K, Johnston M 1997 Validation of the Oswestry low back pain disability questionnaire, its sensitivity as a measure of change following treatment and its relationship with other aspects of the chronic pain experience. Physiother Theory Pract 13: 67–80
Flor H 2003 Cortical reorganisation and chronic pain: implications for rehabilitation. J Rehabil Med 35: 66–72
Flor H, Denke C, Schaefer M, Grusser S 2001 Effect of sensory discrimination training on cortical reorganisation and phantom limb pain. Lancet 357: 1763–1764
Flor H, Nikolajsen L, Jensen TS 2006 Phantom limb pain: a case of maladaptive CNS plasticity? Nature Reviews Neuroscience 7: 873–881
Fordyce WE 1970 Operant conditioning as a treatment method in management of selected chronic pain problems. Northwest Med 69: 580–581
Fordyce WE 1973 An operant conditioning method for managing chronic pain. Postgrad Med 53: 123–128
Gifford L, Thacker M, Jones M 2006 Physiotherapy and pain In: McMahon SB, Koltzenburg M (eds) Textbook of pain. Churchill Livingstone: Edinburgh, pp. 603–618
Goldingay S 2006a Communication and assessment: the skills of information gathering. In: Gifford L (ed.) Topical Issues in Pain. CNS: Falmouth
Goldingay S 2006b Communication and assessment: What are the issues for physiotherapists? In: Gifford L (ed.) Topical Issues in Pain. CNS: Falmouth
Gore M, Brandenburg NA, Dukes E et al. 2005 Pain severity in diabetic peripheral neuropathy is associated with patient functioning, symptom levels of anxiety and depression, and sleep. J Pain Symptom Manage 30: 374–385
Gracely RH, Dubner R, Deeter WR, Wolskee PJ 1985 Clinicians'expectations influence placebo analgesia. Lancet 1: 43
Greenhalgh S, Selfe J 2006 Red Flags. A Guide to Identifying Serious Pathology of the Spine. Churchill Livingstone: Edinburgh, p. 214
Harris AJ 1999 Cortical origin of pathological pain. Lancet 354: 1464–1466
Jensen MP, Karoly P, Huger R 1987 The development and preliminary validation of an instrument to assess patients' attitudes toward pain. J Psychosom Res 31: 393–400
Keller S, Bann CM, Dodd SL et al. 2004 Validity of the brief pain inventory for use in documenting the outcomes of patients with noncancer pain. Clin J Pain 20(5): 309–318
Kelly KG, Cook T, Backonja M-M 2005 Pain ratings at the thresholds are necessary for interpretation of quantitative sensory testing. Muscle Nerve 32: 179–184
Keltner JR, Furst A, Fan C et al. 2006 Isolating the modulatory effect of expectation on pain transmission: a functional magnetic resonance imaging study. J Neurosci 26: 4437–4443
Kendall NAS, Linton SJ, Main C 1998 Psychosocial yellow flags for acute low back pain: 'yellow flags' as an analogue to 'red flags'. Eur J Pain 2: 87–89
Klages U, Kianifard S, Ulusoy O, Wehrbein H 2006 Anxiety sensitivity as predictor of pain in patients undergoing restorative dental procedures. Community Dent Oral Epidemiol 34: 139–145
Kouyanou K, Pither CE, Rabe-Hasketh S, Wessely S 1998 A comparative study of iatrogenesis, medication abuse and psychiatric morbidity in chronic pain patients with and without medically explained symptoms. Pain 76: 417–426
Levine FM, De Simone LL 1991 The effects of experimenter gender on pain report in male and female subjects. Pain 44: 69–72
Maihofner C, Handwerker HO, Neundorfer B, Birklein F 2004 Cortical reorganization during recovery from complex regional pain syndrome. Neurology 63: 693–701
Matthews KA, Schier MF, Brunson BI, Carducci B 1980 Attention, unpredictability, and reports of physical symptoms eliminating the benefits of predictability. J Pers Soc Psychol 38: 525–537
McCracken LM 1997 'Attention' to pain in persons with chronic pain: a behavioral approach. Behav Ther 28: 271–284
McCracken LM, Zayfert C, Gross RT 1992 The pain anxiety symptoms scale: development and validation of a scale to measure fear of pain. Pain 50: 67–73
McQuay HJ, Moore RA, Eccleston C et al. 1997 Systematic review of outpatient services for chronic pain control. Health Technol Assess 1: i–iv, 1–135
Melzack R 1975a Prolonged relief of pain by brief, intense transcutaneous somatic stimulation. Pain 1: 357–373
Melzack R 1975b The McGill pain questionnaire: major properties and scoring methods. Pain 1: 277–299
Melzack R 1990 Phantom limbs and the concept of a neuromatrix. Trends Neurosci 13: 88–92
Melzack R, Wall PD 1965 Pain mechanisms: a new theory. Science 150: 971–979

Merskey H, Bogduk N 1994 Classification of Chronic Pain, 2nd edn. IASP: Seattle, p. 210

Meyer R, Ringkamp M, Campbell JN, Raja SN 2006 Peripheral mechanisms of cutaneous nociception In: McMahon SB, Koltzenburg M (eds) Textbook of Pain, 5th edn. Churchill Livingstone: Edinburgh, pp. 3–35

Miller R, Kori S, Todd D 1991 The Tampa scale for kinesiphobia. Unpublished report. Tampa, FL

Moerman D 2002 Meaning, medicine and the 'placebo effect'. Cambridge University Press: Cambridge, p. 172

Moseley GL 2002 Combined physiotherapy and education is effective for chronic low back pain. A randomised controlled trial. Aus J Physioth 48: 297–302

Moseley GL 2003 Joining forces — combining cognition-targeted motor control training with group or individual pain physiology education: A successful treatment for chronic low back pain. J Man Manip Therap 11: 88–94

Moseley GL 2004 Evidence for a direct relationship between cognitive and physical change during an education intervention in people with chronic low back pain. Euro J Pain 8: 39–45

Moseley GL 2006a Do training diaries affect and reflect adherence to home programs? Arthritis Rheum-Arthritis Care Rese 55: 662–664

Moseley GL 2006b Making sense of S1 mania — are things really that simple? In: Gifford L (ed.) Topical Issues in Pain, vol 5. CNS: Falmouth, pp. 321–340

Moseley GL 2007 Reconceptualising pain according to its underlying biology. Physical Therapy Reviews. In press

Moseley GL, Arntz A 2007 The context of a noxious stimulus affects the pain it evokes. Pain. In press

Moseley GL, Gandevia SC 2005 Sensory-motor incongruence and reports of 'pain'. Rheumatology 44: 1083–1085

Moseley GL, Nicholas MK, Hodges PW 2004 A randomized controlled trial of intensive neurophysiology education in chronic low back pain. Clin J Pain 20: 324–330

Naveteur J, Mars F, Crombez G 2005 The effect of eye orientation on slowly increasing pain. Eur J Pain 9: 79–85

Nicholas M, Sharp TJ 1997 Cognitive-behavioral programs: theory and application. Int Anesthesiol Clin 35: 155–170

Nicholas M, Molloy A, Tonkin L, Beeston L 2003 Manage Your Pain: Practical Ways of Adapting to Chronic Pain. Souvenir: London

Nicholas MK 2010 Cognitive behavioural pain management. In: Moseley GL (ed.) Pain. Do you get it? Butterworth–Heinemann: Oxford

Nicholas MK, Tonkin L 2004 Application of cognitive-behavioural principles to activity-based pain management programs. In: Refshauge K, Gaff E (eds) Musculoskeletal Physiotherapy: Clinical Science and Evidence-based Practice. Butterworth–Heinemann: Oxford, pp. 277–293

Nicholas MK, Wilson PH, Goyen J 1991 Operant-behavioural and cognitive-behavioural treatment for chronic low back pain. Behav Res Ther 29: 225–238

Peters ML, Vlaeyen JW, van Drunen C 2000 Do fibromyalgia patients display hypervigilance for innocuous somatosensory stimuli? Application of a body scanning reaction time paradigm. Pain 86: 283–292

Pleger B, Tegenthoff M, Ragert P et al. 2005 Sensorimotor returning in complex regional pain syndrome parallels pain reduction. Ann Neurol 57: 425–429

Ploghaus A, Tracey I, Gati JS et al. 1999 Dissociating pain from its anticipation in the human brain. Science 284: 1979–1981

Ploghaus A, Becerra L, Borras C, Borsook D 2003 Neural circuitry underlying pain modulation: expectation, hypnosis, placebo. Trends Cogn Sci 7: 197–200

Poiraudeau S, Rannou F, Baron G et al. 2006 Fear-avoidance beliefs about back pain in patients with subacute low back pain. Pain 124: 305–311

Pollo A, Amanzio M, Arslanian A et al. 2001 Response expectancies in placebo analgesia and their clinical relevance. Pain 93: 77–84

Pud D, Amit A 2005 Anxiety as a predictor of pain magnitude following termination of first-trimester pregnancy. Pain Med 6: 143–148

Raja SN, Meyer RA, Ringkamp M et al. 1999 Peripheral Neural Mechanisms of Nociception. In: Wall P, Melzack R (eds) The Textbook of Pain. Churchill Livingstone: Edinburgh, pp. 11–57

Roland M, Morris R 1983 A study of the natural history of back pain. Part I: Development of a reliable and sensitive measure of disability in low-back pain. Spine 8: 141–144

Rommel O, Gehling M, Dertwinkel R et al. 1999 Hemisensory impairment in patients with complex regional pain syndrome. Pain 80: 95–101

Sawamoto N, Honda M, Okada T et al. 2000 Expectation of pain enhances responses to nonpainful somatosensory stimulation in the anterior cingulate cortex and parietal operculum/posterior insula: An event-related functional magnetic resonance imaging study. J Neurosci 20: 7438–7445

Schmeltz M, Schmidt R, Weidner C et al. 2003 Chemical response pattern of different classes of C-nociceptors to pruritogens and algogens. J Neurophys 89: 2441–2448

Schupp CJ, Berbaum K, Berbaum M, Lang EV 2005 Pain and anxiety during interventional radiologic procedures: effect of patients' state anxiety at baseline and modulation by nonpharmacologic analgesia adjuncts. J Vasc Interv Radiol 16: 1585–1592

Sullivan MJL, Bishop SR, Pivik J 1995 The pain catastrophizing scale: development and validation. Psycholog Ass 7: 524–532

Sullivan MJL, Thorn B, Haythornthwaite JA et al. 2001 Theoretical perspectives on the relation between catastrophizing and pain. Clin J Pain 17: 52–64

Tang J, Gibson SJ 2005 A psychophysical evaluation of the relationship between trait anxiety, pain perception, and induced state anxiety. J Pain 6: 612–619

Turk DC, Melzack R (eds) 2001 Handbook of Pain Assessment, 2nd edn.: Guildford: New York

van Griensven H 2005 Pain in Practice: Theory and Treatment Strategies for Manual Therapists. Butterworth–Heinemann: Oxford, p. 17

van Tulder M, Kovacs F, Muller G et al. 2002 European guidelines for the management of low back pain. Acta Orthop Scand 73: 20–25

Vernon H, Mior S 1991 The neck disability index: a study of reliability and validity. J Manipulative Physiol Ther 14: 409–415

Vlaeyen JW, Linton SJ 2000 Fear-avoidance and its consequences in chronic musculoskeletal pain: a state of the art. Pain 85: 317–332

Von Korff M 1994 Studying the natural history of back pain. Spine 19: 2041S–2046S

Waddell G, Newton M, Henderson I et al. 1993 A fear-avoidance beliefs questionnaire (FABQ) and the role of fear-avoidance beliefs in chronic low back pain and disability. Pain 52: 157–168

Wager TD 2005 Expectations and anxiety as mediators of placebo effects in pain. Pain 115: 225–226

Wall P 1999 Pain. The Science of Suffering. Orion: London

Watkins L, Maier S 2000 The pain of being sick: implications of immune-to-brain communication for understanding pain. Ann Rev Psychol 51: 29–57

Watson P, Kendall NAS 2000 Assessing psychosocial yellow flags In: Gifford L (ed.) Topical Issues in Pain. CNS: Falmouth

Williams DA, Robinson ME, Geisser ME 1994 Pain beliefs: assessment and utility. Pain 59: 71–78

Woolf CJ, Costigan M 1999 Transcriptional and posttranslational plascicticity and the generation of inflammatory pain. Proc Natl Accd Sci USA 96(14): 7723–7730

World Health Organization 2002 Towards a common language for functioning, disability and health. http://www3.who.int/icf/icftemplate.cfm?myurl=beginners.html&mytitle=Beginner's%20Guide

Zalucki N, Weich K, Moseley GL 2006 Treating complex regional pain syndrome by cross-modal training of tactile acuity. Eur J Pain 10: S124

Chapter **20**

Common chronic inflammatory polyarthropathies

John A. Goodacre and Chandini Rao

CHAPTER CONTENTS

INTRODUCTION

This chapter provides an introduction to several types of chronic polyarthritis that are common in clinical practice. The main symptoms and signs of these conditions are described, focusing also on the investigations that are most important for diagnosis, clinical monitoring and evaluation of interventions. Key principles of clinical management are also discussed, highlighting issues that have broad relevance to all types of musculoskeletal condition as well as those that apply more specifically to the types of chronic arthritis described here. The need to implement integrated multidisciplinary and multi-agency approaches to clinical management is emphasised as being of paramount importance in order to achieve optimal outcomes in these long-term conditions.

TYPES OF CHRONIC INFLAMMATORY POLYARTHROPATHY

There are many types of chronic inflammatory polyarthritis. They all cause pain, swelling and functional impairment of multiple joints, and all are frequently associated with extra-articular and systemic symptoms and signs.

Development of chronic inflammation in and around the joints is often, although not invariably, accompanied by structural damage to cartilage and bone, as well as to other tissues associated with the joint. The rate and extent of joint damage are highly variable and are determined by a complex array of interacting cellular and molecular pathways and mechanisms, leading to tissue breakdown as well as tissue repair. In recent years, much research aimed at understanding these pathways and mechanisms has led to the identification of an increasing number of promising new molecular targets and medications for treating patients with chronic polyarthropathies. These advances, together with the increasing availability and use of genetic and other clinical information to improve the definition of patient subgroups, have opened up the realistic possibility that in the future it may be possible to use effective programmes of therapies tailored to individual characteristics in these diseases. They have also provided considerable momentum in developing exciting new treatments for people with chronic arthritis.

Categories of symptoms and signs

Knowledge of the key features of the symptoms and signs in chronic arthritis provides a useful framework for distinguishing the different types, based upon:

- characteristics and distribution of joint involvement
- presence and characteristics of extra-articular and systemic features
- presence of previous or current associated diseases
- family history of arthritis or associated conditions
- results from laboratory investigations and bone or joint imaging.

Diagnostic issues

Some types of polyarthropathy display characteristic *patterns of joint involvement*, which provides an important basis for diagnosis. The pattern of joint involvement, combined with other features of the history, examination and results of investigations, enables different diagnostic groups to be distinguished. Other types of polyarthropathy are less distinctive in terms of which joints are involved.

Even within particular diagnostic types, however, there can be a remarkable degree of individual heterogeneity in terms of disease onset, progression and outcome. Furthermore, it is quite commonly the case that the clinical features in individual patients may not conform exactly to the characteristics attributed to recognised diagnostic categories.

20

Clinical note

The clinical features of chronic arthritis may evolve and change over months or years, sometimes requiring the passage of time before the correct diagnosis can be made with certainty.

Irrespective of the type of arthropathy involved, all people with chronic arthritis experience variable and usually unpredictable levels of joint pain and swelling, which leads to various degrees of functional impairment and also engenders significant personal concerns and anxieties about state of health, employment capability, and capacity for independence and social functioning in both the short and long term. The overall effects of chronic polyarthropathies on health almost always, therefore, involve many aspects of physical, psychological and social well-being.

Consequently, clinical assessment and monitoring of patients by health professionals needs to take account of key factors within each of these domains. For example, in addition to the need for careful observation and documentation of physical symptoms and signs, and accurate and appropriate interpretation of investigative findings, it is essential for health professionals to assess aspects of each patient's overall mood and coping capacity, together with the level and effectiveness of external support available. Factors such as personal goals and work or social needs can often have a very important bearing on disease expression and progression, as can knowledge, beliefs and expectations formed by gleaning information from traditional or Internet-based sources of written information, shared experience or anecdote.

The multidisciplinary team and evidence-based therapies

The members of the multidisciplinary care team have the important task of drawing together the different elements of diagnosis and assessment in order to synthesise and formulate a plan for management and monitoring. The plan should be based on goals that are relevant, realistic and feasible.

Whilst it remains the case that some aspects of clinical management of the chronic polyarthropathies must continue to involve decisions based on clinical experience, common sense and general consensus rather than proven evidence, there are now an increasing number of circumstances in which clinicians working in this field can utilise the rapidly developing base of published evidence in order to guide their decisions in clinical management. It is likely that clinical management teams will need to give increasing consideration to the use of new biological therapies for several of these conditions, as well as paying greater attention to ways of identifying patient subgroups to facilitate effective and selective targeting of different medical and non-medical therapies as appropriate, and to ways of synergising the increasing number of different treatment modalities in order to achieve optimal benefit. This era is therefore one of unprecedented excitement and opportunity for all working in the field.

Successful translation into clinical practice of new knowledge from many disciplines within the clinical, health, life and social sciences, and the related technologies, will require tomorrow's health professionals to be able to utilise an advancing base of knowledge across these disciplines, as well as to acquire and maintain specialist knowledge and skills within their chosen area of expertise. Although these issues present major challenges — not only for students and healthcare professionals but also for the different sectors and institutions involved in undergraduate and postgraduate education and healthcare provision — they nevertheless demonstrate how substantial improvement in the health of patients with chronic arthritis is increasingly feasible and attainable.

RHEUMATOID ARTHRITIS

The *multisystem autoimmune diseases*, of which the most common is rheumatoid arthritis (RA), are associated with marked systemic upset and involvement of other organs and tissues in addition to chronic joint disease. These diseases are all characterised by high titres of autoantibodies and other features of immune activation and immunoregulation.

Key point

Rheumatoid arthritis affects about 1 per cent of adults and is characterised by a peripheral, symmetrical erosive polyarthritis, frequently associated with extra-articular tissue involvement. It is the cause of substantial levels of morbidity, disability and economic burden worldwide.

Pathogenesis

RA is a long-term condition, usually involving unpredictable cycles of exacerbation and remission. The causes are unknown, but it is recognised as a type of autoimmune disorder.

The pathogenesis of RA involves chronic synovitis, in which a wide range of types of inflammatory and immune cell migrate into synovial tissue. This process, and its consequences, also involve endothelial cells as well as several different types of cell resident not only in synovium but also in adjacent bone and cartilage, such as fibroblasts, osteoclasts and chondrocytes. Although many of the key molecular pathways that drive and perpetuate this process have been identified in recent years, the fundamental reasons why RA inflammation develops and persists remain unknown. Nevertheless, it is clear that complex cellular and molecular interactions between infiltrating inflammatory cells and resident cells, mediated by a variety of cell surface receptors, cytokines, chemokines, extracellular enzymes and other inflammatory mediators, results in persistent chronic synovitis and breakdown of cartilage and bone.

It is well established that the pathogenesis of RA involves an important component of *genetic susceptibility*, although non-genetic factors, as yet unidentified, play a predominant role. For example, RA disease concordance in identical twins has been reported to be as low as about 15 per cent. Susceptibility to RA involves several genes, of which the highly polymorphic human leucocyte antigen (HLA) DRB1 gene is known to impart the most significant contribution. Detailed structural analyses of the DRB1 gene alleles that confer susceptibility to RA have led to the theory that the key disease mechanisms may depend upon aspects of the activation and function of T lymphocytes, since DRB1 genes are known to have an important role in these pathways. These findings have also provided further support for the concept that RA is an autoimmune disease. This view was based originally on the fact that RA involves the production of various autoantibodies, of which rheumatoid factor is an example. Rheumatoid factors are antibodies that recognise epitopes in the constant regions of immunoglobulin G (IgG) molecules; that is, they are antibodies that recognise and bind to other antibodies. Rheumatoid factors are often found in high concentrations in RA sera (which are consequently termed 'seropositive') and are therefore used as one of the diagnostic criteria for RA. However, some people with RA are termed 'seronegative', since they do not have high concentrations of rheumatoid factor in their sera. Furthermore, rheumatoid factor is quite frequently found in other chronic inflammatory diseases besides RA. Other autoantibodies besides rheumatoid factors can also be found in RA, particularly anti-citrullinated peptide antibodies, which may help provide a better diagnostic marker for RA.

The formal and widely used American College of Rheumatology (ACR) criteria for the diagnosis of RA are shown in Table 20.1.

Clinical features

RA manifests as joint pain, swelling and stiffness, accompanied by severe fatigue and systemic disturbance. The onset can be either rapid or insidious, and usually begins in the hands and/or feet. Elbows, knees and cervical spine are also commonly involved. In the early stages the disease can sometimes undergo quite prolonged periods of remission. Chronic synovitis may be accompanied by effusion, and joint function may be compromised. There may also be an associated lymphadenopathy.

In addition to joint symptoms there is marked systemic upset and severe fatigue. For many patients, fatigue is often the most troublesome and frustrating aspect of the disease. Loss of muscle bulk and strength, loss of appetite, and intermittent fever may also occur.

Outside the joints, rheumatoid nodules may appear — for example, on the extensor surfaces of the elbows — and

Table 20.1 The 1987 American College of Rheumatology diagnostic criteria for rheumatoid arthritis*

Criterion	Comment
1. Morning stiffness	Morning stiffness in and around the joints lasting at least 1 hour
2. Arthritis in three or more joint areas	Arthritis in three or more joint areas, involving the PIP, MCP, wrist, elbow, knee, ankle or MTP joints on the right or left Soft-tissue swelling or fluid (but not bony overgrowth) observed by a physician, present simultaneously for at least 6 weeks
3. Arthritis of the hand joints	Swelling of wrist, MCP or hand joints for at least 6 weeks
4. Symmetrical arthritis	Simultaneous involvement of the same joint areas (defined in 2 above) on both sides of the body (bilateral involvement of PIP, MCP or MTP joints is acceptable without absolute symmetry) for at least 6 weeks
5. Rheumatoid nodules	Subcutaneous nodules over bony prominences, extensor surfaces or in juxta-articular regions, observed by a physician
6. Rheumatoid factor	Detected by a method positive in fewer than 5% of normal controls
7. Radiographic changes	Typical of RA on postero-anterior hand and wrist X-rays These must include erosions or unequivocal bony decalcification localised in or most marked adjacent to the involved joints (OA changes alone do not qualify)

From Arnet FC, Edworthy SM, Bloch DA et al. 1988 The American Rheumatism Association 1987 revised criteria for the classification of rheumatoid arthritis. Arthritis Rheum 31: 315–324.
*At least four criteria must be fulfilled for the diagnosis of RA to be made.
MCP, metacarpophalangeal; MTP, metatarsophalangeal; OA, osteoarthritis; PIP, proximal interphalangeal

other symptoms may result from involvement of extra-articular tissues. A wide range of other tissues and organs may be involved in RA, among which involvement of the lacrimal and salivary glands, leading to dry eyes and dry mouth (Sjögren's syndrome), is particularly common (Table 20.2).

Establishing the diagnosis

The first step is to establish a diagnosis, using information from the history and examination together with the results of laboratory investigations and joint imaging. Classically, the presence of a peripheral and symmetrical polyarthritis, associated with systemic fatigue, nodules, erosive changes on X-rays of the hands or feet, and raised titres of serum rheumatoid factor, would leave the diagnosis in no doubt. However, the absence of one or more of these features can quite often lead to the need to make a provisional, rather than a definite, diagnosis. This may particularly apply in the diagnosis of early RA.

Clinical assessment and monitoring

After the diagnosis has been established, a full medical and social assessment is essential, involving discussions with all the health professionals involved as well as with the patient's family, carers or friends. This should lead to the development of an appropriate treatment plan, following which further assessments should continue to be conducted at regular intervals in order to

Table 20.2 Common extra-articular features of rheumatoid arthritis

Systemic	Nodules Anaemia Lymphadenopathy Amyloidosis[a] Vasculitis[b] Felty's syndrome[c]
Ocular	Keratoconjunctivitis Scleritis and episcleritis
Bone	Osteoporosis
Neurological	Peripheral nerve entrapment Peripheral neuropathy Cervical spine instability Cervical cord compression Nerve root compression
Pulmonary	Pleurisy Pleural effusion Pulmonary alveolitis and fibrosis
Cardiovascular	Pericarditis and myocarditis Pericardial effusion Conduction defects Atherosclerosis

[a]Results when amyloid protein builds up in one or more organs to cause their malfunction. The heart, kidneys, nervous system and gastrointestinal tract are most often affected.
[b]A type of inflammation of the blood vessels.
[c]Includes an enlarged spleen and an abnormally low white blood count.

20

inform discussions about the efficacy of intervention(s), and to enable the treatment plan to be reviewed and modified accordingly.

Observations and investigations

Disease activity and severity is assessed using a range of subjective and objective methods aimed at providing overall measures of the inflammatory, systemic and functional components of the disease. The assessment should include evaluation of active synovitis, as measured by tender and swollen joint counts, and the erythrocyte sedimentation rate (ESR) and concentrations of serum acute-phase proteins such as C-reactive protein (CRP) or ferritin. The acute-phase response in RA is reflected in the raised ESR that is usually present in these patients, and which is a useful objective indicator of the severity of inflammation. Similarly, haemoglobin concentrations are typically reduced, usually reflecting an anaemia of chronic illness (although other possible causes of anaemia should always be considered and sought), and platelet counts are often increased. Although useful diagnostically, rheumatoid factor titres are a relatively poor indicator of the severity of synovitis.

Baseline laboratory investigations should include tests of hepatic and renal function. The assessment should also include measures of severity of pain, morning stiffness and fatigue, and of joint function as reflected by range of movement, instability and deformity. The presence of extra-articular features and comorbid conditions should be sought. Joint imaging should be performed routinely at an early stage, and in current practice this usually involves X-rays of the hands and feet. In the early stages, X-rays may show soft-tissue swelling, periarticular osteoporosis or loss of joint space. These changes may be followed by the development of erosion of cartilage and bone, and subsequently, in severe cases, by complete loss of the structure of the joint. Additional imaging techniques — for example, MRI and high-resolution ultrasound — are now increasingly available and are being extensively evaluated for their potential role in RA assessment.

Clinical assessment scales

A variety of clinical assessment scales to score the severity of joint inflammation have been developed, among which the Ritchie Index, or one of its modified forms, continues to be used commonly, particularly in research settings. For measuring function, several quantitative scales have been developed for use in both research and healthcare settings. These include the Health Assessment Questionnaire (HAQ) and the Arthritis Impact Measurement Scale (AIMS).

A variety of composite methods of expressing overall disease activity as a single score have been developed, of which the Disease Activity Scale (DAS) score is in most frequent use. The DAS score measures disease activity on a scale from 1 to 10 and is based on the number of swollen joints, the number of tender joints, and the ESR.

> **The DAS score**
>
> Since it was first introduced, the score has been modified to the simpler DAS28; this takes account of fewer joints than the original form, which involved assessment of 44 joints.

Furthermore, a variety of methods of quantifying overall change in disease status have been developed, primarily for the purpose of comparing the efficacy of different treatment interventions. The ACR definition of response requires improvement in the tender and swollen joint counts, together with improvement in three of the following five parameters:

- patient's global assessment
- physician's global assessment
- pain severity
- level of disability (as measured, for example, using the HAQ)
- levels of the acute-phase response as measured by the ESR or serum concentrations of CRP.

Responses are defined as ACR 20, ACR 50 or ACR 70, in which the figures denote percentage improvement in clinical scores compared with baseline measurements.

Clinical management

Overall, the major goals of treatment are to minimise joint inflammation and damage, prevent loss of joint function, and reduce symptoms of pain, stiffness and fatigue.

Assessment and discussion by a multidisciplinary team, with active involvement of the patient and the family or carer, leading to the development of a coherent and coordinated plan, provide the optimal basis for long-term clinical management. It is essential that this process be underpinned by clear and effective communication between all members of the team.

> **Consensus guidelines**
>
> Consensus guidelines for the management and monitoring of RA were first developed by the American College of Rheumatology in the mid-1990s and have recently been reviewed and revised. These guidelines provide a useful framework of reference from which practices tailored to local conditions and resources can be developed.

The treatment plan must reflect both the nature and severity of the disease and the views and expectations of the patient. Since predicting the course of the disease and its response to treatment is uncertain, the clinicians in the team should aim to provide support that is optimistic whilst balanced with a level of realism appropriate for each individual patient.

Optimal management of RA is achieved by combining non-pharmacological and pharmacological treatments in a manner tailored to individual patient's needs and disease status.

Non-pharmacological treatments

Maintenance of joint function and overall personal function (at home, at leisure and in the workplace) are vitally important goals, and to this end all patients should, at an early stage, undergo a detailed programme of instruction and advice in the principles of joint protection and splinting, pain management, energy conservation and management, and exercise.

The importance of dynamic and aerobic exercise programmes for maintaining muscle strength and joint mobility has been widely recognised for many years, but this particular aspect of clinical management is currently gaining even more importance in the context of preventing the long-term cardiovascular sequelae of RA. The programme should also cover relevant aspects of activity planning, diet and nutrition, choice and use of appropriate footwear, and the availability of assistive technologies.

Patients should also be given advice and guidance on sources of further information and literature, and details of local, regional and national self-help and other support groups. Opportunities should be sought to involve, as appropriate, other family members or carers so that patients can benefit from informed support in the domestic setting.

The potential educative and therapeutic value of a programme that addresses the issues described here is extremely high, and this approach can often be invaluable in providing an effective means of establishing a secure basis for effective and successful care delivery in this long-term condition.

20

Pharmacological treatments

Pharmacological therapies for RA can be categorised according to whether the medication is aimed primarily at relief of symptoms or at disease modification, and to whether or not the medication is based upon a defined molecular target.

Complementary therapies

Use of complementary therapies is extremely common amongst people with RA. A wide variety of preparations, approaches and dietary supplements are available for use in helping to alleviate the symptoms of pain, stiffness and systemic upset.

Analgesic and anti-inflammatory medications

These include non-steroidal anti-inflammatory drugs (NSAIDs) and selective cyclo-oxygenase 2 (COX-2) inhibitors. The primary role of these medications is to achieve symptomatic improvement, rather than to alter the course of the disease or prevent joint damage. The choice of medication usually takes into account considerations of efficacy, safety and cost, as well as the issue of whether or not the patient has had any side-effects from previous use of such treatments.

Key point

In principle, patients should take only one from this class of medication at any given time. If symptoms are not satisfactorily relieved to an acceptable level, the medication should be stopped before a different drug within this class is tried.

Dyspepsia and gastroduodenal ulceration are common side-effects. If the patient is found to be at risk of an adverse gastrointestinal event, the use of gastroprotective therapies (such as H_2 blockers and proton pump inhibitors) should be considered, although routine concomitant use of gastroprotective therapies is not recommended.

Disease-modifying antirheumatic drugs (DMARDs)

This category of medication includes a diverse array of drugs, which are used because of their potential to reduce joint damage. They are used in people who have persistently active synovitis, persistently elevated ESR, and radiographic joint damage. The trend in recent years has been to commence DMARDs at an early stage in people who fulfil these clinical features. Typically, it takes several weeks or months for clinical benefit to become manifest, and it is important that patients on DMARDs be closely monitored for possible side-effects.

DMARDs commonly used in RA include methotrexate, sulfasalazine and hydroxychloroquine, whilst leflunomide, azathioprine, gold salts, d-penicillamine, minocycline and ciclosporin are still used in some centres. Choice of DMARD is influenced by many factors, including patient preference, physician experience, and convenience of administration and monitoring.

Key point

There has been an increasing trend recently towards exploring the use of combination DMARD therapy in RA.

Glucocorticoids

Low-dose glucocorticoids (that is, prednisolone in doses of less than 10 mg daily) may have disease-modifying effects in RA and patients may feel markedly better within days of commencing such therapy. However, these factors need to be balanced against the known adverse effects of glucocorticoids, particularly osteoporosis. Similarly, glucocorticoid injection of joints and tendons continues to be used in clinical practice and can sometimes provide dramatic local, and even systemic, benefit, albeit often only temporarily. It is important to rule out other possible causes of active synovitis in RA, such as joint infection and crystal-mediated arthritis, before injections are given, and repeated injections into the same joint or tendon should be avoided if at all possible.

Biological therapies

The feasibility of developing and utilising biological therapies in the treatment of RA has arisen from the success of a large body of research aimed at increasing understanding of the molecular mechanisms of the disease. This has led to the identification of several well-defined target molecules, which, allied to the availability of modern techniques in molecular biology and protein chemistry, has for the first time enabled pharmacological therapy in RA to be approached on a rational scientific basis.

The first examples of such therapies to reach the clinic were based on the knowledge that two cytokines — namely, tumour necrosis factor alpha (TNFα) and interleukin 1 (IL-1) — that regulate inflammatory and immune responses, have a key role in RA pathogenesis. This led to the design and development of therapeutic molecules based closely on the known natural structure of these cytokines or their receptors and which could therefore be used to modify their biological effects. Clinical trials in RA using infliximab (a monoclonal antibody which binds TNFα), etanercept (a soluble form of one of the types of TNFα receptor found on cell surfaces), adalimumab (a fully humanised anti-TNFα monoclonal antibody) and anakinra (a soluble form of the IL-1 receptor antagonist) produced promising results, such that the benefits of these therapies appeared markedly stronger and were manifest much earlier than those of traditional DMARDs. More recently, rituximab (a chimeric anti-CD 20 antibody) previously used in the treatment of lymphoma, has been licensed for use in refractory RA.

> **Key point**
> Studies to determine long-term outcome and to investigate possible long-term side-effects of these therapies are in progress. An increasing range of other types of biological therapy based on these and other known key target molecules in RA are currently under development and evaluation.

Surgery

Surgical procedures may be indicated in RA when the effects of severe structural joint damage lead to loss of function and/or intractable pain. Total joint arthroplasty is potentially extremely beneficial, such that many patients experience marked improvement in their function and quality of life. The longevity of joint prostheses is being gradually increased through the use of new materials for manufacturing prostheses and for use in cements, as well as through continuing improvements in surgical and perioperative techniques and experience. Other surgical procedures used in RA include synovectomy, joint fusion, resection of the metatarsal heads, and carpal tunnel release.

PRACTICE POINTS IN THE MANAGEMENT OF RA

This section describes some of the practical issues that frequently arise in the management of RA and which are of direct relevance to allied health professionals involved in the field. Many of the points raised here are not necessarily exclusive to RA and may apply equally to other types of polyarthropathy; nor are they necessarily regarded as being the only available method of treating the problems commonly faced by people with RA.

Joint splinting: general principles

Custom-made and proprietary splints are used frequently in the management of RA. The fabrication of splints often falls into the remit of therapists. Splints can be classified either by their design or by their function. In relation to design, splints are either static (preventing movement and resting affected joints) or dynamic (allowing movement by incorporating hinges, elastic or springs). In relation to function, the majority of splints used in the management of RA fall into three main categories: resting, functional and corrective.

- *Resting splints* are used to relieve pain, decrease inflammation, prevent the development of contractures, maintain proper joint alignment, decrease or alleviate symptoms of nerve entrapment, and support ligaments and joint capsules.
- *Functional splints* are used to relieve pain, support unstable joint structures, accommodate for muscle weakness or atrophy, protect from further damage, assist in controlling inflammation, and protect against nerve entrapment or tenosynovitis.
- *Corrective splints* are used to modify soft-tissue contractures.

Other types of splint are used postoperatively to maintain joint alignment or mobility, to assist with post-operative stretching and to minimise adhesions.

A wide range of thermoplastic materials are available to custom-made splints, the choice of which is influenced by factors such as the specific requirement of the splint, the length of time for which the splint will be used, the place where the splint is being made and the equipment available, the condition of the patient's skin, and the cost of materials.

Key point

The provision of any splint should occur in conjunction with appropriate patient education to ensure that the patient understands the purpose of the splint, the need to carry out relevant exercise programmes, and the need to check for signs of an ill-fitting splint, such as the occurrence of pressure points.

Management of specific joints

Hands

Resting splints are commonly used to treat hand involvement in early and active RA. Fabrication of hand splints should occur only after a detailed hand assessment has been carried out to provide baseline measurements against which changes can be assessed, and to define the aims of splinting. All resting splints should be custom-made in order to ensure correct fit and joint positioning, and to be acceptable to the patient. Short-term use may still offer some symptomatic benefit and help to prevent deformity. Splints may also help to prevent deterioration of features such as ulnar deviation, swan-neck or boutonnière deformities.

Local corticosteroid injections are often used as a means of reducing active synovitis in one or more PIP or MCP joints, or to treat flexor tendon nodules or flexor tenosynovitis, in which there may be limited active flexion of the fingers but nevertheless a good range of passive movement. Treatment of local flexor tendon problems by injection requires highly skilled and accurate infiltration of corticosteroid into the flexor tendon sheath.

20

Key point

There is often cause for concern about the potential for tendon rupture following steroid injection. This is an important issue that should be taken into account when discussing the advantages and disadvantages of this approach with the patient, whilst bearing in mind that tendon rupture may also sometimes occur as a result of the chronic inflammatory process of RA itself.

Wrists

Proprietary splints can be invaluable in helping to maintain function, reducing pain and preventing deformity of the wrists. It is important to appreciate that poor wrist function will undoubtedly contribute significantly to poor overall hand function. More rigid polythene or prefabricated splints may sometimes be considered, particularly if wrist mobility is already reduced. Long-term restriction of movement should not occur, although a stiff wrist held in an optimal position may still be relatively pain-free and functional.

Carpal tunnel syndrome, due to entrapment of the median nerve, is a common associated problem in RA and may lead to hand pain and sensory symptoms. Confirmation of the diagnosis using nerve conduction studies should be obtained if possible. If symptoms do not improve despite the regular use of splints, control of the activity of the rheumatoid disease and a local steroid injection, then surgery to decompress the carpal tunnel may need to be considered.

Elbows

A programme of active exercises and education to encourage movement and prevent flexion deformities of the elbows is of paramount importance in RA. If the elbows are particularly inflamed such that the patient's capacity for conducting the recommended exercise programme is compromised, and if other causes of inflammation have been excluded, a corticosteroid injection into the joint or bursa may be given in an attempt to reduce pain and to enable maintenance of exercises in order to preserve range of movement in the joint.

Rheumatoid nodules occur in approximately 25–30 per cent of patients with RA. Surgical removal may be considered, particularly if infection of the nodule occurs. However, nodules frequently recur after surgical removal.

Shoulders

Shoulder involvement is common in RA, and should be anticipated and addressed in the form of a specific programme of exercise and education in order to prevent loss of movement and function. Restriction of abduction and external rotation of the shoulder should be sought from an early stage and monitored closely, and the patient's exercise programme modified accordingly if the range of movement shows signs of deterioration. A painful arc of movement of the shoulder joint suggests tendonitis, which may, if diagnosed in its early stages, respond to a local steroid injection. As always, accurate localisation of the injection and skilled technique are essential.

Precise diagnosis of the structures producing shoulder pain is often extremely difficult, and imaging with ultrasound or MRI can provide invaluable assistance in identifying the inflamed structure and informing the choice of appropriate therapy.

Key point

Tendon rupture or partial tears should always be assessed by an orthopaedic surgeon.

Cervical spine

The cervical spine is commonly affected in RA and the consequent effects of this on the spinal cord may lead to serious complications or even death. Therefore, before embarking upon any course of physiotherapy, X-rays of the cervical spine should be taken in flexion, in extension and with an open-mouth view. The films should be assessed carefully in order to determine the presence of atlanto-axial or subaxial subluxation and the involvement of the odontoid peg, and the findings should be taken into account when planning the course of treatment. This issue should also be borne in mind when preparing patients for anaesthesia, and during surgery and postoperative management.

Soft and rigid cervical collars may be of symptomatic value for some RA patients with neck problems, although many patients find them uncomfortable.

Dorsal spine and lumbar spine

The lower spine is rarely affected by RA. Any episodes of sudden acute onset of pain should be investigated for possible vertebral collapse, especially if the patient has been treated with glucocorticoids.

Hips

Acute synovitis of the hips in RA is relatively rare unless it forms part of more widespread exacerbation in inflammation involving other joints. Pain arising from the hip joint itself is usually felt in the groin, whilst pain over the lateral aspect of the hip may often arise as referred pain from the lower lumbar spine or pelvis, or may indicate a subtrochanteric bursitis. An ultrasound or MRI scan can be useful in confirming the presence of synovitis in the hip: for example, by demonstrating the presence of fluid in the joint.

An active exercise programme, with hydrotherapy, should be used to help reduce symptoms, maintain hip movement and improve muscle strength.

Knees

Active synovitis in the knee commonly occurs in both early and chronic RA. Pain may cause the knee to adopt a flexed position. Early treatment is essential and may involve resting splints, serial plaster or thermoplastic splinting and active quadriceps exercises in an effort to maintain range of movement. As always, a strong emphasis should be placed on the prevention of deformity as well as symptom management, and the vital importance of this should be explained carefully and repeatedly to the patient from the outset.

Ankles and feet

Ankle pain may often arise from the subtalar joint, for which, if other measures have failed, brief immobilisation in a light weight-bearing plaster of Paris is still sometimes used. Similarly, use of below-knee callipers and orthoses to immobilise the subtalar joint whilst allowing flexion at the ankle joint is still sometimes appropriate for intractable ankle pain prior to surgery.

Key point

Early involvement of a podiatrist for biomechanical assessment and provision of orthoses is an important component of the multidisciplinary management of RA. Consultation with a podiatrist is usually also an excellent opportunity for the patient to receive general advice about the use of appropriate and supportive footwear, and about other aspects of foot care.

The MTP joints are frequently the first joints affected in RA, but despite this the symptoms and signs of MTP involvement are often overlooked.

Prevention of pressure areas is essential as, apart from being focal areas of pain and functional impairment, they may also serve as a portal of entry for infection.

OTHER AUTOIMMUNE POLYARTHROPATHIES

Although RA is the most common type of autoimmune rheumatic disease, there are several other members of this family of disorders. Overall, a wide variety of often-overlapping disease features are found, reflecting the fact that many different tissues and organs can be affected in these conditions.

The diverse array of clinical features is, to some extent, paralleled by the different types of autoantibody present in patients' sera. Broadly speaking, different sets of clinical features can to some extent be matched to different profiles of autoantibodies, and this provides a framework for identifying distinct *diagnostic groups*. The family of autoimmune polyarthropathies includes Sjögren's syndrome, systemic lupus erythematosus (SLE), the vasculitides, systemic sclerosis, dermatomyositis and polymyositis. The main features are listed in Table 20.3.

All the autoimmune polyarthropathies typically undergo a course of exacerbations and remissions, associated with varying degrees of chronic inflammation, tissue damage and repair. In some instances factors that induce disease exacerbation can be identified — for example, exposure to sunlight or certain medications in

Table 20.3 Clinical features and associated autoantibodies in autoimmune rheumatic diseases

	Clinical feature	Associated autoantibodies
Sjögren's syndrome	Dry eyes	Rheumatoid factor
	Dry mouth	Ro, La
	Fatigue	
	Fever	
	Lymphadenopathy	
	Raynaud's phenomenon	
	Organ-specific autoimmune disease	
	Arthralgia/arthritis	
	Pulmonary disease	
	Liver disease	
	Renal disease	
SLE	Malar rash[a]	Antinuclear
	Photosensitivity	DNA binding
	Oral ulcers	Sm
	Alopecia	
	Serositis	
	Arthritis	
	Renal disease	
	Neuropathy	
Antiphospholipid syndrome	Venous or arterial occlusion	Anticardiolipin
	Recurrent fetal loss	
	Livedo reticularis[b]	
	Thrombocytopenia[c]	
Systemic vasculitis	Myalgia	Antineutrophil cytoplasmic
	Arthralgia	Cryoglobulins
	Purpura[d]	
	Skin ulcers	
	Sinusitis	
	Dyspnoea	
	Chest pain	
	Gastrointestinal upset	
	Neuropathy	
Systemic sclerosis	Raynaud's phenomenon	Anticentromere
	Telangiectasia[e]	
	Skin thickening	
	Calcinosis	
	Oesophageal stricture	
	Small bowel malabsorption	
	Pulmonary hypertension	
Polymyositis/dermatomyositis	Proximal muscle weakness	Jo1
	Muscle tenderness	
	Skin rash	
	Arthritis	
	Pulmonary fibrosis	
	Cardiac conduction defects	
	Disturbed gastrointestinal motility	

SLE, systemic lupus erythematosus
[a]Rash over the cheeks which may be butterfly-shaped.
[b]Mottling of the skin.
[c]Low platelet count.
[d]Purplish discolorations in the skin produced by small bleeding vessels.
[e]Persistently dilated blood capillaries.

SLE — but in most circumstances the course is unpredictable. Occasionally, clinical deterioration in SLE, vasculitis and other conditions can be very rapid, and although such situations thankfully occur relatively rarely, it is nevertheless important to appreciate that they can be life-threatening and that deterioration may require urgent medical attention.

Broadly, the management of these conditions is based on principles similar to those applied to the management of RA. Non-pharmacological, as well as pharmacological, therapies have an important role. Traditionally, a wide range of medications and treatment protocols have been used in an attempt to achieve immunosuppression and disease remission. As is also the case for RA, recent identification of specific molecular targets in several of these conditions is currently leading to the development of an increasing number of novel biological therapies, several of which are already at the stage of clinical trial and evaluation.

It is normally the case that the diagnosis and management of these conditions should be based on a multispecialist as well as multidisciplinary approach, and effective communication within and across healthcare sectors is essential. It is particularly important, therefore, that all healthcare professionals involved should work to ensure optimal planning, coordination and delivery of care to people with these complex diseases. This applies not only in the context of therapeutic interventions, both pharmacological and non-pharmacological, but also to the important aspects of education, advice and counselling.

THE SPONDYLOARTHROPATHIES

The group of conditions called *spondyloarthropathies* were at one time thought to be related to RA, but the recognition of characteristic features of spinal involvement and the presence and pathogenic importance of enthesopathy (inflammation at the site of tendon or ligament insertion) allowed the identification of this distinct group of rheumatic diseases. The different types of spondyloarthropathy share particular clinical, epidemiological and genetic features, including associations with HLA B27, which is one of the genes known to be involved in the pathogenesis of these conditions.

The typical pathological feature for these conditions is enthesopathy. The enthesis is the site of tendon, ligament or capsule attachment into bone. The underlying lesion is a focal non-specific chronic inflammation. The cartilaginous layer of the enthesis and adjacent bone are destroyed and replaced by granulation tissue. Enthesopathy is followed by new bone formation and may subsequently lead to ankylosis (fusion) of the joint.

In the spine, changes at the insertion of the outer fibres of annulus fibrosus to the anterior and lateral margins of the vertebral body result in squaring of vertebral bodies, vertebral endplate destruction and syndesmophyte formation (Figure 20.1). These changes can be demonstrated on X-ray (Figure 20.2). Syndesmophytes that completely bridge the vertebral disc eventually form the so-called bamboo spine. These changes may take many years to develop.

> **The spondyloarthropathies**
>
> The major recognised types of spondyloarthropathy are ankylosing spondylitis (AS), reactive arthritis (ReA) and psoriatic arthritis.

ANKYLOSING SPONDYLITIS

Clinical features

The symptoms of AS usually develop in adolescence or early adult life. Although the usual age of presentation is the late teens or early twenties, juvenile onset can occur. The principal symptoms are low back pain and

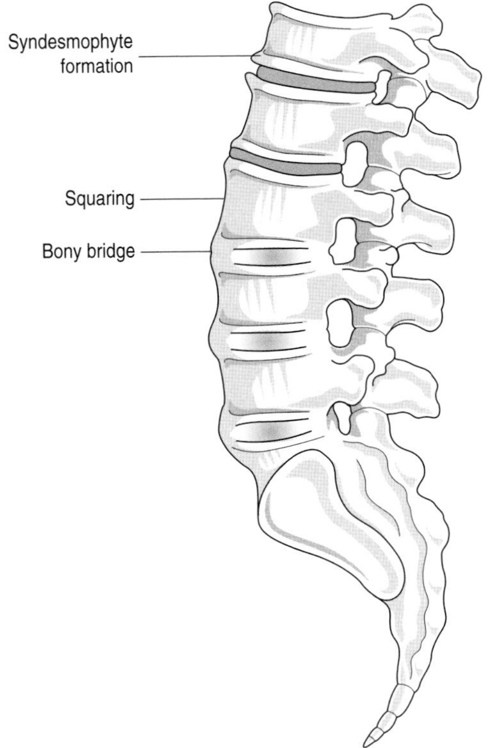

Figure 20.1 Spinal involvement in ankylosing spondylitis. (Adapted from David and Lloyd 1998, with permission.)

20

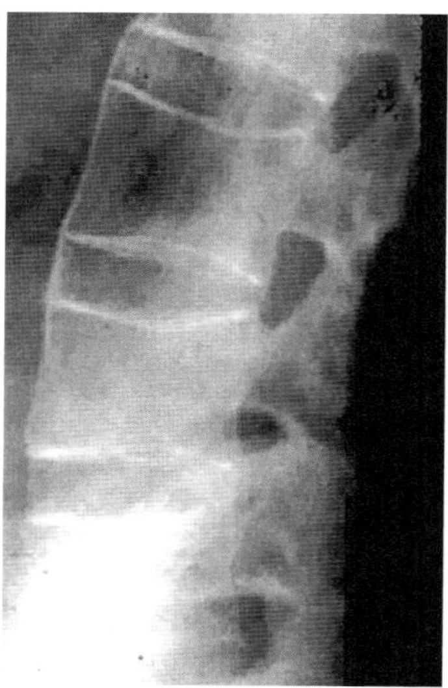

Figure 20.2 The lumbar spine in ankylosing spondylitis. Note the formation of syndesmophytes along the anterior margin of the spine.

stiffness, and the presence of stiffness often helps to distinguish AS from other causes of low back pain, such as vertebral collapse or nerve root inflammation. One or more peripheral joints are often also involved.

> ***Key point***
> Although previously thought to be more common in males, AS has undoubtedly been frequently underdiagnosed in females. Early reports of AS suggested a male/female ratio of 10:1 but more recent studies have suggested a ratio of 2.5:1. Females may have milder disease with more peripheral joint involvement.

The diagnosis of AS should always be considered in a young person presenting with low back pain, buttock pain or occasionally dorsal and chest wall pain. Stiffness is likely to be present in the morning and symptoms are
20 made worse by inactivity and usually improved with exercises. There is often a delay in making the diagnosis, which may be due to the intermittent nature of symptoms and a lack of radiological changes.

Characteristically, involvement of the sacroiliac joints is primarily responsible for the symptoms of low back pain and stiffness. Typical sites of enthesis involvement are at the Achilles tendon, the plantar aspect of the heel, the chest wall and the pelvis. Peripheral joint involvement can be a presenting feature in about 15 per cent, and will occur at some stage in up to 35 per cent of people with AS. Systemic features such as pyrexia, fatigue, weight loss or anaemia should

Table 20.4 Modified New York criteria for the diagnosis of ankylosing spondylitis (1984)

1. Low back pain for at least 3 months, improved by exercise and not relieved by rest
2. Limitation of lumbar spine movement in sagittal and frontal planes
3. Chest expansion decreased relative to normal values for age and sex
4. Bilateral sacroiliitis, grade 2–4
5. Unilateral sacroiliitis, grade 3–4

increase the suspicion for a diagnosis of AS in a young person with back pain. Most of the extra-articular features (Table 20.4) occur in the later stages of the disease, although acute anterior uveitis presenting as a painful red eye may occur at any stage.

Genetic susceptibility

Clinical observations of familial clustering of AS and related conditions, including inflammatory bowel disease, which were subsequently confirmed in twin studies and other family studies, have shown clearly that genetic factors have an important role in AS pathogenesis.

The first and probably the most important gene that was found to be involved is located within the human leucocyte antigen (HLA) class I region on the short arm of chromosome 6. As is the case for many other genes within the HLA region, the HLA B gene is remarkably polymorphic and exists in many different allelic forms within the population. The HLA B27 allele is strongly linked to ankylosing spondylitis; for example, among Caucasians with AS over 95 per cent possess this allele, whereas it is found in only about 6 per cent of the population as whole. Furthermore, the prevalence of AS in different countries broadly reflects the prevalence of HLA B27 within the population.

The fact that HLA B27 is present in such a large proportion of AS patients has led to extensive molecular and epidemiological research in an attempt to elucidate the underlying mechanisms. It is important to appreciate, however, that other genes besides B27 are likely to be involved in ankylosing spondylitis, and that most people with the B27 gene do not develop the disease. For example, HLA B27-positive relatives of HLA B27-positive AS patients are about twenty times more likely to develop AS than HLA B27-positive relatives of healthy B27-positive subjects. In other words, the B27 gene is clearly an important factor for susceptibility to AS, but other factors, both genetic and environmental, have an important role in the pathogenesis.

The mechanisms whereby B27 determines susceptibility to AS remain unknown. There continues to be much interest in the possibility that this may be linked to the normal biological role of B27-encoded molecules: namely, in selecting and binding short peptide fragments from among the pool of intracellular self-proteins or microbial antigens, transporting them to cell surfaces and presenting them to T lymphocytes. This process is fundamentally important in the development and regulation of the immune system and in protective immune responses. Several hypotheses have been proposed to explain how this might lead to disease, including the possibility that B27 molecules might be more likely than others to present microbial peptides that are sufficiently similar to self peptides so as to evoke autoimmune responses by a mechanism termed 'molecular mimicry'. Recent work demonstrating the propensity of B27 molecules to bind each other, and for these complexes to be expressed on cell surfaces for recognition by T lymphocytes, may also be important in AS pathogenesis.

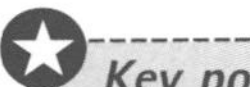

Key point

HLA B27 is also linked with the other types of spondyloarthropathy described later in this chapter, although less strongly than with AS. The associations seem generally stronger when applied to hospital-based, rather than population-based, groups, raising the possibility that the main effect of B27 may be on disease severity.

Establishing the diagnosis

The diagnosis is usually made primarily on clinical grounds, and clinical criteria can also be used to compare different series of patients. The only laboratory tests of use are those which measure inflammatory markers, such as the ESR or serum CRP concentrations. Tissue typing for HLA B27 is not helpful in the routine diagnosis of AS because of the high prevalence of this gene in the population.

The earliest radiological changes may take years to develop and usually manifest as blurring of the margins of the sacroiliac joints. This may be followed by the development of sclerosis, which may be accompanied by characteristic radiological appearances of fusion of the spine due to calcification in chronically inflamed spinal joints and ligaments. Syndesmophytes (Figures 20.1 and 20.2) are the gradual ossification of the superficial layers of the annulus fibrosus following inflammation and reactive sclerosis. Destructive osteitis and repair lead to squaring of the vertebral body. Early changes may be difficult to diagnose, although further information may be obtained from isotope bone scanning or an MRI scan.

Clinical assessment and monitoring

Assessment

Involvement of the sacroiliac joints is assessed by stressing these joints by pressure applied over the sacrum or by cross-compression of the pelvis. These manœuvres may result in pain or discomfort in the presence of active sacroiliitis. The loss of normal lumbar lordosis, with flattening of the lumbar spine in forward flexion, is the earliest clinical sign of lumbar spine involvement. Gradually, lumbar spinal movements may become restricted in all planes.

The most commonly used assessment in the clinic is the modified Schober test. A 10 cm line is drawn upwards from the L5–S1 junction (at the dimples of Venus) and the increase measured during flexion. In the normal spine an increase of 4 or 5 cm would usually be expected. Chest expansion, in the increase following full inspiration, is measured at the fourth intercostal space. Finger–floor distance is a measure of hip movement as well as spinal mobility, and hip involvement can be assessed by the standard methods of measuring ranges of movement, and monitored by measuring the intermalleolar distance. Neck movement is assessed by measuring the tragus to wall distance and rotation of the cervical spine.

Modified Schober test

See Chapter 21 on the physiotherapy management of ankylosing spondylitis for illustrations of how to perform this test.

In the later stages of the disease an abnormal posture with thoracic kyphosis and a flexion deformity of the neck may develop if early treatment has been ineffective. This is now much less common than previously due to improvements in early diagnosis, active physiotherapy and appropriate use of medication.

Monitoring

Regular formal assessments, on at least an annual basis, are very useful to monitor treatment and to determine progression or improvement of the condition. Assessments of spinal mobility, chest expansion, involvement of peripheral joints and entheses should be recorded. Several validated and convenient methods of assessment of disease status in AS are now available for use in both healthcare and research settings. These include the Bath AS Disease Activity Index (BASDAI), which provides a clinical measure of the severity of active inflammation. In addition, assessments of the severity of nocturnal pain and morning stiffness may also serve as useful measures of disease status. Overall disability can also be monitored using scoring systems such as the Bath AS Functional Index (BASFI) and the Health Assessment Questionnaire (HAQ).

Course of the disease

The course of AS is very variable. Some patients continue with the typical inflammatory features over decades, whilst others develop a rigid spine within 10 years. The typical progression is of slowly ascending pain and stiffness with periods of remission and relapse.

The development of spinal pain with movement, eased by rest, suggests the possibility of a mechanical problem, such as a spinal fracture through a syndesmophyte or a destructive lesion of an intervertebral disc. Another possibility would be a mobile segment, which occurs where there is fusion above and below an unfused area such that movement can occur, resulting in pain. Spinal osteoporosis, stenosis and cauda equina syndrome are other late spinal complications of AS. Other recognised systemic complications (Table 20.5) are relatively rare but should be borne in mind if a person with AS becomes generally unwell.

Clinical management

Non-pharmacological treatments

It is now well recognised and widely accepted that the single most important aspect of clinical management of this condition is the practice of a clearly specified programme of regular exercises aimed at preventing the disastrous loss of spinal mobility that used to occur and which is still depicted in many medical textbooks. The potentially catastrophic and irreversible consequences of spinal immobility should be emphasised repeatedly to the patient. Some people have relatively little difficulty in undertaking a regular exercise programme and, following initial instruction and discussion, are able to incorporate such a programme satisfactorily into their domestic, work and social commitments. Others prefer to conduct an exercise programme as part of a group activity, an approach that can provide valuable additional benefits in terms of support and maintenance of morale. Self-help groups are facilitated and supported nationally by the National Ankylosing Spondylitis Society (NASS). Hydrotherapy and swimming are invaluable adjuncts to other exercise programmes.

Table 20.5 Common extra-articular features of ankylosing spondylitis

Ocular	Uveitis
	Conjunctivitis
	Synechiae*
	Glaucoma
Pulmonary	Upper lobe fibrosis
	Cavitation
	Aspergillosis
Cardiovascular	Aortic regurgitation
	Conduction defects
Neurological	Nerve root or cord compression
Systemic	Amyloidosis

*Adhesions, particularly between the iris and the cornea or lens of the eye.

Key point

If exercises are perceived to make a patient worse, particularly in the later stages, then investigations for a fracture or mobile segment should be undertaken and the exercise programme stopped whilst this is done.

Weblink

National Ankylosing Spondylitis Society (NASS): www.nass.co.uk

Individual assessment and advice with regard to pain management and activities of daily living, such as driving, are also a very important part of management and health professionals often play a particularly key role in these aspects.

The use of prismatic spectacles for patients with severe upper spinal deformities can often be extremely beneficial. Spinal orthoses are not routinely used but may sometimes have a place in preventing increasing spinal deformity, and in particular to support the chin where there is a flexion deformity of the neck.

Pharmacological treatments

Many people with AS find analgesics or NSAIDs useful, particularly at times when the inflammation is active. The main aim of using these medications is to obtain relief of nocturnal pain and morning stiffness and thereby to enable the patient to undertake an exercise regimen in the morning. They are therefore usually prescribed for the evening to obtain maximum benefit in the early morning, and their use may be intermittent depending upon the pattern of symptoms.

The benefits of these medications in terms of symptom relief have to be weighed against the potential for side-effects, and their use should be monitored carefully to avoid inappropriate continual or habitual use.

DMARDs

These are rarely used in AS. Sulfasalazine is occasionally added to an NSAID, although most benefit is seen in the peripheral joint features rather than the spinal disease.

Biological therapy

Clinical trials of anti-TNFα therapy in AS have reported extremely promising results, and significant benefits have also been found in the other spondyloarthropathies. The use of anti-TNFα, and perhaps other biological therapies, in the treatment of these conditions is likely to become increasingly commonplace in the future.

Surgery

The indications for joint replacement are similar to those for patients with RA. Hip or knee joint replacement is an appropriate intervention in situations in which joint destruction is severe. Hip involvement is common in severe AS, particularly when the disease starts in early teenage life. Hip replacement, even at an early age, may dramatically reduce pain, improve mobility and improve the postural abnormalities that develop from fixed flexion deformities of the hip.

Osteotomy of the dorsal spine for severe kyphosis is sometimes considered in specialised spinal units, and although atlanto-axial instability is less common than in RA, fusion may sometimes need to be considered, as is also the case for spinal decompression in patients with cauda equina syndrome.

REACTIVE ARTHRITIS

Definition

The term 'reactive arthritis' (ReA) is used to diagnose arthritis that follows a known microbial infection and in which the microbe itself cannot be isolated in viable form from the joints.

Pathogenesis

Reactive arthritis has been described following a large number of bacterial and viral infections, including, for example, *Streptococcus pyogenes*, which can lead to a variety of sequelae such as ReA or rheumatic fever. However, among the wide range of microbes recognised as having arthritogenic potential in humans, some are known to lead to rheumatic sequelae that are very similar to the features of AS and the other spondyloarthropathies. This applies in particular to intracellular enteric bacteria (*Campylobacter*, *Salmonella*, *Yersinia*, *Shigella*), which are common causes of acute enteritis, and to *Chlamydia*, which is a common cause of urethritis. Infection with any of these microbes can lead to ReA, and the clinical features are very similar irrespective of the causal microbe.

Clinical features

Typically, the arthritis develops between 1 and 3 weeks after an episode of infection of the urogenital tract or bowel, although infection may be asymptomatic, particularly with *Chlamydia*. The clinical features of the reactive sequelae bear close similarities to AS, although often with a greater prominence of peripheral joint involvement and enthesopathy and less severe spinal features, although low back pain and stiffness is common. The peripheral arthritis is acute, and the knees are the most commonly involved joints.

Extra-articular features of ReA are common and include sterile conjunctivitis, mouth ulcers, ulcers of the glans penis (circinate balanitis) and keratoderma blenorrhagica, a rash similar to pustular psoriasis. Other features of systemic involvement may be similar to those of AS, particularly in people with persistent or chronic disease.

Diagnosis and management

The diagnosis of ReA is made predominantly on the clinical history and examination. Patients usually present several weeks after the initial infection, and it is therefore relatively uncommon for the microbe to be cultured from stool or urethral cultures. Laboratory tests may reveal raised ESR and CRP levels as non-specific markers of inflammation. Depending on the time of presentation, demonstration of a rise in titre of antibody levels to the inciting microbe may be feasible as a means of confirming the diagnosis.

Although the majority of patients improve over a period of up to 6 months, about 15–20 per cent may experience a recurrence in symptoms and signs, and in some people the arthritis becomes more severe over a period of 10–20 years, particularly in those who have the HLA B27 gene. The extent to which this depends upon repeated infections, either overt or subclinical, following the initial episode is unknown.

Treatment of ReA is aimed at relief of symptoms, involving the standard principles of joint protection, pain management, exercise, and appropriate use of NSAIDs and analgesics as needed. Sulfasalazine, methotrexate or azathioprine is sometimes used to treat severe, persistent joint inflammation. There is evidence to suggest that antibiotic therapy may enhance recovery in post-chlamydia ReA, but there is no evidence of a similar benefit from antibiotics in the treatment of post-enteric ReA.

PSORIATIC ARTHRITIS

It is well recognised that psoriasis can occur in association with rheumatic disease, and that the onset of joint problems can occur at any stage, before or after the onset of dermatological disease.

Patterns of disease

Among the different patterns of joint disease that have been described in psoriasis, dactylitis, enthesopathy and sacroiliitis are commonly found in these groups.

The classical patterns of psoriatic arthropathy have been described as:

- arthritis of the distal interphalangeal joints
- arthritis mutilans
- symmetrical peripheral polyarthritis, similar to RA
- asymmetrical oligoarthritis
- spondyloarthropathy.

The pattern of arthritis in an individual patient may change over time from one group to another. Psoriatic nail changes occur in 40 per cent of people with skin psoriasis and in 90 per cent of those with arthritis. The skin and joint involvement often has no direct relationship, and in 15–20 per cent of cases joint involvement precedes skin psoriasis. The skin involvement may be minimal and careful examination of the scalp, flexures and umbilicus may be required in order to reveal small patches of psoriasis.

X-rays may show erosions with osteolysis and the development of a 'pencil in cup' appearance seen characteristically in arthritis mutilans. Sternoclavicular and manubriosternal joints may also be involved, this being a recognised feature of the seronegative spondyloarthropathies.

Course and management

The course of the arthritis is typically that of periodic relapses and remissions, but fewer than 5 per cent of cases develop very severe deforming arthritis.

The principles of clinical assessment, treatment and management of these conditions are essentially the same as those described above for other types of chronic polyarthritis. Medical treatment involves the use of NSAIDs and disease-modifying drugs as appropriate, including sulfasalazine, methotrexate and ciclosporin A. An increasing amount of clinical trials data suggests that anti-TNFα treatments have efficacy in this condition, and also that biological therapies are likely to have an important role in the treatment of psoriatic arthritis in the future. Surgery also has a place in management in ways similar to those that apply for patients with RA.

USEFUL LINKS

www.jointzone.org.uk
www.cks.library.nhs.uk
www.rheumatology.org.uk
www.arc.org.uk
www.dipex.org.uk

FURTHER READING

Calin A, Taurog JD (eds) 1998 The Spondyloarthritides. Oxford University Press: Oxford

Firestein GS, Panayi GS, Wollheim FA (eds) 2000 Rheumatoid Arthritis: New Frontiers in Pathogenesis and Treatment. Oxford University Press: Oxford

Hochberg MC, Silman AJ, Smolen JS et al. (eds) 2003 Rheumatology, 3rd edn. Mosby: Philadelphia

Maddison PJ, Isenberg DA, Woo P, Glass DN (eds) 1998 Oxford Textbook of Rheumatology. Oxford University Press: Oxford

Chapter 21

Physiotherapy management of ankylosing spondylitis

Juliette O'Hea, with contributions from Julie Barlow

CHAPTER CONTENTS

INTRODUCTION

Physiotherapy is a key component in the management of ankylosing spondylitis (AS) and intervention should take place as early as possible following diagnosis. Owing to the chronic nature of the disease, people with AS must be encouraged to take control and responsibility for their own overall management. The task of the physiotherapist is to empower patients by increasing their knowledge of the disease and self-management principles. The patients need to know and believe that investment of time and energy in an exercise programme will result in a meaningful improvement in their quality of life.

AIMS OF PHYSIOTHERAPY MANAGEMENT

The overall aims are to minimise deformity and disability and to maintain normal function, thereby improving the person's quality of life and well-being. Specifically these aims can be achieved in the following ways, by:

- reduction of pain
- advice on postural awareness and ergonomics
- improvement and maintenance of posture and function by:
    - increasing the mobility of spinal, costovertebral and peripheral joints
    - strengthening the anti-gravity muscles
    - stretching specific muscle groups
- improvement and maintenance of cardiovascular fitness
- monitoring posture, mobility and function through regular assessment
- provision and monitoring of a home programme of specific exercises that are suitable and consistent with long-term compliance
- supporting them in whatever exercise/sports programme that they wish to undertake

- providing information about the disease and its management.

Helping the person to achieve these aims should contribute to improving the person's psychological state, coping strategies and exercise compliance.

PAIN IN ANKYLOSING SPONDYLITIS

Pain may vary from low-grade discomfort to intense pain. Typically, pain is aggravated by inactivity and is often reduced by exercise. The perception of pain can be influenced by several factors, including fatigue (which is a common symptom of AS). Physiotherapy modalities such as ultrasound, acupuncture, transcutaneous nerve stimulation (TENS), megapulse and gentle spinal mobilisations (Bulstrode et al. 1987) can be effective, especially for localised pain. However, this form of treatment should not be allowed to discourage the patient from ongoing participation in an exercise programme.

It is important to remember that from a lay perspective, pain is the body's way of signalling that there is something wrong and this usually means that the individual has to rest. Patients with AS need to know and understand when it is safe for them to continue exercising and when they need to rest the joints involved.

In the early stages of starting up an exercise regimen, pain may be provoked and exercises should therefore be commenced gradually. Wearing supportive shock-absorbing shoes can decrease the jarring effect of walking on hard surfaces and reduce the likelihood of aggravating any pain. If pain wakes the patient at night, gentle exercise, heat and analgesics may be useful. Hot packs, a hot shower, a bath or hydrotherapy can reduce pain by muscle relaxation which enables more movement in the joints and soft tissues affected. In addition, the patient can try cognitive techniques for pain management such as distraction, guided imagery and relaxation.

POSTURE

21

Figure 21.1 shows the typical postural deformities of advanced ankylosing spondylitis. In the early stages of the disease a flattening of the lumbar curve may occur. Then, with increasing pain and a flexed posture (some patients find that assuming a flexed posture reduces the pain), the thoracic curve can become more accentuated. If unchecked, this can be followed by a loss of the cervical curve. The head then protracts in an attempt to compensate for the forward flexion of the thoracic spine. As the hips become more flexed, hip flexion contractures can occur and the knees flex to improve balance and

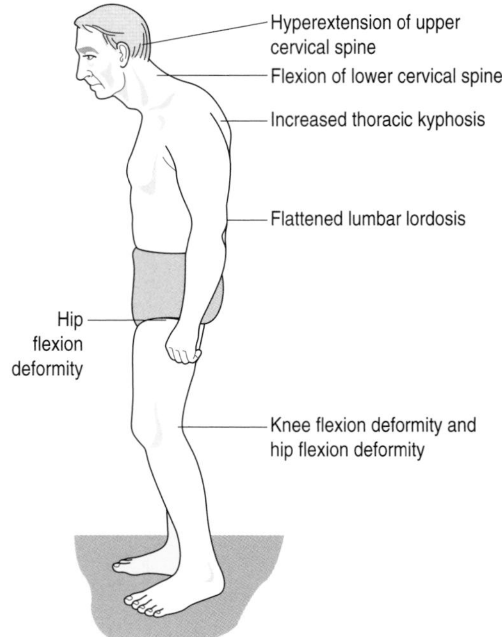

Figure 21.1 The typical postural deformities of advanced ankylosing spondylitis.

vision. This type of posture is biomechanically inefficient because the line of gravity falls outside the base of support. Poor posture results in muscle fatigue, weakness, disability and a poor body image. Good management of the disease should prevent poor posture from occurring, although any fusion may only be delayed and not halted.

> ***Key point***
>
> Scoliosis does not usually exist to any significant degree in AS because pathological changes to the spinal column tend to be symmetrical.

Ergonomic considerations and postural correction

A flexed posture can relieve the pain but should be discouraged. Ergonomic advice on how to maintain good posture at work, in the home and during leisure activities will improve the long-term outcome of the disease. The longer the patient assumes a flexed posture during the day and night, the more likely it is that the spine will assume a flexed position if the vertebrae fuse. Advice is particularly important if the patient has a sedentary job or needs to be in a prolonged stooped position (e.g. a dentist). The advice would be to get up and move around at regular intervals and check the posture regularly. An army officer may not need to check posture so often!

Encourage the patient to maintain a good posture by walking tall and tucking the chin in. It may help to visualise being lifted up by a piece of string from the occiput. The posture can be checked in a mirror or by the patient standing as straight as possible against a wall, tucking the chin in. The person should try to maintain this posture when walking away from the wall.

Many of us lead sedentary lifestyles, so it is important to invest in chairs and car seats that are comfortable and supportive. Ideally, a chair should provide support for the whole spine, including the neck. The hips and knees should be at right angles and the feet should be supported if they do not touch the floor. Forearms supported on arm rests can relieve tension in the neck.

Car seats that support both the neck and the back are more comfortable and could reduce the risk of fracture if the person is involved in a road traffic accident. A close fit between the head and the head restraint, a head restraint that extends a minimum of 7 cm above the level of the eyes, and a restraint and seat that are designed as one system are recommended (Eriendsson 1998). Special internal and external car mirrors that can increase the field of vision may be purchased from the National Ankylosing Spondylitis Society (NASS).

For people who spend a lot of time at a computer, simple alterations such as altering the height of the computer screen and chair can make a significant difference. There are UK and European Union regulations that require employers to assess the health and safety risks to employees (Health & Safety Executive 1994).

For specialist advice on seating (both at home, at work and in the car), on beds and on work stations, referral to an ergonomist, to a specialist health professional or to a Jobcentreplus Disability Employment Advisor (DEA) may be appropriate.

ASSESSMENT

Subjective assessment

Include similar questions to those asked in a musculoskeletal assessment. This demographic data would be followed by a more detailed account of current pain levels, previous medical history, family history, social history and drug history (see Chapter 2). A brief overview of postural considerations is useful. Subjective assessment should be kept up to date by noting any changes to the person's circumstances.

Pain

A body chart can be used to indicate the areas, intensity, frequency and persistence of pain during a typical 24-h period (including night pain). This is particularly useful with enthesitis pain. Enthesitis pain can be measured using a validated enthesitis score (e.g. MASES Heuft-Dorenbosch 2003) and spinal pain is measured using a Visual Analogue scale (VAS). Both pain experienced during the daytime and at night over the last week should be recorded.

Previous medical history

- Date/year of onset of symptoms/diagnosis.
- Radiology results.
- HLAB27: positive, negative or unknown.
- Medical history: skin, eyes, bowels, chest, depression, other.
- Effectiveness of steroid injections: joint/entheses/intramuscular/intravenous.
- Peripheral joint involvement.
- Surgery: joint(s) affected and dates.

Family history

Any family history of AS, iritis, psoriasis or bowel problems should be noted.

Social history

- Main problems: pain, stiffness, fatigue, depression, family, work, hobbies.
- Occupation. Employed/unemployed/student/retired/sickness benefits.
- Any children? Any parental difficulties due to the condition?
- Current exercise regimen/sports: frequency, effect on pain.
- Smoker? Alcohol?
- Member of local NASS group?

Drug history

- Medications: present/past, frequency, side-effects (see Chapter 20).

Ergonomic assessment

- Seating at home, work and in the car (include head restraints).
- Table/desk height at work/home.
- Type of mattress and number of pillows.

Objective assessment

Outcome measures

Traditionally, patient assessment was dominated by a multitude of individual anthropometric measurements that were not necessarily standardised, reliable, valid and responsive to change. Therefore, accurate assessment of improvement or deterioration was difficult to measure.

Key point

As Calin (1994) pointed out, 'without a clear understanding of outcome, we could not know whether physiotherapy or any other modality really "works" in ankylosing spondylitis'. It gives the clinician the ability to decide whether to initiate, terminate, continue or modify a treatment (Bellamy et al. 1998).

Over the years, a number of both disease-specific and generic outcome measures were developed. However, Bellamy et al. (1998, 1999) revealed a lack of standardisation in the selection and use of outcome measurements by rheumatologists in clinical practice. With an increasing interest in AS research and the introduction of biological therapy, it was evident that outcome measures needed to be standardised.

In response to this problem, the Ankylosing Spondylitis Assessment Study group (ASAS) was set up in 1995 as a subcommittee to the larger Outcome Measures in Rheumatology Clinical Trials (OMERACT) initiative (van der Heijde et al. 1999). ASAS comprises experts in the field of spondyloarthritis and its mission is to support and promote translational and clinical research with the ultimate goal being to improve the well-being and outcome of patients with spondyloarthritis of which AS is subgroup. A method of achieving this is via the development and validation of assessment tools.

Based on an extensive literature review and consensus, ASAS decided upon the most acceptable instruments (either generic or disease-specific) that could be used to determine changes of different domains over time (van de Heijde 1999). These instruments could be used in both clinical research and routine practice. The instruments had to measure what was intended, show reliability and sensitivity to change, and be simple to complete. The domains were chosen specifically to reflect the nature of the disease. These included patient global assessment, pain, stiffness, fatigue, peripheral and entheseal involvement, spinal mobility, physical function, and acute phase reactants (such as ESR and CRP).

21

Examples of some of the instruments that are currently used in clinical practice are shown in Table 21.2. New instruments will be developed and some will need modification in due course as further research and the work of the ASAS working group continues.

THE BATH INDICES

The Bath Indices were developed by a research team at the Royal National Hospital for Rheumatic Diseases, in Bath. Rheumatologists, physiotherapists, research associates and patients were involved in the creation of these indices. They are very popular in both research and clinical practice due to their reliability, reproducibility, sensitivity, speed and simplicity. The Bath Indices booklet contains all the Bath Indices and has a detailed account of how to use them. The booklet can be downloaded from the National Ankylosing Spondylitis (NASS) website (see useful links below), or a free copy can be obtained from NASS.

The Bath Ankylosing Spondylitis Metrology Index (BASMI)

It was found that only five objective measurements from an original set of 20 were able to show validity, reliability and sensitivity to change.

These were tragus to wall, cervical rotation, lumbar side-flexion, lumbar flexion (modified Schober's) and intermalleolar distance. The BASMI uses these five measurements to generate a score out of 10. The higher the BASMI score, the more severe the patient's limitation of movement. The BASMI can show clinically significant changes in spinal movement (Jenkinson et al. 1994).

Equipment for assessment should include a neck goniometer (gravity action or spirit level), a long ruler and tape measure. In order to standardise the measurement, the assessment should ideally be made by the same physiotherapist at the same time of day and before hydrotherapy or a gym session. To make the measurement reproducible, standardise the patient's starting position, watch for any 'trick movements', and allow time for the patient to achieve maximum stretch. See Table 21.1.

The Bath Ankylosing Spondylitis Functional Index (BASFI)

The BASFI (Calin 1994) is a quick and easy 10-item self-administered questionnaire that includes eight questions relating to activities that patients with AS find typically difficult and two related to their ability to cope with everyday life. The responses are measured using a 10 cm visual analogue scale (VAS). The final score is a mean of the 10 questions and the higher the score, the higher the disability. A high BASFI is an important predictor of AS-related work disability and a high BASFI at baseline predicts poor response to biologic therapy (Davis et al. 2005).

The Bath Ankylosing Spondylitis Disease Activity Index (BASDAI)

The BASDAI (Garrett 1994) is a useful tool to measure disease activity and includes the domains of fatigue, spinal pain, joint pain and swelling, areas of localised tenderness and two questions relating to early morning stiffness

Table 21.1 Five anthropometric measures commonly used in AS assessment

Measure	Starting position	Method
Tragus to wall (Figure 21.2)	This is a good measurement of posture. The patient stands with bare feet, back to the wall, knees straight and scapulae, buttocks and heels as close to the wall as possible. Keep outer edges of feet 30 cm apart and feet parallel. Keep shoulders level and chin tucked in as far as possible	The tragus to wall distance is measured on both sides with a rigid rule. The average of the two measurements is recorded. Height can be measured at the same time
Cervical rotation	The patient lies supine with head at the end of the plinth and chin tucked in. Ensure shoulders do not move and the head is not tilted back	Place the goniometer lightly on forehead. The patient rotates his/her head. Repeat on other side
Lumbar side-flexion	Maintain same starting position as above. Keep fingers straight	Measure from middle finger tip to floor. The patient then reaches down to the left, keeping shoulders against the wall. Measure from middle finger to tip of floor again. Side flexion is the difference between the two measurements. Repeat on other side
Schober's test (modified) (Figure 21.3)	This measures the amount of lumbar spine flexion. The patient stands with bare feet 30 cm apart and parallel	Draw a line at the L4–L5 junction and mark 10 cm above and 5 cm below this line. The patient bends forwards with knees slightly bent. Hold the end of the tape measure on the upper mark and measure between that and the lowest mark. Any increase beyond 15 cm is the lumbar flexion
Intermalleolar distance (hip abduction)	The patient lies supine on the floor with legs apart, knees straight and feet turned out	Measure between the medial malleoli

(EMS). Again the questionnaire is self-administered and uses a 10 cm VAS. To give each symptom equal weighting, a mean of the two scores relating to EMS is taken. The resulting 0–50 score is divided by five to give a final score of between 0–10. Again, the higher the score, the greater the disease activity. The BASDAI forms part of the screening process for biologic treatment.

EXERCISE IN ANKYLOSING SPONDYLITIS

General issues

Regular, specific exercise is essential and effective in the management of AS and patients should be made aware of its importance. It has a profound influence on how the disease affects the person in the long term. Non-steroidal anti-inflammatory drugs (NSAIDs) should control the pain adequately to encourage exercise. Therefore, an understanding of how these medications work most effectively is important. With regular exercise, it may be possible to reduce the dose of the NSAID or stop it altogether.

Intensive physiotherapy regimens (Tomlinson et al. 1986; Viitanen et al. 1995) in a group situation (Hidding et al. 1993) and during inpatient programmes (Band et al. 1997) have been shown to be the most successful. However, it has been found that, unless the exercise is supervised, intensive and sustained, progressive loss of movement can occur (Lubrano and Helliwell 1999).

Table 21.2 Examples of outcome and anthropometric measurements used in AS assessment

Domain	Instrument	Original reference
Function	Bath Ankylosing Spondylitis Functional Index (BASFI)	Calin et al. (1994)
	Dougados/Spondylitis Function Index	Dougados et al. (1988)
Spinal mobility	Cervical rotation	O'Driscoll et al. (1978)
	Modified Schober	Macrae and Wright (1969)
	Tragus to wall	Tomlinson et al. (1986)
	Lumbar side-flexion	Pile et al. (1991)
	Chest expansion	Tomlinson et al. (1986)
	Bath Ankylosing Spondylitis Metrology Index (BASMI)	Jenkinson et al. (1994)
Disease activity	Bath Ankylosing Spondylitis Disease Activity Index (BASDAI)	Garrett et al. (1994)
Pain	10 cm visual analogue scale	
Enthesitis pain	Validated enthesitis score, e.g. Maastricht AS enthesitis score	Heuft-Dorenbosch 2003
Depression	HAD (generic)	Zigmond and Snaith (1983)
Quality of life/well-being	Bath Ankylosing Spondylitis Global Score (BAS-G)	Jones et al. (1996b)
	Ankylosing Spondylitis Quality of Life (ASQoL)	Reynolds et al. (1999)

Table 21.3 A typical AS exercise record

Date					
	Gym	Pool		Gym	Pool
WARM-UP					
Stretching:			Lumbar spine extensors		
Rectus femoris			Lumbar side flexors		
Psoas			Abdominals		
Hip adductors			Hip extensors		
Hip rotators			Hip abductors		
Hamstrings			Hip rotators		
Calf			Quadriceps		
Pectorals			Ankle and foot		
Thoracic rotators			**Mobilising:**		
Abdominals			Neck		
Neck			Temporomandibular		
Shoulder extensors			Shoulder		
Shoulder adductors			Thoracic rotation		
Shoulder rotators			Lumbar side-flexion		
Strengthening:			Lumbar flexion/extension		
Neck retractor			**Breathing exercises**		
Other neck muscles			**Posture awareness**		
Shoulder elevators			**Cardiovascular**		
Thoracic spine extensors			**Relaxation**		
Thoracic rotators			**COOL DOWN**		

(Reproduced by kind permission of Jane Barefoot.)

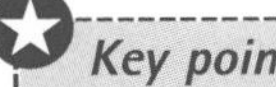

Key point

A regular exercise pattern must start as early as possible following diagnosis and be performed for life. This requires a great deal of motivation on behalf of the patient, particularly given the relatively early age at onset of AS, which means that an individual may be required to exercise every day for most of their adult life. In the early, more acute stages of AS, individual treatment may be preferable. The physiotherapist plays an essential role in providing the patient with ongoing education, stimulus and inspiration, so that exercise becomes part of a daily routine.

Typically, the symptoms of AS fluctuate. The person may experience acute exacerbations of pain and muscle spasm, chronic low-grade pain and quiescent periods. Whatever the symptoms, exercise should be continued regularly in order to prevent deterioration of posture as muscle weakness and shortening of the soft tissues results in a loss of physical function. The person with AS should make the most of the relatively pain-free periods by exercising as vigorously as possible and maintaining a good general fitness level. It is important to note that this strategy differs somewhat from that advocated for most other types of arthritis (e.g. RA) where patients are advised to pace themselves so as not to aggravate their symptoms during times of low disease activity.

To guarantee full participation, the physiotherapist should always be prepared to modify an exercise. A variety of equipment can be used to make the exercises more interesting, such as a gymnastic ball or Theraband but always ensure that the patient is exercising in a safe environment. When exercising supine, the patient's head should be supported with the minimum number of pillows – just enough to prevent the head from tilting back.

For examples of land exercises, see Tables 21.4 to 21.7.

Joint mobility exercises

Flexion, extension, lateral flexion and rotation of the cervical, thoracic and lumbar spines can become limited in a person with AS owing to muscle tension, fibrosis and bony changes (formation of syndesmophytes). Therefore, exercises should be designed to maintain and improve these movements.

Mobility exercises should put a joint through the full range of available movement.

Clinical note

As the person's rib cage mobility can be reduced owing to involvement of the costovertebral and sternocostal joints, breathing exercises should be encouraged. Singing or playing a wind instrument can be both therapeutic and enjoyable.

Strengthening exercises

Loss of muscle strength is a feature of AS. Muscles weaken due to postural deformity and inactivity and the associated pain (Cooper et al. 1991). Strengthening of the antigravity (extensor) muscle groups and abdominal muscles is important to maintain an erect posture, and it enables everyday activities to be undertaken with greater ease. Examples of extensor muscle groups are the cervical, thoracic and lumbar spine extensors (erector spinae) and the glutei. Exercises can be made harder by extending the lever arm (see Chapter 6), using gravity or buoyancy as a resistance, or by adding weights. Strengthening exercises are held for several seconds and repeated at least five times. Strengthening of other muscle groups, such as the lumbar side flexors and thoracic rotators, is also important. These particular muscle groups can be effectively strengthened in the hydrotherapy pool.

Muscle stretches

The muscles most commonly affected by tightness are the sternocleidomastoid and trapezii in the neck, shoulder adductors and flexors, hip flexors and adductors, hamstrings and gastrocnemius. Much of the stiffness that patients experience is due to muscle tension. Stretching the muscles, tendons and ligaments allows more joint movement to occur and improves posture.

The contract–relax method of stretching is commonly used (Bulstrode et al. 1987). This involves a maximal isometric contraction for 3 seconds made in the position of maximum stretch of the muscle, followed by a relaxation of 2 seconds and a further passive stretch of the muscle for 6 seconds. This cycle is repeated at least three times. To improve effectiveness, it is important that the patient can feel the stretch in the correct area. The contraction can be into a firm surface or into a hydrotherapy float. If using a slow, prolonged stretch, this should be maintained for between 30 and 60 seconds (Beaulieu 1981). There are many ways to stretch each muscle group, see Table 21.7 for examples.

Table 21.4 Mr L's mobility exercises

Movement	Starting position	Action
Lumbar extension and flexion	Lie prone with hands under shoulders 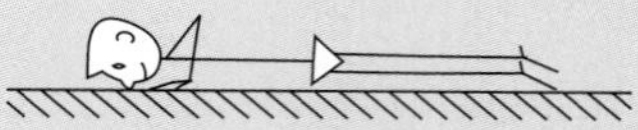	Push up on hands. Keep pelvis flat on floor 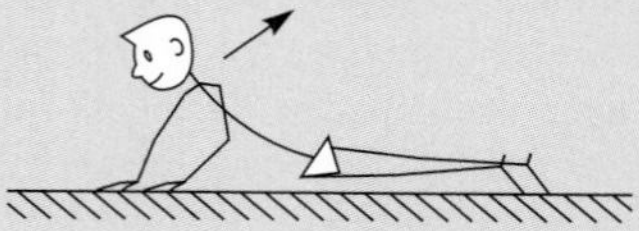
	Four-point kneeling with hands under shoulders, hip and knees at 90 degrees 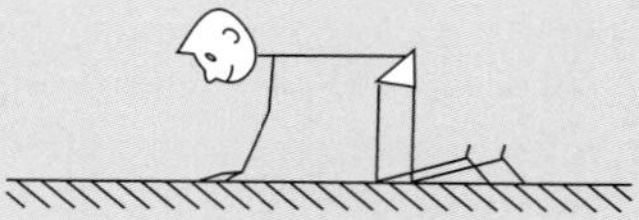	(a) Hump back, clasp knee to chest and look down (b) Hollow back, take leg straight out behind and look straight ahead 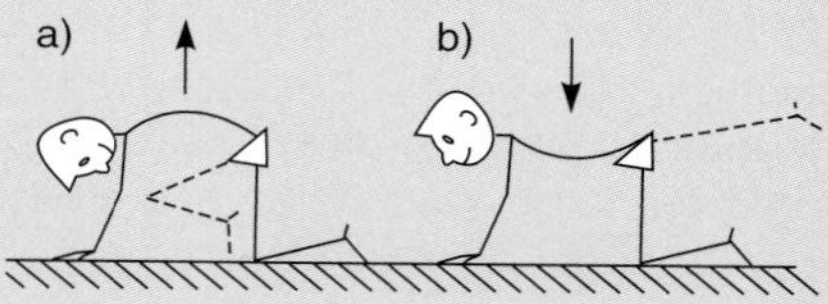 a) b)
	Sit on gym ball with feet flat on floor 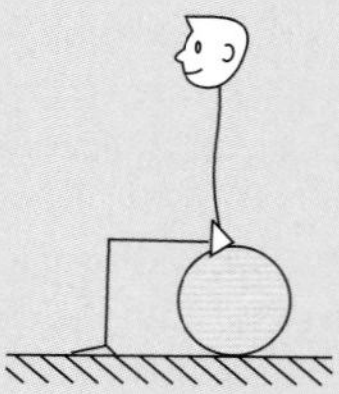	Slump forwards and backwards (pelvic tilt) 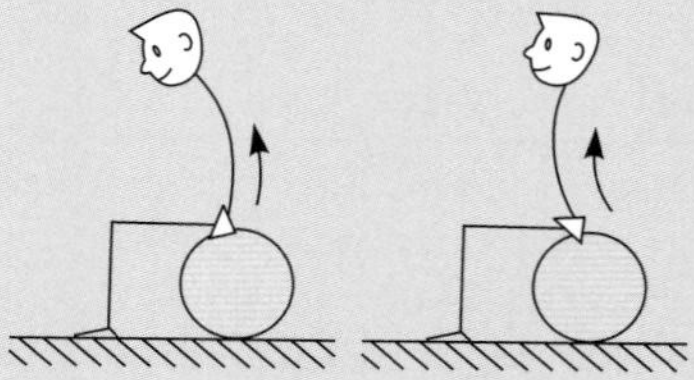

Table 21.4 Mr L's mobility exercises—cont'd

Movement	Starting position	Action
Lumbar side-flexion	Stand sideways to wall bars 1 metre away. Hold wall bar at hip height with inside arm 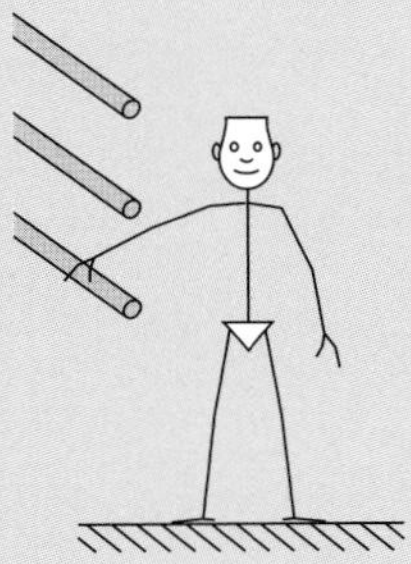	Take outside arm up over head to hold bar at head level. Push hips out to side and then in towards the wall bars 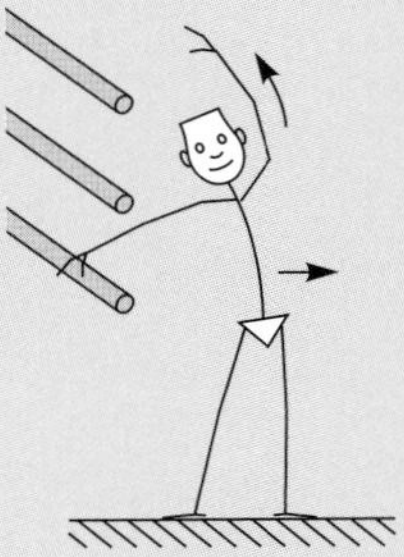
	Lie on side over gym ball at waist level. Rest forearm and lateral side of leg on floor 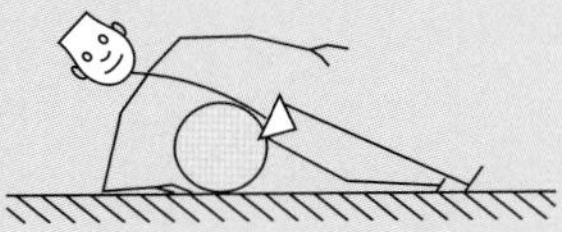	Push up on legs, straightening bottom leg. Stretch top arm over head. Touch floor with hand if possible 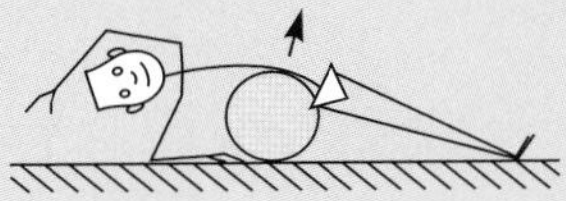
Thoracic rotation	Lie supine with knees bent 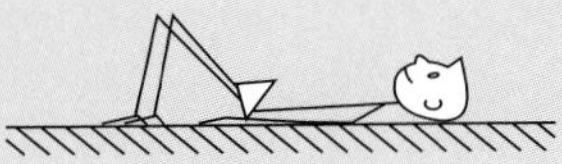	Roll knees together to each side. Take arms to opposite side. Look down arms 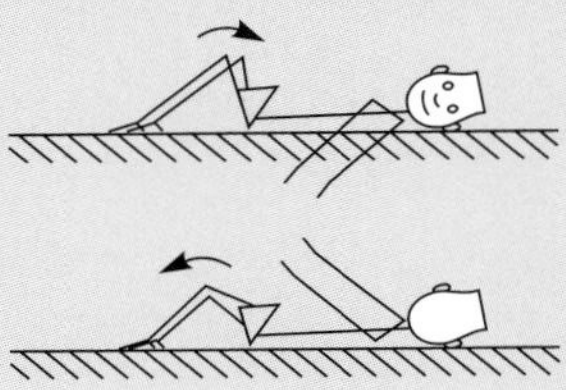

(Continued)

Table 21.4 Mr L's mobility exercises—cont'd

Movement	Starting position	Action
	Stand with back towards wall and a short distance from it. Have feet slightly apart and knees facing forwards and slightly bent 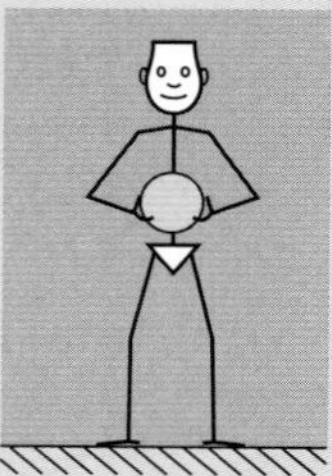	Twist to one side, attempting to touch wall with flat hands. Can twist using ball or partner. Turn head around to look at wall 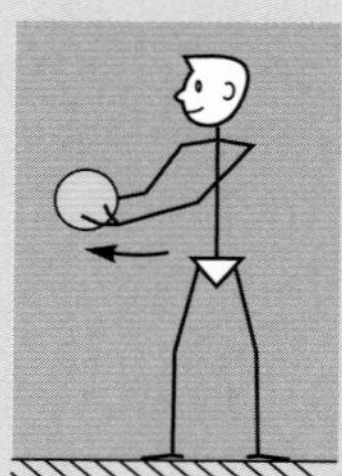
Thoracic extension	Stand with back to wall with arms by side 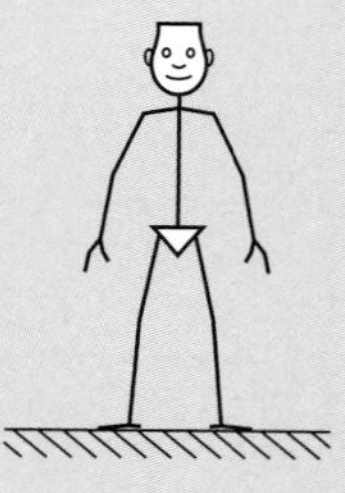	Lift arms up, keeping back of hands in contact with wall. Try to touch hands overhead 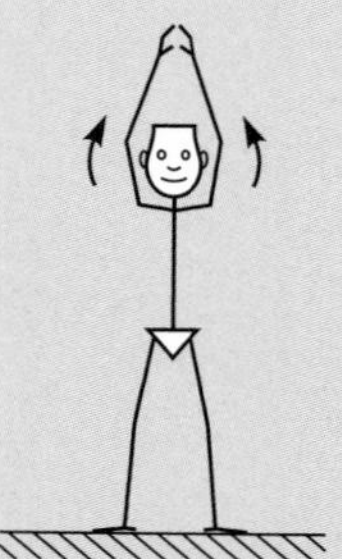
	Sit supported with back to wall and ball behind back. Knees bent and feet on floor 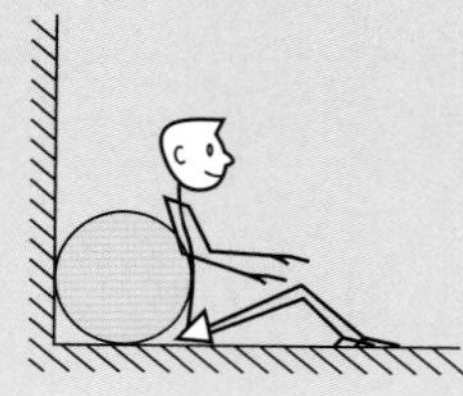	Stretch arms to touch wall with back of hands. Push thoracic spine into ball 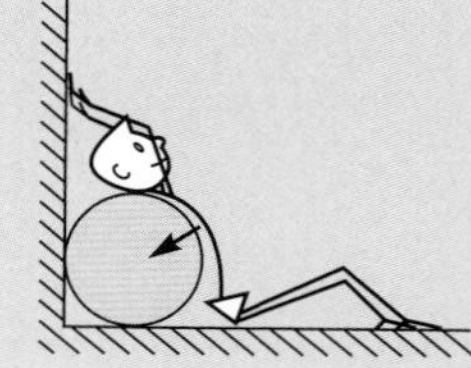

Table 21.5 Mr L's strengthening exercises: thoracic spine extensors

Starting position	Movement
Crook lie. Elbows by side. Shoulders and buttocks on floor 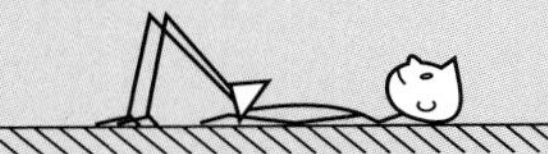	Push down on elbows. Arch thoracic spine. Keep pelvis on floor 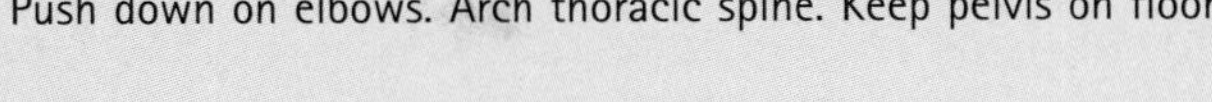 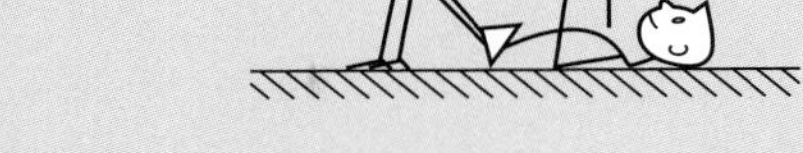
Lie prone, arms by side. Grasp stick in hands behind back 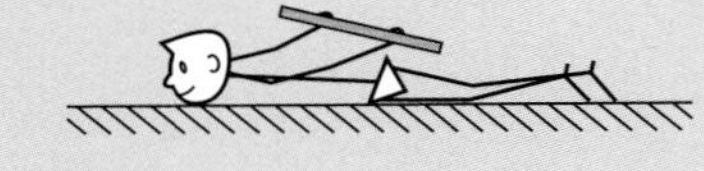	Raise stick behind back. Lift head and shoulders off floor a short distance, looking at floor 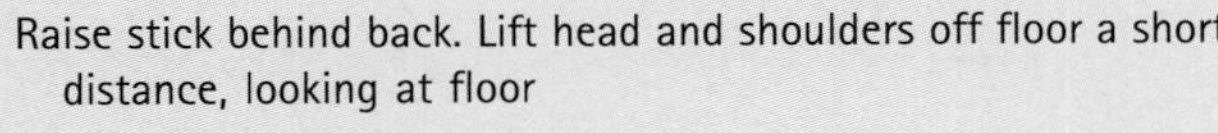 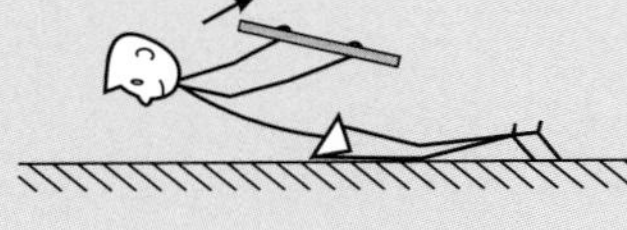
Lie prone. Hold gym ball out in front, elbows as straight as possible 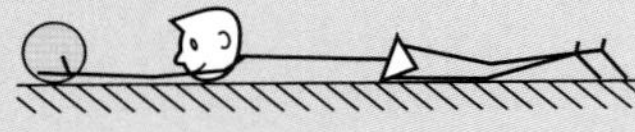	Raise ball off ground 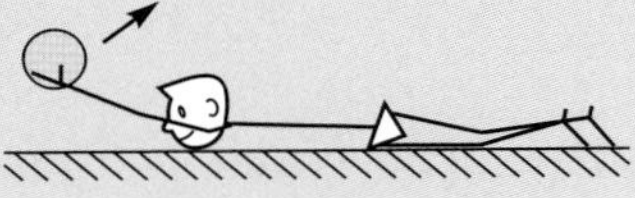

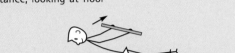

Table 21.6 Mr L's strengthening exercises: lumbar spine extensors/glutei

Starting position	Movement
Supine lie. Knees bent, feet flat on floor 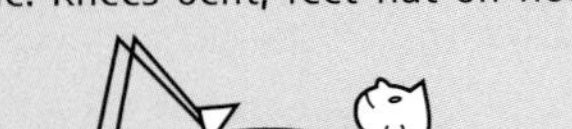	Lift buttocks high off floor (bridging). Move feet further from body and/or lift leg to make more difficult. Can bridge with feet on ball or chair with straight or bent knees 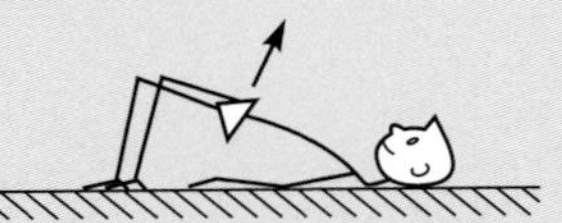
Four-point kneeling 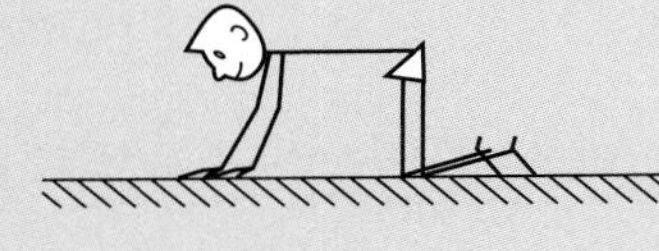	Lift opposite arm and leg at the same time. Keep arm and leg straight. Repeat other side 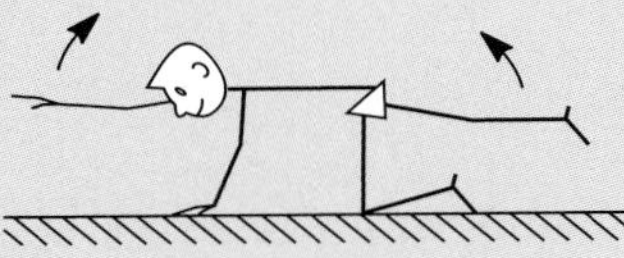
Lie prone 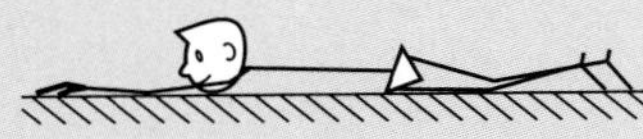	'Skydive position'. Lift head, with straight arms and legs, looking at floor 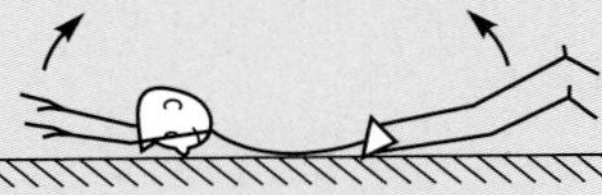

21

Table 21.7 Mr L's stretching exercises

Starting position	Movement
Neck rotators Sit straight in a chair with shoulders back 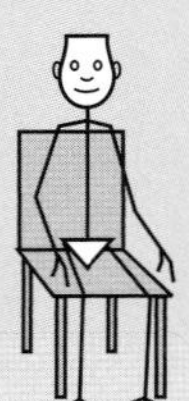	Turn head to right as far as possible. Place chin in palm of right hand with fingers spread along right cheek. Place left hand around back of head. Attempt to turn the head around to the left but resist the movement with the right hand. Relax and turn the head further to the right with both hands. Repeat three times 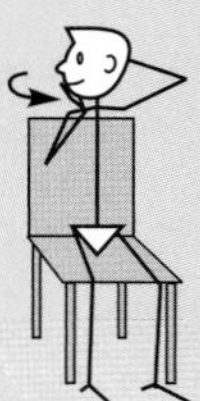
Neck side-flexors Same starting position as above 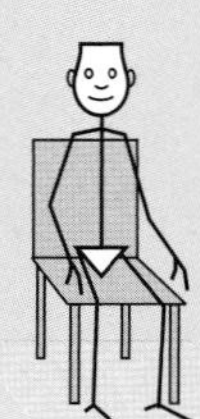	Take neck sideways to right as far as possible. Take right hand across top of head to rest above left ear. Push head up into the hand but do not allow any movement. Relax and stretch the neck side-flexors with the right hand further to the right. Repeat three times 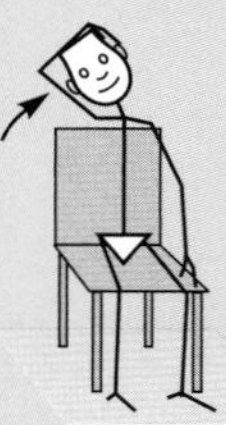
Hamstrings Place heel on chair seat with knees straight and foot dorsiflexed 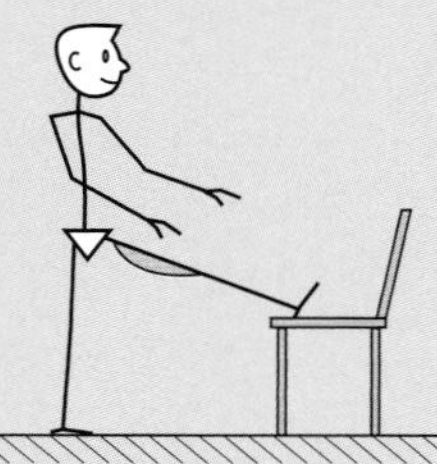	Stretch hamstring to maximum by reaching down leg. Push heel into seat, relax, then stretch hands down leg still further. Repeat three times 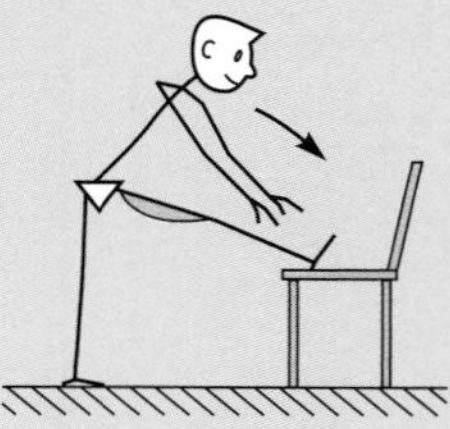
Hip adductors Sit on floor with soles of feet touching and knees out to side. The back may need to be supported. Rest forearms on inside of knees 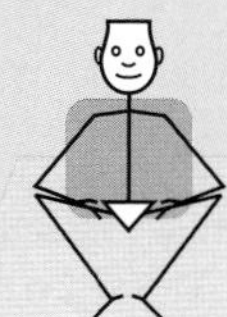	Pull knees towards each other but do not allow them to move by resisting the movement with the forearms. Relax the knees out to the side, then push knees further apart as far as possible. Repeat three times 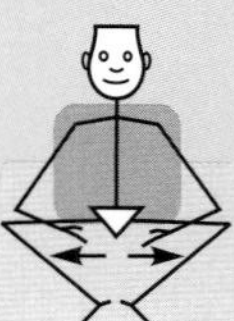

21

Table 21.7 Mr L's stretching exercises—cont'd

Starting position	Movement
Hip flexors/Quadriceps Stand straight, holding right ankle with right hand. Place other hand on wall for balance 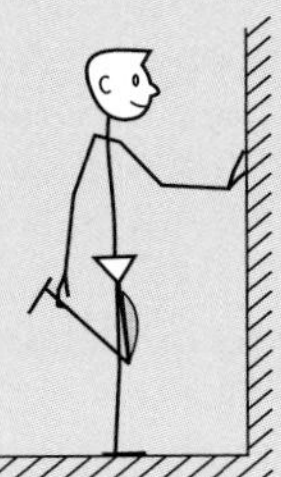	Take right knee back to maximum stretch. Without moving the hip or knee, attempt to pull the knee forward to wall. Then relax and stretch knee back further 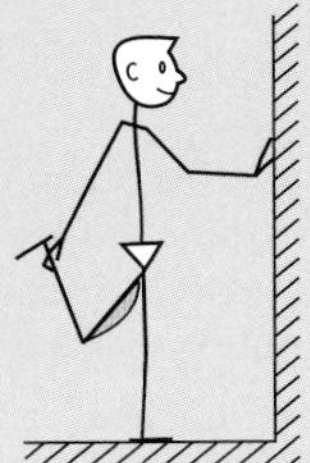
Calf muscles Stand facing wall with left foot a pace back from wall and right foot directly behind in stride stand. Keep right knee straight. Place hands flat on wall 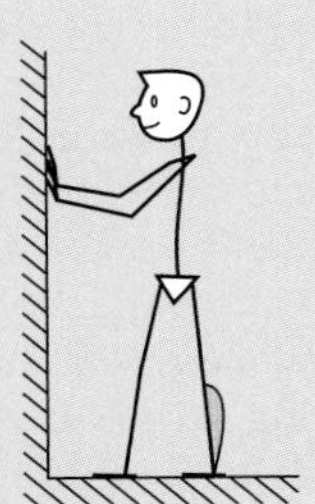	Slowly bend left knee with heels firmly on ground. When maximum stretch of calf muscles of right leg has been achieved, attempt to lift right heel off the ground but resist the movement. Relax and bend left knee further 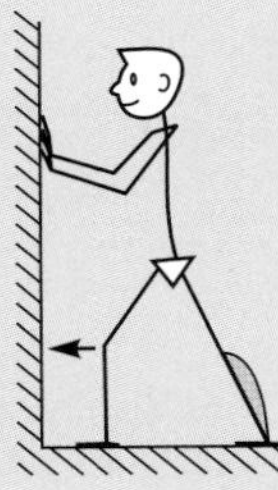

Cardiovascular fitness, stamina and muscle endurance

Physical fitness can be improved by cardiovascular exercise that increases muscle strength and endurance, as well as exercising the heart and lungs. This form of exercise can improve stamina and enables people to pursue their everyday activities with less effort.

Circuits in the gym should include a variety of strengthening and stretching exercises interspersed with low-impact cardiovascular exercises such as the rowing machine and static bike. High-impact activities such as jogging and step-ups can aggravate both the spinal and the weight-bearing joints. Low-impact cardiovascular activities, such as swimming, aquarobics, cycling and walking, increase stamina and muscle endurance with less joint aggravation. Cardiovascular exercise can also be undertaken in the hydrotherapy pool (see Hydrotherapy section). Contact sports such as rugby and football are best avoided, as any sudden impact can worsen joint problems.

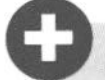

Clinical note

The use of goggles can prevent aggravating the neck while swimming (especially in breaststroke and crawl). Goggles also protect the eyes from chlorine, which can exacerbate uveitis. A snorkel can be used if the neck is very stiff. The use of a variety of swimming strokes prevents stress and fatigue in any one area.

With increased respiratory excursion, cardiovascular exercise helps to mobilise the thoracic joints and maintain or improve chest expansion and vital capacity. Regular cardiovascular exercise has other benefits, including control of bodyweight and protection from heart disease and diabetes. It also can improve sleep, relaxation and well-being.

Key point

Effective cardiovascular exercise should be performed 3–4 times a week and built up slowly. Any prolonged joint pain is an indication that the exercise has been too vigorous.

Hydrotherapy

Hydrotherapy is an effective way of treating AS. The warmth of water can relieve pain and muscle spasm and promote relaxation. Dry-land stretches are most effective directly after hydrotherapy. Buoyancy relieves pressure on the weight-bearing joints (Tinsley 1997), assists with movements that are difficult or painful on dry land and can also provide a resistance to be used in muscle strengthening. Most patients find hydrotherapy enjoyable and it can improve morale. Although hydrotherapy facilities are not always available, it may be possible for people with AS to attend 'disability' swims, where the temperature in the pool is raised to a higher level than usual, at local disabled or sports centres.

Key point

Hydrotherapy pools are expensive to build and maintain, so exercises should be devised to make the most of the properties of water and the time spent in the pool.

To enhance the effect of buoyancy, flotation can be used. Other properties of water such as turbulence, the drag effect and the metacentre effect can all be used to mobilise and stabilise joints and to strengthen muscles. The pool is also a good medium for cardiovascular exercises due to the reduced impact on weight-bearing joints.

The type and amount of exercise should be determined by the amount of pain that the person is experiencing. A patient in flare may find gentle stretching exercises and relaxation to be the most beneficial. Again, the physiotherapist should always be prepared to modify an exercise (see pp. 535–536).

Training

Sufficient specific training is essential before practising hydrotherapy. A good knowledge of the properties of water and precautions is required. It is advisable to attend a foundation course before working unsupervised. Refer to CSP paper 39 and standards 17 and 18 in The Service Standards of Physiotherapy Practice (2005), available free from the CSP.

EFFECTIVE PHYSIOTHERAPY FOR AS

General issues

Patients are more likely to perform an exercise effectively if it is clearly demonstrated, its rationale is explained, and they have the opportunity to carry out the exercise in a safe environment (for example, under the supervision of a physiotherapist). The last of these is known as mastery experience and is the main way of enhancing individuals' self-efficacy (confidence) (Bandura 1977) in their own ability to carry out a behaviour that will lead to desired outcomes. Intentions to perform behaviours such as exercises are influenced by beliefs about their consequences (Duran and Trafimow 2000). Observing the person with constant attention to detail ensures accuracy and optimum patient effort. If targets are set, enquire about the results. Be aware of the individual's capabilities and give praise and encouragement appropriately. As exercise adherence is more likely if the patient has been part of the goal setting process, offer choice wherever possible. For example, the patient could decide whether to exercise in the morning or evening, or whether to do 5 or 6 or 7 repeats. In a group setting, certain exercises may have to be adapted for the stiffer patients in order to ensure full participation. By using a variety of different equipment (e.g. gymnastic balls and sticks), exercise can be made more interesting for the patient and there is no limit to the variety of new exercises that can be created. In the hospital setting, a mixture of both gym and hydrotherapy can be used, according to availability.

The physiotherapist should consider:

- What the exercise is achieving.
- How to make the exercise harder.
- How to adapt the exercise for the stiffer patient.
- How to avoid trick movements.
- How to fixate in order to achieve a more specific movement.
- The patient's confidence levels and their safety.

Partnered exercises can be fun and effective, as long as both people are exercising simultaneously. They could be done at home with a family member; thus training for the family member is important.

If you are involved in regular exercise sessions, record the muscle groups that were exercised to make sure that important mobility, strengthening or stretching exercises are not omitted. Poor performance by an individual should also be documented. See Table 21.3 for an example of a typical record.

Self-management in AS and the role of the physiotherapist

Home programmes

AS is a chronic, potentially disabling condition that patients can learn to manage for themselves. NHS resources are not limitless and people often want to take control of their own lives, rather than be ruled by their illness and disability. Therefore, the majority of AS disease management will be controlled by the patient and undertaken at home, local sports clubs and so on.

A home programme of exercises and posture awareness should be devised to be specific to the needs and the abilities of the patient and to suit that person's lifestyle and home environment. Realistic goals should be agreed between the physiotherapist and the patient to take into account fatigue and personal circumstances. Memory aids, such as an exercise DVD, exercise sheets and a radio cassette, are available from NASS. If appropriate, family members could be encouraged to familiarise themselves with the exercises by participating in the exercise classes.

To improve compliance, the exercise routine should be slotted into the most convenient time of the day, depending on the patient's schedule and when the patient is the most relaxed and mobile. Exercise can also be integrated into the daily activities: for example, reaching up to cupboards and twisting around in a static chair to a waste paper bin behind.

Patients should check posture (see home checks, p. 537), and stretch out the spine and hip flexors on a regular basis. This can be achieved by lying supine on a bed with minimal pillows under the head, the knees bent off the edge of the bed and feet dangling towards the floor.

Education

The physiotherapist should provide advice on the disease, fatigue, pain relief, footwear, postural issues (e.g. chairs, beds, sleeping, driving, etc.) and recommended sports and activities. Literature and memory aids should be provided to patients wherever possible. Guidebooks can be obtained from NASS free of charge. When a person becomes a member of NASS, further support and advice can be offered through direct communication with the organisation and from their twice-yearly newsletter. Encourage the patient to attend regular exercise sessions, by becoming a member of the local NASS group, to partake in daytime hospital sessions or intensive residential educational programmes (held at certain specialist centres) and to attend their local leisure centre.

Key point

People who take an active interest in their condition can positively influence its outcome.

PSYCHOSOCIAL EFFECTS

Like other chronic diseases, patients may have to go through several stages before they can accept that their recovery is in their own hands and then start to do something about it. Emotions may include grief, fear, denial, anger and depression. Giving up work, a hobby that they enjoy or social activities, may feel like bereavement. After diagnosis, they may change from someone who feels that they are in control of their destiny to someone with a feeling of loss of control over their life. Coping with these emotions consumes energy and any of these emotions can come back to haunt the patient at any time.

Barriers to exercise

Barlow (1998) conducted three focus groups with AS patients and found that the main barriers cited were pain, fatigue, boredom, time pressures, lack of education regarding 'safe' exercises, lack of support from family and friends, lack of space/facilities, and the stigma experienced when exercising in group settings. Solutions generated by the groups included varying exercise regimes, exercising in groups with similar others, support from family and friends, time management, pain management, establishing exercise as a feature of daily life and increasing confidence that exercise is a safe activity for each individual. Other barriers to exercise include lack of short-term gain, poor body image, lack of knowledge, aversion to exercise and denial.

For patients new to an exercise regimen, it is important to explain that exercise may increase pain levels or they may not want to pursue it. Conversely, those patients with mild pain may need to be more motivated to exercise.

Santos et al. (1998) found that, with regard to AS, adherence to a regular exercise regimen is associated with rheumatologist follow-up, belief in the benefits of exercise, and a higher education level. Santos et al. maintain that those who are less educated and are followed by GPs should be targeted for additional support. Consistency of exercise, rather than quantity, is of most importance. On the whole, compliance with exercise is improved when people with AS find that their pain is eased by active exercises and they can reduce their medication.

Disease duration need not be a barrier to exercise, since Viitanen et al. (1995) concluded that it was possible by means of an intensive rehabilitation course to prevent, for over 1 year, the deterioration of spinal function and fitness in AS patients irrespective of their disease duration.

Fatigue

Persistent fatigue is now accepted as a common symptom of AS, and it is in many ways more debilitating than the pain itself. Fatigue can be all consuming with an enduring sensation of general tiredness and exhaustion. It is considered such an important domain that it is included in the BASDAI along with axial pain, peripheral pain, enthesopathy pain and stiffness.

Fatigue can be the consequence of pain, anaemia, disturbed sleep, poor posture, stress and chemicals released in the body during the inflammatory process. It can affect concentration and increase irritability and frustration, which can impact on relationships and cause anxiety and depression (Barlow 1994).

Management of this fatigue is still something of an enigma (Jones et al. 1996a).

First attempts at exercise may worsen the fatigue. However, an increase in general, aerobic and leisure time activities (e.g. swimming and cycling), has been associated with lower levels of fatigue and an improvement in the mental health of AS patients (Da Costa et al. 2004).

Such findings serve to highlight the importance of taking a global 'look' at patients' well-being including psychosocial factors.

The National Ankylosing Spondylitis Society (NASS)

NASS was founded in 1975 by a group of patients who were keen to attend regular exercise sessions. The membership includes patients, their families and health professionals. NASS provides support, education and information in the management of social and medical aspects of the disease. It also funds research into AS. Currently, NASS has 105 local branches around Britain. Most of the branches meet on a weekly basis at a local hospital where hydrotherapy and gym work are normally on offer. Physiotherapists with a special interest in AS supervise the sessions. The day-to-day running of the branch is organised by a committee consisting of members.

Apart from ongoing education and exercise, the NASS group offers other advantages, such as improving morale and encouraging individuals to take control of their disease by providing support, understanding, encouragement, motivation and fun. The groups are cost-effective, in terms of both time and money, for the hospital, patient and physiotherapists. NASS self-help group members appear to comply more with exercise treatment and also receive a valuable source of social support from fellow members.

See also the section of useful links towards the end of the chapter.

21

CASE STUDY ANKYLOSING SPONDYLITIS

Subjective assessment

Mr L is a non-complaining 22-year-old software designer who spends most of his working day sitting at a desk and most evenings slouching on the sofa. He still lives with his parents. He does not particularly enjoy exercise but enjoys watching sport on TV. He has no specific hobbies but enjoys going out to the cinema and socialising.

He had experienced intermittent low-grade unilateral buttock pain since he was 15. He was occasionally off games at school and although he had seen his GP at the time, his symptoms were put down to 'growing pains'. More recently, pain had developed in the mid-thoracic spine and around the costosternal joints. It was beginning to limit his breathing and made it painful for him to turn in bed at night. His back was stiff in the morning for about 1 h and eased off as the day progressed. He admitted to having an old soft mattress and sleeping curled up on his side. He also had pain under the heel of his right foot and this was making it difficult for him to walk. He was concerned about feeling exhausted most of the time, as this was affecting his social life. His mother had recently dragged him along to his GP as she was concerned that the chest pains might herald heart problems and also worried that her son was spiralling into depression. The GP found that his ECG was normal and referred him to a rheumatologist who made a diagnosis of AS following a detailed history and an X-ray of the sacroiliac joints which revealed sacroiliits. He was also found to be HLA B27 positive but there was no known family history of the disease. He was started immediately on the maximum dose of a NSAID and an analgesic. He was then referred to physiotherapy for assessment, advice and exercises.

Although better, when measured using a 10 cm VAS, his pain levels were found to be moderate at 5 and 4 out of 10, respectively. An enthesitis index to measure enthesitis pain was not used in this case, as the physiotherapist was not familiar with its use but the thoracic, chest and plantar fasciitis entheseal pain was marked on a body chart and given a score of 2, when 1 is the least pain and 4 is the worst pain.

He completed an Ankylosing Spondylitis Quality of Life Questionnaire (ASQOL), which gave a score of 10 (out of a maximum of 18), indicating that the AS was having a moderate impact on his quality of life.

Objective assessment

Mr L's posture was very poor in both standing, walking and sitting. However, most of this could be corrected and apart from a decreased lumbar flexion (Schober's) of 4 cm, his neck, lumbar side-flexion and hip abduction were within normal limits. His height was recorded and as he was experiencing thoracic and referred chest pain, his chest expansion was also measured and this was found to be reduced. The overall BASMI score put him in the mild category. However, both his BASFI and BASDAI scores were moderate at 3.8 and 4.4, respectively, indicating that his disease was fairly active and that he was having difficulties performing normal activities of daily living.

Aims of treatment

- Decrease pain, fatigue and depression.
- Improve posture.

Motivate him to exercise in order to:

- Increase extensor muscle strength.
- Increase mobility of spinal joints especially in the thoracic region.
- Increase and maintain length of flexor muscle groups and calf muscles.
- Increase cardiovascular fitness.
- Keep him in employment.

Treatment

In order to motivate him, he was immediately enrolled in a 1-week-long intensive daytime course of gym exercises and hydrotherapy at the hospital (for examples of hydrotherapy exercises, see below). The classes also included open discussion sessions on the pathology of AS and a variety of related subjects including medication, the benefits of exercise and ergonomics.

Following the detailed assessment, he was given a home program of exercises and stretches (see Tables 21.4–21.7) that were specific to his needs and he was encouraged to take up a form of exercise that he really enjoyed. He chose swimming and joined his local leisure centre. He was told that he would be reassessed in 6 months time unless he wanted to be seen earlier. He was also encouraged to attend the evening NASS class as soon as the course had finished.

He was referred to an orthotist for full length foot orthoses to be put in his shoes to ease the plantar fasciitis.

He was advised to move around at work and not to sit still in one position for too long. An appointment was made with the local Disability Employment advisor (DEA) for a full ergonomic assessment of his workplace. Meanwhile, he was advised to change his mattress for a more supportive one and to try to sleep on his back with minimal pillows under his head. If he did wake in the night with pain, he was advised to get out of bed and to move around and to take analgesics or use some form of heat if necessary.

After 6 months, he was able to stop his daytime NSAID dose. This motivated him to exercise still further and he increased his swimming to 3 times a week and started cycling to work. All of his outcome measurements showed significant improvement.

Hydrotherapy

As with any exercise programme, it is advisable to start the hydrotherapy session with a warm-up and to finish with a stretch and cool-down. In order to achieve maximum effort, exercises can be carried out using a variety of starting positions and flotation devices. The exercise should be repeated at least 5 times.

The following are a few examples of exercises that can be done. It is by no means a comprehensive list.

Warm-up

Keep the neck and shoulders under water as much as possible by standing in the correct depth of water. If necessary, bend the knees and hips. Faster movement causes more turbulence and therefore produces greater resistance. Count aloud and perform the activity at least 10 times to increase the CV content and respiratory exertion.

1. Walk with big strides forwards, backwards or sideways around the edge of the pool. Exaggerate the arm swing and trunk movements. Change direction quickly into the turbulence created.
2. Clasp the hands together under the water straight out in front and quickly swish the arms as far round as possible to right and left.
3. Bend the right knee and reach down to the outside of the right heel with the right hand. Repeat to other side.
4. Hop, touching the right elbow with the bent left knee. Repeat using the opposite legs and arms.
5. Jump, punching the right arm forwards and the left leg backwards. Repeat to the other side.

Mobilising

Lumbar and thoracic spine flexion and extension

Hold the rail with both hands straight out in front and the elbows extended. Stand two paces back facing the pool rail and with the buttocks back as far as possible. The feet should be slightly apart.

1. Push the hips forwards towards the wall (into extension) and then back out to the starting position. Keep the elbows and knees straight.
2. Using the same starting position as above, bring one foot up towards the wall with an extended knee. Leading with the heel and keeping the knee straight, take the heel backwards as high as possible. Repeat using the other leg.

Thoracic and cervical spine rotation

1. Use the same starting position as above but with legs astride. Bend the left elbow and twist to the left reaching under the elbow with the right arm. Repeat to the other side.
2. Face the wall and rest the arms on the bar. Bend the knees to 90 degrees and keep the trunk, pelvis and thighs flat against the wall. Keep the knees together. Fix the shoulders by holding on to the pool rail with the hands and forearms. Swing both knees up to the right as far as possible until the outside of the left thigh is flat on the wall. Repeat to the other side.

Strengthening exercises: supine with hands holding the rail

Make sure that the neck is supported in a neck float and push the occiput into the water during the exercise. Place a hip-float tightly around the hips or position a woggle under the buttocks to keep them elevated. Hold the rail to fix the trunk but not so tight that the shoulders and neck are aggravated.

Spinal and hip extensors/quadraceps

With straight knees, take both heels down towards the bottom of the pool (hip and lumbar spine extension).

A float can be used around the ankle to increase buoyancy.

Lumbar side-flexors

Swing the legs as far as possible to each side, side-bending at the waist and keeping knees straight and the pelvis in neutral.

Thoracic rotators

Bend the knees to 90 degrees, put a float under the soles of the feet and keep the hips in neutral. Keep the knees just under the surface of the water, while swinging the feet up towards the surface of the water to each side.

Hip abductors

Float in side lie using both waist and neck floats. Hold onto the bars with both hands. Put a small float around the ankle of the lower leg and take this leg down towards the bottom of the pool.

Strengthening exercises: supine with feet tucked under the rail

Float supine with the neck and pelvis supported in floats. Keep the backs of hands in the water.

Shoulder abductors, adductors and flexors

Take straight arms out from the sides of the body to above the head, keeping the backs of hands in the water. Then bring the arms back quickly to the sides.

Thoracic and shoulder extensors

Take the arms out to 90 degrees from the body, keeping the elbows straight. Hold bats in both hands and take the backs of hands down towards the bottom of the pool.

Strengthening exercise: prone

Abdominals

Put a float around the feet and hold the rail with both hands. Stretch both legs straight out behind, allowing the float to bring the feet up to the surface of the water. Push the feet down in the float to contract the abdominal muscles and then relax.

Fun and games

Take care to match patients equally and ensure safety in the pool at all times.

1. Race each other across pool forwards, backwards and sideways.
2. Two opponents face each other prone with a ring or a woggle held at arms length between them. Using any swimming kick, the winner is the person who pushes the ring over to the partner's side.
3. As a race, pass a large ring over the body starting at either the head or the feet.
4. Sit with a woggle between the legs. Use legs in a cycling action to race across the pool.

Stretching exercises

Key points

Trunk and leg stretches are particularly effective in the hydrotherapy pool due to the relaxing effects of the warm water. The effects of buoyancy ensures a firm passive stretch. The amount of flotation should be adjusted for each patient by either adding or removing air from the float. Again, the contract-relax method can be used.

Hamstrings

Stand straight with back to the wall and arms resting on the rail. Keeping the knees straight, put a float behind the ankle. Allow the leg to float up towards the surface of the water to maximum stretch. To add stretch for the calf muscles, dorsiflex the ankle.

Push the heel down into the float a short distance, relax and allow the float to take the heel back up to the surface of the water. Reach down the leg with the hands for a greater stretch. Repeat to the other side.

Hip adductors

Start as for the hamstring exercise above. Take the right leg out to the side with toes pointing forwards. Put a float around the right ankle and allow a full passive stretch. Stay in an upright position.

Push down the right leg into the float a short distance, relax and allow the float to take the leg up further into abduction.

Quadriceps

Stand facing the wall and hold on to the rail. Keep the left leg straight and touching the wall. Bend the right knee, put a float around the right ankle and keep the right thigh against the wall.

Push the foot down into the float, relax and allow the float to take the foot up behind still further. The right knee may come away from the wall a short distance but avoid leaning forward.

Pectorals and abdominals

Lean backwards against the wall with the hips flexed and feet 1 metre away from the wall. Take the arms overhead to hold the rail.

Arch the back and lift the sternum to take the back away from the wall. A float can be placed behind the back at scapula level.

Trunk rotators

Face the wall with hips bent at 90 degrees and feet apart and away from the wall. Have the right arm out straight, holding onto the rail. Hold a float with the left hand.

Twist the trunk and head by taking the float under the right elbow. At the position of maximum stretch, press the float down into the water a short distance, relax and allow the float to take the hand further up to the surface of the water.

Cooling down

Finish the session with a cool-down. Stand with the back to the wall, the knees bent and the neck under water. Allow the arms to float up to the surface of the water to encourage relaxation of the shoulders. Do some gentle neck and breathing exercises. Relaxation while totally supported with floats is very enjoyable.

HOME CHECKS

With regard to exercises, patients can record their own measurements at home. On each occasion, the patient should try to improve on the last attempt. This section contains some examples of how this might be achieved.

Fingertips-to-floor

This gives a composite measurement of lumbar and hip flexion and hamstring length. The patient grips a long ruler vertically between the feet and bends forwards, running the fingers down the ruler, keeping the knees straight. The distance from the fingertips to the floor is recorded.

Posture check

The patient stands straight with the feet back against a wall and the chin tucked in to keep a book (minimum thickness) in place between occiput and wall. Ensure that the same thickness of book can be held in place on each occasion. Height can be measured in this position.

Thoracic and neck rotation

The patient is seated with their buttocks pushed firmly into the back of the chair which is in a fixed position. They then turn trunk and head around as far as possible. The eye nearest to the wall is closed and at the point where the tip of the nose appears to meet the wall, a point is marked on the wall.

Lumbar side-flexion

The patient is seated with their buttocks pushed firmly into the back of the chair and runs the fingertips of one hand down the back leg of the chair. This is repeated to the other side. A piece of blue tack can be put on the chair leg to mark how far they are able to reach.

CONCLUSION

The quality of life of AS patients can be determined by their understanding of the condition and how much exercise they are prepared to undertake in their lifetime. As physiotherapists, we play a crucial role in their journey and should not take our responsibilities lightly.

USEFUL LINKS

National Ankylosing Spondylitis Society (NASS)
Unit 0.2, One Victoria Villas, Richmond, Surrey TW9 2GW
Tel: 020 8948 9117
E-mail:nass@nass.co.uk
Web:www.nass.co.uk

Arthritis Care
18–20 Stephenson Way, London NW1 2HD
Tel: 080 8800 4050
Web:www.arthritiscare.org.uk

Arthritis Research Campaign (ARC)
Copeman House, St Mary's Court, St Mary's Gate, Chesterfield, Derbyshire S41 7TD
Tel: 0870 850 5000
Web:www.arc.org.uk

Hydrotherapy Association of Chartered Physiotherapists (HACP)
Web:www.csp.org.uk/membergroups/clinicalinterestgroups

Website for Physiotherapists with a special interest in AS
Web:www.astretch.co.uk

National Association for Colitis and Crohn's Disease (NACC)
4 Beaumont House, Sutton Road, St Albans, Herts AL1 5HH
Tel: 0845 1302233
Web:www.nacc.org.uk

Psoriasis Association
Dick Coles house 2, Queensbridge, Northampton, Northants NN4 7BF
Tel: 08456 760076
Web:www.psoriasis-association.org.uk

FURTHER READING

Calin A 1991 Ankylosing spondylitis and other inflammatory disorders of the spine. In: Schlapbach P, Gerber N (eds) Physiotherapy: Controlled Trials and Facts. Karger: Bern

David C, Lloyd J 1999 Rheumatological Physiotherapy. Mosby: London

Haywood K 2000 Health outcomes in ankylosing spondylitis: an evaluation of patient-based and anthropometric measures. DPhil thesis, University of York

NASS (online) A Positive Response to Ankylosing Spondylitis: the Guidebook for Patients. The Bath Indices. Outcome Measures for Use with Ankylosing Spondylitis Patients. Download both from: www.nass.co.uk

Russell A 1998 Ankylosing spondylitis: history. In: Klippel J, Dieppe P (eds) Rheumatology Mosby: London, pp. 1–2 vol. 1, 2nd edn.

21

REFERENCES

Band D, Jones S, Kennedy G et al. 1997 Which patients with ankylosing spondylitis derive most benefit from an inpatient management programme? J Rheumatol 24: 2381–2384

Bandura A. (1977). Self efficacy: Toward a unifying theory of behavioral change. Psychological Review 84: 191–215

Barlow J 1994 Fatigue in ankylosing spondylitis: a personal perspective. NASS Newsletter autumn/winter: 5–8

Barlow JH 1998 Understanding exercise in the context of chronic disease: an exploratory investigation of self-efficacy. Percept Mot Skills 87(2): 439–446

Beaulieu JG 1981 Developing a stretching program. Phys Sports Med 9(11): 59–69

Bellamy N, Kaloni S, Pope J et al. 1998 Quantitative rheumatology: a survey of outcome measurement procedures in routine rheumatology outpatient practice in Canada. J Rheumatol 25(5): 852–858

Bellamy N, Muirden K, Brooks P et al. 1999 A survey of outcome measurement procedures in routine rheumatology outpatient practice in Australia. J Rheumatol 26(7): 1593–1599

Bulstrode SJ, Barefoot J, Harrison R, Clarke A 1987 The role of passive stretching in the treatment of ankylosing spondylitis. Br J Rheumatol 26: 40–42

Calin A 1994 Can we define the outcome of ankylosing spondylitis and the effect of physiotherapy management? J Rheumatol 21(2): 184–185

Calin A, Garrett S, Whitelock H et al. 1994 A new approach to defining functional ability in ankylosing spondylitis: the development of the Bath Ankylosing Spondylitis Functional Index. J Rheumatol 21(12): 2281–2285

Cooper R, Freemont A, Fitzmaurice R et al. 1991 Paraspinal muscle fibrosis: a specific pathological component in ankylosing spondylitis. Ann Rheum Dis 50(11): 755–759

Da Costa D, Dritsa M, Ring A, Fitzcharles M-A 2004 Mental health status and leisure-time physical activity contribute to fatigue intensity in patients with spondyloarthropathy. Arthritis Rheum 51(6): 1004–1008

Davis JC, van der Heijde DM, Dougados M et al. 2005 Baseline factors that influence ASAS 20 response in patients with ankylosing spondylitis treated with etanercept. J Rheumatol 32(9): 1751–1754

Dougados M, Gueguen A, Nakache J et al. 1988 Evaluation of functional index and an articular index in ankylosing spondylitis. Br J Rheumatol 15(2): 302–307

Duran A, Trafimow D 2000 Cognitive organization of favorable and unfavorable beliefs about performing a behavior. J Soc Psychol 140(2): 179–187

Eriendsson J 1998 Car Driving with Ankylosing Spondylitis. Publication available from the National Ankylosing Spondylitis Society

Garrett S, Jenkinson T, Kennedy LG et al. 1994 A new approach to defining disease status in ankylosing spondylitis: the Bath Ankylosing Spondylitis Disease Activity Index. J Rheumatol 21(12): 2286–2291

Health & Safety Executive 1994 A pain in your work place? Ergonomic problems and solutions. HSE: London

Heuft-Dorenbosch L, Spoorenberg A, van Tubergen A et al. 2003 Assessment of enthesitis in ankylosing spondylitis. Ann rheum Dis 62(2): 127–132

Hidding A, van der Linden S, Boers M et al. 1993 Is group physical therapy superior to individualised therapy in ankylosing spondylitis? A randomised controlled trial. Arthr Care Res 6(3): 117–125

Jenkinson T, Mallorie H et al. 1994 Defining spinal mobility in ankylosing spondylitis: the Bath Metrology Index. J Rheumatol 21(9): 1694–1698

Jones SD, Koh WH, Steiner A et al. 1996a Fatigue in ankylosing spondylitis: its prevalence and relationship to disease activity, sleep, and other factors. J Rheumatol 23(3): 487–490

Jones SD, Steiner A, Garrett SL, Calin A 1996b The Bath Ankylosing Spondylitis Patient Global Score (BAS-G). Br J Rheumatol 35(1): 66–71

Lubrano E, Helliwell P 1999 Deterioration in anthropometric measures over six years in patients with ankylosing spondylitis. Physiotherapy 85(3): 138–143

Macrae I, Wright V 1969 Measurement of back movement. Ann Rheum Dis 28: 584–589

O'Driscoll S, Jayson M, Baddeley H 1978 Neck movements in ankylosing spondylitis and their response to physiotherapy. Ann Rheum Dis 37: 64–66

Pile K, Laurent M, Salmond C et al. 1991 Clinical assessment of ankylosing spondylitis: a study of observer variation in spinal measurements. Br J Rheumatol 30(1): 29–34

Reynolds S, Doward L, Spoorenberg A et al. 1999 The development of the Ankylosing Spondylitis Quality of Life questionnaire. Qual Life Res 8(7): 651

Santos H, Brophy S, Calin A 1998 Exercise in ankylosing spondylitis: how much is optimum? J Rheumatol 25(11): 2156–2160

Tinsley M 1997 Rheumatic diseases. In: Campion MR (ed.) Hydrotherapy. Butterworth–Heinemann: Oxford, pp. 255–268

Tomlinson M, Barefoot J, Dixon A 1986 Intensive inpatient physiotherapy courses improve movement and posture in ankylosing spondylitis. Physiotherapy 72(5): 238–240

van der Heijde D, van der Linden S, Bellamy N et al. 1999 Which domains should be included in a core set for endpoints in ankylosing spondylitis? Introduction to the ankylosing spondylitis module of OMERACT IV. JRheumatol 26(4): 945–947

Viitanen JV, Lehtinen K, Suni J, Kautiainen H 1995 Fifteen months' follow-up of intensive inpatient physiotherapy and exercise in ankylosing spondylitis. Clin Rheumatol 14(4): 413–419

Zigmond A, Snaith R 1983 The hospital anxiety and depression scale. Acta Psych Scand 67: 361–370

Chapter 22

The research process

Lynne Goodacre

CHAPTER CONTENTS

INTRODUCTION

The word 'research' is prone to cause anxiety and panic in students approaching their dissertation. But if you think about it, we all undertake research every day. You probably undertook research when deciding which textbook to buy for your course. You had a question in mind: 'Which book is the most suitable to help my studies?' You then set about the research process and, by asking colleagues, looking on the Internet, speaking to your lecturers or looking in the library, you came to your conclusion.

Physiotherapy students are usually required to undertake a research project or a critical evaluation of a research paper as part of their programme of undergraduate study. This chapter takes you through some of the aspects of the research process that students often find confusing.

Whilst there are different approaches to research, the research process comprises a sequence of steps designed to increase the sum of what is known about a certain phenomenon (Hockey 1996). The steps within the process apply to all research, whether conducted by healthcare professionals in a clinical setting or by scientists in a laboratory. The aim of the chapter is to provide an overview of this systematic process with an emphasis on the completion of a research project appropriate for an undergraduate dissertation.

The chapter starts by focusing on the development of a research question and moves on to explore the relationship between the question asked, the methodological approach taken, and the specific methods used to collect data. It then describes how all of the stages in the process are brought together within the context of a research proposal.

> **Student's note**
>
> It is not within the scope of a single chapter to provide in-depth information about specific methods of data collection and data analysis. However, an introduction is provided to some of the main methods used in undergraduate research projects. To enable readers to access more detailed information, a further reading list is provided at the end of the chapter.

It is likely that you will be approaching your dissertation with preconceived ideas about what it means to 'do research' and about the distinctions between data that are expressed by numbers (quantitative) and data that are expressed by words (qualitative). You may already have opinions about which approach you wish to adopt in your own project, or perceive one methodological approach to be 'better' than another.

The approach taken in this chapter is to advocate that, at undergraduate level, it is important to develop an understanding of the relationship between the research question, the methodological approach and the methods used, and not to develop a blinkered view about the perceived supremacy of one approach over another. Research skills, like any clinical skill, are learnt and developed over time. The focus of learning at undergraduate level should be to develop an understanding of the strengths and weaknesses of different approaches and the way in which different methods produce different kinds of data. Therefore the real focus of your thinking should be on 'What is my research question?' and 'What is the best approach to answering this question?'

An undergraduate dissertation provides you with an opportunity to conduct a small study and to use one or two methods of data collection. It provides a platform from which research skills can be developed and built upon in a clinical setting.

> ***Key point***
>
> Research is not just the pursuit of academics within universities but should be viewed as a central component of clinical practice, whether related to the critical appraisal of evidence to inform practice or the conduct of a study to contribute to the evidence base of physiotherapy. *Best Research for Best Health* (DoH 2006) outlines the Department of Health's strategic approach to the development of a thriving research culture *within* the NHS.

DEVELOPING A RESEARCH QUESTION

Getting started

The first decision you are required to make relates to the area in which you wish to develop your project. This decision should be made as a result of careful consideration rather than last-minute panic. For most new researchers the identification of a research area and, more specifically, the development of a research question are the result of a process that can take several weeks of refinement. It is therefore unwise to leave this decision until a day or two before a supervisory meeting in which you are expected to have your research question defined.

The area chosen should be one that is personally stimulating and hopefully exciting, as you will be living with the chosen project for a considerable amount of time and it will be demanding in terms of time, intellect and energy. The research process is rarely smooth and your chosen topic should be of enough interest and importance to sustain you through times when your project may not be going well and your enthusiasm might be waning. Many factors can influence the choice of an area of research (Figure 22.1).

> ***Key point***
>
> Before undertaking a great deal of work on a proposal, it is important to discuss potential areas of research with your supervisor to ensure that he or she feels the chosen area to be relevant and one in which a project can be conducted and completed within the time and resources available.

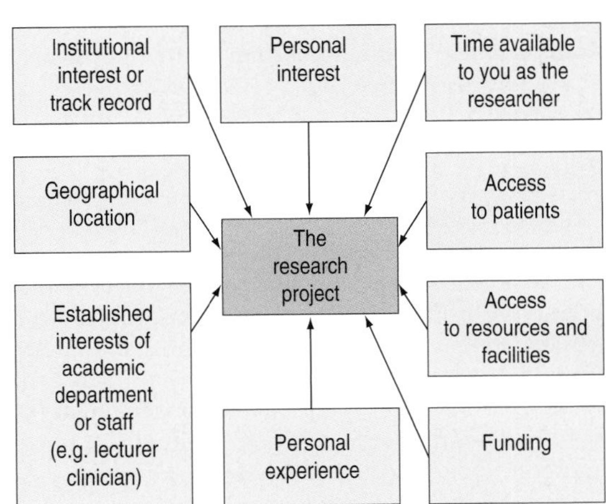

Figure 22.1 Factors that can influence the choice of area of research.

Having identified an area of research, the next stage is to develop a specific research question. Many students, when asked about the research they are undertaking, answer with a description of the area of research rather than a research question. Moving from a research area to a research question requires you to become focused in your thinking to enable you to state quite specifically what you are trying to address in your project.

To define your research question, it is helpful to undertake a broad review of the literature within your chosen topic. This means identifying, within current publications, the main research questions being addressed, different theoretical positions being adopted and the main arguments/positions being taken. Familiarising yourself with the literature in this way will also help you to identify key papers that are referenced or referred to consistently, the main methodological approaches being taken and the different methods being used.

Whilst you are reading, it will be helpful to start drawing up a list of potential research questions. At this stage do not worry too much about the specificity of the questions but write down all of the potential research questions that come to mind. When you feel you have developed a broad understanding of your chosen area you can then start to develop your research question by refining the general questions you have noted. It may be helpful to do this in conjunction with other students, as the process of verbalising and explaining your question helps to clarify your thinking. If you are unable to explain clearly and concisely, without going into lengthy descriptions, what you want to do, it is likely that you need to do more work on the question. Over time your list of potential questions should be refined and honed to identify what you feel may be two or three potential research questions. These can be used to inform discussion with your supervisor to identify a single research question that will become the focus of your investigation.

What makes a good research question?

As suggested, developing a research question is a process of becoming focused on the specific issue you are trying to address. Most new researchers need help and guidance with this process, as some questions are not amenable to research. This can be because the question posed relates to a philosophical or ethical issue, which can be debated extensively but not answered. Whilst it may be tempting to ask a complex question, success at undergraduate level is achieved by asking a very clear and straightforward question that is *answerable*.

As well as focusing on the question, it is also important to think about the amount of time and the kinds of resource that will be needed to complete the project. If, for example, you want to evaluate the impact of a specific intervention, do you have access to a clinical setting or participants? Are you being realistic in terms of the time required to complete the study and write up your dissertation? Trying to assess the amount of time taken to conduct a project is difficult if you have no previous research experience, but your supervisor will guide you on the feasibility of completing the project within the time available and the resources that you are able to access within your department.

THE METHODOLOGICAL APPROACH

Many students undertaking research for the first time want to move quickly on to learning about methods, to enable them to start data collection. Whilst it may be tempting to skip over the first few chapters in research textbooks, which usually contain what can seem to be complex philosophical debates about the nature of truth and different ways of gaining knowledge, don't! At undergraduate level it is important in your dissertation to demonstrate an understanding of the different methodological approaches and, more importantly, to be able to explain the link between your research question, the methodological approach you have taken and the methods you have used.

Methodology can be a difficult concept to understand, as it is used to describe a philosophical position being taken by a researcher. Methodological approaches are often presented as being founded upon a person's beliefs about the nature of truth and different ways of knowing and, in the past, this has led to researchers being described as either 'positivists' or 'naturalists'. Whilst some researchers always work within either a positivist or a naturalist paradigm, an increasing number of researchers within health contexts are using a mixed methods approach and combining both quantitative and qualitative approaches within the same study.

The positivist paradigm

A positivist paradigm is perhaps best understood by reflecting upon the kinds of philosophical assumption that underpin the scientific or experimental method. This approach is guided by the belief that knowledge can be gained by the measurement and quantification of a phenomenon in a way that can be replicated by an independent observer. Within this paradigm, research questions are usually framed as hypotheses. It focuses on the discovery of a single 'truth', which is generalisable and is achieved by breaking a phenomenon down into its constituent parts and understanding them and their relationships to each other. For this reason it is sometimes described as *reductionist* in approach. Central to this approach are the notions of objectivity and control, which lead to researchers being seen as detached from the research process and their influence being eliminated as far as is possible.

The naturalistic paradigm

Within this paradigm the approach to research is based on the belief that human experience is affected by the interpretation placed on it by individuals, and influenced by such things as previous experience and personal beliefs. The focus of research is therefore on describing or understanding the meanings people attach to these experiences and how they make sense of the social world.

Key point

Owing to the emphasis on how human experience is interpreted, it should be possible to see that, within naturalistic research, the notion of a single truth that is generalisable to a whole population is not relevant. There may be a number of realities or truths.

The notion of objective value-free research is contested strongly. In contrast to conducting research in a controlled environment, researchers emphasise the relevance of the wider social context, and research often takes place within this wider context rather than being removed from it. The notion of a detached researcher is also challenged. The researcher is seen as central to, not detached from, the research process; he or she seeks to become involved in the world of the participants, sometimes, in the case of observational studies, literally in order to gain as much insight as possible into the lived experiences of participants.

Given the different focus of positivist and naturalist methodologies it should seem logical that different methods are used within each paradigm to generate data. The term *method* is used to refer to data-generation techniques and procedures, the selection of data 'sources' and sampling (Mason 2002).

Mixed method approach

In recent years there has been an increasing use of a mixed methods approach in health research. In using this approach, research is designed to collect and analyse data derived from quantitative and qualitative approaches in a single study (Creswell and Plano Clarke 2007). Three approaches to mixing methods have been proposed:

- where the data converge and results from each approach are compared side by side
- where the data connect and one kind of data builds upon another
- where data are embedded and one kind of data is used in a supporting role for the other kind of data (Creswell and Plano Clarke 2007).

Student's note

The next section will familiarise you with some of the techniques of data collection used frequently in undergraduate dissertations. More in-depth information about these and other methods can be found in the references provided at the end of the chapter.

QUANTITATIVE RESEARCH

Hypothesis testing

It is usual for the research question in an experimental design to be expressed in terms of a *hypothesis*, described as 'a predicted answer to a research question' (Punch 2005), in which the predicted effect of the intervention to be tested is defined. A hypothesis may be worded as a general statement of an effect using words like 'influence' (a two-tailed hypothesis, as the influence may be either positive or negative), or it may be specific and indicate the direction of the effect using words like 'increase' or 'decrease' (a one-tailed hypothesis).

An alternative way of expressing a hypothesis is as a *null hypothesis*. This acknowledges an important philosophical premise that it is never possible to obtain absolute proof that a biological factor or a clinical intervention is having a significant effect in a given experiment. A null hypothesis embodies the notion that, strictly speaking, the results of an experiment can be interpreted only in terms of the likelihood that an intervention has *no* effect on the outcome under study. For example, if the effect of an intervention was being tested in a clinical situation, the null hypothesis would state that there would be no difference between the test group and the control group. The analysis of the data would enable the likelihood of this to be calculated, thereby providing an expression of the level of certainty with which the null hypothesis could be rejected.

Key point

In clinical research, most hypotheses are structured as null hypotheses, and the statistical methods used for data analysis are designed to test null hypotheses.

Experimental studies

Whilst different experimental designs exist, the focus of this section will be on the basic experimental design of a study comprising two groups, one of which (the *experimental* group) is exposed to an intervention and the other (the *control* group) which is not. The experiment is based on comparisons made between the groups and achieved by the collection of data prior to the intervention taking place (*pre-test*), which provides baseline data, and after the intervention has taken place (*post-test*), which provides data on differences in effect between the groups. The effect of an intervention is determined by comparisons of the data derived from the pre-test and post-test measurements and comparisons of data between the two groups.

Two fundamental aspects of an experimental design are randomisation and control.

Randomisation

Randomisation refers to the way in which participants are allocated to either the experimental or control group in order to create groups that are as similar as possible. This is necessary to ensure that the results of the experiment are attributable to the intervention rather than to some other variable such as age, disease duration or socioeconomic status.

There are many different methods of randomisation. Two methods used frequently in health research are the use of computer-generated numbers and stratification.

- *Computer-generated numbers* randomly allocate participants to either the treatment or control group on the basis of, for example, all odd numbers being allocated to the treatment group and all even numbers to the control group.
- In *stratification*, participants are divided into groups according to a baseline variable such as gender and then allocated from each group. A group stratified by gender would ensure that the experimental and control groups had equal numbers of men and women in them. This method is used to ensure that the groups are equally balanced in relation to variables that have been identified as having a potential impact on the results — such as gender, disease duration or age. Such a balance would not be achieved by using computer-generated numbers.

Controls

The concept of control has several applications. As has already been described, it can refer to a group of participants who do not receive an intervention. But there are other factors that a researcher may seek to control; these are known as confounding variables, as they have the potential to confound (confuse) the results. Here are some examples:

- *Variables relating to the therapist.* If the outcome measure used is an assessment of joint range of movement and several therapists take measurements, there could be variability in the measurements arising from the different ways in which the therapists assess range of movement. It would therefore be important to ensure that all the therapists are using the same approach to measurement, or that the same person collects all of the measurements.
- *Variables relating to treatment method.* If a research question focuses on the impact of a treatment and several different pieces of equipment are used to produce measurements, there could be variability in the measurements arising from the use of different equipment. It would therefore be important to make sure that all of the equipment is measuring with the same degree of accuracy and all departments taking part in the research are using the same equipment.
- *Variables relating to the environment.* If people recruited to a study are from different hospitals, one hospital may be in an area of social deprivation, it may have a higher proportion of people from different cultural groups, or the GPs may have different approaches to referring patients to the hospital. It would therefore be important to make sure that this is taken into account when people are allocated to experimental or control groups.

The creation of an environment in which all confounding variables can be controlled is extremely difficult in most clinical settings. It is important, however, for researchers to demonstrate that they have identified the potential confounding variables and taken steps to minimise their effects.

Measurement

As the aim of an experiment is to explore the effect of an intervention, a method of measuring the effect is required. The method used will be influenced by the variable being measured but may include assessment of range of movement, physiological measures such as cardiovascular output and respiration, or standardised questionnaires assessing pain, fatigue, activity limitation or psychological status. Whichever approach you use, it is important to think carefully about the accuracy of your system of measurement.

Before embarking upon the development of a new questionnaire it is sensible to check whether an existing questionnaire can be used. An immense amount of time and expertise is invested in the development of reliable and valid questionnaires and, once validated, they enable you to conduct more sophisticated statistical analysis than a questionnaire you have developed yourself for the purpose of your study.

In choosing a questionnaire it is important to understand the concepts of reliability, validity and responsiveness:

- *Reliability* is used to describe the consistency and reproducibility of a measure. Therefore, when it is used with the same group of people whose clinical condition is stable under the same experimental conditions, it should produce the same score. If different scores are obtained, this is an indication that the measure in not reliable.
- A *valid* measure is one that measures what it is supposed to measure.
- A *responsive* measure is one that has the ability to detect change when change has occurred or is present.

A word of caution is necessary about the reliability and validity of questionnaires published in journal articles. Not all questionnaires described in research papers have been tested for reliability and validity. Some questionnaires will have been developed by the researchers for their own study without them undertaking testing of the questionnaire; in critically appraising research papers, this is one of the factors you should be looking for. Just because someone has used a questionnaire and published results from it does *not* mean it is reliable and valid. In choosing a measure that has been psychometrically tested, you should be able to identify papers describing the process of development and how the items were identified as well ,as reporting on its reliability, validity and sensitivity.

A common reason given for not using existing measures is that they do not address all of the issues of relevance. However, it is permissible to ask additional questions alongside a standardised questionnaire, as long as you are clear about the limitations of the information you obtain from these questions and how the data can be treated in your analysis. You should not change the wording, ordering or method of scoring of a standardised questionnaire or omit questions; if you do so, you will change the psychometric properties of the questionnaire.

Surveys

In some studies there will be a need to develop your own questionnaire and the most likely situation is when you are undertaking a survey. Surveys can be used to describe certain phenomena (*descriptive surveys*) within a population of interest, or to investigate associations between variables (Bowling 2002). Information is collected from a sample of the population: for example, a sample of physiotherapists using a specific treatment modality in a specific area of clinical practice. Common methods of data collection are face-to-face or telephone interviews or self-complete questionnaires that may be posted to participants. Descriptive surveys usually involve the collection of data at a single point in time and are therefore 'cross-sectional' in nature. Analytical surveys analyse events at more than one point in time and can be used to explore the direction of cause and effect (Bowling 2002). Such surveys are therefore described as 'longitudinal'. Most longitudinal surveys are prospective, which means that data are collected as people progress through, for example, an illness trajectory, with surveys being completed 6 months, 1 year and 2 years after diagnosis.

Key point

The time and resource constraints of undergraduate projects dictate that the most likely survey method used will be descriptive.

Developing the questions

To ensure that a questionnaire remains focused on the research question, every question should have a purpose and use simple and unambiguous language. Questions used in questionnaires are either open or closed.

1. *Open questions* require respondents to provide their own answer and are a way of finding out about peoples' views or experiences. They are, however, more demanding for the person completing the questionnaire and this should be borne in mind, especially if they are being used in an environment where time may be short, or filled in by people who have, for example, poor grip or hand coordination or cognitive impairments.
2. *Closed questions* provide a predefined list of responses and ask the respondent to choose one — or in some instances, more than one — answer. They impose a structure for the respondents, who have to choose a response that best reflects their experiences.

The most common response options used in closed questions are:

- *dichotomous* — which enable a respondent to choose between two answers (e.g. yes/no)
- *multiple-choice* — which provide respondents with a number of options from which to select an answer (e.g. a Likert scale asks people to rate agreement with a statement, usually on a scale of 1 to 5).

Some questionnaires use a mixture of open and closed questions (for example, starting with a closed question and then asking the respondent to explain the answer).

Key point

Whichever form of questionnaire you choose, think carefully about the questions included and make sure that they are all focused on answering an aspect of your research question. It is usual to produce several drafts of a questionnaire before you think about piloting it.

Formatting your questionnaire

The appearance of a questionnaire is important, especially if it is being sent by post, as this is one of the factors that will influence a person's decision as to whether or not to complete it. If it is very long, uses a small font size, is full of spelling mistakes and muddled in appearance, people will be deterred from filling it in! The tools available on modern word-processing packages should enable you to produce a professional layout and print quality.

Once you feel you have produced a questionnaire that addresses the key issues, seek the opinions of your supervisor and (if possible) other people who have knowledge of your research area.

Piloting your questionnaire

Piloting a questionnaire involves more than asking a couple of people to complete the questionnaire and looking at the answers they have written. A structured approach is needed, which requires forethought and preparation. It is usual to adopt a semi-structured interview approach to the discussion, starting with an explanation of what you are trying to achieve, to encourage participants to give you constructive feedback. The issues to explore include:

- clarity of the instructions
- clarity and understanding of the questions
- identification of questions that may be left consistently unanswered or about which respondents ask for advice before answering
- respondents' views on the content of the questionnaire (e.g. whether anything has been omitted, views on the length and time taken to complete, whether enough response categories have been provided).

Feedback from these discussions can then be used to inform a revision of the questionnaire.

22

Methods of questionnaire administration

The three common methods of administering questionnaires are by post, face-to-face and over the phone. The method of administration will be influenced by issues such as the geographical area within which participants live, access to participants, and your time and resources.

If, for example, you want to obtain data from a patient group who meet on a regular basis in your local area, it may be feasible to attend the group and administer the questionnaire face-to-face. If you are trying to elicit the views of a group of therapists and recruiting them via a national database, a postal or phone-based method of administration would be more appropriate.

Preparing questionnaire data for analysis

The first step in analysing questionnaire data is the allocation of numeric values to answers or coding. If closed questions are used, it is possible to develop the coding framework whilst the questionnaire is being developed. Dichotomous questions may be coded with 1 being given to all 'yes' answers and 2 to all 'no' responses. In questions providing information about the respondents you may need to allocate more codes; for example, in asking about marital status 'single' is coded as 1, 'married' as 2, 'cohabiting' as 3 and so on. In scale questions a 1–5 code may be used where 1 is extremely satisfied, 2 is moderately satisfied and so on.

Key point

It is usual to analyse statistical data using a software package such as Statistical Package for the Social Sciences (SPSS) or Minitab. The coded data are entered into such a package in preparation for analysis.

If open questions have been included, a coding framework is needed for each of the questions. The approach to this will depend on whether data are being analysed within a quantitative or qualitative paradigm. This will involve firstly grouping together all of the answers for the same question and identifying the common themes contained within the answers. If a quantitative approach is being used, categories within each question are given numbers; if a qualitative approach is being used, categories are described and explained.

ANALYSING QUANTITATIVE DATA

Within the context of research, statistics have two main functions:

- *Descriptive statistics* are used to convey information about and interpret large sets of numbers in an efficient way (Clegg 1983).
- *Inferential statistics* are used to make inferences from the data you have collected and express the confidence with which we can generalise from a sample to a whole population (Howitt and Cramer 2004).

Explanations of specific statistical tests can be obtained from the Further reading list provided at the end of the chapter.

Descriptive statistics

Commonly used examples of descriptive statistics relevant to undergraduate research are measures of central tendency, dispersion and frequencies.

- *Measures of central tendency* include calculating the mean (adding together all the values and dividing by the number of values), the median (ordering all the numbers and identifying the number which falls in the middle) and the mode (identifying the number which is the most popular). They provide an indication of where the mid-point of a set of numbers lies but do not tell you how wide the range of numbers is. For example, if describing the age of a group of patients these measures will not tell you how old the youngest or oldest people are.
- *Measures of spread or dispersion* describe over how many numbers the data are spread and how much variation there is in the scores. Two measures of dispersion encountered frequently are the range and the standard deviation:

  The *range* describes the difference between the smallest and largest number and is calculated by subtracting the smallest number from the largest.

  The *standard deviation* describes the variability of the scores about the mean.
- *Frequencies* are another way of summarising and describing data. Individual scores are tabulated to show how many participants have, for example, given a particular response to a question or fall within a specific category. Frequencies are often expressed in terms of percentages and, if used, should always be used in conjunction with the actual value to give people an idea of what, for example, 28% means in the context of your sample.

Distribution

Measures of central tendency and dispersion enable you to examine the distribution of data. Plotting all of the scores on a graph will illustrate the kind of curve they produce. If data are *normally distributed*, they will be symmetrical and form a bell-shaped curve. For normally distributed data, the mean, the mode and the median all have the same or similar values. Some scores, however, may not be evenly distributed and the scores may fall predominantly above or below the mean. When scores fall mainly below the mean, they are described as *positively skewed*; when they fall mainly above, they are known as *negatively skewed*.

The relevance of understanding the concept of the normal distribution is that many statistical methods can only be applied reliably to normally distributed data.

Inferential statistics

The aim of conducting an experiment, as discussed earlier, is to examine the relationship between two variables. If your data indicate that an intervention has had an effect and the statistical tests conducted indicate a difference, there are two questions you will probably like answered:

1. How likely is it that the results can be attributed to the intervention rather than that they happened by chance?
2. With what degree of confidence can I generalise the results I obtained from my sample to the population as a whole?

These two questions are addressed in terms of significance and confidence intervals.

Significance

Significance is expressed as a '*p*-value' and is the one thing that most people, however limited their statistical knowledge, will know to look for when reading a research paper.

Key point

The significance level indicates the probability of an effect happening by chance.

One of the things that can be confusing is that there is more than one *p*-value. The lowest level of confidence that is acceptable is a *p*-value of 0.05, indicating that there is a 5% likelihood of the result occurring by chance (5 times in a 100). Other *p*-values seen frequently are 0.01 (1% or 1 in 100) and 0.001 (0.1% or 1 in 1000).

Confidence

If it were possible to conduct an experiment on a whole population, the results achieved would not be the same as those achieved from conducting the same experiment on a sample of the population. *Confidence intervals* are used to express the values between which a researcher is 'confident' that the true value for a population can be found. As well as the range, an indication of the level of confidence is given — usually 95%.

Levels of measurement

There are various ways in which numbers are used to measure things. The main types of measurement encountered in health research are classified as:

- nominal
- ordinal
- interval
- ratio.

It is important to understand the difference between these levels of measurement, as the degree of precision varies from category to category and influences the type of statistical analysis you can conduct on your data.

- *Nominal data* are used to classify things and can be binary (with only two possible choices, such as dead or alive) or have several values (such as ethnic origin). The numbers given to each category are arbitrary and could just as easily be letters. When coding data you could use 1 and 2 or A and B to represent dead and alive — it would make no difference.
- *Ordinal data* refers to scales where the numbers are ordered or ranked but there is no assumption that the distance between the numbers is equal. An example is a question relating to pain, in which the respondent is asked to tick one box on a linear scale that is marked from 1 to 5, where 1 = severe, 2 = moderate and so on, in answer to the invitation 'Please rate your pain over the last week. 1 = severe, 2 = moderate, 3 = mild and so on.'
- *Interval data* refers to scales where the numbers are ordered, as in an ordinal scale, but the intervals between the numbers are known to be equal. For example, in the question above we do not know whether the distance between 'severe' and 'moderate' pain is the same as between 'moderate' and 'mild'. Each person answering the question may have a different perception of this. However, in an interval scale we know that the distance is always the same. (For example, the distance between 1 cm and 2 cm is always the same as between 2 cm and 3 cm.)
- *Ratio scales* are the same as interval scales in that the numbers have an order and the distance between them is the same, but ratio scales also have an absolute zero. Examples of ratio scales include weight and height.

The importance of data type

The importance of being able to identify the kind of data you are generating and the distribution of these data is that this will influence the kind of analysis you can conduct.

22

A distinction is made in statistical tests between parametric and non-parametric statistics:

- *Non-parametric statistics* refer to statistical tests that can be conducted on data for which no assumptions are made regarding the Normal distribution of the data. Examples of non-parametric tests include the Mann–Whitney U test and the Wilcoxon signed-rank test.
- The use of *parametric statistics* is based on the assumption that the data have a Normal distribution, that they are derived from interval or ratio scales, and that the variance within the data is approximately the same. Parametric statistics are more powerful statistically than non-parametric tests.

Key point

It is not possible to enter into discussion here about specific statistical tests, but further references are supplied at the end of the chapter. It is important to stress that discussing your proposal with a statistician at an early stage will help to identify the kind of data you will generate from your work and the tests that will be relevant.

QUALITATIVE RESEARCH

Qualitative methods are used to make sense of the meanings that people give to their experiences and how they understand their world (Pope and Mays 2000). The focus of the research may be a group of people who have a shared experience or it may be gaining insight into the culture of a group or an organisation. Qualitative research does not set out to test a hypothesis but to explore and develop a greater understanding of the area being studied based on the descriptions and explanations provided by participants.

Ritchie and Lewis (2003) summarise the key elements of qualitative research as follows:

- Research aims that are focused on providing in-depth and interpreted understandings of the social world of research participants by learning about their social and material circumstances, their experiences, perspectives and histories
- Small samples purposively selected using relevant criteria
- Interactive methods of data collection that usually involve close contact between the researcher and participants
- Data that are detailed, rich in information and extensive
- Analysis that is open to emergent concepts and ideas
- Results that focus on the interpretation of meaning through mapping and 're-presenting' the social world of participants.

Interviews

Interviews are probably one of the mostly commonly used methods of data collection for undergraduate dissertations. An interview is a guided conversation between a researcher and a participant, which provides an environment in which the participant can tell a story in his or her own words. They are usually conducted face to face but can also be conducted by telephone or via the Internet.

Interview structure

Interviews range from being highly structured and following a predefined list of questions asked in a systematic way to being unstructured with the researcher introducing a small number of topics and facilitating the discussion with minimum guidance.

Highly structured interviews are usually associated with survey questionnaires in which the questionnaire is being administered face to face. The approach used most commonly in qualitative research is described as 'semi-structured'. Such interviews are guided by an interview schedule (a predefined list of questions) but encourage flexibility so that the researcher can follow lines of enquiry raised by the participants and adapt their questions as the project progresses. Three characteristics of qualitative interviews are that:

- They are modifications of ordinary conversations.
- Interviewers are more interested in people's understanding, knowledge and insights than in categorising people and events into academic theories.
- The content of interviews, as well as the flow of discussion and choice of topics, changes to match the experiences of the interviewee (Rubin and Rubin 2004).

Whilst interviews are similar to conversations, several distinctions should be made. An interview requires careful preparation, thinking about the questions that will be asked, the order in which they will be asked and ways of asking what may be perceived as sensitive questions. Before you embark upon interviews you need to be clear and focused about what you are hoping to achieve. During the interview you need to spend time probing what you are being told to make sure that your data have depth, clarifying the experiences that are being described, and checking that you both have the same understanding of what is being discussed. This requires you to listen carefully to make sure that important points are not missed or that points raised by the interviewee that are not on the schedule but are of relevance are followed up.

Key point

If you have not prepared well for the interview, it is likely that you will be so focused on remembering the questions or checking the tape machine that you will not actually listen to what is being said.

The interview questions

In preparing for an interview it is important to think carefully about the questions that will be asked and the order in which they will be asked. Whilst it is tempting to include as many questions as possible, it is important to remember that you are seeking to obtain a detailed understanding of your topic; asking numerous questions will probably mean that you obtain limited insights. If people are faced with a long stream of questions, it is likely that they will give short answers and feel that they are being subjected to an interrogation rather than participating in a discussion. You need to develop the skill of listening rather than talking.

Three kinds of question have been described (Rubin and Rubin 2004):

- main questions
- probing questions
- follow-up questions.

Having identified your research question, you need to break the topic down into a series of main questions, the wording of which should encourage discussion: for example, 'Can you tell me how you felt after your treatment?'

Probing questions are a way of increasing the depth of a person's explanation and finding out more: for example, 'Could you tell me a little more about that?' They can also be used to clarify something that you are unsure about: 'Could you explain that, please? I don't quite understand what you mean by ....'

Follow-up questions are used to follow up themes that emerge during the interview. A person may make a comment that throws a new light on the area you are interested in and you may want to explore this new line of thought with other people you are interviewing: for example, 'Another person mentioned that .... Was this your experience?'

The potential to vary questions within the schedule is something that new researchers often worry about. However, after conducting several interviews, your understanding of the area of interest will have changed. People may have identified issues that you had not thought about and introduced new lines of enquiry, and you may wish to explore these issues in subsequent interviews. It would be unusual if this did not happen.

Question order

Most people participating in an interview are keen to help but are nervous at the start of the discussion, especially if the interview is being recorded. Therefore it is helpful to start by asking them to talk about something with which they are familiar. This gives them the opportunity to talk for a little while to get used to being in a situation where their personal experience is the focus of attention, the discussion is being recorded and they are being questioned by a stranger. Some researchers send their questions to participants prior to the interview to enable them to think about the questions in advance and prepare their thoughts.

As the interview progresses, the interviewee's confidence usually increases and therefore it is towards the middle of an interview that more sensitive or probing questions are asked.

Interviews can be an emotionally draining experience for the interviewee and therefore it is important to think about how you end the discussion. If a person has become upset or emotional during an interview or has been asked to discuss a personally challenging topic, the interview needs to end on a lighter note. Therefore think about what questions can be asked to bring the discussion to an end whilst leaving the person in a positive frame of mind.

Before conducting an interview you should be clear in your own mind about the content of your interview schedule to enable you to steer a smooth course through the discussion without having to keep referring to notes to remind yourself of the next question.

Recording the interview

Interviews are usually recorded to enable a full transcript of the discussion to be made.

Key point

If a recorder is being used, it is wise to practise using it before any interviews take place. The production of a recorder at the start of an interview can make people nervous, and if you are nervous about using it and need to keep checking that it is switched on and working, you will constantly draw attention to the fact that a recording is being made.

It is important to check as soon as possible after the interview that you have actually recorded the discussion. If a problem has arisen with the recording, you will be able to make detailed notes of the discussion whilst it is fresh in your memory. You should also allow enough time between interviews to listen to each one and reflect not only on the information you have obtained but also on how well the interview went. For example, did the person find specific questions difficult to understand? Were new areas of discussion identified that you had not thought about? Did you talk too much? and so on. This will help you to refine your questions and your interview technique as the project progresses.

Once completed, interviews are then transcribed (see later).

22

Focus groups

Focus groups are carefully planned group discussions designed to obtain participants' perceptions of a predefined area of interest. The group setting provides an environment in which group members interact with and influence each other as they exchange experiences and points of view, ask questions of each other and respond to ideas and points raised by other members of the group (Krueger 1994).

Conducting a focus group

As with interviews, it is necessary to prepare for the group both in terms of practical arrangements like the organisation of time, venue, transport and refreshments, and developing the questions to be asked during the session.

Focus groups should be held in an environment that is accessible and comfortable and creates a relaxed and welcoming feel. Most sessions last between 1 and 2 hours. Groups usually comprise between six and ten people to ensure that everyone has an opportunity to be actively involved in the discussion. Larger groups tend to put some people off talking and also provide the opportunity for some people to take a more passive role.

Given the emphasis on the group discussion and interaction, the role of the researcher should be limited to asking a few questions and facilitating discussion. Four or five questions should really be the maximum number of main questions posed in a group, but as with interviews, probing questions may also be used to explore a point further.

The researcher usually introduces the session by explaining the purpose of the group, emphasising the discursive nature of the group and establishing any ground rules for the session, such as a no-smoking policy and issues of confidentiality regarding what is said. In the introduction it is also helpful to explain that the aim of the group is to obtain different views and that, if a person disagrees with what is being said, to say so. Before moving on to asking your first question, it is important to ask each member of the group to introduce themselves. This ensures that everyone has an opportunity to get used to speaking in the group, that they know who they are sharing the discussion with and that when it comes to transcribing you are able to match a voice to a name.

It is difficult for one person to welcome participants, provide refreshments, facilitate the discussion and keep a track of all of the group dynamics taking place. Therefore it is usual for groups to be facilitated by two people: one person to facilitate the discussion and the other to make notes about the group dynamics and interactions.

As with interviews, you need to give careful thought to the questions that you are going to ask and the order in which you are going to ask them. In addition to asking questions, your role as a researcher is also to facilitate the group process by trying to make sure that everyone has an equal opportunity to contribute, that one person does not dominate the discussion and that the conversation flows as smoothly as possible. Focus groups are usually tape-recorded, as long as all participants consent to this happening, and transcribed in preparation for analysis.

Observational studies

Observational studies involve the 'systematic, detailed observation of behavior and talk' (Pope and Mays 2000). The setting of observational studies can vary. A psychologist may choose to undertake an observational study in a clinical or laboratory setting, whereas a sociologist is more likely to observe the phenomenon of interest in the context in which it occurs. Within the social sciences, observational studies are usually called 'ethnography' and are closely associated with anthropology. Both are built upon the premise that, to understand a group of people, a researcher needs to observe their daily lives, usually by living like or working with them. A number of approaches can be taken in observational studies, one factor being the level of participation of the researcher:

- Participant observation requires the researcher to participate in the activity or group being observed.
- In non-participative studies the researcher observes rather than participates.

Another distinction is whether the participation of the researcher is known about by other members of the group or is concealed.

The term 'observation' can be misleading, as data collection in observational studies tends to be derived from a number of methods, including interviews and documentary research. The processes involved in observational studies include: negotiating access to the area of study, determining methods of collecting observational data, watching, recording events taking place, and analysing data.

Case studies

This method of research focuses on one case (a single case study) or a small number of cases (multiple case studies). A 'case' may be a person or an environment such as a place of work or an institution. The number of cases is usually small, owing to the detail that is required in such studies. This method may be used to explore an issue retrospectively, at a single point in time, or over a period of time: for example, the impact of a new management structure on an organisation. A number of methods are usually used to collect data about each case and include interviews, analysis of documents and observation. Such studies are often undertaken to understand complex social situations or to develop our understanding about a specific phenomena.

Consensus methods

These methods are used to assess the extent of agreement or resolve disagreement where there may be contradictory evidence. Two consensus methods are the *Delphi technique* and the *nominal group technique*. Both seek to estimate the degree of consensus on a given issue and data are derived from panels of 'experts'.

Within normal group discussion a very persuasive individual or group of individuals with a strong point of view or vested interest can dominate the group and influence the outcome of a decision. Consensus techniques have been developed to overcome this problem.

The Delphi technique

The Delphi technique uses a group of people identified as experts in the field of interest and comprises a number of stages. Once they have been identified, the individual experts are invited to give their opinions on a specific issue using a postal questionnaire comprising open and closed questions. The questionnaires are analysed and data are then grouped into a series of statements. The statements are then sent back to the participants, who are asked to indicate their level of agreement with each statement. These are returned to the researcher who, based on all of the responses, provides a ranking of the statements; the ranking is then recirculated. Participants are given the opportunity to review the ranking they gave each statement and these responses are returned to the researcher. These data are then re-analysed to assess the level of consensus. If, at this stage, consensus is reached, the process stops and the results are fed back to the participants. If consensus is not reached, then the process is repeated.

Nominal groups

This method, like the Delphi method, uses a group of experts but in this instance they are brought together in a group context. Unlike focus groups, nominal groups are highly structured by the researcher. Participants may have been asked to prepare for the meeting by being given the topic of interest in advance or may spend time writing down key points about a given topic at the start of the group. Each person is then asked to contribute one point that is written on a flip chart by the researcher and this continues until all points have been covered. Each person is then asked to rank the points on the flip chart privately to ensure that the views of other group members do not influence the ranking. Again, in contrast to the focus group, the level of group interaction at this stage of a nominal group is minimal. Once this task is completed, the researcher collects the rankings and combines them to calculate an overall ranking of issues raised by the group. This ranking is then discussed by the group. Following the discussion, participants are asked to re-rank the issues and once again an overall group ranking is worked out and fed back to the group.

Using multiple methods

More than one method can be used within a single project: for example, interviews and focus groups. The use of different methods can increase the validity of the findings by demonstrating that the same conclusions can be drawn when a number of methods are used to observe the same phenomena. Using more than one method can also provide the opportunity to highlight different phenomena relevant to the research question by providing different versions or levels of answer (Mason 2002).

> ***Key point***
> If you decide to use more than one method within your project, it is important to think about how the methods will be combined, in terms of both the study design and the data analysis.

ANALYSING QUALITATIVE DATA

Analysis of quantitative data usually takes place when all of the data have been collected. In qualitative research the processes of data collection and analysis are often intertwined and a more interactive approach is adopted. This approach to data analysis provides the researcher with the opportunity to explore new insights as they occur during data collection and follow leads that emerge during the course of the interviews. Therefore, by the end of the process of data collection, you should have a good level of familiarity with your data.

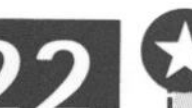

> ***Key point***
> A qualitative study can produce a large amount of data from which sense needs to be made. There are a number of ways in which qualitative data can be analysed.

It is important to understand that there are a number of ways in which qualitative data are analysed and the approach taken will be dependent on the theoretical approach taken in the research. Ritchie and Lewis (2003) describe an analytical hierarchy that can be applied to different approaches of analysis; it comprises the three stages of data management, the production of descriptive accounts and the production of explanatory accounts.

Transcribing

Before detailed analysis can begin, the recordings from interviews or discussions need to be transcribed. A transcript usually refers to a verbatim (exact word by word) reproduction of the conversation. Transcription is a lengthy process, a rough guide being that it takes 4 or 5 hours of typing for 1 hour of discussion. Access to a transcription machine can significantly reduce the time required to produce a transcript. Whilst time-consuming to produce, transcripts enable you to locate a segment of text within the wider context of the conversation and provide an accurate account of what was said, and helps to ensure that coding reflects the meaning derived from participants rather than a researcher's recollection of what was said.

Data management

Once transcripts have been produced, the first stage of analysis is, in effect, to reduce and fragment the data. This involves identifying themes within your data and allocating descriptive labels (codes) to the segments of text. The segments will vary in size and one segment can be given more than one code. For example, 'my pain was excruciating and I was unable to concentrate on anything' could be coded as a description of pain ('excruciating') and as an effect of being in pain ('unable to concentrate on anything'). You need to work through each interview transcript and assign labels in this way.

The production of descriptive and explanatory accounts

Once all of the transcripts have been coded, the process of analysis moves from data management to the production of descriptive accounts. To enable this to happen, the data are reorganised and all of the data relating to each theme are brought together. It is then possible to conduct a more focused analysis of each theme, looking for similarities and differences, and identifying different dimensions of the theme. It is also important at this stage to question whether the dimensions are common to everyone or whether there are differences in what is being said. If, for example, your sample comprises men and women, do they have different perspectives on the theme? The same questions should be asked of people from different background or of different ages and so on. This level of interrogation can only occur when you are familiar with your data and with the characteristics of the people who participated in your project.

Once descriptive accounts of each theme have been made, the process of analysis then moves into a phase where the focus of attention is on creating explanatory accounts of your data.

Computer-assisted coding

The use of dedicated software packages in qualitative analysis has increased significantly in recent years. However, the use of such software to aid analysis is a source of debate amongst qualitative researchers.

Software packages such as ATLAS.ti and QSR NVivo have been developed to facilitate analysis, but it must be stressed that they do not analyse data for you. Such packages enable you to code segments of text on the screen and then sort data automatically into themes. They also enable you to set up enquiries about data: for example, to ask for all the discourse relating to a specific issue derived from men living in London or women over 40. These comparisons can be made far more easily using a computer package than by conducting the same process manually. The software also includes tools to build diagrammatic representations of relationships between themes to help build theory, and to write and organise analytical memos whilst you are conducting your analysis.

These packages require a significant investment of time to learn how to use them. Given the quantity of data generated from an undergraduate project, it is likely to be more efficient to analyse the data using the cut and paste options of a word processor, unless someone in your department is familiar with such packages and willing to provide advice and assistance. With many software packages it is easy to get carried away with the tools and facilities they offer and the speed at which they produce outputs, without really understanding the rationale for what you are doing or the meaning and relevance of the outputs you have obtained. Developing and understanding the processes involved in analysis and *then* using software to facilitate the process is perhaps a more meaningful use of software packages.

RECRUITMENT AND SAMPLING

Having identified a research question, chosen your methodological approach and identified the relevant methods of collecting data, the next stage of the research process focuses on deciding on the number and type of people to involve in the study and how they will be identified.

Sampling strategies

Sampling strategies are divided into:

- *random sampling*, whereby every person in a population of interest has an equal chance of being chosen for the study
- *non-probability sampling*, in which the selection is not random.

The main methods of random sampling include 'simple' random sampling using computer-generated numbers, and 'stratified' sampling; these have been described previously in relation to the experimental method. Another form of random sampling is 'cluster' sampling, which focuses on sampling from clusters of the population.

Non-probability sampling is often used in qualitative research and there are a number of different approaches that can be adopted. In a convenience sample, the sample is derived from people who are easy to access or most likely to respond. Purposive sampling is undertaken when researchers have specific characteristics or experiences they want to represent in their sample. Other approaches to sampling include quota sampling, which is used by market researchers who have specific targets for their study population (such as numbers of people required from different sociodemographic or age groups), and snowballing, which occurs when the researcher has identified a small group of participants and then asks them to recruit other people they know who would be in the target group. These people are contacted and asked if they would be willing to take part in the project, and are likewise asked for potential contacts.

Sample size

'How many people do I need to recruit for my study?' is an obvious question to ask, but the answer is not at all straightforward. The statistical approach to calculating sample size is a *power calculation*. This method is used to calculate the number of people needed in a study to detect a true difference between two groups. However, it is unlikely that the size of an undergraduate project would warrant such an approach.

Key point

In the written account of your work you will need to describe and justify the sampling strategy you used, the size of the sample, and how it was selected.

In relation to qualitative research at undergraduate level the most common approach will probably be purposive sampling, and the number of participants will probably be influenced by the time and resources available, as well as factors like access to participants. Given the diversity of methods, it would be wise to obtain guidance on determining the sample size once you have identified your question and methods.

PREPARATORY WORK

You may be keen to embark upon the actual process of 'doing the research', but time should be allocated at the start of a project to doing some preparatory work. This might seem to be an unnecessary distraction but it is guaranteed to be time well spent. Experienced researchers will testify to the frustration of losing a crucial reference or of not having made careful note of the source of a key quotation as the submission deadline looms. The *'eureka'* moment you had — and thought you would never forget — fades rapidly as the focus of a project moves through the various stages and the research develops.

Keeping a research diary

Key point

Research or fieldwork diaries are closely associated with qualitative research but are of equal value in quantitative research.

The aim of keeping a diary is to provide a record of the development of a research project from inception to completion. It enables you to keep personal memos and reflections about your research in one place that is easy to locate as the project develops. The diary usually takes the form of handwritten or word-processed notes. The structure varies from researcher to researcher. Some people choose to keep notes in chronological order, as in a personal diary, whilst others organise their diary under headings such as 'literature', 'methods', 'data collection' and 'personal thoughts'.

The diary provides a place in which you can keep track of how the research question has evolved. You can note methodological issues arising throughout the data collection process, such as your thoughts on the different kinds of standardised measure that could be used and why you chose one measure over another. You can record particular papers or discussions that may have stimulated a specific train of thought. Once the process of data collection begins, the diary may be used to record personal profiles of the participants. If you are conducting interviews, you may note information about the actual process of the interview — questions that elicited a good discussion or those that people found hard to understand or engage with, or issues that have been raised by a participant that you thought were really important.

Research is a reflective process and a research diary provides a place in which this reflection can be recorded.

Keeping track of references

The development of a systematic method of recording and referencing is as much a research skill as that of conducting an interview or undertaking an experiment. At the start of a project it is easy to underestimate the time taken to compile the reference section of a dissertation, so develop a systematic method of recording and filing references from day one. Developing a system will save an immense amount of effort towards the end of your dissertation, when time, energy and resources will be challenged considerably.

Student's note

It is a common experience to have a memory of reading a crucial piece of information or writing down a quotation but not being able to locate the exact source!

There are several methods of managing references, the most common being the use of a card index system or dedicated computer software such as Reference Manager or Endnote. Whichever system is used, the *minimum* amount of information recorded should be as follows:

For a journal or magazine:

- author (or authors), including surname and initials
- name of the journal or magazine
- title of the article
- date of publication
- volume number, and issue number if relevant
- the pages where the article can be found (e.g. 331–338).

For a book or report:

- author (or authors) including surname and initials
- title of the book
- date of publication
- name of publisher
- place of publication.

For a chapter in an edited book:

- editor (or editors), including surname and initials
- author (or authors), including surname and initials
- title of the book
- title of the chapter
- page numbers of the chapter
- date of publication
- name of publisher
- place of publication.

It is helpful also to write a short summary of the relevant points of the paper or chapter and to note, carefully, any quotations that you feel you may wish to use in the dissertation. If you are noting direct quotations, keep a record of the page on which the quotation can be found, to save having to check through the whole publication to find, for example, a two-sentence quotation.

If a card index system is used, separate cards should be made out for each publication and a filing system developed to help with retrieval. Software packages have several advantages over card indexes, as they offer a number of tools helpful in the management of references, including:

- a mechanism for importing full reference details and abstracts from literature searches conducted without having to enter individual references
- scope to input summaries and key words alongside the reference details
- the incorporation of references into text whilst word-processing
- automatic formatting of reference sections in a specified style (e.g. Harvard, Vancouver).

A filing system is needed for storage and retrieval of papers. These may be stored alphabetically or under subject headings.

Regulations

The regulations for dissertations vary from college to college, so make sure you are familiar with and understand the regulations that apply to your dissertation before starting work. They will set out the format of your dissertation and procedures for issues such as gaining ethical approval for your project. The regulations will have been produced for a reason and must be followed. At undergraduate level, ignoring such guidance can result in the need to revise and resubmit the work. In the context of proposals written for funding applications, failure to follow the regulations and guidance can result in the application being rejected. It is therefore worth getting used to reading and following any guidance or regulations provided, at an early stage in your research career.

As well as understanding the regulations of your college, you may also need to give careful consideration to other regulations such as the Ethical Approval Data Protection Act, Codes of Professional Conduct and Codes of Research for your college. Your supervisor will be able to advise you on the regulations that apply to your chosen project, including the issue of research governance.

Supervision

An important component of conducting any research project is the quality of supervision provided throughout the work and the relationship between you and your supervisor. The supervisory process is two-way, with the onus on both parties to create an informative, discursive and supportive environment. As dissertations usually come at the end of a programme of study, you will be expected to have reached a stage in your academic and professional development whereby you are able to assume more responsibility for the development and conduct of your project. Your supervisor will not expect to keep telling you what to do next.

Your supervisor may not have in-depth knowledge and clinical expertise in your chosen area of study but is likely to have extensive experience in the supervision and successful completion of dissertations, and experience of the methodological approach and methods being used.

Here are some key points to remember:

1. Plan ahead for your supervision. Prior to your meetings make a list of the issues you wish to discuss and make sure that at the start of supervision you agree an agenda.
2. If the aim of a session is to discuss work that needs to be submitted prior to the meeting, make sure you give your supervisor plenty of time to read the work. It is not uncommon for students to push deadlines to the limit, leading to work being handed in a day or two before supervision, or being brought to the meeting. Such an approach is unlikely to generate high-quality discussion about your work, as supervisors need to have time to read and reflect on the work and prepare for the meeting in the same way that you do.
3. Keep notes of the key issues discussed during supervision. These notes can form part of the fieldwork diary. Write notes either during the meeting or straight afterwards. It is easy to forget key issues discussed or lines of enquiry recommended, as supervisory meetings can cover several topics in one session.
4. At the end of the meeting, make sure you are clear about the next stage of your work and expectations regarding work that needs to be completed before the next meeting.
5. If you are encountering problems with your research, bring them to the attention of the supervisor as soon as possible. Research is rarely a process that is smooth and problem-free. Things not going to plan should be seen as part of the process rather than a failing on your part.

Key point

Completing your dissertation on time requires planning — not only based on your own time but also taking into consideration the time of others involved in the project.

Time management

The reality of many research projects is that completion is often dependent on the time commitments of other people over which you will have no control. These will include research and ethics committees, people or groups involved in the recruitment of participants, participants themselves, and your supervisor. Whilst your project may be your number one priority, it will not be given the same priority by others. You therefore need to develop an understanding of the time constraints within which other people are operating, and to be prepared to give people realistic timescales for the things you are asking them to do.

At the start of the project draw up a calendar divided into weeks and also a list of the key milestones in your research process. Then start marking on the calendar the time required for each task. Be realistic, and if you are not sure how long some things will take, discuss it with your supervisor. Allow time for slippage in the plan, as this is bound to occur. As your project progresses, keep going back to your timeframe and make revisions if necessary. This will also help when you are asking other people to be involved in the project, as you will be able to give them an indication of when things need to be done. For example, if someone is sending out questionnaires on your behalf, you will know when this has to be done by, rather than plucking a date out of the air.

Personal presentation

It is as important to think about how you are going to present yourself in a research setting as it is in a clinical setting. Your research will be carried out either in person or in writing. Whichever form it may take, you need to convey your professionalism and communicate the importance of your work. The manner in which you approach people will have a direct impact upon their willingness to engage with your study.

If you are approaching potential participants in person, think about your appearance, plan the way in which you will present your project, and allow time to give a proper explanation of who you are, what you want to do and why you want to do it. These may seem obvious points, but the successful completion of your project will, in some instances, be influenced by your ability to present yourself and communicate your work. You will usually have only one opportunity with each person to do this.

If you are contacting potential participants by post, spend time working on the letter you intend to send, not only in relation to content but also in terms of format. Try to keep to a minimum the amount of medical terminology used, if writing to potential participants, and explain the relevance of the project and the exact implications for a person taking part in the study. A useful aid for checking the language you have used in your letter is the readability tool provided in some software packages. Readability scores provide an indication of the reading level of the document and can assess the ease of reading, rated on a 100-point scale; they also indicate the school grade level in relation to reading level.

Student's note

The issues outlined so far in this chapter should help in the planning and implementation of a research project. The focus will now move on to considering how all of the different components discussed in this chapter are brought together within the context of writing a research proposal.

WRITING A RESEARCH PROPOSAL

The role of the proposal is to 'describe what the research is about, what specifically it is trying to achieve, how you will go about doing this, what will be learnt from the research, and the contribution it will make to existing knowledge' (Punch 2006). The components of a proposal are fairly standard but it is essential to check the specific regulations governing your dissertation.

Writing a research proposal provides a clear plan of action for conducting your project as well as the structure for your dissertation, with the addition of a results section.

Components of the proposal

A research proposal should have the following elements:

- title
- abstract
- introduction
- literature review
- statement of the research question
- methodology and methods to be used
- recruitment and sampling
- analysis intended
- initial references
- appendices.

The title and abstract

Think carefully about the title of your proposal. Try to convey the key points of your project in a clear and concise manner. An abstract provides a summary of the project and is usually the last section of the proposal written. It is normally limited to around 250 words. At the proposal stage the abstract should enable the reader to understand the context of the research, the research question and the methods used to address the question. Once the research has been completed, the revised abstract will also include the main results and conclusions. Whilst the word length of an abstract is small, the skill required to write it should not be underestimated — considerable effort is required to summarise a project in 250 words.

The introduction

A distinction needs to be made between an introduction and a literature review, as they perform two different functions. An introduction should provide the reader with an understanding of how the study fits into what is already known about the research topic and provides a justification as to why this particular piece of research is important. Introductions need not be lengthy but they should locate your study within the broad context of your chosen topic. The literature review then moves on to focus on the specific area of the proposed research, culminating with a statement of the research question.

The literature review

Key point

The literature review has been described as 'a systematic, explicit, and reproducible method for identifying, evaluating and interpreting the existing body of recorded work produced by researchers, scholars and practitioners' (Fink 2004).

The function of a literature review is to locate your work within the context of the work already conducted in the chosen area. It should demonstrate that you have an understanding of your area of research by providing the reader with an overview of the state of knowledge in the field and the major questions being asked.

The definition provided by Fink provides insight into the core elements of conducting a comprehensive literature review. It requires two very different skills:

- searching the literature
- appraising the literature.

The literature review should also identify the theoretical base of the project and, if you are studying an area where several theoretical positions exist, should justify the particular perspective you have chosen to adopt. The methods used to undertake the review should be made explicit by detailing the major databases or information sources used. The literature reviewed can take many forms and may include journal articles, books, reports and government circulars.

The main focus of searching for most undergraduate dissertations will be via computer-based systems, primarily accessed via a college network (e.g. Medline or CINAHL, Cumulative Index of Nursing and Allied Health Literature). The process of conducting a search begins with the identification of key words. Most databases contain a thesaurus that enables you to check that the key word or terms you have chosen actually appear in the database. You need to put time and effort into planning the literature search before starting to use the databases. Keep a record of the key words you have used, the searches that you have carried out and the results of each search. It is likely that this process will take place over a number of sessions and it may be difficult to remember exactly what you have done and how you refined the searches.

Having identified key words you may find that one of two things occurs:

1. You are presented with a list of hundreds of references, which probably indicates that the terms you have used are too general.
2. You are presented with only a few references, which may indicate that your search was too narrow.

The majority of databases make use of what are known as 'Boolean operators' to enable you to refine or expand your search by combining words by using the keyword AND, or excluding words by using the keyword OR.

The results of your search will be a list of articles of potential relevance to your project. It is likely that not all of the references will be relevant, so you need to read the abstracts to check on the relevance before locating the articles within the library or requesting them via inter-library loans. Photocopying and requesting articles is expensive for you and the college, so you should be convinced of the relevance of an article before obtaining the full text. Most databases enable you to move back and forth between the reference list and abstracts marking the references of interest and thus refining your initial search further.

Not all of the literature you review will come from journal publications; a large amount of information is to be gained from books, government departments and professional organisations, as well as voluntary organisations and websites. Conducting an Internet search requires a systematic approach similar to that used to search databases, as the potential to identify sources of information is immense. It is important to remember that you will also need to develop and demonstrate an understanding of literature to support your methodology and methods.

Key point

An important distinction to understand is the difference between describing the literature and evaluating and appraising it. Many students conducting a literature review for the first time present a description of the papers they have obtained rather than an evaluation and appraisal of them.

Evaluating and appraising literature is a skill that needs to be developed. Being able to critique research papers when you are developing your own understanding of the research process is difficult, but further reading has been provided at the end of the chapter to provide you with guidance. Developing a critical approach to literature will help you to understand the criteria that will be used to judge your own work once it is completed.

Whilst the literature review is normally one of the first tasks in developing your research proposal, it should not be viewed as complete until the project has been completed. The majority of undergraduate dissertations are typically conducted over a 12-month period, during which time new papers of relevance will be published. Having conducted a systematic review, you will develop an understanding of the specific journals in which new papers are likely to be published. During the period of your research you should keep up to date and, where appropriate, incorporate new papers into your review. This can be difficult to achieve once you have embarked upon the process of data collection, as time and resources will be focused elsewhere. However, if you have access to the Internet it is worth setting up journal alerts for key publications. This will ensure that, each time a new journal issue is published, the contents page will be e-mailed to you.

The research question

Whilst the research question may have been introduced in a general way at the end of the introduction, it is worth restating it before the methods section to refocus the reader's attention on the specific question being addressed.

Methods to be used

The methods section should explain the methodological approach you are taking and the specific methods you are using. It is usual to begin with an explanation of the relevance of the methodological approach to your research question. Is a quantitative or qualitative approach appropriate to address the specified question? Or has a mixed methods approach been chosen? Rather than just describing which approach you are using, you need to provide a justification as to why this is the most appropriate approach to use.

This section should describe the way in which you are going to address your question (the study design) and give a detailed account of the specific methods of data collection being used. If you have chosen to use standardised measures or treatment interventions, they should be explained and referenced and details of their validity and reliability provided. If you have chosen to develop your own method of measurement, you need to explain the steps you plan to take to develop your measure.

It should also include details of the ethical considerations of the project, whether or not ethical committee approval will be obtained, and details of how you will obtain informed consent, if appropriate. The method of recruitment you intend to use should be described and your sample and sample size provided and justified, along with the sampling strategy you intend to use. You should also describe any inclusion or exclusion criteria you have determined for the study.

The intended analysis

In this section you should demonstrate that you have considered the analysis of data and provide insight into the techniques you are going to use. For a quantitative study you will need to specify any statistical package you intend to use (e.g. SPSS or Minitab), as well as the statistical tests. For a qualitative study, again you need to detail the process of analysis you will be using and whether or not you will use software such as ATLAS.ti or NVivo.

It may be helpful to include at the end of this section a time plan that identifies key milestones for the project and a target for completion.

The references

Your college regulations may specify the format in which the reference section is to be compiled. Make sure that you check this and comply with the relevant requirements.

Appendices

One or more appendix sections can provide additional information of relevance to the study. You might wish to include examples of standardised questionnaires, and a copy of the interview schedule that will guide qualitative interviews.

The dissertation

When the project has been completed and you start writing it up, the structure of your dissertation will be very similar to that of the proposal. There will, of course, be additional sections: one for the results, which is placed after the analysis, and one for the discussion and conclusions, which comes after the results section.

CONCLUSION

By the time you are preparing to start writing your dissertation you will already have been introduced to the importance of research in informing the evidence base of clinical practice in physiotherapy. For a newly qualified therapist, the grounding you will have developed in understanding the research process should not be underestimated. As a new member of a department, with research experience, you have a great deal to offer to help demystify research and facilitate its integration into clinical practice.

If you are stimulated by the practice of research, do not underestimate the potential of your first dissertation. Unfortunately, many dissertations collect dust in cupboards or on shelves, even though they could possibly form the basis of a journal article or a presentation at a seminar — so do explore this prospect with your supervisor.

To end where we started: many people are overwhelmed by the prospect of research and tend to diminish what they have achieved in dissertations. Your dissertation could be the first building block of a research career.

FURTHER READING

General

Bell J 2005 Doing Your Research Project: a Guide for First-Time Researchers in Education and Social Science, 4th edn. Open University Press: Buckingham.

Blaxter L, Hughes C, Tight M 2006 How to Research, 3rd edn. Open University Press: Buckingham.

Bowling A 2002 Research Methods in Health: Investigating Health and Health Services, 2nd edn. Open University Press: Buckingham.

Brett Davies B 2007 Doing a Successful Research Project Using Qualitative or Quantitative Methods. Palgrave Macmillan: Basingstoke.

Punch KF 2005 Introduction to Social Research: Quantitative and Qualitative Approaches, 2nd edn. Sage: London.

Punch KF 2006 Developing Effective Research Proposals, 2nd edn. Sage: London.

Walliman N 2004 Your Undergraduate Dissertation. The Essential Guide for Success. Sage: London.

Research ethics

Oliver P 2003 The Student's Guide to Research Ethics. Oxford University Press: Maidenhead.

Literature reviews

Fink A 2004 Conducting Research Literature Reviews: From the Internet to Paper, 2nd edn. Sage: Thousand Oaks, CA.

Hart C 1998 Doing a Literature Search. A Comprehensive Guide for the Social Sciences. Sage: London.

Hart C 2001 Doing a Literature Review: A Comprehensive Guide for the Social Sciences. Sage: London.

Questionnaires and measurement scales

Bowling A 2001 Measuring Disease: a Review of Disease-Specific Quality of Life Measurement Scales. Open University Press: Buckingham.

Bowling A 2004 Measuring Health: a Review of Quality of Life Measurement Scales. Open University Press: Buckingham.

Buckingham A, Saunder P 2004 The Survey Methods Workbook. Polity: Cambridge.

Streiner D, Norman G 2003 Health Measurement Scales: a Practical Guide to their Development and Use, 2nd edn. Oxford University Press: Oxford.

Statistics

Altman D 1990 Practical Statistics for Medical Research. Chapman & Hall: London.

Clegg F 1983 Simple Statistics: a Course Book for the Social Sciences. Cambridge University Press: Cambridge.

Hart A 2001 Making Sense of Statistics in Healthcare. Radcliffe Medical: Abingdon.

Howitt D, Cramer D 2004 An Introduction to Statistics in Psychology: a Complete Guide for Students, 3rd edn. Pearson Education: Harlow.

Mixed methods

Creswell J, Plano Clark V 2007 Designing and Conducting Mixed Methods Research. Sage: London.

Qualitative methods

Flick U 2006 An Introduction to Qualitative Research, 3rd edn. Sage: London.

Hammersley M, Atkinson P 2004 Ethnography: Principles in Practice, 2nd edn. Routledge: London.

Krueger R, Casey M 2002 Focus Groups: a Practical Guide for Applied Research, 3rd edn. Sage: London.

Mason J 2002 Qualitative Researching, 2nd edn. Sage: London.

Morgan D 1997 Focus Groups as Qualitative Research, 2nd edn. Sage: London.

Morgan D 1998 The Focus Group Guidebook. Sage: London.

Renzetti CM, & Lee RM (eds) *1993* Researching Sensitive Topics. Sage: London.

Ritchie J, & Lewis J (eds) *2003* Qualitative Research Practice. A guide for social science students and researchers. Sage: London.

Rubin H, Rubin I 2004 Qualitative Interviewing: the Art of Hearing Data. 2nd edn. Sage: London.

Strauss A, Corbin J 1998 Basics of Qualitative Research. Techniques and Procedures for Developing Grounded Theory. 2nd edn. Sage: London.

REFERENCES

Bowling A 2002 Research Methods in Health: Investigating Health and Health Services. 2nd edn. Open University Press: Buckingham.

Clegg F 1983 Simple Statistics: a Course Book for the Social Sciences. Cambridge University Press: Cambridge.

Creswell JW, Plano Clark VL 2007 Designing and Conducting Mixed Methods Research. Sage: Thousand Oaks, CA.

Department of Health 2006 Best Research for Best Health. Department of Health: London. Crown copyright.

Fink A 2004 Conducting Research Literature Reviews: From the Internet to Paper. Sage: Thousand Oaks, CA.

Glaser B, Strauss A 1967 The Discovery of Grounded Theory: Strategies for Qualitative Research. Aldine: Chicago.

Hockey L 1996 The nature and purpose of research. In: Cormack DF (ed.) The Research Process in Nursing, 3rd edn. Blackwell Science: Oxford.

Howitt D, Cramer D 2004 An Introduction to Statistics in Psychology: a Complete Guide for Students, 3rd edn. Pearson Education: Harlow.

Krueger RK 1994 Focus Groups: a Practical Guide for Applied Research, 2nd edn. Sage: Thousand Oaks, CA.

Mason J 2002 Qualitative Researching, 2nd edn. Sage: London.

Pope C, Mays N (eds) 2000 Qualitative Research in Health Care, 2nd edn. BMJ Books: London.

Punch KF 2005 Introduction to Social Research: Quantitative and Qualitative Approaches, 2nd edn. Sage: London.

Punch KF 2006 Developing Effective Research Proposals, 2nd edn. Sage: London.

Ritchie J, & Lewis J (eds) 2003 Qualitative Research Practice. A Guide for Social Science Students and researchers. Sage: London.

Rubin H, Rubin I 2004 Qualitative Interviewing: the Art of Hearing Data. Sage: Thousand Oaks, CA.

Chapter **23**

Changing relationships for promoting health

Sally French and John Swain

CHAPTER CONTENTS

INTRODUCTION

Our focus for this chapter is 'changing relationships'. The chapter is divided into three sections.

- The first, 'between people', focuses on the dynamics of relationships within therapy practice, at the interpersonal level, and also broadens the discussion to the group level, looking at questions of culture.
- The second section, 'context of relationships', considers the social context of relationships, particularly as regards inequalities in health and health care, and the various ideologies and viewpoints that prevail in therapy practice.
- Finally, in 'changing relationships', we look towards possibilities for changing the dynamics of relationships by focusing first on the notion of partnership and then on health promotion itself.

We both work in the field of disability studies and will draw examples from our own work and that of others in this field. Thus the chapter is particularly orientated towards disability and therapy with disabled people. The processes we are examining, however, are general and, overall, we hope to demonstrate the interrelationships between the interpersonal, personal, cultural and societal in the dynamics of changing relationships to improve and promote health.

BETWEEN PEOPLE

Labelling people

Various terms are used to refer to disabled people in relation to services. All are being challenged by disabled people themselves.

Patient This term clearly labels people in medical terms and is derived from 'pati', meaning 'suffer'.

Client This refers to a person using the services of a professional (lawyer, architect, medical practitioner and so on). In recent times the term 'customer' has also been used.

Service user This is perhaps the most neutral term, although it still labels people according to their relationship with services.

Communication

The provision of physiotherapy can be thought of as a form of communication and the whole process as one of communication between the client and the physiotherapist, between the physiotherapist and colleagues (including other physiotherapists, doctors and so on), and between the physiotherapist and members of the client's family. The purpose of this section, then, is to examine interpersonal communication in the particular context of physiotherapy practice.

Models of communication

Linear models

Linear models of communication seem to accord with common sense, as communication is viewed as a process of sending and receiving messages. A popular communication model that is used in the literature is as follows:

- sender (self)
- encoder (converting thought into message)
- channel (verbal, non-verbal, both verbal and non-verbal)
- decoder (interpretation of message)
- receiver (other/others) (Rungapadiachy 1999).

Social models

A social view of communication posits a dynamic model in the sense that communication is seen as a transaction constructed between people.

Social models concentrate more on the communication process itself, rather than the notion of message-sending (Pearce 1994). From this perspective, improving communication is not a simple matter of improving physiotherapists' skills of expressing and listening to information. Communication is 'meaning-making' rather than 'information-processing' and meanings are constructed between people. Communication is both based on and generates our perceptions, descriptions and understandings of the world or, more specifically, physiotherapy.

There are a number of important aspects to a social model of communication. Interpersonal communication is viewed as an interplay between people, in which participants are both active agents, affecting the interplay, and reactive agents, affected by the interplay. There is no simple one-to-one correspondence between acts of communication and the meaning expressed. The context is all-important. Silence, for instance, can 'say' more than words, but has no meaning outside the particular interpersonal and social context. It could be taken to mean the person is experiencing boredom, fear, respect, deep mutual understanding, passion, hatred — the list is potentially endless. Even signals that usually have a well-defined meaning, such as raising the hand to signal 'stop', depend on the context of the two-way flow. If accompanied by a smile, for instance, the raising of the hand could be meant as and understood to be a joke. Furthermore, this model is holistic. Meaning-making is constituted through the organisation and system of a conversation, with the whole being greater than the sum of the parts. Physiotherapist–client communication is not just a means for undertaking physiotherapy practice; the participants are *creating* physiotherapy practice through their communication.

Barriers to communication from the viewpoint of clients

- Inequality of professional–patient relationships
- Attitudinal barriers
- Barriers to access to services
- Barriers to access to information
- Lack of concern on the part of professionals with emotional issues
- Lack of disabled professionals

This takes us into clients' experiences of services, concentrating on barriers to communication, recognising that any analysis of barriers to communication needs to identify the complexities of the communication process itself and the diversity of clients' experiences (Figure 23.1). Such an analysis also needs to recognise the inequality of professional–client relationships. Professional dominance can be seen in assessment procedures where, for example, the professional's observations are viewed as 'objective' whereas the patient's perceptions are viewed as 'subjective', and where pseudoscientific language serves to mystify and confuse service-users (French 1993). Because of the specialisation of the various professional groups, definitions of need tend to be narrow, their

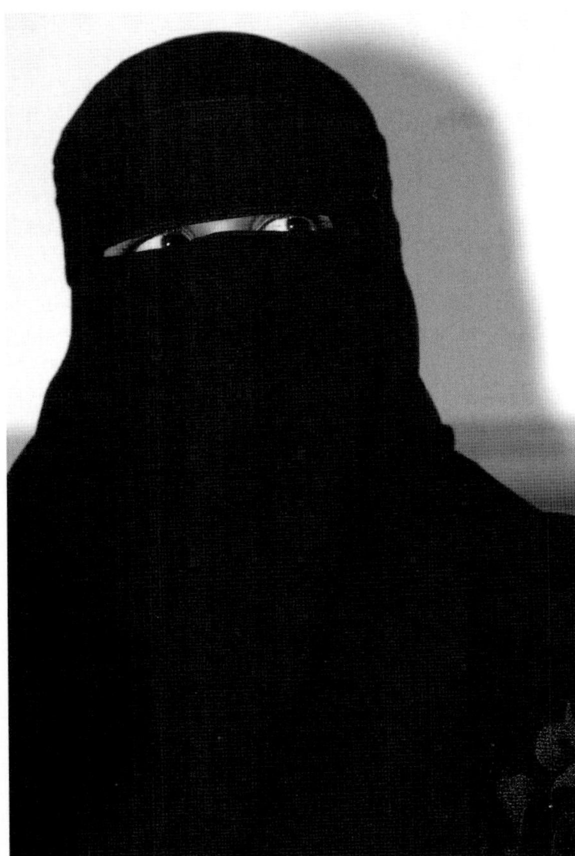

Figure 23.1 Barriers to communication, a means of oppressing women, or a symbol of personal, cultural and religious identity?

scope being dictated by specialised knowledge and interests. The needs of disabled people, on the other hand, tend to be multifaceted. As Marsh and Fisher (1992) point out:

> *If the process of assessment becomes one of professional discovery of 'need', rather than a negotiation of problems, then users tend to feel hemmed in by the definitions used to describe their circumstances and trapped by the choices they are faced with.*

Attitudinal barriers are commonly referred to by disabled clients. Boazman (1999), for instance, had mixed responses from health professionals when she became aphasic following a brain hemorrhage:

> *Their responses towards me varied greatly; some showed great compassion, while others showed complete indifference. I had no way of communicating the fact that I was a bright, intelligent, whole human being. That is what hurt the most.*

Similar mixed experiences were reported by people with aphasia interviewed by Parr and Byng (1997). One person, talking of doctors, said:

> *When you can't communicate they treat you like a kid and that is just so frustrating . . . A handful of doctors were just awful. You just wanted to say, 'Do you know what this is like?'*

Pound and Hewitt (2004) write of the equation of communication disability with 'having nothing to say' and 'being stupid', which, they believe, illustrates the 'Does he take sugar?' syndrome (Figure 23.2). In another small-scale study involving people with speech impairments, it was found that most difficulties were encountered within medical services and doctors' and dentists' receptionists were singled out for particular criticism (Knight et al. 2002). Mary, one participant, recalled:

> *My most embarrassing incidents have been with my doctor's and dentist's receptionists. I have had more trouble with them than with any other group. They were impatient and rude when I tried to make appointments, and would talk to my carer when I was trying to ask questions.*

Another participant described his encounters with hospital consultants (Knight et al. 2002):

> *They have excluded my carer from any discussion despite me indicating that I preferred to have my carer lip-read to avoid having to use my oesophageal voice.*

Another common complaint of the research participants in this study was the means of access to services that generally depended on the telephone.

People with speech and language impairments are often compelled to wait long periods of time for the communication equipment they need. A survey conducted by *Scope* (Ford 2000) found that nearly one-fifth

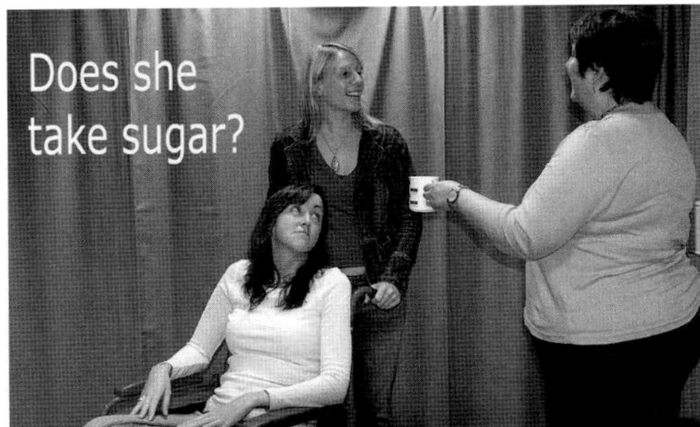

Figure 23.2 Does she take sugar?

of people waited for more than a year. Professionals may also have control of when the equipment can be used. One of the research participants said:

> *Physiotherapists at school have recommended the Delta Talker be removed from situ during travelling because of possible safety problems. They also used to request removal of the talker at meal times.*

Deaf people have complained about the insistence of professionals that they use speech rather than sign language. A deaf person interviewed by Corker (1996) states:

> *I hated learning speech — hated it — I felt so stupid having to repeat the s,s,s . . . I was asking myself 'Why do I have to keep going over and over it? I don't understand what it all means.' . . . It was just so stupid, a waste of time, when I could have been learning more important things.*

In interviews conducted by French (2004a), two participants spoke of their experiences of occupational therapy:

> *I've often thought about OTs in rehab, if only they could think about the context from which their patients came. I was received as head of department of a girls' comprehensive school, head of physical education, and this OT said to me, 'Now you've really got to learn to type because that's what you'll be doing.' She negated the whole context of my professional life — I was just a patient. Just because someone has had an accident or an illness doesn't mean that they've changed one iota. I went in as a gymnast and a sports person; that hadn't changed, it was just that I couldn't do it anymore. There was no acknowledgement of what my life was about or how to shape my new future. They had a routine. It was almost like, 'She's got fingers, she can type.' I couldn't identify with it, there was no link with anything to do with me.*

> *It was a case of being treated like a patient. I felt like my feelings were being ignored, that they were just going through a routine and they would give me exercises to do which I couldn't understand the purpose of because they didn't explain. I had enough speech to ask, but I didn't ask, because I didn't have the confidence to ask.*

Information can also be given in an insensitive way, as Joan (interviewed by French et al. 1997) explained:

> *When I came back for the negatives, oh it was terrible. He lifted them up to the light and he said to the nurse 'Macula degeneration in both eyes, sign a BDS form' or whatever it is. Then he turned to me and he said 'There's nothing we can do about it . . . You'll always be able to see sideways but you've got no central vision' . . . So I came home feeling very upset about it.*

Being unable to access information is a problem faced in all areas of life by visually impaired people, with potentially hazardous consequences of unreadable notices and loss of privacy when documents are unreadable by the intended recipient. Vale (2001) reports that appointment letters continue to be sent out in standard-size print, even by many hospital eye clinics, and only one-third of NHS hospitals offer general patient information in large print.

It is important to recognise that social divisions — for example, gender, age and ethnicity — intersect disability, and also produce communication barriers in some instances. Summarising the evidence from several studies of the experiences of disabled people from ethnic minority communities, Butt and Mirza (1996) state:

> *The fact that major surveys of the experience of disability persist in hardly mentioning the experience of black disabled people should not deter us from appreciating the messages that emerge from existing work. Racism, sexism and disablism intermingle to amplify the need for supportive social care. However, these same factors sometimes mean that black disabled people and their carers get a less than adequate service.*

In their study of young black disabled people's experiences and views, Bignall and Butt (2000) conclude:

> *Our interviews revealed that most of these young people did not have the relevant information to help them achieve independence. Hardly any knew of new provisions, such as Direct Payments, which would help with independent living. Most people did not know where to get help or information they wanted, for example, to move into their own place or go to university.*

Begum (1996) takes institutionalised discrimination as her basis for analysing difficulties in the relationship between disabled women and their GPs. She explored physical, communication and attitudinal barriers and found that they deny opportunities to women with impairments and can impede access to the services they require. Disabled women, for instance, often find that information is withheld from them. One of her respondents explained that she had not initially been told that multiple sclerosis had been diagnosed, yet her husband had been told 2 years before she was informed. It seems too that the flow of information from disabled people to GPs is liable to distortion and failure. This is, at least in part, due to GPs' responses to impairment. One respondent in the research (Begum 1996) said

> *Sometimes I find that a GP — particularly one who is only here for a short time and fairly new — is more*

interested in my sight problem, or my child's sight problem, than in what I've come to ask about.

Age can also be a factor that distorts communication. Olwen (interviewed by French et al. 1997), talking about the attitude of professionals to her loss of sight, said:

> *Even though I'm older, they were 'At your age what can you expect?' You know they talk to you like that.*

Henwood (1993) makes the point that:

> *Services for people with disabilities have been a low priority over many years, and the inadequacy of provision — both in quantity and in quality — is well known. Older people are particularly disadvantaged by this situation because of their greater likelihood of disability.*

Disabled professionals stand in an interesting position in an analysis of communication between professionals and disabled people. It can be argued both that the barriers to communication have discriminated against disabled people wishing to be service providers and also that the acceptance of more disabled people into the professions would be a significant factor in developing inclusive communication. A visually impaired physiotherapist interviewed by French (2001) spoke of poor communication with her colleagues:

> *I'm a registered blind person but they haven't got a clue ... If I stay in one building I'm fine, it's only when I go over to G ... that I get really lost ... and one of the physios says, 'So you're not talking today!' because I've walked right past them ... and I've worked with them for years; oh dear ... I just say 'I didn't see you' but they don't seem to learn.*

Other health professionals have spoken of the advantages they have when communicating with ill and disabled clients. A disabled doctor explains (French 1988):

> *Very many people have told me they can talk to me because I know what it feels like to have an illness. Once you get over that hump of being accepted for training then you can use your disability.*

Cultural differences

Definition

Culture is a general term for the symbolic and learned aspects of human society, a set of basic assumptions – shared solutions to universal problems of external adaptation (how to survive) and internal integration (how to stay together) – which have evolved over time and are handed down from one generation to the next.

Here our focus is on inequality of power, locating culture within its socioeconomic, political and historical context. One layer of power is provided by the wider social relationships in which everyone in health and social care — service users and service providers — are embedded. In this broader social context, there are significant and constantly changing differences in power between people belonging to different groups embedded in different cultures. Some groups have greater power, resources and status, and better health. Others — including members of ethnic minority groups, disabled and older people — can face discrimination in a variety of areas, including access to required services.

Definition

Institutionalised discrimination is unfair or unequal treatment of individuals or groups, which is built into institutional organisations and can result from the majority simply adhering unthinkingly to the existing organisational rules or social norms.

Language, in terms of cultural issues, is often seen as the main barrier to effective service provision. It is, therefore, assumed that an adequate supply of leaflets in appropriate languages and interpreters would solve the problem. However, communication consists of more than language skills and literacy. Research by Banton and Hirsch (2000) suggests that, even among British-born, English-speaking Asians, there is considerable lack of knowledge of what services are on offer. They state:

> *Communication problems are identified in all work in this area. Such problems are partly to do with language differences, but also arise from the separate lives led by different ethnic groups in our society and the consequent unlikely coincidence of communications about services arising through informal contacts.*

Perhaps the most consistent recommendation from research has been the necessity for the direct involvement of disabled clients, including Black disabled clients, in the planning of services (Butt and Box 1997). Again, this needs to be understood within the context of multiple discrimination. Concluding their study with Asian deaf young people and their families, Jones et al. (2001) state:

> *Identities are not closely tied to single issues and young people and their families simultaneously held on to different identity claims. To this extent, it is not a question of forsaking one claim for another and choosing, for instance, 'deafness' over 'ethnicity', but*

to negotiate the space to be deaf and other things as well. It is only through addressing these tensions that services will adequately respond to the needs of Asian deaf people and their families.

In 1991 Hill drew attention to the extremes of oppression faced by Black disabled people. She stated that the cumulative effect of discrimination is such that Black disabled people are 'the most socially, economically and educationally deprived and oppressed members of society.'

Studies of the families of Asian people with learning difficulties also provide evidence of high levels of poverty with 69 per cent of families having no full-time wage-earner and half of the families being on income support (Nadirshaw 1997). Significant language barriers were found in the same study, with 95 per cent of carers being born outside Britain and only a minority able to speak or write English.

There are dangers, however, in such statistics. Firstly, they can feed presumptions and stereotyping which belie diversity. In her study of Asian parents, for instance, Shah (1998) found that 'the majority of parents had a good command of English and, for some, English was their first language.' She also cites language barriers as an example of preconceived notions of discrimination experienced by Asian families. Secondly, there is a danger of oversimplifying language barriers. Language engages us in freedom of expression, release of emotion, developing cultural identity and sharing values. A common language, therefore, is no guarantee of shared understanding. At the attitudinal level of institutional discrimination, there is a lack of understanding among the majority population concerning the lifestyle, social customs and religious practices of people from ethnic minority groups (Atkin et al. 2004). Discrimination has sometimes been denied and rationalised through myths that, for instance, Black families prefer 'to look after their own'.

Comparable analyses of the experiences of the interaction of other social divisions — for example disabled and old, disabled and female, disabled and gay or lesbian, and disabled and working-class — indicate that there are parallels. For instance, in the most extensive research into the views and experiences of disabled lesbians and bisexual women, there was evidence that they felt marginalised by lesbian and gay groups: 'many disabled lesbian and bisexual women have experienced alienation rather than nurturing and support from the lesbian and gay community' (Gillespie-Sells et al. 1998).

23

Another more recent addition to the list of groups with fragmented identities whose interests are not fully taken into account by single-issue movements is disabled refugees and asylum-seekers, who 'constitute one of the most disadvantaged groups within our society' (Roberts 2000). Disabled refugees and asylum-seekers are 'lost in the system' because both 'the disability movement and the refugee community focus their attention ... on issues affecting the majority of their populations and fail to engage adequately with issues which affect a small minority' (Roberts 2000).

CONTEXT OF RELATIONSHIPS

Inequalities in health

To the busy physiotherapist with many patients to treat and assess, it may seem that illness, impairment and accidents 'just happen' and that whether somebody has a fractured hip, a chest infection or a stroke is largely a matter of chance. All the major research reports over the years, however, demonstrate that mortality, morbidity and life expectancy are strongly correlated with socioeconomic class, with those in the lower social classes being at a considerable disadvantage (Townsend et al. 1982; Whitehead 1988). Although Britain has become healthier and wealthier over the years, health inequalities persist; in fact, the gap between the richest and poorest sectors of society has widened (Talley 2004).

Definition

Socioeconomic status is the structural position in society of an individual or a group compared with other individuals and groups. It is a central term in the social sciences and a subject of considerable controversy. In official statistics people are generally classified on the basis of their occupation and income.

Certain groups within society, such as women, old people, people from ethnic minorities and disabled people, are also disadvantaged partly because of their over-representation in the lower socioeconomic groups (Swain and French 2004). This section of the chapter will examine the meaning of health inequalities. In order to do this it is necessary to consider what is meant by 'health'.

Definition

Definitions of health differ between individuals, cultural groups and social classes. One view is that health is the absence of disease or illness. From broader perspectives, health includes the physical, psychological, behavioural, social and spiritual aspects of a state of well-being and recognises the importance to individuals of realising aspirations and needs.

In 1946 the World Health Organization (WHO) defined health as 'a state of complete physical, psychological and social well-being and not merely the absence of disease or infirmity' (WHO 1946, cited in Ewles and Simnett 2003). Although this definition moved the concept of health away from a biological view and towards a more holistic understanding, it was criticised for being idealistic and unrealistic and for failing to recognise that people define their health in a variety of ways based on their knowledge, values and expectations and whether or not they can fulfil roles of importance to them (Jones 2000a). In 1984 WHO (cited in Ewles and Simnett 2003) re-defined health as:

> *the extent to which an individual or group is able, on the one hand, to realise aspirations and satisfy needs; and, on the other hand, to change or cope with the environment. Health is, therefore, seen as a resource for everyday life, not the objective of living; it is a positive concept emphasising social and personal resources as well as physical capacities.*

This holistic definition of health is reflected in the book, *Meeting the Health Needs of People who have a Learning Disability* (Thompson and Pickering 2001), which contains chapters on self-concept, meaningful occupation and life transitions. It can be argued that, unless we feel good about ourselves and have meaning in our lives, such as going to work, raising a family, learning new skills, visiting friends or pursuing hobbies and interests, we cannot be fully healthy.

There are many influences on all aspects of our health. Dahlgren and Whitehead (1995) depict these as layers piled on top of each other. At the bottom of the pile are biological factors over which we have limited, or no, control. These include our sex and age and the genes we inherit from our parents. Many diseases become more common as we grow older (for example, cancer and cardiovascular disease), some diseases are specific to men or women (for example, prostate and ovarian cancer), while others are genetic or congenital in origin (for example, cystic fibrosis and congenital heart disease). When the NHS was established in 1948, it concentrated on this biological layer. It was hoped that improvements in health would eliminate health inequalities (Smith and Goldblatt 2004), but although the overall health of the population gradually improved (mainly through improved living conditions), the gap between the social classes widened (Department of Health 2001).

The second layer focuses on our personal behaviour. This includes whether or not we smoke cigarettes or eat too much, the amount of exercise we take and how well we attend to our health needs in the broadest sense. Most policy initiatives from government have focused on this layer, where attempts have been made to change peoples' behaviour in order to improve their health (Jones 2000b; Owen Hutchinson 2004): for example, in the form of anti-smoking campaigns.

The next layer concerns social and community influences. The people around us, including family members, neighbours, colleagues and friends, can influence our health by giving meaning to our lives and providing assistance and support in times of illness, difficulty and stress. Organisations such as the church and self-help groups may also be important. Conversely, these people can have a detrimental effect on our health by neglect, abuse or failing to take account of our needs. Communication with the people around us does, therefore, have an effect on our health, even if they are not particularly close.

Living and working conditions comprise the next layer of influence. It is well known, for example, that the type of house in which we live and our environment at work can affect our health. Work pressure or noisy neighbours may cause depression and anxiety that can lead to physical ill health (Leon and Walt 2001) and physical hazards, such as dampness, poor architectural design and dangerous work practices, can cause disease and accidents (Talley 2004). Much of the legislation passed by the Victorians improved people's health by tackling problems at this level (Brunton 2004). Various factory, housing and sanitation Acts, for example, reduced the incidence of serious diseases, such as tuberculosis and typhoid, as well as improving the quality of people's lives generally (Gray 2001). Le Fanu (1999) claims that there was a 92 per cent decline in tuberculosis before the introduction of curative drugs. Similar evidence has been put forward by McKeown (1984), who notes that many life-threatening and disabling diseases, such as poliomyelitis and diphtheria, had radically declined before the introduction of inoculation.

The outermost layer affecting our health concerns general socioeconomic, cultural and environmental conditions. This includes the economic state of the country, the level of employment, the tax system, the degree of environmental pollution and our attitudes, for example, towards women, old people, ethnic minorities and disabled people. Increasingly, these factors have taken on an international dimension as globalisation accelerates (Held 2004). It is at this level that government can be particularly influential by implementing policy and passing legislation to bring about wide social change: for instance, seat belt legislation, restrictions on cigarette advertising and equality legislation such as the Sex Discrimination Act (1975), the Disability Discrimination Act (1995) and the Human Rights Act (1998). Despite the individualistic stance of most health policy, the present government has taken some heed of the social determinants of health in, for example, attempting to improve education, housing and transport (Department of Health 1999).

It is clear that these levels all interact and influence each other. If the economic state of the country is favourable, for example, people are likely to have more disposable income, which may improve their health by allowing them to buy good-quality food and housing of a better standard, engage in leisure pursuits, give their children more opportunities and enjoy relaxing holidays to reduce stress. Similarly, if a person is attempting to give up drugs, success is more likely if community support is strong and if government is willing to act by establishing and financing supportive policies. As Whitehead (1995) states:

> *If one health hazard or risk factor is focused upon, it is important to examine how it fits in with other layers of influence and whether it could be considered a primary cause or merely a symptom of a much larger problem represented in some other layer.*

Despite the various influences on our health, the evidence overwhelmingly suggests that broad social factors concerning housing, income, educational level, employment and social integration are more important than our individual behaviour or medical practice and advances (Benzeval et al. 1995; Ewles and Simmett 2003). People of the lowest socioeconomic status are at far higher risk, not only of physical illness and early death, but also of accidents, premature births, mental illness and suicide. Smith and Goldblatt (2004) report that in 1997 the infant mortality rate was one and a half times higher for babies born into the lowest social class than those born into the highest social class and that there was a 5-year difference in longevity between the two social classes. Furthermore, of the 66 major causes of death, 62 were found to be more prevalent in the lowest two social classes. A similar pattern has been found with regard to accident rates among children (Green 2001).

It can be disconcerting for healthcare professionals to realise that there is no obvious correlation between healthcare and health status in any population; indeed, the health service has sometimes been referred to as an 'ill health' service, as it tends to respond when the damage has been done.

This is not to imply that inequalities in health and healthcare facilities should be tolerated. Healthcare should be distributed fairly and in accordance with need. There is evidence, for example, that the uptake of preventative services, such as birth control and screening, is low among poor people (Independent Inquiry into Inequalities in Health 1998). This is due to a range of factors that were summed up by Tudor Hart (1971) in his notion of the 'inverse care' law.

The inverse care law

This law states that those who are most at risk of acquiring illness and disease are least likely to receive medical and social services. This is due to a wide variety of factors relating to social inequalities and the availability of services.

People with low incomes find it harder to access healthcare services because of social isolation and lack of facilities such as a car. It is also the case that the areas in which they live tend to have poor facilities and that health professionals tend to give them less time and attention than people who are perceived to be culturally similar to themselves (French 1997).

There are still many people in Britain who do not fully benefit from the facilities of the NHS. People from ethnic minorities are not well served (Atkin et al. 2004); nor are people with learning difficulties (Shaughnessy and Cruse 2001). As noted in the section on culture, this is due to a variety of factors, which include poor and inadequate communication, racism, disablism and lack of cultural sensitivity.

Different models

Definition

Disability can be defined from an individual model or a social model. The individual model is dominant and assumes that the difficulties faced by disabled people are a direct result of their individual impairments or lack or loss of functioning. The social model of disability recognises the social origin of disability in a society geared by and for non-disabled people. The disadvantages and restrictions, often referred to as barriers, permeate every aspect of the physical and social environment. Disability can, therefore, be defined as a form of social oppression.

In this section of the chapter we will examine two central models of disability — the individual model and the social model — to illustrate the ways in which underlying ideas and concepts can shape physiotherapy practice and wider medical and social policy. A model can be defined as a set of assumptions about how an event or process operates; it usually lies within the framework of a broader theory (French 2004b). Within every society there are competing models of disability, with some being more dominant than others at different times (Oliver 2004; Wilder 2006). In earlier centuries, for example, models of disability were based upon religion (Stiker 1997; Whalley Hammell 2006). Although often in conflict, models of disability may gradually influence and modify each other. The models put forward by powerful groups within society, such as the medical profession, tend to dominate the models of less powerful groups, such as disabled people themselves (Russell 1998; French and Swain 2002).

It is essential to explore these models of disability, for attitudes and behaviour towards disabled people, policy, professional practice and the running of institutions, including hospitals and rehabilitation centres, are based, at least in part, upon them. As Oliver (1993) states:

> *The 'lack of fit' between able-bodied and disabled people's definitions is more than just a semantic quibble for it has important implications both for the provision of services and the ability to control one's life.*

Even the ways in which single words are defined can shape both policy and practice. The work 'independence' is an example.

Definition

The predominant meaning of independence is the ability to do things for oneself. This definition has, however, been challenged by disabled people who view independence in terms of self-determination, control and managing and organising any assistance that is required. Some cultures have a collectivist orientation and do not value independence as much as others. In a very real sense we are all dependent on each other for our survival, so nobody is independent.

Health professionals tend to define independence as 'doing things for yourself,' whereas disabled people define it as having control of your life. Ryan and Holman (1998) state that 'independence is not necessarily about what you can do for yourself, but rather about what others can do for you, in ways that you want it done.'

The individual model of disability

The most widespread view of disability at the present time, at least in the Western world, is based upon the assumption that the difficulties disabled people experience are a direct result of their individual physical, sensory or intellectual impairments (French 2004b; Whalley Hammell 2006; Oliver and Sapey 2006). Thus, the blind person who falls down a hole in the pavement does so because he or she cannot see it, and the person with a motor impairment fails to get into the building because of his or her inability to walk. Problems are thus viewed as residing *within* the individual. The individual model of disability is deeply ingrained and 'taken as given' in the medical, psychological and sociological literature. Even in the literature on the sociology of health and illness, disability as a social problem is rarely acknowledged (Barnes and Mercer 1996; Swain et al. 2003).

The medical model can be regarded as a subcategory of the overarching individual model of disability where disability is conceived as part of the disease process, abnormality and individual tragedy — something that happens to unfortunate individuals on a more or less random basis. Treatment, in turn, is based upon the idea that the problem resides within the individual and must be overcome by the individual's own efforts. Disabled people have, for example, been critical of the countless hours they have spent attempting to learn to walk or talk at the expense of their education and leisure and the way their lives have been dominated by medicine, especially when they were young (Sutherland 1981; Oliver 1996). Mason and Rieser (1992) state:

> *For young people the disadvantages of medical treatment need to be weighted against the possible advantages. Children are not usually asked if they want speech therapy, physiotherapy, orthopaedic surgery, hospitalisation, drugs or cumbersome and ugly 'aids and appliances'. We are not asked whether we want to be put on daily regimes or programmes which use hours of precious play-time. All these things are just imposed on us with the assumption that we share our parents' or therapists' desire for us to be more 'normal' at all costs. We are not even consulted as adults as to whether we think those things had been necessary or useful.*

None of these arguments implies that considering the medical or individual needs of disabled individuals is wrong; the argument is that the individual model has tended to view disability *only* in those terms, focusing almost exclusively on attempts to modify people's impairments and return them or approximate them to 'normal'. The effect of the physical, attitudinal and social environment on disabled people has been largely ignored or regarded as relatively fixed, which has maintained the status quo and kept disabled people in their disadvantaged state within society (Oliver and Sapey 2006). Thus the onus is on disabled people to adapt to a disabling environment (Swain and French 2004). This is something that disabled people are increasingly joining forces to challenge. As Oliver (1996) states:

> *The disability movement throughout the world is rejecting approaches based upon the restoration of*

normality and insisting on approaches based upon the celebration of difference.

Definition

Normality is a dominant, shared expectation of behaviour and personal characteristics that defines what is considered culturally desirable and appropriate.

Individualistic definitions of disability certainly have the potential to do serious harm. The medicalisation of learning disability, whereby people were institutionalised and abused, is one example (Ryan and Thomas 1987; Potts and Fido 1991; Atkinson et al. 2000). Other examples are the practice of oralism, where deaf children were prevented from using sign language and punished for using it (Humphries and Gordon 1992; Dimmock 1993; Corker 1996), and 'sight-saving' school where visually impaired children were prevented from using their sight and, in consequence, were denied a full education (French 2005). All of these policies and practices were rooted in an individual model of disability.

The social model of disability

The social model of disability is often referred to as the 'barriers approach', where disability is viewed not in terms of the individual's impairment, but in terms of environmental, structural and attitudinal barriers that impinge upon the lives of disabled people and which have the potential to impede their inclusion and progress in many areas of life, including employment, education and leisure, unless they are minimised or removed (Oliver 1996). The social model of disability has arisen from the thinking, writings and growing cultural identity of disabled people themselves (Swain and French 2004).

The following definition of impairment and disability is that of the Union of the Physically Impaired Against Segregation (UPIAS), an early radical group of the Disabled People's Movement. Its major importance is that it breaks the link between impairment and disability:

Definitions

Impairment Lacking part or all of a limb, or having a defective limb, organ or mechanism of the body.

Disability The disadvantage or restriction of activity caused by a contemporary social organisation which takes no or little account of people who have physical impairments and thus excludes them from participation in the mainstream of social activities. Physical disability is therefore a particular form of social oppression. (UPIAS 1976)

23

The word 'physical' is now frequently removed from this definition so as to include people with learning difficulties and users of the mental health system (Oliver and Barnes 1998). This, and similar definitions, break the connection between impairment and disability, which are viewed as separate entities with no causal link. This is similar to the distinction made between sex (a biological entity) and gender (a social entity) in the women's movement (Saraga 1998). In recent years, however, it has been recognised that the body is more than a biological entity. Just as height, weight, age and physique have social and cultural dimensions and consequences, so too does impairment (Hughes and Paterson 1997).

The WHO's International Classification of Impairment, Disability and Handicap (ICIDH, 1980) and the revised version, ICIDH-2 (2000), have been rejected by the Disabled People's Movement because, despite taking social and environmental factors into account, the meaning of disability is still underpinned by the medical model and the causal link between impairment and disability remains intact (Pfeiffer 2000; Hurst 2000).

Disability is viewed within the social model in terms of barriers (French 2004b). There are three types of barrier, which all interact:

- *Structural barriers* — which refer to the underlying norms, mores and ideologies of organisations and institutions which are based on judgements of 'normality' and which are sustained by hierarchies of power
- *Environmental barriers* — which refer to physical barriers within the environment (for example, steps, holes in the pavement) and lack of resources for disabled people (for example, lack of Braille and lack of sign language interpreters). It also refers to the ways things are done which may exclude disabled people (for example, the way meetings are conducted and the time allowed for tasks).
- *Attitudinal barriers* — which refer to the adverse attitudes and behaviour of people towards disabled people.

It can be seen that the social model of disability locates disability not within the individual disabled person, but within society. Thus the person who uses a wheelchair is not disabled by paralysis but by building design, lack of lifts, rigid work practices, and the attitudes and behaviour of others (Figures 23.3 and 23.4). Similarly, the visually impaired person is not disabled by lack of sight, but by lack of Braille and large print, cluttered pavements, and stereotypical ideas about blindness. Finkelstein (1981, 1998) has argued that non-disabled people would be equally disabled if the environment were not designed with their needs in mind: for example, if the height of doorways only accommodated wheelchair users. Human beings fashion

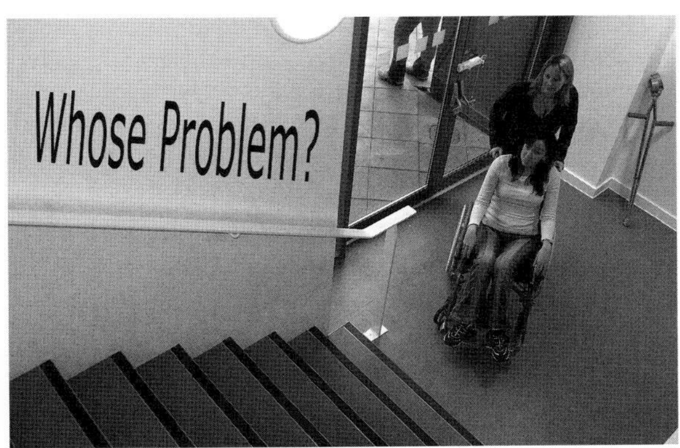

Figure 23.3 Whose problem?

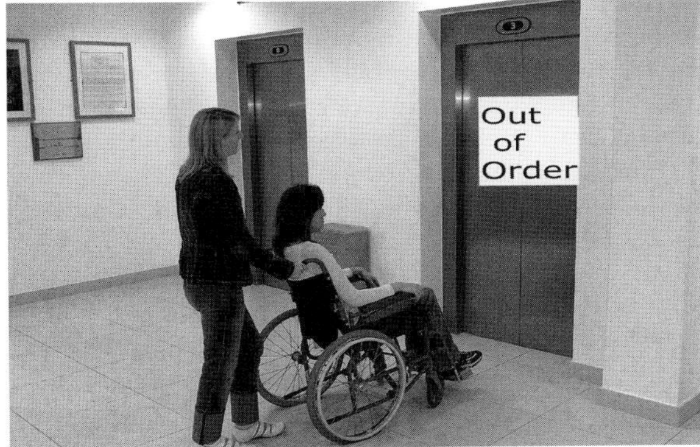

Figure 23.4 Out of order.

the world to suit their own capabilities and limitations and disabled people want nothing more than that.

CHANGING RELATIONSHIPS

Partnership and user involvement

Definition

Looked at broadly, partnership refers to organisations or individuals working together or acting jointly.

In recent policy developments partnership has been a dominant concept signifying the attainment of greater equality in professional–client relations generally. At a policy level, partnership and collaborative working are considered to be 'good' things. Governments of all persuasions have placed emphasis on the need for different agencies to work together to provide more 'seamless' and 'joined-up' service provision by moving towards more integrated health and social care provision (Department of Health 2000a).

Partnership-associated terms

- Inter-agency collaboration
- Joint working
- Multiprofessional practice
- Service user involvement
- Client-centred practice

Partnership in terms of policy, practice and provision has become a buzz-word, widely accepted as an imperative in the development of services for disabled people (and other service users). Defining the concept of partnership, however, is difficult because partnership means different things to different groups of people. It is associated with numerous other terms such as 'participation' and 'empowerment' and also encompasses different relationships.

1. Partnership refers to the relationship between professionals and professional organisations. Associated terms include 'inter-agency collaboration', 'joint working' and 'multi-professional practice'. Cohen (2005) states:

   'Joining-up' is used here in a generic sense to denote the development of a wide range of relationships intended to promote closer and more effective working between services. 'Inter-agency collaboration' is used to refer to a relationship between agencies and services which may involve collaboration in planning, working together on specific issues or projects, or the sharing of posts.

2. Partnership refers to the relationship between service users and the service system. A key term here is 'service user involvement'. This is again mandated within policy. For instance, one of the Department of Health's six medium-term priorities was that health authorities should:

   give greater voice and emphasis to users of NHS services and their carers in their own care, the development and definition of standards set for NHS services locally and the development of NHS policy both locally and nationally (Department of Health 1995:9).

3. Though much less recognised, the term 'partnership' can be applied to relationships between disabled people and other service users, to include partnerships within and between organisations of disabled people. Barnes and Mercer (2006) state:

   The gap between disabled people's expectations and their actual involvement in the statutory and voluntary sectors has reinforced claims from disabled people's organisations that the move to a more equal and democratic society demands a bottom-up approach to politics and policy making. Its potential is realised by the emergence of active user-led organisations.

4. The term 'partnership' also refers to the more immediate relationship between a professional and a service user. This again can encompass different terms such as 'client-centred practice'. Sumsion (2005) defines this as follows:

In the UK client-centred occupational therapy is a partnership between the client and the therapist that empowers the client to engage in functional performance and fulfil their occupational roles in a variety of environments. The clients participate actively in negotiating goals that are given priority and are at the centre of assessment, intervention and evaluation.

In terms of more detailed breakdowns of the meaning of the term partnership, Reynolds (2004) suggests that a partnership approach to healthcare makes the following assumptions:

- Both professionals and service users are regarded as bringing strengths or resources to the therapeutic process and the therapeutic relationship.
- Both professionals and service users are part of the team that will openly share information and make decisions about the ways forward in therapy.
- The relationship is respectful and affirmative, rather than shaped by dependency, submissiveness or power struggles.
- The relationship is based on adult strategies of communication, rather than infantilising, manipulation or stereotyping, with both partners having a respected voice in the interaction.
- The service user is motivated to share responsibility with the therapist for the therapy process and outcome.
- The purpose of the partnership is to promote the service user's self-actualisation, development and quality of life rather than pressurising specifically for better compliance with treatment.

Partnership in therapy practice could include the service users' voices in the following decision-making processes:

- identifying problems to be tackled, issues to be addressed, goals to be achieved
- deciding what steps are to be taken and who needs to do what
- undertaking the necessary work through collaboration and consultation
- reviewing progress and agreeing any changes that need to be made to the agreed course of action
- bringing the work to a close, if and when necessary
- evaluating the work done, highlighting strengths, weaknesses and lessons to be learned (Thompson 1998).

Definition

Inclusive communication is the valuing and celebration of differences and empowerment through the power of communication. The following factors are central:

- participation
- accessible communication
- diversity and flexibility
- human relations
- inclusive language.

The term 'inclusion' has been seen by many as a process of social change, rather than a particular state (Ballard 1999), and this can be seen to apply equally to communication and relationships. To develop this notion of an inclusive communication environment, we shall conclude this section by tentatively offering some general principles based on our previous discussion.

Participation

Priority needs to be given to the participation of service users in the planning and evaluation of changing policy, provision and practice in developing inclusive communication. The onus is on service providers to face the challenges of enabling true participation of service users in decision-making processes, recognising that service users wish to participate in different ways. These include the democratic representation of the views of organisations of service users. Participation also includes as wide a consultation process as possible. Service users often continue to be treated as passively dependent on the expertise of others, yet control has become increasingly central to social change for service users. As a disabled man interviewed by French (2004a), with a great deal of experience of therapy treatment, states:

Users should have more power. Until you give users real power, real control, we'll get nowhere . . . there's an awful lot of people with a lot of vested interests. The more we shout about rights, the more people get afraid. I'd like to see therapy training following the social model rather than the medical model. The only way to do it is to get much more input from disabled people into the training.

The relationship between disabled people and health professionals has never been an easy one, for it is an unequal relationship with the professional holding most of the power. Traditionally, the professional worker has defined, planned and delivered the services while the disabled person has been a passive recipient, with little if any opportunity to exercise control (French and Swain 2001) Disabled people's definitions of the problems they face, and the appropriate solutions to such problems, have generally been given insufficient weight, thereby seriously hampering the rehabilitation process, for if there is no consensus, little real progress can be made.

While physiotherapists may feel constrained by their working role, there usually remains some degree of flexibility in which they can work in partnership with disabled people and other patients and clients. For example, they can share power by sharing 'expert' knowledge and information, and they can encourage patients and clients to participate actively in the writing of reports and case files, so that their voices are heard and their viewpoints represented in official documents.

Awareness of disability on the part of all those who work in physiotherapy departments can be encouraged and developed through disability equality training, run by skilled disabled people. Disability equality training:

> *is primarily about changing the meaning of disability from individual tragedy to social oppression; it emphasises the politics of disability, the social and physical barriers that disabled people face, and the links with other oppressed groups. (French 1996)*

Another way in which physiotherapists can work in partnership is by recognising and acknowledging the disabled person's expertise in relation to the meaning and experience of being disabled and his or her particular impairment. This means encouraging disabled people to exercise choice of services appropriate to their desired lifestyles. Physiotherapists can work in partnership with disabled people by regarding themselves as a resource (expertise, information, advocacy) so that disabled people can work towards achieving their own goals. This would include clarifying the goals to which the disabled person aspires, identifying the barriers that may prevent the realisation of those goals, and working towards removing the barriers.

From the perspective of the social model of disability, professional power can be used to highlight the shortfall in resources for disabled people, to ensure that the voices of disabled people are heard and responded to, and to encourage and support disabled people to assert themselves so that their expertise in disability is at the centre of the development of services and support. It is important that physiotherapists, and all other staff in physiotherapy departments, make a conscious decision to heighten their awareness of disability as an area of enquiry.

Accessible communication

The issues around language and ethnicity are complex but there are many examples of good practice. The Sandwell Integrated Language and Communication Service (SILCS) in the West Midlands, for instance, involves a range of local health organisations — health authorities, NHS Direct, primary care groups, local authorities and voluntary agencies — working together to provide a pooled resource for spoken, written and telephone translation and interpreting, as well as sign language interpreters (Douglas et al. 2004). Accessibility of communication, however, needs management beyond such a resource, including training for staff on using interpreters. The provision of written information in a range of languages must ensure that translations meet the information needs of Black and ethnic minority communities and are culturally relevant. There are, of course, many social factors within the diversity of the needs of people from Black and ethnic minority communities. As Dominelli (1997) argues, for instance, 'translation services should be publicly funded and provide interpreters matched to clients' ethnic grouping, language, religion, class and gender.'

Much is known about the accessibility of information based on the views expressed by disabled people. Clarke (2002) offers wide-ranging recommendations which cover such things as alternative formats — for example, large print, Braille, accessible websites, videotape and British Sign Language, suggestions for plain written language, layout, typeface and font size. For some people, particularly those with communication disabilities, the issue of time can be crucial to an inclusive communication environment. For people with communication disabilities a slower tempo can be the only accessible pace to ensure understanding. A participant within the research by Knight et al. (2002) explains:

> *I would rather repeat myself ten times than have someone finish a sentence for me. This is why I won't use a communication aid. I prefer to speak for myself and I would rather repeat myself several times than have someone say they understood me when they did not.*

Along similar lines, Pound and Hewitt (2004) emphasise that access in meetings requires attention to their length and timing.

Diversity and flexibility

Responding to diversity and being flexible are complex issues, as Douglas et al. (2004) point out:

> *Interpreting is extremely complex in that interpreters must ensure that the patient or client easily understands the language they use. Again other factors, such as class, region, religion and geography,*

may impinge on the process of interpreting and communication — such that just speaking the same language may not necessarily mean the same understanding will follow.

A disabled client interviewed by French (2004a) provides the foundation for this by questioning the focus on 'normality', rather than being flexible and taking the client's perspective into account:

> *What concerns me most of all is this focus on trying to make me 'normal'. I get that from all the therapists. I get a lot of referrals of 'this may help' and 'that may help'. They had a massive case conference before the adaptations — it was a case of 'how normal can we make her first? Are the adaptations necessary?'*

The lists of recommendations for communication access, as produced by Clarke (2002) and others, clearly challenge the imperatives of 'normality' and emphasise the diversity of communication styles and formats (Figure 23.5). Nevertheless, there are diverse needs even within specific groups of people with impairments, which again puts the emphasis on listening to individual people and giving them control. Sally French, as a person with a visual impairment, has found, for example, that she is often presented with large print even though it is the depth, font and colour contrast that are more important to her.

Human relations

Communication is constructed and embedded in relationships between people. The notion of personal relationships can be seen as irrevocably intertwined with communication. Communication is a means of expressing a relationship; it constitutes the initiation, maintenance and ending of a relationship; and it is the medium and substance through which the relationship is defined and given meaning. A disabled client (French 2004a) offered advice to therapists on the basis of her experience:

> *Forget you're a therapist — just be yourself. I don't mean forget all your training — but be yourself. Don't be afraid of showing the real you because that's what makes people respond; when they're ill they respond more easily if the therapist is being real.*

Use of inclusive language

Inclusive language reflects the idea that language controls or constructs thinking. Sexism, ageism, homophobia, racism and disablism are framed within the very

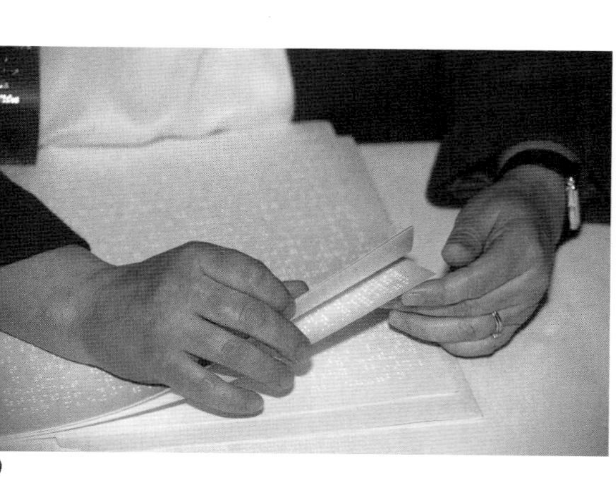

(a)

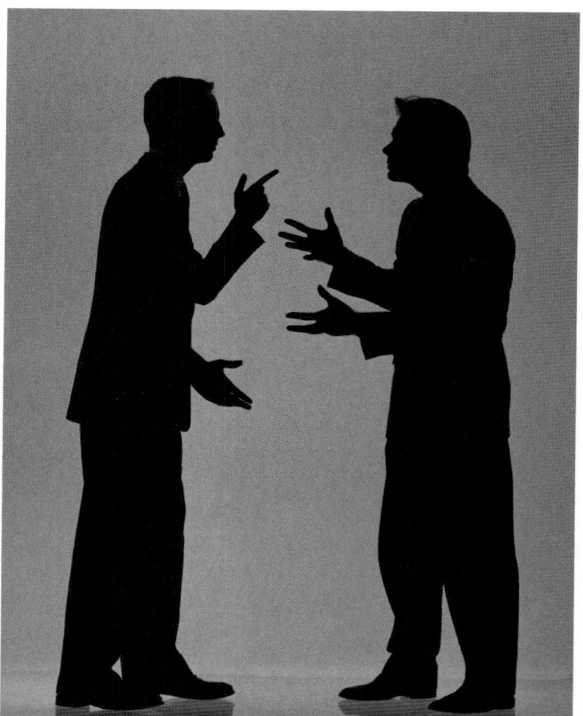

(b)

Figure 23.5 There are many ways to communicate.

23

language we use. This has been characterised and degraded by some people as 'political correctness' (PC), often with reference to examples seen as trivial or fatuous (for example, being criticised for offering black or white coffee). Use of language, however, is not simply about the legitimacy of words or phrases — what we are allowed to say or not say. As Thompson (1998) explains, language is a powerful vehicle within interactions between health and social care professionals and clients. He identifies a number of key issues:

- *Jargon* — the use of specialised language, creating barriers and mystification and reinforcing power differences
- *Stereotypes* — terms used to refer to people that reinforce presumptions: for example, disabled people as 'sufferers'
- *Stigma* — terms that are derogatory and insulting: for example, 'mentally handicapped'
- *Exclusion* — terms that exclude, overlook or marginalise certain groups: for example, the term 'Christian name'
- *Depersonalisation* — terms that are reductionist and dehumanizing: for example, 'the elderly', 'the disabled' and even 'CPs' (to denote people with cerebral palsy).

In this light, questioning the use of language goes well beyond listing acceptable and unacceptable words to examining ways of thinking that rationalise, legitimise and underline unequal therapist–client power relations.

Definition

Service user involvement is a general term that covers service user consultation and collaboration in service policy-making, planning, delivery and evaluation. It can involve:

- giving users information about what others have decided
- consulting users
- making joint decisions with users
- users doing things for themselves and taking control.

In terms of partnership encompassed within the notion of service user involvement, the literature suggests that methods of involving users of services can take many forms. For instance, Brown (2000) lists the following methods with particular reference to residential care for disabled people:

- residents' committees
- user panels
- customer surveys
- suggestion boxes
- involvement in management committees
- involvement in forums and working parties
- focus groups
- public meetings.

Bewley and Glendinning (1994) warn against relying heavily on any one method, as none is perfect and a variety are needed to reach all disabled people. They state:

> *There are a range of methods by which disabled people and voluntary organisations are involved in community care planning and there is nothing necessarily inappropriate about using any of them. What disabled people involved in this project criticised was the reliance by social and health services on a small range of methods to reach and consult all disabled people on all matters; the burdens that involvement placed on individuals; the exclusion of more marginalised groups and communities; and the lack of clarity and debate about the purpose of each method and its suitability for achieving that purpose.*

The following principles do not rely on any particular method but focus on general principles to provide both the foundations for development and a framework for monitoring change through user involvement.

- There is a clear and absolute requirement that the effective development of user involvement must be generated by and controlled by service users themselves.
- The development of user involvement needs to be seen as embedded in all decision-making within the organisation, including financial and management decision-making at all levels (local, regional and national).
- User involvement is embedded in service users' lives. It is part of defining the quality of life for service users. Quality of life is determined within the say that people have over their lives, from day-to-day decisions over basic needs (sleep, eating, toilet and so on) to control over their own finances, and over the support they receive.
- There is no existing model of user involvement that has been developed that can or should be adopted for general usage. Any attempt to do so is more likely to be retrograde than to enhance user involvement.
- There is no body of concern that can be seen as 'user involvement' that is separate or isolated from all decision-making structures and processes within an organisation — finance, management and so on.

- User involvement in policy-making is crucial. Firstly, service users should be involved in the writing of policy, rather than simply being consulted about drafts of policy statements. Secondly, the least restrictive possible policies and practices arising from legislation need to be implemented. Thirdly, in adopting the least restrictive response, policy-making should, as far as possible, be made at a local level, with full user involvement.
- Approaches to user involvement also need to be open, flexible and individual (or client-centred).
- Effective communication is fundamental to user involvement. This includes increased support, communication workers and use of communication equipment at an individual level. It also includes a creative and flexible approach to group meetings, including video conferencing, to open opportunities.

Looking towards inclusion, Bewley and Glendinning (1994) note a heavy reliance on formal meetings in service user involvement and point out that in order to reach Black disabled people, people living in rural areas and other marginalised groups, such as travellers and people with learning difficulties, a community development approach, working with local networks, needs to be adopted on a sustained basis. Carr (2004), in her review of the literature, found that little attention was paid to the diversity of users, even though those from ethnic minorities were often in most need of services. She also found that the belief that disabled people from ethnic minorities 'look after their own' (and therefore do not need services) is still prevalent. Physiotherapists and managers need to ensure that meetings are held in accessible venues and that disabled people are not excluded by lack of transport. Some disabled people may also need support in the form of advocacy to express their views and concerns.

Turning to the standpoint of disabled people, or 'service users', Beresford et al. (1997) note that organisations of disabled people have influenced mainstream services by collaborating on projects and by training professionals in disability issues. Some disabled people feel that this collaboration is strategically important to ensure their involvement in community care, though others are more cautious, fearing that professionals will become too dominant. In their research into self-organised user groups of social and health care services, Barnes et al. (1999) found that the representation of disabled people within key decision-making forums was seen as both an end in itself and a means for achieving other objectives. One participant, for instance, stated:

> *I think the patients' council works well because it does work on the principle that it's not one or two of our service users . . . sitting on the edge of a meeting or whatever; it is managers, senior managers, coming to meetings of service users to be accountable and really they have to account on the spot.*

A very important component of user involvement has been the development of services that are run and controlled by disabled people for disabled people. Drake (1996) states that:

> *disabled people have been increasingly active not only in policy debates but also in producing self-governed groups and projects such as CILs which have proved a cogent and powerful alternative to the traditional gamut of projects like day centres and social clubs.*

Centres for Independent (or Integrated) Living provide a range of services which are designed to meet the needs of disabled people as they define them. These include the provision of information, advice and associated support services; training in the employment of personal assistants; repair services; peer counselling; independent advocacy; and disability equality training. Mercer (2004) believes that:

> *There is a broad consensus that user-led organisations offer a distinctive approach to service provision. This encompasses adherence to a social model, democratic accountability, promoting independent/integrated living through wider user choice and control and including all disabled people.*

From her review of the literature on user involvement Carr (2004) states:

> *Evaluation of user-led organisations for disabled people has shown that there was overwhelming agreement that user-led organisations were far more responsive to disabled people's support needs both in terms of what was on offer and how it was delivered, with peer support a major consideration.*

It is not surprising, then, that Thompson (2001) argues that CILs can act as a model for service provision. If we return to the four relationships or types of partnership outlined above, they can be viewed as interrelated. The partnership between disabled people themselves is a key to shifting the power relations between service providers and service users.

Disability studies (the social, political and cultural analysis of disability) have barely touched the curriculum of health professionals, including physiotherapists, but with the growing impact of the social model of disability, and changes such as the implementation of the Disability Discrimination Act (1995), physiotherapists will need to extend their viewpoint beyond the individual model of disability and to work with disabled people as equal partners. This may mean moving away from the traditional approach of 'helping' and 'treating', towards a much broader brief that involves joining forces with disabled people and using their professional power, in collaboration and partnership with disabled people, to dismantle every aspect of disablism and to further the fight for full citizenship for all disabled people.

Health promotion

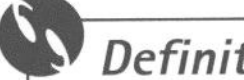

Definition

Health promotion is a broad range of activities that aim to improve health. These include health education, such as teaching correct lifting techniques; environmental measures, such as the control of pollution; preventative medicine, such as cervical screening; fiscal measures, such as financial benefits; and legal measures, such as seat belt legislation.

The profession of physiotherapy has largely taken a biomedical approach to patient and client care. This is strongly reflected in physiotherapy literature and research and the undergraduate curriculum. Over the years, however, education in the social sciences has been included and more physiotherapists now work in the community rather than hospitals, reflecting changes in NHS structure and policy (Department of Heath 2000b). Physiotherapy has, until recent times, been under the control of doctors and physiotherapy practice, with its biomedical orientation, has reflected this control. Tones and Tilford (2001) point out that medicine has focused on the individual and that this has been perpetuated by the greater power of medical professionals when compared with those who work in health promotion. Looking outwards to wide social, political, cultural and economic factors that may impact on people's health and well-being has not been encouraged and, even today, education in the social sciences within physiotherapy is somewhat marginalised and focused on micro-issues such as interpersonal communication (Swain 2004).

This section of the chapter aims to uncover the meaning of health promotion in physiotherapy practice. Health promotion is a complex and contested concept that is defined in many ways (Katz et al. 2000; Scriven 2005). This is not surprising, given that the notion of health itself has a wide range of meanings. Tones and Tilford (2001) state that health promotion:

> *means different things to different people. Since health itself is a multi-dimensional notion — open to multiple interpretations — it is unsurprising that the definition of health promotion is itself problematic.*

Ewles and Simnett (2003) trace the development of health promotion throughout the 20th century. In the first half of the century the main concern was 'public health', which saw, for example, the clearance of the slums, the building of new towns and legislation aimed at reducing environmental pollution. Between 1950 and 1970 the emphasis changed to health education, whereby people were given information designed to persuade them to change their 'unhealthy' behaviours as a way of preventing disease. Schoolchildren, for example, were provided with information about a balanced diet in order to prevent diseases such as diabetes and coronary heart disease in later life. Women were given prenatal and postnatal advice and instruction by physiotherapists, including pelvic floor exercises, in order to reduce complications such as stress incontinence after birth. People were urged to take part in screening programmes and to have their children inoculated against diseases such as poliomyelitis and diphtheria, which can lead to impairment or death. Health education came under criticism on the grounds that it leads to a 'victim-blaming' approach (Naidoo and Wills 1998).

Definition

Victim-blaming may be defined as a tendency to blame the person who is experiencing ill health or other difficulties. A heavy smoker, for example, may be blamed for contracting lung cancer. Victim-blaming denies the influence of wide social, economic, cultural and political factors on people's behaviour, over which they may have little control.

As noted in the discussion on health inequalities, people in deprived circumstances have the fewest choices, including those concerning their health. It may, for example, be more difficult or impossible for them to find the time to exercise regularly, to attend health-screening and health education programmes or to afford a balanced diet. Furthermore, environmental factors, such as noise, pollution and poor housing, impact on their physical and mental health to a greater extent than their more affluent peers. Tones and Tilford (2001) state:

> *a focus on individual sins of omission and commission characterised the approach of preventive medicine and health education for the better part of the 20th century. Increasingly, however, explanations of the determinants of health and disease is shifting away from this narrow orientation on individual behaviours and beginning to emphasise the importance of environmental factors.*

Behaviours labelled unhealthy may be rational strategies to reduce stress caused by wider social and economic factors. Thus the single mother who lives in a high-rise flat in a run-down part of town may smoke in order to cope with her difficult situation. Trying to prevent her from smoking may be both counter-productive and damaging because, for her, the emotional gains outweigh the physical costs. Ewles and Simnett (2003) state:

> *We cannot assume that individual behaviour is the primary cause of ill health . . . There is a danger that focusing on the individual detracts attention from the more significant (and, of course, politically sensitive) determinants of health, such as the social and economic factors of racism, relative deprivation, poverty, housing and unemployment.*

From the 1980s, what is sometimes known as the 'new public health' has emerged. This focuses on both public health and health education and aims to involve people and their communities (Nutbeam and Harris 1999). It encompasses traditional healthcare, personal social services, preventative healthcare, community-based work (for example, the establishment of self-help groups, pressure groups, community facilities and activities), organisational development (for example, equal opportunity policies and measures to reduce stress), public policies (such as education, housing and transport), environmental policies (such as smoke-free zones and noise control) and legislative change (such as the labelling of food and the control of advertising). Nutbeam and Harris (1999) claim that a broad approach to health promotion is likely to be more successful than focusing on one particular area such as education. Broad programmes operate at multiple levels and address a wide range of health-related problems that can be present in a population.

The term 'health promotion' refers to strategies that not only attempt to prevent ill-health and disease in its broadest sense, but also to improve quality of life and well-being (Bunton and Macdonald 2002; Seedhouse 2004). This is in contrast to the biomedical approach, where the emphasis is on finding a cure or managing a condition once it has occurred (Talley 2004). Most definitions of health promotion emphasise the need to empower people to have more choice and control over those aspects of their lives that affect their health, including the communities in which they live. There is a recognition that medicine and professional practice have had little effect on health and that health can be improved more successfully by investing in the physical and social fabric of society and reducing inequalities (Ewles and Simnett 2003). Tones (2001) argues that health services need to be reshaped away from medicalisation and towards the empowerment of patients and clients.

23

Naidoo and Wills (1998) see health promotion as encompassing disease prevention, health education and health information, public health reform and community development. They view the work of those involved in health promotion as emphasising a focus on health not illness, the empowerment of clients, recognising that health is multidimensional, and acknowledging the influence of factors external to individuals that impinge upon their health. They state that, 'Health promotion can take place at the level of individuals, communities, policies and structures.' When attempting to deal with a health issue such as smoking, for example, a wide range of health-promoting activities are necessary, such as health education, developing assertiveness skills, community development such as organising an anti-smoking campaign, and structural adjustments such as legislation to ban cigarette advertising and smoking in public places. They emphasise that a diverse range of information and theories is needed in the practice of health promotion drawn from epidemiology, demography and the social sciences, as well as information about particular community needs and priorities. Ewles and Simmett (2003) list the following approaches to health promotion, which are not necessarily mutually exclusive:

- *The medical approach.* This approach values preventative measures and patient compliance.
- *The behavioural change approach.* This approach seeks to change people's attitudes and behaviour in ways defined by the professional.
- *The educational approach.* In this approach people are given information but their values and choices are respected. The role of the professional is to help people to gain the skills to make well-informed decisions and to offer their help and support.
- *The client-centred approach.* In this approach patients and clients identify what they want to know and what actions, if any, to take. Self-empowerment is central and the professional acts as a facilitator.
- *The social change approach.* In this approach the focus is overtly political and is on changing society rather than changing individuals.

It would seem from the literature and from first-hand accounts from physiotherapists (French and Swain 2005) that physiotherapy practice reflects most strongly the first three approaches listed above. In the *Curriculum Framework for Qualifying Programmes in Physiotherapy* (2002), for instance, the Chartered Society of Physiotherapy defines health promotion in terms of providing advice and health education to patients, carers, support workers and other healthcare professionals. Some disabled people have criticised this apolitical stance, which, they claim, maintains the status quo. Davis (2004), a disabled activist, for example, is fervent in his criticism of health professionals' lack of interest and involvement in the disability rights agenda. Similar critiques of medical professionals and healthcare services have been voiced by sociologists such as Illich (1976) and McKnight (1995), and feminists such as Doyal (1995). Talking of clients with learning difficulties, however, Standing (1999), a physiotherapist, moves towards the client-centred approach. She advocates working in partnership with patients and clients in order to fulfil their unique goals and aspirations and, in consequence, to improve their health and well-being.

Health promotion is a broad and complex concept that demands of physiotherapists a comprehensive understanding of the meaning of health and well-being, both within individual lives and within the communities in which people live. Physiotherapists are playing their part in many aspects of health promotion (Scriven 2005), though mostly in the areas of preventative medicine and health education. Central to moving towards more health-promoting practice is shifting the emphasis from medical and behavioural change approaches towards more client-centred and social change approaches. This shift would involve a broadening of the physiotherapist's role and working in partnership with those engaged in health promotion outside 'traditional' health and social services such as architects, community workers and political campaigners. This will involve many skills, not least those of communicating with a wide range of people from diverse disciplines. As Scriven (2005) points out, this is no easy task within the NHS, where resources are restricted and where curing disease takes precedence over promoting health. An holistic approach towards health and well-being challenges a medicalised view of individuals and extends thinking and activity beyond the individual to the broad social, economic, cultural and political context (Figure 23.6).

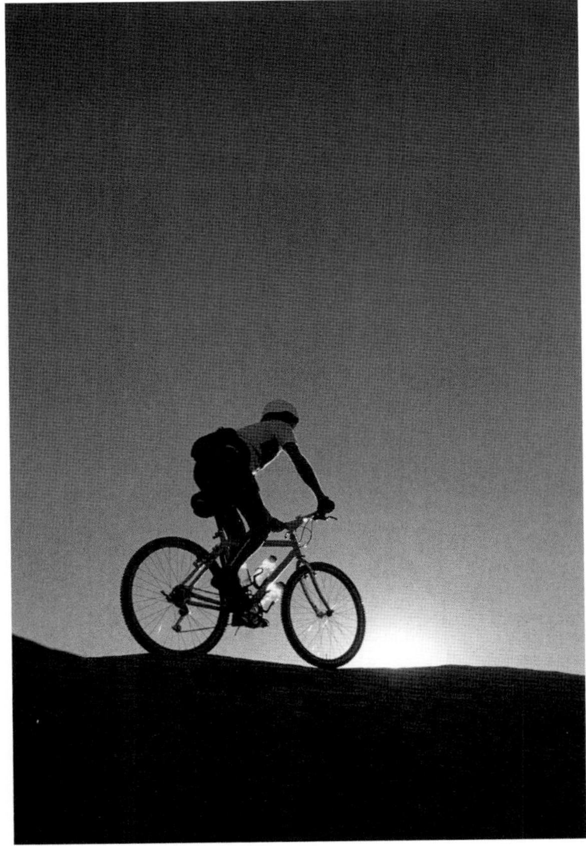

(a)

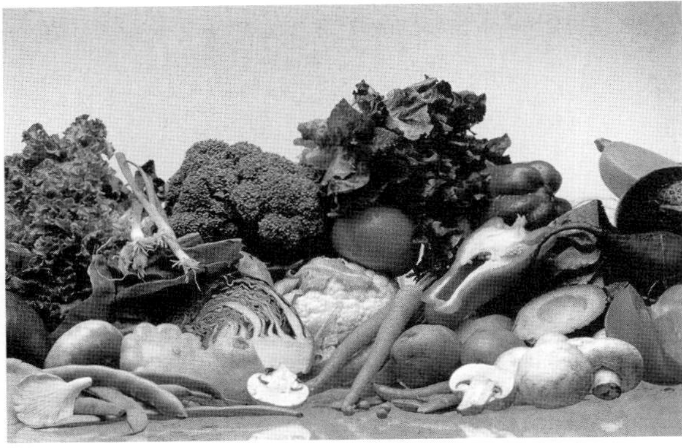

(b)

Figure 23.6 What does this have to do with health?

CONCLUSION

In this chapter we have examined relationships within physiotherapy practice and have discussed how these relationships might change to encompass current reasoning, knowledge, policy and legislation. As front-line workers in the NHS, it is vital that physiotherapists understand the meaning of health, illness and disability from the perspective of patients and clients, and that the physiotherapy service is run flexibly and imaginatively so that people who may benefit from it can use it with ease and convenience and in ways that facilitate their aspirations and goals. Improving health, in its broadest sense, is not just about medicine; it necessitates involvement in areas such as housing, employment, education, leisure, out-reach services and community regeneration. It also demands working *with* rather than *on* or *for* people.

REFERENCES

Atkin K, French S, Vernon A 2004 Health care for people from ethnic minority groups. In: French S, Sim J (eds) Physiotherapy: a psychosocial approach, 3rd edn. Butterworth–Heinemann: Oxford

Atkinson D, McCarthy M, Walmsley J et al. (eds) 2000 Good Times, Bad Times: Women with Learning Difficulties Telling their Stories. British Institute of Learning Disability: Kidderminster

Ballard K 1999 Concluding thoughts. In: Ballard K (ed.) Inclusive Education: International Voices on Disability and Justice. Falmer: London

Banton M, Hirsch M 2000 Double Invisibility: Report on Research into the Needs of Black Disabled People in Coventry, Warwickshire County Council, p. 32

Barnes C, Mercer G (eds) 1996 Exploring the Divide: Illness and Disability. Disability Press: Leeds

Barnes, C, Mercer G 2006 Independent Futures: Creating User-led Disability Services in a Disabling Society. Policy Press: Bristol, pp. 91–92

Barnes M, Harrison S, Mort M, Shardlow P 1999 Unequal Partners: User Group and Community Care. Policy Press: Bristol, p. 24

Begum N 1996 Doctor, doctor … disabled women's experiences of general practitioners. In: Morris J. (ed.) Encounters With Strangers: Feminism and Disability. Women's Press: London, pp. 83–84

Benzeval M, Judge K, Whitehead M 1995 Introduction. In: Benzeval M, Judge K, Whitehead M (eds) Tackling Inequalities in Health: An Agenda for Action. King's Fund: London

Beresford P, Croft S, Evans C, Harding T 1997 Quality in personal social services: the developing role of user involvement in the UK. In: Evans A, Haverinen K, Leichsering K, Wistow G (eds) Developing Quality in Personal Social Services. Ashgate: Aldershot

Bewley C, Glendinning C 1994 Involving Disabled People in Community Care Planning. Joseph Rowntree Foundation: York, p. 16

Bignall T, Butt J 2000 Between Ambition and Achievement: Young Black Disabled People's Views and Experiences of Independence and Independent Living. Policy Press: Bristol, p. 49

Boazman S 1999 Inside aphasia. In: Corker M, French S (eds) Disability Discourse. Open University: Buckingham, pp. 18–19

Brown H 2000 Challenges from service users. In: Brechin A, Brown H, Ely MA (eds) Critical Practice in Health and Social Care. Sage: London

Brunton D 2004 Dealing with disease in populations: public health, 1830–1880. In: Brunton D (ed.) Medicine Transformed: Health, Disease and Society in Europe 1800–1930. Manchester University Press: Manchester

Bunton R, Macdonald G 2002 Health Promotion: Disciplines, Diversity and Developments. Routledge: London

Butt J, Box L 1997 Supportive Services, Effective Strategies: The views of black-led organisations and social care agencies on the future of social care for black communities. Race Equality Unit: London

Butt J, Mirza K 1996 Social Care and Black Communities. Race Equality Unit: London, p. 94

Carr S 2004 Has Service User Involvement Made a Difference to Social Care Services? Social Institute for Excellence: London, p. 12

Clarke L 2002 Liverpool Central Primary Care Trust Accessible Health Information: Project Report: www.leeds.ac.uk/disability-studies

Cohen B 2005 Inter-agency collaboration in context: the 'joining-up agenda'. In: Glaister A, Glaister B (eds) Inter-Agency Collaboration: Providing for Children. Dundee Academic Press: Edinburgh, p. 2

Corker M 1996 Deaf Transitions: Images and Origins of Deaf Families, Deaf Communities and Deaf Identities. Jessica Kingsley: London, p. 29

Curriculum Framework for Qualifying Programmes in Physiotherapy 2002 Chartered Society of Physiotherapy: London

Dahlgren G, Whitehead M 1995 Policies and strategies to promote social equity in health. In: Benzeval M, Judge K, Whitehead M (eds) Tackling Inequalities in Health: an Agenda for Action. King's Fund: London

Davis K 2004 The crafting of good clients. In: Swain J, French S, Barnes C, Thomas C 2004 Disabling Barriers — Enabling Environments, 2nd edn. Sage: London

Department of Health 1995 Priorities and Planning Guidance for the NHS: 1996/97. NHS Executive: London

Department of Health 1999 Saving Lives: Our Healthier Nation. HMSO: London

Department of Health 2000a The Health and Social Care Bill. HMSO: London

Department of Health 2000b The NHS Plan: a Plan for Investment, a Plan for Reform. HMSO: London

Department of Health 2001 The National Health Inequalities Targets. HMSO: London

Dimmock AF 1993 Cruel Legacy: an Introduction to the Record of Deaf People in History. Scottish Workshop: Edinburgh

Dominelli L 1997 Anti-Racist Social Work, 2nd edn. Macmillan: Houndmills, p. 107

Douglas J, Komaromy C, Robb M 2004 Diversity and Difference in Communication, Unit 6 K205. Open University: Milton Keynes, p. 74

Doyal L 1995 What Makes Women Sick: Gender and the Political Economy of Health. Basingstoke. Macmillan.

Drake RF 1996 Understanding Disability Policies. Macmillan: Basingstoke, p. 190

Ewles L, Simnett I 2003 Promoting Health: A Practical Guide, 5th edn. Baillière Tindall, London, pp. 6–7, 41

Finkelstein V 1981 To Deny or Not to Deny Disability. In: Brechin A, Liddiard P, Swain J (eds) Handicap in a Social World. Hodder & Stoughton: Sevenoaks

Finkelstein V 1998 Emancipating disability studies. In: Shakespeare T (ed.) The Disability Reader: Social Science Perspectives. Cassell: London

Ford J 2000 Speak For Yourself. Scope: London, p. 29

French S 1988 Experiences of Disabled Health and Caring Professionals. Sociology of Health and Illness 10(2): 170–188

French S 1993 Setting a record straight. In: Swain J, Finkelstein V, French S, Oliver M (eds) Disabling Barriers — Enabling Environments. Sage: London

French S 1996 Simulation exercises in disability awareness training: a critique. In: Hales G (ed.) Beyond Disability: Towards an Enabling Society. Sage: London, p. 121

French S 1997 Why do people become patients? In: French S (ed.) Physiotherapy: a Psychosocial Approach, 2nd edn. Butterworth–Heinemann: Oxford, pp. 35, 37

French S 2001 Disabled People and Employment: a Study of the Working Lives of Visually Impaired Physiotherapists. Ashgate: Aldershot, p. 140

French S 2004a Enabling relationships in therapy practice. In: Swain J, Clark J, Parry K et al (eds) Enabling Relationships in Health and Social Care: A Guide for Therapists. Butterworth–Heinemann: Oxford, pp. 99, 103, 106

French S 2004b Defining disability: implications for physiotherapy practice. In: French S, Sim J (eds) Physiotherapy: a Psychosocial Approach, 3rd edn. Butterworth–Heinemann: Oxford

French S 2005 Don't look! The history of education for partially sighted children. Br J Visual Impairment 23(3): 108–103

French S, Swain J 2001 The relationship between disabled people and health and welfare professionals. In: Albrecht G, Seelman KD, Bury M (eds) Handbook of Disability Studies. Sage: London

French S, Swain J 2002 The perspective of the disabled people's movement. In: Davies M (ed) The Blackwell Companion to Social Work, 2nd edn. Blackwell: Oxford

French S, Swain J 2005 The culture and context for promoting health through physiotherapy practice. In: Scriven A (ed.) Health Promoting Practice: the Contribution of Nurses and Allied Health Professionals. Palgrave Macmillan: Basingstoke

French S, Gillman M, Swain J 1997 Working with Visually Disabled People: Bridging Theory and Practice. Venture: Birmingham

Gillespie-Sells K, Hill M, Robbins B 1998 She Dances to Different Drums: Research into Disabled Women's Sexuality. London: King's Fund, p. 57

Gray A 2001 The decline of infectious diseases: the case of England. In: Gray A (ed.) World Health and Disease. Open University: Buckingham

Green J 2001 Children and accidents. In: Davey B (ed.) Birth to Old Age: Health in Transition. Open University: Buckingham

Held D (ed.) 2004 A Globalizing World? Culture, Economics, Politics, 2nd edn. Routledge: London

Henwood M 1993 Age discrimination in health care. In: Johnson J, Slater R (eds) Ageing and Later Life. Sage: London, p. 113

Hill M 1991 Race and disability. In: Open University (ed.) Disability — Identity, Sexuality and Relationships: Readings, K665Y course. Open University: Milton Keynes, p. 6

Hughes B, Paterson K 1997 The social model of disability and the disappearing body: towards a sociology of impairment. Disability and Society 12: 225–240

Humphries S, Gordon P 1992 Out of Sight: the Experience of Disability 1900–1950. Northcote House: Plymouth

Hurst R 2000 To revise or not to revise. Disability and Society 15: 1083–1087

Illich I 1976 Limits to Medicine: Medical Nemesis, the Expropriation of Health. Penguin: Harmondsworth

Independent Inquiry into Inequalities in Health 1998 Report. HMSO: London

Jones L 2000a Promoting health: everybody's business? In: Katz J, Peberdy A, Douglas J (eds) Promoting Health: Knowledge and Practice, 2nd edn. Palgrave: Basingstoke

Jones L 2000b Behavioural and environmental influences on health. In: Katz J, Peberdy A, Douglas J (eds) Promoting Health: Knowledge and Practice, 2nd edn. Palgrave: Basingstoke

Jones L, Atkin K, Ahmad WIU 2001 Supporting Asian deaf young people and their families: The role of professionals and services. Disability and Society 16(1): 51–70

Katz J, Peberdy A, Douglas J (eds) 2000 Promoting Health: Knowledge and Practice, 2nd edn. Palgrave: Basingstoke

Knight B, Sked A, Garrill J 2002 Breaking the Silence: Identification of the Communication and Support Needs of Adults with Speech Disabilities in Newcastle. CENTRIS: Newcastle, pp. 17, 19

Le Fanu J 1999 The Rise and Fall of Modern Medicine. Little, Brown: London

Leon D, Walt G 2001 Poverty, Inequality and health in international perspective: a divided world? In: Leon D, Walt G (eds) Poverty, Inequality and Health: an International Perspective. Oxford University Press: Oxford

Marsh P, Fisher M 1992 Good Intentions: Developing Partnership in Social Services. Joseph Rowntree Foundation, London, p. 50

Mason M, Rieser R 1992 The limits of 'medicine'. In: Rieser R, Mason M (eds) Disability Equality in the Classroom: a Human Rights Issue, 2nd edn. Disability Equality in Education: London, p. 82

McKeown T 1984 The medical contribution. In Black N, Boswell D, Gray A et al. (eds) Health and Disease: a Reader. Open University: Buckingham

McKnight J 1995 The Careless Society. Basic Books: London

Mercer G 2004 User-led organisations: facilitating independent living. In: Swain J, French S, Barnes C, Thomas C (eds) Disabling Barriers — Enabling Environments, 2nd edn. Sage: London, p. 179

Nadirshaw Z 1997 Cultural issues. In: O'Hara J, Sperlinger A (eds) Adults with Learning Difficulties. John Wiley: London

Naidoo J, Wills J 1998 Practising Health Promotion: Dilemmas and Challenges. Baillière Tindall: London, p. 4

Nutbeam D, Harris E 1999 Theory in a Nutshell: A Guide to Health Promotion Theory. McGraw-Hill: London

Oliver M 1993 Re-defining disability: a challenge to research. In: Swain J, French S, Barnes C, Thomas C (eds) Disabling Barriers — Enabling Environments, 2nd edn. Sage: London, p. 61

Oliver M 1996 Understanding Disability: From Theory to Practice. Macmillan: London, p. 44

Oliver M 2004 If I had a hammer: the social model in action. In: Swain J, French S, Barnes C, Thomas C (eds) Disabling Barriers — Enabling Environments, 2nd edn. Sage: London

Oliver M, Barnes C 1998 Disabled People and Social Policy: from Exclusion to Inclusion. Longman: London

Oliver M, Sapey B 2006 Social Work with Disabled People, 3rd edn. Macmillan: London

Owen Hutchinson J 2004 Health, Health Education and Physiotherapy Practice. In: French S, Sim J (eds) Physiotherapy: a Psychosocial Approach, 3rd edn. Butterworth–Heinemann: Oxford

Parr S, Byng S 1997 Talking about Aphasia. Open University: Buckingham, p. 74

Pearce WB 1994 Interpersonal Communication: Making Social Worlds. HarperCollins: New York

Pfeiffer D 2000 The Devils are in the Details: the ICIDH2 and the disability movement. Disability and Society 15: 1079–1082

Potts M, Fido R 1991 A Fit Person to be Removed: Personal Accounts of Life in a Mental Deficiency Institution. Northcote House: Plymouth

Pound C, Hewitt A 2004 Communication barriers: building access and identity. In: Swain J, Barnes C, French S, Thomas C (eds) Disabling Barriers — Enabling Environments. Sage: London

Reynolds F 2004 The professional context. In: Swain J, Clark J, Parry K et al. Enabling Relationships in Health and Social Care: A Guide for Therapists. Butterworth–Heinemann: Oxford

Roberts K 2000 Lost in the system: disabled refugees and asylum seekers in Britain. Disability and Society 15(6): 943–948

Rungapadiachy DV 1999 Interpersonal Communication and Psychology for Health Care Professionals: Theory and Practice. Butterworth–Heinemann: Oxford

Russell M 1998 Beyond Ramps: Disability at the End of the Social Contract. Common Courage: Monroe, ME

Ryan J, Thomas F 1987 The Politics of Mental Handicap, 2nd edn. Free Association: London

Ryan T, Holman A 1998 Able and Willing: Supporting People with Learning Difficulties to use Direct Payments. Values into Action: London, p. 19

Saraga E 1998 Embodying the Social: Constructions of Difference. Routledge: London

Scriven A 2005 Health promoting practice: a context and overview. In: Scriven A (ed.) Health Promoting Practice: the Contribution of Nurses and Allied Health Professionals. Palgrave Macmillan: Basingstoke

Seedhouse D 2004 Health Promotion: Philosophy, Prejudice and Practice, 2nd edn. Wiley: Chichester

Shah R 1998 'He's our child and we shall always love him' — Mental handicap: the parents' response. In: Allott M, Robb M (eds) Understanding Health and Social Care: An Introductory Reader. Sage: London, p. 186

Shaughnessy P, Cruse S 2001 Health Promotion with people who have a learning disability. In: Thompson J, Pickering S (eds) Meeting the Health Needs of People who have a Learning Disability. Baillière Tindall: London

Smith B, Goldblatt D 2004 Whose health is it anyway? In: Hitchliffe S, Woodward K (eds) The Natural and the Social: Uncertainty, Risk, Change, 2nd edn. Routledge: London

Standing S 1999 The practice of working in partnership. In: Swain J, French S (eds) Therapy and Learning Difficulties: Advocacy, Partnership and Participation. Butterworth–Heinemann: Oxford

Stiker H 1997 A History of Disability. University of Michigan Press: Michigan

Sumsion T 2005 Promoting health through client centred occupational therapy practice. In: Scriven A (ed.) Health Promoting Practice: The Contribution of Nurses and Allied Health Professionals. Palgrave Macmillan: Houndmills, p. 100

Sutherland AT (1981) Disabled We Stand. Souvenir: London

Swain J 2004 Interpersonal communication. In: French S, Sim J (eds) Physiotherapy: a Psychosocial Approach, 3rd edn. Butterworth–Heinemann: Oxford

Swain J, French S 2004 Understanding inequality and power. In: Swain J, Clark J, French S (eds) Enabling Relationships in Health and Social Care: a Guide for Therapists. Butterworth–Heinemann: Oxford

Swain J, French S, Cameron C 2003 Controversial Issues in a Disabling Society. Buckingham: Open University

Talley J 2004 Change, diversity and influences on patterns of health and ill health. In: French S, Sim J (eds) Physiotherapy: A Psychosocial Approach, 3rd edn. Butterworth–Heinemann: Oxford

Thompson N 1998 Promoting Equality. Macmillan: Basingstoke, p. 213

Thompson N 2001 Anti-Discrimination Practice, 3rd edn. Palgrave: Houndmills

Thompson J, Pickering S (eds) 2001 Meeting the Health Needs of People who have a Learning Disability. Baillière Tindall: London

Tones K 2001 Health promotion: the empowerment imperative. In: Scriven A, Orme J (eds) Health Promotion: Professionals' Perspectives, 2nd edn. Palgrave: Basingstoke

Tones K, Tilford S 2001 Health Promotion: Effectiveness, Efficiency and Equity, 3rd edn. Nelson Thormes: Cheltenham, pp. 2, 7

Townsend P, Davidson N eds 1982 Inequalities in Health: the Black Report. Penguin: Harmondsworth

Tudor Hart J 1971 The Inverse Care Law. Lancet 401–412

Union of the Physically Impaired Against Segregation 1976 Fundamental Principles of Disability. UPIAS: London, p. 14

Vale D 2001 Improving Lives: Priorities in health social care for blind and partially sighted people. On behalf of the Improving Lives Coalition by the Royal National Institute for the Blind: London

Whalley Hammell K 2006 Perspectives on Disability and Rehabilitation: Contesting Assumptions; Challenging Practice. Elsevier: Oxford

Whitehead M 1988 The Health Divide. Penguin: Harmondsworth

Whitehead M 1995 Tackling inequalities: a review of inequalities. In: Benzeval M, Judge K, Whitehead M (eds) Tackling Inequalities in Health: an Agenda for Action. King's Fund: London, p. 24

Wilder EI 2006 Wheeling and Dealing: Living with Spinal Cord Injury. Wanderbilt University Press: Nashville

Chapter **24**

Upper and lower limb joint arthroplasty

Ann Birch and Ann Price

CHAPTER CONTENTS

INTRODUCTION

There is no 'typical' patient who is appropriate for a joint arthroplasty. As with all modern medicine, a decision has to be made that balances the risks of surgery against the potential improvements.

Patient age per se is no longer an acceptable clinical decision-making tool (Brander et al. 1997). Generally, the surgical team will wait until pain or disability is severe enough to cause a significant impact on the person's quality of life, where surgery would make things significantly better or prevent a major deterioration. It is quite feasible, for example, to replace the hips of a 16-year-old with severe rheumatoid arthritis. An artificial joint is not as efficient as its organic counterpart. If a synthetic joint becomes worn or damaged, it does not repair itself as a normal joint does. It will also not be as efficient at absorbing the stresses and strains of daily life as an organic joint. The field of joint prosthetics is making remarkable improvements, however.

UPPER LIMB ARTHROPLASTY

There are prostheses available for every joint in the upper limb. Elbow, wrist and finger arthroplasties are mainly performed for patients with rheumatoid arthritis, although metacarpophalangeal (MCP) and proximal interphalangeal (PIP) joints are now being developed for patients with osteoarthritis and following trauma. The carpometacarpal joint of the thumb is the most common joint replacement for osteoarthritis. There are also prostheses available to replace the ulnar head and the radial head; these are normally used for reconstruction following difficult forearm and elbow fractures.

This part of the chapter will look at the two most common upper limb joint arthroplasties in some detail:

shoulder and MCP joints. It also includes a selection of illustrations of other upper limb arthroplasties.

SHOULDER ARTHROPLASTY

Developments

The first shoulder arthroplasty is thought to have been carried out in 1894 (Hamblen 1984) but it was in 1951 that the modern story of shoulder replacement began.

In 1951 Charles Neer developed a hemi-arthroplasty, primarily for the reconstruction of severe proximal humerus fractures. However, it was also used for people suffering from osteoarthritis, with surprisingly good results. In 1973 Neer redesigned the humeral component and added a glenoid to make the first unconstrained total shoulder arthroplasty (TSR) — known as the Neer II. The basis of the design was to produce as near to an anatomical replacement as possible. Neer published his early results in 1982 (Neer et al. 1982). This principle is followed in most modern prostheses.

A single-piece prosthesis, such as the Neer, would require a huge number of sizes to be kept in stock, in order to cater for the variety of dimensions encountered in the population. To attempt to address this problem, modular systems such as the 'global shoulder' have been developed, in which different sizes of shaft, head and glenoid can be interchanged (Figures 24.1 and 24.2).

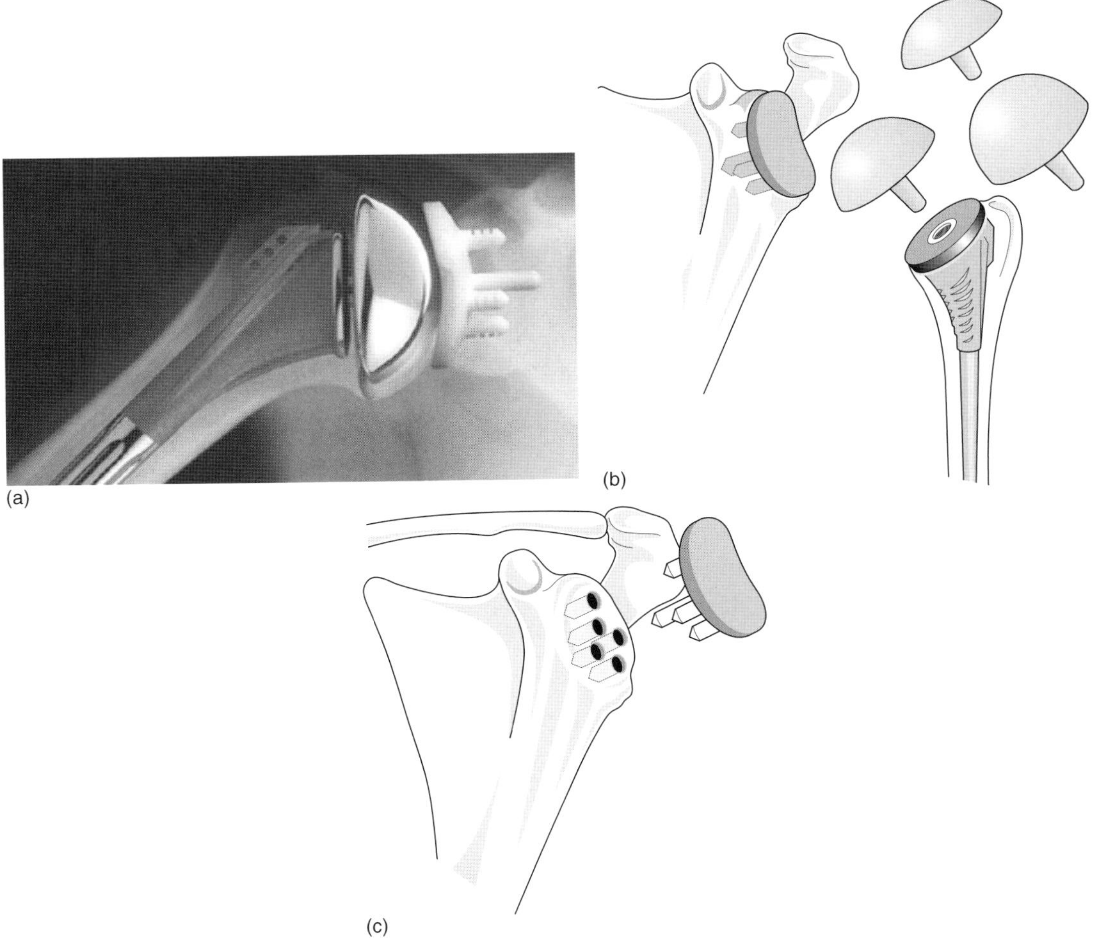

Figure 24.1 (a) The global shoulder implant. (b) Sketch to demonstrate the different heights of humeral head available. (c) Sketch to show how the glenoid component is attached to the glenoid fossa. (Reproduced by kind permission of De Puy Orthopaedics Inc., IN, USA.)

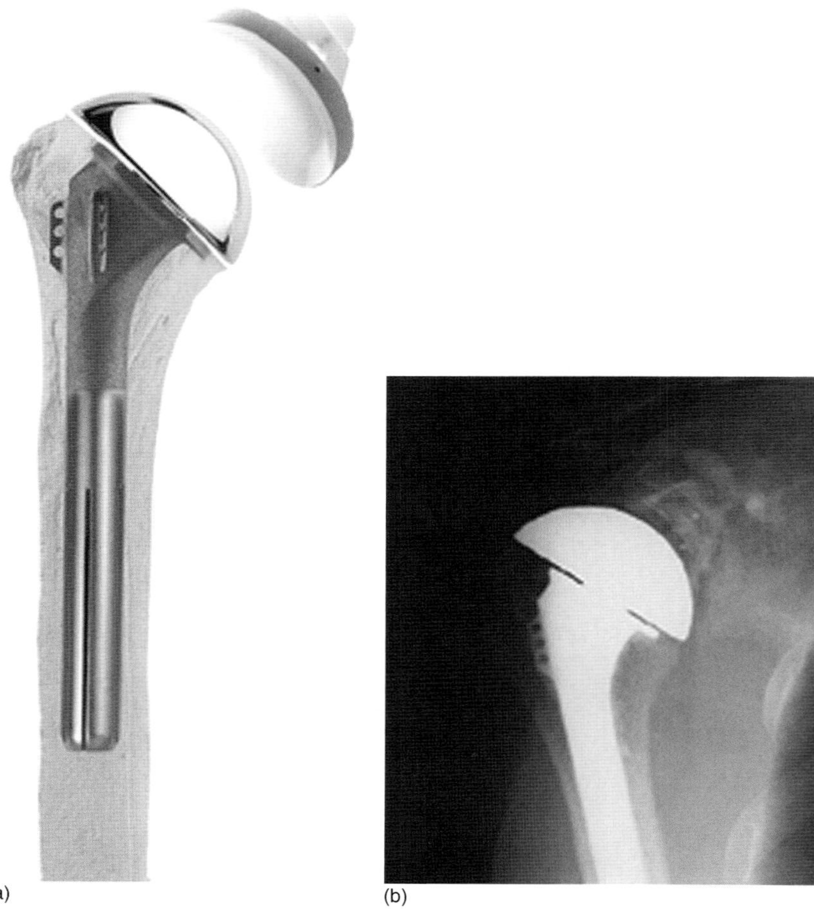

(a) (b)

Figure 24.2 Shoulder replacement showing humeral and glenoid components and the appearance on X-ray. (Reproduced by kind permission of Adam C. Gaines.)

Key point

There are currently 20 different prosthetic systems in use in the UK (Mackay et al. 2001). A survey carried out by Mackay and Williams (1999) suggested that around 2800 shoulder replacements were carried out in the UK in 1998.

Factors influencing outcome of shoulder arthroplasty

There are many factors influencing the outcome of shoulder arthroplasty (Iannotti and Williams 1998; Table 24.1). It is mainly in the last section, that of the rehabilitation programme, that physiotherapists have influence, but practitioners need to know as much about the other factors as possible so that realistic goals can be set. We do not want patients to be given unrealistic expectations, but neither do we want them to fail to achieve their full potential. Good communication with the surgical team is therefore very important.

Key point

There are three main situations in which a shoulder arthroplasty operation is performed: in osteoarthritis, in rheumatoid arthritis, and following a complex fracture.

Table 24.1 Factors affecting outcome of prosthetic shoulder reconstruction

Pathology
- Rotator cuff disease
- Glenoid erosion bone loss
- Humeral bone loss
- Bone loss
- Bone density

Surgical technique
- Prosthetic placement
- Prosthetic–cement–bone interface
- Soft-tissue balancing

Prosthetic design
- Size selection
  Glenoid
  Humeral head
  Humeral stem
- Offsets
- Material properties

Rehabilitation programme
- Range of motion
- Strength
- Stability

Table 24.2 Example of postoperative routine following primary total shoulder arthroplasty for osteoarthritis

Day 1
- Usual postoperative check, maintenance of range of movement in hand and wrist

Day 2
- Assisted active flexion and abduction, first by physiotherapist followed by teaching patient-assisted active of same movements using pulleys and exercise stick
- Patient is taught to do exercises × 4 daily

Day 3 to 3 weeks
- Continue with exercises as above and add extension, internal rotation and lateral rotation to 30 degrees, with the arm by the side. Abduction should always be with the arm in neutral as the combined movement of abduction and lateral rotation should not be attempted until 6 weeks post-op
- The patient can progress from assisted active to active movement as able. Once the person is comfortable he or she may begin to use the arm for self-care activities within the limits of pain and strength

3 weeks to 6 weeks
- The patient should now have discarded the sling completely during the day and should be progressing from assisted active to active movement. The physiotherapist will be showing appropriate ways to do this
- Active external rotation can be progressed beyond 30 degrees but stretching should still be avoided

6 weeks to 3 months
- Progressive strengthening exercises in all ranges should be encouraged according to the patient's individual capabilities. Rotator cuff strengthening should be emphasised, using a progressive system such as Theraband

3 months onwards
- Many patients are discharged from treatment but should be encouraged to continue with strengthening exercises until optimum function has been achieved

Primary osteoarthritis (OA)

This is the indication for TSR from which the best results can be expected. Godenèche et al. (2002) reviewed a series of 267 operations for osteoarthritis and found that 77 per cent of them had results that were classed as good or excellent. They found that the result was dependent on the severity of the degenerative changes that had taken place prior to surgery. It seems, therefore, that for patients who have primary osteoarthritis without gross soft-tissue damage or loss of bone, we can expect to achieve near-normal range of movement and strength. Patients who start off with rotator cuff disease or glenoid erosion should have less high expectations.

Procedure

The most common surgical approach is known as the 'deltopectoral approach'. The incision passes between the deltoid and pectoralis major, and access to the shoulder joint is via the subscapularis muscle and the anterior part of the capsule. Thus the subscapularis muscle is the only active structure that will need to be protected in the early postoperative period.

Table 24.2 shows a typical postoperative protocol. Details will vary, depending on surgeon preference. As always, the postoperative regimen must be agreed between the surgeon and the physiotherapy team.

Rheumatoid arthritis (RA)

People with RA who undergo shoulder arthroplasty are likely to have a number of the adverse pathological factors listed in Table 24.1. The expected results will depend on how many and how severe they are.

People with rheumatoid arthritis do not tend to be referred for replacement arthroplasty until these factors are fairly advanced, so the results are generally not as good as in osteoarthritic patients. The surgical approach and basic postoperative management are the same.

In advanced disease of either the osteoarthritis or rheumatoid arthritis type, it is not always possible to insert a glenoid component. If there is gross bone loss around the glenoid fossa, it is not possible to attach the implant securely enough. Also, the lack of rotator cuff function causes the humeral head to 'rock' the glenoid component, causing loosening. The problem of glenoid fixation is one of the ongoing dilemmas in shoulder arthroplasty.

Complex fracture

Following a complex fracture, it is normally a hemiarthroplasty that is performed, as the glenoid is intact.

The operation can be performed either acutely as the primary treatment for the fracture, or later as a secondary procedure. The results are better if it is performed acutely. This is a different operation from the one performed as an elective procedure, as there is disruption of the tuberosities to which the rotator cuff muscles are attached. The challenge to the surgeon is to restore the anatomy to as close to normal as possible and to attach the tuberosities securely enough so that mobilisation can be commenced early.

The trauma that caused the fracture will also have caused soft-tissue damage, so the physiotherapy regimen must take this into account as well. Once again, details may vary from surgeon to surgeon, and individual patients will have different concurrent injuries, so the regimen will have to be personalised to take account of these.

METACARPOPHALANGEAL JOINT REPLACEMENT

Rheumatoid arthritis can affect any joint in the body, but it is particularly devastating to the complex collection of joints and intricate soft tissues that make up the hand. The most obvious aspect of the deformity, shown in Figure 24.3, is the ulnar deviation of the fingers referred to by the French as *coup de vent* or windswept; the more functionally debilitating deformity, however, is the volar subluxation of the metacarpal heads, as this robs the flexor tendons of a proportion of their power, thus weakening grip.

24

Key point

A principal role of the upper limb is to allow for maximum use of the hand. Without a functioning hand, the rest of the upper limb becomes mainly a component of balance.

The factors influencing the development of deformities at the MCP joint are complex. They have been well described in rheumatology and hand therapy textbooks.

Surgical procedures

There are many reconstructive and preventative procedures that can be performed for this condition, but by far the most common is the replacement of the MCP joint by a silastic flexible hinge (Figure 24.4). Swanson developed this in the 1960s when he saw that the results of simple resection arthroplasty were unsatisfactory (Swanson et al. 2000). There have been other attempts at designing MCP joint replacements, but none so far has stood the test of time like the Swanson version.

Key point

Swanson devised an equation to explain the process: bone resection + implant + encapsulation = new joint (Swanson et al. 1978).

A flexible implant arthroplasty is different in principle from other joint arthroplasties in that the implant acts as an inert flexible spacer, which is quickly

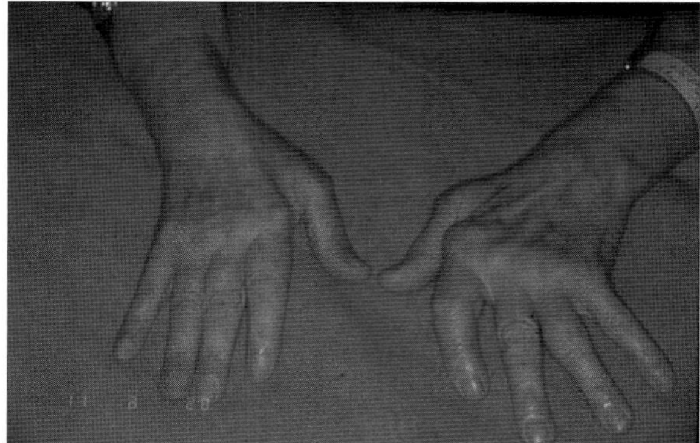

Figure 24.3 The hands of a person with rheumatoid arthritis showing the common deformities of ulnar drift and subluxation of the MCP joints.

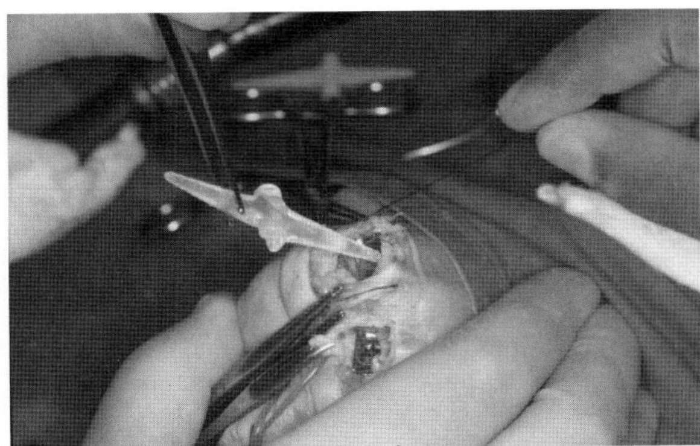

Figure 24.4 Insertion of a Swanson silastic MCP flexible implant. (Reproduced courtesy of Wright Medical Inc.)

surrounded by a layer of synovial tissue. The new tissue remains in contact with the implant and surrounding this a stronger capsule develops.

As well as excising the destroyed joint surfaces and inserting the flexible hinge, the surgeon must release and rebalance the soft tissues crossing the joint if function is to be restored.

Postoperative management

The short-term aims are:

- to achieve a functional arc of movement
- to protect soft tissue repairs
- to prevent further deformity at the affected joint and the development of secondary deformities/pathological change in the related musculoskeletal system
- to strengthen weak muscles
- to re-educate function
- to teach specific joint protection techniques.

The short-term aims are achieved by early controlled movement, which stimulates the formation of a strong but flexible capsule around the implant. The pattern of collagen formation is influenced by the forces applied to it. The dynamic splint allows movement to take place only in a flexion–extension arc, which influences the collagen to be laid down in straight parallel lines rather than in a haphazard manner (Swanson et al. 1978).

The most common way of controlling the movement is by the use of a dynamic extension splint (DES), often referred to as an 'outrigger' (Figure 24.5a). This provides proprioceptive input for the patient to carry out flexion at the MCP joint and provides assistance for the weak extensor muscles. In recent years, static splinting regimes have also been developed, which involve the patient taking the splint off for exercise but wearing it all the time in between (Burr and Pratt 2003).

Longer-term aims are achieved by strengthening exercises, re-education of pulp–pulp pinch, and education in joint protection techniques. When the outrigger is first removed, patients are fitted with a splint to wear when doing heavier functional activities, to protect against the ulnar deviation forces that are inherent in strong gripping (Figure 24.6).

An example of a postoperative regimen is given in Table 24.3. An example of how two static splints can be used instead of a dynamic splint is shown in Figure 24.7. These are examples; details will vary greatly from unit to unit.

Static regime

This involves the use of two static splints:

- Splint1:
  Wrist extension 30 degrees
  MCPs flexed, ideally 60–70 degrees
  IPs extended 0 degrees
- Splint 2:
  Wrist extension 30 degrees
  MCPs extended 0 degrees
  IPs extended 0 degrees

The splints are alternated every 24 hours.
Splints are removed hourly during the day for active exercise:

- isolated MCP joint flexion
- isolated IP joint flexion
- mass flexion
- passive MCP joint extension
- active MCP joint extension
- radial finger walking.

Clinical note

When treating rheumatoid patients following surgery, always remember that they have a systemic disease; postoperative regimens often need to be individually tailored to take account of other deformities.

Expected outcome

The patient normally attends the department for treatment and education until 3 months after surgery. By that time it is hoped that the person will have gained:

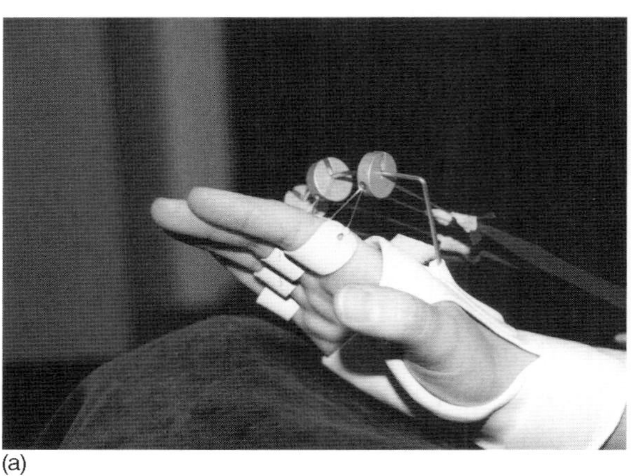

(a)

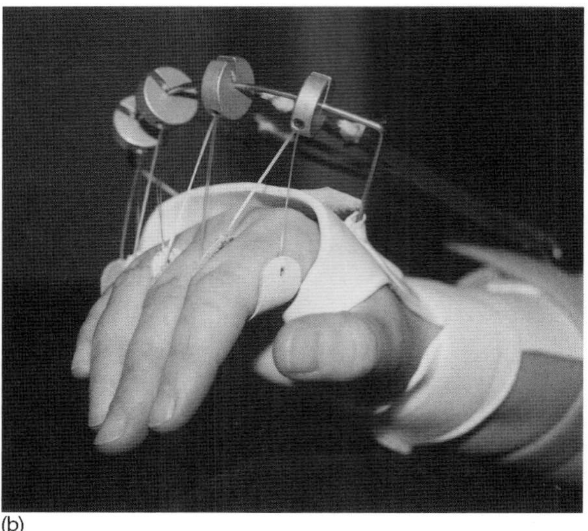

(b)

Figure 24.5 (a) Dynamic extension splint (outrigger) in the resting position. (b) Flexion at the MCP joints against the resistance of the elastic bands.

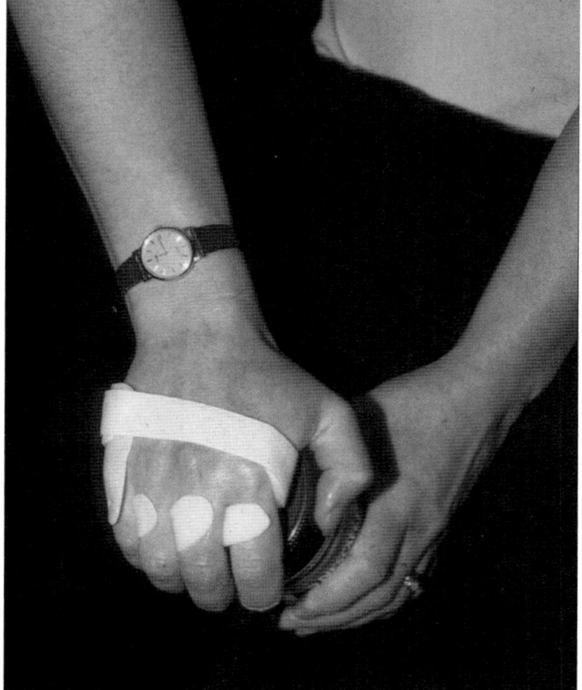

Figure 24.6 Splint to protect against recurrence of ulnar drift. Protection is particularly important in strong gripping activities.

- a functional grip
- the ability to open the hand wide enough to grasp jars and glasses
- the ability to manipulate small objects such as coins or buttons with pulp-to-pulp pinch.

Delaney and Stanley (2000) have shown that the range of movement, particularly into extension, can continue to increase for up to 12 months following surgery. The average range of movement from this study was from 20 degrees of flexion to 70 degrees of flexion, although the enhanced stability of the joints and the functional factors listed above are far more important than the actual range of movement.

EXAMPLES OF OTHER UPPER LIMB ARTHROPLASTIES

Figures 24.8–24.11 show photographs of radial head, wrist, finger and trapezium arthroplasty photographs and X-rays.

LOWER LIMB ARTHROPLASTY

Modern successful joint replacements are based on appropriate patient selection, selection of the appropriate implant, specific surgical technique and expertise, and multidisciplinary patient preparation and rehabilitation.

Table 24.3 Metacarpophalangeal (MCP) Joint Replacement Postoperative Regimen

Days 0–1
- Elevation, antibiotics, pain relief

Day 2
- Immediate post-op dressing removed, wound inspection, drain removed
- Plaster of Paris slab replaced by thermoplastic night resting splint

Days 3–5
- Patient maintains elevation of the hand, pain relief as appropriate

Day 5
- Construction of dynamic extension splint
- Commencement of exercise programme

Day 6
- Supervision of exercise regimen
- Arrangements for discharge, including assessment of activities of daily living
- Patient discharged home when needs have been met

Day 14
- Removal of sutures, splint check and adjustment if necessary, exercises checked

Day 21
- Attendance at therapy as outpatient
- Commence scar massage
- Teach new exercises:
  Active flexion/extension with forearm mid-prone, hand resting on the table
  Radial abduction of fingers one by one with hand resting palm down on table (finger walking)

3–6 weeks
- Patient attends minimum of once weekly to check/progress exercise, carry out adjustments on splint, addition of extra splints to aid flexion range if necessary

6 weeks
- Cease use of dynamic splint if joints stable
- Commence light function
- Provision of ulnar drift protection splint
- Joint protection advice

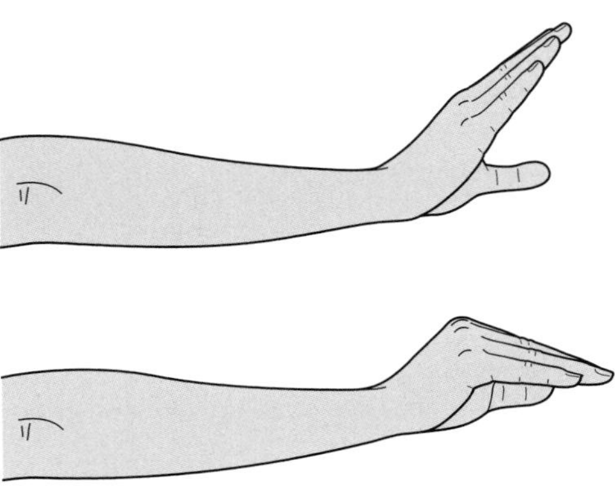

Figure 24.7 Static regime. (Reproduced from Burr and Pratt 2003, with permission.)

Key point

Lower limb joint replacement began in the 1950s. Sir John Charnley refined and researched the low-friction hip arthroplasty that today is the gold standard against which all other joint arthroplasty is compared. Bizot et al. (2000) claim 90.4 per cent 10-year survival rates for certain types of hip prostheses.

The aims of lower limb joint replacement are:

- to relieve pain
- to improve the range of motion at the joint
- to improve the functional ability of the individual
- to improve the person's quality of life
- to prevent further deformity.

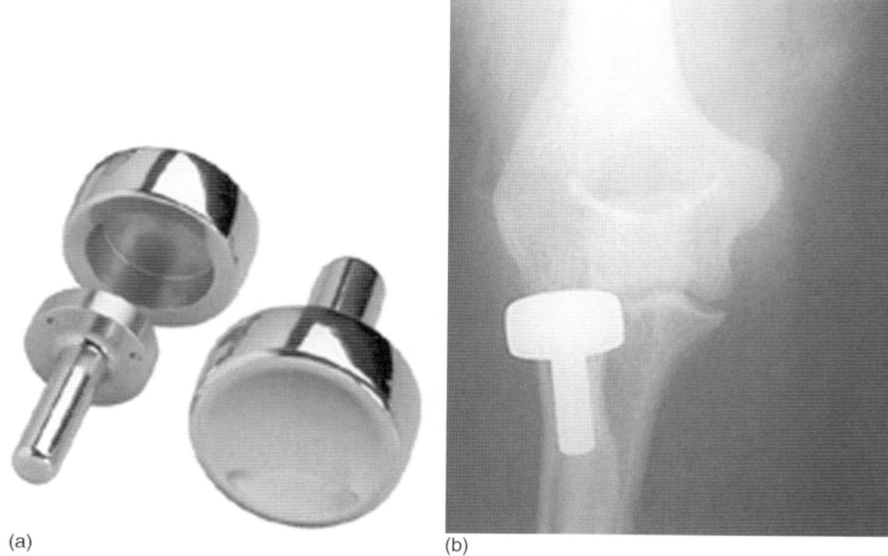

(a) (b)

Figure 24.8 Radial head arthroplasty and the appearance on X-ray. (Reproduced by kind permission of Adam C. Gaines, Wright Medical Technology, TN, USA.)

Indications for lower limb joint replacement

Hip joint replacement is a major yet commonplace orthopaedic procedure. The two main pathologies that lead to replacement surgery are osteoarthritis (primary and secondary) and rheumatoid arthritis, although other indications include congenital dislocation of the hip (CDH), trauma, necrosis of the femoral head and infection. Specialist centres offer more complex procedures, including arthrodesis to implant conversions. Previously, the majority of these patients would be in marked pain with encroaching severe disability.

These pathologies and their respective drug therapies can lead to varying bone structure that the surgeon has to allow for at operation. For example, in the rheumatoid joint the bone tends to be 'soft', whereas if the patient has had previous surgery (such as upper tibial osteotomy), then the bone is 'harder'.

An increasing number of patients are requiring revision surgery owing to implant failure from wear. The minimum life of a joint replacement should be 10 years, and many hip replacements can last over 20 years. The main factors determining implant life are surgical skill, bodyweight, life demands (working/not working) and levels of high-impact stress. There are many functional replacement hip joints that have been in place for up to 30 years. Hip replacements are now being used that have ceramic components; these do not wear as quickly.

General principles

Patient selection

Many objective assessments have been devised, particularly for the hip and knee, to quantify the severity of a patient's problem. None is used universally or routinely, but they are valid tools for research purposes.

To manage their condition, most patients will have had drug therapy, minor procedures where indicated (particularly in the knee) and physiotherapy, including self-management programmes. Joint replacement is then the only option that will allow a return to an improved quality of life that is on the whole pain-free with good function.

Factors taken into account by the surgeon when listing a patient for surgery include:

- severity of disease — onset, progress, other joints affected, investigations
- pain and sleep disturbance
- disability — effect on work and lifestyle
- age — given the life expectancy of the implants
- weight — keeping the implant stresses as low as possible
- emotional stability — less successful after shock or bereavement
- cognitive function.

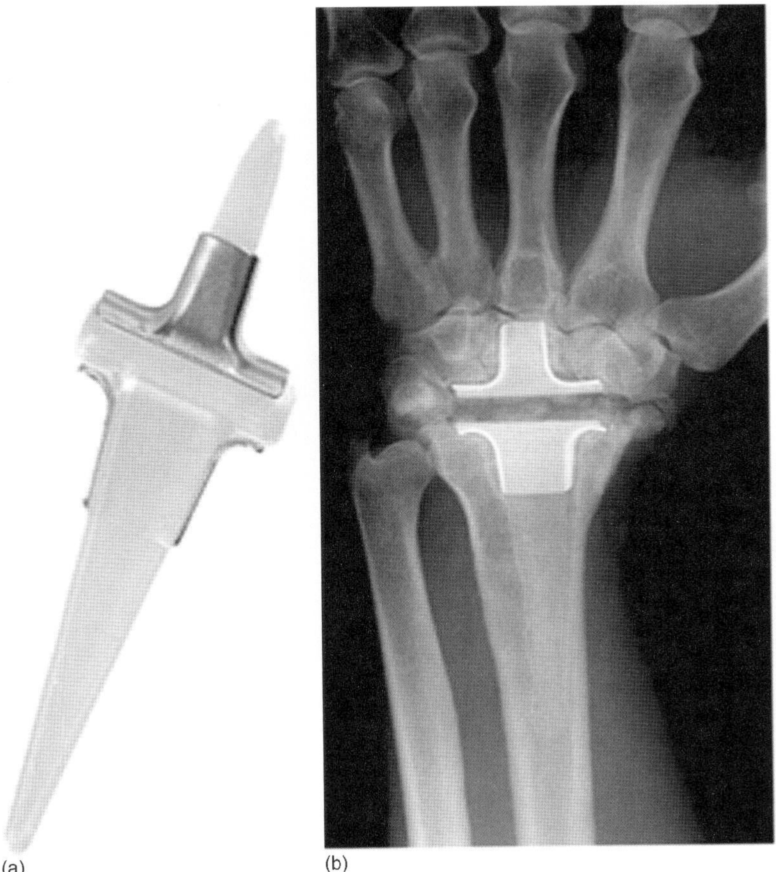

Figure 24.9 Wrist joint arthroplasty and the appearance on X-ray. (Reproduced by kind permission of Adam C. Gaines, Wright Medical Technology, TN, USA.)

Cognitive function needs to be assessed in relation to the pain relief gained by surgery set against the significant problem of potential failure.

Pre-operative patient preparation

Any underlying medical condition must be stabilised prior to surgery. The GP is informed so that the appropriate steps can be taken, such as referral to a specialist for cardiac pathology.

The anaesthetist will review patients with significant medical history, decide the level of anaesthetic risk and, if possible, plan appropriate anaesthesia for the given procedure. Frequently, spinal anaesthesia with peripheral blocks is used instead of a general anaesthetic and this does facilitate postoperative mobilisation, as the patient usually feels less unwell in the first couple of postoperative days.

As the date for surgery approaches, the patient is again reviewed by the pre-operative staff to ascertain fitness for surgery. The physiotherapist assesses the patient for rehabilitation needs and walking aids, and gives instruction in movement procedures and exercises to practise. The occupational therapist will assess the patient for managing at home following discharge and can start the liaison with other agencies that can provide equipment and home help if required.

In specialist centres where the volume of patients is high, the multidisciplinary team may invite patients and their relatives to group information and preparation sessions that are more informal. The less medical environment reduces anxiety and facilitates learning. This preparation allows for speedy successful rehabilitation.

Biomechanical considerations

Modern implants aim as far as possible to replicate the surfaces of the joint to be replaced. Experience has

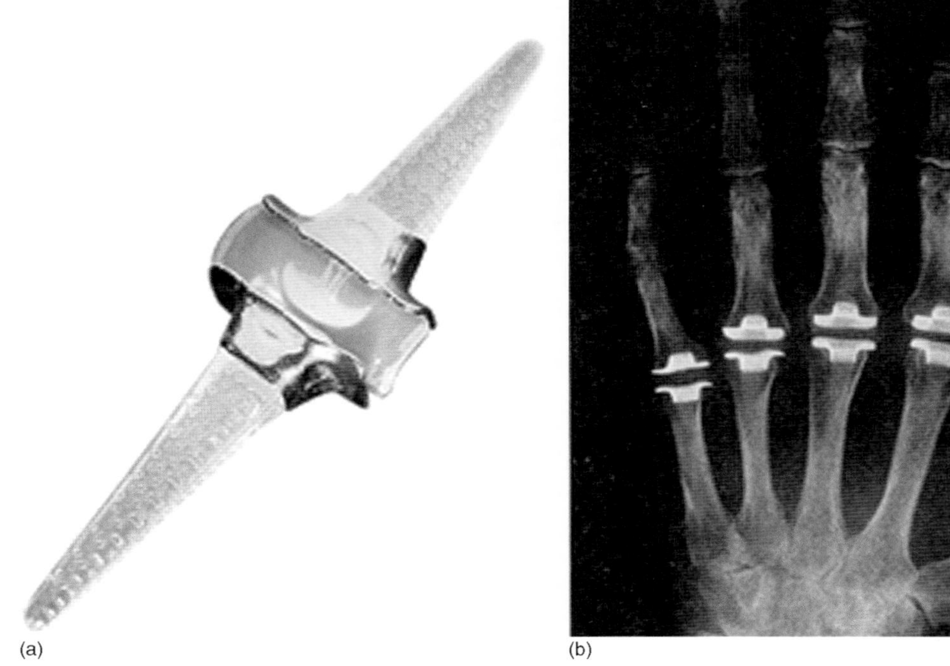

Figure 24.10 Swanson finger replacement and the appearance on X-ray. (Reproduced by kind permission of Adam C. Gaines, Wright Medical Technology, TN, USA.)

shown that failure to understand joint motion fully and to engineer components capable of tolerating the complex interplay of forces generated by muscle pull (a three-dimensional effect), ligaments, acceleration, deceleration, weight and gravity, will result in implant failure, pain and disability.

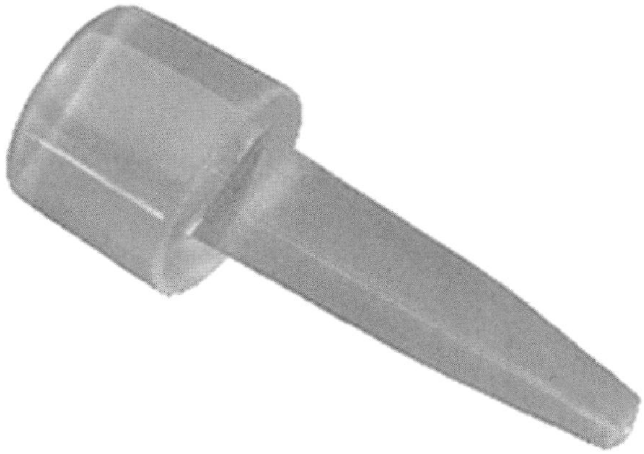

Figure 24.11 Trapezium replacement. (Reproduced by kind permission of Adam C. Gaines, Wright Medical Technology, TN, USA.)

There has been much research into materials that are biologically inert and hard-wearing, with minimum coefficient of friction. This has led to the use today of components manufactured from metal alloys and high-density polyethylene.

Fixation of the components within the bone is again a complex issue, but most success is through pressurised cementing techniques or the use of hydroxyapatite-coated implants that enable a fibro-osseous fixation to develop as part of the bone healing process.

Complications of surgery

Complications of joint replacement can be divided postoperatively into short-term (up to 8 weeks) and long-term (up to 18 months).

In the short term, complications are likely to be secondary to having a surgical intervention: deep-vein thrombosis (DVT), pulmonary embolism, chest infection, wound infection, heart dysfunction, paralytic ileus and bleeding. Specific early orthopaedic complications include dislocation, deep infection, neuropraxia and haematoma.

In the long term, complications include dislocation, joint infection and procedure failure.

TOTAL HIP REPLACEMENT (THR)

The hip is the largest and deepest joint in the body. It takes the form of a multiaxial spheroidal joint with three degrees of freedom of movement, high levels of congruency (stability and surface area for stress transmission) and extensive range of movement.

The implant

The modern hip implant is a metal-alloy femoral head and stem (e.g. stainless steel, chromium cobalt) with a high molecular weight (high-density) polyethylene cup (Figure 24.12). Where the small head of the Charnley prosthesis is used, the procedure is known as the 'low-friction arthroplasty' (LFA).

The operation

The surgical approach to the hip joint depends on the surgeon's preference and impacts upon postoperative rehabilitation. Commonly used approaches include the lateral transtrochanteric division, necessitating trochanteric rewiring at closure, and posterolateral intermuscular division. The femoral neck is divided, the joint dislocated (where possible) and the head removed.

The femoral canal and acetabulum are reamed down to fresh bleeding bone and prepared for component implantation. Cavity size depends on the fixation technique.

If the components are to be cemented in situ, trial cups and stems are inserted to ensure biomechanically correct size and alignment. These are then removed and quick-setting cement, available impregnated with antibiotics, is pushed into the cavities. The implants (with their surfaces protected) are pushed into the cement; a complete cement mantle between the implant and the bone is essential for even distribution of forces, one of the essentials for long-term success in joint replacement. Significant pressure is applied to ensure this.

The joint is then relocated and tested for stability. Once the surgeon is satisfied, the joint is adducted, flexed and medially rotated to dislocate the joint. The surface protection is removed from the implant, the joint relocated and closure commenced.

If access to the hip joint is lateral, then the required trochanteric osteotomy is repaired by a specialised wiring technique, developed to resist breakage. If access to the hip is through soft tissues, these are sutured in layers. Deep and/or superficial drains may or may not be used. Depending on the type of anaesthesia given and patient medical history, a urinary catheter may be used. The operating time is about 1 hour or less and the patient is nursed postoperatively in the recovery ward for 4–6 hours before returning to

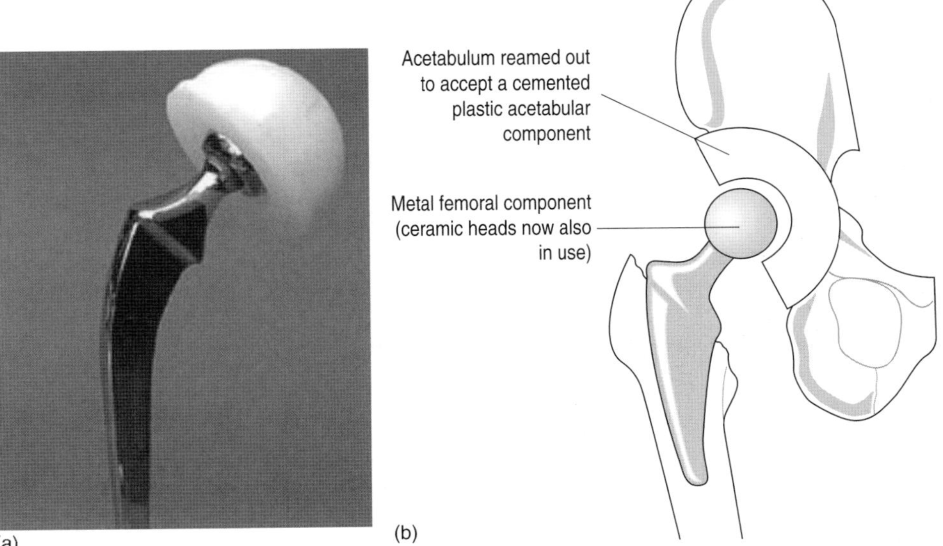

Figure 24.12 Total hip replacement. (Reproduced by kind permission of Medical Models Ltd, UK.)

the ward, providing a satisfactory recovery is made and observations are stable. Pain relief is given through a wide variety of means; it is usually patient-controlled for the first 24–48 hours before oral medication will suffice. Effective pain management enables swift rehabilitation and safe discharge home within 2–4 days.

Figure 24.13 shows an X-ray of a total hip replacement.

Complications of hip replacement

All surgery is not without potential complications. Hip replacement surgery constitutes major surgery and the general major risks apply. Specific complications can be intraoperative, early postoperative and late:

- During surgery there is a risk of nerve and blood vessel damage
- Early postoperative complications include dislocation (3.9 per cent), embolism (0.9 per cent) and deep infection (0.2 per cent) (Heisel et al. 2003).
- Late complications (that is, after 6 months) include aseptic loosening (4.3 per cent), recurrent dislocation (1.1 per cent) and deep infection (0.3 per cent) (Franklin et al. 2003).

Table 24.4 lists other complications and their possible solutions.

The role of the physiotherapist

The preoperative period

The physiotherapist should provide education in preparation for postoperative rehabilitation and effective self-management after discharge from hospital. An assessment should be made for any special needs and to predict rehabilitation requirements. The patient can also be taught correct use of walking aids and simple movement techniques that protect the joint whilst standing up and sitting down, getting in and out of bed and moving up and down stairs. Other tasks may include pre-operative respiratory physiotherapy as necessary.

Many centres provide education through a multidisciplinary approach, employing multiskilled generic assistants to supply routine pre-operative information. Now that hospital length of stay is minimal, written information is vital for the patient and family. As part of the multidisciplinary team, the physiotherapist is involved in providing up-to-date information to the patient through a variety of media such as written booklets, DVDs, Web pages and so on.

This is a busy time for all staff involved in patient care and a stressful time for the patient. Nevertheless, there are many benefits to seeing the patient before surgery, and even a brief visit will often be enough to allay the person's fears.

Hip replacement is now very commonplace and most people who undergo the operation will know or will have spoken to someone who has already had a hip replaced. However, the fact that it is commonplace does not detract from the fact that it is still a major orthopaedic operation. People often have unrealistically high or unrealistically low expectations of the surgery. It is essential to avoid making unrealistic claims about the person's subsequent rehabilitation.

Explain the operation only if necessary. Some people want to know a lot of detail about what is to follow, but others would rather not — you must respect their wishes.

Key point

It is vital for the physiotherapist to understand the procedure that the person is about to undergo and the likely routine to be followed. Watching the operation at least once is useful.

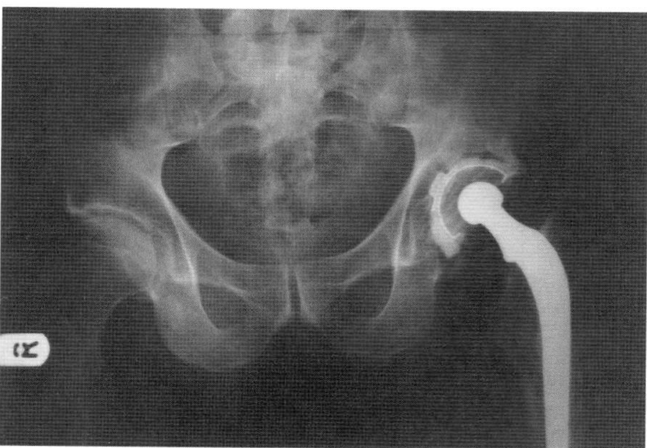

Figure 24.13 X-ray of a hip replacement.

Common questions asked by people about to undergo surgery

Will it hurt me?

Take care when answering this question. Although most people mobilise remarkably quickly, a hip or knee joint replacement constitutes major orthopaedic surgery and it is unreasonable to say that the person will have no pain at all. A suggested answer is: 'You will probably experience some discomfort after your operation but your pain will be closely monitored by all staff, and you should not be afraid to call for attention if your pain does become severe.'

Typically, a person who has undergone a joint replacement will not experience pain until the

Table 24.4 Complications of hip arthroplasty

Complication	Caused by	Solution
Anaesthetic risk (chest, heart)	General anaesthetic	Careful pre-operative anaesthetic assessment, spinal anaesthetic/epidural if necessary Appropriate respiratory physiotherapy
Infection	Open surgery	Prophylactic antibiotics postoperatively Laminar flow theatres and exhaust suits
Dislocation	Difficult surgery, poor surgical technique, complex case, inherently unstable, e.g. if patient has had a cerebrovascular accident, the risk of subsequent dislocation may be higher owing to decreased muscular stability at the hip joint	Abduction wedge, no adduction/flexion beyond 90 degrees, special restraining acetabulum may be used in cases of previous dislocation
Deep vein thrombosis/ pulmonary embolism	Pelvic surgery, immobility	DVT prophylaxis usually chemical, e.g. clexane (low molecular weight heparin) for up to 28 days post-operatively alongside early mobilisation
	Damage to blood vessels during surgery	Prophylactic anticoagulants, early mobilisation by physiotherapists, release leg periodically during surgery to restore blood flow
Anaemia	Blood loss during/after surgery	Blood transfusion now usually only if haemoglobin (Hb) below 8 or on clinical findings
Swollen ankle	Ineffective muscle pump	Reassure, walk little and often, frequent rest in bed, compression stockings may help
Back pain	Unequal leg length or perceived by pelvis as unequal leg length	Reassure
Arm pain	Crutch walking	Time
Neck pain	Neck trauma due to neck being held in an extended position during intubation	Time
Stiffness after immobility	Inflammatory exudate builds at rest	Reassure, walk little and often

physiotherapist appears at the bedside! It is therefore in the best interests of patient, physiotherapist and other members of the healthcare team that the person's pain be controlled adequately. The timing of analgesia should be such that maximum pain relief occurs during mobilisation by the physiotherapist, and this requires close liaison between nursing staff and the physiotherapist.

Will the joint come out of its socket?

There is a small risk that a dislocation will occur following hip replacement. (Knee replacements do not carry the same potential problems of dislocation.) Reassure the person that you are aware of the risks and that you will take all appropriate steps to minimise them.

How long will I be in hospital?

The average stay for a first total hip replacement is probably between a week and 10 days. A person who is on bed rest following a revision (redo) will not fall into this category.

Clinical note

After a few years in clinical practice, physiotherapists and allied health professionals may become blasé about procedures such as hip replacement. Never forget that most patients are very apprehensive.

How will I manage to walk again?

Patients are understandably very anxious about how they are going to manage, especially after the first time out of bed when they might not do as well as hoped or as well as the patient in the next bed. Encouragement is vital. Set realistic goals and explain the psychological benefits of walking slightly further each time. It may be necessary to explain that the person in the next bed had different surgery or that it was performed earlier.

Do not underestimate the psychological benefit to the patient of a positive attitude on the part of the physiotherapist. Patients watch their therapist very closely for signs of impatience or dissatisfaction with progress.

Can I put my weight on it?

This depends on the operation, the prosthesis and the surgeon's instructions. The physiotherapist must know the routine for the unit and should certainly not guess.

Will the physiotherapy hurt me?

The nature of physiotherapy means that what we do often causes some discomfort. An important skill is to gain the confidence of the patient, and strike a balance between pushing the patient and being compassionate.

Will I be allowed to use my frame?

If a person has used a frame for many years and only feels comfortable with it, then he or she should be allowed to use it, as long as it is not contraindicated.

The immediate postoperative period

The patient usually returns from the theatre to the recovery ward and stays there until medically stable. There will be a drip in situ for a day or so, and this is usually removed once the patient is drinking properly. The patient sometimes has drainage tubes coming away from the operation site that are connected to vacuum drainage bottles; the purpose of these is to remove any haematoma from the area. These usually stay in for 48 hours and are simply pulled out with no need for anaesthetic.

The patient will have an abduction pillow in place to encourage the tissues to heal in the most stable position. Gallay et al. (1997) advocate use of anticoagulation therapy and this can be given up to 30 days after the operation. However, use of pneumatic compression devices may rival the effectiveness of pharmacological prophylaxis (Hooker et al. 1999). The thromboprophylaxis debate continues. Deep tension sutures are rarely used nowadays.

Physiotherapy includes active exercises for feet and ankles, isometric hip and knee contractions of all muscle groups, chest physiotherapy as necessary, advice on positioning, and mobility in the bed.

Patients are assessed as ready to mobilise once they are orientated, their observations are satisfactory, their pain is controlled and motor control is established (for those patients with epidural/peripheral nerve blocks). To start with, they are helped out of bed by two staff and instructed in movement techniques that prevent excess hip flexion, adduction and medial rotation and that ensure safe mobilisation. Weight-bearing is usually partial and involves the use of an appropriate aid — a walking frame or a pair of elbow crutches.

Initially, the patient will stand out of bed and take a few steps with crutches or another aid. Walking distance is progressed daily until the patient is walking independently with crutches or a frame.

Routines vary, but patients usually commence sitting at 2–7 days (no adduction or flexion beyond 90 degrees), with stair practice before discharge if needed. Usually patients remain on crutches for 6 weeks, at which time they progress to sticks, then full weight-bearing.

Dos and don'ts must be stressed to the patient (Table 24.5), and an educational booklet provided as a

Table 24.5 Dos and don'ts following total hip replacement

Don't

- Pick up any objects from the floor or reach into low cupboards. Use a reaching aid if possible
- Cross your legs
- Force your hip to less than a right angle (knee towards chest)
- Sit on low chairs, low stools or low toilets
- Sit on chairs without arms. You may need to use the arms of the chair to help you to rise
- Allow your hip to rotate when sitting, standing or lying down; keep your leg in a neutral position with toes pointing forwards
- Move to the edge of the chair before you stand up; keep your operated leg straight at the knee
- Lie on your side without a pillow placed between your legs

Do

- Take your time when you get home
- Rotate your activities, i.e. lie for short periods if you are very tired, walk little and often, sit for short periods
- Set yourself small achievable targets with your walking
- Pace yourself
- Remember that you will have good days and bad days
- Keep a progress diary so that you can reflect on your achievements

reminder. It is also important that occupational therapists and other members of the multidisciplinary team see the patient.

Rehabilitation protocol following THR

> ***Key point***
> All activity should be documented to the CSP documentation standards. Multidisciplinary team care pathways can also be completed. These aid effective communication between all staff, ensure all goals are met and allow for ease of service audit.

Day 1

There should be assessment by the physiotherapist of neurovasculomotor and respiratory systems. Active exercises for circulation and static exercises for muscle tone around the hip can be started, along with deep breathing exercises. Notes and X-rays should be studied as soon as available. Note the surgical approach and any non-standard procedure.

Day 2

Provided the surgeon is satisfied, mobilisation starts with the physiotherapist and assistant. The routine protocol can be followed.

The assistant prepares the environment and the patient, and assists the patient from behind in bed transfers with the physiotherapist. A sliding sheet may be used in accordance with the moving and handling policy if the patient is heavy and/or has difficulty with transfers. Drains, catheters and drips are dealt with appropriately, according to nursing policy.

The physiotherapist assists with the operated leg and ensures hip protection at all times. The patient is taught and reminded throughout the procedure of the hip protection measures required:

- partial weight-bearing
- limited flexion
- maintenance of some abduction
- no rotation.

Perch-sitting balance and standing balance are assessed. Mobilisation starts with three-point gait on elbow crutches, using a walking frame only if necessary initially. Distance is not important, patients being taken as far as their ability allows. Constant monitoring of the patient by observation and questioning is essential, as faintness is common and hazardous. The patient is returned to bed. This is done at least once per day, twice ideally.

Functional activities such as toilet procedure and sitting are taught in accordance with the surgeon's routine, usually from day 2 or 3. Advice as to length of time in sitting is given — no more than an hour at a time, perhaps at mealtimes — to try to limit leg swelling and subsequent discomfort in the initial weeks of recovery. Techniques to manage stairs, steps and ramps safely are taught according to individual home circumstances.

Day 3 onwards

Mobility is progressed on a daily basis. The patient may be walked and instructed by two assistants, if his or her condition allows, then with one assistant until the patient is safe to mobilise unsupervised — that is, has good dynamic balance, has correct gait with walking aids, and is competent at hip protection. Advice is given as to the right amount of activity/rest to take; walking hourly and taking bed rest morning and afternoon constitute the usual level for discharge.

Advice is given prior to discharge concerning expected levels of activity until clinic review. No other specific exercises are recommended during this period. Regular and gradually extended walking practice is necessary indoors and out. The emphasis is on hip protection and recovery (effective capsular scarring). There are three simple golden rules:

1. Do not overbend the hip (flex beyond a right angle).
2. Do not cross the leg over the mid-line (adduct beyond neutral).
3. Do not twist in either standing or sitting.

These rules apply for 6 weeks in all cases. If the trochanter is to be protected, then the rules apply for longer and it is generally accepted that the patient can return to normal activities at 3 months.

After discharge

If the soft-tissue approach was used during surgery, the patient may be issued with sticks and advised to increase weight-bearing gradually over the next 6 weeks. If the transtrochanteric approach was used, then the site of bony union must be protected for 12 weeks. The patient remains on elbow crutches for a minimum of 6 weeks but then can start to increase weight-bearing gradually until ready for full weight-bearing at 12 weeks, weaning from crutches to sticks/stick over that time. If the surgeon has used a cementless implantation, then the patient is non-weight-bearing (toe touch with elbow crutches — hopping is not safe) for 6 weeks, then partial weight-bearing for at least another 6 weeks. This allows for the ingrowth of fibroblasts into the hydroxyapatite coating.

A long-term rule is to avoid high-impact activities, as sudden high pressures cause the most wear to the plastic. Plastic particulates have an exponential wear action that involves the alloy head and the cement mantle/bone interface. This process eventually means the patient needs a new hip arthroplasty — a revision procedure.

The patient may ring with queries following discharge but must contact the GP if there is any sudden significant pain or swelling.

Further physiotherapy/exercise may be required following clinic review and the appropriate referral can made. Some centres offer outpatient rehabilitation programmes.

Rehabilitation following revision surgery

Depending on the reason for revision (commonly wear and loosening, fracture, infection or dislocation) and the complexity of the procedure, the physiotherapy as outlined above is modified appropriately in accordance with the surgeon's instructions.

Augmentation of the bone is frequently required on the acetabular side — by bone grafting and in some cases the use of screws to hold the graft in place. The graft acts as scaffolding for migrating osteocytes, which then lay down new bone.

Following any procedure that subsequently requires bony healing or union, the patient is mobilised following the non-weight-bearing protocol outlined above. It is common for the revision patient to need longer bed rest prior to mobilisation and a slower rate of progression.

TOTAL KNEE REPLACEMENT (TKR)

The knee is a complex joint whose stability is dependent on extra-articular ligaments and muscular control. Knee problems usually present with gross biomechanical deformity requiring soft-tissue release at operation in order to regain biomechanical alignment and normal soft-tissue lengths.

In the case of a severely deformed joint, physical constraint to movement can be incorporated by use of a moulded tibial implant. This will give increased inherent stability. The risk of failure secondary to its inability to move freely is less likely in the patient with low functional demand.

> **The implant**
>
> The implant uses metal-alloy components over the distal femur and proximal tibia. A high molecular weight (high-density) polyethylene bearing is inserted between the two. The patella may be resurfaced with a metal alloy articulating button, if necessary.

The operation

Commonly, a tourniquet is applied, the leg exsanguinated and the tourniquet tightened for a timed period.

With the knee in flexion, the surgical approach is on the whole by anterior skin incision followed by medial parapatellar incision through quadriceps expansion. The patella is reflected laterally and the joint exposed. Very rarely (and this is seen more in revision surgery), the tibial tuberosity has to be sawn off with a large piece of anterior tibial bone. This allows better access to the joint.

The femoral component is held in place by two short pegs cemented into each condyle and the tibial component by a large single peg into the tibia. The pressurised cementing technique, as described previously for the hip replacement operation, is used. Bone cuts and preparation followed by component trial are carried out. Closure of the joint is in layers.

The patient may or may not have drains inserted. A wool and crêpe bandage is applied to control oedema and a backsplint applied to maintain the knee in extension until quadriceps function is regained. The operating time is about 90 minutes.

Figure 24.14 shows knee replacements.

Rehabilitation protocol following TKR

The general postoperative physiotherapy is as previously described for hip replacement, except that the emphasis is on regaining quadriceps control. If the patient has had a femoral block for pain relief, active quadriceps function may take up to 24 hours to return.

Mobilisation and the start of the exercise programme commence on day 2. The patient starts to walk with two crutches, partial weight-bearing for 6 weeks. Transfer on to sticks is possible at any point during this time. It is a weaning process to full weight-bearing depending on the level of pain, bruising, swelling, muscle function and range of movement.

Exercises are prescribed according to the surgeon's routine and the physiotherapeutic assessment of the patient. The splint and bandage must be removed prior to physiotherapy. It is vital that exercises are practised very regularly — little and often, almost hourly at first, progressing to several times per day of additional differing exercises. It is paramount that quadriceps function be regained and therefore the control and protection of the joint established.

Common in the early phase is the use of simple equipment: closed-chain quadriceps over a sponge ball or in prone with toes tucked under, progressing to open-chain quadriceps over a wedge, and sliding boards for hamstrings. It is useful to provide the

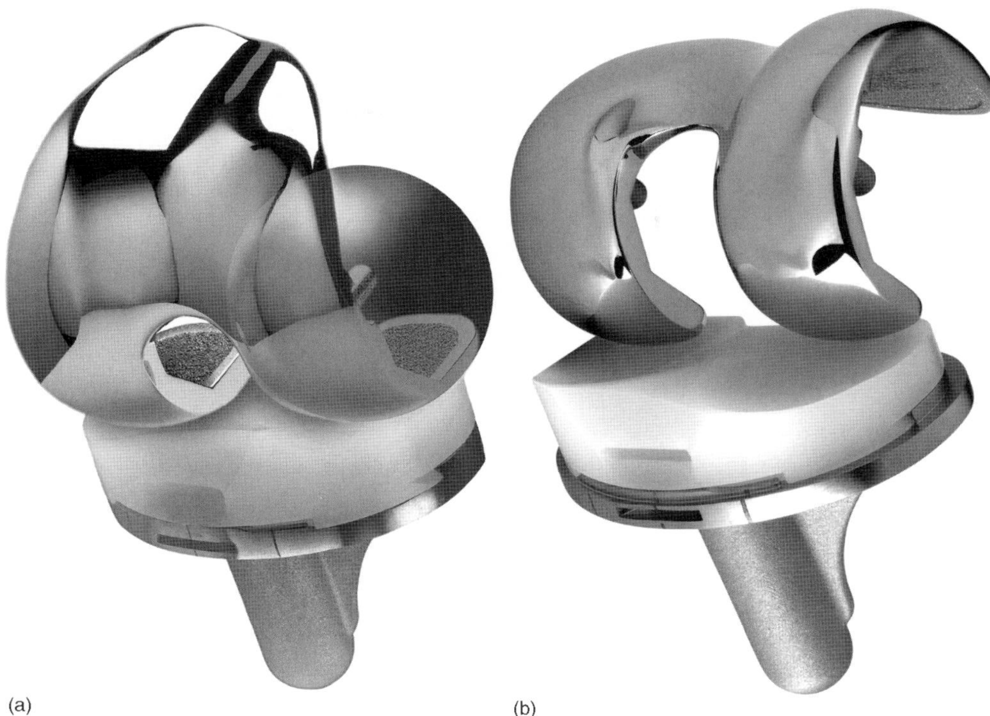

Figure 24.14 Total knee replacements. (Reproduced courtesy of Wright Medical Technology, Inc.)

patient with a written exercise programme tailored to the individual's needs, which can be adjusted and reviewed as progress continues.

Flexion is usually hampered by pain, fear, bruising and swelling. Physiotherapy should therefore include help in the control of these symptoms by reassurance, coordination with analgesia, cryotherapy and careful massage leading into assisted flexion. The patient can be instructed in the safe application of ice and massage at home. Do not forget that full extension is a vital component of knee joint function.

Length of hospital stay is usually 7–8 days, by which time the patient should be functionally independent and progressing with rehabilitation. Ideally, the range of movement should be 0–90 degrees with active quadriceps; a straight leg raise should be performed with minimal lag.

On discharge, most patients are referred for outpatient physiotherapy to review progress, continue with assisted exercises or start more advanced strengthening and mobilising workouts.

TOTAL ANKLE REPLACEMENT (TAR)

Total ankle replacement is the 'youngest' of the lower limb joint replacements. Attempts were made in the 1970s but were unsuccessful. There is now a semi-constrained implant that is working very successfully, although as yet there are insufficient numbers to compare outcomes with the knee or hip replacements.

Hind foot function and pain are closely related to both the function of the ankle joint and the subtalar joint. The success of a TAR will depend on the health of the subtalar joint below it. Often, particularly in people with rheumatoid arthritis, the diseased subtalar joint is fused prior to the TAR (no replacement is currently available) to give the optimum outcome.

The ankle joint is an anatomically constrained hinge joint. Particularly in this region, the integrity of the circulation is vital and great care is taken in the selection of a patient in whom both circulation and skin can withstand the stress of operation and support the demands of the healing process.

The articular surfaces of the tibia and the talus are replaced with metal-alloy implants. The talar implant is centrally ridged forward to back to accommodate the sulcus on the inferior surface of the polyethylene bearing inserted between them (Figure 24.15). This allows for flexion and extension and decreases the risk of malleolar fracture by medial slip of the bearing.

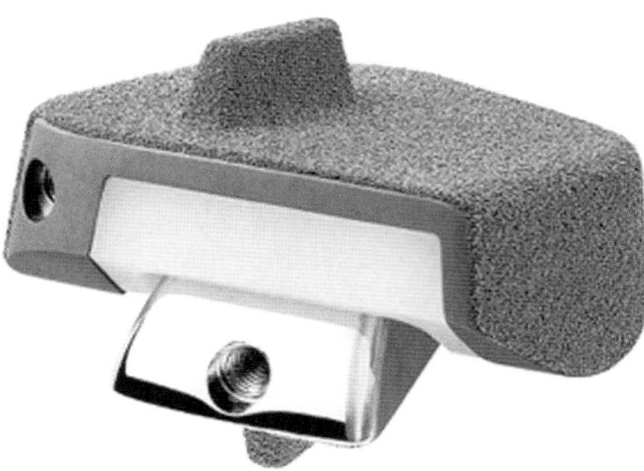

Figure 24.15 Ankle joint replacement. (Reproduced by kind permission of De Puy Orthopaedics Inc., IN, USA.)

The operation

Approach to the joint is via a 10 cm anterior incision. Care is taken to avoid the anterior tibial neurovascular bundle. The bones are cut and prepared, as previously described. The implant is usually uncemented, the components being hammered into place. The tissues are closed in layers and compression dressing is applied.

The patient is roused and nursed as previously described, with the limb maintained in elevation.

Rehabilitation protocol following TAR

Postoperative physiotherapy is as previously described for hip and knee replacements, except that routine ankle exercises are avoided and toe exercises substituted. The physiotherapist must ensure dorsiflexion to a right angle (plantigrade); where this is difficult, the patient should be shown an appropriate stretch exercise with a strap.

Mobilisation is usually on day 3 or 4 when the swelling is controlled and the compression dressings are removed, according to the surgeon's instructions. A protective knee-length plastic boot that can be removed for wound inspection can be fitted and the patient mobilised in partial weight-bearing with elbow crutches for functional requirements only. (The leg is rested in elevation otherwise.) Techniques to manage stairs/steps/ramps are taught.

The length of stay is usually 5–6 days. The patient is reviewed in clinic at 3 weeks for removal of sutures and the plastic boot. Exercises can be started at this point to facilitate rehabilitation, including Achilles tendon stretches, muscle strengthening and balance function. Specific mobilisation of the ankle is avoided.

FURTHER READING

Atkinson K, Coutts F, Hassenkamp A-M 1999 Physiotherapy in Orthopaedics: a Problem Solving Approach. Churchill Livingstone: Edinburgh

Birch A, Gwillian L 2000 Rheumatoid arthritis and its effects on the hand. In: Salter M, Cheshire L (eds) Hand Therapy Principle and Practice. Butterworth–Heinemann: Oxford

Mackin JM, Callahan AD, Skirven TM et al. (eds) Rehabilitation of the Hand and Upper Extermity, 5th edn. Mosby: St Louis

Simmen BR, Allieu Y, Luch A, Stanley J (eds) 2001 Hand Arthroplasties. Martin Dunitz: London

REFERENCES

Bizot P, Banallec L et al. 2000 Alumina-on-alumina total hip prostheses in patients 40 years of age or younger. Clin Orthop 379: 68–76

Brander VA, Malhotra S et al. 1997 Outcome of hip and knee arthroplasty in persons aged 80 years and older. Clin Orthop 345: 67–78

Burr N, Pratt A 2003 MCP Joint arthroplasty case study: the Mount Vernon static regime. Br J Hand Ther 4(4): 137–140

Delaney R, Stanley JK 2000 A prospective study of range of movement following metacarpophalangeal joint replacements: optimum time of recovery. Br J Hand Ther 5(3): 85–87

Franklin J, Robertsson O, Gestsson J et al. 2003 Revision and complication rates in 654 Exeter total hip replacements, with a maximum follow-up of 20 years. BMC Musculoskelet Disord 4: 6

Gallay S, Waddell JP et al. 1997 A short course of low-molecular-weight heparin to prevent deep venous thrombosis after elective total hip replacement. Can J Surg 40(2): 119–123

Godenèche A, Boileau P, Favard L et al. 2002 Prosthetic replacement in the treatment of osteoarthritis of the shoulder: early results of 268 cases. J Shoulder Elbow Surg 11(1): 11–18

Hamblen DL 1984 History of Shoulder Replacement. University of Glasgow Department of Orthopaedics Study Day, 13 January 1984, printed by 3M Healthcare: Bracknell

Heisel C, Schmalzried TP 2003 Incidence rates of serious complications after total hip replacement. J Bone Joint Surg Am 85: 20–26

Hooker JA, Lachiewicz PF et al. 1999 Efficacy of prophylaxis against thromboembolism with intermittent pneumatic compression after primary and revision total hip arthroplasty. J Bone Joint Surg Am 81: 690–696

Iannotti JP, Williams GR 1998 Total shoulder arthroplasty: factors influencing prosthetic design. Orthop Clin North Am 29: 377–391

Mackay DC, Williams J 1999 A Survey of Elbow and Shoulder Surgeons in the UK. British Elbow & Shoulder Society: Sheffield

Mackay DC, Hudson B, Williams JR 2001 Which primary shoulder and elbow replacement? A review of the results of prostheses available in the UK. Ann R Coll Surg Engl 83: 258–265

Neer CS, Watson KC, Stanto FJ 1982 Recent experience in total shoulder replacement. J Bone Joint Surg 64A: 319–337

Swanson AB, Swanson G de G, Leonard J 1978 Postoperative rehabilitation program in flexible implant arthroplasty of the digits. In: Hunter JM, Schneider LH, Mackin EJ, Bell JA (eds) Rehabilitation of the Hand. Mosby: St Louis, pp. 477–481

Swanson AB, Swanson G de G, DeHeer DH 2000 Small joint implant arthroplasty: 38 years of research experience. In: Simmen BR, Allieu Y, Luch A, Stanley J (eds) Hand Arthroplasties. Martin Dunitz: London

Chapter **25**

Physiotherapy for people with amputation

Carolyn A. Hale

CHAPTER CONTENTS

INTRODUCTION

Rehabilitation following amputation is the responsibility of the multidisciplinary team (MDT), with the patient focused at the centre. Working with a specialist team will produce the best outcome for the individual who has undergone life-changing amputation surgery (Pernot et al. 1997). The physiotherapist is a key member of this team, involved at all stages of the process from the pre-operative phase, through amputation, into prosthetic training and during life thereafter.

This chapter provides an overview of the physiotherapy management of people with amputation, outlining the role and importance of the physiotherapist's intervention. Readers will need to refer to the appropriate texts for details of specific treatment modalities and knowledge of causative factors, surgical techniques, prosthetic components and associated equipment. The list of reading material and resources will help you source this information. This chapter will predominantly address the management of a lower limb amputation.

Amputation is performed for life-threatening disease or pain, when all other treatments have failed. The goal is to preserve life and improve function and general health. Having a limb amputated is a life-changing episode with potentially devastating consequences for every aspect of living, not just physical functioning. Becoming disabled in this way can affect a person's personality, altering relationships and body image, and sometimes challenging the family unit. If amputation occurs when someone is of a young age, it can affect earning potential and ambition, and in most cases result in the person having to move home to accommodate the new circumstances. For many, this is the incentive that gives them the determination to achieve great things.

CAUSES AND LEVELS OF AMPUTATION

Over 85 per cent of lower limb amputations performed in the UK are the result of vascular deficiencies caused by peripheral arterial disease and diabetes (Van de Ven and Engstrom 1999). In fact, this is the case for the majority of lower limb amputations performed in the Western world (Ebskov 1999). Most patients in this category will be over the age of 65 and may have other comorbidities associated with the ageing process, such as arthritis and cardiac disease (Fyfe 1992; Ham and McCreadie 1992). As most vascular pathologies are progressive in nature, the patient may have undergone earlier intervention in the form of bypass operations or toe amputations prior to a major amputation. When planning a treatment regime, these concurrent pathologies and history must be taken into account.

The next most common cause is trauma, where an individual has often been involved in a road traffic accident or crush injury and the musculoskeletal system cannot be saved or is non-viable after surgery. Amputation may be at the time of the accident, or in some cases, days, months or even years afterwards. Trauma is the major cause of upper limb amputation, which is often the result of a work-related accident. This population of patients are usually therefore young and of working age.

Other reasons for amputation of an arm or leg are tumours, infection and congenital deficiency. Children born with limb absences or deformity do not always have an amputation; however, their limb dysfunction is often managed like an amputation.

The decision regarding amputation level is determined in the removal of all non-viable tissue whilst creating a functional and prosthetically suitable residuum (stump), also called residual limb. Incidentally, many patients do not like their leg being referred to as a 'stump' and appropriate references should be found. Tables 25.1 and 25.2 list the causes of amputation seen in the developed world and the recognised levels of surgical amputation.

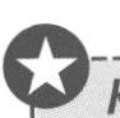

Key point

The multidisciplinary team consists of surgeons, nurses, physiotherapists, occupational therapists, counsellors and psychologists, prosthetists and orthotists, wheelchair therapists, rehabilitation doctors, podiatrists and chiropodists, social workers and homecare agencies. Specialist regional units, known as Disablement Services Centres (DSCs) are the usual hub of management. Services are provided by primary, secondary and tertiary establishments. The patient will meet numerous clinicians throughout their rehabilitation. The physiotherapist has a key role, often providing the link between all these professionals.

Table 25.1 Causes of amputation in the developed world

Cause	Relative percentage (%)
Lower limb	
Peripheral arterial disease (25–50% of which also have diabetes mellitus)	85–90
Trauma	9
Tumour	4
Congenital deficiency	3
Infection	1
Upper limb	
Trauma	29
Disease	30
Congenital deficiency	15
Tumour	26

(Reproduced from Van De Ven and Engstrom 1999, with permission.)

Table 25.2 Levels of amputation

Lower limb	Upper limb
■ Hemipelvectomy	■ Forequarter
■ Hip disarticulation	■ Shoulder disarticulation
■ Transfemoral*	■ Transhumeral*
■ Supracondylar, transcondylar and Gritti–Stokes	■ Elbow disarticulation
■ Knee disarticulation	■ Transradial*
■ Transtibial*	■ Wrist disarticulation
■ Symes	■ Transmetacarpal
■ Chopart/Lisfranc	■ Interphalangeal
■ Transmetatarsal	
■ Interphalangeal	

*The most commonly seen levels in clinical practice. (Reproduced from Van De Ven and Engstrom 1999, with permission.)

THE PSYCHOSOCIAL IMPACT OF AMPUTATION

The physiotherapist and all team members must have an understanding of the psychological implications associated with having a limb amputated. This will help in building a rapport with the patient, aiding agreed goal-planning and facilitating a motivating rehabilitation regime for the individual.

The person will undergo a grief process associated with loss. Loss of a body part and altered body image can potentially lead to loss of confidence, loss of function, loss of a lifestyle, loss of role, income and status, and loss of independence and control. Having an amputation can leave people feeling vulnerable, worthless and isolated. Individuals will be affected by each of these to a different degree, and their ability to accept their new situation will vary greatly too. The normal reactions to grief and bereavement are well documented (Kubler-Ross 1969; Parkes 1972, 1975; Campling 1981); for some patients, the reaction is transient and minor, whilst for others it is profound, disabling and longer-lasting (Bridway et al. 1984; Butler et al. 1992; Krueger 1984; Bradway et al. 1984).

Key point

Models of grief and bereavement offer frameworks for understanding grief associated with loss. It must be recognised that grief affects people in different ways and does not always manifest itself in a set pattern to a set timeframe. The physiotherapist must be sensitive to patients' emotional needs at all stages of the rehabilitation process.

Anyone who has an amputation needs to be given time to adjust. Patients need to be given accurate information about their rehabilitation programme and realistic ideas of what they can expect. Amputation affects the whole family and loved ones should be included in any rehabilitation process (Caron 1989). A successful outcome in restoring independence and self-worth is dependent on adjustment and acceptance on the part of the individual and their close support network. People with disability often lack choice and other people make decisions on their behalf (O'Shea and Kennelly 1996). This has the impact of denying them a role in society. Physiotherapists must take time to talk with their patients, to understand their fears and their hopes, to recognise barriers to progress and to work together to set goals. Recovering after an amputation is not just about functional recovery: being able to 'walk' or make a cup of tea.

PAIN AND PAIN RELIEF

There are two potential types of pain following amputation:

- residual limb pain
- phantom pain and sensations.

Residual limb pain

Amputation surgery creates tissue disruption and trauma. This produces a natural inflammatory response resulting in oedema (swelling). This pressure on and injury to the nerve endings causes pain. This pain is usually managed postoperatively with analgesics and

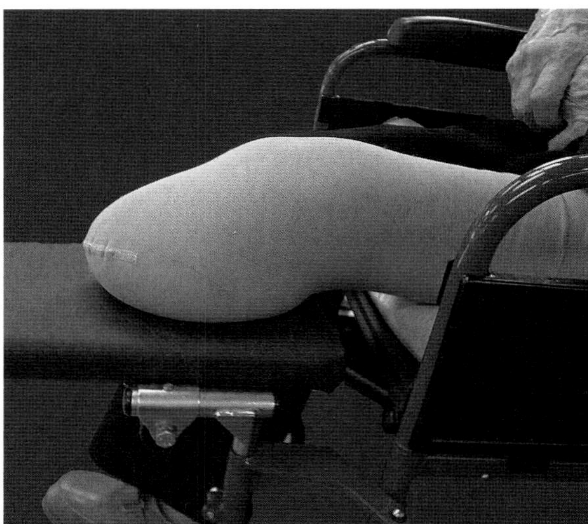

Figure 25.1 Elevation with a wheelchair stump board and compression garment.

possibly epidurals. Managing the oedema will also help with pain relief. The physiotherapist can use elevation (Figure 25.1), elastic and intermittent compression and exercise to improve the circulation, thereby promoting the healing process, reducing swelling and thus pain. Normal healing takes around 3 weeks. Any delays in healing can result in greater scar tissue, which can be painful if adherent to the underlying bone. Massage and ultrasound can be helpful for relieving this type of pain.

Later on, use of a prosthesis can sometimes cause pain in the residual limb and the physiotherapist must check that the user has put it on correctly and ensure a correct fit. Liaison with the prosthetist is essential.

Phantom pain and sensations

Phantom pain is described as pain experienced in the missing limb part. It is well documented; symptoms are well recognised, if poorly understood (Fraser et al. 2001), and it is a feature that can impact significantly on the life of a patient (Weiss and Lindell 1996; Williams and Deaton 1997; Hill et al. 1995).

There are two reasons why someone will still perceive the amputated body part:

- Firstly, the nerves have been severed, causing injury to nerve tissue, and therefore pain messages are sent to the brain.
- Secondly, the brain has an area of tissue dedicated to that body part and will expect sensory information. This area of the brain is not removed during limb amputation and thus still tries to process information. Often this is perceived as pain.

Phantom pain can be described as 'burning', 'electric', 'shooting', 'twisting', 'cramping', 'crushing' and 'sharp'. It may be intermittent or constant, and can be felt in any part of the removed limb. This can take a long time to settle down and, in a few cases, never resolves.

Key point

Phantom pains are often exacerbated by stressful life events, such as illness, changing house or job, or divorce and bereavement.

Phantom pain should not be confused with phantom sensations, which are sensations in the missing limb that are not painful. These are often sensations of the limb as it was before amputation, in normal orientation but sometimes in a strange position. People have described such sensations as 'foot facing backwards', 'tight shoes', 'itching' and 'pins and needles,' as well as feeling that their hand or foot is now at the end of the residual limb, known as a telescoping affect. These sensations can be equally distressing and as distracting as phantom pain.

It is important that the physiotherapist assesses pain carefully to determine its cause and allay patient fears that something is wrong. Effective pain-relieving modalities for phantom pain include TENS, acupuncture, relaxation, massage, exercise, compression and analgesia. Alternative methods can include reflexology, counselling and hypnotherapy.

THE ROLE OF THE PHYSIOTHERAPIST FOLLOWING LOWER LIMB AMPUTATION

Physiotherapy involves the continuous assessment of patients' goals, needs and abilities, in order to set realistic and agreed treatment plans.

The physiotherapist re-educates movement patterns to optimise independent function for activities of daily life, such as self-care, wheelchair and prosthetic use, and normal occupation.

Physiotherapy aims

Rehabilitation following lower limb amputation is a continual process, involving all aspects of a person's life: physical, mental, emotional and socioeconomic. For a successful physiotherapeutic outcome, all these aspects must be addressed.

The final goal should be optimal independence, with or without a prosthesis, to return to as normal a life as possible. Ideally, the person should achieve:

- independent self-caring
- independent indoor mobility
- independent outdoor mobility
- ability to get into/out of car or other transport
- return to leisure/hobbies/work/society.

Considerations

The following are reasons why some patients have difficulties achieving goals:

- *poor residual limb condition* — for example: adherent scar tissue, unhealed, bulbous, failed myodesis, neuroma, bony prominences, pain, hypersensitivity, poor vascularity, short leverage
- *concurrent pathology* — leading to: inability to learn, reduced range of motion, reduced strength and stamina, pain, poor balance, poor dexterity, socket intolerance
- *social and environmental difficulties* — for example: living alone, unsuitable accommodation for wheelchairs, poor access to accommodation, unhealthy lifestyle, dominant carers
- *lack of motivation* — fear, fatigue, emotional barriers to achieving success
- *inappropriate equipment* — for example: prosthetic socket fit or alignment, wheelchair too big or too small, incorrect prescriptions
- *lack of specialist rehabilitation services.*

The inability to learn new skills is probably the largest determining factor to successful outcome. Sometimes this can be influenced by physiotherapy intervention but not in every case.

Patients must be involved in coordinating aspects of their treatment planning, goal-setting and monitoring, as self-responsibility and self-management are the foundations of rehabilitation (Watson 1996).

PHYSIOTHERAPY ASSESSMENT

A thorough subjective and objective assessment will ensure accurate and realistic goal planning. Table 25.3 outlines the content of both a subjective and an objective assessment. It is important during the assessment that the physiotherapist gains an understanding of what patients have been through, their current situation and their goals for the future. This needs to be in terms of both their physical and their psychosocial well-being. The objective assessment needs to look at any musculoskeletal or neurological dysfunction and movement control patterns carefully.

Following amputation, the skeletal system makes compensations for the imbalance caused by the missing anatomy or the restrictions caused by the prosthesis. Joint alignment and soft tissues adapt to new prolonged postures. Muscles can start to work inefficiently and in an uncoordinated manner, affecting a person's ability

Table 25.3 Recommended content of assessment following amputation

Subjective assessment	
Present complaint	Level of amputation and cause, time since amputation Current symptoms
History of present complaint	Ulcers, gangrene, bypass surgery, intermittent claudication, rest pain, sympathectomy, embolectomy, heparinisation, stages of amputation Accident details and orthopaedic history, salvage operations, oncology treatment
Past medical history	Related: diabetes, myocardial infarction, cerebrovascular accident, angina, renal status, eyesight, neuropathy, concurrent injuries Other: respiratory disorders, osteoarthritis, rheumatoid arthritis, major surgery, old injuries, hearing and sight, depression, epilepsy, low back or peripheral joint pain
Social history	Home environment, cohabiters, family support and dependents, home care package, district nurse, access (ramps), doorways, bathroom upstairs, rails/stair lift, employment, school and education, hobbies, finances, compensation claim status (related to trauma), driving, smoking and lifestyle, attitude to exercise and fitness
Drug history	Drugs that may affect rehabilitation programme
Mobility	Pre-amputation – distance covered, walking aids used, stairs, outdoors, wheelchair, exercise and sports, limiting factors Post-amputation – as above plus transfers and bed mobility. Type of wheelchair, walking aids and prosthesis
Function	Self-care, domestic tasks, shopping, laundry, carrying objects, picking up objects, stairs, steps/kerbs, slopes, energy expenditure, limiting factors, compensations, safety, falls, aids used
Prosthetic rehabilitation history	Current and previous prostheses: prescription, delivery date, socket fit, ability to don/doff, maintenance, pattern of use (how long, daily, how far) and reasons for no prosthesis. Current and previous physiotherapy intervention.
Psychological status	Attitudes, emotions, depression, goals and aspirations
Objective assessment	
Residual limb	Wound, scar, healing status, dressings, oedema, pain (VAS 0–10*), sensation, colour, temperature, compression therapy, reflexes, joint range, contractures, weakness, strength, coordination
Remaining limb	Vascularity, strength, joint range, scars, wounds, risk level, temperature, ulcers, footwear, colour, pulse, pain, oedema, numbness, joint dysfunction and adaptations, sensation, reflexes, motor control
Trunk and balance	Sitting, standing, pain, trunk range and control of movement, alignment, posture and core stability, abdominal strength, compensation reactions (Figure 25.2)
Gait/function with prosthesis	Gait pattern, deviations and possible causes, speed, indoor and outdoor use, varying surfaces, exercise tolerance

*Visual analogue scale (VAS), where 0 denotes no pain and 10 denotes worst pain imaginable.

to move safely (Comerford et al. 2005). Figure 25.2 shows the likely postural shift in someone with a lower limb amputation. The head centralises over the remaining heel and the foot has rotated outwards for increased stability. In some cases, such postural changes can result in pain. The altered biomechanics can result in increased energy expenditure and loss of confidence when moving.

Problem list

Based on findings from the assessment, a problem list is formulated, to include agreed and realistic goals, both short- and long-term.

Treatment plan

A treatment plan is drawn up in order to achieve the goals based on the assessment findings.

> ***Key point***
> Frequent reassessment will guide any revision of goals. Physiotherapy treatment is concerned with teaching people new skills. It is a partnership, not related to 'doing to patients' but related to patients learning to do things for themselves.

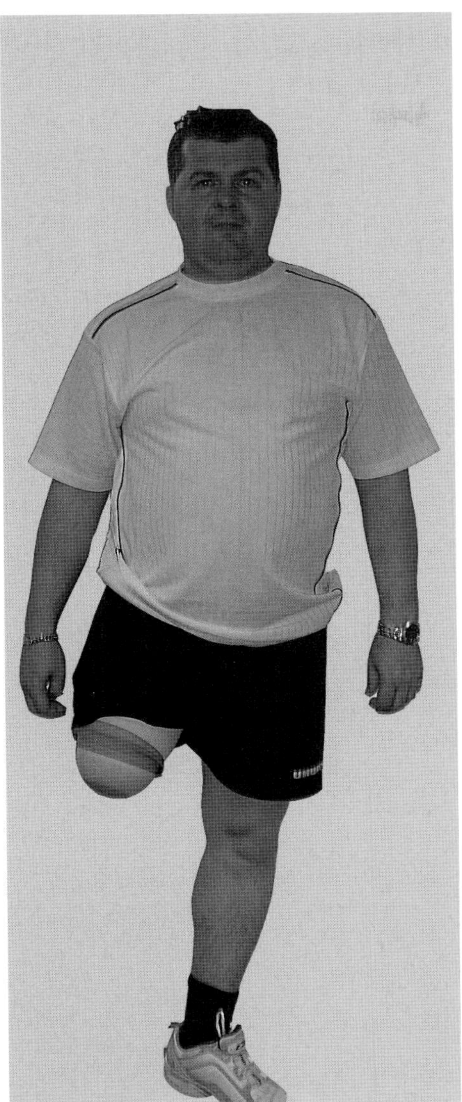

Figure 25.2 Common postural changes following amputation.

STAGES OF PHYSIOTHERAPY MANAGEMENT

The physiotherapist acts as part of the MDT and is involved at all stages of the amputation management, as summarised in Table 25.4. It is important that the physiotherapist liaises with all members of the team at the different stages of the rehabilitation process in order to gain best outcome for the patient and to establish common agreed goals.

Pre-operative stage

The physiotherapist should assess the patient before the amputation. This should always be possible in cases of planned surgery. The physiotherapy assessment should look at:

- physical status, including respiratory status as well as sensory and motor performance
- functional performance, addressing current and pre-morbid levels of independence
- psychological wellbeing.

As part of the MDT, the physiotherapist should be involved in the decision as to what level to amputate and in the preparation of the patient for surgery (Cutson and Bougiorni 1996). Exercises and wheelchair or crutch use can be taught at this stage, if the patient is not in too much pain. The quality of the amputation surgery can influence final rehabilitation outcome; therefore the surgeon is an integral member of the team.

Both the patient and his or her family will benefit from information about the rehabilitation process and what to expect (Yetzer et al. 1994). At this time it is helpful to spend time with the patient, giving reassurance and building a rapport. This will be advantageous in the postoperative stage.

Postoperative stage

Once patients have had their amputation, they are usually brought back to the main ward. Only if there are comorbidities or complications are they transferred to high-dependency or intensive care units.

Ongoing physiotherapy assessment needs to take place at all stages. At many operating hospitals a care pathway is in place, which will outline how the immediate postoperative phase should be managed. The physiotherapist can be guided by this, applying it to the individual patient's needs. An example of such a pathway can be found in Table 25.5.

Early mobility is important to prevent weakening, stiffness, loss of balance and confidence, especially in the elderly. It is common practice to get out of bed on day two after amputation. This immediate re-education of posture and balance provides a big psychological boost.

Controlling residual limb oedema is vital to postoperative progress. A reduction in swelling will lessen pain, improve compliance, aid healing and prevent delays to rehabilitation. Compression, exercise and positioning in elevation will aid oedema control.

Table 25.4 Summary of stages of physiotherapy management

Stage of management	Aspects
Pre-operative	Carry out physical, functional and psychological assessment prior to surgery to inform decision of level to amputate
	Provide pre-operative exercises in preparation for postoperative period
	Provide information about rehabilitation process
	Give wheelchair and mobility practice
Postoperative	Carry out physical and functional assessment
	Address pain and oedema control
	Practise transfers and independent function
	Practise use of walking aids and wheelchairs
	Promote wound healing, pressure care and good nutritional intake
	Provide exercises for strengthening, stretching and balance, in order to aid independent mobility
	Provide education and information for patient and carers
	Liaise with MDT within the hospital and community
	Refer to appropriate agencies for discharge
Pre-prosthetic	Do prosthetic preparation: compression and shaping of the residual limb using elasticated stocking, elevation, exercise and early walking aids
	Improve cardiovascular fitness
	Provide education and information for patient and carers
	Liaise with MDT within the hospital and community
	Refer to appropriate agencies for prosthetic provision
Prosthetic	Carry out physical, psychological and functional assessment
	Provide exercises for strengthening, stretching, stability and balance
	Give gait re-education to minimise gait deviations, achieve safe mobility and promote energy-efficient function
	Continue pain control measures
	Progress walking aids and skills with the prosthesis
	Practise activities of daily living (dressing, cooking, walking outdoors, shopping) as part of MDT
	Provide information regarding care of the residual and remaining limbs, and prosthesis
Life-long	Prescribe maintenance exercises
	Provide further intervention when the situation changes
	Organise review appointments to reassess
	Liaise with community agencies
	Facilitate reintegration to normal living
	Act as long-term resource for patients, families and carers

Key point

Residual limb shape is important for making a prosthetic socket and can be determined by using a JUZO compression garment, which controls the oedema. The correct sizing of such a garment is essential and should be measured by a suitably qualified practitioner (Lambert et al. 1995; www.juzousa.com).

As integral members of the team and using a holistic approach, physiotherapists should also play their part in pressure management of vulnerable tissues at this time of relative immobility and encourage adequate nutrition to aid postoperative recovery.

An essential role of the physiotherapist at this stage is to encourage normal movement patterns and prevent joint contracture. Reduced joint range can be painful, delaying rehabilitation, and in severe cases can prevent prosthetic fitment. The physiotherapist educates the patient in exercises for joint stretching and posture care. The common contractures in lower limb amputation affect both the hip and the knee joints, and are associated with pain and prolonged sitting positions:

Table 25.5 Example care pathway for early rehabilitation following lower limb amputation

Day 1 – in bed
- Respiratory care, pain control, exercises for bed mobility and joint range

Day 2 – sit out in chair
- Range of movement and strength for all limbs and trunk
- Balance training
- Transfer practice and wheelchair provision
- Oedema control

Day 3 – independence
- Continue exercises for strength, range and balance
- Pain and oedema control
- Functional exercises, i.e. bridging and supported standing, wheelchair, personal care
- Posture correction

Days 4–7 – discharge planning
- Plan home visit with occupational therapist
- Monitor oedema control
- Continue exercise programme and mobility
- Ensure appropriate clothing for rehabilitation

Days 7–14 – prosthetic assessment
- Attend gym environment, individual and group exercise sessions
- Assess and practise with early walking aid, i.e. PPAM aid*
- Prepare for prosthetic rehabilitation: stump shape, balance, proprioception and strength
- Refer to regional prosthetic centre
- Discharge or transfer to rehabilitation ward or intermediate care

Days 14–28 – develop appropriate plan
- Progress rehabilitation programme: prosthetic or non-prosthetic

Weeks 4–6 – outpatient or community
- Cast for prosthesis
- Start prosthetic training
- Ensure reintegration into home environment

*PPAM, pneumatic post-amputation mobility.

- Transtibial level — contracture of the knee into a flexed position. Active knee extension should be encouraged, with passive stretching provided by elevation on the bed or stump board, as shown in Figure 25.1.
- Transfemoral level — contracture of the hip into a flexed position. There may also be a contracture into abduction, where the hip flexors and abductors are unopposed by weakened extensors and adductors. Active exercise of the weak muscles and positioning will help to address this imbalance.

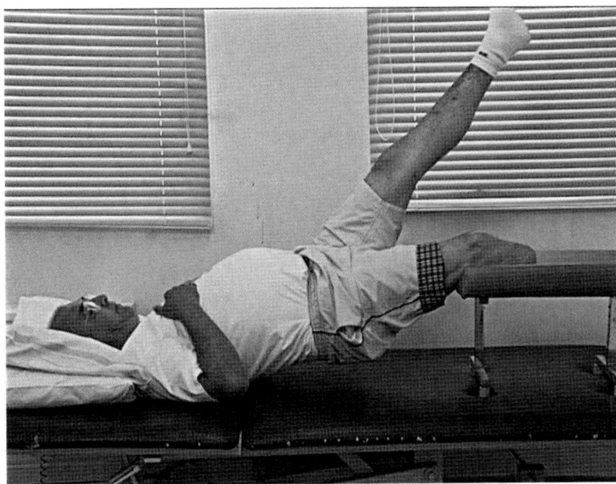

Figure 25.3 Combined muscle strengthening to control joint range.

- Hip flexion contractures. These can also commonly occur in transtibial amputations. Figure 25.3 shows how a small stool can be used to strengthen groups of muscles, creating better balance between opposing muscles, and therefore reducing the incidence of joint contractures.

Re-educating postural balance and control will contribute to safe mobility, whether with a wheelchair, crutches or prosthesis. A gym ball is a great adjunct for developing a person's core stability and control, as Figure 25.4 demonstrates.

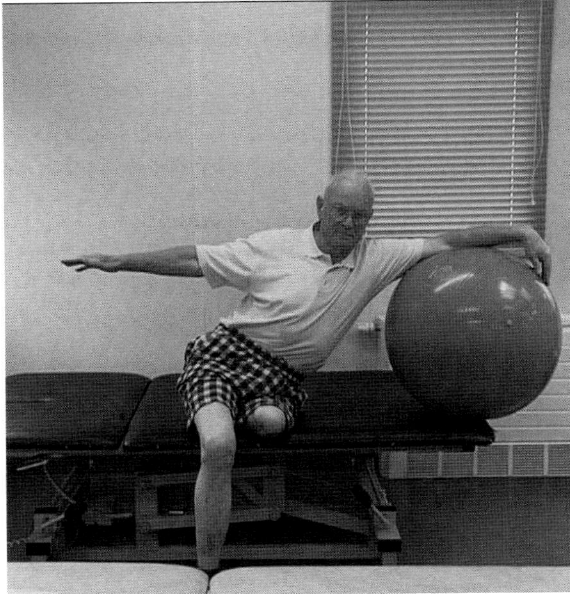

Figure 25.4 Use of a gym ball to aid trunk rehabilitation.

Reassuring patients and repeating information will allay fears and help them to concentrate on their rehabilitation programme. Liaison with colleagues and discharge agencies is necessary to facilitate smooth progress. Continuing rehabilitation into the community will encourage adaptation to new skills of independence aided by the familiar surroundings (Park et al. 1994).

Pre-prosthetic stage

Once it has been decided that a person has the ability to use a prosthesis, pre-prosthetic preparation should start. Exercises should be progressed to challenge the posture and balance in a more upright position. Use of early walking aids, equipment that offers bipedal gait without a prosthesis, promotes oedema reduction and wound healing and provides an insight for patients and therapists as to how well someone will progress. Over 80 per cent of UK physiotherapy departments have early walking aids called PPAM aids, manufactured by a company called Ortho-europe (Lein 1992; www.ortho-europe.com). PPAM stands for pneumatic post-amputation mobility, whereby the patient's residual limb is surrounded by an inflatable bag within a metal frame, which enables some weight to be carried on the amputated side. The bags are inflated to 40 mmHg in a non-weight-bearing position; it is known that this pressure will not cause tissue damage when applied in a constant manner. Walking with a PPAM aid should be partial weight-bearing and should always be initiated within the parallel bars (Figure 25.5). In vascular cases this should be introduced at days 7–10 post-operation. The physiotherapist should always follow the manufacturer's instructions and national guidelines.

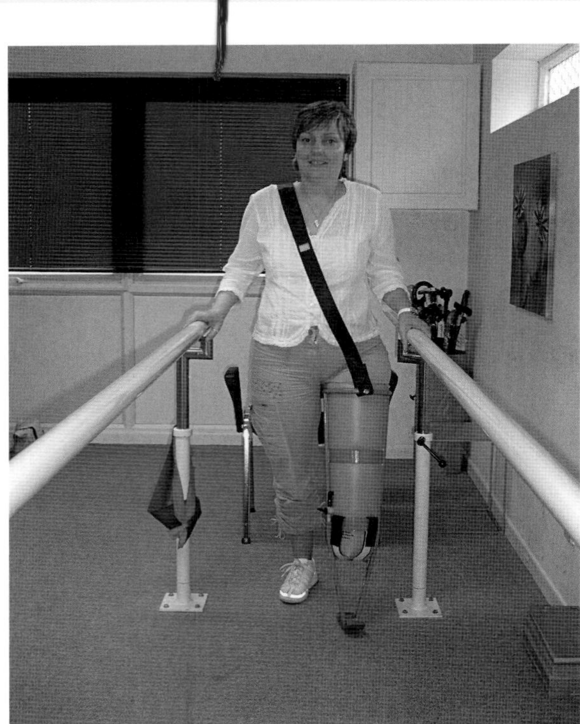

Figure 25.5 Use of PPAM aid within parallel bars.

Prosthetic stage

The ability to use a prosthesis can allow a person to enjoy a better quality of life, possibly being rid of years of pain and poor function, and being able to return to work and leisure activities. At this stage of rehabilitation an intensive gait re-education programme is necessary. Early prosthetic fitting and rehabilitation are vital to successful physical, emotional and psychological recovery, in the short and long term (Bradway et al. 1984).

Using a prosthesis well is about learning a new motor skill, similar to learning to play the piano, play tennis or ride a bicycle. The prosthetic user needs to move with the equipment. It takes hours of practice to become and remain competent. Natural ability influences the final outcome to some degree; however, effective training by a physiotherapist makes a huge impact.

The safe environment of the parallel bars is provided initially for walking, progressing from here so as not to encourage dependence on the bars for partial weight-bearing and for fear of walking beyond this environment. Tension increases fatigue, so patients are always advised about what is happening and what is expected from them. All movement is observed carefully to assess anything that is not normal.

An essential aspect to using a prosthesis is being able to weight-bear fully through the socket. In addition, the user must develop his or her proprioception to feel contact with the ground through the socket, in order to move confidently over the prosthetic foot. Appropriate motor output relies on sensory input. Learning to recognise stimuli at low thresholds forms effective proprioception, leading to normal recruitment of muscle activity and balance reactions. A comfortable socket is vital to achieving this. Exercises should be used to facilitate correct muscle recruitment, in particular to create pelvic excursion and to stabilise body segments. Figure 25.6 shows how stepping on to a block with the remaining leg can encourage weight-bearing through weight transfer over the prosthesis, using hip abductors and extensors. Figure 25.7 shows how the physiotherapist can facilitate rotation of the pelvis around the longitudinal axis necessary for forward progression. Being able to stabilise the body whilst standing on the prosthesis is also necessary for safe, confident movement

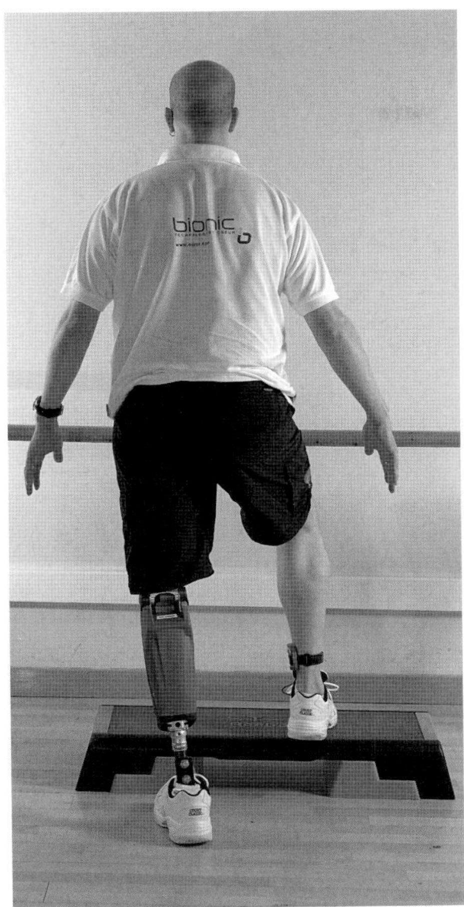

Figure 25.6 Exercise for controlling weight-bearing and weight transference.

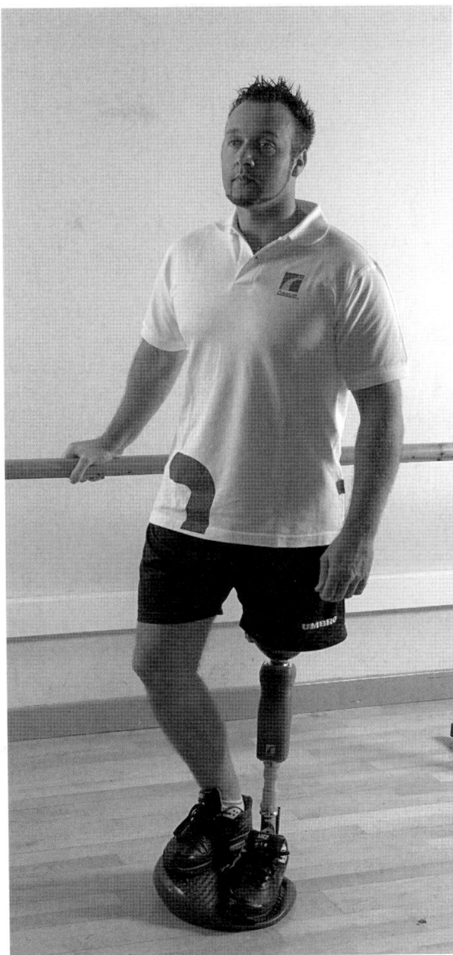

Figure 25.8 Hip stabilisation exercises.

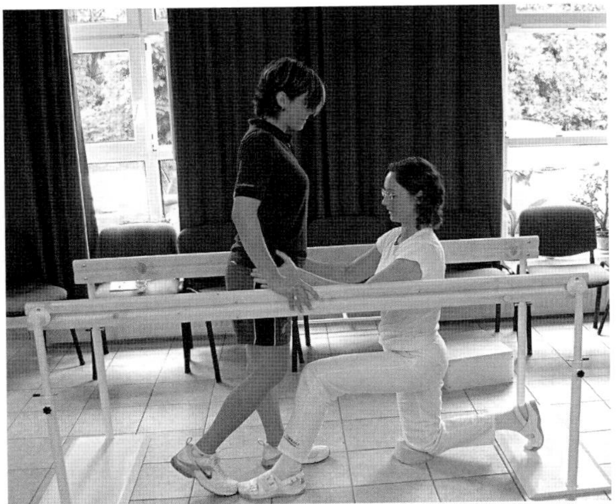

Figure 25.7 Facilitation of pelvic rotation.

and can be encouraged using dynamic surfaces such as a wobble cushion (Figure 25.8).

During prosthetic training, the physiotherapist is responsible for teaching users how to care for their residual and remaining limbs. This is particularly important for people with diabetes, whose lack of foot sensation puts them at great risk of a second amputation. Learning how to care for the prosthesis, understanding how the components function and knowing how to don the socket properly are key to successful use. Prevention of pressure sores will ensure continued use of the prosthesis. The physiotherapist must also make the prosthetic rehabilitation programme functional and orientated to the individual's lifestyle. Where appropriate, getting down on and up off the floor, using transport and walking outdoors over uneven ground, slopes, stairs and kerbs should be included, as should tasks around the home.

Key point

Specialist prosthetic training is essential to the success of the rehabilitation programme. Readers are directed to the numerous texts that contain specific knowledge of prosthetic products, the normal gait cycle and gait training techniques.

For some people, having a prosthesis can be more of a hindrance than a help. Learning to use a prosthesis requires strength, coordination, cardiovascular fitness, motivation and cognitive ability. Prosthetic abandonment is common. At long-term post-amputation evaluation, approximately half of transtibial and less than a third of transfemoral amputees are still using the prosthesis full-time (De Luccia et al. 1992; Davies and Datta 2003). Wheelchair independence is a more appropriate option for many elderly amputees.

Life-long stage

The physiotherapist should be involved in the long-term management of a person with an amputation. Maintenance exercises should be issued and monitored to minimise secondary dysfunctions that can occur as a result of compensation made by the skeleton. Review appointments can promote independence and continued use of the prosthesis.

As people progress through life, their needs will change, necessitating the further input of the physiotherapist. Examples of such events are when the prosthetic prescription changes, return to work and/or sport, issues related to the aging process or change in health status, and problems occurring due to compensations.

Regular reassessments will highlight when the physiotherapist needs to refer on to other professionals, and a working link should be maintained with key MDT members.

PROSTHESES

The prosthetist is primarily responsible for deciding on the type of prosthesis to be provided and its manufacture. The rehabilitation doctor and physiotherapist are also key in deciding what functions are most appropriate for the user.

A prosthesis comprises a bespoke socket, a form of suspension, joint and interjoint segments, a foot or hand, and a cosmetic cover. Examples of transtibial and transfemoral prostheses can be seen in Figures 25.9 and 25.10. The socket must contain the remaining musculoskeletal tissues (muscle, fascia and bone) and transmit the internal and external forces involved in movement to the ground. A comfortable socket is critical to a successful prosthesis. Weight should be loaded on weight-tolerant tissues and offloaded in areas of pressure intolerance, such as bony structures and nerves. Peak pressures and friction will cause tissue damage and make the user reluctant to wear the prosthesis. Teaching the user to don the prosthesis correctly cannot be stressed enough.

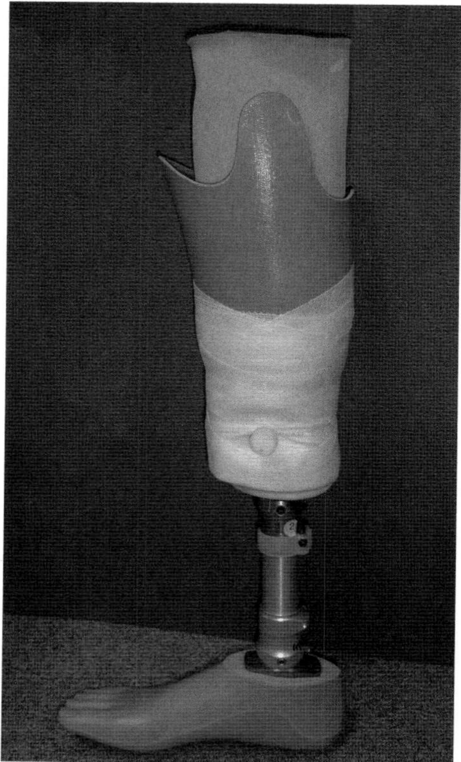

Figure 25.9 Example of a transtibial prosthesis.

The mechanics of the prosthesis can cause the user to move in a certain manner. This can be very disconcerting and it is the role of the physiotherapist to teach the user to control the prosthesis and not be controlled by it. The physiotherapist must be familiar with different facets of prosthetic components and their provision in order to teach best use. Close liaison with the prosthetist will ensure an optimal outcome.

GAIT DEVIATIONS

A sound understanding of normal gait will allow the physiotherapist to analyse prosthetic gait and diagnose any deviations. Gait abnormalities are caused by the

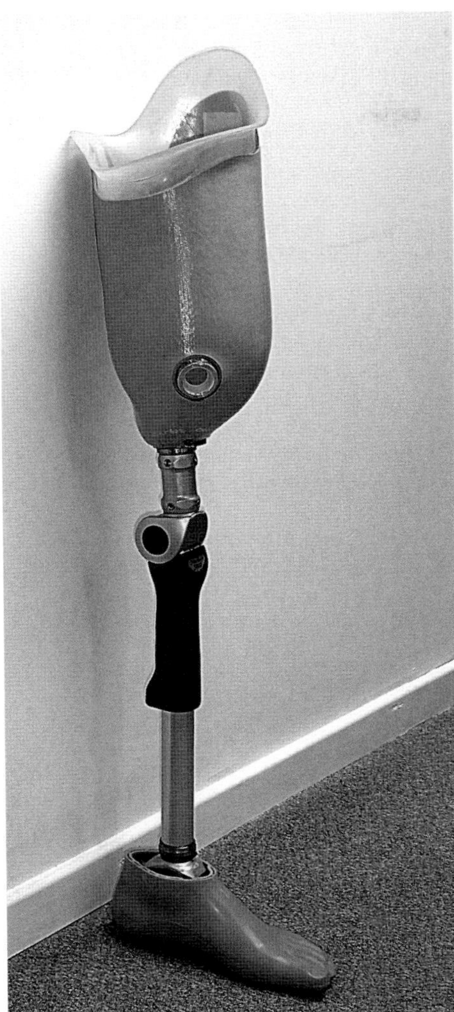

Figure 25.10 Example of a transfemoral prosthesis.

user's movement patterns or the prosthesis, or can be a combination of both.

The most common gait deviations are described in brief below. This list is not exhaustive.

Transtibial-level deviations

- Excessive knee flexion during stance — due to weak quadriceps and gluteals, fixed flexion at hip or knee, excessive dorsiflexion at prosthetic ankle, short prosthetic foot lever.
- Insufficient knee flexion during stance — due to poor hip and knee control, socket discomfort, excessive plantar flexion at prosthetic ankle.
- Lateral bending of the trunk to prosthetic side during stance — due to socket discomfort, lack of hip stability, too short a prosthesis.

Transfemoral-level deviations

- Abducted prosthesis, a wide base of support throughout stance and swing — due to abduction contracture, weak hip stabilisers, socket discomfort, too long a prosthesis, insufficient lateral socket wall support, poor knee control.
- Lateral bending of the trunk to prosthetic side during stance — due to abduction contracture, short residual limb, poor hip stability, insufficient lateral socket wall support, too short a prosthesis.
- Circumduction, abduction through prosthetic swing only — due to weak adductors, too long a prosthesis, inadequate suspension, unstable prosthetic knee, poor knee control.
- Vaulting, rising into plantar flexion through stance on sound side — due to short residual limb, poor prosthetic swing control, too long a prosthesis, inadequate suspension.
- Excessive lumbar lordosis during prosthetic stance — due to hip flexion contracture, weak abdominals and hip extensors, unstable prosthetic knee, insufficient socket flexion.

General observations

General observed deviations are uneven step length, uneven timing and uneven arm swing. Using a prosthesis requires energy expenditure in excess of normal walking with two intact limbs. This can be very tiring. To compensate, users will walk more slowly.

The physiotherapist plays a pivotal role in training and can influence the following causes of deviation: fear, weakness, poor range of movement, poor weightbearing, pain, poor fit/donning, incorrect use, poor movement patterns from incorrect muscle recruitment, fatigue, inappropriate walking aids or their use, poor balance, change in footwear and bad habit/technique.

Prosthetic length and alignment issues are best identified and resolved with the physiotherapist and prosthetist working together as a team. With respect to energy levels and proprioception, it is far easier to rehabilitate with a transtibial level amputation than a transfemoral level, greater mobility can be achieved.

OUTCOME MEASURES

A physiotherapist should always have a benchmark by which to measure whether a physiotherapy intervention has been successful or not. This can be level of pain, range of joint motion or level of function. Rehabilitation after amputation is complex and multifaceted, and measuring the outcome can be problematic. There are a number of outcome tools for disability that can be applied to amputees. Described here are the tools validated specifically for prosthetic rehabilitation.

- *SIGAM Algorithm* (Special Interest Group in Amputee Medicine; based on the Harold Wood scale). This offers a simple, valid and reliable means of measuring mobility in lower limb amputees. SIGAM can be used throughout the stages of rehabilitation to identify changes in mobility, making it useful for both new and established amputees (Ryall et al. 2003).
- *Locomotor Capabilities Index* (LCI). The index was designed to trace a comprehensive profile of locomotor capabilities of the lower limb amputee with the prosthesis and to evaluate the level of independence while performing these activities. The LCI is part of the Prosthetic Profile of the Amputee (Grisé 1993; Gauthier-Gagnon et al. 1998).
- *Trinity Amputee Prosthetic Evaluation Scale* (TAPES). This questionnaire was designed to investigate different aspects of having an artificial limb (Gallagher and MacLachlan 2004).
- *Functional Measure of the Amputee* (FMA) (Callaghan 2002). The FMA questionnaire was developed from the Prosthetic Profile of the Amputee (PPA) questionnaire, to collect long-term functional and prosthetic use information following discharge. It contains the LCI.
- *Video*. Simple video recordings can be taken at stages of rehabilitation as an aide-mémoire and a tool for comparing change.

SPECIAL CONSIDERATIONS

Children with amputation

Children with acquired amputation or congenital deficiency represent a highly specialised area in the field of prosthetic rehabilitation, as the numbers are relatively small. Much of the physiotherapist's time will be spent reassuring, informing and teaching the parents, who may be feeling very distressed and guilty about their child. A child cannot be forced into using a prosthesis and many manage very adequately in life without one, especially at upper limb levels. Adaptation throughout their life is dependent on acceptance of the deformity by those around them, such as family, friends and teachers. Bipedal and bimanual activities should be encouraged as early as possible, to facilitate normal child development. Acquired amputations pose different challenges from birth defects. Each person is unique. When involved in training a child, the therapist must make sessions fun and challenging.

Trauma and tumour amputation

People who undergo amputation for accidental injury are often of working age. Amputation can be the result of a road traffic accident, industrial injury, domestic accident or gunshot wounds. These patients can usually compensate well and adapt physically to amputation but it can be a huge psychological blow. Rehabilitation plans must address their emotional needs, as many suffer from post-traumatic stress disorder following horrific experiences. As this patient group is young and active, there are high expectations for recovery and it can be a challenge for the MDT to meet their activity demands. Many need to return to work and sport (Figure 25.11).

Patients involved in accidents can claim compensation and may purchase their prosthetic rehabilitation from private clinics. A claim can take many years to settle, and this can be a trying time for the amputee.

Those who have an amputation for cancerous tumours often face arduous treatment for the cancer at the same time. Rehabilitation needs to be quick in cases where life expectancy is shortened. An understanding of emotional status is imperative, as, coupled with the trauma of limb loss, the individual must deal with the life-threatening condition of malignancy.

Upper limb amputation

Amputation at this level is most frequently seen in young adults and the working population, in whom exposure to trauma is more likely. It tends to affect men more than women. The second distinct group of

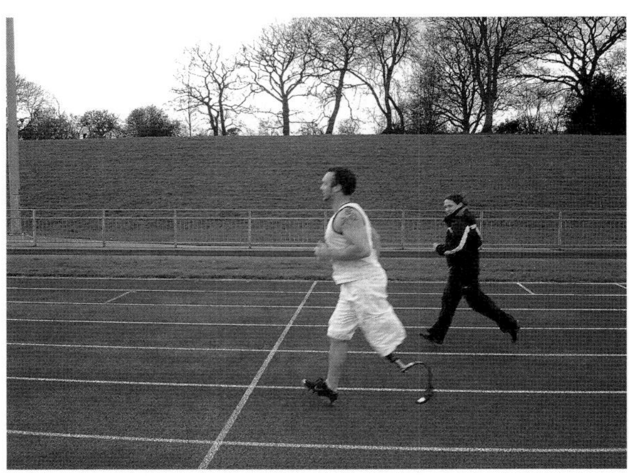

Figure 25.11 Running with transfemoral prosthesis.

patients requiring upper limb amputations is those with congenital limb absence. In these cases, complete amputation is not always indicated and a prosthetic socket can be fitted to the limb remnant.

Traditionally, prosthetic training is undertaken by an occupational therapist. If the amputation is on the dominant side, occupational therapy intervention must be instrumental in promoting a change in hand dominance. The physiotherapist's role relates more to exercising for strength, range and coordination, managing oedema and offering pain-relieving modalities. Phantom pain is as common in upper limb amputation as lower limb, where people describe feeling their hand in the last position prior to the traumatic event.

Arms and hands are used in social interaction, as tools of expression and embrace. They are essential for providing comfort and for intimate self-care. It can be very difficult to adjust to an upper limb amputation. People with upper limb amputations desire effective cosmetic replacements as well as functional tools, and usually more than one prosthesis is provided to meet these separate goals. Figure 25.12 shows a transradial prosthesis prior to completion. Some upper limb prostheses use body power to move prosthetic joints, whereas others can use myoelectric signals, sensed by electrodes within the socket, for hand control. Skin care and pressure management within the prosthetic socket, due to gravity dependence rather than loading as in the lower limb cases, require equal care and attention.

Complex cases

Due to the progressive nature of vascular disease, a third to a half of people with amputations of this origin will undergo a second amputation of their remaining leg within a few years. Bilateral amputation is difficult at any age and requires considerable environmental adaptations when the person is older and often wheelchair-dependent.

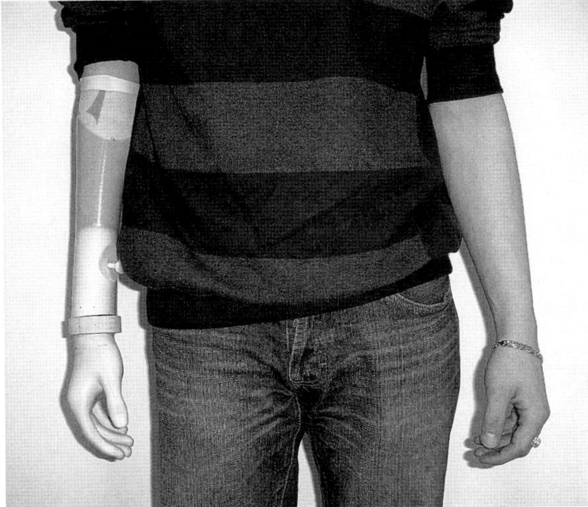

Figure 25.12 Transradial prosthesis at the fitting stage.

People presenting with multiple amputations, including extensive orthopaedic or neurological involvement, pose a real challenge to the physiotherapist. All the therapist's skills are required to teach independence in activities of personal care and daily living. The whole MDT will need to work together to address all aspects. Causes of multiple limb loss are burns, meningococcal septicaemia, accidents and combat. Often rehabilitation programmes must be modified to accommodate associated skin damage and muscle loss. Energy levels for ambulation are immense and sometimes prosthetically prohibitive.

Key point

Amputation is a life-long, life-changing event. The physiotherapist plays a key role in optimising a person's independence and reintegration into normal life experiences.

Weblinks

British Association of Chartered Physiotherapists in Amputee Rehabilitation (BACPAR): www.bacpar.org.uk

International Society for Prosthetics and Orthotics (ISPO): www.ispo.org.uk

Limbless Association: www.limbless-association.org

Limb Loss Information Centre: www.limblossinformationcentre.com

Scottish Physiotherapy Amputee Research Group (SPARG)/National Centre for Training and Education in Prosthetics and Orthotics (NCTEPO), University of Strathclyde, Glasgow: www.strath.ac.uk/prosthetics

FURTHER READING

BACPAR 2001 Evidence-Based Guidelines: The Physiotherapy Management of Adults using Lower Limb Prostheses. www.bacpar.org.uk

BACPAR 2006 Evidence-Based Guidelines: Pre- and Post-operative Physiotherapy Management of Adults with Lower Limb Amputation. www.bacpar.org.uk

Butler DS, Moseley GL 2003 Explain Pain. NOI: Adelaide

Disability Information Trust 1994 Employment and the Workplace. Disability Information Trust: Oxford

Disability Information Trust 1996 Sport and Leisure — Equipment for Disabled People. Disability Information Trust: Oxford

Disability Information Trust 1998 Powered Wheelchairs and Scooters — a Practical Guide. Disability Information Trust: Oxford

Disability Information Trust 1999 Outdoor Transport. Disability Information Trust: Oxford

Day HJB, Kulkarni JR, Datta D 1993 Prescribing Upper Limb Prostheses. Amputee Medical Rehabilitation Society: London

Ham R, Cotton L 1991 Limb Amputation. Chapman & Hall: London

Ham R, Barsby P, Lumley C, Roberts C 1995 Amputee Rehabilitation: a Handbook. Lumbley: York

Lusardi MM, Nielson 2000 CC Orthotic and Prosthetics in Rehabilitation. Butterworth–Heinemann: Oxford

Mensch E, Ellis PM 1987 Physical Therapy Management of Lower Extremity Amputations. Heinemann: London

Redhead RG, Day HJB, Marks LJ, Lackmann SL 1993 Prescribing Lower Limb Prostheses. Disability Services Authority:

Rose J, Gamble J 1992 Human Walking, 2nd edn. Lippincott, Williams & Wilkins: Philadelphia

Söderberg B 2001 Partial Foot Amputations: Guidelines to Prosthetic and Surgical Solutions, 2nd edn. Helsingborg: Swedish Orthopaedic Association

Turner A, Foster M, Johnson SE (eds) 2002 Occupational Therapy and Physical Dysfunction: Principles, Skills and Practice. Churchill Livingstone: Edinburgh

Van de Ven C, Engstrom B 1999 Therapy for Amputees, 3rd edn. Churchill Livingstone: Edinburgh

Vitali M, Robinson KP, Andrews BG, Harris EE 1978 Amputations and Prostheses. Baillière Tindall: London

Whittle MW 1991 Gait Analysis — an Introduction. Butterworth–Heinemann: Oxford

Winchell E 1995 Coping with Limb Loss: a Practical Guide to Living with Amputation for You and Your Family. Avery: New York

REFERENCES

Bradway JK, Malone JM, Racy J et al. 1984 Psychological adaptation to amputation: an overview. Orthot Prosthet 38: 46–50

Butler DJ, Turkal NW, Seidl JJ 1992 Amputation: preoperative psychological preparation. J Am Board Fam Pract 5: 69–73

Callaghan BG, Sockalingam S, Treweek SP, Condie ME 2002 'A post-discharge functional outcome measure for lower limb amputees: test-retest reliability with transtibial amputees. Prosthet Orthot Int 26(2): 113–119

Campling J 1981 Images of ourselves: Women with Disabilities Talking. Routledge: London

Caron C 1989 Study on predictive factors for adjustment to chronic haemodialysis: a literature review and discussion of future directions. Can J Psych 34(7): 654–661

Comerford MJ, Mottram SL, Gibbons SGT 2005 Understanding Movement and Function. Kinetic Control: Shropshire

Cutson TM, Bougiorni DR 1996 rehabilitation of the older lower limb amputee: a brief review. J Am Geriatr Soc 44: 1388–1393

Davies B, Datta D 2003 Mobility outcome following unilateral lower limb amputation. Pros and Orthot Int 27: 186–190

De Luccia N, De Souza Pinto MAG, Guedes JPB, Albers MTV 1992 Rehabilitation after amputation for vascular disease: a follow-up study. Pros and Orthot Int 16: 124–128

Ebskov B 1999 Relative mortality and long-term survival for the non-diabetic lower limb amputee with vascular insufficiency. Prosthet Orthot Int 23: 209–216

Fraser CM, Halligan PW, Robertson IH, Kirker SGB 2001 Characterising phantom limb phenomena in upper limb amputees. Pros and Orthot Int 25: 235–242

Fyfe NCM 1992 Assessment of the rehabilitation of amputees. Current Pract Surg 4: 90–98

Gallagher P, MacLachlan M 2004 The Trinity amputation and prosthesis experience scales and quality of life in people with lower limb amputation. Arch Phys Med Rehabil 85: 730–736

Gauthier-Gagnon C, Grisé M, Lepage Y 1998 The locomotor capabilities index: content validity. J Rehabil Outcome Measures 2(4): 40–46

Grisé MC, Gauthier-Gagnon C 1993 Prosthetic profile of people with lower extremity amputation: conception and design of a follow-up questionnaire. Arch Phys Med Rehabil 74: 862–870

Ham R, McCreadie M 1992 Rehabilitation of elderly patients in the United Kingdom following lower limb amputation. Top Geriatric Rehabil 8(1): 64–71

Hill A, Niven CA, Knussen C 1995 The role of coping in adjustment to phantom limb pain. Pain 62: 79–86

Krueger DW 1984 Rehabilitation Psychology — a Comprehensive Textbook. Aspen: Maryland

Kubler-Ross E 1969 On Death and Dying. Macmillan: London

Lambert A, Johnson J 1995 Stump shrinkers: a survey of their use. Physiotherapy 81: 234–236

Lein S 1992 How are physiotherapists using the Vessa Pneumatic Post Amputation Mobility Aid? Physiotherapy 78(5): 318–322

O'Shea E, Kennelly B 1996 The economics of independent living: efficiency, equity and ethics. Int J Rehabil Research 19(1): 13–26

Park S, Fisher AG, Velozo CA 1994 Using the assessment of motor and process skills to compare occupational performance between clinic and home settings. Am J Occup Ther 48(8): 697–709

Parkes CM 1972 Bereavement Studies of Grief in Adult Life. Tavistock: London

Parkes CM 1975 Psychological transition comparison between reactions of loss of limb to loss of spouse. Br J Psychol 127: 204–210

Pernot HF 1997 Daily functioning of the lower extremity amputee: an overview of the literature. Clin Rehabil 11(2): 93–106

Ryall NH, Eyres SB, Neumann VC et al. 2003 The SIGAM mobility grades: a new population-specific measure for lower limb amputees. Disability Rehabil 25(5): 833–844

Van de Ven C, Engstrom B 1999 Therapy for Amputees, 3rd edn. Churchill Livingstone: Edinburgh

Watson G 1996 Neuromusculoskeletal physiotherapy: encouraging self-management. Physiotherapy 82(6): 352–357

Weiss SA, Lindell B 1996 Phantom limb pain and etiology of amputation in unilateral lower extremity amputees. J Pain Symptom Manage 11(11): 3–7

Williams AM, Deaton SB 1997 Phantom pain, elusive yet real. Rehabil Nurs 22(2): 73–77

Yetzer EA, Kauffman K, Sopp F, Talley L 1994 Development of a patient education programme for new amputees. Rehabil Nursing 19(6): 355–358

Index

Note: Figures and tables are comprehensively referred to from the text. Therefore, significant material in figures and tables have only been given a page reference in the absence of their concommitant mention in the text referring to that figure.

A

B

C

D

E

G

H

I

J

K

M

N

O

P

Q

R

S

T

U

V

W

X

Y

Z

ELSEVIER DVD-ROM LICENCE AGREEMENT

Minimum system requirements

Windows®

Windows 2000 or higher
1.4Ghz processor
128 MB RAM
4x DVD-ROM drive
VGA Monitor supporting 800x600 at millions of colours

Macintosh®

Apple G4 Macintosh
Mac OS 9.1 or later
128 MB RAM
4x DVD-ROM drive
VGA Monitor supporting 800x600 at millions of colours

NB: No data is transferred to the hard disk.
The DVD-ROM is self-contained and the application runs directly from the DVD-ROM.

Installation instructions

Windows®
If your system does not support Autorun, navigate to your DVD drive and double click on 'Start.exe' to begin.

Alternatively, click Start, Run and type 'D:Start.exe' to begin. If D: is not your DVD drive, substitute D: with the appropriate drive letter.

Macintosh®
If the DVD does not autorun, open the DVD icon that appears on the desktop and select 'Start' to begin.

Using this Product

This product is designed to run with Internet Explorer 6.0 or later (PC) and Netscape 4.5 or later (Mac). Please refer to the help files on those programs for problems specific to the browser.

To use some of the functions on the DVD, the user must have the following:

a. DVD requires "Java Runtime Environment" to be installed in your system to use "Export" and "Slide Show" features. DVD automatically checks for "Java Runtime Environment" version 1.4.1 or later (PC) and MRJ 2.2.5 (Mac) if not available, it starts installing from the DVD. Please complete the installation process. Then click on the license agreement to proceed. "Java Runtime Environment" is available in the DVD Software folder. If the user manually install the software, please make sure that the user start the application by clicking the appropriate exe file.
b. Your browser needs to be Java-enabled. If the user did not enable Java when installing your browser, the user may need to download some additional files from your browser manufacturer.
c. If your system does not support Autorun, then please explore the DVD contents click on 'Start.exe' to start.

Acrobat Reader can be installed from the Software folder of the DVD.

Viewing Images
You can view images by chapter and export images to PowerPoint or an HTML presentation. Full details are available in the Help section of the DVD-ROM.

Frequently Asked Questions (FAQ)

Do I need to have internet connection to run this program?
No. The program is designed to run entirely from the DVD-ROM, independent of the Internet. However the disk may contain some links to material on the Internet (website link) and to view this material you will require an Internet connection.

When I launch the application, I get messages after Netscape starts. What do I do?
TCP/IP is required to run any browserbased application. TCP/IP is included with Windows 95, 98 and NT. To add TCP/IP in Windows 95/98/NT, go to Network in the Control Panel. Click the Add button. Click the protocol option and click Add. Under manufacturers, select Microsoft and under Network Protrocols, select TCP/IP and click OK. Click OK again and Windows will start to install TCP/IP. When finished you will have to restart your machine.

What should I do if when I launch the application my ISP starts to dial out?
This application is able to run with or without a connection to the Internet. If your ISP starts to dial out, you can cancel this and the program will still run. Many ISPs will automatically dial out when a browser is launched. You may be able to turn this option off in the properties for your ISP.

When opening the DVD-ROM in Internet Explorer on the Mac my default home page opens. What should I do?
When you run the DVD-ROM in Internet Explorer on the Mac two windows are opened – your default home page and the opening page of the DVD-ROM. Simply close the window that contains your default home page. We recommend, however, that Mac users view the DVD-ROM in Netscape.

The export function is not working properly. What should I do?
The Export feature requires the DVD-ROM Server to run in the background. The Server application requires the "Java Runtime Environment" to be installed in the system. The Server can be started manually by selecting 'server.exe' in Windows and 'server' application in MacOS.

Technical Support
Technical support for this product is available between 7.30 a.m. and 7.00 p.m. CST, Monday through Friday. Before calling, be sure that your computer meets the minimum system requirements to run this software.
Inside the United States and Canada, call 1-800-692-9010.
Inside the United Kingdom, call 00-800-692-90100.
Outside North America, call +1-314-872-8370.
You may also fax your questions to +1-314-997-5080,
or contact Technical Support through e-mail: technical.support@elsevier.com.